TEXTBOOK OF
DIAGNOSTIC SONOGRAPHY

SEVENTH EDITION   VOLUME TWO

TEXTBOOK OF
DIAGNOSTIC SONOGRAPHY

Sandra L. Hagen-Ansert,
MS, RDMS, RDCS, FASE, FSDMS

Cardiology Department
Supervisor, Echo Lab
Scripps Clinic—Torrey Pines, California

with 3,463 illustrations

ELSEVIER
MOSBY

ELSEVIER
MOSBY

3251 Riverport Lane
St. Louis, Missouri 63043

TEXTBOOK OF DIAGNOSTIC SONOGRAPHY   ISBN: 978-0-323-07301-1
Copyright © 2012 by Mosby, Inc., an affiliate of Elsevier Inc.

Notices

Previous editions copyrighted 2006, 2001, 1995, 1989, 1983, 1978

Publisher: Andrew Allen
Executive Editor: Jeanne Olson
Developmental Editor: Linda Woodard
Publishing Services Manager: Julie Eddy
Project Manager: Richard Barber
Design Direction: Paula Catalano

Printed in the United States

Last digit is the print number: 9 8 7 6 5 4 3 2

To my daughters,
Becca, Aly, *and* **Kati,**
who are changing the world one day at a time

Joan Baker, MSR., RDMS, RDCS
President, Sound Ergonomics
Kenmore, Washington

Carolyn Coffin, MPH, RDMS, RDCS, RVT
CEO, Sound Ergonomics
Kenmore, Washington

Marveen Craig, RDMS
Diagnostic Ultrasound Consultant
Tucson, Arizona

M. Robert De Jong, RDMS, RDCS, RVT
Radiology Technical Manager, Ultrasound
The Russell H. Morgan Department of Radiology
and Radiological Science
The Johns Hopkins Hospital
Baltimore, Maryland

Terry J. DuBose, MS, RDMS
Associate Professor and Director
Diagnostic Medical Sonography Program
University of Arkansas for Medical Sciences
Little Rock, Arkansas

Pamela Foy, M.S., RDMS
Clinical Instructor, Department OB/GYN
The Ohio State University Medical Center
Columbus, Ohio

Candace Goldstein, BS, RDMS
Sonographer Educator
Scripps Clinic Carmel Valley
San Diego, California

Charlotte G. Henningsen, MS, RT (R), RDMS, RVT
Chair and Professor
Diagnostic Medical Sonography Department
Florida Hospital College of Health Sciences
Orlando, Florida

Mira L. Katz, PhD, MPH
Associate Professor
Division of Health Behavior and Health Promotion
School of Public Health
The Ohio State University
Columbus, Ohio

Fredrick Kremkau, PhD
Professor & Director
Center for Medical Ultrasound
Wake Forest University School of Medicine
Winston-Salem, North Carolina

Salvatore LaRusso, MEd, RDMS, RT (R)
Technical Director
Penn State Hershey/ Hershey Medical Center
Department of Radiology
Hershey, Pennsylvania

Daniel A. Merton, BS, RDMS
Technical Coordinator of Research
The Jefferson Ultrasound Research and Educational Institute
Thomas Jefferson University
Philadelphia, Pennsylvania

Carol Mitchell, PhD, RDMS, RDCS, RVT, RT(R)
Quality Assurance Coordinator, UW AIRP
Program Director, University of Wisconsin School of Diagnostic Medical Ultrasound
University of Wisconsin Hospitals & Clinics
Madison, Wisconsin

Cindy A. Owen, RT, RDMS, RVT
Global Luminary and Research Manager
Radiology & Vascular Ultrasound
GE Healthcare
Memphis, Tennessee

Mitzi Roberts, BS, RDMS, RVT
Chair, Assistant Professor
Diagnostic Medical Sonography Program
Baptist College of Health Science
Memphis, Tennessee

Jean Lea Spitz, MPH, RDMS
Maternal Fetal Medicine Foundation
Nuchal Translucency Quality Review Program
Oklahoma City, Oklahoma

Susan Raatz Stephenson, MEd, BSRT-U, RDMS, RT(R)(C)
International Foundation for Sonography Education & Research
AIUM communities.org
Sandy, Utah

Diana M. Strickland, BS, RDMS, RDCS
Clinical Assistant Professor and Co-Director
Ultrasound Program
Department of Obstetrics and Gynecology
Brody School of Medicine
East Carolina University
Greenville, North Carolina

Shpetim Telegrafi, M.D.
Assistant Professor
Director, Diagnostic Ultrasound
NYU School of Medicine, Department of Urology
New York City, New York

Barbara Trampe, RN, RDMS
Chief Sonographer
Meriter/University of Wisconsin Perinatal Ultrasound
Madison, Wisconsin

Barbara J. Vander Werff, RDMS,
  RDCS, RVT
Chief Sonographer
University of Wisconsin-Madison
  Hospitals and Clinics
Madison, Wisconsin

Kerry Weinberg, MS, RDMS,
  RDCS
Director
Diagnostic Medical Sonography
  Program
New York University
New York, New York

Ann Willis, MS, RDMS, RVT
Assistant Professor, Diagnostic
  Medical Sonography Program
Baptist College of Health Sciences
Memphis, Tennessee

Dennis Wisher, BS, RDMS, RVT
Director of Education and Product
  Management
Medison America, Inc.
Cypress, California

Jan Blend, MS, RT(R), RDMS, ARDMS
Program Coordinator, Diagnostic Medical Sonography
El Centro College
Dallas, Texas

Katherine K. Borok, BS, RDMS, RDCS
Clinical Coordinator
American Institute of Ultrasound in Medicine
Laurel, Maryland

Joie Burns, MS, RT(R)(S), RDMS, RVT
Associate Professor, Program Director, Diagnostic Medical Sonography
Boise State University
Boise, Idaho

Saretta C. Craft, MS, RDCS, RVT
Program Director, Diagnostic Sonography
St. Catharine College
St. Catharine, Kentucky

Laura L. Currie, BS, RT(R), RDMS, RVT
Clinical Coordinator
Cape Fear Community College
Wilmington, North Carolina

Marianna C. Desmond, BS, RT(R), RDMS
Clinical Coordinator, Diagnostic Medical Sonography Program
Triton College
River Grove, Illinois

Jann Dolk, MA, RT(R), RDMS
Adjunct Faculty, Diagnostic Medical Sonography Program
Palm Beach State College
Palm Beach Gardens, Florida

Ken Galbraith, MS, RT(R), RDMS, RVT
State University of New York
Syracuse, New York

Karen M. Having, MS Ed, RT, RDMS
Associate Professor, School of Allied Health
Southern Illinois University-Carbondale
Carbondale, Illinois

Bridgette Lunsford, BS, RDMS, RVT
Adjunct Faculty, George Washington University
Washington, D.C.

Kasey L. Moore, ARRT, RDMS, RT(R) (M) (RDMS)
Sonography Instructor
Danville Area Community College
Danville, Illinois

Susan M. Perry, BS, ARDMS
Program Director, Diagnostic Medical Sonography
Owens Community College
Toledo, Ohio

Kellee Ann Stacks, BS, RTR, RDMS, RVT
Program Director, Medical Sonography
Cape Fear Community College
Wilmington, North Carolina

PREFACE

INTRODUCING THE SEVENTH EDITION

The seventh edition of *Textbook of Diagnostic Sonography* continues the tradition of excellence that began when the first edition published in 1978. Like other medical imaging fields, diagnostic sonography has seen dramatic changes and innovations since its first experimental days. Phenomenal strides in transducer design, instrumentation, color-flow Doppler, tissue harmonics, contrast agents, and 3D imaging continue to improve image resolution and the diagnostic value of sonography. The seventh edition has kept abreast of advancements in the field by having each chapter reviewed by numerous sonographers currently working in different areas of medical sonography throughout the country. Their critiques and suggestions have helped ensure that this edition includes the most complete and up-to-date information needed to meet the requirements of the modern student of sonography.

Distinctive Approach

This textbook can serve as an in-depth resource both for students of sonography and for practitioners in any number of clinical settings, including hospitals, clinics, and private practices. Care has been taken to cultivate readers' understanding of the patient's total clinical picture even as they study sonographic examination protocol and technique. To this end, each chapter covers the following:

- Normal anatomy (including cross-sectional anatomy)
- Normal physiology
- Laboratory data and values
- Pathology
- Sonographic evaluation of an organ
- Sonographic findings
- Pitfalls in sonography
- Clinical findings
- Differential considerations

The full-color art program is of great value to the student of anatomy and pathology for sonography. Detailed line drawings illustrate the anatomic information a sonographer must know to successfully perform specific sonographic examinations. Color photographs of gross pathology help the reader visualize some of the pathology presented, and color Doppler illustrations are included where relevant.

To make important information easy to find, key points are pulled out into numerous boxes; tables throughout the chapters summarize the pathology under discussion and break the information down into Clinical Findings, Sonographic Findings, and Differential Considerations.

Sonographic findings for particular pathologic conditions are always preceded in the text by the following special heading:

Sonographic Findings. This icon makes it very easy for students and practicing sonographers to locate this clinical information quickly.

Study and review are also essential to gaining a solid grasp of the concepts and information presented in this textbook. Learning objectives, chapter outlines, comprehensive glossaries of key terms, full references for cited material, and a list of common medical abbreviations printed on the back inside cover all help students learn the material in an organized and thorough manner.

Scope and Organization of Topics

The *Textbook of Diagnostic Sonography* is divided into eight parts:

Part I introduces the reader to the foundations of sonography and patient care and includes the following:
- Basic principles of ultrasound physics and medical sonography
- Terminology frequently encountered by the sonographer
- Overview of physical findings, physiology, and laboratory data
- Patient care for the sonographer
- Ergonomics and musculoskeletal issues for practitioners
- Basics of other imaging modalities
- Image artifacts

Part II presents the abdomen in depth. The following topics are discussed:
- Anatomic relationships and physiology
- Abdominal scanning techniques and protocols
- Abdominal applications of ultrasound contrast agents
- Ultrasound-guided interventional techniques
- Emergent abdominal ultrasound procedures
- Separate chapters for the vascular system, the liver, gallbladder and biliary system, pancreas, gastrointestinal tract, urinary system, spleen, retroperitoneum, and peritoneal cavity and abdominal wall

Part III focuses on the superficial structures in the body including the breast, thyroid and parathyroid glands, scrotum, and musculoskeletal system.

Part IV explores sonographic examination of the neonate and pediatric patient.

Part V focuses on the thoracic cavity and includes:
- Anatomic and physiologic relationships within the thoracic cavity
- Echocardiographic evaluation and techniques
- Fetal echocardiography

Part VI comprises four chapters on extracranial and intracranial cerebrovascular imaging and peripheral arterial and venous sonographic evaluation.

Part VII is devoted to gynecology and includes the following topics:
- Normal anatomy and physiology of the female pelvis
- Sonographic and Doppler evaluation of the female pelvis
- Separate chapters on the pathologic conditions of the uterus, ovaries, and adnexa
- Updated chapter on the role of sonography in evaluating female infertility

Part VIII takes a thorough look at obstetric sonography. The following topics are discussed:
- The role of sonography in obstetrics
- Clinical ethics for obstetric sonography
- Normal first trimester and first-trimester complications
- Sonography of the second and third trimesters
- Obstetric measurements and gestational age
- Fetal growth assessment
- Prenatal diagnosis of congenital anomalies, with a separate chapter on 3D and 4D evaluation of fetal anomalies
- Chapters devoted to the placenta, umbilical cord, and amniotic fluid, as well as to the fetal face and neck, neural axis, thorax, anterior abdominal wall, abdomen, urogenital system, and skeleton

New to This Edition

Ten new contributors joined the seventh edition to update and expand existing content, bringing with them a fresh perspective and an impressive knowledge base. They also helped contribute the more than 1000 images new to this edition, including color Doppler, 3D, and contrast-enhanced images. More than 30 new line drawings complement the new chapters found in the seventh edition.

Essentials of Patient Care for the Sonographer (Chapter 3) covers all aspects of patient care the sonographer may encounter, including taking and understanding vital signs, handling patients on strict bed rest, patients with tubes and oxygen, patient transfer techniques, infection control, isolation techniques, emergency medical situations, assisting patients with special needs, and patient rights.

Ergonomics and Musculoskeletal Issues in Sonography (Chapter 4) outlines the importance of proper technique and positioning throughout the sonographic examination as a way to avoid long-term disability problems that may be acquired with repetitive scanning.

Understanding Other Imaging Modalities (Chapter 5) is a comparative overview of the multiple imaging modalities frequently encountered by the sonographer: computerized tomography, magnetic resonance, positron emission tomography (PET), nuclear medicine, and radiography.

Artifacts in Scanning (Chapter 6) is an outstanding review of all the artifacts commonly encountered by sonographers. There are numerous examples of the various artifacts and detailed explanations of how these artifacts are produced and how to avoid them.

3D and 4D Evaluation of Fetal Anomalies (Chapter 54) has a three-fold focus: (1) to introduce the sonographer to the technical concepts of 3D ultrasound; (2) to acquaint the sonographer with the 3D tools currently available; and (3) to provide clinical examples of the integration of 3D ultrasound into conventional sonographic examinations. Although a chapter with this title appeared in the last edition, this chapter has been entirely rewritten and includes all new illustrations.

Student Resources

Workbook. Available for separate purchase, *Workbook for Textbook of Diagnostic Sonography* has also been completely updated and expanded. This resource gives the learner ample opportunity to practice and apply the information presented in the textbook.

- Each workbook chapter covers all the material presented in the textbook.
- Each chapter includes exercises on image identification, anatomy identification, key term definitions, and sonographic technique.
- A set of 30 case studies using images from the textbook invites students to test their skills at identifying key anatomy and pathology and describing and interpreting sonographic findings.
- Students can also test their knowledge with the hundreds of multiple choice questions found in the four exams covering different content areas: General Sonography, Pediatric, Cardiovascular Anatomy, and Obstetrics and Gynecology.

Evolve. On the *Evolve* site, students will find a printable list of the key terms and definitions for each chapter; a printable selected bibliography for each chapter, and Weblinks.

Instructor Resources

Resources for instructors are also provided on the *Evolve* site to assist in the preparation of classroom lectures and activities.

- PowerPoint lectures for each chapter that include illustrations
- Test bank of 1500 multiple-choice questions in Examview and Word
- Electronic image collection that includes all the images from the textbook both in PowerPoint and in jpeg format

Evolve Online Course Management. *Evolve* is an interactive learning environment designed to work in coordination with *Textbook of Diagnostic Sonography.* Instructors may use *Evolve* to include an Internet-based course component that reinforces and expands upon the concepts delivered in class. *Evolve* may be used to:

- Publish the class syllabus, outlines, and lecture notes
- Set up virtual office hours and email communication
- Share important dates and information on the online class calendar
- Encourage student participation with chat rooms and discussion boards
- Post exams and manage grade books

For more information, visit http://www.evolve.elsevier.com/HagenAnsert/diagnostic/ or contact an Elsevier sales representative.

ACKNOWLEDGMENTS

I would like to express my gratitude and appreciation to a number of individuals who have served as mentors and guides throughout my years in sonography. Of course it all began with Dr. George Leopold at UCSD Medical Center. His quest for knowledge and his perseverance for excellence have been the mainstay of my career in sonography. I would also like to recognize Drs. Dolores Pretorius, Nancy Budorick, Wanda Miller-Hance, and David Sahn for their encouragement throughout the years at the UCSD Medical Center in both Radiology and Pediatric Cardiology.

I would also like to acknowledge Dr. Barry Goldberg for the opportunity he gave me to develop countless numbers of educational programs in sonography in an independent fashion and for his encouragement to pursue advancement. I would also like to thank Dr. Daniel Yellon for his early-hour anatomy dissection and instruction; Dr. Carson Schneck, for his excellent instruction in gross anatomy and sections of "Geraldine;" and Dr. Jacob Zutuchni, for his enthusiasm for the field of cardiology.

I am grateful to Dr. Harry Rakowski for his continued support in teaching fellows and students while I was at the Toronto Hospital. Dr. William Zwiebel encouraged me to continue writing and teaching while I was at the University of Wisconsin Medical Center, and I appreciate his knowledge, which found its way into the liver physiology section of this textbook.

My good fortune in learning about and understanding the *total patient* must be attributed to a very dedicated cardiologist, James Glenn, with whom I had the pleasure of working while I was at MUSC in Charleston, South Carolina. It was through his compassion and knowledge that I grew to appreciate the total patient beyond the transducer, and for this I am grateful.

For their continual support, feedback, and challenges, I would like to thank and recognize all the students I have taught in the various diagnostic medical sonography programs: Episcopal Hospital, Thomas Jefferson University Medical Center, University of Wisconsin-Madison Medical Center, UCSD Medical Center, and Baptist College of Health Science. These students continually work toward the development of quality sonography techniques and protocols and have given back to the sonography community tenfold.

The continual push towards excellence has been encouraged on a daily basis by our Scripps Clinic Cardiologists and David Rubenson, Medical Director of the Echo Lab at Scripps Clinic.

The sonographers at Scripps Clinic have been invaluable in their excellent image acquisition. Special thanks to Ewa Pikulski, Megan Marks and Kristen Billick for their echocardiographic images. The general sonographers at Scripps Clinic have been invaluable in providing the excellent images for the Obstetrics and Gynecology chapters.

I would like to thank the very supportive and capable staff at Elsevier who have guided me though yet another edition of this textbook. Jeanne Olson and her excellent staff are to be commended on their perseverance to make this an outstanding textbook. Linda Woodard was a constant reminder to me to stay on task and was there to offer assistance when needed. Jennifer Moorhead has been the mainstay of this project from the beginning and has done an excellent job with the manuscript. She is to be commended on her eye for detail.

I would like to thank my family, Art, Becca, Aly, and Kati, for their patience and understanding, as I thought this edition would never come to an end.

I think that you will find the 7th Edition of the *Textbook of Diagnostic Sonography* reflects the contribution of so many individuals with attention to detail and a dedication to excellence. I hope you will find this educational experience in sonography as rewarding as I have.

Sandra L. Hagen-Ansert
MS, RDMS, RDCS, FSDMS, FASE

CONTENTS

TEXTBOOK OF
DIAGNOSTIC SONOGRAPHY

PART V

The Thoracic Cavity

Anatomic and Physiologic Relationships within the Thoracic Cavity

Sandra L. Hagen-Ansert

OBJECTIVES

On completion of this chapter, you should be able to:
- Describe the landmarks of the thoracic cavity
- Define the relational landmarks of the heart
- Discuss the function of the pericardial sac
- Differentiate the three layers of the heart wall
- Describe the anatomic landmarks of the cardiac chambers, valves, and interventricular septum

OUTLINE

The Thorax and the Thoracic Cavity
The Heart and Great Vessels
 Pericardial Sac
 Linings of the Heart Wall
 Right Atrium and Interatrial Septum
 Tricuspid Valve
 Right Ventricle
 Pulmonary Valve and Trunk

Left Atrium
Mitral Valve
Left Ventricle
Interventricular Septum
Aortic Valve
Aortic Arch and Branches
The Cardiac Cycle
The Electrical Conduction System
 Bundle of His
 Cardiac Nerves

The Mechanical Conduction System
Electrocardiography
 P Wave
 QRS Complex
 P-R Interval
 T Wave
Auscultation of the Heart Valves
Principles of Blood Flow
 Ventricular Ejection
 Coronary Circulation

The cardiovascular system delivers oxygenated blood to tissues in the body and removes waste products from these tissues. The heart pumps blood to all the organs and tissues of the body. The autonomic nervous system controls how the heart pumps, and the vascular network (arteries and veins) carries blood throughout the body, keeps the heart filled with blood, and maintains blood pressure.

THE THORAX AND THE THORACIC CAVITY

The thorax constitutes the upper part of the body (Figure 31-1). There are eight external landmarks of the thorax. The *costal margin* is the lower boundary of the thorax; it is formed by the cartilages of the seventh through tenth ribs and the ends of the eleventh and twelfth cartilages. The *midaxillary line* runs vertically from a point midway between the anterior and posterior axillary folds. The *midclavicular line* is a vertical line from the midpoint of the clavicle. The *midsternal line* lies in the median plane over the sternum. The *sternal angle* is the angle between the manubrium and the body of the sternum; it is also known as the angle of Louis. The *suprasternal notch* is the superior margin of the manubrium sterni, lying opposite the lower border of the body of the second thoracic vertebra. The *xiphisternal joint* is the junction between the xiphoid and the sternum. The final external landmark of the thorax is the *xiphoid*, the lowest point of the sternum.

The thoracic cavity lies within the thorax and is separated from the abdominal cavity by the diaphragm. The diaphragm reaches upward as high as the midaxillary level of the seventh rib. The mediastinum is the medial portion of the thorax, and the pleurae and lungs are the lateral components (Figure 31-2).

Superiorly the upper thoracic cavity gives access to the root of the neck. It is bounded by the upper part of

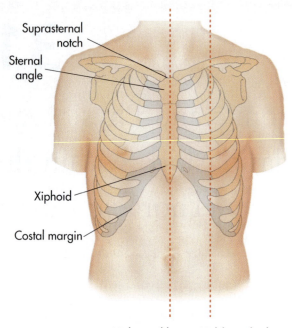

FIGURE 31-1 External landmarks of the thorax.

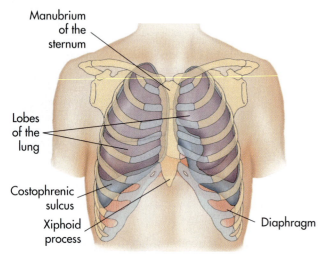

FIGURE 31-2 Anterior view of the thorax.

BOX 31-1	Major Mediastinal Structures from Anterior to Posterior

Superior Mediastinum
- Thymus
- Great veins
- Great arteries
- Trachea
- Esophagus and thoracic duct
- Sympathetic trunks

Inferior Mediastinum
- Thymus
- Heart within the pericardium with the phrenic nerves on either side
- Esophagus and thoracic duct
- Descending aorta
- Sympathetic trunks

lung. The external layer, or parietal pleura, is adherent to the inner surface of the chest wall (costal pleura), diaphragm (diaphragmatic pleura), and mediastinum (mediastinal pleura). The two layers become continuous with each other by a "cuff" of pleura that surrounds the structures at the hilum of the lung.

The costophrenic sinus is the pleural reflection between the costal and diaphragmatic portions of the parietal pleura. This space lies lower than the edge of the lung and, in most cases, is never occupied by the lung. When pleural fluid accumulates, its most common location is in the costophrenic sinus. On a radiographic examination, the costophrenic angle is blunted by the presence of pleural effusion.

The mediastinum is the median partition of the thoracic cavity. The mediastinum is a movable, thick structure and extends superiorly to the thoracic inlet and the root of the neck and inferiorly to the diaphragm. It extends anteriorly to the sternum and posteriorly to the 12th thoracic vertebra. Within the mediastinum are found the remains of the thymus, the heart and great vessels, the trachea and esophagus, the thoracic duct and lymph nodes, the vagus and phrenic nerves, and the sympathetic trunks.

The mediastinum may be divided into a superior and inferior mediastinum by an imaginary plane from the sternal angle to the lower body of the fourth thoracic vertebra (Box 31-1). The inferior mediastinum is subdivided into three parts: (1) middle, which contains the pericardium and the heart; (2) anterior, which is a space between the pericardium and sternum; and (3) posterior, which lies between the pericardium and vertebral column.

THE HEART AND GREAT VESSELS

The heart lies obliquely in the chest, posterior to the sternum, with the greater portion of its muscular mass lying slightly to the left of midline. The heart is protected within the chest by the sternum and rib cage anteriorly

the sternum, the first ribs, and the body of the first thoracic vertebra.

Anteriorly the sternum consists of the manubrium, the corpus sterni (body), and the xiphoid process. The junction between the manubrium and the body of the sternum is a prominent ridge; together they form the angle of Louis. This palpable landmark is important in locating the superior mediastinum or the second rib cartilages, which articulate with the sternum at this point.

The greater part of the thoracic cavity is occupied by the two lungs, which are enclosed by the pleural sac. To understand the pleural sac, imagine a deflated plastic bag covering your fist. Your fist should be enveloped by both sides of the bag to simulate the pleural sac. The internal layer, or visceral pleura, is adherent to each lobe of the and the vertebral column and rib cage posteriorly. The other structures within the thoracic cavity in close approximation to the heart are the lungs, esophagus, and descending thoracic aorta.

Contrary to most simplified anatomic illustrations, the heart is not situated with its right chambers lying to the right and its left chambers to the left. It may be better considered as an anteroposterior structure, with its right-side chambers located more anterior than its left-side chambers. As we look at the embryologic development, the heart forms as a tubular right-to-left structure. However, as development continues, the right side becomes more ventral and the left side remains dorsal.

In addition, another change in axis causes the apex (or the inferior surface of the heart) to tilt anteriorly. The final development of the heart presents the right atrium anterior to the left atrium and to the right of the sternum, whereas the right ventricle presents anterior to the left ventricle and slightly to the left of the sternum. The left atrium becomes the most posterior chamber to the left of the sternum, whereas the left ventricle swings its posterior axis slightly toward the anterior chest wall.

The heart has three surfaces: sternocostal (anterior), diaphragmatic (inferior or apex), and base (posterior)

(Figure 31-3). The right atrium forms the right border of the heart to the right of the sternum. The vertical atrioventricular groove separates these two structures.

The left border is formed by the left ventricle and left atrial appendage. The right and left ventricles are separated by the anterior interventricular groove. The diaphragmatic surface of the heart is formed principally by the right and left ventricles, separated by the posterior interventricular groove (Figure 31-4). A small part of the inferior surface of the right atrium also forms this surface.

The base of the heart is formed by the left atrium, into which the four pulmonary veins enter from the lungs. The right atrium contributes a small part to this posterior surface (Figure 31-5). The left ventricle forms the apex of the heart, which can be palpated at the level of the fifth intercostal space, about 9 cm from the midline.

Pericardial Sac

The heart and roots of the great vessels lie within the pericardial sac (see Figure 31-3). Like the pleura of the lungs, the pericardium is a double sac. The fibrous pericardium limits the movement of the heart by attaching to the central tendon of the diaphragm below and the

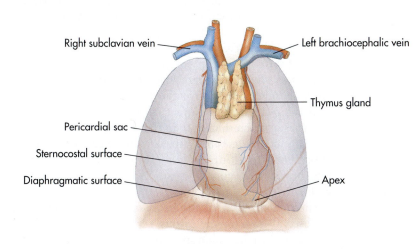

Right subclavian vein

Left brachiocephalic vein

Thymus gland

Pericardial sac

Sternocostal surface

Diaphragmatic surface

Apex

FIGURE 31-3 The heart and great vessels.

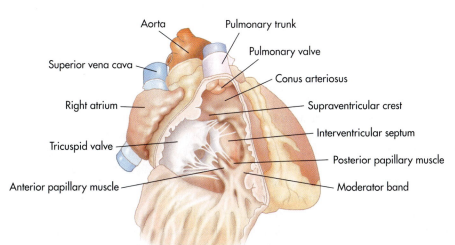

Aorta

Pulmonary trunk

Pulmonary valve

Superior vena cava

Conus arteriosus

Right atrium

Supraventricular crest

Interventricular septum

Tricuspid valve

Posterior papillary muscle

Anterior papillary muscle

Moderator band

FIGURE 31-4 Anterior view of the right ventricle.

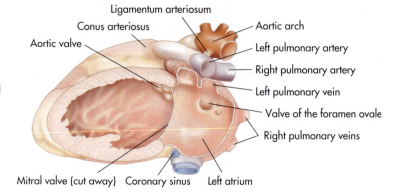

FIGURE 31-5 Posterolateral view of the left atrium and ventricle.

outer coat of the great vessels above. The sternopericardial ligaments attach to it in the front. The serous pericardium is divided into parietal and visceral layers. The parietal layer lines the fibrous pericardium and is reflected around the roots of the great vessels to become continuous with the visceral layer of serous pericardium. The visceral layer is closely applied to the heart and is often called the **epicardium.** The slit between the parietal and visceral layers is the pericardial cavity. This cavity normally contains a small amount of fluid that lubricates the heart as it moves.

The pericardial sac protects the heart against friction. If the serous pericardium becomes inflamed, pericarditis will develop, or if too much pericardial fluid, fibrin, or pus develops in the pericardial space, the visceral and parietal layers may adhere to one another.

The pericardial sac does not totally encompass the heart. On the posterior left atrial surface of the heart, the reflection of serous pericardium around the pulmonary veins forms the recess of the oblique sinus. This may be an important landmark in the echocardiographic separation of pericardial effusion from pleural effusion. The transverse sinus lies between the reflection of serous pericardium around the aorta and pulmonary arteries and between the reflection around the pulmonary veins.

Linings of the Heart Wall

The chambers of the heart are lined by the endocardium, myocardium, and epicardium. The **endocardium** is the intimal lining of the heart and is continuous with the intima of the vessels connecting to it. The endocardium is similar to the intima of blood vessels. It also forms the valves that lie between the filling (atria) and pumping (ventricle) chambers of the heart and along each base of the two great arterial trunks leaving the heart (the aorta and pulmonary artery).

The muscular part of the heart, the **myocardium,** is a special type of muscle found only in the heart and great vessels. This cardiac muscle is equivalent to the media of a blood vessel. The cardiac muscle is complex compared with other muscular fibers. Although it is striated like voluntary muscle, the fibers of the cardiac muscle branch

and anastomose so that it is impossible to determine the limits of a fiber. The myocardium of both ventricles is one continuous muscle mass, as is the myocardium of both atria. Because of this continuity, an impulse for contraction originating in the atrium can spread throughout the atrial musculature; similarly, an impulse originating in a ventricle can spread throughout the ventricular musculature. A special bundle of fibers connects the atria to the ventricles. The unique feature of cardiac muscle is the ability to possess intrinsic rhythmic contractility. It is this rhythmicity that keeps the heart contracting, with nerve impulses modifying rather than initiating the heartbeat.

Because the atria work at low pressures, the musculature of the atria is thin compared with the ventricular wall mass. The primary purpose of the atria is to act as filling chambers that drive the blood into the relaxed ventricular cavity. In contrast, the myocardium of the ventricles is much thicker than that of the atria. The left ventricle has the greatest muscle mass, because it must pump blood to all of the body, whereas the right ventricle needs only enough pressure to pump the blood to the lungs.

The outside layer of the heart is the epicardium, or the visceral layer of the serous pericardium. The outer surface of the epicardium is a single layer of mesothelial cells continuous with the serous (inner) surface of the pericardium.

Right Atrium and Interatrial Septum

The right atrium forms the right border of the heart (Figure 31-6). The superior vena cava enters the upper posterior border, and the inferior vena cava enters the lower posterolateral border. The posterior wall of the right atrium is directly related to the pulmonary veins (which flow from the lungs to empty into the left atrium). The medial wall of the right atrium is formed by the interatrial septum. The septum angles slightly posterior and to the patient's right, so the atrium lies in front and to the right of the left atrium. The central ovale portion of the septum is thin and fibrous. Just superior and in front of the opening of the inferior vena cava lies a shallow depression, the fossa ovalis. Its borders are the limbus fossae ovalis and the primitive septum primum. The foramen ovale lies under the most superior part of the limbus fossae. The limbus fossae ovalis is the remainder of the atrial septum and forms a ridge around the fossa ovalis.

The atrioventricular part of the membranous septum separates the right atrium and left ventricle. Atrial septal defects can occur in this area, causing blood to flow from the high-pressured left ventricle into the right atrial cavity.

The anterior and lateral walls of the right atrium are ridged by the pectinate muscles. The superior portion of the right atrium, the right atrial appendage, contains the most prominent pectinate muscles. The posterior and medial walls are smooth, probably because of the continual flow of blood from the inferior and superior vena cavas and coronary sinus.

The inferior vena cava is guarded by a fold of tissue called the eustachian valve, and the coronary sinus is guarded by the thebesian valve.

The coronary sinus drains the blood supply from the heart wall. It is bordered by the fossa ovalis and the tricuspid valve.

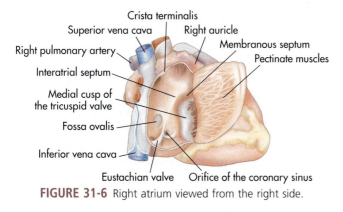

FIGURE 31-6 Right atrium viewed from the right side.

Tricuspid Valve

The tricuspid valve separates the right atrium from the right ventricle. It has three leaflets: anterior, septal, and inferior (or mural) (Figure 31-7). The septal leaflet may be maldeveloped in association with such conditions as ostium primum defect or ventricular septal defect. The leaflets are attached by their base to the fibrous atrioventricular ring. The chordae tendineae attach the leaflets to the papillary muscles. As these muscles contract with ventricular contraction, the leaflets are pulled together to prevent their being pulled into the atrial cavity. The septal and anterior leaflets are connected to the same papillary muscle, which helps in this process.

Right Ventricle

The base of the right ventricle lies on the diaphragm, and the roof is occupied by the crista supraventricularis, which lies between the tricuspid and pulmonary orifices. The right ventricle is essentially divided into two parts—the posteroinferior inflow portion (containing the tricuspid valve) and the anterosuperior outflow portion (containing the origin of the pulmonary trunk). The demarcation between these two parts is several prominent bands—the parietal band, supraventricular crest, septal band, and moderator band (see Figure 31-4). Together these bands form an almost circular orifice that normally is wide and forms no impediment to flow.

The inflow tract of the right ventricle is short and heavily trabeculated. It extends from the tricuspid valve and merges into the trabecular zone. This zone is the body of the right ventricle. The trabeculae carneae enclose an elongated ovoid opening. The inflow tract unites with the outflow tract, which extends to the pulmonary valve. The outflow portion of the right ventricle, or infundibulum, is smooth-walled and contains few trabeculae.

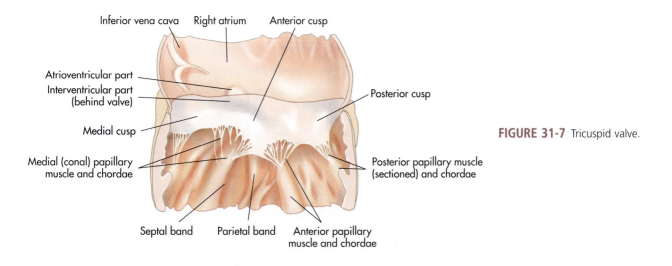

FIGURE 31-7 Tricuspid valve.

The right ventricle has two walls, an anterior wall (corresponding to the sternocostal surface) and a posterior wall (formed by the ventricular septum).

Pulmonary Valve and Trunk

The pulmonary valve lies at the upper anterior aspect of the right ventricle. It has three cusps: anterior, right, and left (Figure 31-8). The wall of the pulmonary artery bulges out adjacent to each cusp to form pockets known as the pulmonary sinuses of Valsalva.

The pulmonary trunk passes posterior and slightly upward from the right ventricle. It bifurcates into the right and left pulmonary arteries just after leaving the pericardial cavity. The ligamentum arteriosum connects the upper aspect of the bifurcation to the anterior surface of the aortic arch. (The ligamentum arteriosum is a remnant of the fetal ductus arteriosus.)

Left Atrium

The left atrium is a smooth-walled, circular sac that lies posterior in the base of the heart. Two pulmonary veins enter posteriorly on either side of the cavity (see Figure 31-5). Occasionally, these veins unite before entering the atrium, and sometimes there are more than two veins on either side. The veins may also be congenitally defective and enter the right atrium or other areas in the thoracic cavity. This absence of pulmonary veins entering the left atrial cavity is known as *total anomalous pulmonary venous return*.

The septal surface of the atrium is fairly smooth. A somewhat irregular area indicates the position of the fetal valve of the foramen ovale. The left auricle, or left atrial appendage, is a continuation of the left upper anterior part of the left atrium. Small pectinate muscles are located within its lumen.

Mitral Valve

The mitral valve separates the left atrium from the left ventricle. It consists of two large principal leaflets (anterior and posterior) and two small commissural cusps (which usually merge with the posterior leaflet). The anterior leaflet is much longer and larger than the posterior leaflet. It projects downward into the left ventricular cavity. The leaflets are thick membranes that are trapezoidal with fine irregular edges (Figure 31-9). They originate from the anulus fibrosus and are attached to the papillary muscles by chordae tendineae. The functions of the chordae tendineae are to prevent the opposing borders of the leaflets from inverting into the atrial cavity, to act as mainstays of the valves, and to form bands or foldlike structures that may contain muscle.

Left Ventricle

The left ventricle is conical or egg shaped. The smaller end of the ventricle represents the apex of the heart, and the larger end, near the orifice of the mitral valve, is near the base of the heart (Figure 31-10). The left ventricle has a short inflow tract from the mitral valve to the trabecular zone that merges with the outflow tract extending to the aortic valve. Unlike the right side of the heart (where there is no continuity between the tricuspid and pulmonary valves), the anterior leaflet of the mitral valve is continuous with the posterior aortic wall, and the left side of the interventricular septum is continuous with the anterior aortic wall.

The left ventricle has several wall segments that can be recognized in relation to their surrounding structures. The medial wall is formed by the ventricular septum. The lateral wall, posterior wall, posterior-basal wall, and apex are all formed by their relative locations in the heart. The lateral wall is covered with trabeculae, which

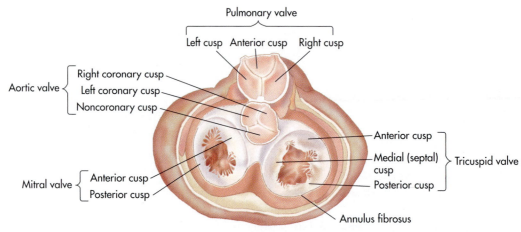

FIGURE 31-8 Heart viewed from the base with the atria removed.

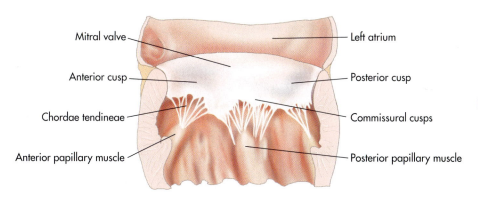

FIGURE 31-9 Mitral valve.

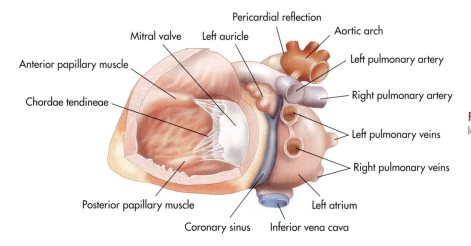

FIGURE 31-10 Posterolateral view of the left ventricle.

are finer and more numerous than those found in the right ventricle.

As mentioned previously, the wall of the ventricle consists of the endocardium, the myocardium, and the epicardium. This wall thickness is two to three times thicker than the right ventricular wall because it must handle the increased pressures in the left ventricular cavity.

Interventricular Septum

The septum is somewhat triangular in shape, with its apex corresponding to the apex of the heart and its base fusing posteriorly and superiorly with the atrial septum. The ventricular septum is formed of membranous, inflow, trabecular, and infundibular parts. These parts arise from the endocardial cushions, the primitive ventricle, and the bulbus cordis. The membranous septum varies in size and shape. It merges into the tissue at the aortic root and infundibular septum, but is sharply demarcated from the muscular portion of the septum.

Most of the interventricular septum is muscular and thicker than the membranous portion of the septum (Figure 31-11). The muscular septum makes up about two thirds of the septal length, with the membranous septum located just inferior to the aortic root in the area of the left ventricular outflow tract. Most interventricu-

lar septal defects occur in this thin, membranous part of the septum.

The muscular septum consists of two layers: a thin layer on the right side and a thicker layer on the left side. The major septal arteries run between these layers. The muscular portion of the septum has approximately the same thickness as the left ventricular wall.

Aortic Valve

The aortic valve lies at the root of the aorta and has right, left, and posterior (or noncoronary) cusps (Figure 31-12). The wall of the aorta bulges slightly at each cusp to form the sinus of Valsalva. The main coronary arteries arise from the right and left coronary cusps. At the center of each cusp is a small fibrous nodule, Arantius' nodule, which aids in preventing leakage of blood from the left ventricle when the aortic cusps are closed. Often it becomes the site of calcification in patients in whom arteriosclerosis develops.

Aortic Arch and Branches

The aortic arch is a continuation of the ascending aorta (Figure 31-13). The arch lies behind the manubrium sterni and runs upward, backward, and to the left in front of the trachea. It then passes downward to the left

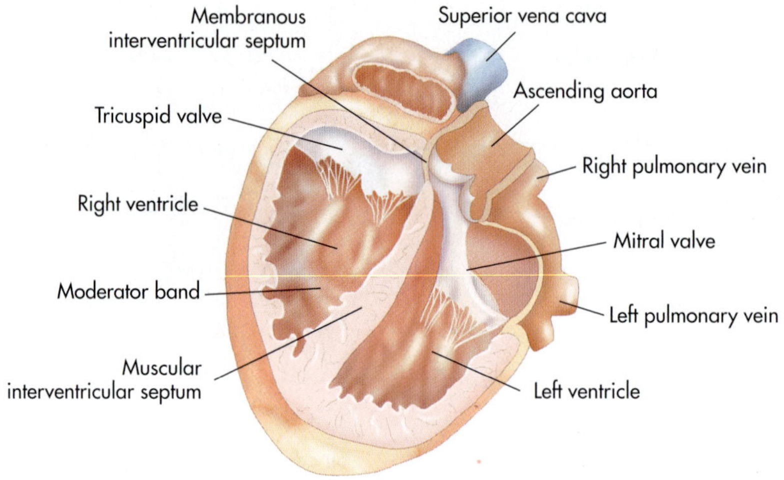

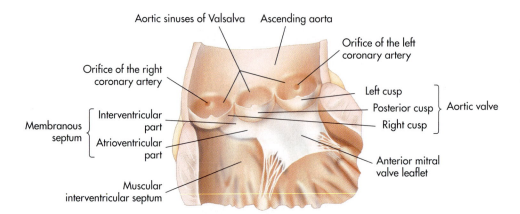

FIGURE 31-11 Long-axis view of the heart.

Membranous interventricular septum
Superior vena cava
Tricuspid valve
Ascending aorta
Right pulmonary vein
Right ventricle
Mitral valve
Moderator band
Left pulmonary vein
Muscular interventricular septum
Left ventricle

FIGURE 31-12 Aortic valve.

Aortic sinuses of Valsalva
Ascending aorta
Orifice of the left coronary artery
Orifice of the right coronary artery
Left cusp
Posterior cusp
Aortic valve
Membranous septum
Interventricular part
Right cusp
Atrioventricular part
Anterior mitral valve leaflet
Muscular interventricular septum

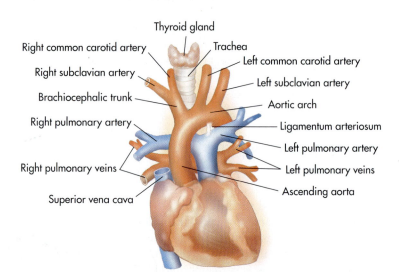

FIGURE 31-13 Aortic arch and branches.

Thyroid gland
Right common carotid artery
Trachea
Left common carotid artery
Right subclavian artery
Left subclavian artery
Brachiocephalic trunk
Aortic arch
Right pulmonary artery
Ligamentum arteriosum
Left pulmonary artery
Right pulmonary veins
Left pulmonary veins
Ascending aorta
Superior vena cava

of the trachea to become continuous with the descending aorta at the sternal angle.

The brachiocephalic artery arises from the convex surface of the arch. It passes upward and to the right of the trachea and divides into the right subclavian and common carotid arteries. The left common carotid artery arises from the aortic arch on the left side of the bra-chiocephalic artery. It runs upward and to the left of the trachea and enters the neck behind the left sternoclavicu-lar joint.

The left subclavian artery arises from the arch behind the left common carotid artery. It runs upward along the right side of the trachea and the esophagus to enter the root of the neck.

THE CARDIAC CYCLE

The heart is a muscular pump that propels blood to all parts of the body. It is able to act in definite strokes, or beats, and in the normal adult usually beats in sinus rhythm at 70 times per minute. The cardiac cycle is the series of changes that the heart undergoes as it fills with blood and empties (Box 31-2). Rhythmic contraction of the heart causes blood to be pumped through the chambers of the heart and out through the great vessels. The forceful contraction of the cardiac chambers is "systole," and the relaxed phase of the cycle is "diastole."

During diastole the venous blood enters the right atrium from the superior and inferior vena cavae. At the same time, the oxygenated blood returns from the lungs through the pulmonary veins to enter the left atrium. At this point the **atrioventricular valves** (tricuspid and mitral) between the atria and ventricles are open so that the blood may flow from the atria into the ventricles. The next phase allows atrial contraction to squeeze the remaining blood from the atria into the ventricles. The combination of atrial contraction and increased pressure of the full atrial cavities ultimately drains the atrial blood into the ventricles.

Shortly after this phase, the ventricles contract (ventricular systole). The rising pressure in the ventricular cavity closes the atrioventricular valves. As the pressure increases in the ventricles, the **semilunar valves** (pulmonary and aortic) open so that blood can be forced into the lungs and body, respectively.

The ventricles relax when contraction is completed (ventricular diastole). The blood in the aorta is under very high pressure, and the decreased pressure in the ventricles would cause it to flow backward into the ventricle. However, the semilunar valves prevent this reverse flow. The blood fills the sinuses of Valsalva and forces the valves to close. During ventricular contraction, the atria relax and the venous blood starts to fill them again. When the ventricles are completely relaxed, the atrioventricular valves open and blood flows into the ventricles to begin the next cardiac cycle.

THE ELECTRICAL CONDUCTION SYSTEM

The heart consists of a syncytium of striated muscle cells held together with fibrous tissue. The specialized muscle cells with a high degree of inherent rhythmicity are present in conduction tissue in the areas concerned with the generation and propagation of excitatory electrical activity.

The electrical conduction system of the heart consists of specialized cardiac muscle in the sinoatrial node, atrioventricular node, atrioventricular bundle and its right and left terminal branches, and subendocardial plexus of Purkinje fibers (Figure 31-14). The sinoatrial node initiates the normal cardiac impulse and is often called the pacemaker of the heart. It is situated on the lateral wall of the right atrium, at the upper part of the sulcus terminalis just to the right of the opening of the superior vena cava. Once activated, the cardiac impulse spreads through the atrial myocardium to reach the atrioventricular node. The atrioventricular node is located in the right posterior portion of the interatrial septum. It lies subendocardially in the medial wall of the right atrium to the left of the ostium of the coronary sinus and immediately posterior to the basal attachment of the septal cusp of the tricuspid valve.

Bundle of His

The atrioventricular node is continuous with the bundle of His, which forms the common bundle that passes along the posterior edge of the membranous septum. The bundle branches include the common bundle, and right and left branches. The common bundle divides into the right and left bundle branch and extends subendocardially along both septal surfaces. The left branch divides into anterior and posterior branches that run along the left interventricular septal surface into the Purkinje fibers, which spread to all parts of the ventricular myocardium.

Cardiac Nerves

The heart is innervated by cholinergic fibers from the vagus nerve and by adrenergic fibers arising from the thoracolumbar sympathetic system and passing through the superior, middle, and inferior cervical ganglions.

BOX 31-2	Phases of the Cardiac Cycle (Electromechanical Events)

1. Passive Filling Phase (Ventricular Diastole)
Early diastole, blood enters ventricles through AV valves
Venous blood continues to enter atria during this phase
Ventricles expand and pressure slowly rises as ventricular volume increases
Inflow volume diminishes in middiastole

2. Atrial Systole (P Wave on EKG, Late Diastole)
Active contraction of atria stops venous inflow
Rapid push of blood into ventricles
Causes pressure rise in both atria and ventricles (a wave)

3. Isovolumetric Contraction
Part of preejection period from onset of QRS complex to onset of ventricular ejection
Occurs from closure of AV valves to onset of ventricular ejection (opening of semilunar valves)
Ventricles contract isovolumetrically:
  a. Pressure rises in ventricles until pressure reaches that of corresponding great vessel
  b. Pulling down of mitral/tricuspid valve ring causes fall in atrial pressure
  c. Rate of change in LV pressure during isometric ventricular contraction is dp/dt

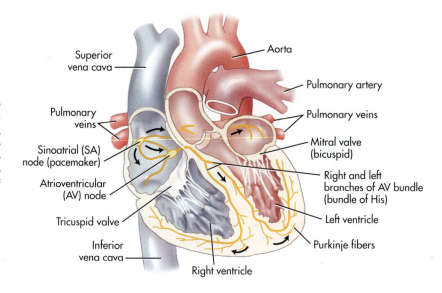

FIGURE 31-14 Conducting system of the heart. Specialized cardiac muscle cells in the wall of the heart rapidly conduct an electrical impulse through the myocardium. The signal is initiated by the SA node (pacemaker) and spreads to the rest of the atrial myocardium and to the AV node. The AV node then initiates a signal that is conducted through the ventricular myocardium by way of the AV bundle of His and Purkinje fibers.

THE MECHANICAL CONDUCTION SYSTEM

The Frank-Starling law of the heart states that the output of the heart increases in proportion to the degree of diastolic stretch of the muscle fibers. When a sarcomere is maximally shortened, the actin filaments overlap in the middle, covering up and eliminating from cross-linkage a number of active sites. As the sarcomere is stretched, more sites are uncovered and made available for cross-linkage, increasing the force that is developed. The longer the initial resting length of the cardiac muscle (preload), the greater the strength of contraction of the following beat. A further stretch beyond the normal range cuts the amount of overlap and the force of contraction by reducing the number of cross-bridges.

The shortening velocity of cardiac muscle is inversely related to *afterload*, or the force opposing ventricular ejection. The long interval between beats increases the strength of the next cardiac contraction. Tachycardia causes increased strength of contraction. The intracellular calcium ion concentration is probably involved in cellular mechanism.

ELECTROCARDIOGRAPHY

Electrocardiography is a method of recording the heart's electrical activity. It is used to assess cardiac function and disorders of the heart. The contraction of the heart muscle is accompanied by electrical changes, which can be detected by electrodes placed on the skin's surface, and they can be recorded as an electrocardiogram on a sheet of graphic paper. On stimulation of a muscle or nerve, the cell membranes are **depolarized,** and on recovery they are **repolarized.** These electrical events are spread throughout the body and can be detected with suitable instruments applied to the skin's surface at considerable distances from the sites of origin. There are various standard positions on the front of the chest on which the electrodes are placed to obtain an adequate electrical signal.

The heart's electrical activity is propagated in the following manner:

- It starts with firing of the SA node.
- Electrical events precede mechanical events: atrial contraction follows the P wave on EKG and generates the atrial systolic activity (a wave). Activation proceeds in an orderly, repetitive fashion as the impulse spreads by several internodal pathways through both atria.
- When the impulse reaches the AV node near the tricuspid valve, the cells of the bundle of His are activated and the impulse passes via the right and left bundle branches, the latter splitting into the anterior and posterior divisions.
- The impulse spreads via the Purkinje fibers to activate the ventricles, generating the Q, R, and S waves of the ECG (ventricular depolarization).
- After the ventricles depolarize, they begin to repolarize; this repolarization is demarcated by the T wave on the ECG.

In echocardiography examinations, three ECG lead wires are used for the electrocardiogram (ECG) tracing. Two ECG leads are placed on the patient's right and left shoulders and a ground lead on the right hip. The ECG has three components: P, QRS, and T waves (Figure 31-15).

P Wave

The impulse is initiated by the sinoatrial (SA) node and spreads over the atria. The P wave represents the electrical activity associated with the spread of the impulse over the atria (i.e., the wave of depolarization or activity of the atria).

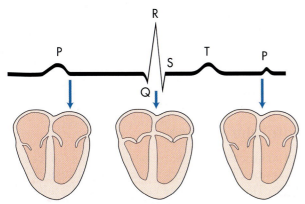

FIGURE 31-15 Components of the ECG as seen on the real-time image. The P wave represents the depolarization of cardiac muscle tissue in the SA node and atrial walls. Before the QRS complex is observed, the AV node and AV bundle depolarize. The QRS complex occurs as the atrial walls repolarize and the ventricular walls depolarize. The T wave occurs as the ventricular walls repolarize. Depolarization triggers contraction in the affected muscle tissue. Cardiac muscle contraction occurs after depolarization.

QRS Complex

The wave of depolarization spreads from the SA node over the bundle branches (bundle of His) and Purkinje system to activate both ventricles simultaneously. The QRS complex is the result of all electrical activity occurring in the ventricles.

P-R Interval

The P-R interval is measured from the beginning of the P wave to the beginning of the QRS complex. It indicates the time that elapses between activation of the SA node and activation of the AV node.

T Wave

The T wave represents ventricular repolarization. The echocardiographic examination is always performed with an ECG. This allows the cardiac sonographer to assess cardiac events as they occur in systole and diastole.

Excitation Contraction Coupling. The cardiac muscle is a type of striated muscle tissue. The cells are joined by intercalated disks. The calcium ions are stored and released in response to electrical activity.

AUSCULTATION OF THE HEART VALVES

Heart sounds are associated with the initiation of ventricular systole, closing of the atrioventricular valves, and opening of the semilunar valves (Figure 31-16). The first sound is lower in pitch and longer in duration than the second. Both sounds can be heard over the entire area of the heart, but the first sound, "lub," is heard most clearly in the region of the apex of the heart.

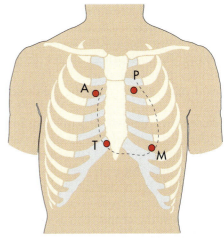

FIGURE 31-16 The valve opening and closing sounds may be heard best with the least interference at the location of the circles. *A,* Aortic valve; *M,* mitral valve; *P,* pulmonic valve; *T,* tricuspid valve.

The second sound, "dub," is sharper and shorter and has a higher pitch. It is heard best over the second right rib because the aorta approaches nearest to the surface at this point. The second sound is caused mainly by the closing of the semilunar valves during ventricular diastole. Following the second sound, there is a period of silence. Thus, the sequence sounds like this: lub, dub, silence, lub, dub, silence, and so on.

Defects in the valves can cause excessive turbulence or regurgitation of the blood. These are extra abnormal sounds and are called **murmurs** or *clicks*. If the valves fail to close tightly and blood leaks back, a hissing murmur is heard in the area of the affected valve; thus, if the mitral valve is affected, it will be heard in the first sound. Another condition giving rise to an abnormal sound is stenosis or stiffening of a valve orifice. In this case, a rumble is heard in the area of the affected valve. A **diastolic murmur** begins with or after the time of the second heart sound and ends at or before the time of the first heart sound. A **systolic murmur** begins with or after the time of the first heart sound and ends at or before the time of the second heart sound. A **continuous murmur** begins in systole and continues without interruption through the time of the second heart sound into all or part of diastole. Murmurs are graded according to **frequency** and **intensity**.

It is beyond the scope of this text to present an in-depth approach to auscultation, and the reader is referred to the Selected Bibliography on the Evolve site for additional reading on this subject. An understanding of auscultation will help in understanding cardiac physiology and echocardiographic differential considerations.

PRINCIPLES OF BLOOD FLOW

Blood flow may be described in terms of laminar flow or disturbed flow. *Laminar flow* means that blood moves in smooth layers that slide against each other. The blood cells move with similar velocities and directions in an organized manner. *Disturbed flow* means that blood cells move in different directions with varying velocities (disorganized flow). The turbulence denotes the presence of random vortices (flow eddies).

The flow dynamics depend on the fluid viscosity and the momentum of molecules in the fluid. The velocity profile indicates two pathways: parabolic flow or flat flow. The *parabolic flow velocity profile* is such that as fluid moves through a tube, fluid layers in the center have a higher velocity than those on outer surfaces. The *flat flow velocity profile* states that as flow accelerates and converges, more fluid travels at velocities closer to peak velocity as layers in the center. This is characteristic of high-velocity flow and at the inlets of the great vessels.

The heart is a pulsatile pump. In systole the ventricles eject blood into the aorta and pulmonary artery. In diastole, the ventricles fill with blood from the atria and flow to the body organs. The damping effect is achieved because of the elasticity of great vessels as they absorb high flow pulsatility of the heart and smooth it out before sending it to the blood downstream. The blood vessels stretch in response to an increase in pressure (compliance). The increase in fluid pressure during systole causes the aorta and pulmonary artery to expand and store some of the ejected blood. Blood is prevented from reentering the ventricles by the closure of the valves. Stored blood is pushed downstream into circulation when the aorta and pulmonary artery begin to return to normal dimensions in diastole. The hardening of the arteries results in loss of vessel compliance. The circulatory impedance occurs because of resistance to flow downstream in small vessels and capillaries. Flow is produced when a pressure gradient exists. The blood flow through a constriction creates a high fluid pressure upstream from constriction. The high fluid pressure forces blood through the constriction in the form of a laminar high-velocity jet. The fluid pressure gradually decreases as it goes downstream. Flow velocity through the constriction is higher than the velocity upstream. The normal resting cardiac output is 5 L/min.

Ventricular Ejection

Both ventricles eject the same proportion of contents with systole. The normal left ventricular ejection fraction is 67%. The normal stroke volume is 45 ± 13 ml/m^2. The amount of filling (preload) influences the pressure developed during the next systole via the Frank Starling mechanism. The output of the ventricle depends on resistance encountered by the contracting ventricle when the aortic valve opens during systole (afterload). The most important indicator of cardiac work is the metabolic cost of cardiac activity, which is given by the oxygen consumption of the myocardium.

Coronary Circulation

The coronary flow is essential to myocardial performance. The right and left coronary arteries arise from the base of the ascending aorta. The left coronary artery flow is mainly diastolic. The right coronary artery flow is more evenly spread through systole and diastole. The flow goes from the epicardium to the endocardium. The diastolic aortic pressure is a major factor in coronary perfusion. Myocardial ischemia may occur in situations in which blood pressure is acutely lowered. The arteries and arterioles anastomose with one another and the small collateral channels increase in number when vessels are occluded.

Introduction to Echocardiographic Evaluation and Technique

Sandra L. Hagen-Ansert

The evaluation of cardiac structures by echocardiography is regarded as an essential diagnostic tool in clinical cardiology. The reason for its widespread use in the evaluation of cardiac disease is its noninvasive, reproducible, and accurate assessment of cardiac structures. Early evaluation of the cardiac structures was initially performed with A-mode assessment of the mitral valve. The development of motion mode (M-mode) allowed the clinician to observe the diastolic and systolic components of the valve motion over time. The M-mode technique was limited in that it provided only a one-dimensional or "ice pick" view of the heart. Echocardiography exploded when two-dimensional (2D) echocardiography was developed, which allowed the cardiac structures to be dynamically visualized in real-time. Thus, the echocardiographer can now assess the four chambers of the heart, all the cardiac valves, the intracardiac anatomy, and the intracardiac lesions; observe contractility; deter-mine valvular function; and assess hemodynamics. The combination of real-time, Doppler, and color flow analysis provides an extremely accurate means to evaluate wall or valve thickness, valvular orifice and chamber size, and contractility of the cardiac structures. The introduction of transesophageal echocardiography (TEE) and three-dimensional (3D) echocardiography has enabled exquisite visualization of the heart while the transducer is guided through the mouth and into the esophagus to image the cardiac anatomy. Contrast injected into the bloodstream has provided an additional pathway to enhance cardiac endocardial borders, whereas saline bubble injections have been a clinical aid to determine the presence and direction of septal shunt flow. Exercise echocardiography and dobutamine-injection echocardiography have provided information about the contractility and performance of the left ventricle in a simulated stress situation.

To perform an echocardiographic examination of good diagnostic quality, the sonographer must understand the anatomic, hemodynamic, and pathophysiologic parameters of the heart and be able to incorporate the physical principles of sonography into the routine examination. This chapter introduces the reader to the basic concepts of echocardiography through two-dimensional, M-mode, Doppler, and color Doppler imaging. Emphasis will be on common findings the general sonographer may encounter "above the diaphragm."

TRANSDUCERS

Several types of transducers are available for echocardiographic techniques. Ideally, one should use as high a frequency as possible to improve the resolution of returning echoes. However, the higher the frequency, the less the penetration; therefore, compromises have to be made to obtain the best possible image. Many echocardiographers working with adults use a 2.5- to 5.0-MHz transducer with a medium focus. A pediatric patient generally requires a 5.0- or 7.5-MHz transducer for improved resolution and near-field definition.

EXAMINATION TECHNIQUES

The patient is generally examined in the left lateral semidecubitus position. This position allows the heart to move away from the sternum and closer to the chest wall, thus allowing a better cardiac window. The cardiac window is found between the third and fifth intercostal spaces, slightly to the left of the sternal border. The cardiac window may be considered that area on the anterior chest where the heart is just beneath the skin surface, free of lung interference.

The cardiac sonographer must keep in mind that different body shapes require variations in transducer position. An obese patient may have a horizontal transverse heart, and thus a slight lateral movement from the sternal border may be needed to record cardiac structures. A thin patient may have a long and slender heart, requiring a lower, more medial transducer position. Barrel-chested patients may have echocardiographic difficulties because of the lung absorption interference. It may be necessary to turn these patients completely on their left sides or even prone to eliminate the interference. Sometimes the upright or slightly forward-bent position is useful in forcing the heart closer to the anterior chest wall.

The following techniques are guidelines for the average patient. In the initial echocardiographic study, moving the transducer freely along the left sternal border until all the cardiac structures are easily identified is a better practice than restricting the transducer to one interspace. This procedure saves time and gives the examiner a better understanding of cardiac relationships. If the heart is actually medial, the best study is performed with the patient completely on his or her left side. If too much lung interference clouds the study, the patient should exhale for as long as possible. This usually gives the examiner enough time to record valid information.

TWO-DIMENSIONAL ECHOCARDIOGRAPHY

The widespread clinical acceptance of real-time, two-dimensional imaging has tremendously aided the diagnostic results of a typical echocardiographic examination. Improved transducer design, resolution capabilities, focus parameters, gray-scale differentiation, gain control factors, cine loop functions, and other computer capabilities have aided the cardiac sonographer in the attempt to record consistent, high-quality images from the multiple scan planes necessary to obtain a composite image of the cardiac structures.

In addition, two-dimensional transducers have the combined function of imaging and performing an M-mode or a Doppler study simultaneously. The introduction of color flow Doppler has added a new dimension for the cardiac sonographer in detecting intracardiac shunt flow, mapping regurgitant pathways, and determining obstructive flow pathways. This chapter presents two-dimensional echo with Doppler and color flow Doppler techniques together.

Transducer Location and Imaging Planes

The Committee on Nomenclature and Standards in Two-Dimensional Echocardiography of the American Society of Echocardiography recommends the following nomenclature and image orientation standards for transducer locations (Figure 32-1):

- *Suprasternal.* Transducer placed in the suprasternal notch.
- *Subcostal.* Transducer located near the body midline and beneath the costal margin.
- *Apical.* Transducer located over the cardiac apex (at the point of maximal impulse).
- *Parasternal.* Transducer placed over the area bounded superiorly by the left clavicle, medially by the sternum, and inferiorly by the apical region.

The imaging planes are described by the manner in which the two-dimensional transducer transects the heart (Figure 32-2):

- *Long axis.* Transects the heart perpendicular to the dorsal and ventral surfaces of the body and parallel with the long axis of the heart.
- *Short axis.* Transects the heart perpendicular to the dorsal and ventral surfaces of the body and perpendicular to the long axis of the heart.
- *Four chamber.* Transects the heart approximately parallel with the dorsal and ventral surfaces of the body.

CARDIAC COLOR FLOW EXAMINATION

The **color flow mapping (CFM)** examination is generally performed along with the conventional two-dimensional examination. The advantage of CFM is its ability to rapidly investigate flow direction and movement within the cardiac chambers (Box 32-1). Flow toward the transducer is recorded in red, and flow away from the transducer is blue (Figure 32-3). As the velocities increase, the flow pattern in the variance mode turns from red to various shades of red, orange, and yellow before it aliases. Likewise flow away from the transducer is recorded in blue; this color turns to various shades of blue, turquoise, and green before it aliases. Depending on the location of the transducer, the flow signals from various structures within the heart appear as different colors. An understanding of cardiac hemodynamics helps the examiner understand the flow patterns.

Although normal cardiac flows are difficult to accurately time during the CFM examination because of its slow frame rate, the use of color M-mode (with a faster

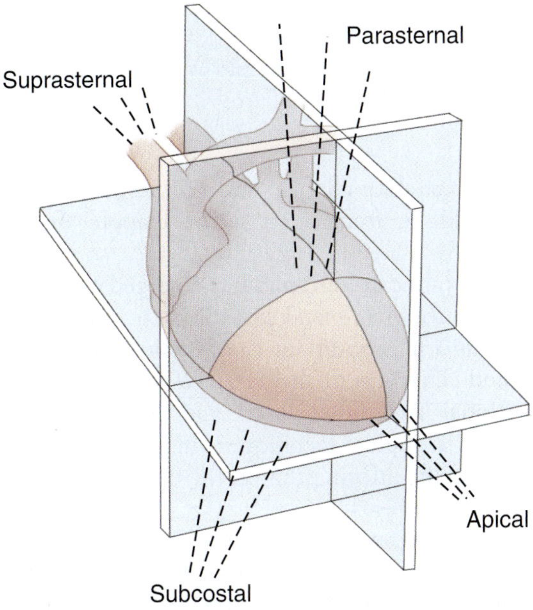

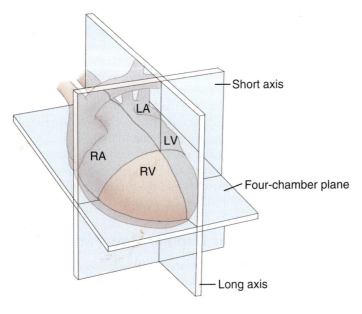

FIGURE 32-1 Schema of the four transducer positions for the two-dimensional echocardiogram: suprasternal transducer is placed in the suprasternal notch, subcostal transducer is located near the midline and beneath the costal margin, apical transducer is located over the cardiac apex, and parasternal transducer is located in the fourth intercostal space just to the left of midline.

BOX 32-1	Normal Color Flow Mapping Examination and Techniques

- The color flow mapping examination is generally performed in the same planes used for conventional Doppler examination.
- Parasternal long-axis view: MV, TV, AO
- Parasternal short-axis view: AO, PA, RVOT, IAS, TV
- Parasternal short-axis view: MV, TV, AO, PV
- Apical four-chamber plane: MV, TV
- Apical five-chamber plane: LVOT, AV
- Apical long-axis, two-chamber view: LV, MV, LA
- Subcostal four-chamber view: IAS, IVS, RV, LV, RA, LA
- Subcostal view: IVC, hepatic veins
- Subcostal 5 chamber view: AO, LVOT
- Subcostal short-axis view: AO, PA, RVOT
- Suprasternal view (long axis): ascending and descending aorta, SVC
- Suprasternal view (short axis): arch, RPA, LA, SVC, pulmonary veins

AO, Aorta; *AV,* aortic valve; *IAS,* interatrial septum; *LA,* left atrium; *LV,* left ventricle; *RA,* right atrium; *RV,* right ventricle; *IVS,* interventricular septum; *LA,* left atrium; *LV,* left ventricle; *LVOT,* left ventricular outflow tract; *MV,* mitral valve; *PA,* pulmonary artery; *PV,* pulmonary valve; *RA,* right atrium; *RPA,* right pulmonary artery; *RV,* right ventricle; *RVOT,* right ventricular outflow tract; *SVC,* superior vena cava; *TV,* tricuspid valve.

FIGURE 32-2 Schema of the parasternal long and short axis, and apical four-chamber views of the heart. *LA,* Left atrium; *LV,* left ventricle; *RA,* right atrium; *RV,* right ventricle.

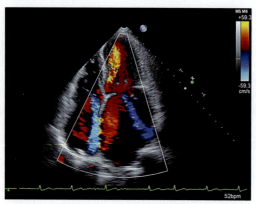

FIGURE 32-3 Apical four-chamber view with color. The color bar is shown along the right margin; yellow and red indicate flow toward the transducer, and blue and turquoise indicate flow away from the transducer. This patient has both mitral and tricuspid regurgitation. Note the blue flow in the right and left atria from the regurgitant jet.

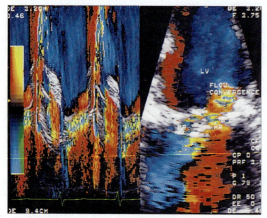

FIGURE 32-4 Flow convergence as imaged in the four-chamber view and M-mode/color flow mapping image. The red inflow is from the pulmonary veins into the left atrium, the blue is swirling flow within the left atrium, and the multicolored flow at the level of the mitral valve is regurgitant flow. *LV,* Left ventricle; *MR,* mitral regurgitation.

frame rate) allows one to precisely determine specific cardiac events in correlation with the ECG. The color M-mode is made in the same manner as a conventional M-mode study (Figure 32-4). The cursor is placed through the area of interest, and the flow is evaluated using an autocorrelation technique. The operator must thoroughly understand the color instrument settings to produce a high-quality image. Familiarity with the color flow maps provided in the software of the equipment is necessary to understand the alias patterns and turbulent flow parameters.

DOPPLER APPLICATIONS AND TECHNIQUE

The Doppler effect (see Chapter 1) is demonstrated on an echocardiogram as red blood cells move from a lower-frequency sound source at rest toward a higher-frequency

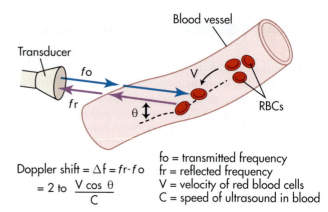

$$\text{Doppler shift} = \Delta f = fr - fo$$
$$= 2 \, to \, \frac{V \cos \theta}{C}$$

fo = transmitted frequency
fr = reflected frequency
V = velocity of red blood cells
C = speed of ultrasound in blood

FIGURE 32-5 The Doppler effect. The Doppler shift depends on the transmitted frequency *(fo),* the velocity of the moving target *(V),* and the angle *(θ)* between the ultrasound beam and the direction of the moving target.

sound source. The change in frequency is called the Doppler shift in frequency, or the **Doppler frequency** (Figure 32-5).

Doppler echocardiography has emerged as a valuable noninvasive tool in clinical cardiology to provide hemodynamic information about the function of the cardiac valves and chambers of the heart. When combined with conventional two-dimensional and M-mode echocardiography, Doppler techniques may be focused to produce specific information on the flows of a particular area within the heart.

Advances in Doppler technology have made it possible to provide steerable continuous wave and pulsed wave Doppler. The ability to be qualitative and quantitative in evaluating valvular function, intracardiac shunts, dysfunction of a prosthetic valve, and obstruction of a surgically inserted shunt and to record normal cardiac blood flow patterns has contributed to the understanding and diagnostic capability of the Doppler technique in cardiology. However, to record this information, the cardiac sonographer and physician should master cardiac physiology and hemodynamics. In addition, the operator must clearly understand Doppler principles, artifacts, and pitfalls to produce a quality study. Although cardiac instrumentation is fundamentally similar to imaging echocardiography, the approach to Doppler, especially color Doppler, varies considerably from one company to another. A solid understanding of the instrumentation is necessary to produce a valid examination.

This section on the normal Doppler examination is presented so the reader may become familiar with the normal Doppler patterns and the pitfalls in both recording and listening to Doppler signals.

Normal Cardiac Doppler Flow Patterns

It is important to understand the relationship between the two-dimensional study and the Doppler flow study. Real-time two-dimensional imaging allows assessment of cardiac anatomy and function. On the other hand, Doppler flow analysis allows examination of blood flow rather than cardiac anatomy. The Doppler principle on which this technique is based involves the backscatter of transmitted ultrasonic waves from circulating red blood cells. The difference in frequency between transmitted and backscattered sound waves (Doppler shift) is used to quantify forward or backward blood flow velocity.

Quality Doppler studies require the patient to be still for several seconds. In adult patients this usually is not difficult, but in pediatric patients it may be a challenge. Therefore, it is necessary that the instrumentation used in pediatrics respond quickly to changes in the menu or Doppler format. It is essential to be able to change back and forth between the real-time image and the Doppler image or to image the real-time and Doppler images simultaneously. The ability to simultaneously perform the Doppler and two-dimensional study allows the sonographer to image cardiac structures and to place the sample volume in the proper location.

The best-quality Doppler signals are obtained when the sample volume is parallel to the direction of flow. The flow of blood occurs in three-dimensional space, whereas the real-time image is only in two dimensions. Therefore, the two-dimensional image serves as a guide to the operator as small adjustments of the transducer and sample volume are made in the valve orifice to record the optimal Doppler signals. The key is to produce a spectral signal to show a well-defined velocity envelope along with a clearly defined audio tone. The clarity of the audio tone cannot be emphasized enough. Frequently the clarity of tone is used to guide the Doppler cursor into the correct plane to record the maximum velocity.

Blood flow toward the transducer is displayed by a time velocity waveform above the baseline at point zero, or a positive deflection (Figure 32-6). Flow away from the Doppler signal is displayed below the baseline or as a negative deflection. A simultaneous ECG should be displayed to help time the cardiac cycle.

Pulsed Wave Doppler

A **pulsed wave transducer** is constructed with a single crystal that sends bursts of ultrasound at a rate called the *pulsed repetition frequency*. The transducer receives sound waves backscattered from moving red blood cells during a limited time between transmitted pulses. A time gating device is then used to select the precise depth from which the returning signal has originated because the signals return from the heart at different times.

The particular area of interest undergoing Doppler evaluation is referred to as the *sample volume*. The sample volume and directional line placement of the beam are moved by use of the trackball. The exact size and location of the sample volume can be adjusted at the area of interest. Some instruments have a fixed sample volume size. Others allow the operator to select the size appropriate for the particular study.

Velocities under 2 m/sec are recorded without an alias pattern (Figure 32-7). However, pulsed Doppler is limited in its ability to record high-velocity patterns. The maximum frequency shift that can be measured by a pulsed Doppler system is called the Nyquist limit, and is one half the pulsed repetition frequency. Velocities that exceed this limit are known to produce an aliasing pattern (Figure 32-8). Normal cardiac structures do not exceed the Nyquist limit and are easily measured with the pulsed Doppler system.

Continuous Wave Doppler

The **continuous wave probe** differs from the pulsed wave probe in that it requires two crystals (Figure 32-9). One crystal continuously emits sound; the other receives sound as it is backscattered to the transducer. This probe may be part of a phased or annular array imaging probe or may be a stand-alone independent probe. If it is part of a two-dimensional imaging transducer, the sample direction can sometimes be steered by use of the

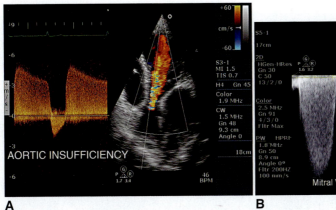
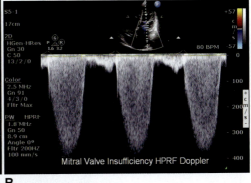

FIGURE 32-6 A, Flow above the baseline represents forward flow (as seen in this patient with aortic insufficiency). **B,** Flow below the baseline represents flow moving away from the transducer (as seen in this patient with mitral regurgitation).

trackball. This method has many advantages in the Doppler study; it is quicker and more efficient to be able to image a structure and then move the Doppler cursor to obtain the best audio and spectral signals.

Some instruments have a fixed continuous wave sample direction, which means that the area of interest must be aligned with a stationary line on the screen to obtain the best signal. This method is tedious and difficult to maintain for a good tracing.

The independent continuous wave probe is smaller than the imaging probe and thus has advantages in obtaining a good Doppler study. Because the diameter of the probe is smaller, it allows greater flexibility to reach in between small rib interspaces or to obtain signals from the suprasternal notch. Many patients will allow the small independent probe to be angled within their suprasternal notch but not the bulky imaging probe. The independent probe is often more sensitive and therefore produces better Doppler signals. The audio portion of the Doppler examination becomes a critical factor in this study because there is no two-dimensional image to guide in the transducer location.

It is often beneficial to use both probes to perform the study. Once the proper transducer position is found with the imaging transducer, the angulation and window are marked for proper placement of the continuous wave transducer (see Figure 32-8). The audio sound and spectral wave pattern are then used to guide the correction angulation of the beam for maximum-velocity recordings. There is not a particular sample volume site within the continuous wave beam. Velocities are recorded from several points along the linear beam. This technique has the ability to record maximum velocities without alias patterns. The recording ability is especially useful for very high-velocity patterns.

Audio Signals and Spectral Display of Doppler Signals

The best Doppler signals are obtained when the ultrasound beam is parallel or nearly parallel to the flow of

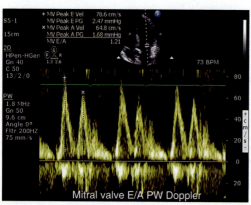

FIGURE 32-7 Pulsed wave flow pattern at the mitral valve level in a patient demonstrates the biphasic inflow pattern of the mitral valve.

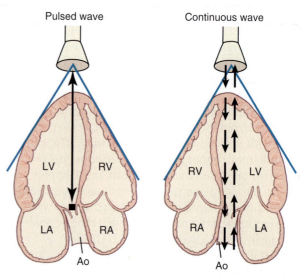

FIGURE 32-9 Drawing of pulsed-wave and continuous-wave Doppler echocardiography with the transducer placed in the PMI at the apex of the heart.

FIGURE 32-8 The sample volume (SV) is placed in the left ventricular outflow tract. There is aortic insufficiency that exceeds the Nyquist limit of the pulsed wave Doppler (flow is seen above and below the baseline).

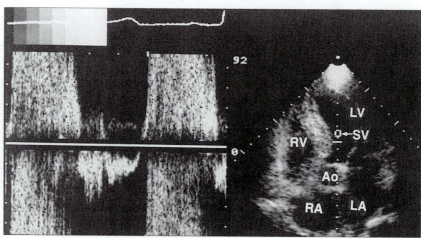

blood. Therefore, the best windows used to record the two-dimensional images may not be the best windows to record Doppler flow patterns. This section discusses the technique for recording quality Doppler signals from the inflow and outflow tracts through the cardiac valves.

Audio Signals. The audio signal from the frequency shift, as recorded in the Doppler study, is in the audible range, which is conveyed through a headphone or through dual speakers. (Dual speakers allow the operator to differentiate forward and reverse flow.) The recognition of Doppler signals does take experience. The signal from the arterial flow is very different from that of the venous flow; likewise, mitral and tricuspid patterns differ from the aortic and pulmonary valve patterns. The blood flow velocity determines the pitch or frequency of the audio signal. As the velocity becomes higher, the pitch becomes higher; as the velocity decreases, so does the pitch.

Normal blood flow across the cardiac valves demonstrates a narrow range of velocity with a smooth and even Doppler audio signal. When the flow becomes disturbed, as occurs distal to an obstruction or regurgitation of the valve, the tone becomes harsh. Very-high-velocity flows produce a very-high-frequency signal with a sharp whistling-hissing tone. This signal may be found in obstruction and regurgitant lesions.

Other movements within the cardiac chambers produce audio signals, but these signals are not as well defined. The valve opening and closure can be heard as a discrete click when the Doppler window is located too close to the valve. The normal cardiac function causes the valve to move in and out of the Doppler beam, producing a lower-frequency signal. Therefore, careful angulation along with the audio signal helps the operator observe the dynamics of the cardiac cycle for correct beam placement to obtain the best quality Doppler signal.

To record accurate velocity measurements, the ideal position of the Doppler beam is along a line of sight in which the angle of the beam is parallel to the transducer. As the angle decreases, the clarity of the audio signal increases, indicating that a quality signal is being recorded.

Spectral Analysis. The spectral analysis waveform allows the operator to print a graphic display of what the audio signal is recording because it provides a representation of blood flow velocities over time. The velocity on the vertical axis is measured in centimeters per second or meters per second, whereas time is shown on the horizontal axis. Therefore, the direction and velocity of flow may be measured very accurately when the beam is parallel to the flow. Flow toward the transducer is above the baseline. Flow away from the transducer is below the baseline. Multiple velocity measurements are used to quantify valvular function, stroke volume, and intracardiac shunts and pressures.

A normal spectral display pattern has a typical appearance. In normal blood flow, the cells generally have a uniform direction with similar velocities. The spectral tracing appears as a smooth mitral velocity pattern bordered by a narrow band of velocities. As the velocity increases, so does the turbulence within the border of the narrow-band velocities, producing a filling of the velocity curve. As the cardiac structure moves in and out of the beam, the Doppler frequency shift is recorded as tall artifact spikes.

Gray-scale imaging is used to display the amplitude of the velocity signal, with the highest velocities appearing as the darkest shade (if a black-on-white spectral analysis is used) or white (if a white-on-black spectral analysis is used).

Doppler Quantitation

Quantitation of the Doppler signal to obtain hemodynamic information is derived from the measurement of blood flow velocity (Table 32-1). As explained previously, it is critical that the angle of the Doppler signal be as parallel to flow as possible. The Doppler equation is based on the principle that the velocity of blood flow is directly proportional to the Doppler frequency shift and the speed of sound in tissue, and it is inversely related to twice the frequency of transmitted ultrasound and the cosine of the angle of incidence between the ultrasound beam and the direction of blood flow. Therefore, the relationship between the angle and its cosine becomes significant and can be a source of error if ignored. If the angle is less than 20 degrees, the cosine is close to 1 and can be ignored. If the angle increases beyond 20 degrees, the cosine becomes less than 1 and may produce an underestimation of velocity.

Doppler Examination

The Doppler examination is also performed along with the two-dimensional study of the cardiac structures. During this conventional study, the sonographer notes structures that may need special attention during the Doppler examination (e.g., a redundant mitral valve leaflet may indicate the need to search for mitral regurgitation). Throughout the Doppler study, various patient positions and transducer rotations are necessary to place the sample volume parallel to blood flow (Box 32-2).

TABLE 32-1	Maximal Velocities Recorded with Doppler in Normal Individuals	
	Children (cm/sec)	**Adults (cm/sec)**
Mitral flow	80–130	60–130
Tricuspid flow	50–80	30–70
Pulmonary artery	70–110	60–90
Left ventricle	70–120	70–110
Aorta	120–180	100–170

BOX 32-2	**Doppler Windows**

Apical Window

Mitral valve, tricuspid valve, left ventricular outflow tract, aortic valve, pulmonary vein inflow, superior vena cava inflow, interventricular septum, interatrial septum

Parasternal Short-Axis Window

Pulmonary valve, main pulmonary artery, right and left branches pulmonary artery (patent ductus arteriosus flow), tricuspid valve

Suprasternal Notch Window

Ascending aorta, descending aorta, patent ductus arteriosus flow, right pulmonary artery

Subcostal Window

Interatrial septum, interventricular septum, inferior vena cava flow, superior vena cava flow

Parasternal Long-Axis Window

Mitral regurgitation, tricuspid regurgitation, aortic regurgitation

Right Parasternal Window

Ascending aorta

There are basically five transducer positions used to record quality Doppler flow patterns: the apical four chamber, the left parasternal, subcostal, suprasternal, and the right parasternal. The patient should be forewarned about the audio sounds produced by the Doppler signal because some find the sound alarming if the volume is set too high.

THE ECHOCARDIOGRAPHIC EXAMINATION

The protocol for the evaluation cardiac structures begins with the parasternal long- and short-axis views, followed by the apical four-chamber, long-axis, and two-chamber views. The subcostal and suprasternal views complete the study (Box 32-3).

It is the responsibility of the cardiac sonographer to acquire the patient's blood pressure and height/weight (to calibrate the body surface area) of each patient.

Ideally, the sonographer should digitally acquire one or more cardiac cycles as needed for quantification and analysis. If an irregular rhythm is present (i.e., atrial fibrillation, flutter, or frequent ectopy), the sonographer should acquire 2 to 3 consecutive cardiac cycles for 2D; Doppler will need 4 to 10 consecutive beats averaged. If two or more myocardial segments of the left ventricle are not well visualized, the use of an approved injectable contrast agent should be considered if no

BOX 32-3	**Transducer Position and Cardiac Protocol** (Figure 32-10)

Parasternal

Long-axis view: LV in sagittal plane

RV inflow

LV outflow

Short-axis view: LV apex

Papillary muscles (midlevel)

Mitral valve (basal level)

Aortic valve—RV outflow tract

Pulmonary trunk bifurcation

Apical

Four-chamber view

Five-chamber view (including aorta)

Two-chamber view

Subcostal Window

Inferior vena cava

Hepatic veins

RV and LV inflow

LV aorta

RV outflow

Suprasternal Notch Window

Ascending aorta

Descending aorta

Right pulmonary artery

Left atrium

Right Parasternal Window

Ascending aorta

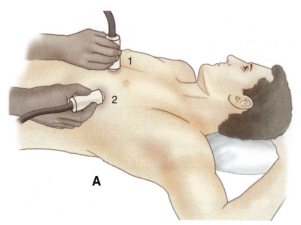

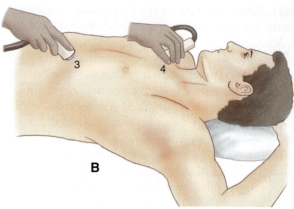

FIGURE 32-10 The patient is rolled into a left decubitus position. There are four standard transthoracic positions: **A,** *(1)* parasternal, *(2)* apical; **B,** *(3)* subcostal and *(4)* suprasternal.

contraindications are present. The sonographer should always compare the echocardiographic images to the previous study when preparing the preliminary report.

The sonographer should acquire the respective loop(s) for 2D and color flow Doppler and acquire the representative still frames for M-modes and PW/CW Doppler. The color Doppler *sector* should be long, spanning the entire cardiac image from top to bottom. This sector should be narrow enough to get the frame rate (FR) ≥17 Hz. The following is a *minimum* standard to be performed for all complete 2D/M-mode, color flow Doppler, and spectral Doppler exams. Additional views are often required and are based on presence of disease and clinical indications.

The order of acquisition is important and should always follow this sequence: (1) 2D image, then (2) full screen color flow Doppler of same image, followed by (3) spectral Doppler of the same view. The intent is to show anatomy first (zoom as needed), then color flow of that anatomy (zoom as needed), then spectral. This makes digital exams easier to read because transition between views is lost on the digital exam versus videotape. Labeling views or structures is strongly recommended whenever there is an interruption in the 2D/CFD/Spectral format or if nonstandard images are used. All 2D images should be full screen first and then, if needed, zoomed. All color flow Doppler (CFD) images should be full screen first and then, if needed, zoomed. Zoomed images are preferred to narrow sector imaging. Either mode may not increase frame rate depending on harmonic frequency selection. Digitally acquire the following views in the order listed here.

Parasternal Views

Parasternal Long-Axis Two-Dimensional View. The parasternal long-axis view is the initial image in the echographic examination. An attempt should be made to record as many of the cardiac structures as possible, from the base of the heart to the apex. Generally, this is accomplished by placing the long axis of the transducer slightly to the left of the sternum in about the fourth intercostal space. When the bright echo reflection of the pericardium is noted, the transducer is gradually rotated until a long-axis view of the heart is obtained. If it is not possible to record the entire long axis on a single scan, the transducer should be gently rocked cephalad to caudad in an "ice pick" fashion to record all the information from the base to the apex of the heart. See Boxes 32-4 and 32-5 for protocols.

The cardiac sonographer should observe the following structures and functions in the parasternal long-axis view:

1. Composite size of the cardiac chambers
2. Contractility of the right and left ventricles
3. Thickness of the right ventricular wall

BOX 32-4 Parasternal Long-Axis View
(Figure 32-11)

1. Record deep PS LAX view (regardless of presence of effusion); typical depths are 20 to 24 cm. Far field should not be dark unless there is effusion; TGC gain accordingly
2. PS LAX full screen (not zoomed)
3. Color Doppler full screen of aortic, mitral valve, LVOT, and include RVOT in color Doppler
4. PS LAX 2D zoom as needed to show anatomy/pathology better and then zoom of same image with color
5. M-Mode cursor through the minor axis of the aorta and left atrium
6. M-Mode cursor through mitral valve leaflet tips
7. M-Mode cursor through minor axis of LV just superior to papillary muscle
8. High PS LAX window to assess ascending aorta; CFD as needed to differentiate between artifact and a dissection; also high PS SAX 2D and with CFD if needed to help differentiate between an artifact and a dissection

BOX 32-5 Right Ventricular Inflow View
(Figure 32-12)

1. RA/RV, full screen
2. Color Doppler of RA/RV
3. Whether or not tricuspid regurgitation is seen, attempt CW Doppler for peak tricuspid regurgitation velocity and record

---

4. Continuity of the interventricular septum with the anterior wall of the aorta
5. Pliability of the atrioventricular and semilunar valves
6. Coaptation of the atrioventricular valves
7. Presence of increased echoes on the atrioventricular and semilunar valves
8. Systolic clearance of the aortic cusps
9. Presence of abnormal echo collections in the chambers or attached to the valve orifice
10. Presence and movement of chordal-papillary muscle structure
11. Thickness of the septum and posterior wall of the left ventricle
12. Uniform texture of the endocardium and myocardium
13. Size of the aortic root and left atrium

Parasternal Long-Axis View for Color Flow Mapping. In **diastole,** the parasternal long-axis view shows the left atrium filled with various shades of red as the pulmonary venous flow enters the atrial cavity from the right and left branches. While the blood is pushed toward the mitral leaflets, some turbulence is shown when the flow enters into the left ventricle.

During **systole,** the mitral leaflets close and the ventricle contracts to push the blood through the left ventricular outflow tract through the open aortic cusps. The blood is now flowing toward the transducer and is

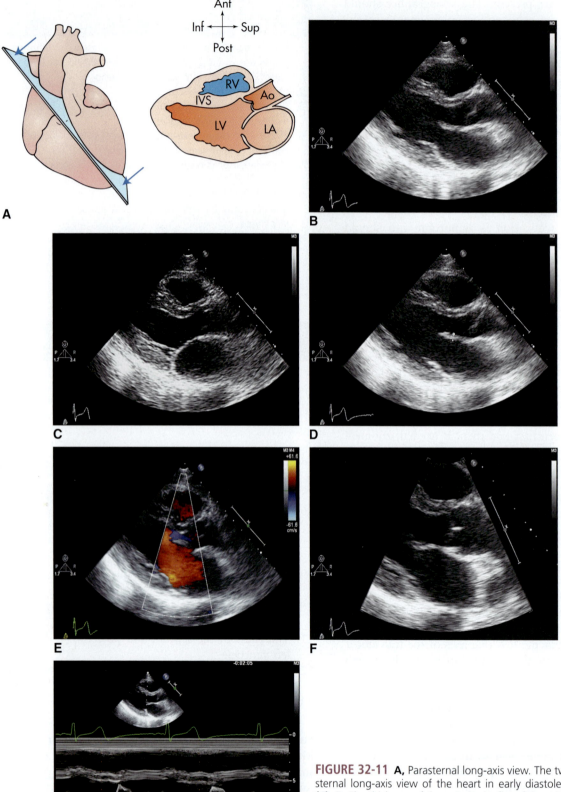

FIGURE 32-11 A, Parasternal long-axis view. The two-dimensional parasternal long-axis view of the heart in early diastole **(B)** and end systole **(C). D,** The thickness of the anterior leaflet of the mitral valve is measured. **E,** Color Doppler shows the mitral valve open (diastole) with red flowing from the left atrium into the left ventricle. **F,** Magnified image of the mitral valve apparatus. **G,** M-mode representation of the mitral valve as it opens in diastole and closes in systole. *Ao,* Aortic root; *IVS,* interventricular septum; *LA,* left atrium; *LV,* left ventricle; *RV,* right ventricle.

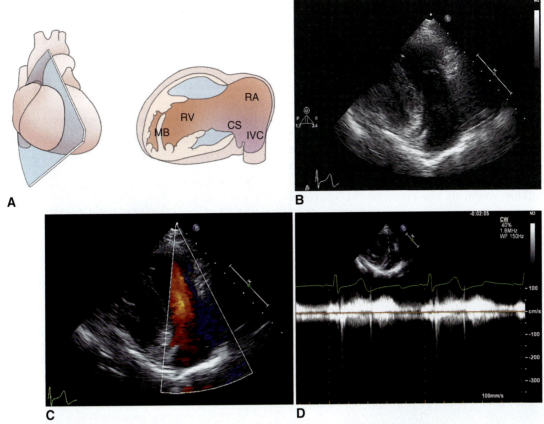

FIGURE 32-12 A, Parasternal long-axis view of the tricuspid valve as it separates the right ventricle *(RV)* from the right atrium *(RA)* in diastole **(B). C,** The inflow pattern of filling *(red)* as blood empties from the right atrium, across the tricuspid valve, into the right ventricle. **D,** The continuous wave flow pattern of the tricuspid valve inflow.

shown as a shade of red with some yellow highlights as it approaches the aortic root. Aliasing can occur when the Nyquist limit is lower than the maximum velocity of the flow. No color flow is seen to cross at the level of the membranous septum in the normal patient.

If mitral regurgitation is present, a turquoise flow arising from the mitral valve is seen in the left atrial cavity during systole (Figure 32-13). If aortic insufficiency is present, a yellowish mosaic flow pattern is seen during diastole (this generally hugs the left side of the interventricular septum, but the amount of calcification or thickening present in the aortic cusps determines which direction the regurgitant jet takes) (Figure 32-14). **Left Parasternal Window for Doppler.** The parasternal long-axis view with the patient rolled in a left lateral decubitus position has limited applications with Doppler. The transducer is more perpendicular to the cardiac structures than parallel, so the maximum velocity is difficult to record. However, disturbances in flow, especially mitral, aortic, and tricuspid (with the transducer angled medial) regurgitation, may be recorded in some patients with this view. Thickened cusps may direct the regurgitant flow in a pathway not typically seen as well on the apical view as on the parasternal long-axis view (Figure 32-15). A ventricular septal defect may be visualized on this view because the flow of blood is more parallel to

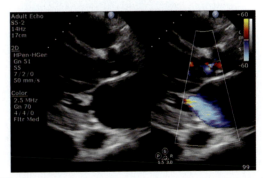

FIGURE 32-13 Parasternal long-axis view showing disturbed blue and yellow flow representing severe mitral regurgitation in the left atrial cavity.

the beam. Both muscular and membranous defects may be imaged from this view along with the apical and subcostal views.

Right Parasternal View for Color Flow Mapping. The right parasternal view is performed after the patient has been rolled into a steep right decubitus position. The transducer is placed along the right sternal border in the second intercostal space. This view may be useful for visualization of the entrance of the superior vena cava into the right atrium. The caval flow appears red as it enters the right atrium. This view also provides another window to image the entrance of the pulmonary veins into the left atrium. Flow patterns from the veins may be seen, whereas the actual veins are difficult to image on the two-dimensional study.

Right Parasternal Window for Doppler. The right parasternal position is most useful in the difficult-to-image adult or older pediatric patient after surgery who has a jet of aortic stenosis directed more to the right. The patient is rolled into a steep right decubitus position and the transducer placed in the first, second, or third intercostal space to the right of the sternum. Often the independent probe is easier to position in this patient, with the audible sound as the guide to the maximal velocity jet.

Parasternal Short-Axis Two-Dimensional View. The transducer should be rotated 90 degrees from the parasternal long-axis view to obtain multiple transverse short-axis views of the heart, particularly at the following four levels. See Box 32-6 for the protocol.

1. The low parasternal short-axis view should demonstrate the right ventricle, left ventricle, and papillary muscles (chordal echoes may also be seen):
   a. Contractility of the septum and posterior wall of the left ventricle
   b. Thickness of the septum and posterior wall

BOX 32-6   Parasternal Short-Axis View

1. PS SAX at level of papillary muscles, full screen (Figure 32-16, *A* and *B*)
2. PS SAX at level of left ventricular apex, full screen (Figure 32-16, *C*)
3. PS SAX at level of mitral leaflet tips, full screen (Figure 32-17, *A* and *B*)
4. PS SAX color flow Doppler of mitral valve; include entire annulus and if MVR include entire ring to assess for paravalvular leak (Figure 32-17, *C*)
5. PS SAX at level of aortic valve and left atrium, full screen (Figure 32-18, *A* and *B*)
6. Zoom of aortic valve and then with CFD if AI present (Figure 32-18, *C*)
7. Often, PA, TV, and RV are not well visualized from PS SAX AO/LA; take additional loops separately emphasizing PA, RV, and TV by 2D
8. PS SAX of pulmonary artery down to bifurcation (without color Doppler) (Figure 32-19, *A* and *B*)
9. PS SAX with long color flow Doppler sector of the right ventricular outflow tract and pulmonary artery including the bifurcation (Figure 32-19, *C*)
10. PW Doppler of RVOT at the level of the pulmonic annulus with closing click seen for PVR application; if PS, also get prestenosis PW Doppler whether this be in the RVOT or RV (Figure 32-19, *D*)
11. CW Doppler through pulmonary artery as needed to asses for pulmonic stenosis or if PS not ruled out by color Doppler screen; also, CW Doppler of PI signal
12. PS SAX of tricuspid valve, right atrium, and right ventricle
13. PS SAX color flow Doppler of tricuspid valve, right atrium, right ventricle, and interatrial septum
14. Whether or not tricuspid regurgitation is seen, attempt continuous wave Doppler for peak tricuspid regurgitation velocity and record

---

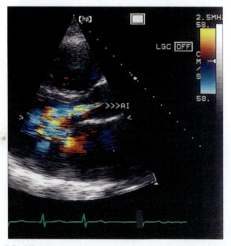

FIGURE 32-14 Parasternal long-axis view showing flow reversal through the aortic leaflets during ventricular diastole in a patient with aortic insufficiency.

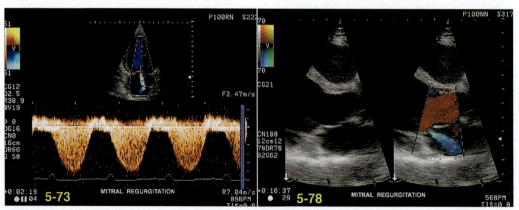

FIGURE 32-15 Parasternal long-axis view in a patient with mitral regurgitation (blue flow in the left atrium). The continuous wave flow is recorded in the apical position to measure 5 m/sec.

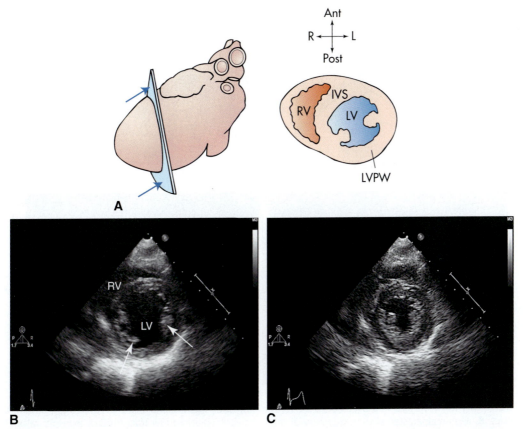

FIGURE 32-16 **A,** Parasternal short-axis view of the left ventricle. *IVS,* Interventricular septum; *LV,* left ventricle; *LVPW,* left ventricular posterior wall; *RV,* right ventricle. **B,** Low parasternal short-axis view of the right ventricle *(RV),* left ventricle *(LV),* and posterior papillary muscle *(arrows)* in end diastole. **C,** End-systolic squeeze of the left ventricle.

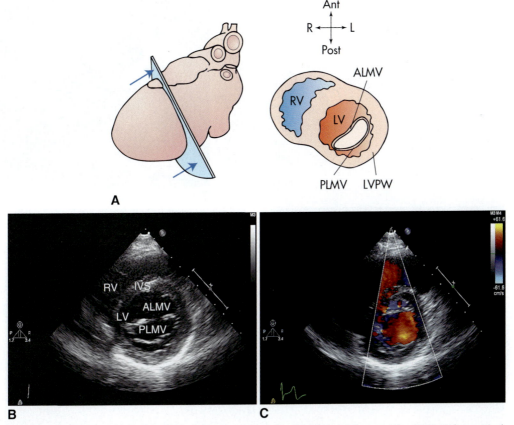

FIGURE 32-17 **A,** Parasternal short-axis view. *ALMV,* Anterior leaflet mitral valve; *LV,* left ventricle; *LVPW,* left ventricular posterior wall; *PLMV,* posterior leaflet mitral valve; *RV,* right ventricle. **B,** Midparasternal short-axis view of the right ventricle *(RV),* interventricular septum *(IVS),* anterior leaflet mitral valve *(ALMV),* posterior leaflet mitral valve *(PLMV),* and left ventricle *(LV).* **C,** Color Doppler of the filling of the ventricular cavities *(red).*

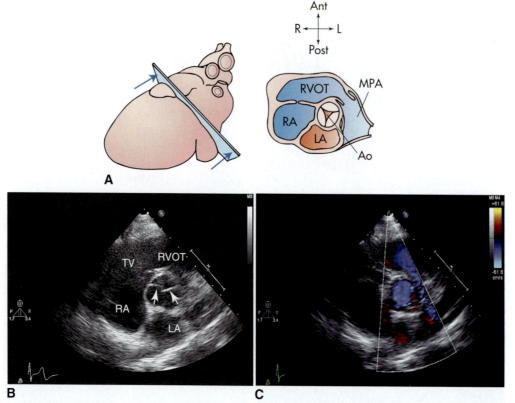

FIGURE 32-18 A, Parasternal short-axis view. *Ao,* Aorta; *LA,* left atrium; *MPA,* main pulmonary artery; *RA,* right atrium; *RVOT,* right ventricular outflow tract. **B,** High midparasternal short-axis view of the right ventricular outflow tract *(RVOT),* tricuspid valve *(TV),* right atrium *(RA),* aortic cusp *(arrows),* and left atrium *(LA).* **C,** Color Doppler of the end-diastolic phase.

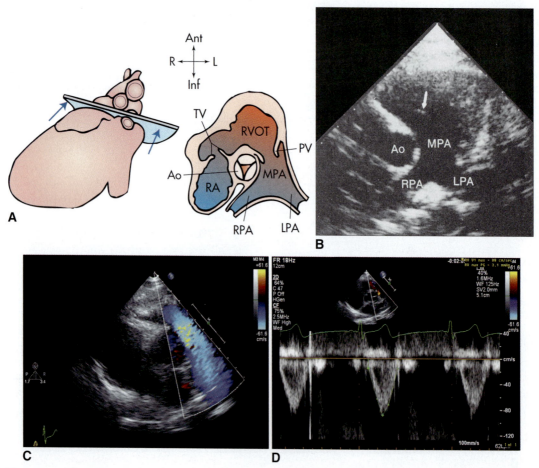

FIGURE 32-19 A, Parasternal short-axis view. *Ao,* Aorta; *LPA,* left pulmonary artery; *MPA,* main pulmonary artery; *PV,* pulmonary valve; *RA,* right atrium; *RPA,* right pulmonary artery; *RVOT,* right ventricular outflow tract; *TV,* tricuspid valve. **B,** High parasternal short-axis view of the aorta pulmonary cusp *(arrow),* main pulmonary artery *(MPA),* right pulmonary artery *(RPA),* and left pulmonary artery *(LPA).* **C,** Color *(blue)* shows the flow leaving the right ventricle through the pulmonary valve into the main pulmonary artery. **D,** Pulsed Doppler taken at the level of the right ventricular outflow tract.

c. Size of the left ventricle

d. Presence or absence of mural thrombus or other mass

e. Presence or absence of pericardial fluid, constriction, or restriction

f. Presence of increased echo density in posterior wall

g. Number of papillary muscles and their location within the left ventricular cavity

2. The midparasternal short-axis view should demonstrate the right ventricle, left ventricular outflow tract, and anterior and posterior leaflets of the mitral valve:

a. Size of the left ventricular outflow tract

b. Size of the septum and posterior wall

c. Presence of mass lesions in left or right ventricle

d. Mobility and thickness of the mitral valve

e. Presence of a flutter on the septum or anterior leaflet of the mitral valve or both

f. Systolic apposition of mitral valve leaflets

g. Contractility of septum and posterior wall

3. The moderate to high parasternal short-axis view should demonstrate the right ventricle, tricuspid valve, aortic cusps, coronary arteries, right and left atria:

a. Size of right ventricle and left atrium

b. Presence of mass lesions in right or left atrium

c. Mobility and thickness of tricuspid and aortic valves

d. Continuity of interatrial septum

e. Right ventricular wall thickness

f. Presence of trileaflet aortic valve

4. The high parasternal short-axis view should demonstrate the pulmonary valve, right ventricular outflow tract, and aorta:

a. Typical sausage-shaped right ventricular outflow tract and pulmonary artery draped anterior to circular aorta

b. Semilunar cusp thickness and mobility

c. Presence of calcification, extraneous echoes, or both in right ventricle or valve areas

d. Pulmonary valve mobility and thickness

Parasternal Short-Axis View for Color Flow Mapping. At the level of the aortic valve, the blood flow appears as a red signal moving toward the transducer from the right atrium into the right ventricle through the open tricuspid valve in diastole. Flow into the coronary arteries is sometimes seen in the right coronary, left main coronary, and circumflex and proximal left anterior descending arteries. Depending on the orientation of the coronary arteries, the blood flow appears yellow-red or bluish.

With slight angulation of the transducer, flow from the inferior vena cava can be seen while it flows into the right atrium. This flow appears red. When atrial systole occurs, blue signals can be seen moving from the right atrium into the inferior vena cava. Blue signals can also be seen as blood leaves the right ventricular outflow tract

to enter the pulmonary valve and main pulmonary artery in systole. While the transducer is angled slightly, the flow from the main pulmonary artery is seen to move into the bifurcation of the right and left pulmonary arteries. This flow is still primarily blue while it moves away from the transducer.

Pulmonary insufficiency is shown easily with CFM as a yellow and red high-velocity flow pattern (Figure 32-20). Pulmonary stenosis would appear as a high-velocity disturbed pattern through the narrowed pulmonic orifice.

A short-axis view at the level of the mitral valve in diastole may show flow signals in the mitral orifice and the right ventricle. When the transducer is angled medially, the right ventricular inflow plane may show flow signals while they arise from the coronary sinus into the right heart during diastole.

Parasternal Short-Axis Window for Doppler. The parasternal short-axis view is very useful for recording flow from the right ventricular outflow tract and pulmonary artery. The sample volume should be placed distal to the pulmonary cusps to record flow in the main pulmonary artery. The flow pattern is similar to that obtained from the aortic flow when the transducer is placed in the apical position but with a slightly slower upstroke. The spectral display shows a velocity curve below the baseline with a narrow band of frequencies. Normal pulmonary flow velocities range from 60 to 90 cm/sec in adults and 70 to 110 cm/sec in children. This view is useful for recording pulmonary regurgitation and stenosis, as well as abnormal patent ductus arteriosus flow that may be present in the neonate or child.

As the sample volume is positioned closer to the bifurcation of the pulmonary artery, the flow velocity increases slightly. To record velocities in the right ventricular outflow tract, the sample volume is placed just proximal to the pulmonary valve. The flow pattern is similar to the pulmonary outflow but has a slightly lower velocity. This view is especially useful for detecting a left-to-right

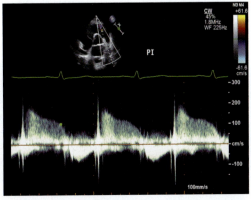

FIGURE 32-20 CW Doppler from the parasternal short-axis view of pulmonic insufficiency as it leaks into the right ventricular outflow tract.

shunt at the membranous ventricular septum, a coronary artery fistula, or a muscle bundle in the right ventricular outflow tract.

Sometimes the parasternal short-axis view with the transducer angled slightly to the right is useful for recording increased flow from tricuspid regurgitation. In this view, the sample volume is placed just inferior to the tricuspid leaflets in the right atrial cavity (Figure 32-21). If the interatrial septum is well seen, the increased flow pattern from a patent ductus arteriosus or atrial septal defect may be recorded.

Apical Views

Apical Two-Dimensional Views. Three apical views are very useful: the four-chamber view, the two-chamber view, and the apical long-axis view. The cardiac sonographer should palpate the patient's chest to detect the point of maximal impulse (PMI) (Figure 32-22). The transducer should then be directed in a transverse plane at the PMI and angled sharply cephalad to record the four chambers of the heart. If there is too much lung interference, then the proper cardiac window has not been found and care should be taken to adjust the patient's position or the transducer position to adequately see all four chambers of the heart. Many laboratories

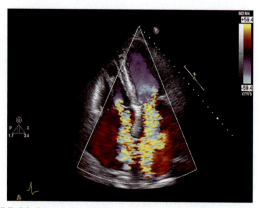

FIGURE 32-21 Apical four-chamber view of tricuspid and mitral regurgitation as it leaks into the right atrial cavity.

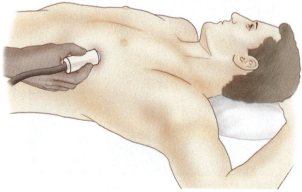

FIGURE 32-22 The transducer is placed at the PMI for the apical images.

have found it useful to use the special echocardiographic bed in which a dropout enables the sonographer to readily access the cardiac apex. This allows the transducer more flexibility for recording the apical views.

The apical views are excellent for assessing cardiac contractility, size of cardiac chambers, presence of mass lesions, alignment of atrioventricular valves, coaptation of atrioventricular valves, septal or posterior wall hypertrophy, chordal attachments, and the presence of pericardial effusion. It is not a good view from which to evaluate the presence of an atrial septal defect because the beam is parallel to the thin foramen ovale and the septum commonly appears as a defect in this view. The subcostal four-chamber view is much better for evaluating the presence of such a defect. See Boxes 32-7 through 32-11 for apical protocols.

The cardiac sonographer should observe the following structures:

1. Size of the cardiac chambers
2. Contractility of right and left ventricles
3. Septal and posterior wall thickness, contractility, and continuity
4. Coaptation of atrioventricular valves
5. Alignment of atrioventricular valves
6. Presence of increased echoes on valve apparatus
7. Presence of mass or thrombus in cardiac chambers
8. Entrance of pulmonary veins into left atrial cavity

BOX 32-7	Apical Four-Chamber View (Figure 32-23)

1. Ap4C showing all four chambers and A-V valves, full screen
2. If right heart and left heart are not well visualized from one Ap4C view, take left heart images now; additional full screen Ap4C loops of the right heart will be taken later
3. Ap4C color flow Doppler of the mitral valve (long sector from the apex through the mitral valve and the entire left atrium)
4. Zoom on left heart structures as needed to better define anatomy/pathology then zoomed CFD if needed for MR (PISA, VC)
5. If MR present, CW Doppler of mitral regurgitation for dP/dt and peak velocity should be taken here
6. PW/CW Doppler of MV inflow, DTI lateral and septal MV annulus, and R. pulm vein and, if needed, IVRT, and MV Valsalva

BOX 32-8	Apical Five-Chamber View (Figure 32-24)

1. Ap5C full screen then zoom AoV as needed to show anatomy/pathology better
2. Ap5C color flow Doppler of the aortic valve with color sector box from apex through aortic valve and aorta; if there is aortic insufficiency, record CW Doppler signal
3. If there is LVOT obstruction, show PW before obstruction and then CW through obstruction; also, PW/CW Doppler of LVOT and then AoV

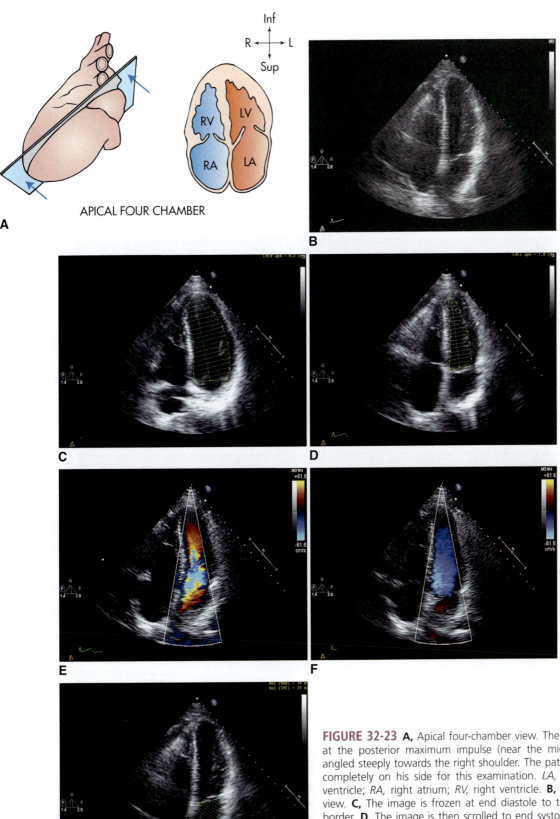

FIGURE 32-23 A, Apical four-chamber view. The transducer is placed at the posterior maximum impulse (near the midcoronal plane) and angled steeply towards the right shoulder. The patient should be rolled completely on his side for this examination. *LA,* Left atrium; *LV,* left ventricle; *RA,* right atrium; *RV,* right ventricle. **B,** Apical four-chamber view. **C,** The image is frozen at end diastole to trace the endocardial border. **D,** The image is then scrolled to end systole to again trace the endocardial border to determine the ejection fraction of the left ventricle. **E,** Color Doppler at end diastole shows the high velocity flow as blood empties from the left atrium into the left ventricular cavity. **F,** Color Doppler at end systole demonstrates the blood flow leaving the ventricle in blue. **G,** The maximum volume of the left atrial cavity is traced.

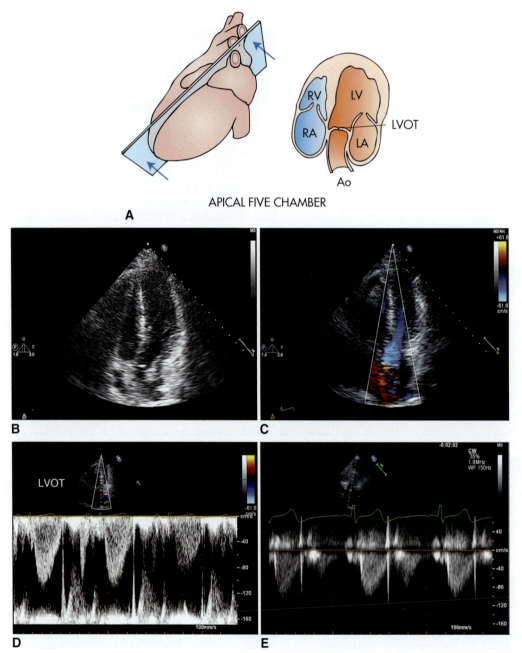

APICAL FIVE CHAMBER

FIGURE 32-24 **A,** Apical five-chamber view (left ventricular outflow tract). Anterior angulation from the four-chamber view will demonstrate the left ventricular outflow tract and the ascending aorta *(Ao)*. *LA,* Left atrium; *LV,* left ventricle; *RA,* right atrium; *RV,* right ventricle. **B,** End-diastolic frame of the left ventricular outflow tract with the aortic cusps closed. **C,** Color Doppler shows the blue flow leaving the left ventricle into the ascending aorta. **D,** PW Doppler taken at the level of the left ventricular outflow tract. **E,** CW Doppler is taken in the ascending aorta.

9. Size of left ventricular outflow tract, signs of obstruction, mobility of aortic cusps, absence of subaortic membrane
10. Entrance of inferior and superior vena cava into the right atrium

The apical long-axis view is very useful for evaluation of the left ventricular cavity and aortic outflow tract. Once the apical four-chamber view is obtained, the transducer should be rotated 90 degrees to visualize the left ventricle, left atrium, and aorta with cusps. This view permits the cardiac sonographer to evaluate the wall motion of the posterior basal segment of the left ventricle, the anterior wall, and the apex of the left ventricle. It also permits another view of the left ventricular outflow tract, which may be useful in determining aortic cusp motion or the presence of a subvalvular membrane.

Apical View for Color Flow Mapping. The apical four-chamber view is one of the most useful views in color flow mapping. In the typical four-chamber view,

the operator can follow blood flow as it enters the atrial cavities and flows through the atrioventricular valves in diastole to enter the ventricular chambers before it exits through the great arteries.

The right-side events appear slightly earlier as the tricuspid valve opens before the mitral valve. When

blood fills the atrial cavities, it appears red as it flows toward the transducer. Pulmonary venous inflow to the left atrial cavity may be seen in this four-chamber view. Flow from the right and left upper veins appears reddish with some yellow, whereas flow from the lower left pulmonary vein appears blue as it moves away from the transducer. Although the transducer is angled more posterior and medial, inflow from the superior vena cava is red when it enters the medial aspect of the right atrium along the border of the interatrial septum.

Diastolic flow through the atrioventricular orifice occurs at a slightly higher velocity, giving rise to changes in colors from red to yellow. The flow returns to red as the inflow chamber of the ventricles fills. When the flow reaches the apex, it begins to swirl toward the ventricular outflow tract and the color changes to blue. Again the velocity increases as the flow moves toward the leaflets of the aorta in systole, changing the color into more intense blue shades. Flow in the ascending aorta should

BOX 32-9	Apical Four-Chamber View: Right Heart (Figure 32-25)

1. Ap4C emphasizing RV, TV, and RA (do not use narrow sector)
2. Perform and measure TAPSE (TAM) and TA DTI at this time
3. Ap4C color flow Doppler of tricuspid valve from RV apex through tricuspid valve and entire RA; include interatrial septal interrogation here or perform separately
4. Whether or not tricuspid regurgitation is seen, attempt CW Doppler for peak tricuspid regurgitation velocity and record
5. Coronal RV view is not routinely mandatory, but if performed should be done now; if RV or TV case, do coronal RV view

BOX 32-10	Apical Two-Chamber View (Figure 32-26)

1. Ap2C, full screen
2. Ap2C color flow Doppler of the mitral valve from the apex through the MV and entire LA

BOX 32-11	Apical Long-Axis View (Figure 32-27)

1. Ap LAX, full screen
2. Ap LAX color flow Doppler of mitral and aortic valves from apex through valves and beyond

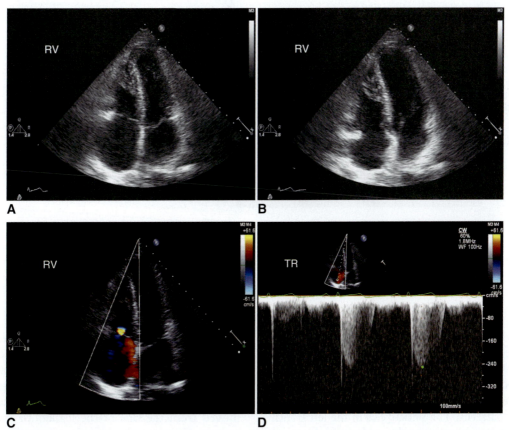

FIGURE 32-25 A, Apical four-chamber view of the right ventricle and right atrium at end systole. **B,** End diastole shows the tricuspid valve open. **C,** Color Doppler at end systole shows a small yellow flow representing trace tricuspid regurgitation. **D,** CW through the tricuspid regurgitation.

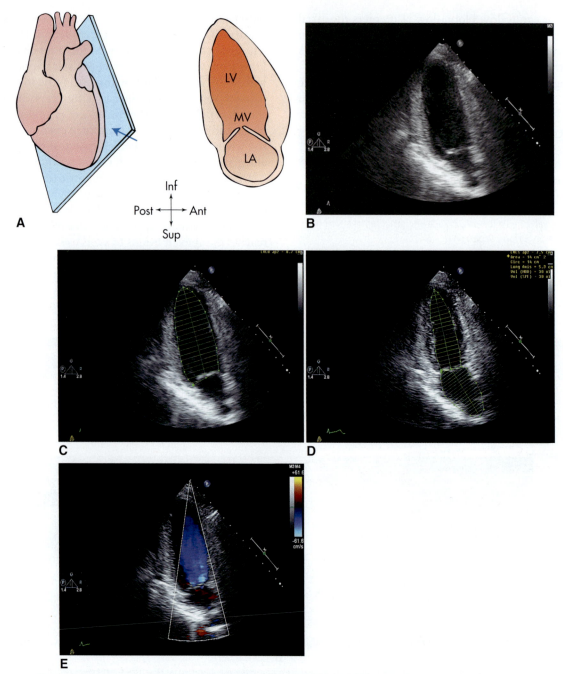

FIGURE 32-26 A, Apical two-chamber view. The transducer is rotated 90 degrees from the apical four-chamber view to show only the left ventricle *(LV),* mitral valve *(MV),* and left atrium *(LA).* **B,** Apical two-chamber view. **C,** End-diastolic frame with tracing along the endocardial border. **D,** End-systolic frame with tracing along the endocardial border to determine the ejection fraction by method of discs. **E,** Color Doppler at end systole shows the blue flow as it leaves the left ventricle into the ascending aorta.

be a uniform blue. Regurgitant flow into the left atrium from the incompetent mitral or tricuspid valve will appear as a blue-green mixed pattern.

Apical Window for Doppler. The apical four-chamber position is one of the most widely used for recording multiple Doppler patterns. The patient lies in the left lateral decubitus position with the transducer placed at the apical impulse and directed toward the patient's right shoulder. This position allows sampling of flow through the mitral, tricuspid, and aortic valves at nearly parallel angles to the beam. See Boxes 32-12 and 32-13 for protocols.

Inflow through the mitral valve leaflets may be recorded by placing the Doppler signal at the level of the tips of the leaflets. The pulsed sample volume may be moved from the tips of the leaflets to the level of the mitral annulus to obtain a clean recording. The normal mitral flow velocity tracing is similar to that found on an M-mode recording.

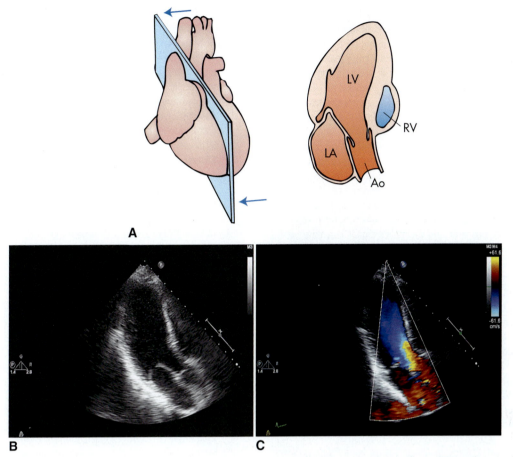

FIGURE 32-27 A, Medial angulation from the two-chamber view will show the left ventricular outflow tract and aorta *(Ao)*. **B,** Three-chamber view; the parasternal short-axis and apical two-chamber views are used to show abnormal motion in the posterobasal segment of the left ventricular wall. **C,** Color Doppler shows the red inflow from the pulmonary veins and the blue flow through the ascending aorta.

The initial peak occurs during the rapid-filling phase of diastole. The smaller second peak occurs late in diastole (with atrial contraction). In patients with decreased left ventricular compliance, the first peak may be lower and the second peak higher. Normal flow velocity across the mitral valve ranges from 60 to 130 cm/sec in adults and similar velocities in children. Mitral regurgitation can be recognized as the sample volume is moved into the left atrial cavity. Careful angulation of the Doppler beam is necessary to sweep across the level of the annulus. An abnormal, high-pitched systolic flow pattern below the baseline represents regurgitation.

The tricuspid valve flow may be recorded in the apical position while the transducer is angled slightly to the right. With the transducer position at the level of the leaflets, a pattern similar to mitral valve flow is recorded with two peaks during diastole. The first occurs during ventricular filling and the second with the onset of atrial contraction. The velocity pattern is much lower in the tricuspid valve, with significant respiratory changes that increase during inspiration and decrease during expiration. The normal velocity range is 30 to 70 cm/sec for adults and is similar for children (see Table 32-1).

In the apical position, the transducer may be angled slightly anterior or rotated into a long-axis view to record blood flow from the left ventricular outflow tract as it enters the aortic root and ascending aorta. With the pulsed-wave sample volume placed just proximal to the aortic root (in the left ventricular outflow tract), the flow is away from the transducer during systole. The spectral display shows a narrow band of frequencies below the baseline.

The normal velocity pattern in the left ventricular outflow tract in the adult is 70 to 110 cm/sec, and it is similar in children. As the sample volume is moved across the aortic valve, flow can be recorded within the ascending aorta. This velocity pattern is slightly higher and peaks earlier. Normal velocities range from 100 to 170 cm/sec in adults and 120 to 180 cm/sec in children.

Subcostal Views

Subcostal Two-Dimensional View. The subcostal view also has multiple windows in the four-chamber and short-axis planes (Figure 32-30). Many of the views are

BOX 32-12 | Spectral Doppler

Every effort should be made to avoid measuring postectopic beats. Average 3 to 10 consecutive beats if frequent ectopy (i.e., bigeminy) or atrial fib/flutter is present. Every effort should be made to align Doppler parallel to flow. Doppler should be recorded at 100 mm/s sweep speed except for when needing to average consecutive beats or when documenting for respiratory variations. Acquire spectral signal at end-expiration or during quiet breathing. All signals should be set with minimal "wall filter" to show signal intersecting with baseline to allow for more accurate time measurements. PW Doppler should be recorded with gains/reject set to show clear envelope. Sample volume size should be between 2 and 5 mm.

1. PW Doppler transmitral flow recording with sample volume at the leaflet (Figure 32-28); tips during opening; sample volume beyond leaflet tips and into LV makes signal less crisp; MV sample volume at annulus for regurgitant fraction calculations and to better see A kick for A duration measurement
2. PW DTI is recorded from lateral and septal mitral annulus; septal velocity should be slightly smaller; use clinical eye if big discrepancy exists (Figure 32-29, A and B)
3. PW Doppler of pulmonary veins with sample volume >1 cm in the pulm vein for cleanest signal; signal should be free of MR jet signal and truly reflect pulm vein S, D, and AR flow (Figure 32-29, C)
4. CW Doppler between MV and LVOT for IVRT; avoid AI and MR signals (PW may be necessary)
5. PW Doppler of MV with Valsalva as needed for differentiation between stage 3 and 4 diastolic dysfunction and stage 2 from normal
6. PW Doppler of LVOT about 0.5 to 1.0 cm below AoV; if LVOT obstruction present, show pre- and postobstruction Doppler signals
7. CW Doppler through AoV

BOX 32-13 | 2D and Doppler Measurements and Calculations

1. LV diastolic and systolic volumes from Ap4C and Ap2C for biplane-MOD EF%. May substitute Ap LAX for Ap2C if Ap2C is technically inadequate. May use Definity to trace volumes. Keep in mind apex does not move inward towards annulus; rather, annulus moves toward apex. This will provide a more accurate LAX length for biplane-MOD. Begin trace at MV annulus and not in LV cavity.
2. LA biplane-MOD volume from Ap4C and Ap2C. May need to optimize a separate image to visualize LA. Exclude LAA, pulmonary vein ostium, and atrial septal anomalies (i.e., aneurysm) from trace. Stop trace at MV annulus (i.e., do not include area under leaflet tips). Correct LAX dimension.
3. RVSP = TR gradient + CVP where CVP equals:
   5 mmHg if IVC is normal size and collapses ≥ 50% with inspiration
   10 mmHg if IVC is normal size and collapses ≤ 50% with inspiration
   15 mmHg if IVC is large and collapses ≤ 50% with inspiration
   20 mmHg if IVC is large, shows no collapse, and presence of significant TR and RA enlargement
4. Normal RVd2 measurement per ASE poster mandatory for all RV cases. IVC size is <2.0 cm although athletic individuals are an exception.
5. For all Aortic Stenosis and Prosthetic AoV cases, report the following in Aortic Valve section of Echo report: AoV area by continuity, AoV peak/mean pressure gradient, and Dimensionless index. Use AVA(I,D) calculation for AVA area. Do not label LV V1 Max as it will put a second AVA on report. Use the previous Echo's LVOT diameter when present. For prosthetic valves, use preprosthetic valve LVOT diameter when present. Otherwise, LVOT diameters are generally between 1.9 and 2.3 cm. For serial echo comparisons, compare only AoV area changes in Interpretation Summary section of report.
6. LAP using simplified E/E' + 4 mmHg. E' is lateral MV annulus; however, averaging with septal E' may be warranted if there is a significant difference between lateral and medial velocities. Clinical eye needed.
7. Measure and label MV deceleration time.
8. Measure and label MV E and A waves.

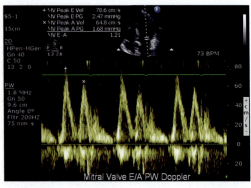

FIGURE 32-28 PW Doppler of the mitral valve inflow. The initial peak occurs during the rapid-filling phase of diastole. The smaller second peak occurs late in diastole with atrial contraction.

only available in the pediatric patient (because of the flexible abdominal muscles). The subcostal four-chamber view is generally useful in many adults and may serve as an alternative view if the apical four-chamber view is unobtainable. The transducer should be placed in the subcostal space and, with moderate pressure applied, angled steeply toward the patient's left shoulder. The plane of the transducer is transverse for visualization of

the four chambers of the heart. See Box 32-14 for the subcostal protocol.

It is usually easy to follow the inferior vena cava into the right atrium of the heart. With careful angulation, the interatrial septum may be visualized between the anterior right atrial chamber and the posterior left atrial chamber. It is usually more difficult to open the right ventricular cavity in this view; therefore, no size assessment should be made. This view is usually very good for assessing the presence of pericardial effusion, especially because it surrounds the anterior segment of the right side of the heart.

Subcostal View for Color Flow Mapping. The subcostal view is a long-axis view that shows the inferior vena cava inflow pattern as primarily red as it enters the right atrial cavity. The flow from the hepatic veins appears

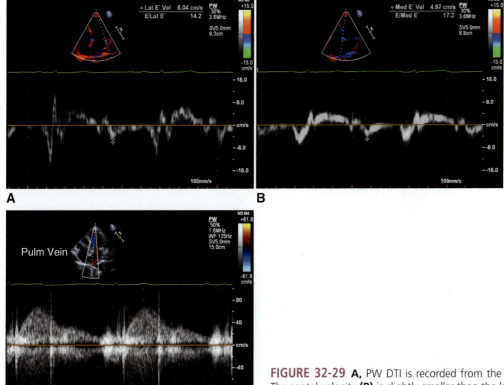

FIGURE 32-29 A, PW DTI is recorded from the lateral and septal mitral annulus. The septal velocity **(B)** is slightly smaller than the lateral wall velocity. **C,** PW Doppler at the level of the pulmonary veins is taken with the sample volume placed 1 cm into the pulmonary vein. The systolic, diastolic, and AR flow is observed.

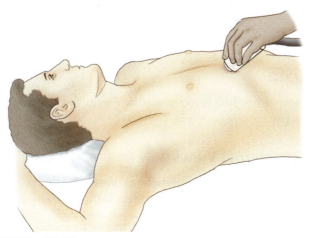

FIGURE 32-30 Subcostal four-chamber view. The transducer is placed below the costal margin and angled steeply toward the head to record the four-chamber view.

BOX 32-14 | **Subcostal View** (Figure 32-31)

1. SC4C, full screen
2. SC4C color flow Doppler of interatrial septum; may be necessary to zoom IAS in order to keep FR ≥17 Hz
3. SC SAX showing IVC and hepatic veins; demonstrate IVC with inspiration or sniff maneuver; hepatic vein interrogation if unsure of TR grade (TDS) or if ≥moderate TR present
4. Show any additional structures not well interrogated from other views because of poor image quality; include 2D as well as color flow Doppler and spectral Doppler (usual digital format order); deep SC4C toward right pleural space for R pleural effusion on all CHF cardiomyopathy patients to assess for decompensation

---

blue when blood enters the inferior vena cava at the level of the diaphragm throughout diastole and systole. During atrial systole, some retrograde flow is seen as it moves from the right atrium into the inferior vena cava and hepatic veins. With the transducer angled slightly to the left, blue pulsatile flow signals through the descending and abdominal aorta may be seen in systole.

In the subcostal short-axis view, the right ventricular outflow tract and pulmonary artery may be demonstrated. The right ventricular outflow tract appears blue as it leaves the right ventricle to enter through the pulmonary cusps. The velocity increases slightly, causing some color change from blue to turquoise and green before returning to blue when it enters the main pulmonary artery. Some aliasing may be experienced as the flow bounces off the tricuspid leaflets and right ventricular walls. Red and yellow flow can be seen arising from the coronary artery along the posterior wall of the right ventricle. Superior vena cava inflow appears as red and orange flow as it enters the right atrium.

Subcostal Window for Doppler. The subcostal position is especially useful in the neonatal and pediatric population because the transducer is placed in the subcostal region and, with gentle pressure applied, the

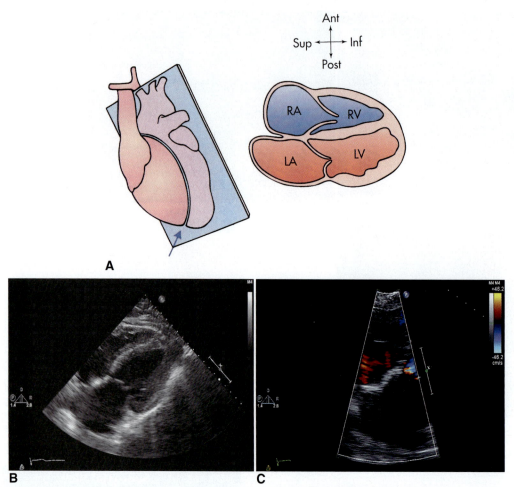

FIGURE 32-31 **A,** Subcostal view shows the four chambers of the heart, interatrial and interventricular septa. *LA,* Left atrium; *LV,* left ventricle; *RA,* right atrium; *RV,* right ventricle. **B,** Subcostal four-chamber view. **C,** Color Doppler with low PRF is taken in the subcostal view of the atrial cavities to look for the presence of intraatrial shunt flow.

transducer is angled superiorly to record the four chambers of the heart. In adults with pulmonary obstructive disease, this view is useful because the increased size of the lungs pushes the heart into the view of the transducer without too much pressure on the diaphragm.

In this position the interatrial and interventricular septa are perpendicular to the transducer, so the presence of a left-to-right defect shows positive high-velocity flow from the baseline on the spectral display and the flow is parallel to the beam. A right-to-left flow shows as a negative deflection on the spectral display. This view may also be useful for recording the flow pattern from the pulmonary veins (upper right and left and lower left) when they enter the left atrium.

The superior vena cava flow is shown as a high-pitched, low-velocity, positive deflection from the baseline on the spectral display. The inferior vena cava flow may be recorded as a negative display on the spectral display. A better view of the inferior vena cava flow is made in the subcostal long-axis view through the right lobe of the liver. The inferior vena cava may be well seen as it moves slightly anterior to pierce the diaphragm before it enters the right atrial cavity. This display would

project as a low-velocity positive reflection from the baseline.

Suprasternal Views

Suprasternal Two-Dimensional View. In the suprasternal view, the transducer is directed transversely in the patient's suprasternal notch and angled steeply toward the arch of the aorta (Figure 32-32). This view is only useful if the transducer is small enough to fit well into the suprasternal notch. The patient is best prepared if several towels or a pillow are placed under the shoulders. In this position the patient's neck should flex, avoiding interference with the neck of the transducer and cable. The patient's head should be turned to the right, again to avoid interference with the cable. With careful angulation, the cardiac structures visualized are the aortic arch, brachiocephalic vessels, right pulmonary artery, left atrium, and left main bronchus. This view is especially useful in determining supravalvular enlargement of the aorta, coarctation of the aorta, or dissection of the aorta. See Boxes 32-15 and 32-16 for the suprasternal notch and right parasternal border protocols.

Suprasternal View for Color Flow Mapping. In the suprasternal long-axis plane of the ascending aorta, arch, and descending aorta, flow signals begin as red in the ascending aorta and turn to blue when flow moves into the arch (some aliasing and reversal of color is seen along this point as the flow bounces off the walls in the arch). When the flow enters the descending aorta, a bright blue color is seen. The atrial and ventricular septa are well seen on this view, and adequate visualization of a possible defect may be made in this imaging plane.

In the short-axis plane, the superior vena cava flow is blue when it enters the right atrium. Flow within the aortic arch and right pulmonary artery is also seen. In some patients, pulmonary venous inflow may be seen in the suprasternal view.

Suprasternal Window for Doppler. The suprasternal position is used to record velocities in the ascending and descending aorta, right pulmonary artery, superior vena cava inflow, and pulmonary venous return into the left atrium. Initially the patient's shoulders are elevated by a pillow, the neck extended, and the transducer placed in the suprasternal notch with an inferior angulation of the beam.

The transducer sample volume is placed in the ascending aorta when the walls of the aorta are as nearly perpendicular to the beam as possible. The flow is then

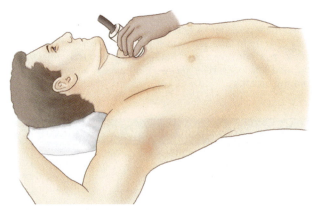

FIGURE 32-32 Suprasternal view. The transducer is placed in the suprasternal notch and angled steeply toward the arch of the aorta.

> **BOX 32-15   Suprasternal Notch** (Figure 32-33)
>
> This view is mandatory for AS, AI, aorta disease, CVA/TIA, and PDA.
> 1. SSN LAX of aortic arch and descending aorta
> 2. SSN LAX color flow Doppler
> 3. Aortic stenosis cases must have Pedoff AoV CW Doppler signal recorded
>   If no signal is obtainable, attempt must be digitally acquired nonetheless.

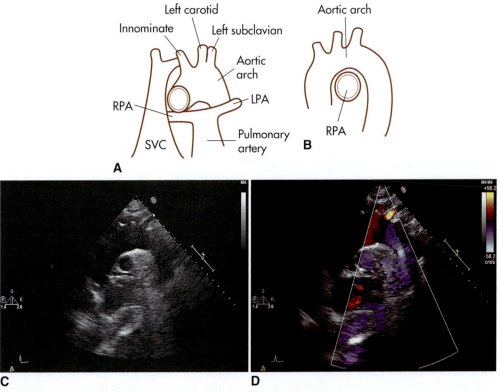

FIGURE 32-33 A, Transverse suprasternal notch view of the superior vena cava *(SVC)* as it lies to the right of the arch of the aorta. The right pulmonary artery *(RPA)* is posterior to the arch of the aorta. *LPA,* Left pulmonary artery. **B,** Longitudinal suprasternal notch view of the ascending aorta and right pulmonary artery. **C,** Suprasternal long view of the ascending, arch, and descending aorta. The right pulmonary artery is posterior to the arch. **D,** Color Doppler at the level of the arch shows the flow in red in the ascending aorta/arch and blue in the arch/descending aorta.

BOX 32-16	**Right Parasternal Border**

(This view is mandatory for AS and Aorta disease).
   Patient should be in right lateral decubitus position
1. RPS LAX of ascending aorta
2. RPS color flow Doppler of ascending aorta and through AoV
3. Aortic stenosis cases must have Pedoff AoV CW Doppler signal recorded; if no signal is obtainable, attempt must be digitally acquired nonetheless

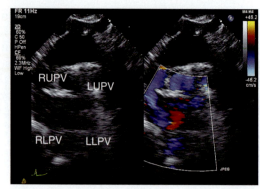

FIGURE 32-34 Suprasternal view of the pulmonary veins. The transducer is aligned with the ascending aorta, the beam is then angled more posterior to record the dorsal aspect of the left atrial cavity. The right and left upper pulmonary veins (RUPV, LUPV) appear as a negative flow away from the baseline, whereas the right and left lower veins (RLPV, RLPV) appear as a positive flow from the baseline.

parallel to the pulsed Doppler cursor, and a positive deflection with a narrow band of frequencies is shown above the baseline. Careful sweeping back and forth allows the operator to determine the highest velocity possible. The audio sound helps direct the probe to the maximal jet flow. If high velocities are suspected, the continuous wave probe is used.

The spectral tracing from this probe contains a wider range of frequencies with the same peak velocity measurements as the pulsed wave. As the transducer is angled to the left and posterior, velocity from the descending aorta is recorded. Generally with the pulsed Doppler, the sample volume is placed near the level of the left subclavian artery to record the maximum flow away from the transducer as it flows down the descending aorta to the abdominal aorta.

The suprasternal notch position is extremely useful for recording abnormal velocities, such as those found in aortic stenosis, coarctation of the aorta, and patent ductus arteriosus. In aortic stenosis, the harsh systolic velocities increase in the ascending and descending aorta. In coarctation of the aorta, the velocity increases slightly proximal to the area of narrowing, and velocity increases dramatically throughout systole as the beam traverses the area of coarctation. In patients with a patent ductus arteriosus, a positive, high-pitched, high-velocity flow will be seen on the spectral display at the level of the subclavian artery.

The flow pattern of the superior vena cava may be recorded from the suprasternal position while the transducer is directed inferiorly and to the right (medial) of the ascending aorta. Flow away from the transducer is recorded with two low-velocity peaks in systole and diastole, which may increase in height during inspiration. This view is useful for recording flow patterns that may be obstructed in the area of the superior vena cava.

The demonstration of the pulmonary veins from the suprasternal notch is more difficult to obtain. With the transducer aligned with the ascending aorta, the beam is angled more posterior to record the dorsal aspect of the left atrial cavity (Figure 32-34). The right and left upper pulmonary veins appear as a negative flow away from the baseline, whereas the right and left lower veins appear as a positive flow from the baseline. The velocity is low, with changes in respiration and cardiac motion.

BOX 32-17	**Normal M-Mode Measurements**

Aortic Root Dimension	1.9–4.0 cm
Aortic cusp separation	1.5–2.6 cm
Left atrial dimension	1.9–4.0 cm
Mitral valve excursion	1.6–3.0 cm
Left ventricular end-diastolic dimension	3.5–5.7 cm
Left ventricular end-systolic dimension	2.5–4.0 cm
Left ventricular ejection fraction	>55%
Interventricular septal thickness	0.6–1.2 cm
Posterior left ventricular thickness	0.6–1.2 cm
Right ventricular dimension	0.7–2.7 cm

M-MODE IMAGING OF THE CARDIAC STRUCTURES

Box 32-17 lists normal M-mode measurements for cardiac structures and left ventricular ejection fraction.

Mitral Valve

Echographically, the mitral valve is one of the easiest cardiac structures to recognize. With M-mode, the mitral valve has the greatest amplitude and excursion and can be unquestionably recognized by its "double," or biphasic, kick. This kick is caused by the initial opening of the valve in ventricular diastole and the atrial contraction at end diastole (Figure 32-35).

When diastole begins, the anterior mitral leaflet executes a rapid anterior motion, coming to a peak at point *e*. While the ventricle fills rapidly with blood from the left atrium, the valve drifts closed at point *f*. The rate at which this movement takes place represents the rate of left atrial emptying and serves as an important indicator of altered mitral function. As the left atrium contracts, the mitral valve opens in a shorter anterior excursion and terminates at point *a*, which occurs just after the P

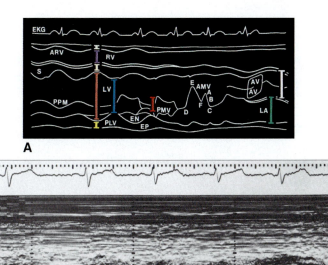

A

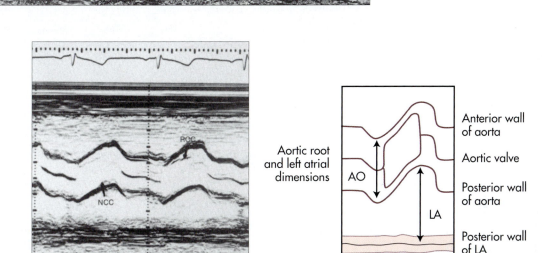

B

FIGURE 32-35 A, Illustration of the M-mode sweep. *AMV,* Anterior leaflet mitral valve; *ARV,* anterior wall right ventricular wall; *AV,* aortic cusp; *EN,* endocardium; *EP,* epicardium; *LA,* left atrium; *LV,* left ventricle; *PLV,* posterior wall left ventricle; *PMV,* posterior leaflet mitral valve; *PPM,* posterior papillary muscle; *RV,* right ventricle; *S,* septum. **B,** Both leaflets of the mitral valve are clearly seen in this patient. The systolic segment moves slightly anteriorly until diastole begins, which causes the anterior leaflet *(ALMV)* to sweep anteriorly while the posterior leaflet *(PLMV)* dips posteriorly. Atrial contraction gives rise to the smaller *"a"* kick until the valve closes at end diastole.

A   **B**

FIGURE 32-36 A, The right coronary cusp *(RCC)* is the most anterior cusp seen in the aortic sweep, and the noncoronary cusp *(NCC)* is the most posterior. The left coronary cusp is sometimes seen in the middle of the other two cusps. **B,** Measurements of the aortic root diameter and size of the left atrium may be made.

wave on the electrocardiogram. This motion is followed by a rapid posterior movement from point *b* to point *c*, which coincides with the QRS systolic component on the electrocardiogram produced by the left ventricular contractility closing the valve.

Aortic Valve and Left Atrium

The echoes recorded from the aortic root on M-mode should be parallel, moving anteriorly in systole and posteriorly in diastole. When the transducer is angled slightly medial, two of the three semilunar cusps can be visualized. The right coronary cusp is shown anterior and the

noncoronary cusp posterior (Figure 32-36). When seen, the left coronary cusp is shown in the midline between the other two cusps. The onset of systole causes the cusps to open to the full extent of the aortic root. The extreme force of blood through this opening causes a fine flutter to occur during systole. As the pressure relents in the ventricle, the cusps begin to drift to a closed position until they are fully closed in diastole.

The chamber posterior to the aortic root is the left atrium, which can be recognized by its immobile posterior wall. As one sweeps from the mitral apparatus medially and superiorly, the left ventricular wall blends into the atrioventricular groove and finally into the left atrial

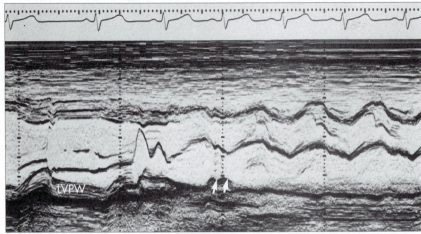

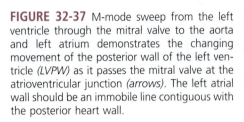

FIGURE 32-37 M-mode sweep from the left ventricle through the mitral valve to the aorta and left atrium demonstrates the changing movement of the posterior wall of the left ventricle (*LVPW*) as it passes the mitral valve at the atrioventricular junction (*arrows*). The left atrial wall should be an immobile line contiguous with the posterior heart wall.

wall (Figure 32-37). Thus, the sweep demonstrates good contractility in the left ventricle, with anterior wall motion in systole to the atrioventricular area, where the posterior wall starts to move posteriorly in systole, and then to the left atrium, where there is no movement.

Other structures posterior to the left atrial cavity that may lead to confusion in the identification of the left atrial wall are the left atrial appendage and descending aorta. The left atrial appendage may appear prominent posterior to the left atrial wall if there is severe enlargement of the left atrial cavity (especially seen in patients with severe mitral valve disease). Real-time evaluation with the transducer in the apical four-chamber position clarifies the atrial appendage as a separate structure. The descending aorta may also be recognized as a parallel, pulsating, tubular structure posterior to the left atrial cavity. The aorta is not continuous with the left ventricular wall, but the left atrial wall is. Thus, the cardiac sonographer should be able to distinguish this echo reflection as normal anatomy.

Interventricular Septum

The septum thickens in systole at the midportion of the ventricular cavity (Figure 32-38). The measurement and evaluation of septal thickness and motion should be made at this point. Normal septal thickness should match that of the posterior left ventricular wall and not exceed 1.2 cm.

Left Ventricle

Correct identification of the left ventricle may be made when both sides of the septum are seen to contract with the posterior heart wall. If the septum is not well defined or does not appear to move well, a more medial placement of the transducer along the sternal border with a lateral angulation may permit better visualization of this structure.

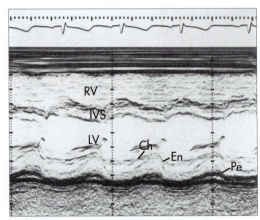

FIGURE 32-38 M-mode recording in the left ventricular cavity. *Ch*, Chordae; *En*, endocardium; *IVS*, interventricular septum; *LV*, left ventricle; *Pe*, pericardium; *RV*, right ventricle.

The three layers of the posterior heart wall—the endocardium (inner layer), myocardium (middle layer), and epicardium (outer layer)—should be identified separately from the pericardium (Figure 32-39). Sometimes it is difficult to separate the epicardium from the pericardium until the gain is reduced. The myocardium usually has a fine scattering of echoes throughout its muscular layer. The endocardium may be a more difficult structure to record because it reflects a weak echo pattern. The chordae are much denser structures than the endocardium. They generally are shown in the systolic segment along the anterior surface of the endocardium. As the ventricle contracts, the endocardial velocity is greater than the chordae tendineae velocity.

Tricuspid Valve

When the transducer has recorded the mitral apparatus, the beam should be angled slightly medially under the sternum to record the tricuspid valve (Figure 32-40). It is fairly easy to identify the whipping motion of the

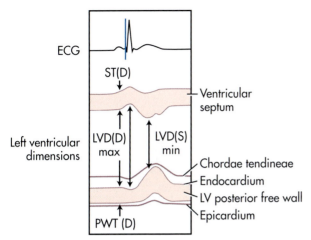

FIGURE 32-39 Measurements of the interventricular septum, left ventricle in diastole and systole, and the posterior wall are made. M-mode recording in the left ventricular cavity demonstrates the layers of the posterior heart wall: endocardium *(En)*, myocardium *(Myo)*, epicardium *(Ep)*, pericardium *(Pe)*, and chordae *(Ch)*. The distinction between the endocardium and chordal structures may be made by assessing the velocity of the two structures. The normal endocardial velocity is always much greater than the chordal velocity.

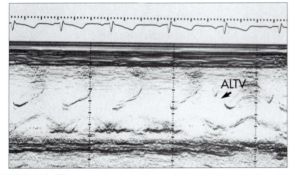

FIGURE 32-40 M-mode recording of the anterior leaflet of the tricuspid valve *(ALTV)*.

anterior valve in systole and early diastole. However, the complete diastolic period reveals the pathologic changes of stenosis and regurgitation; careful angulation may allow this phase to be recorded.

Pulmonary Valve

The anterior aortic root forms the posterior boundary of the pulmonary valve area. The appearance of the pulmonic cusp is similar to the aortic cusp and requires very slight angulations of the beam to demonstrate fully. With two-dimensional capabilities, the optimal view is generally a high-parasternal short-axis view with a slight angulation of the beam toward the left shoulder.

At the beginning of diastole, the pulmonary valve is displaced downward and is represented anteriorly on the ultrasound recording. The low transducer position with upward beam angulation, together with the vertical inclination of the pulmonary ring, results in the examination

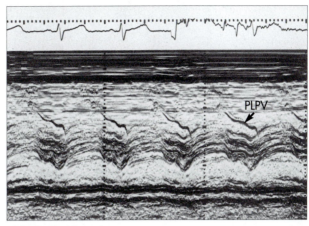

FIGURE 32-41 M-mode recording of the posterior cusp of the pulmonary valve. The cusp opens in systole and closes in diastole. *PLPV,* Posterior leaflet of the pulmonary valve.

BOX 32-18	M-Mode/2D Measurements and Calculations

If M-mode angles are oblique, measurements should be made using 2D with 2D calipers placed along minor axis. Even if oblique, include M-mode in study for motion of structures.

   Measure: LVIDd, LVIDs*, IVSd** , LVPWd, LA***, Ao root diameter****, and Ascending aorta*****.

*Measure LVIDs for all patients with ≥mod AI but do not label; use dropdown in LV Size/Shape section to report. Include only one EF% on the report. Multiple EFs% on a report are confusing to our clinicians. Calculate EF% by biplane-MOD if wall motion abnormalities are present (segmental or global), Chemo/pre-Chemo, and/or ≥ mild valve disease (stenosis and/or regurgitation). Otherwise, calculating EF% by Teicholz is okay. Strongly recommend EF% by biplane-MOD on all patients. It is okay to give EF% as range for atrial fib/flutter or frequent ectopy, but range should agree with calculated EF%. Visual estimation of EF% is not recommended and is only used as a last resort for technically extremely difficult cases; Echo contrast should be attempted. 3D EF% does not substitute for 2D derived EF% at this time as not all machines are 3D capable thus making serial Echo comparisons subject to methodological inaccuracies.
**IVSd measurements may be made from Ap4C view when not clearly seen in PS LAX. It is okay to measure (but do not label) discrete septal thickening separately so as not to misrepresent LV mass.
***Omit LA single plain dimension from report if it does not agree with LA biplane volume.
****Aortic root measurement is performed at sinus of Valsalva.
*****Asc Ao measurement is done at biggest minor axis seen (not necessarily at sinotubular junction).

of the valve from below. All elevations of the pulmonary valve in the stream of flow are represented as posterior movements on the echo. Likewise, downward movements are represented by anterior cusp positions on the trace.

   The pulmonary valve begins to move posteriorly (points *e* to *f*) in a gradual manner as the right ventricle fills in diastole (Figure 32-41). Atrial systole elevates the valve and produces a 3- to 7-mm posterior movement *a (dip)*. The valve completes the opening (points *b* and *c*), and, at the *c* to *d* point, the valve moves upward with ventricular systole.

Fetal Echocardiography: Beyond the Four Chambers

Sandra L. Hagen-Ansert

OBJECTIVES

On completion of this chapter, you should be able to:
- Describe embryologic development of the fetal heart
- Discuss fetal circulation
- List the risks factors that indicate fetal echocardiography
- Describe how to evaluate the fetus with two-dimensional, M-mode, pulsed Doppler, and color-flow Doppler imaging
- Discuss fetal ultrasound landmarks
- Describe normal anatomy seen in the views discussed in this chapter

OUTLINE

The continued development and improvement of high-resolution, real-time sonography has enabled the sonographer to visualize fetal cardiac activity with transvaginal transducers early in the first trimester. (Detailed visualization of all the anatomic structures of the fetal heart is better imaged in the second and third trimesters.) This ability to visualize cardiac anatomy has aided in the prenatal diagnosis of congenital heart disease. The incidence of congenital heart disease is about 8%, or 30,000 infants per year in the United States. Sonographic visualization allows the sonographer and clinician to image the small cardiac structures and obtain hemodynamic information from the fetal heart.

Conditions such as small cardiac defects, abnormal size or location of cardiac structures, arrhythmias, or abnormal cardiac function may all be observed with fetal echocardiography. The information obtained from the sonogram regarding the congenital heart defect is then managed through a team effort of multiple clinicians—including the pediatric cardiologist, geneticist, cardiovascular surgeon, and imaging specialists—to allow the patient to make educated decisions regarding the opportunities and outcomes for her fetus with a congenital heart defect.

Improvement in high-resolution transducers has permitted good resolution and visualization of even the smallest structures within the fetal cardiac chambers. These transducers and dedicated cardiac instrumentation, complete with motion mode (M-mode), 2D, 3D, color and Doppler capabilities, enable the sonographer to perform a complete fetal echocardiogram on obstetric patients between their sixteenth week of pregnancy and the time of delivery. Although fetal heart motion may be seen within the gestational sac as early as 4 to 5 weeks, structural information is better seen at 14 to 16 weeks of gestation, with even more detailed information available after 18 weeks of gestation.

Fetal echocardiography has been a tremendous clinical aid for the high-risk obstetric patient. The ability to map normal cardiac structures and ventricular function in a patient who has had a previous child with congenital heart disease helps relieve the pregnant patient of worry. Moreover, if a congenital heart condition is found, arrangements may be made to deliver the patient in a facility with the appropriate staff to manage such a neonate.

The addition of Doppler and color flow imaging has aided the diagnosis of congenital heart disease and has helped in the understanding of flow dynamics in the fetus. These two modalities, Doppler and color flow imaging, are used with discretion in the fetus with congenital heart disease. Three-dimensional echocardiography has been introduced in fetal echocardiography to allow more intricate visualization of the cardiac structures. This technique still requires a good axis of the fetal heart to be obtained before adequate interpolation of the data is made.

EMBRYOLOGY OF THE CARDIOVASCULAR SYSTEM

A single major error in the genetic constitution is the basis of congenital malformations. Human teratogens produce or raise the incidence of congenital malformations; 7% are caused by environmental agents or teratogens. A spontaneous abortion usually occurs if the genetic malformation is severe.

The most sensitive period in the first trimester for cardiac development is between 3.5 to 6.5 weeks. The cardiovascular system is the first organ system to reach a functional state; by the end of the third week, circulation of blood has begun.

Development of Blood Vessels

The primitive heart is a tubular structure that forms like a large blood vessel from the mesenchymal cells in the cardiogenic area of the embryo. Paired endocardial heart tubes develop before the end of the third week and begin to fuse, thus forming the primitive heart.

The circulation of blood starts by the end of the third week as the tubular heart begins to beat. The embryo obtains sufficient nourishment during the second week of development by diffusion of nutrients from maternal blood flow. The vascular system begins during the third week in the wall of the yolk sac, the connecting stalk, and the chorion. The blood vessels begin to develop 2 days later. Blood islands are formed; cavities develop in the islands to form primitive blood cells and vessels. These primitive vessels form a vascular network in the wall of the yolk sac. Blood vessels form in the mesenchyme associated with the connecting stalk and chorion. Blood vessels also form in the embryo toward the end of the third week and join to form a continuous system of vessels on each side.

Blood vessels from the embryo join those on the yolk sac, connecting stalk, and chorion to form a primitive cardiovascular system (Figure 33-1). The cardinal veins return blood from the embryo, and the vitelline veins return blood from the yolk sac. The umbilical veins return oxygenated blood from the placenta (only one umbilical vein persists). Two dorsal aortas fuse in the caudal half of the embryo to form a single dorsal aorta. Blood formation in the embryo begins at the fifth week.

Aortic Arches

Each branchial arch is supplied by an aortic arch (Figure 33-2). The arteries to the fifth pair are rudimentary or absent. The third pair of aortic arches becomes the common carotid artery and the proximal parts of the internal carotid arteries. The left fourth arch forms part of the arch of the aorta. The right fourth arch forms the proximal part of the right subclavian artery. The right sixth aortic arch becomes the right pulmonary artery. The left sixth aortic arch forms the left pulmonary artery and the ductus arteriosus (Box 33-1).

Development of the Heart

The heart tube grows rapidly, bending on itself because it is fixed at its cranial and caudal ends. The bending forms a U-shaped bulboventricular loop. The sinus

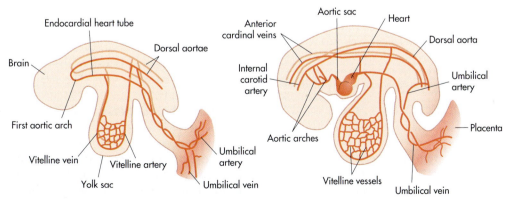

FIGURE 33-1 Cardiovascular system in a 26-day-old embryo. The two endocardial heart tubes have fused to form a tubular heart ring. The umbilical vein carries oxygenated blood and nutrients to the embryo from the placenta.

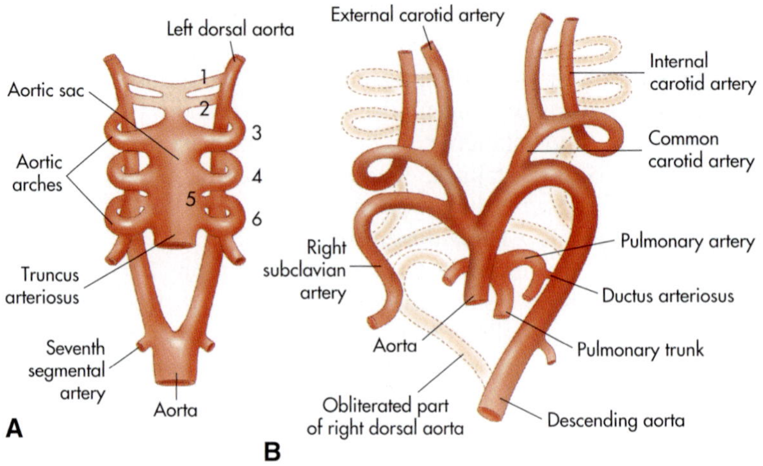

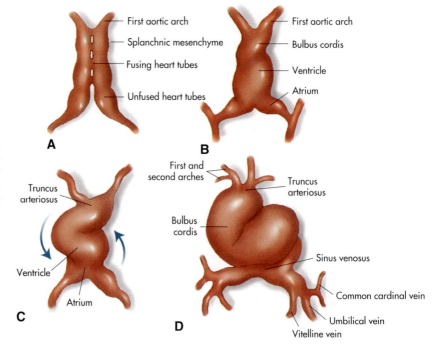

FIGURE 33-2 Aortic arches in a 6-week embryo **(A)** and in an 8-week embryo **(B)**.

FIGURE 33-3 The heart during the fourth week of development. The paired endocardial heart tubes **(A)** gradually fuse to form a single tubular heart **(B)**. The fusion begins at the cranial end of the tubes and extends caudally until a single tubular heart is formed. As the heart elongates, it bends on itself **(C** and **D)**.

BOX 33-1 | Cardiac Development

- *Sinus venosus.* The caudal region of the primitive heart, which receives all blood returning to the heart from common cardinal veins, vitelline veins, and umbilical veins.
- *Primitive atrium.* Develops into the right and left atria.
- *Primitive ventricle.* Develops into the left ventricle.
- *Bulbus cordis.* Develops into the right ventricle.
- *Truncus arteriosus.* Dilates to form the aortic sac from which the aortic arches arise.

---

venosus is initially a separate chamber that opens into the **right atrium** (Figure 33-3).

Right Atrium. The left horn of the sinus becomes the coronary sinus. The right horn is incorporated into the wall of the right atrium (forms a smooth portion of the adult right atrial wall). The right half of the primitive atrium persists as the right auricle.

Left Atrium. The **left atrium** is formed by incorporation of the primitive pulmonary vein. As the atrium grows, parts of this vein and its branches are absorbed. Four pulmonary veins eventually enter the left atrium from the lungs. The smooth wall of the left atrium is from the absorbed pulmonary vein. The left auricle is from the primitive heart.

Four-Chambered Heart. During the fourth and fifth weeks of fetal development, the division of the four chambers occurs.

Division of the Atrioventricular Canal. Endocardial cushions develop in the atrioventricular region of the heart. The cushions grow toward each other and fuse to divide the atrioventricular canal into right and left canals.

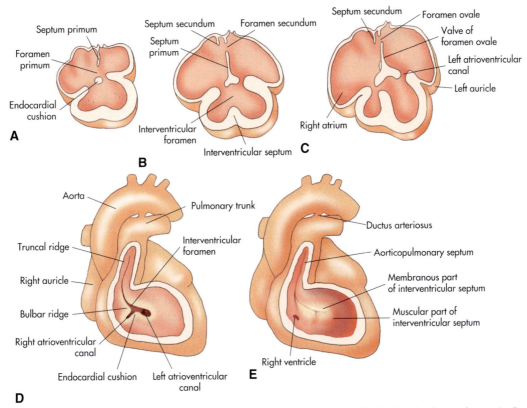

FIGURE 33-4 The partitioning of the primitive atrioventricular canal, atrium, and ventricle in the developing heart. **A, B,** and **C,** Frontal sections of the embryonic heart during the fourth week. **D** (5 weeks) and **E** (7 weeks) show schematic drawings of the heart illustrating closure of the interventricular foramen and formation of the interventricular septum. Note that the interventricular foramen is closed by tissues from three sources.

Division of the Primitive Atrium. The **septum primum** grows from the dorsal wall of the primitive atrium and fuses with the endocardial cushions (Figure 33-4, A and B). Before the fusion of the septum primum, a communication exists between the right and left halves of the primum atrium through the ostium primum or foramen primum. As the septum primum fuses with the endocardial cushions (obliterating the foramen primum), the superior part of the septum primum breaks down, creating an opening called the *foramen secundum* (see Figure 33-4, A and B). As this foramen develops, another membranous fold, the **septum secundum,** grows into the atrium to the right of the septum primum. The septum secundum overlaps the foramen secundum and the opening of the septum primum. There is also an opening between the free edge of the septum secundum and the dorsal wall of the atrium called the **foramen ovale** (Figure 33-4, C).

Formation of the Ventricles. The **left ventricle** is formed from the primitive vein. The right ventricle is formed from the **bulbus cordis.** The interventricular septum begins as a ridge in the floor of the primitive ventricle and slowly grows toward the endocardial cushions (see Figure 33-4, B and C). Until the seventh week, the right and left ventricles communicate through a large interventricular foramen. Closure of the interventricular foramen results in formation of the membranous part of the interventricular septum.

Partitioning of Bulbus Cordis and Truncus Arteriosus. The division of this part of the heart results from the development and fusions of the truncal ridges and bulbar ridges (Figure 33-4, D and E). Fused mesenchymal ridges form the aorticopulmonary septum, which divides the truncus arteriosus and bulbus cordis into the ascending aorta and pulmonary trunk.

Development of the Conduction System. The **sinoatrial node** forms in the wall of the sinus venosus near its opening into the right atrium; later it is incorporated into the right atrium with the right horn of the sinus venosus. The **atrioventricular node** and bundle are derived from cells in the walls of the sinus venosus and atrioventricular canal.

FETAL CIRCULATION

Blood flow in the fetus varies in two respects from the neonatal stage (Figure 33-5). Communication is open between the right and left sides of the heart through the **fossa ovale** and between the aorta and the pulmonary artery via the **ductus arteriosus.** It is useful to know these important communications to appreciate the fetal physiology of the cardiac structures.

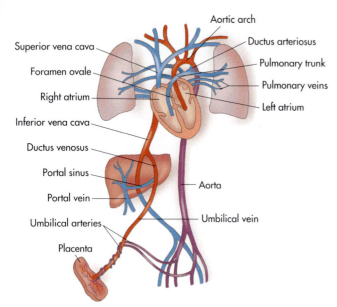

FIGURE 33-5 Fetal circulation.

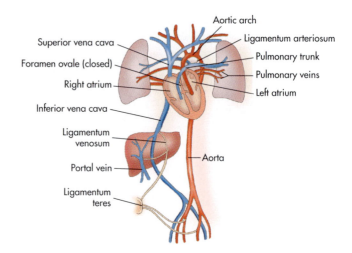

FIGURE 33-6 Neonatal circulation.

Before birth the oxygenated blood is given to the fetus by way of the umbilical vein from the placenta to the heart. Approximately half of the blood passes through the hepatic sinusoids, whereas the remainder bypasses the liver to go through the ductus venosus into the inferior vena cava. Blood flows from the **inferior vena cava** and **superior vena cava** and enters the right atrium. Blood in the right atrium is less oxygenated than blood in the umbilical vein.

A small amount of oxygenated blood from the inferior vena cava is diverted by the crista dividens and remains in the right atrium to mix with deoxygenated blood from the superior vena cava and coronary sinus. Some of the blood from the inferior vena cava is directed by the lower border of the septum secundum (the crista dividens) through the foramen ovale into the left atrium.

The blood in the right atrium flows through the three-leaflet **tricuspid valve** into the **right ventricle** and leaves the right ventricle through the **main pulmonary artery.** This artery bifurcates into right and left pulmonary artery branches that lead to their respective lungs. However, most of this blood passes through the connection of the ductus arteriosus into the descending aorta; only a very small amount goes to the lungs.

The blood mixes with a small amount of deoxygenated blood as it returns from the lungs via the four **pulmonary veins** into the left atrium. The pulmonary veins enter the posterior of the left atrium. The four veins are named according to their locations: right upper, left upper, right lower, and left lower. The blood then flows from the left atrium into the left ventricle through the bicuspid **mitral valve** and leaves the heart through the ascending aorta. The head, neck, and upper torso of the fetus are fed via the three branches off the ascending aorta. These branches are the innominate, left carotid, and left subclavian arteries. The rest of the mixed blood

in the descending aorta passes into the umbilical arteries and is returned to the placenta for reoxygenation. The remainder of the blood circulates through the lower part of the body.

After birth, the circulation of the fetal blood through the placenta ceases, and the neonatal lungs begin to function. The fetal cardiac structures no longer necessary are the foramen ovale, the ductus arteriosus, the ductus venosus, and the umbilical vessels (Figure 33-6).

Omission of the placental circulation causes an immediate fall of blood pressure in the newborn's inferior vena cava and right atrium. As the lungs expand with air, there is a fall in the pulmonary vascular resistance. This causes an increase in pulmonary blood flow and a progressive thinning of the walls of the pulmonary arteries. Thus, the pressure in the left atrium becomes higher than that in the right atrium. This causes the foramen ovale to close. With time, complete closure of the foramen occurs from adhesion of the septum primum to the left margin of the septum secundum. The septum primum forms the floor of the fossa ovalis. The lower edge of the septum secundum forms the limbus fossae ovalis, which demarcates the former cranial boundary of the foramen ovale.

The ductus arteriosus usually constricts shortly after birth (usually within 24 to 48 hours) once the left-sided pressures exceed the right-sided pressures. Often there is a small shunt of blood from the aorta to the pulmonary artery until these pressures adjust to neonatal life. The ductus turns into the ligamentum arteriosum in the neonate. If this communication persists, it is called a **patent ductus arteriosus.** This ligament passes from the left pulmonary artery to the arch of the aorta.

The umbilical arteries also constrict after birth to prevent blood loss from the neonate. The umbilical vein may remain patent for some time after birth.

Heart Rate

The normal fetal heart rate is between 120 and 160 beats per minute. In the first trimester of pregnancy, the heart rate begins around 90 beats per minute and increases to 170 beats per minute before returning to a normal rate and sinus rhythm. If the heart rate is too slow (less than 60 beats per minute), it is called *bradycardia*; a heart rate more than 200 beats per minute is termed *tachycardia*.

A very slow fetal heart rate, under 60 beats per minute, places the fetus at high risk of associated heart disease; fetal echocardiography should be performed to rule out the presence of a structural heart defect. The association of complete heart block with structural cardiac defects appears to have a poor prognosis, presumably because of their adverse interaction and the atrioventricular valve regurgitation that commonly complicates the condition. Connective tissue disorder (e.g., systemic lupus erythematosus) is associated with heart block and pericardial effusion.

RISK FACTORS INDICATING FETAL ECHOCARDIOGRAPHY

Specific risk factors indicate that the fetus is at a higher than normal risk for congenital heart disease and warrants a fetal echocardiogram. These may be divided into the following three categories: fetal risk factors, maternal risk factors, and familial risk factors.

Fetal Risk Factors

Fetal risk factors include the presence of intrauterine growth restriction, cardiac arrhythmias, abnormal amniocentesis indicating a trisomy, abnormal amniotic fluid collections, abnormal heart rate, and other anomalies as detected by the sonogram, such as hydrops fetalis.

The presence of extracardiac abnormalities (renal anomalies, gastrointestinal anomalies, single umbilical artery, etc.) in the fetus is frequently associated with congenital heart disease. If the abnormality is found in more than one organ system, the incidence of congenital heart disease increases further. Nonimmune hydrops may be cardiac related (heart failure) or related to other problems in the fetus.

Cardiac arrhythmias in the fetus may be a common finding if they are simply extrasystoles (premature atrial beats secondary to the immature conducting system). A small percentage of arrhythmias are associated with significant heart disease. However, a fetus with congenital heart block is usually associated with structural abnormalities in about half of the cases, most commonly atrioventricular septal defect as found in trisomy 21.

Maternal Risk Factors

Maternal risk factors include the previous occurrence of congenital heart disease in siblings or parents; a maternal disease known to affect the fetus, such as diabetes mellitus or connective tissue disease (e.g., lupus erythematosus); and maternal use of drugs, such as lithium or alcohol.

The incidence of congenital heart disease in fetuses whose mothers have uncontrolled diabetes is much higher than when the diabetes is controlled. The most common anomalies are ventricular septal defect, transposition of the great arteries, and tetralogy of Fallot.

Excessive alcohol during pregnancy has known effects of fetal alcohol syndrome, which includes facial abnormalities, growth restriction, mental retardation, and cardiac abnormalities (ventricular septal defect).

Indomethacin, a nonsteroidal antiinflammatory drug, has been used in the treatment of preterm labor. This drug has an effect on early closure of the patent ductus arteriosus. Evaluation of the fetus may be monitored with ultrasound to measure velocities across the patent ductus to detect if early closure is evident.

Familial Risk Factors

Familial risk factors include genetic syndromes or the presence of congenital heart disease in a previous sibling. The recurrence risk cited given a sibling with one of the most common cardiovascular abnormalities (ventricular septal defect, atrial septal defect, patent ductus arteriosus, tetralogy of Fallot) varies from 2.5% to 3%. Similar data given one parent with a congenital heart defect suggest that for the common defects listed, the recurrence risk ranges from 2.5% (atrial septal defect) to 4% (ventricular septal defect, patent ductus arteriosus, tetralogy of Fallot).

BEYOND THE FOUR-CHAMBER VIEW

Transducer Requirements

The ideal transducer for fetal echocardiography is a multi-frequency transducer that can be quickly and easily changed from a low to a high frequency. This is especially useful when the fetus is located in a position far from the transducer face or when a lower-frequency Doppler signal is necessary to obtain a high-velocity flow profile.

The following guidelines may be used in selecting the proper multihertz transducer for the fetal echocardiogram:

1. A 5.0-MHz transducer or higher with a medium focus is generally ideal for the typical pregnancy in a small to average-size patient in the second trimester.
2. A 3.5-MHz transducer with a medium-to-long focus may be used on patients of average to large build and on patients in the third trimester.
3. A 2.25-MHz transducer with medium-to-long focus is used for the obese patient in the second or third trimester.
4. The higher-frequency transvaginal probe is useful when the fetus is directed in a transverse lie. The probe is placed transabdominally in the mother's

umbilicus with gentle pressure and angled toward the fetal heart.

5. The size of the transducer varies. The early second trimester fetus may be adequately imaged with a curved array transducer; however, some laboratories prefer the small-sector, high-frequency probe.

Instrumentation

Other features useful on the ultrasound equipment include the following: cine-loop feature that allows imaging of the heart in frame-by-frame analysis, digital or disk recordings for later playback or comparison evaluation, high-power resolution zoom capability, simultaneous M-mode with range expansion (for cardiac arrhythmias), simultaneous Doppler capability with pulsed and continuous wave (to record high-velocity flow), and color Doppler.

Motion Mode Imaging

Motion mode (M-mode) is used to evaluate cardiac motion. Once the two-dimensional image is made, a single vertical line of information can be obtained from the face of the transducer through the fetal cardiac structures (Table 33-1). This image is electronically rotated 90 degrees so the depth of the image is along the vertical axis and the time display is shown along the horizontal axis (Figure 33-7). Acquisition of heart wall motion, septal and valve movement, and cavity size may be easily obtained from this technique. Heart rate is measured by counting the number of beats that occur within a specific time frame, usually more than 1 second. If 2.5 beats were shown in a 1-second time period, the heart rate would be 2.5 beats × 60 seconds = 150 beats per minute.

Pulsed Doppler Imaging

Pulsed Doppler demonstrates the direction and characteristics of blood flow within the fetal heart and great vessels and allows the qualitative and quantitative defini-

tion of flow disturbances, such as those that occur with valvular stenotic or regurgitant lesions. Doppler uses the principle of the Doppler shift, or sound waves reflected from the red blood cells within the fetal heart: If the cells are moving toward the transducer, the pitch increases; if the cells are traveling away, the pitch decreases. On the spectral display, the flow is displayed above (toward) or below (away) from the baseline. The sample volume may be gated or moved to the area of interest to record the optimum signal as the transducer is parallel to the flow of blood (Figure 33-8).

Higher levels of ultrasound energy are used with Doppler, and although no harmful effects have been reported on the fetal heart, the American Institute of Ultrasound in Medicine (AIUM) recommends keeping the Doppler ultrasonic energy at or below 100 mW/cm² spatial peak-temporal average, and Doppler interrogation should be limited to as short a time as possible (Table 33-2).

Color Flow Doppler Imaging

Color flow Doppler may help detect flow disturbances and flow direction (to check whether vessels or chambers

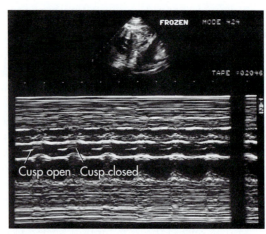

FIGURE 33-7 M-mode of the aorta and left atrial cavity. Time is depicted along the horizontal axis (dots along the top of the image). The distance between two dots represents 1 second. Distance is located along the vertical axis. The aorta is shown as the two parallel lines moving as a "unit" through systole (pumping) and diastole (resting). The aortic cusps open and remain open during ventricular systole. The left atrial cavity is shown posterior to the aorta. The left atrial wall motion may be seen within the left atrial cavity.

TABLE 33-1	Normal Fetal M-Mode Cardiac Measurements			
Cardiac Structure				
Weeks of Gestation	LV/RV	IVS	AO/PA	LA
20	6	1.5	4	5
22	8	1.7	4.8	6
24	9	2	5	6.5
28	10	2.3	6	8
32	12	3	7	10
36	14	3.5	8	11
40	16	3.8	9	12.5

AO, Aorta; *IVS*, interventricular septum; *LA*, left atrium; *LV*, left ventricle; *PA*, pulmonary artery; *RV*, right ventricle.

TABLE 33-2	Normal Doppler Measurements (Peak Systole)
Mitral valve	40–60–80 cm/sec
Tricuspid valve	45–65–87 cm/sec
Aortic valve	40–60–100 cm/sec
Pulmonic valve	25–55–80 cm/sec
Foramen ovale	20–30 cm/sec
Aortic arch, level of ductal insertion	120–150 cm/sec

are patent) and should be integrated into the fetal echocardiogram. Color Doppler flow mapping is a multigated Doppler technique in which sampling along all of the scan lines and depths in the field occurs simultaneously. Color displays are usually oriented so that flow toward the transducer is projected in shades of red and orange, and flow away is projected in cool blue colors. Disturbed flow is seen as a mixture of red, orange, and yellow or blues and greens.

Three-Dimensional Imaging

Clinical investigation of three-dimensional echocardiography has been performed both with and without cardiac gating. The gated acquisition showed improved resolution of structures compared with the nongated acquisition. Clarity of images is still the primary problem in this technique: the fetal heart is beating so quickly and the volume is too small to acquire enough data points to display an image better than the current real-time two-dimensional images.

FETAL ULTRASOUND LANDMARKS

In most cases, the obstetric patient has had a previous ultrasound and is referred for a dedicated or "target" fetal echocardiographic examination. Generally a dedicated fetal echocardiographic study may take from 30 to more than 60 minutes, depending on the type of pathologic condition present.

The cardiac sonographer must know certain characteristics that will help in the cardiac evaluation. (The reader is referred to Chapter 32 for illustration of these normal structures.)

The fetal survey should demonstrate the following structures before focusing on the fetal heart:

1. The position of the fetus (vertex, breech, transverse)
2. The position of the fetal thorax (spine up or down; determine right side and left side)
3. The position of the fetal stomach (right or left)
4. The location of the apex of the heart (left, right, or midline) (Figure 33-9)

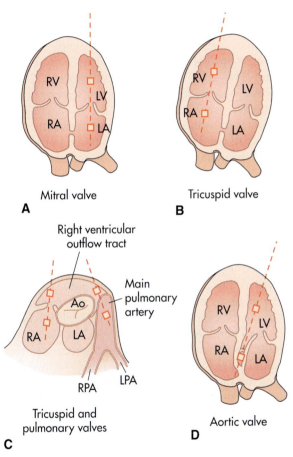

Mitral valve — **A**

Tricuspid valve — **B**

Right ventricular outflow tract

Main pulmonary artery

Ao

RA LA

RPA LPA

Tricuspid and pulmonary valves — **C**

Aortic valve — **D**

FIGURE 33-8 Pulsed Doppler sample volume placement for fetal echo. **A** and **B**, The four-chamber view is ideal to sample the velocity flow patterns of the mitral and tricuspid valves. The sample volume is initially placed at the annulus of the valve. To record regurgitation, the volume is moved into the atrial chamber; to record inflow of the valves, the sample volume is moved into the ventricular cavity. *LA,* Left atrium; *LV,* left ventricle; *RA,* right atrium; *RV,* right ventricle. **C,** The high short-axis view is best to obtain velocities from the tricuspid and pulmonary valves. The same procedure is used for the tricuspid valve as described in the four-chamber view. To record flow in the main pulmonary artery, the sample volume is placed at the level of the cusps and then moved back into the right ventricular outflow tract, then into the main pulmonary artery to look for abnormal flow patterns. *AO,* Aorta; *LPA,* left pulmonary artery; *RPA,* right pulmonary artery. **D,** The five-chamber view is good to record velocity flow in the left ventricular outflow tract and the ascending aorta. The sample volume should be placed below the aortic leaflets in the left ventricular outflow tract and then slowly moved through the cusps into the ascending aorta to see flow velocities.

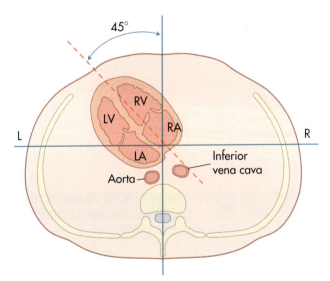

FIGURE 33-9 Measurement of the cardiac axis from a four-chamber view plane of the fetal chest. *LA,* left atrium; *LV,* left ventricle; *RA,* right atrium; *RV,* right ventricle. The apex of the heart should not exceed a 45-degree angle from the line drawn perpendicular to the fetal spine.

5. The location of the fetal abdominal aorta and inferior vena cava (aorta left, close to spine, inferior vena cava right, and elevated from spine)
6. The position of the fetal placenta (anterior placenta may cause noise that interferes with visualization of the cardiac structures if the thorax is adjacent to the placenta)
7. The biparietal diameter or femur length for measurement correlation

Obstacles to obtaining an adequate image include decreased amniotic fluid (oligohydramnios), unusual fetal position (spine up, transverse, or low lie in the maternal pelvis), and maternal obesity. The diabetic mother is generally more difficult to scan; these patients image best in the middle of the second trimester, between 20 and 22 weeks of gestation.

When the fetus is in a difficult-to-image position, the sonographer may ask the mother to get up, use the restroom, walk the hall for a few minutes, or do toe touches or jumping jacks to encourage the fetus to change positions. This technique usually works.

ECHOCARDIOGRAPHIC EVALUATION OF THE FETUS

A normal cardiac study should include the following views: four-chamber, outflow tracts, and oblique long-axis view for the aortic arch and ductus arteriosus.

Four-Chamber View

The four-chamber view is probably one of the easiest views to demonstrate cardiac anatomy (Box 33-2). Remember, the fetal heart lies in a horizontal position within the thorax, and the apex of the heart (the left ventricle) is directed toward the left hip (Figure 33-10). The transducer is angled in a cephalic direction through the fetal liver, which serves as a good window to visualize cardiac structures.

The sonographer should note the relative size and function of the atria and inflow ventricular cavities (see Figure 33-10, *D* and *E*). The right heart is slightly larger in utero than the left heart. The right and left sides may

be identified by the opening flap of the patent foramen ovale: in utero the foramen opens toward the left atrium. After birth the pressure in the left heart forces the foramen to close; failure to close results in an atrial septal defect. The moderator band can also be used to identify the right ventricle. It stretches horizontally across the right ventricle near the apex. The right ventricle is also more trabeculated than the left ventricle at the apex.

The position of the mitral and tricuspid leaflets (atrioventricular leaflets) should be assessed. Normally the tricuspid valve is located just slightly inferior to the mitral valve.

The left atrial cavity is generally about the same size as the right atrial cavity and is hypoechoic. The four pulmonic veins enter into the posterior wall of the left atrium. The right upper enters into the medial-posterosuperior wall; the left upper enters into the lateral-posterosuperior wall; the left lower enters the lateral inferior wall; and the right lower enters the medial inferior wall (see Figure 33-10, *F*). On the four-chamber view, all the pulmonary veins are imaged except for the right lower vein.

The inferior and superior vena cava may be seen to enter the right atrium. The inferior vena cava enters the posterior wall along the inferior lateral margin; the superior vena cava enters the medial posterosuperior wall.

The right and left ventricular width measurements are performed in the four-chamber view at the level of the atrioventricular annulus. The sonographer should clean up the image as much as possible for this measurement by turning the gain down. The right ventricle is measured from the lateral wall, across the level of the tricuspid annulus, to the midportion of the septum (see Figure 33-10, *G*). The left ventricle is measured from the midportion of the septum, across the level of the mitral annulus, to the endocardial surface of the lateral wall of the ventricle (see Figure 33-10, *H*). Normal values have been established to correspond to appropriate gestational ages. At 18 weeks of gestation, the ventricles should each measure approximately 6 mm.

If any abnormality exists in the atrioventricular valves or if the atria are enlarged, the four-chamber view is excellent to record Doppler tracings of blood flow (Figure 33-11). The transducer should be parallel to the four-chamber view, with the cursor placed at the level of the annulus and slowly moved into the ventricular cavity to record atrioventricular inflow patterns. To record regurgitation of the atrioventricular valves, the cursor is slowly moved into the atrial cavity to map the flow pattern and assess flow dynamics. Normally there is no backward flow through the orifice. The sonographer can assess the atrial size as an additional determinant of the presence of regurgitation.

The atrioventricular valves have a "double peak" of blood flow on the Doppler tracing. The first peak, *e*, is termed the *passive filling phase*. (This increases with fetal

---

BOX 33-2	Four-Chamber View Anatomy

- Right atrium and ventricle (with moderator band)
- Tricuspid valve
- Left atrium and ventricle
- Mitral valve
- Interventricular septum
- Interatrial septum
- Foramen ovale
- Pulmonary veins as they enter the left atrium

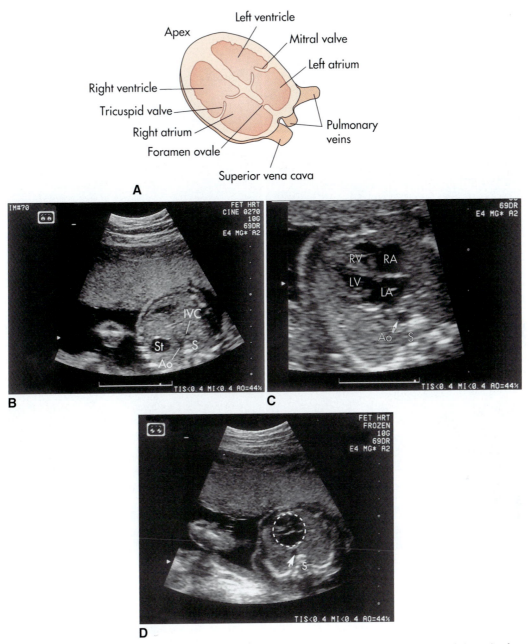

FIGURE 33-10 A, The normal fetal heart lies horizontal in the fetal thorax, with the apex pointing to the left hip. The four-chamber view shows the superior vena cava as it enters the right atrium. The two upper pulmonary veins enter the left atrium. The foramen ovale opens into the left atrium during fetal life. **B,** Transverse view of the 18-week fetus. The fetus is vertex with the spine *(S)* posterior, aorta *(Ao)* and anterior and inferior vena cavas *(IVC)* anterior and to the right; the stomach *(St)* lies to the left. **C,** As the transducer is angled cephalad, the four-chamber view of the heart is seen within the thorax. The spine *(S)* is posterior with the aorta *(arrow)*, anterior to the spine. The left atrium lies directly anterior to the aorta. *LA,* Left atrium; *LV,* left ventricle; *RA,* right atrium; *RV,* right ventricle. **D,** Four-chamber view of the heart with a normal axis.   *Continued*

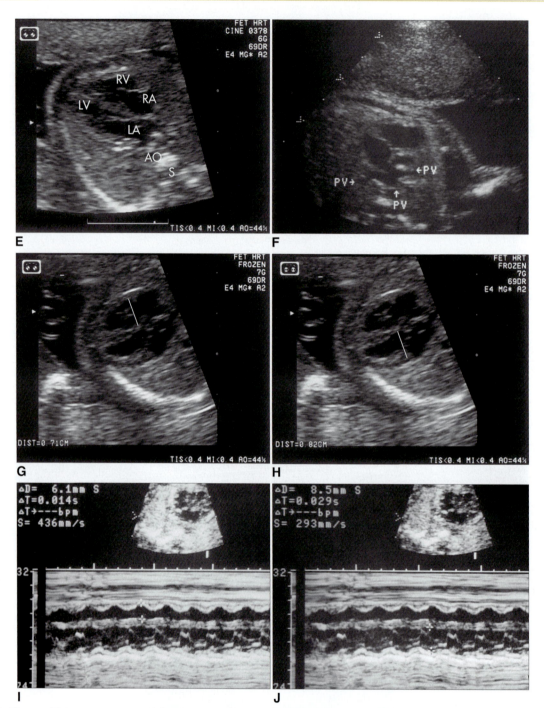

FIGURE 33-10, cont'd E, *AO,* Aorta; *LA,* left atrium; *LV,* left ventricle; *RA,* right atrium; *RV,* right ventricle; *S,* spine. **F,** Three of the four pulmonary veins *(PV)* enter the left atrial cavity. Measurements of the left ventricle **(G)** and right ventricle **(H)** are made on two-dimensional views at the level of the mitral annulus. **I,** M-mode measurements may also be made at the level of the annulus for the RV and LV **(J).**

breathing and with gestational age.) This peak is smaller than the second peak because the fetal heart is less compliant than the neonatal heart. The second, taller peak, *a,* is termed the *active atrial phase.* In later pregnancy the *e* point equals or exceeds the *a* point on the Doppler tracing as the pressure on the left side exceeds the right-side pressure. The mean tricuspid valve velocity is 65 cm/ sec; the mean mitral valve velocity is 60 cm/sec.[2]

Color flow Doppler (Figure 33-12, *A* and *B*) may be useful in demonstrating the amount and path of regurgitation. A multicolored jet would be present in the atrial cavity posterior to the atrioventricular valve. Remember, the pressures in the fetal heart are different than after birth; therefore, the color and Doppler flow patterns will not be truly representative of the velocities obtained after birth.

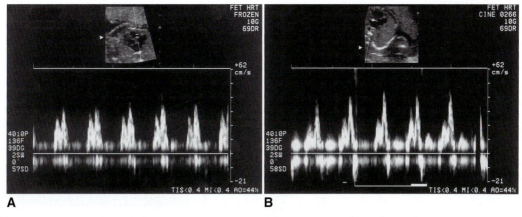

FIGURE 33-11 Normal Doppler flow patterns made in the four-chamber view of the mitral **(A)** and tricuspid **(B)** leaflets. The smaller first peak is the *e* wave; the second higher peak is the *a* wave.

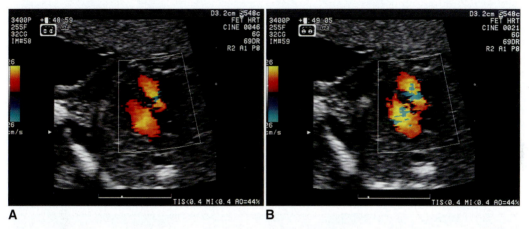

FIGURE 33-12 Color Doppler inflow patterns of the normal heart in a four-chamber view. **A** corresponds to early diastole at the *e* wave (early inflow filling of the ventricle), and **B** represents the *a* wave.

Left and Right Ventricular Outflow Tracts

Five-Chamber View. Aortic flow may be recorded in the five-chamber view (Box 33-3); to obtain this view, the transducer should be angled slightly anterior from the four-chamber view to include the left ventricular and aortic outflow tract (Figure 33-13). Doppler flow patterns of the aorta are recorded with the transducer again parallel to flow and the cursor placed first at the level of the aortic cusps and then moved into the ascending aorta. The mean velocity in the aorta is 60 cm/sec.

Crisscross View. As the transducer is angled from the aorta slightly to the left, the pulmonary artery may be seen as it arises from the right ventricular outflow tract (Figure 33-14). The pulmonary artery normally is anterior and to the left of the aorta. This "sweep" from the aorta to the pulmonary artery is called the crisscross view and allows the sonographer to see the normal relationship of the great arteries to one another (Box 33-4). Pulmonary flow patterns may be obtained in this view if the cursor is parallel with the flow. The cursor is moved into the main pulmonary artery to record the flow pat-

BOX 33-3	Five-Chamber View Anatomy

- Left atrium
- Left ventricular outflow tract
- Aortic root
- Right ventricle

BOX 33-4	Crisscross View of Great Arteries

- Sweep from aorta (located posterior) to pulmonic vessel (located anterior)
- Left ventricular outflow tract
- Right ventricular outflow tract

terns. The mean velocity in the pulmonary artery is 55 cm/sec.

Long-Axis View. In the long-axis view (Figure 33-15, *A* and *B*), the sizes of the right and left ventricles and the left atrial cavity should be assessed to obtain an overview of cardiac disease and contractility (Box 33-5). The left atrial cavity in this view is generally about the same size as the aorta and is hypoechoic. The

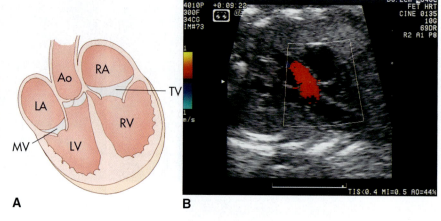

FIGURE 33-13 Aortic outflow is shown in red in this four-chamber view. *Ao,* Aorta; *LA,* left atrium; *LV,* left ventricle; *MV,* mitral valve; *RA,* right atrium; *RV,* right ventricle; *TV,* tricuspid valve.

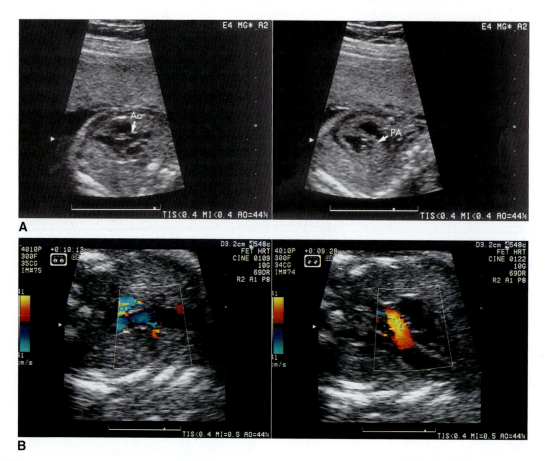

FIGURE 33-14 A, Crisscross view of the heart shows the aorta *(Ao)* posterior in continuity with the ventricular septum. The transducer is angled medial and anterior to image the pulmonic artery *(PA)*. **B,** Color Doppler image of the pulmonary artery outflow is blue as it leaves the right ventricular cavity. The aortic outflow is red as the blood leaves the left ventricle.

BOX 33-5	Long-Axis View

- Right ventricle
- Interventricular septum
- Left ventricle
- Mitral valve leaflets
- Aorta with aortic cusps
- Left atrium

crescent-shaped right ventricle is anterior to the left ventricle.

The thickness of the interventricular septum may be assessed from the parasternal long-axis view when the transducer is perpendicular to the septum. The septum is divided into membranous and muscular segments. The membranous portion is located just inferior to the aorta. This part of the septum is the last to develop and is very thin; it must be examined in several planes to evaluate

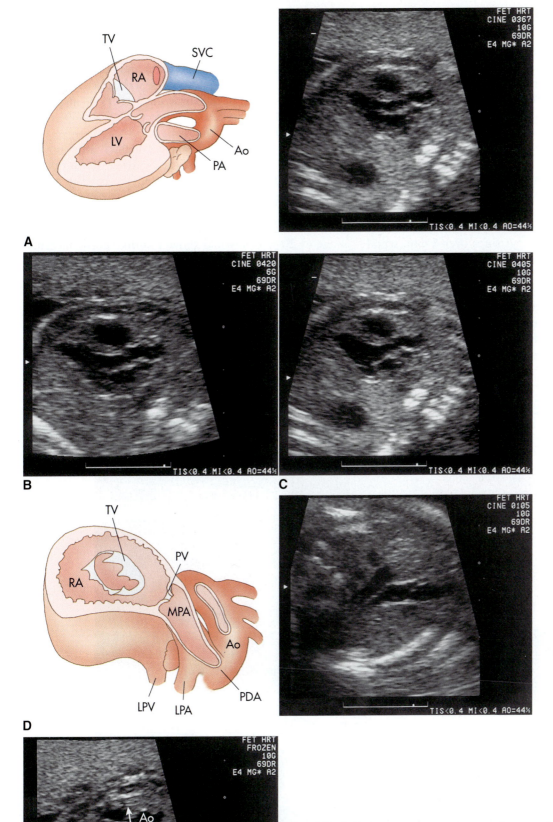

FIGURE 33-15 A, Long-axis view of the left ventricular outflow tract shows the crescent right ventricle, the interventricular septum and its continuity with the anterior wall of the aorta, and the posterior wall of the aorta and its continuity with the anterior leaflet of the mitral valve. The fetal echo was imaged at early diastole, mitral valve open fully, aortic valve closed. **B,** Mid-diastole, mitral valve begins to close. **C,** End-diastole, mitral valve closed, aortic valve opens. **D,** As the transducer is angled medial and slightly anterior, the right ventricular outflow tract with the pulmonary artery *(PA)* is seen on the fetal echo. *Ao,* Aorta; *LPA,* left pulmonary artery; *LPV,* left pulmonary vein; *MPA,* main pulmonary artery; *PDA,* posterior descending artery; *PV,* pulmonary valve; *TV,* tricuspid valve. **E,** The size of the aorta *(Ao)* and left atrium *(LA)* may be measured in this long-axis view.

its inflow and outflow sections. The inflow membranous septum is best seen on the apical four-chamber view at the level of the atrioventricular valves, whereas the outflow may be seen on the long-axis view.

The septum thickens along its muscular component, which makes up the remaining two thirds of the septum. The septum and the posterior left ventricular wall are generally the same thickness at the end of ventricular systole. Normal septal thickness should correspond to the gestational age; a good rule of thumb is that the second-trimester septum should measure about 2 to 2.5 mm and the third-trimester septum should measure under 4 mm. If the septum measures over 5 mm, septal hypertrophy or concentric ventricular hypertrophy should be considered.

On the long-axis view (see Figure 33-15, C), the continuity of the right side of the septum with the anterior wall of the aortic root is important to rule out the presence of a membranous ventricular septal defect (VSD), conal truncal abnormality (such as truncus arteriosus), endocardial cushion defect, or tetralogy of Fallot. A very

small VSD may not be visualized at this stage, depending on the resolution of the equipment and quality visualization of the fetus. Generally the septal defect must be at least half the size of the aortic diameter to be imaged by ultrasound. Multiple septal defects may be difficult to image in the second trimester.

As the transducer is angled slightly anterior and medial from the aortic root, the right ventricular outflow tract may be imaged (see Figure 33-15, D). The pulmonary artery is slightly wider at its origin than the aorta.

The size of the aorta should be assessed. A gestational age of 20 weeks would show a normal aortic measurement of 4 mm. The aortic cusp motion should be assessed on the long- and short-axis views (see Figure 33-15, E). Normally the three cusps open in systole to the full extent of the aortic root and close in a midposition in diastole. The cusps do not "flop" into the left ventricular outflow tract, as is sometimes seen to varying degrees with a bicuspid or unicuspid valve. The aortic root should be anechoic from its base throughout the arch

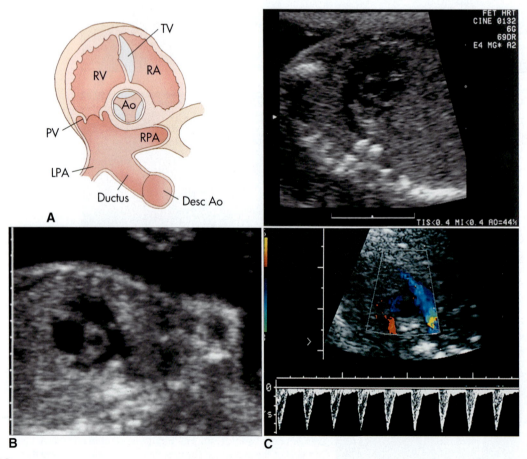

FIGURE 33-16 A, High, short-axis view of the great vessels. The right ventricular outflow tract wraps anterior to the aorta. The pulmonary artery arises from the right ventricle and bifurcates into right and left branches. The ductal insertion occurs midway between the bifurcation of the pulmonary vessels. Measurement of the great vessel diameters may be made at the level of the cusps. *Ao,* Aorta; *Desc Ao,* descending aorta; *LPA,* left pulmonary artery; *PV,* pulmonary vein; *RA,* right atrium; *RPA,* right pulmonary artery; *RV,* right ventricle; *TV,* tricuspid valve. **B,** Normal relationship of the pulmonary artery (tubular) with the bifurcation into right and left pulmonary arteries as it lies anterior to the aorta. **C,** Color Doppler shows the increased velocity in the main pulmonary artery *(blue)* at the ductal insertion *(yellow). AO,* Aorta; *PA,* pulmonary artery.

and descending aorta. The presence of interluminal echoes with dilation may indicate some degree of aortic stenosis (with poststenotic dilation). The presence of a membrane inferior to the aortic cusps may indicate subvalvular aortic obstruction.

Short-Axis View. Once the long-axis view has been obtained, the transducer is rotated 90 degrees to the transverse or short-axis view. Generally the transducer is angled in a cephalic direction to make this a high parasternal short-axis view (Figure 33-16, *A*). The structures listed in Box 33-6 should be visualized.

BOX 33-6 | Short-Axis View

- Right ventricular outflow tract
- Pulmonary cusps
- Main pulmonary artery
- Right and left pulmonary arteries
- Aorta with cusps
- Left atrial cavity

The high short-axis is the view we use to measure the diameter of the pulmonary artery and the aorta (see Figure 33-16, *B*). It is also important to visualize the bifurcation of the main pulmonary artery into the right and left pulmonary arteries to demonstrate the normal relationship of the pulmonary artery as it lies anterior and to the left of the aorta. On the short-axis view, normally the right ventricular outflow tract and pulmonary artery "drape" anterior to the circular aorta (see Figure 33-16, *A*). The great vessels are measured two-dimensionally at the level of the semilunar cusps. At 20 weeks of gestation, both arteries should measure approximately 4 mm each.

The trileaflet aortic cusps may be visualized in this short-axis view. A two-leaflet or **bicuspid aortic valve** appears as two cusps with or without eccentric closure, depending on the equal distribution of cusp tissue.

Pulmonic flow patterns are obtained parallel to flow in the high short-axis plane with the Doppler cursor at the level of the pulmonic cusps. The cursor is moved into the main pulmonary artery to map any changes in the

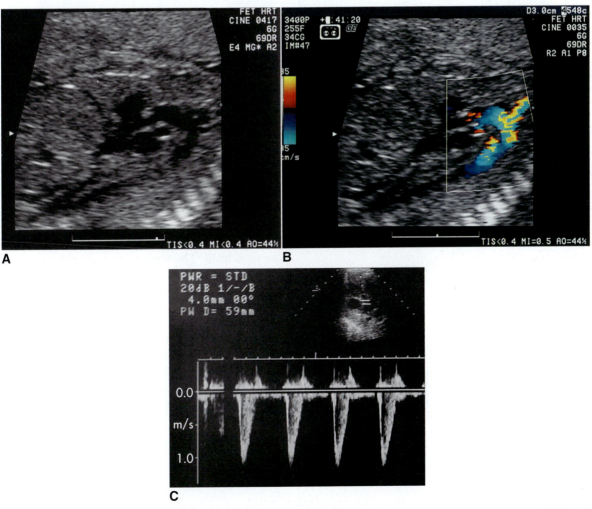

FIGURE 33-17 Normal gray scale **(A)** and color Doppler **(B)** images of the ascending aorta, arch, and descending aorta. The left subclavian is one of the three vessels that arise from the arch of the aorta and is well seen on the color image. **C,** Normal velocity in the aorta.

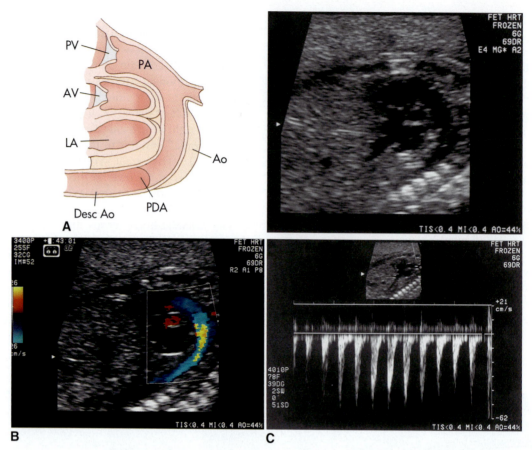

FIGURE 33-18 The ductal arch is found slightly inferior to the aortic arch. **A,** The short-axis view shows the main pulmonary artery and ductal arch as it empties into the descending aorta. *Ao,* Aorta; *AV,* aortic valve; *Desc Ao,* descending aorta; *LA,* left atrium; *PA,* pulmonary artery; *PDA,* patent ductus arteriosus; *PV,* pulmonary valve. **B,** Color shows the increased velocity *(yellow)* at the level of the ductus. **C,** Pulsed Doppler flow velocity shows the normal pattern of 50 cm/sec in the main pulmonary artery. This velocity may more than double at the level of the ductal insertion.

flow pattern. The mean velocity in the pulmonary artery ranges from 60 to 80 cm/sec; when the cursor reaches the level of ductal insertion, near the left pulmonary branch artery, the flow dramatically increases to nearly double the velocity in the main pulmonary artery (150 cm/sec) (Figure 33-16, C).

Ductal and Aortic Arch Views: Oblique Long Axis

With careful angulation of the transducer to an oblique longitudinal plane, the root of the aorta, the ascending aorta, the arch, and the descending aorta may be assessed (Figure 33-17). The sonographer may find the fetal spine in the sagittal plane and angle slightly inward toward the left chest to search for the descending aorta and arch. The tubular dimension of this vessel should be somewhat uniform as one follows the aorta from its base into the

thorax and abdomen. As the sonographer carefully sweeps back and forth, the inner core should be anechoic. The three head and neck branch arteries (innominate, carotid, and left subclavian) may be seen to arise from the perfect curve of the aortic arch as they ascend into the fetal head. The sonographer should be able to demonstrate the candy cane appearance of the ascending aorta, arch, and descending aorta in one image plane.

A second arch-type pattern (which appears as large as the aorta) is shown as the transducer is angled inferior from the aortic arch. This represents the patent ductus arteriosus, a communication between the pulmonary artery and the aorta that is patent during fetal life but closes shortly after birth. The ductus is slightly larger than the aortic arch and has a sharper angle ("hockey stick") as it drains into the descending aorta (Figure 33-18). The ductus does not have arterial structures arising from its wall as the aorta does.

Fetal Echocardiography: Congenital Heart Disease

Sandra L. Hagen-Ansert

This chapter presents the sonographer's approach to evaluating congenital heart disease with examples of many of the more common heart abnormalities. The development of the fetal heart is completed by the eighth week of embryonic life. The presence of congenital heart disease is a result of abnormal cardiac development during this period.

The most common types of congenital heart disease are the ventricular septal defect, atrial septal defects, and **pulmonary stenosis**. The development of congenital heart disease is multifaceted. Environmental factors, chromosomal factors, and hereditary factors may influence the development of congenital heart disease in the fetus. Fetal echocardiography can help to establish the presence and severity of the cardiac abnormality.

RELATIONSHIP OF GENETICS TO CONGENITAL HEART DISEASE

Chromosomal Abnormalities

The frequency of chromosomal abnormalities in infants with congenital heart disease is estimated as 5% to 10% from postnatal data. In a control study of 2100 live-born infants with cardiovascular malformations, chromosomal abnormalities were found in 13%.[1] In this study, Down syndrome occurred in more than 10% of the infants, with the other trisomies each constituting the remaining 1%.

The frequency of abnormal karyotypes in fetuses with cardiac defects has been commonly found at 30% to 40%. Of these fetuses, most have trisomy 21, followed by trisomy 13, trisomy 18, and Turner's syndrome. The association of congenital heart defects and chromosomal abnormalities is lower in live-born infants than in fetuses because of the high in utero mortality of the fetus with trisomy 18, trisomy 13, and Turner's syndrome (45X).

The occurrence of associated extracardiac abnormalities in fetuses with cardiac defects and chromosomal abnormalities is in the order of 50% to 70%. In the fetus with a single cardiac abnormality, the incidence of chromosomal abnormalities is still increased (15% to 30%). The most common single cardiac abnormality is the ventricular septal defect.

Certain cardiac abnormalities are more likely associated with chromosomal defects. In general, malformations of the right side of the heart are rarely associated with karyotypic abnormalities (e.g., pulmonic stenosis and tricuspid atresia). On the other hand, abnormalities such as atrioventricular septal defect, perimembranous ventricular septal defect, tetralogy of Fallot, double outlet right ventricle, coarctation of the aorta, and hypoplastic left heart are often associated with chromosomal abnormalities.

The incidence of cardiac defects in the fetus with trisomy is increased, with trisomy 21 showing the highest rate at 40% to 50%, Turner's syndrome (45X) showing 25% to 40%, and more than 90% having cardiac defects with trisomies 13 and 18 (Table 34-1).

Familial Risks of Congenital Heart Disease

Most congenital heart defects have more than one cause, with genetic and environmental factors both playing a role. Only about 10% to 15% of all congenital heart defects have been attributed to known chromosomal abnormalities, genetic syndromes, and teratogenic embryopathies.

The recurrence risk for an isolated congenital cardiovascular malformation is modified for each family based on the number of affected relatives and the severity of the abnormality. In general, a recurrence risk of 1% to 5% is estimated for the majority of congenital cardiac abnormalities.

Studies have shown that the contribution of genetic factors increases the risk of congenital heart disease significantly. For example, a mother who has had a child with a left heart abnormality (mitral atresia or aortic atresia) has a significantly higher risk (13%) of delivering another child with a form of left heart disease. This risk increases significantly with each pregnancy.

INCIDENCE OF CONGENITAL HEART DISEASE

Congenital heart disease is the most common severe congenital abnormality, with an incidence of 8% in live births. Approximately half of these defects are minor and may be corrected easily with surgery; the other half are responsible for more than 50% of the deaths from congenital abnormalities in childhood. Cardiac defects may account for as much as 4% of congenital heart disease in live births. Common cardiac defects include the **bicuspid aortic valve**, patent ductus arteriosus (common in premature infants), and ventricular septal defects. The incidence of the bicuspid aortic valve defect is 10 in 10,000 births; it may lead to cardiac problems in adulthood.

TABLE 34-1	Congenital Heart Disease and Chromosomal Abnormality		
Chromosomal Abnormality	Incidence at Live Birth	Associated Cardiac Abnormality	Common Cardiac Abnormalities
Trisomy 21	1:800	40%–50%	Atrioventricular septal defect Ventricular septal defect Cleft mitral valve Heart block
Trisomy 18	1:8000	>90%	Ventricular septal defect Double-outlet right ventricle
Trisomy 13	1:20,000	>80%	Ventricular septal defect Atrial septal defect
Turner's Syndrome (Trisomy 45X)	1:10,000	25%–45%	Coarctation of aorta Bicuspid aortic valve

PRENATAL EVALUATION OF CONGENITAL HEART DISEASE

The Four-Chamber View

All sonographers should be familiar with the routine four-chamber view that is part of the normal obstetric examination. This view is easily obtainable after 16 weeks of gestation, although the anatomy becomes more distinctly imaged with ultrasound at 19 to 20 weeks of gestation. The four-chamber view is normal when the following conditions are seen:

1. The fetal situs is normal. (The heart is in the left chest and its apex points to the left, the stomach is to the left, the aorta is anterior and to the left of the spine, and the inferior vena cava is anterior and to the right of the spine; (Figure 34-1, *A*).
2. The size of the heart in relation to the chest is normal (ratio of heart to thorax = 1:3) (Figure 34-1, *B*).

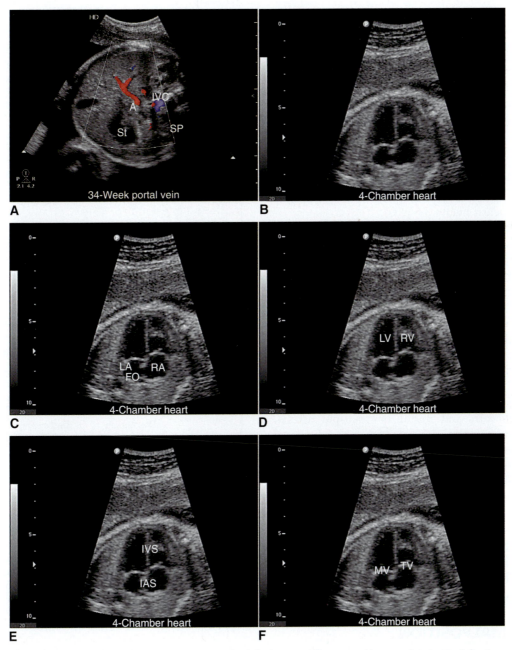

FIGURE 34-1 A, The fetal situs is normal. (Heart position is in the left chest and the apex of heart points to the left; stomach is to the left; aorta is anterior and to the left of the spine; and inferior vena cava is anterior and to the right of the spine.) **B,** The size of the heart in relation to the chest is normal. (Ratio of heart to thorax = 1:3.) **C,** The two atria are equal in size and the flap of the foramen ovale is seen to move toward the left atrium. (The atrium should comprise about one third the size of the heart.) **D,** The two ventricles are equal in size and contractility. (The ventricles should comprise about two thirds the size of the heart.) **E,** The interatrial and interventricular septa are completely formed and normal in thickness. **F,** The atrioventricular valves are normal in thickness, position, and opening.

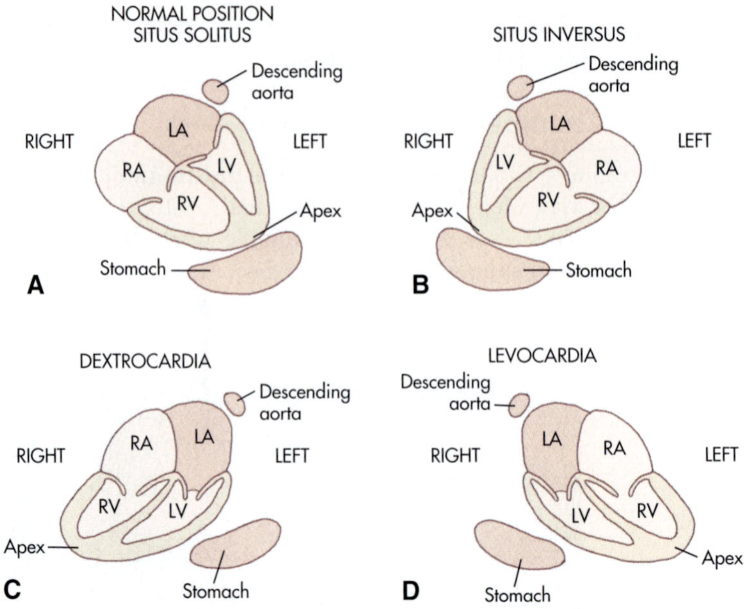

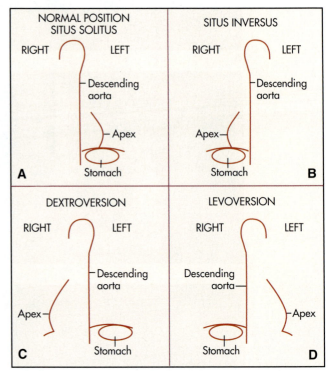

FIGURE 34-2 The anatomic relationship of the descending aorta, left atrium, apex, and stomach in the four cardiac positions. **A,** Normal position, situs solitus. **B,** Situs inversus. **C,** Dextrocardia; and **D,** Levocardia. *RA,* Right atrium; *LV,* left ventricle; *RV,* right ventricle.

3. The two atria are equal in size, and the flap of the foramen ovale is seen to move toward the left atrium. (The atria should constitute about one third of the size of the heart; Figure 34-1, *C*).
4. The two ventricles are equal in size and contractility. (The ventricles should constitute about two thirds of the size of the heart; Figure 34-1, *D*).
5. The interatrial and interventricular septa are completely formed and normal in thickness (Figure 34-1, *E*).
6. The atrioventricular valves are normal in thickness, position, and opening (Figure 34-1, *F*).

Several cardiac abnormalities may be recognized with the four-chamber view alone, such as a large ventricular septal defect, atrioventricular septal defect, hypoplastic left or right heart, and mitral or tricuspid atresia. However, many cardiac abnormalities may be missed with only the four-chamber view. Abnormalities of the cardiac structure (especially the great vessels) that are not located in the four-chamber plane may show a normal four-chamber view, but the specific abnormality will be missed if a complete study is not conducted (e.g., transposition of the great arteries, truncus arteriosus, coarctation of the aorta, small outlet ventricular septal defect, tetralogy of Fallot, and others). The reader is referred to Chapter 33, which covers the normal fetal echocardiographic examination.

CARDIAC MALPOSITION

When the heart is out of its normal position, several terms may be used to describe the exact position of the heart relative to location and position of the cardiac apex (Figures 34-2 and 34-3). **Dextrocardia** means the heart is in the right chest with the apex pointed to the right of

FIGURE 34-3 The alignment of the descending aorta, apex, and stomach in the four basic cardiac positions from the frontal projection. **A,** In situs solitus, the descending aorta, apex, and stomach are all on the left. **B,** In situs inversus, the descending aorta, apex, and stomach are all on the right. **C,** In dextroversion, the descending aorta and stomach are on the left, but the apex is on the right. **D,** In levoversion, the descending aorta and stomach are on the right, but the apex is on the left.

the thorax (Figure 34-4, *A*). Dextrocardia can be associated with a normal visceral situs, situs inversus, or situs ambiguous. **Dextroposition** of the heart refers to a condition in which the heart is located in the right side of the chest and the cardiac apex points medially or to the left.

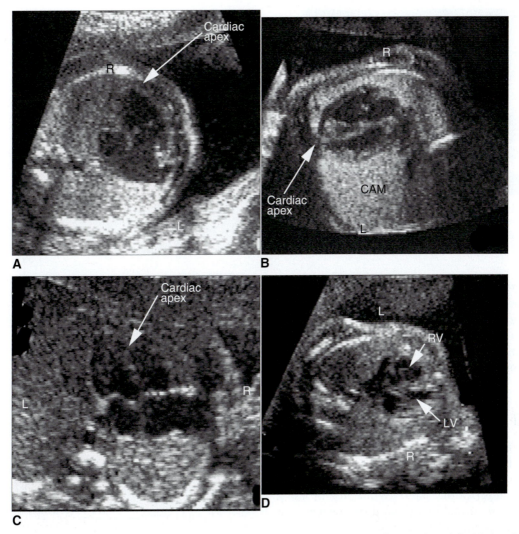

FIGURE 34-4 Abnormal cardiac axis and position. **A,** True dextrocardia. **B,** Dextroposition secondary to a large left-sided cystic adenomatous malformation that pushes the heart into the right chest. **C,** Dextroposition caused by the presence of right lung hypoplasia. The heart shifts into the space lacking lung tissue but maintains a near normal axis. **D,** Mesocardia.

This condition is usually found when extrinsic factors, such as a space-occupying large diaphragmatic hernia or hypoplasia of the right lung, are present (Figure 34-4, *B* and *C*).

Levocardia is the term used to denote the normal position of the heart in the left chest (with the cardiac apex pointed to the left) and is often used when visceral situs abnormalities are present. Levocardia can be associated with normal situs, situs inversus (abdominal organs are located on the opposite side of normal), or situs ambiguous. **Levoposition** of the heart refers to the condition in which the heart is displaced further toward the left chest, usually in association with a space-occupying lesion (Figure 34-4).

Mesocardia indicates an atypical location of the heart, with the cardiac apex pointing toward the midline of the chest. Usually the heart is located more toward the midline. This may be found with the presence of an extracardiac mass or lung abnormalities (Figure 34-4, *D*).

CARDIAC ENLARGEMENT

Cardiomyopathy

Cardiomyopathy is a condition of the myocardial tissue in the heart. This disease process may be caused by exposure to a virus (Coxsackie or mumps) or to bacteria, which leads to an infection that causes cardiomyopathy. Errors of metabolism may also cause cardiomyopathy. Endocardial fibroelastosis has also been associated with cardiomyopathies and hypoplastic left-heart syndrome. Asymmetric septal hypertrophy (as seen in patients with hereditary idiopathic subaortic stenosis) and concentric hypertrophy (as seen in some uncontrolled diabetic mothers) have been reported.

Myocarditis is characterized by necrosis and destruction of myocardial cells and an inflammatory infiltrate. In a viral cardiomyopathy, all four chambers are dilated, with thinning of the myocardial walls (Figure 34-5). Gross valvular regurgitation may be present, resulting

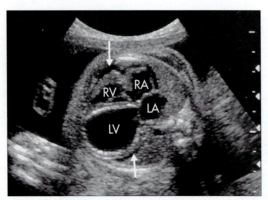

FIGURE 34-5 Four-chamber view of the heart shows dilation of all four chambers. Regurgitation was present in the mitral and tricuspid valves. Pericardial effusion *(arrow)*. *RV,* Right ventricle; *RA,* right atrium; *LV,* left ventricle; *LA,* left atrium.

from the stretched mitral and tricuspid anulus. Cardiac function is decreased severely, leading to congestive heart failure with pericardial effusion, bradycardia, and death.

The general prognosis for a fetus with evidence for a cardiomyopathy is poor. Serial fetal echoes are performed to monitor chamber size, regurgitation, and contractility.

Pericardial Effusion

Pericardial effusion is an abnormal collection of fluid surrounding the epicardial layer of the heart. In the four-chamber view, a hypoechoic area in the peripheral part of the epicardial/pericardial interface of 2 mm or less is considered within normal limits and does not represent a pericardial effusion. The separation must be seen on the M-mode to separate both in systole and in diastole and be greater than 2 mm. A separation that surrounds the heart (from the atrioventricular junction around the apex of the heart) may be associated with hydrops fetalis (Figure 34-6).

With a small pericardial effusion, the separation of the pericardium from the epicardium may localize toward the posterolateral and apical walls of the heart. The larger effusion will extend to the atrioventricular groove posteriorly and around the anterior right ventricular wall.

Pericardial effusion may be seen secondary to indomethacin therapy with premature closure of the patent ductus arteriosus. Pericardial effusion has also been associated with coxsackievirus, cytomegalovirus, parvovirus, human immunodeficiency virus, intrauterine growth restriction, and aneuploidy.

SEPTAL DEFECTS

Atrial Septal Defect

Atrial septal defects allow communication between the left atrium and right atrium. The locations of three

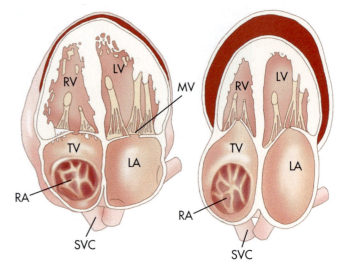

FIGURE 34-6 A, Apical view of a small pericardial effusion. **B,** Apical view of a large pericardial effusion involving the right ventricle, apex, and left ventricle. *RV,* Right ventricle; *LV,* left ventricle; *MV,* mitral valve; *LA,* left atrium; *SVC,* superior vena cava; *RA* right atrium; *TV,* tricuspid valve.

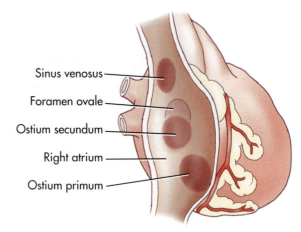

FIGURE 34-7 Atrial septal defects: ostium secundum, ostium primum, and sinus venosus defects viewed from the right atrium.

common atrial septal defects are shown in Figure 34-7. There are three common forms of atrial septal defects: ostium secundum, ostium primum, and sinus venosus. The ostium secundum defect is the defect in the central atrial septum near the foramen ovale and is the most difficult to see in utero, as the flap of the foramen ovale is mobile at this period of development. The ostium primum defect is usually associated with the chromosomal abnormality of trisomy 21 and often will have a cleft mitral valve and abnormalities of the atrioventricular septum. The least common septal defect is the sinus venosus defect that is seen near the entrance of the superior vena cava into the right atrium. This may be associated with a **partial anomalous pulmonary venous return.**

The atrial septal defect is not always recognized during fetal life unless part of the intraatrial septum is missing. The foramen ovale remains open in the fetal heart until after birth, and the pressures change between the right and left heart to force the foramen to close completely. Failure of the foramen to close may result in atrial septal defect, secundum type. An atrial septal defect provides communication between the right and left atrium. The defect must be quite large in the fetus to be identified by ultrasound.

The area of the foramen ovale is thinner in the fetus than the surrounding atrial tissue; therefore, with echocardiography, the area is prone to signal dropout, particularly in the apical four-chamber view when the transducer is parallel to the septum. Any break in the atrial septum in this view must be confirmed by the short-axis or "subcostal" view (the transducer is inferior to the heart and angled cephalad in a transverse or short-axis plane), in which the septum is more perpendicular to the transducer. Because of beam-width artifacts, the edges of the defect may be slightly blunted and appear brighter than the remaining septum.

In utero the natural flow in the atrium is right to left across the foramen (as the pressures are slightly higher on the right). A small reversal flow may be present. The foramen should flap into the left atrial cavity. The flap should not be so large as to touch the lateral wall of the atrium; when this redundancy of the foramen occurs, the sinoatrial node may become agitated in the right atrium and cause fetal arrhythmias. The sonographer should be sure to sweep inferior to superior along the atrial septum to identify the three parts of the septum: the primum septum, fossa ovalis, and septum secundum.

Ostium Secundum Atrial Septal Defect. The most common atrial defect is the secundum atrial septal defect, which occurs in the area of the fossa ovalis (Figure 34-8). Usually an absence of the foramen ovale flap is noted, with the fossa ovalis opening larger than normal.

▶ Sonographic Findings. Doppler tracings of the septal defect with the sample volume placed at the site of the defect show a right-to-left flow with a velocity of 20 to 30 cm/sec. Color flow Doppler is performed in the apical four-chamber and subcostal views and may be useful to outline the size and direction of flow as it crosses the foramen ovale (Figure 34-9). The flow patterns of the mitral and tricuspid valves are slightly increased with the elevated shunt flow.

Ostium Primum Septal Defect. The primum septal defect is deficient in the lower (inferior) portion of the septum, near the crux of the heart (Figure 34-10). It may be seen in atrioventricular septal defect malformation in which there is malalignment of the atrioventricular valves secondary to the defect. In addition, a cleft of the mitral valve is present, causing mitral regurgitation into the left atrial cavity.

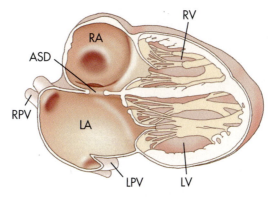

FIGURE 34-8 Four-chamber view of the heart illustrating the absence of the flap of the foramen ovale. *RV,* Right ventricle; *RA,* right atrium; *ASD,* atrial septal defect; *RPV,* right pulmonary vein; *LA,* left atrium; *LPV,* left pulmonary vein; *LV,* left ventricle.

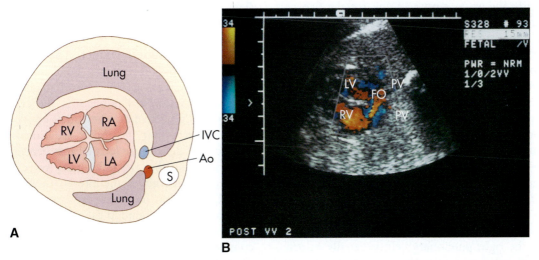

FIGURE 34-9 A, The most common type of atrial septal defects occur in the area of the fossa ovalis, known as the secundum defect. *Ao,* Aorta; *IVC,* inferior vena cava; *LA,* left atrium; *LV,* left ventricle; *RA,* right atrium; *RV,* right ventricle. **B,** In the fetus, normal flow should occur at the level of the foramen ovale *(FO). PV,* Pulmonary vein.

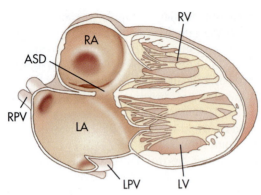

FIGURE 34-10 The ostium primum atrial septal defect in the four-chamber view. *RV,* Right ventricle; *RA,* right atrium; *PRV,* right pulmonary vein; *LA,* left atrium; *LPV,* left pulmonary vein; *LV,* left ventricle; *ASD,* atrial septal defect.

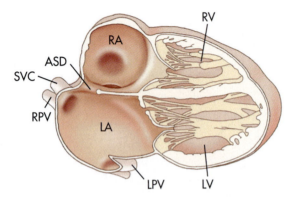

FIGURE 34-11 The sinus venosus atrial septal defect near the entrance of the superior vena cava and right upper pulmonary vein *(RPV). RV,* Right ventricle; *RA,* right atrium; *RPV,* right pulmonary vein; *LA,* left atrium; *LPV,* left pulmonary vein; *LV,* left ventricle; *SVC,* superior vena cava; *ASD,* atrial septal defect.

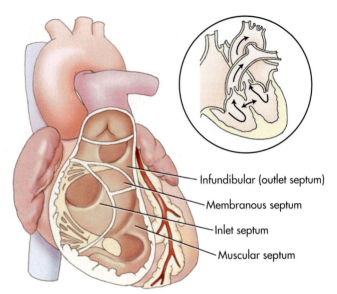

FIGURE 34-12 Ventricular septal defect. Portions of the ventricular septum showing the infundibular (outlet septum), membranous septum, inlet septum, and muscular septa.

◼ **Sonographic Findings.** The primum septal defect is best imaged in the four-chamber plane that is parallel to the transducer beam. The gain should be reduced to clearly identify the atrial septum. Look for the flap of the foramen ovale. This defect may be part of an atrioventricular septal defect or it may be a primary defect with or without a cleft mitral valve.

Sinus Venosus Septal Defect. The sinus venosus atrial septal defect is technically more difficult to visualize with echocardiography. This defect lies in the superior portion of the atrial septum, close to the inflow pattern of the superior vena cava (Figure 34-11).

◼ **Sonographic Findings.** Sinus venosus septal defects are best visualized with the subxiphoid four-chamber view. If signs of right ventricular volume overload are present, with no atrial septal defect obvious, care should be taken to study the septum in search of a sinus venosus type of defect. Partial anomalous pulmonary venous drainage of the right pulmonary vein is usually associated with this type of defect; thus, it is important to identify the entry site of the pulmonary veins into the left atrial cavity. Color flow mapping is useful in this type

of problem because it allows the sonographer to actually visualize the venous return to the left atrium and a flow pattern crossing into the right atrial cavity.

Ventricular Septal Defect

Ventricular septal defect is the most common congenital lesion of the heart, accounting for 30% of all structural heart defects. The septum is divided into two basic segments: the membranous and muscular areas (Figure 34-12). The septum lies in a curvilinear plane and has different areas of thickness. There are a number of sites where ventricular septal defects may occur within the septum. Muscular defects occur more inferior in the septum, usually are very small, and may be multiple (Figure 34-13). Often, smaller defects will close spontaneously shortly after birth. This type of muscular defect is more difficult to image with echocardiography.

Membranous Septal Defect. The (perimembranous) ventricular septal defect may be classified as membranous, aneurysmal, or supracristal (Figure 34-14). The significant anatomic landmark is the crista supraventricularis ridge. The defect lies either above or below this ridge. Defects that lie above are called *supracristal.* Supracristal defects are located just beneath the pulmonary orifice so that the pulmonary valve forms part of the superior margin of the interventricular communication. Defects that lie below the crista are called *infracristal* and may be found in the membranous or muscular part of the septum. Infracristal defects are the most common.

◼ **Sonographic Findings.** The lesion may be partially covered by the tricuspid septal leaflet, and care must be taken to carefully evaluate this area with Doppler and

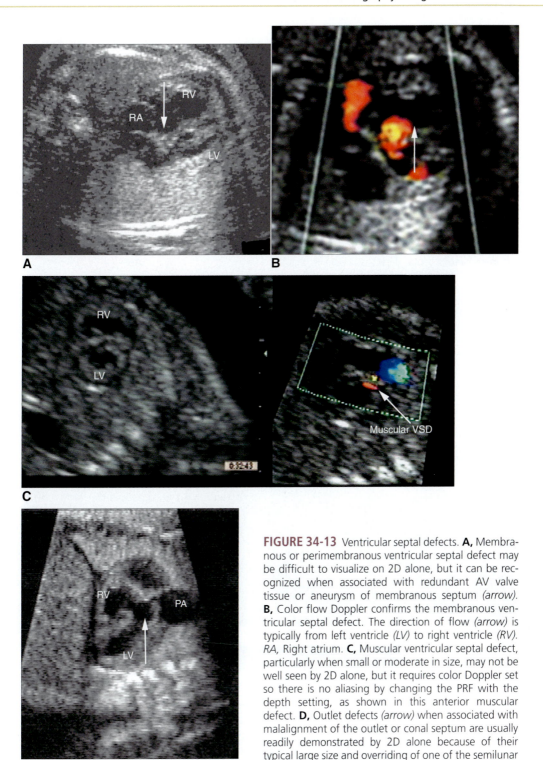

FIGURE 34-13 Ventricular septal defects. **A,** Membranous or perimembranous ventricular septal defect may be difficult to visualize on 2D alone, but it can be recognized when associated with redundant AV valve tissue or aneurysm of membranous septum *(arrow)*. **B,** Color flow Doppler confirms the membranous ventricular septal defect. The direction of flow *(arrow)* is typically from left ventricle *(LV)* to right ventricle *(RV)*. *RA,* Right atrium. **C,** Muscular ventricular septal defect, particularly when small or moderate in size, may not be well seen by 2D alone, but it requires color Doppler set so there is no aliasing by changing the PRF with the depth setting, as shown in this anterior muscular defect. **D,** Outlet defects *(arrow)* when associated with malalignment of the outlet or conal septum are usually readily demonstrated by 2D alone because of their typical large size and overriding of one of the semilunar valves. *PA,* Pulmonary artery.

color flow tracings. The membranous defect is found just below the aortic leaflets; sometimes the aortic leaflet is sucked into this defect (Figure 34-15).

The presence of an isolated ventricular septal defect in utero usually does not change the hemodynamics of the fetus. Defects smaller than 2 mm are not detected by fetal echocardiography. Care must be taken in the four-chamber view to carefully sweep the transducer posterior (to record the inlet part of the septum) to anterior (to record the outlet part of the septum).

Ventricular septal defects may close with the formation of aneurysm tissue, which is commonly found along the right side of the septal defect (Figure 34-16). These aneurysms generally protrude into the right heart in one of the following three directions: (1) above the tricuspid valve and into the right atrium, (2) directly into the

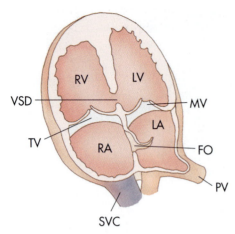

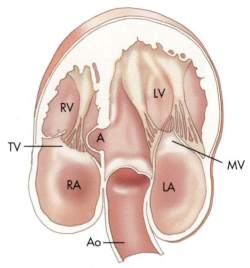

FIGURE 34-14 The membranous septal defect is shown in this four-chamber view. This is located in the inflow of the ventricles. The muscular defect in this four-chamber view may be large, small, or multiple along the thicker part of the septum. *FO*, Foramen ovale; *LA*, left atrium; *LV*, left ventricle; *MV*, mitral valve; *PV*, pulmonary vein; *RA*, right atrium; *RV*, right ventricle; *SVC*, superior vena cava; *TV*, tricuspid valve; *VSD*, ventricular septal defect.

FIGURE 34-16 Five-chamber view of the heart illustrating the presence of a ventricular septal aneurysm inferior to the aortic cusps near the septal leaflet of the tricuspid valve. *RV*, Right ventricle; *LV*, left ventricle; *MV*, mitral valve; *LA*, left atrium; *RA*, right atrium; *A*, atrium; *TV*, tricuspid valve; *Ao*, aorta.

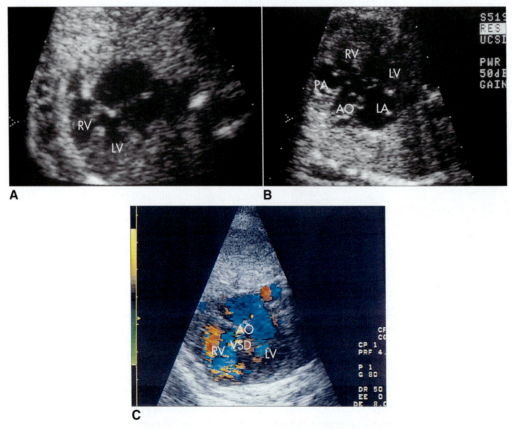

FIGURE 34-15 Ventricular septal defects. **A,** Large isolated membranous septal defect shown in this four-chamber view. The edges of the defect are slightly brighter than the rest of the septum. *LV*, Left ventricle; *RV*, right ventricle. **B,** A patient with trisomy 18 shows a large septal defect involving the membranous and muscular areas. *AO*, Aorta; *PA*, pulmonary artery; *LA*, left atrium. **C,** Color Doppler is helpful when the ventricular septal defect *(VSD)* is large enough to allow crossover of flow from the higher-pressure right side of the heart into the left side of the heart.

septal leaflet of the tricuspid valve, or (3) below the tricuspid leaflets and into the right ventricular cavity. Usually these aneurysms are small, but when they become large, obstruction may occur in the right ventricular outflow tract.

Muscular Defect. A less common infracristal defect is located in the muscular septum. These defects may be large or small, or they may be multiple fenestrated holes (see Figure 34-15, *B* and *C*). The multiple defects are more difficult to repair, and their combination may have the same ventricular overload effect as a single large communication. Small muscular defects are usually found in the neonatal stage and often close spontaneously.

The prognosis is good for a patient with a single ventricular septal defect. However, the association with other cardiac anomalies, such as tetralogy of Fallot, single ventricle, transposition of the great arteries, and endocardial cushion defect, is increased when a ventricular septal defect is found.

One study reported that 40% of ventricular septal defects are closed within 2 years of life and that 60% close by 5 years. The incidence of closure for membranous defects is 25% by 5 years and 65% for muscular defects by 5 years.[2]

Sonographic Findings. The best echocardiographic views to image the septal defect in the outflow tract are the long-axis, short-axis, and five-chamber views. The septal defect in the inflow tract is best seen on the four-chamber view.

Evaluation of shunt flow and direction is made with color flow mapping. Remember that pressures between the right and left heart are almost the same in utero, so a small defect will probably not show a velocity change. If the defect is large, the sample volume should be placed alongside the defect in the left ventricle to see the jet flow.

Atrioventricular Septal Defect

The endocardial cushion defect is also called *ostium primum atrial septal defect, atrioventricular canal malformation, endocardial cushion defect*, and **atrioventricular septal defect** (**AVSD**) (Figure 34-17). These defects are subdivided into complete, incomplete, and partial forms.

Incomplete Atrioventricular Septal Defect. The failure of the endocardial cushion to fuse is termed an incomplete atrioventricular septal defect. This condition results in a membranous ventricular septal defect, abnormal tricuspid valve, primum atrial septal defect, and cleft

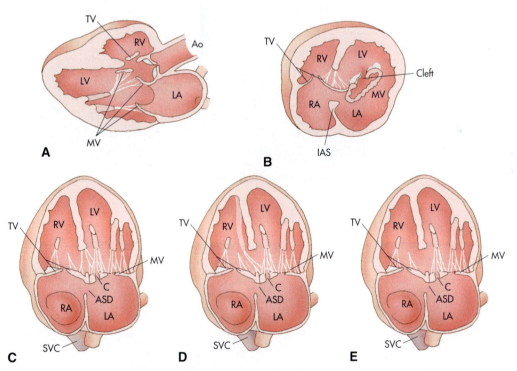

FIGURE 34-17 Atrioventricular septal defect. **A,** Long-axis view shows the discontinuity of the anterior leaflet of the mitral valve with the posterior wall of the aorta. The membranous septal defect is seen. *Ao,* Aorta; *LA,* left atrium; *LV,* left ventricle; *MV,* mitral valve; *RV,* right ventricle; *TV,* tricuspid valve. **B,** Short-axis through the atrioventricular valves shows the cleft in the anterior leaflet of the mitral valve *(MV)*. The primum septal defect is seen. *IAS,* Interarterial septum. **C,** Four-chamber view showing the Rastelli type A large defect in the center (crux) of the heart. The membranous and primum septal defects are seen with the cleft mitral valve. There is a common leaflet from the anterior mitral leaflet to the septal tricuspid leaflet. *ASD,* Atrial septal defect; *SVC,* superior vena cava. **D,** Rastelli type B defect shows the chordal attachments from the medial portion of the cleft mitral leaflet related to the papillary muscle on the right side of the septal defect. **E,** Rastelli type C defect shows a free-floating common atrioventricular leaflet *(C)*.

mitral valve (Figure 34-18). A cleft mitral valve means that the anterior part of the leaflet is divided into two parts (medial and lateral). When the leaflet closes, blood leaks through this hole into the left atrial cavity. The leaflet is usually somewhat malformed, further causing regurgitation into the atrium. In addition, there is a communication between the left ventricle and right atrium (left ventricular to right atrial shunt) because of the absent primum atrial septum and membranous interventricular septum. The ventricular septal defect occurs just below the mitral ring and is continuous with the primum atrial septal defect.

Complete Atrioventricular Septal Defect.

The endocardial defect is characterized by the insertion of the chordae from the cleft mitral and tricuspid valve into the crest of the ventricular septum or a right ventricular papillary muscle (Figure 34-19). The most primitive form is called a complete atrioventricular septal defect. This defect has a single, undivided, free-floating leaflet stretching across both ventricles. A 2D sweep from the mitral to the aortic valves would show the anterior mitral leaflet swinging through the ventricular septal defect in continuity with the tricuspid valve. The

tricuspid valve is said to *cap* the mitral valve. The anterior and posterior leaflets are on both sides of the interventricular septum, causing the valve to override or straddle the septum. This is a more complex abnormality to repair because the defect is larger and the single atrioventricular valve is more difficult to manage clinically, depending on the amount of regurgitation present. The regurgitant jet may extend from the right ventricle to left atrium secondary to the valve deformity and increased right heart pressures. Complete AVSDs are frequently associated with malpositions of the heart (mesocardia and dextrocardia) and atrioventricular block (abnormal rhythm secondary to distortion of the conduction tissues).

AVSDs are frequently associated with other cardiac defects, including truncoconal abnormalities, coarctation of the aorta, and pulmonary stenosis or atresia. There is an increased incidence of Down syndrome (50% of trisomy 21 babies have congenital heart disease) and asplenia and polysplenia syndromes.

Occasionally, complete absence of the interatrial septum is noted in the fetal four-chamber view. With color flow, the entire atria are completely filled throughout systole and diastole. This is termed *common atria*.

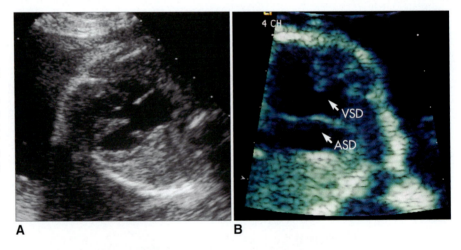

FIGURE 34-18 Atrioventricular septal defect. **A,** A patient with trisomy 21 had 2 : 1 heart block secondary to the complete atrioventricular septal defect, which included the membranous and atrial septa. **B,** A patient with trisomy 21 had a huge atrioventricular defect. The membranous and part of the muscular septum is not present (VSD); the primum septum is also absent (ASD).

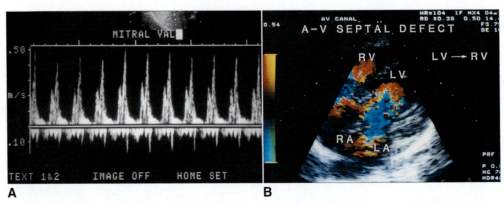

FIGURE 34-19 Atrioventricular septal defect. **A,** Prominent inflow velocities are seen across the mitral valve. There is a small regurgitant flow into the left atrium seen as flow reversal at the end of diastole below the baseline. **B,** Color flow imaging is helpful to map the flow across the defect and to track regurgitation into the atria. *LA,* Left atrium; *LV,* left ventricle; *RA,* right atrium; *RV,* right ventricle.

With a partial AVSD, the fetus has only some of the previously described findings, usually an absent primum atrial septum and a cleft mitral valve.

▶ **Sonographic Findings.** Echocardiographically the ideal views are the long-axis, short-axis (to search for abnormalities in the atrioventricular valves, such as presence of cleft), and four-chamber views (to search for chordal attachment, overriding, or straddling of the valves). The atrioventricular valves share a superior and inferior bridging leaflet that results in a functional single large valve. This may be well demonstrated in the short-axis view of the ventricle as the single large valve appears as a wide circle "8" sign. The crux of the heart is carefully analyzed by slowly sweeping the transducer anterior (toward the aorta outlet) to posterior (toward the atrioventricular valve inlet) to record the outlet and inlet portions of the membranous septum.

Doppler and color flow techniques are extremely useful in determining the direction and degree of regurgitation present in the atrioventricular valves and the direction of shunt flow (increased right heart pressure causes a right ventricular to left atrial shunt in the fetus) (Figure 34-19).

RIGHT VENTRICULAR INFLOW DISTURBANCE

Abnormalities that affect primarily the right side of the heart are listed as inflow or outflow tract disturbances. Each lesion is presented, along with technical advice on how to obtain the ideal fetal cardiac image.

Tricuspid Atresia/Stenosis

Tricuspid atresia is the interruption of the growth of the tricuspid leaflet that begins early in cardiac embryology. This interruption involves the growth of the tricuspid apparatus, causing the valve to be hypoplastic or atretic.

In tricuspid atresia, the inflow portion of the right ventricle has failed to form, and a membrane or dimple in the floor of the right atrium represents the position where the tricuspid valve should have originated (Figure 34-20). A ventricular septal defect may be present to help shunt blood into the hypertrophied right ventricle. The right ventricular outflow tract and pulmonary artery are generally diminished in size.

▶ **Sonographic Findings.** Echocardiographically the tricuspid valve is best visualized on the four-chamber view (Figure 34-21). The findings in tricuspid atresia are a large dilated left ventricular cavity with a small, underdeveloped right ventricular cavity. The echogenic tricuspid annulus is seen with no valvular movement. The mitral valve is clearly the dominant atrioventricular valve. On the long- and short-axis views, the right ventricle is seen as a slitlike cavity just anterior to the interventricular septum.

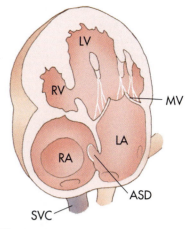

FIGURE 34-20 The hypoplastic right ventricle and immobile echogenic tricuspid valve apparatus are key factors in the four-chamber view in the patient with tricuspid atresia. The right atrium *(RA)* is enlarged. *ASD,* Atrial septal defect; *LA,* left atrium; *LV,* left ventricle; *MV,* mitral valve; *RV,* right ventricle; *SVC,* superior vena cava.

Color flow imaging shows the incoming blood entering the right atrium and crossing the patent foramen ovale to enter the left heart. If no blood flow passes the tricuspid orifice, then pulmonary stenosis is present. However, if a ventricular septal defect is present, the blood flows from the high-pressure left ventricle across the defect into the hypertrophied right ventricle and out the pulmonary outflow tract.

Ebstein's Anomaly of the Tricuspid Valve

Ebstein's anomaly of the tricuspid valve is an abnormal displacement of the septal leaflet of the tricuspid valve toward the apex of the right ventricle (Figure 34-22, *A*). Tricuspid valvular tissue may adhere directly to the ventricular endocardium or may be closely attached to the ventricular wall by multiple, anomalous, short chordae tendineae. The portion of the right ventricle underlying the adherent tricuspid valvular tissue is quite thin and functions as a receiving chamber analogous to the right atrium. This is referred to as the *atrialized chamber* because it registers a right atrial pressure pulse.

The anterior leaflet of the tricuspid valve is the least affected of the three leaflets. The septal and posterior leaflets show the greatest deformity, and the posterior cusp may be rudimentary or entirely absent. The right atrium is usually massively dilated. Often these patients have an incompetent or fenestrated foramen ovale or a secundum atrial septal defect.

The abnormal function of the right heart is related to the following three factors: (1) the malformed tricuspid valve, (2) the "atrialized" portion of the right ventricle, and (3) the reduced capacity of the pumping portion of the right ventricle.

▶ **Sonographic Findings.** Echocardiographically, there is apical displacement of the septal leaflet of the tricuspid

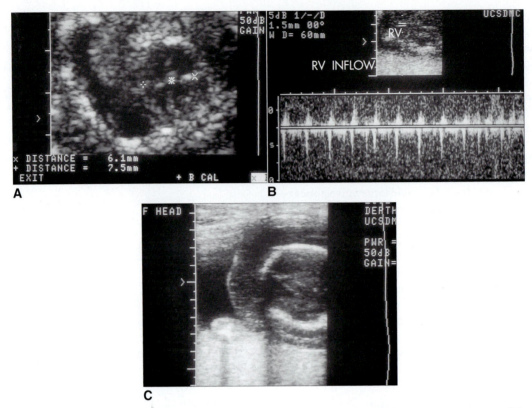

FIGURE 34-21 Tricuspid atresia. **A,** This patient presented in her 22nd week with the fetus demonstrating asymmetry of the ventricles. The annulus of the tricuspid valve was echogenic and immobile. The right ventricle was smaller than the left ventricle. The right atrium was enlarged. **B,** Pulsed Doppler imaging shows decreased inflow through the immobile tricuspid valve. There is mild to moderate tricuspid regurgitation seen at the end of diastole as flow reversal below the baseline. **C,** The patient developed severe hydrops with edema surrounding the scalp and abdomen, pleural effusion, and ascites.

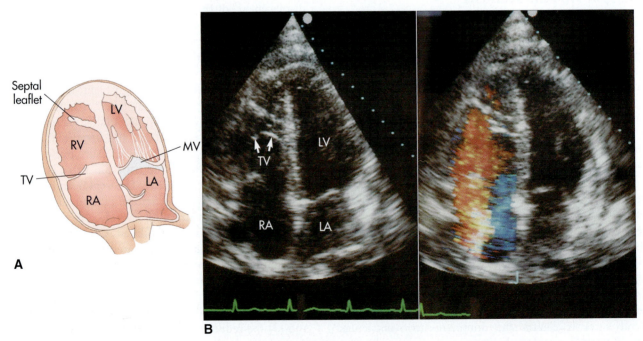

FIGURE 34-22 A, Four-chamber view of Ebstein's anomaly shows the septal leaflet of the tricuspid valve *(TV)* inferiorly displaced from its normal insertion point. The right atrium *(RA)* is markedly enlarged. *LA,* Left atrium; *LV,* left ventricle; *MV,* mitral valve; *RV,* right ventricle. **B,** Inferior displacement of the tricuspid valve into the apex of the right ventricle. This valve is usually dysplastic and regurgitation is present.

valve with resultant insufficiency (as seen on the apical four-chamber view) (Figure 34-22, *B*). The atrialized right ventricle is well seen. Generally, right ventricular dysfunction is present, which results in an overload pattern of wall motion with paradoxical or anterior septal motion in systole. This right ventricular overload also shows flattening of the septum when viewed in the short-axis plane.

Doppler tracings are useful to record the amount of insufficiency present from the abnormal tricuspid valve. The sample volume should be placed at the annulus of the tricuspid valve and then mapped through the atrialized right ventricle into the right atrial cavity to record the maximum jet of insufficiency. One should note how far the regurgitant jet extends and the width of the jet to determine the degree of insufficiency.

RIGHT VENTRICULAR OUTFLOW DISTURBANCE

The normal pulmonic valve comprises three semilunar cusps that open in systole and close completely in diastole just like the aortic cusps. These cusps are best imaged in the high short-axis plane or right long-axis plane of the right ventricular outflow tract.

Hypoplastic Right Heart

There are several forms of **hypoplastic right heart syndrome**: pulmonary atresia with an intact interventricular septum, pulmonary valve fusion with an intact interventricular septum and atrial septal defect, and pulmonary atresia with a normal aortic root diameter.

The right heart is underdeveloped because of obstruction of the right ventricular outflow tract secondary to pulmonary stenosis. The tricuspid valve is small and the pulmonary infundibulum is atretic (see Figure 34-20).

Sonographic Findings. The sonographer must be careful not to call a hypoplastic right heart a hypoplastic left heart (which may be a lethal situation) (Figure 34-23). Careful assessment of the situs of the fetus, great vessel relationships, and trabeculation pattern helps the sonographer determine right from left heart (the right heart is more trabeculated than the left). Care must also be taken to avoid mistaking the papillary muscle for the septum when a large membranous defect is present. In a fetus with a single ventricle (and essentially a hypoplastic right heart), it may be easy to confuse a large papillary muscle with the septum. In this case, it would be difficult to figure out the great vessel origin. A single ventricle usually has an associated transposition of the great arteries with a small pulmonary artery and large aorta.

Tetralogy of Fallot

Tetralogy of Fallot is the most common form of cyanotic heart disease in infants and children. The severity of the disease varies according to the degree of pulmonary stenosis present—the more stenosis, the greater the cyanosis. It is possible to have a mild form of pulmonary stenosis and not have any cyanosis after birth.

In tetralogy of Fallot, the outlet or conal septum is anteriorly and leftward deviated, resulting in impingement of flow through the pulmonary outflow tract. There is a large subaortic ventricular septal defect caused by the large aorta overriding the interventricular septum. This override of the aorta is best seen with a gradual sweep of the outflow tracts. If the pulmonary artery is stenotic, it may be hypoplastic and difficult to recognize as one sweeps from the large aorta to the area of the pulmonary artery. The enlarged aorta is usually more anterior than in the normal heart. The hypoplasia of the pulmonary artery may extend into the branch pulmonary arteries with progressive pulmonary outflow tract obstruction. Color Doppler is often useful to demonstrate patency of flow in the outflow tracts, particularly if there is patency in the pulmonary outflow tract and the direction of flow through the main pulmonary artery. Patency of the ductus arteriosus is critical in planning the postnatal management. If reversed flow is present in the ductus, severe pulmonary outflow obstruction may be present.

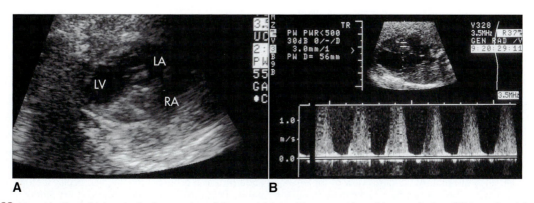

A   **B**

FIGURE 34-23 Hypoplastic right heart. **A,** Asymmetry of the ventricles with severe tricuspid regurgitation **(B)** into the right atrium *(RA)*. *LA,* Left atrium; *LV,* left ventricle.

Tetralogy of Fallot has the following four characteristics (Figure 34-24):

1. High, membranous ventricular septal defect
2. Large, anteriorly displaced aorta, which overrides the septal defect
3. Pulmonary stenosis
4. Right ventricular hypertrophy (not seen in fetal life; occurs after birth when pulmonary stenosis causes increased pressure in the right ventricle)

A large septal defect with mild to moderate pulmonary stenosis is classified as acyanotic disease, whereas a large septal defect with severe pulmonary stenosis is considered cyanotic disease ("blue baby" at birth).

In addition to the association of trisomy abnormalities (13, 18, and 21), other congenital cardiac malformations may occur in patients with pulmonic stenosis and ventricular septal defect, including the following:

- Right aortic arch
- Persistent left superior vena cava
- Anomalies of the pulmonary artery and its branches
- Absence of the pulmonary valve
- Incompetence of the aortic valve
- Variations in coronary arterial anatomy

The prognosis for a fetus with tetralogy of Fallot is good with surgical intervention. One of the first surgical approaches was developed to obviate the underperfusion of the lungs. The Blalock-Taussig shunt was performed to anastomose the subclavian artery to the pulmonary artery.

The prognosis for tetralogy of Fallot with pulmonary atresia or an absent pulmonary valve is not as good. In the fetus shown in Figure 34-25, *A*, a single large great vessel is identified (aorta) without a significant second great vessel. The aortic override is readily apparent on the long axis view. The hypoplastic branch pulmonary arteries may be contiguous or discontinuous. When they are contiguous, they can be demonstrated as the "seagull sign." The lungs and pulmonary arteries receive their blood supply through a tortuous and small ductus arteriosus or collateral vessels that arise from the descending aorta or other systemic arteries. The absent pulmonary valve may cause congestive heart failure in the fetus. Aneurysmal dilation of the pulmonary artery and its branches may be a cause of pulmonary distress.

Sonographic Findings. Echocardiographically the demonstration of tetralogy of Fallot is distinguished on the parasternal long-axis view (see Figure 34-25). The large aorta overrides the ventricular septum. If the override is greater than 50%, the condition is called a *double-outlet right ventricle*, meaning that both great vessels arise from the right side of the heart. A septal defect is present; the size may vary from small to large. The parasternal short-axis view shows the small, hypertrophied right ventricle (if significant pulmonary stenosis is present). The pulmonary artery is usually small, and the cusps may be thickened and domed or difficult to image well.

A sample volume should be made in the high parasternal short-axis view to determine the turbulence of the right ventricular outflow tract and pulmonary valve stenosis (see Figure 34-25, *C*). Color flow is helpful in this condition to actually delineate the abnormal high-velocity pattern and to direct the sample volume into the proper jet flow. If the ventricular septal defect is large, increased flow is seen in the right side of the heart (increased tricuspid velocity, right ventricular outflow tract velocity, and increased pulmonic velocity). The best view for imaging the subvalvular portion of the right ventricular outflow tract is obtained with the subcostal short-axis plane. This view allows extensive visualization of the subpulmonary area so often affected in tetralogy of Fallot. In the fetus the pulmonic obstructive flow patterns are not as pronounced as in the neonatal period.

Pulmonic Stenosis

The most common form of the right ventricular outflow tract obstruction is pulmonary valve stenosis. In pulmonic stenosis, the abnormal pulmonic cusps become

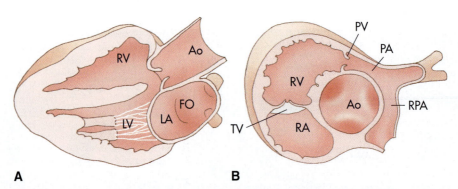

A   **B**

FIGURE 34-24 Tetralogy of Fallot. **A,** Long-axis view of the enlarged aorta *(Ao)* as it overrides the interventricular septum. The amount of aortic enlargement depends on the degree of pulmonary stenosis or atresia present. *FO,* Foramen ovale; *LA,* left atrium; *LV,* left ventricle; *RV,* right ventricle. **B,** Short-axis view of the small pulmonary artery *(PA)* displaced anteriorly by the enlarged aorta *(Ao)*. *PV,* Pulmonary valve; *RA,* right atrium; *RPA,* right pulmonary artery; *TV,* tricuspid valve.

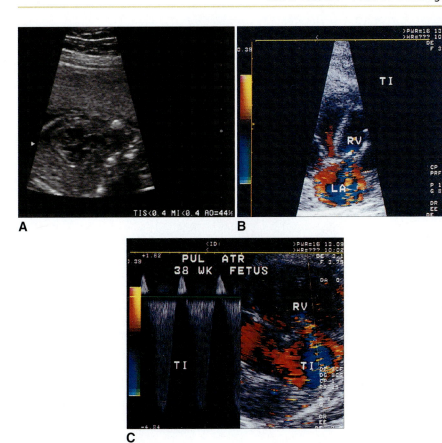

A   **B**   **C**

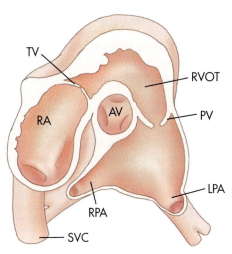

FIGURE 34-25 Tetralogy of Fallot. **A,** Long axis of the heart shows the aorta as it overrides the septum. **B,** Pulmonary stenosis may cause severe tricuspid regurgitation into the right atrium as the blood flow is obstructed in the right ventricular outflow tract. *LA,* Left atrium. **C,** Pulmonary atresia with tricuspid insufficiency *(TI)* is the most severe form of stenosis. *RV,* Right ventricle.

thickened and domed during diastole (Figure 34-26). The main pulmonary artery may be hypoplastic or there may be poststenotic dilation of the pulmonary artery. Other forms of pulmonary stenosis may show subvalvular thickening just inferior to the cusp opening.

▧ **Sonographic Findings.** The domed effect is not quite as noticeable on the fetal echocardiogram, but with careful evaluation the thickness of the cusp may be compared with that of the aortic cusp. An M-mode image may be made through the area to further define cusp mobility and thickness. As with the aortic cusps, multiple degrees of stenosis and atresia may develop in the right ventricular outflow tract. The more atretic the cusp, the more hypoplastic the pulmonary artery becomes. Critical pulmonary atresia may be difficult to image in the early second-trimester fetus because the pulmonary outflow becomes so hypoplastic that it is difficult to recognize.

When pulmonary stenosis is associated with another cardiac anomaly, such as transposition, double-outlet right ventricle, or tetralogy of Fallot, it becomes even more difficult to diagnose. Secondary findings of dilation of the right ventricular cavity and right atrial cavity (secondary to tricuspid insufficiency) usually lead the investigator to the principal cause of the overload of the right side of the heart (pulmonic stenosis).

Color flow Doppler evaluation of the velocity is useful not only to assess the degree of obstruction but also to monitor the fetus in terms of following the course of disease (see Figure 34-25, *B*).

FIGURE 34-26 Pulmonary stenosis. The parasternal short-axis view of the domed pulmonary leaflets and some right ventricular hypertrophy are shown. *TV,* Tricuspid valve; *AV,* aortic valve; *RVOT,* right ventricular outflow tract; *PV,* pulmonary valve; *LPA,* left pulmonary artery; *RPA,* right pulmonary artery; *SVC,* superior vena cava; *RA,* right atrium.

Subpulmonic Stenosis

Subpulmonic stenosis occurs when a membrane or muscle bundle obstructs the outflow tract into the pulmonary artery (Figure 34-27).

▧ **Sonographic Findings.** If the right ventricular outflow tract can be imaged adequately, the actual obstruction

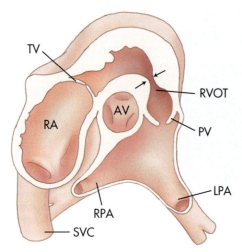

FIGURE 34-27 Subvalvular pulmonary stenosis. The parasternal short-axis view shows the right ventricular hypertrophy *(arrows)* with thickening of the bands of the crista supraventricularis. *TV,* Tricuspid valve; *AV,* aortic valve; *RVOT,* right ventricular outflow tract; *PV,* pulmonary valve; *LPA,* left pulmonary artery; *RPA,* right pulmonary artery; *SVC,* superior vena cava; *RA,* right atrium.

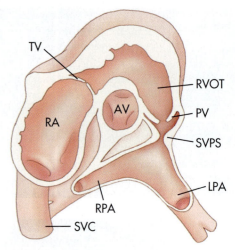

FIGURE 34-28 Supravalvular pulmonary stenosis. Domed pulmonary leaflets and a small pulmonary valve annulus as compared with the normal-sized aortic root. There is poststenotic dilation in the main pulmonary artery. *TV,* Tricuspid valve; *AV,* aortic valve; *RVOT,* right ventricular outflow tract; *PV,* pulmonary valve; *LPA,* left pulmonary artery; *RPA,* right pulmonary artery; *SVC,* superior vena cava; *RA,* right atrium.

may be imaged. The Doppler and color flow pattern shows a turbulent obstructive pattern just before the pulmonary cusps. The velocity would not be as high as in the neonatal period but would measure at least 1.8 to 2 m/sec.

Supravalvular Pulmonic Stenosis

Supravalvular pulmonic stenosis is an abnormal narrowing in the main pulmonary artery. It usually is associated with Williams' syndrome and is hereditary (Figure 34-28).

Sonographic Findings. The parasternal short-axis view is best to image this condition. Prominent, dilated right and left pulmonary branch arteries may be present. Again, color flow will show a turbulent high-velocity flow pattern across the narrowed vessel.

LEFT VENTRICULAR INFLOW DISTURBANCE

Abnormalities that affect primarily the left side of the heart are listed as inflow or outflow tract disturbances. Each of these lesions is presented along with technical advice on how to obtain the ideal fetal cardiac image.

Congenital Mitral Stenosis

In normal cardiac development, the endocardial cushion forms the anterior and posterior mitral apparatus with chordae tendineae attached to two papillary muscles on the left side of the heart. When this development is interrupted in the first trimester, the mitral valve apparatus may not fully develop, causing mitral atresia or stenosis (Figure 34-29). Mitral valve stenosis and regurgitation

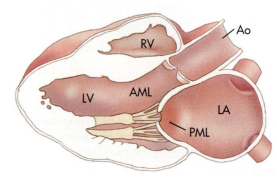

FIGURE 34-29 Mitral stenosis. The parasternal long-axis view shows the thickened chordae and the doming of the mitral valve apparatus. *Ao,* Aorta; *LA,* left atrium; *PML,* posterior mitral leaflet; *AML,* anterior mitral leaflet; *LV,* left ventricle; *RV,* right ventricle.

rarely occur in isolation. They are usually associated with other forms of left heart obstruction.

There are several anatomic varieties of congenital mitral stenosis. In one variety, the leaflets are thickened, nodular, and fibrotic; the commissures are rudimentary or absent; the chordae tendineae are shortened, thickened, and fused; and the papillary muscles are fibrosed. The mitral valve is a funnel-shaped, flat, or diaphragm-like structure.

The second variety consists of a "parachute" deformity of the valve. This occurs when the normal leaflets are drawn into close apposition by shortened chordae tendineae, which converge and insert into a single large papillary muscle.

The third variety of mitral stenosis consists of an anomalous arcade with obstructing papillary muscles that extend between the papillary muscles. The papillary muscles are so large that they encroach on the subvalvular area.

The last form of mitral stenosis occurs when the valve and its supporting structure are anatomically normal but the mitral inlet is encroached upon by a circumferential supravalvular ridge of connective tissue, which arises at the base of the atrial aspect of the mitral leaflets.

Sonographic Findings. The mitral valve should be evaluated from at least two cardiac windows: the long-axis and the four-chamber views. The long-axis view allows the examiner to evaluate the mobility of the anterior and posterior mitral valve leaflets as they open into the left ventricular cavity. The four-chamber view allows comparison of the placement of the mitral valve with the normal, slightly apical displacement of the tricuspid valve. It also allows observation of the pliability of the thin leaflets as they open in diastole and close in systole. The ideal Doppler waveform should be recorded from this apical position.

Mitral Atresia. In a fetus with **mitral atresia** or congenital mitral stenosis, the examiner sees a thickened mitral orifice with restriction of leaflet amplitude. The left ventricular cavity is reduced in volume because of decreased inflow (Figure 34-30). The myocardial thickness is increased (secondary to increased left ventricular pressure overload) if associated aortic atresia is present.

Sonographic Findings. The mitral apparatus may appear thickened and dysplastic with shortened chordae and closely spaced papillary muscles or a single papillary muscle. The left ventricle is small relative to the right. Flow is usually redirected through the foramen; therefore, the flow through the obstructed mitral valve is laminar. Color Doppler can be helpful to determine how much, if any, mitral inflow is present. The apical four-chamber view is again best to obtain this assessment.

Mitral Regurgitation

In fetal life the presence of **mitral regurgitation** is probably from a cleft mitral valve (endocardial cushion defect) or a congenital mitral stenosis. In the presence of mitral regurgitation, the left atrial cavity would become enlarged because of the leakage of blood from the defective mitral valve.

Sonographic Findings. The color Doppler flow pattern of disturbed flow in the left atrial cavity would be seen on the apical four-chamber and probably on the parasternal long-axis view.

LEFT VENTRICULAR OUTFLOW TRACT DISTURBANCE

The normal aortic valve comprises three semilunar cusps that open in systole and close completely in diastole. The cusps are best imaged in the long-axis and short-axis planes. The aortic root is measured in the short-axis plane as the transducer bisects the right ventricular outflow tract, the pulmonary artery, and the aortic root.

Normal Doppler flow is recorded in the aortic outflow tract (either from a five-chamber view or a modified long- or short-axis view).

Bicuspid Aortic Valve

If the development is interrupted during the first trimester, the three aortic cusps may not fully separate. In this instance, the valve may be a *unicuspid* valve with a central opening and aortic stenosis or a *bicuspid* (two-leaflet) valve with asymmetric cusps (Figure 34-31).

Sonographic Findings. In this case, the raphe between the cusp tissue has not separated; thus, the leaflet opens asymmetrically and may show doming on the parasternal long-axis view. In the fetus a bicuspid valve may be difficult to image at 18 weeks, but it should be well visualized in the late second trimester at 27 weeks.

Aortic Stenosis

Critical Aortic Stenosis
Aortic stenosis is an abnormal development of the cusps of the aortic valve that results in thickened and domed leaflets. Critical aortic stenosis signifies end-stage left ventricular dysfunction. At some point in the second or third trimester, an infection or other viral process has

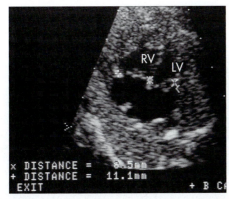

FIGURE 34-30 Mitral atresia. Four-chamber view shows a thickened, immobile mitral leaflet with a small left ventricular cavity. Mitral regurgitation was present. *LV,* Left ventricle; *RV,* right ventricle.

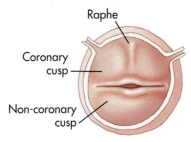

FIGURE 34-31 Bicuspid aortic valve showing the noncoronary cusp, and fused right and left coronary cusps with a raphe.

caused the aortic leaflet to thicken and close prematurely. The fetus shows a normal ascending and descending aorta with abnormal opening of the aortic cusps. The enlarged, dysfunctional left ventricle then "billows" from the increased pressure in the ventricle because the left ventricular outflow tract is blocked (Figures 34-32 and 34-33, *A*). The ventricular walls would be thin and bulge into the right ventricular cavity. The parasternal long-axis and apical four-chamber views are the most helpful to image this disease.

◀ **Sonographic Findings.** Color flow helps to assess the severity of the aortic stenosis to determine how much, if any, blood is flowing through the stenotic aortic leaflets (Figure 34-33, *B*).

Subvalvular or Supravalvular Aortic Stenosis. Subvalvular aortic stenosis occurs when a membrane covers the left ventricular outflow tract (Figure 34-34, *A* and *B*). Supravalvular aortic stenosis is a narrowing of the ascending aortic root.

Supravalvular aortic stenosis may be related to the Williams' syndrome (Figure 34-35). Subaortic stenosis has been described in patients with Turner's syndrome, Noonan's syndrome, and congenital rubella.

◀ **Sonographic Findings.** The left ventricular outflow tract should be carefully evaluated in the parasternal long-axis, apical five-chamber, and aortic arch views to image this thin membrane. The Doppler view shows increased velocity across the obstructive membrane, whereas color flow imaging shows increased turbulence at the area of narrowing.

Hypoplastic Left Heart Syndrome

Hypoplastic left heart syndrome is characterized by a small, hypertrophied left ventricle with aortic or mitral dysplasia or atresia (Figure 34-36). This syndrome has been found to be an autosomal-recessive condition. If a couple has had one child with hypoplastic left heart syndrome, the recurrence is 4%; if two births have been affected, recurrence increases to 25%.

Although the cause of the hypoplastic left heart is unknown, it is thought to be decreased filling and perfusion of the left ventricle during embryologic development. It also may be associated with premature closure of the foramen ovale. When this closure occurs, the blood cannot cross the foramen to help the left ventricle grow. The real-time image shows a reduction in the size of the foramen ovale (the foramen should measure at least 0.6 multiplied by the diameter of the aortic root). Premature closure of the foramen would also show increased velocities across the interatrial septum (around 40 to 50 cm/sec).

The right ventricle supplies both the pulmonic and systemic circulations. The pulmonary venous return is diverted from the left atrium to the right atrium through the interatrial communication. Through the pulmonary artery and ductus arteriosus, the right ventricle supplies the descending aorta, along with retrograde flow to the aortic arch and the ascending aorta. Overload on the right ventricle may lead to congestive heart failure in

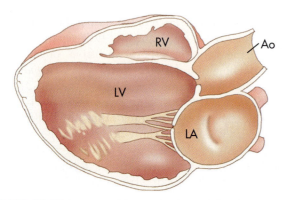

FIGURE 34-32 Parasternal long-axis view of the domed aortic valve, dilated left ventricle, and poststenotic dilation of the ascending aorta. *Ao,* Aorta; *RV,* right ventricle; *LV,* left ventricle; *LA,* left atrium.

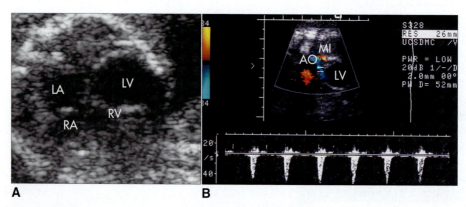

FIGURE 34-33 Critical aortic stenosis. **A,** Critical aortic stenosis appears in the second or third trimester. The four-chamber view shows a dilated left ventricular cavity (assumes the shape of a balloon). The ventricle is tense and quickly becomes noncompliant. *LA,* Left atrium; *LV,* left ventricle; *RA,* right atrium; *RV,* right ventricle. **B,** Color Doppler imaging shows aortic insufficiency *(blue)* and mitral insufficiency *(MI, red)*. *AO,* Aorta; *LV,* left ventricle.

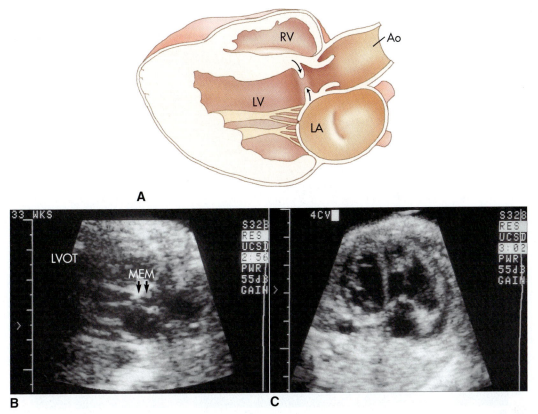

FIGURE 34-34 Submembranous aortic stenosis. **A,** A discrete membrane inferior to the aortic valve is shown in the parasternal long-axis view *(arrows)*. *Ao,* Aorta; *RV,* right ventricle; *LV,* left ventricle; *LA,* left atrium. **B,** Submembranous aortic obstruction. Long-axis view of the ascending aorta and left ventricle shows the thick membrane *(MEM, arrows)* that is located above the aortic cusps to cause obstruction to the left ventricular outflow tract *(LVOT).* **C,** This outflow obstruction causes the left ventricle to enlarge, as seen on this four-chamber view, and go into failure. A small pericardial effusion is seen around the heart.

utero with the development of pericardial effusion and hydrops.

The ascending aorta is often hypoplastic and thread-like, with the distal arch having a slightly larger, and more normal diameter. There is always retrograde flow in the distal aortic arch and left to right atrial flow across the foramen. The evaluation of the right ventricle should be made to ascertain normal function and competency of the tricuspid and pulmonic valve. If these valves are incompetent, cardiovascular compromise may occur. Flow across the atrial septum and pulmonary venous inflow should be assessed. If the foramen ovale flow is restricted, this could result in severe hypoxemia and respiratory distress after birth.

Sonographic Findings. A fetus with major disturbance to the development of the mitral valve or aortic valve shows dramatic changes in the development of the left ventricle. The amount of hypoplasia depends on when the left-sided atresia developed in the valvular area (Figure 34-37). If the mitral atresia is the cause, the blood cannot fill the left ventricle to provide volume, and thus the aortic valve becomes atretic as well, with concentric hypertrophy of the small left ventricular cavity. If the cause is aortic stenosis, the myocardium shows

extreme hypertrophy from the increased pressure overload (Figure 34-38).

M-mode imaging may be used to further define the ventricular disproportion. The sonographer must be aware that even in normal fetuses, the M-mode and real-time measurements of the ventricles depend totally on the position of the fetus, position of the transducer, and angle of the cursor. Therefore, it is important to make sure the transducer is directly perpendicular to the right and left ventricles before making an M-mode measurement. This measurement is always slightly smaller than the real-time direct measurement because the detail of the endocardium is better visualized on the M-mode than on the real-time image.

The prognosis for a fetus with a hypoplastic left heart has improved with cardiac transplantation. Norwood has developed a series of surgical repairs for the hypoplastic left heart patient. His repairs are based on the development of the aorta and aortic arch. Initial palliative procedures are done, including atrial balloon septostomy, banding of the pulmonary artery (to protect the potential volume overload to the lungs), and creation of an aortopulmonary shunt. The modified Fontan surgical procedure is done to connect the left atrium to the

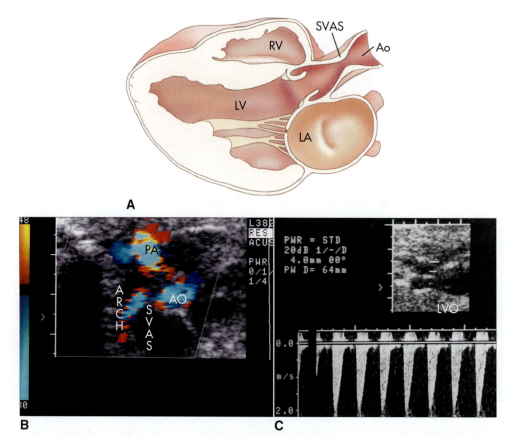

FIGURE 34-35 Supravalvular aortic stenosis. **A,** The parasternal long-axis view shows the hourglass narrowing of the ascending aorta superior to the aortic valve. **B,** Long-axis view of the ascending aorta *(AO)* and arch with the supravalvular narrowing *(SVAS)*. *PA,* Pulmonary artery. **C,** Doppler velocities measure 200 cm/sec, well above the normal range.

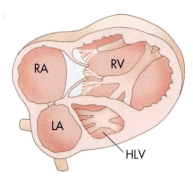

FIGURE 34-36 Hypoplastic left heart syndrome is characterized by a small, hypertrophied left ventricle *(HLV)* with aortic and/or mitral atresia. *LA,* Left atrium; *RA,* right atrium; *RV,* right ventricle.

tricuspid valve and the right atrium to the pulmonary artery. Norwood's challenge is to rebuild the hypoplastic aorta to improve blood flow into the left ventricle.

GREAT VESSEL ABNORMALITIES

Great vessel abnormalities include interruption in the spiraling that occurs during early embryonic development. These anomalies also include complete transposition of the great arteries, corrected transposition of the great arteries, and truncus arteriosus.

Transposition of the Great Arteries

Transposition of the great arteries is an abnormal condition that exists when the aorta is connected to the right ventricle and the pulmonary artery is connected to the left ventricle (Figure 34-39). The atrioventricular valves are normally attached and related. This occurs because of an abnormal completion of the "loop" in embryology. The great vessels originate as a common truncus and undergo rotation and spiraling; if this development is interrupted, the great arteries do not complete their spiral and thus transposition occurs. Usually the aorta is anterior and to the right of the pulmonary artery. Less frequently the two arteries are side by side or the aorta is posterior.

In the fetal heart, no hemodynamic compromise is seen in the fetus when the great arteries are transposed. The problems occur in the neonatal period when there is inadequate mixing of oxygenated and unoxygenated blood.

The prognosis for a neonate with transposition of the great arteries is quite good with surgical intervention.

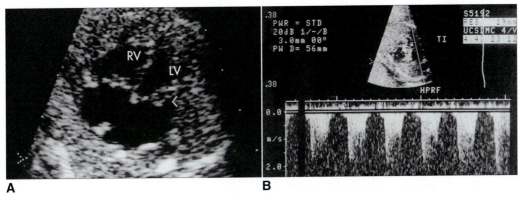

FIGURE 34-37 Hypoplastic left heart. **A,** Four-chamber view shows asymmetry between the right *(RV)* and left *(LV)* ventricles. The aorta and ascending aorta were also hypertrophied. **B,** Backflow of pressures from the left ventricular outflow obstruction results in severe tricuspid regurgitation.

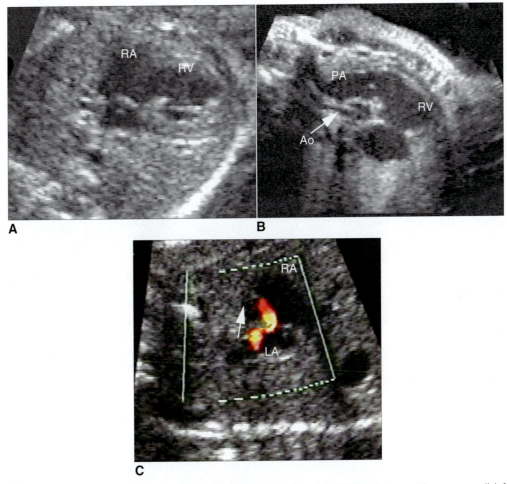

FIGURE 34-38 Hypoplastic left heart syndrome. **A,** Typical four-chamber view seen in this disease with a very small left atrium and left ventricle and prominent right atrium *(RA)* and right ventricle *(RV).* **B,** Sagittal image demonstrates a large pulmonary artery *(PA)* arising from the right ventricle and a diminutive ascending aorta *(Ao).* **C,** There is left *(LA)* to right atrial flow *(arrow),* demonstrated by color Doppler.

The survival rate is 92% at 1 year with surgical correction. Survival depends on other cardiac anomalies that may also be present.

Other associated cardiac anomalies include atrial septal defects, anomalies of the atrioventricular valves, and underdevelopment of the right or left ventricles.

◤ **Sonographic Findings.** The parasternal short-axis view is the key view to image the great arteries and their normal relationship (Figure 34-40). The right ventricular outflow tract, pulmonary artery, and bifurcation should be seen anterior to the aorta in the parasternal short-axis view. In transposition this relationship is not present; it

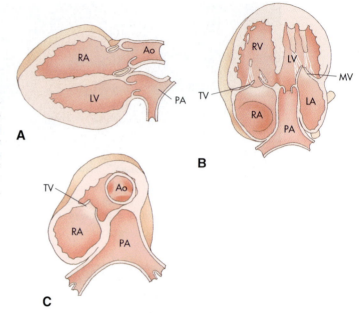

FIGURE 34-39 Transposition of the great arteries. **A,** Four-chamber view shows the aorta *(Ao)* anteriorly, arising from the right ventricle, and the pulmonary artery *(PA)* posteriorly, arising from the left ventricle *(LV)*. *RA,* Right atrium. **B,** Five-chamber view shows the pulmonary artery *(PA)* arising from the left ventricle *(LV)*; as the transducer follows the great artery, the bifurcation of the branch arteries is seen. *LA,* Left atrium; *MV,* mitral valve; *TV,* tricuspid valve. **C,** Short-axis view shows the aorta *(Ao)* anterior to the pulmonary artery *(PA)*.

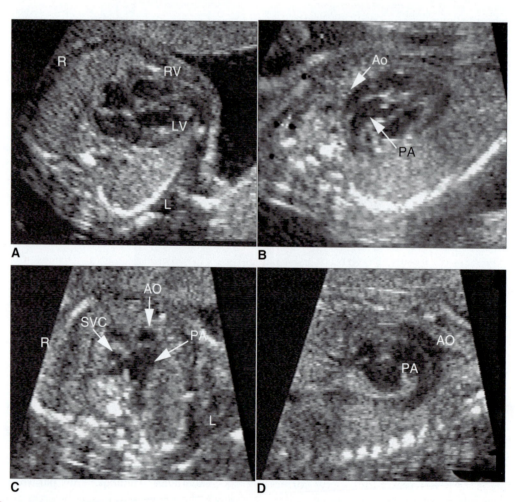

FIGURE 34-40 D-transposition of the great arteries. **A,** Four-chamber view and cardiac axis are usually normal. **B,** Sweeping to the outflow tracts, the great arteries arise in a parallel fashion so they both can be imaged in their long-axis in the same plane. **C,** In the three-vessel view, the aorta *(Ao)* is the most anterior structure and the pulmonary artery *(PA)* is posterior and to the left. **D,** Arches can both be demonstrated in a single plane as a result of the parallel proximal origins of the great arteries. *L,* Left; *LV,* left ventricle; *R,* right; *RV,* right ventricle.

is impossible to demonstrate the bifurcation of the pulmonary artery because the aorta would be the anterior vessel. Sometimes the double circles of the great arteries can be seen in this view.

On the modified long-axis view, the normal crisscross pattern obtained from a normal fetal echocardiogram occurs when the transducer is swept from the left ventricular outflow tract anterior and medial into the right ventricular outflow tract. In a fetus with transposition, this crisscross sweep of the great arteries is not possible. The parallel great arteries are sometimes seen in this view as they both arise from the ventricles.

Corrected Transposition of the Great Arteries.

Corrected transposition of the great arteries is a cardiac condition in which the right atrium and left atrium are connected to the morphologic left and right ventricle, respectively, and the great arteries are transposed. Therefore, these two defects essentially cancel each other out without hemodynamic consequences.

Sonographic Findings. Corrected transposition is associated with malpositions of the heart and sometimes with situs inversus. A ventricular perimembranous septal defect may be present in half of the fetuses. The pulmonary artery may be seen to override the septal defect, with pulmonary stenosis in 50%. Abnormalities of the atrioventricular valves, such as an Ebstein type of malformation and straddling of the tricuspid valve, may be present. Atrioventricular heart block may also be recorded.

Truncus Arteriosus

Truncus arteriosus is a complex congenital heart lesion in which only one great artery arises from the base of the heart (Figure 34-41). From this single great artery arise the pulmonary trunk, the systemic arteries, and the coronary arteries. This defect occurs in the early embryologic period when the conotruncus fails to separate into two great arteries. The conus corresponds to the middle third of the bulbus cordis. It gives rise to the outflow tract of both ventricles and to the muscular portion of the ventricles located between the atrioventricular and semilunar valves. The truncus is the distal part of the bulbus cordis. This structure rotates and divides into the two great semilunar valvular structures that represent the aortic and pulmonic leaflets. Failure of the bulbus to divide causes a single great artery with multiple cusps within.

Associated anomalies include mitral atresia, atrial septal defect, univentricular heart, and aortic arch abnormalities. In the neonatal stage, the prognosis is poor for truncus arteriosus.

Sonographic Findings. The fetal echo shows an abnormal, large, single great vessel arising from the ventricles (Figure 34-42). Usually an infundibular ventricular septal defect is present. Significant septal override is present. The truncal valve is usually dysplastic, thick, and domed. Multiple cusps are seen within the great artery. If truncal regurgitation is present, the prognosis is grim; the fetus usually develops congestive heart failure, pericardial effusion, and hydrops. Truncus arteriosus may be difficult to separate from a severe tetralogy of Fallot with pulmonary atresia (small pulmonary artery and large aorta overriding septal defect).

Coarctation of the Aorta

Coarctation of the aorta is a discrete shelflike lesion present in the isthmus of the arch or, more commonly at the site of the ductal insertion near the left subclavian artery (Figure 34-43, A). The coarctation may be discrete, long segment, or tubular.

Intracardiac associated malformations are present in 90% of cases. These include aortic stenosis, aortic insufficiency, septal defects, transposition of the great arteries, truncus arteriosus, and double-outlet right ventricle. In Turner's syndrome, coarctation of the aorta and ventricular septal defects are the most common cardiac defects found.

Sonographic Findings. If a bicuspid aortic valve is suspected, the aortic arch should be carefully searched for a narrowing or coarctation of the aorta. There is a 25% association of bicuspid aortic valves in fetuses with coarctation of the aorta. It is important to keep in mind

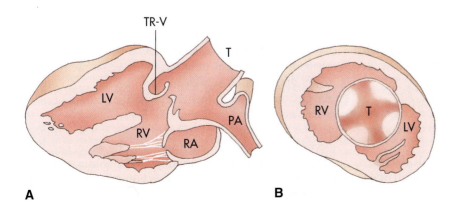

A   **B**

FIGURE 34-41 Truncus arteriosus results when the aorta and pulmonary arteries *(PA)* fail to complete their rotations and divisions early in development. A single large great artery is shown as it arises from the center of the heart on the long-axis view **(A)**. *LV,* Left ventricle; *RA,* right atrium; *RV,* right ventricle; *T,* truncus; *TR-V,* truncal valve. The short-axis view **(B)** shows the single great artery with multiple cusps within.

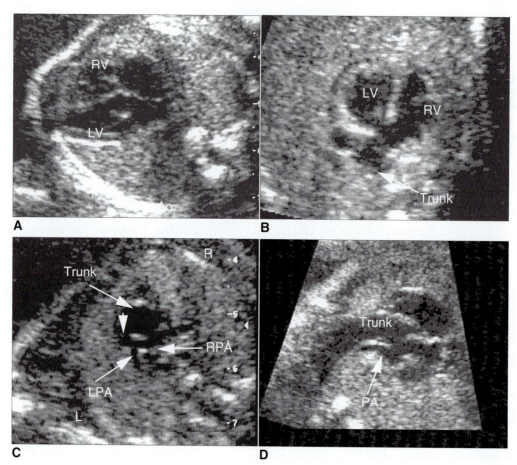

FIGURE 34-42 Truncus arteriosus. **A,** The four-chamber view may not be so abnormal in truncus arteriosus, other than the leftward axis. **B,** Sweeping toward the outflow tract, only a single semilunar valve can be demonstrated, which overrides the ventricular septal defect. **C,** Three-vessel view reveals one very large great artery, the trunk from which both brachiocephalic arteries and the main and branch pulmonary arteries *(LPA and RPA)* arise. **D,** Communication between the trunk and pulmonary artery is demonstrated with an arrow. The pulmonary artery *(PA)* arises from the posterior or leftward aspect of the trunk. *LPA,* Left pulmonary artery; *RPA,* right pulmonary artery.

that coarctation may be difficult to evaluate in the fetus because the ductus arteriosus is patent, so some of the blood may flow into the arch during fetal life (see Figure 34-43, *B*). Once the fetus is delivered and the ductus closes, however, the narrowed portion of the arch becomes evident.

Interrupted Aortic Arch

Interruption of the aortic arch is characterized by complete anatomic interruption of the arch or, rarely, by an atretic fibrous remnant connecting the proximal arch with the descending aorta. The interruption occurs at one of three sites:

1. Distal to the left common carotid artery, so that the left subclavian artery originates from the descending aorta
2. Just beyond the left subclavian, so that all the brachiocephalic arteries arise from the arch and none from the descending aorta

3. Distal to the innominate artery, so that the left common carotid and left subclavian arteries originate from the descending aorta

The descending aorta is really a continuation of the main pulmonary artery via the patent ductus. A ventricular septal defect is almost always present. After birth, these three items make a distinct congenital triad: interruption of the aortic arch, patent ductus arteriosus, and ventricular septal defect. In this condition, the conal septum is posteriorly deviated, thus restricting flow through the aortic outflow tract. A large, more subpulmonary ventricular septal defect, with or without true override of the main pulmonary artery, is the first clue to its diagnosis. A significant size discrepancy between the greater arteries is apparent, with the main pulmonary artery appearing larger than the aorta.

The interruption of the aortic arch also tends to occur with a bicuspid or deformed aortic valve, subaortic stenosis, biventricular origin of the pulmonary trunk, or anomalous origin of the major branches of the ascending aorta.

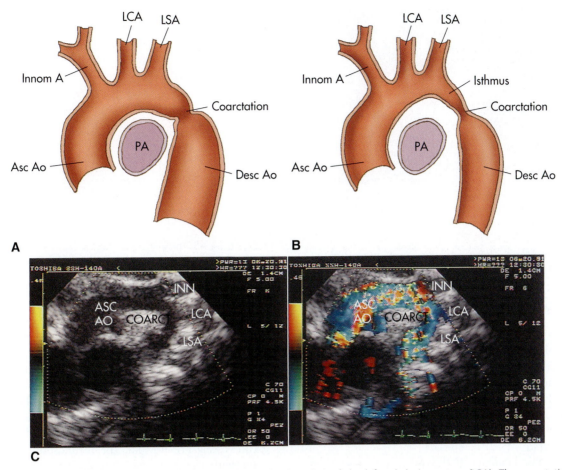

FIGURE 34-43 Coarctation of the aorta occurs just inferior to the insertion of the left subclavian artery (*LSA*). The coarctation may be discrete **(A)** with mild poststenotic dilation in the fetus. This narrowing usually is near the point of ductal insertion. *Asc Ao,* Ascending aorta; *Innom A,* innominate artery; *LCA,* left carotid artery. **B,** A long-segment narrowing of the isthmus is more likely to be found by echocardiography. **C,** A discrete narrowing was found in this 32-week fetus. Long-axis view of the aortic arch shows the narrowing at the level of the left subclavian artery. Pulsed Doppler imaging recorded velocities of 190 cm/sec. *COARCT,* Coarctation; *INN,* innominate artery.

Ductal Constriction

Ductal constriction occurs when flow is diverted from the ductus secondary to tricuspid or pulmonary atresia or secondary to maternal medications (indomethacin therapy) given to stop early contractions. In the normal fetus, the ductus arteriosus transmits about 55% to 60% of combined ventricular output from the pulmonary artery to the aorta. It joins the aorta at an obtuse inferior angle, presumably because flow is directed down to the descending aorta. If aortic atresia or aortic isthmus interruption were present, a much larger proportion of the output would have to flow through the ductus to maintain ventricular output; in fact, in aortic atresia, the total output—excluding pulmonary flow—would cross the ductus. Thus, about 90% of combined ventricular output would be carried by the ductus, which could be considerably wider than normal (no change in Doppler velocities at the ductus).

In tricuspid or pulmonary atresia, no blood would be ejected from the right ventricle into the pulmonary artery. The flow through the ductus would occur from the aorta to the pulmonary arteries. Because this normally represents only about 10% of the combined ventricular output, the ductus may be quite narrow and underdeveloped (with high-velocity Doppler recordings at the level of the ductus). Furthermore, because flow is from the aorta to the pulmonary artery, the connection of the ductus with the aorta has an acute inferior angle.

The primary signs of ductal constriction include right atrial and ventricular dilatation, right ventricular dysfunction, and pulmonary and tricuspid insufficiency. The Doppler flow pattern at the ductus increases in systolic and diastolic velocities. The diastolic velocity may reach peak velocities of greater than 30 cm/sec, and there is continuous flow in diastole, rather than the more pulsatile flow as seen in the normal ductus arteriosus. Heart failure may develop if the ductal constriction is not reversed by the discontinuation of maternal oral therapy or through delivery of the infant.

CARDIAC TUMORS

Cardiac tumors are very unusual. Most of these tumors are benign and isolated. The most common tumors are rhabdomyoma (58%) and teratoma (20%), followed by

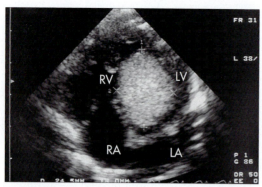

FIGURE 34-44 Four-chamber view of a fetus with a huge rhabdomyoma completely filling the left ventricular cavity. *LA,* Left artery; *LV,* left ventricle; *RA,* right artery; *RV,* right ventricle.

fibroma, myxoma, hemangioma, and mesothelioma. Less than 10% of cardiac tumors are malignant.

Rhabdomyomas

Rhabdomyomas tend to be multiple and involve the septum. This tumor is associated with tuberous sclerosis (50% to 86%) (Figure 34-44). The fetus becomes symptomatic when the tumor is large and causes obstruction to the outflow tract, leading to congestive heart failure, pericardial effusion, hydrops, and death. The prognosis depends on the size of the tumor, its location, and its histologic type.

▶ **Sonographic Findings.** If this mass is suspected, the sonographer should also look for associated tumor mass abnormalities in the kidneys and fetal head. The teratoma may be intrapericardial and extracardiac. The fibroma tumors account for 12% of all cardiac tumors in the neonate. This tumor is pedunculated and may calcify.

The fetal echo shows the tumor best in the four-chamber view. Close analysis should be made to search for regurgitation and obstruction. The right and left ventricular outflow tracts should be carefully studied with Doppler to record velocities in the subvalvular and supravalvular area. Serial evaluation may be made with fetal echocardiography to follow the ventricular function and Doppler flow patterns.

COMPLEX CARDIAC ABNORMALITIES

Single Ventricle

Single ventricle is a congenital anomaly in which there are two atria but only one ventricular chamber, which receives both the mitral and tricuspid valves (Figure 34-45). Both valves are patent, so mitral and tricuspid atresia can be excluded. (Occasionally the mitral and tricuspid valves join to form a common atrioventricular valve.)

▶ **Sonographic Findings.** The most common form of a single ventricle heart is a morphologic left ventricle with

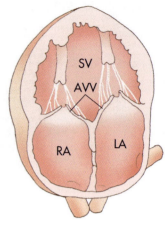

FIGURE 34-45 Three-chamber view shows a single inflow cavity (single ventricle *[SV]*). Two atrial cavities and atrioventricular valves *(AVV)* are present. *LA,* Left atrium; *RA,* right atrium.

a small outlet chamber that represents the infundibular portion of the right ventricle. The right or left atrioventricular connection may be absent and the great arteries may be transposed, with the aorta arising above the small outlet chamber. If transposition is present, the pulmonary artery lies posterior to the aorta. The infundibulum lies at the base of the ventricle, communicating with the aorta above and the single ventricle below. If the great vessels are normal, the infundibulum communicates with the pulmonary trunk. The outlet chambers may be left-side and anterior or right-side and anterior, but they commonly lie high on the cardiac silhouette.

Pulmonary stenosis may or may not coexist. If present, the pulmonary stenosis is usually valvular or subvalvular. The pulmonary trunk is usually slightly smaller than the aortic trunk.

The four-chamber view is the most useful window in delineating the cardiac anatomy (Figure 34-46). The prominent papillary muscles should not be confused with the interventricular septum. In a single ventricle, the papillary muscles may be quite prominent. With careful transducer angulation, the chordal structures may be traced to these structures for correct delineation. The right ventricle may be just a slitlike cavity as seen on the apical four-chamber view. The position of the great arteries should be assessed, and the aorta and pulmonary arteries should be delineated clearly. Regurgitant jets may be associated with abnormal chordal connections of the atrioventricular valves. Doppler evaluation of these valves is useful in depicting any regurgitation present. Color flow imaging is especially useful in outlining the direction of jet flow for proper Doppler evaluation.

Cor Triatriatum

Cor triatriatum occurs when the left atrial cavity is partitioned into two compartments. This anomaly is

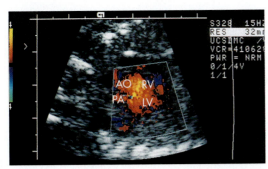

FIGURE 34-46 Color flow image demonstrates complete filling of the essentially "single ventricle" in a patient with transposition of the great arteries and a huge ventricular septal defect. *AO,* Aorta; *LV,* left ventricle; *PA,* pulmonary artery; *RV,* right ventricle.

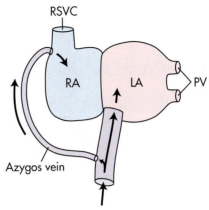

FIGURE 34-48 The inferior vena cava *(IVC)* communicates directly with the left atrium *(LA).* An enlarged azygous vein arises from the anomalous IVC and communicates with the right atrium *(RA)* via a normal right superior vena cava *(RSVC).* Inferior caval blood flows directly into the left atrium *(large arrow);* a portion of the IVC blood is diverted through the azygous vein into the right superior cava and right heart *(small arrow). PV,* Pulmonary veins.

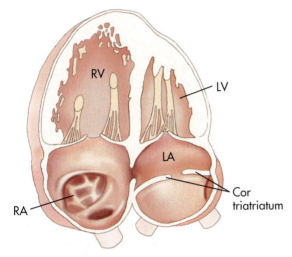

FIGURE 34-47 Cor triatriatum. Four-chamber view of the heart shows the pulmonary veins draining into a segment of the left atrial cavity, separated from the mitral inflow by the subdividing membrane. The amount of obstruction into the left ventricle will depend on how tight the orifice of the cor triatriatum is.

characterized by drainage of the pulmonary veins into an accessory left atrial chamber that lies proximal to the true left atrium (Figure 34-47). The accessory chamber is believed to represent the dilated common pulmonary vein of the embryo. (This lesion has also been called stenosis of the common pulmonary vein.) The distal compartment communicates with the mitral valve and contains the left atrial appendage and usually the fossa ovalis. The fibrous or fibromuscular diaphragm that partitions the left atrium possesses one or more openings, and the size of these openings determines the degree of left atrial obstruction.

Congenital Vena Cava to Left Atrial Communication

Isolated connection of the superior or inferior vena cava to the left atrium is a rare congenital malformation. The left atrium occasionally receives other systemic veins,

such as the coronary sinus, the azygous vein, or the hepatic vein.

Inferior Vena Cava. When the inferior vena cava communicates with the left atrium, the vessel usually has a normal abdominal course and penetrates the diaphragm at the expected site. An enlarged azygous vein may arise from the anomalous inferior cava and ultimately communicate with the right atrium (Figure 34-48). Normally the azygous vein begins as a branch of the inferior vena cava, then proceeds upward through the aortic hiatus of the diaphragm, passes along the right side of the vertebral column, and finally arches forward to enter the superior vena cava. An enlarged azygous system can serve an important function as a conveyor of inferior vena caval blood to the right atrium even though the inferior cava itself communicates with the left atrium. Occasionally the inferior vena cava is absent and infradiaphragmatic blood reaches the right atrium entirely via the azygous system.

Superior Vena Cava. Congenital abnormalities of the superior vena cava generally fall into two categories: anomalies of position and anomalies of drainage (Figure 34-49). Anomalies of position, especially persistent left superior vena cava, are more frequent than those of drainage. A left superior vena cava itself causes no physiologic disturbance because it harmlessly drains into the right atrium via the coronary sinus. However, a persistent left superior vena cava assumes particular significance when it communicates with the left atrium. It also follows that when a superior vena cava drains into the left atrium, the anomalously draining vessel is likely to be a persistent left cava. A right superior vena cava usually coexists and enters the right atrium in normal fashion.

When two superior cavas are present, the right and left may be completely separate from each other or may

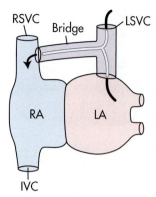

FIGURE 34-49 Persistent left superior vena cava *(LSVC)* communicating with the left atrium *(LA)*. The size of the bridge may vary; when very small, the LSVC blood flows entirely into the left atrium. *RSVC,* Right superior vena cava; *IVC,* inferior vena cava; *RA,* right atrium; *LA,* left atrium.

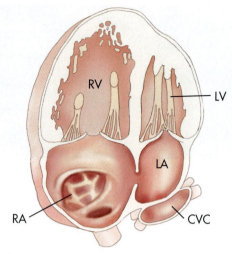

FIGURE 34-50 Four-chamber view of the heart showing total anomalous pulmonary venous return. In this view the veins are shown to enter the anomalous common venous chamber *(CVC)* superior to the left atrial cavity *(LA)*. *RA,* Right atrium; *RV,* right ventricle; *LV,* left ventricle.

be joined by means of an innominate vein. This "innominate bridge" can be widely patent, small, or atretic.

The intracardiac defects that may accompany caval drainage into the left atrium include atrial or ventricular septal defects, single atrium or ventricle, tetralogy of Fallot, transposition of great vessels, and complex positional anomalies of the heart. The extracardiac anomalies that have been associated with this condition include coarctation of the aorta, pulmonary arteriovenous fistula, and inferior vena cava malformations.

Total Anomalous Pulmonary Venous Return

The four pulmonary veins normally return blood into the left atrium from the lungs. When this fails to occur, the condition is termed **total anomalous pulmonary venous return (TAPVR)**. The venous return may be totally into the right atrium or into a "common chamber" posterior to the left atrium, into the superior or inferior vena cava, or into the left subclavian vein, azygos vein, or portal vein. The venous drainage may be total or partial (Figure 34-50).

Sonographic Findings. In the fetus, TAPVR may not be evident unless the pulmonary veins are carefully recorded. The sonographer may image an enlarged right atrial cavity with the atrial septum bulging into the small left atrium. The normal pulmonary veins are seen on the four-chamber view (Figure 34-51). The right upper vein is seen near the base of the heart at the level of the septum secundum, the left upper vein is seen at the lateral atrial wall near the base of the heart, and the left lower vein is seen just above the atrioventricular junction, along the lateral atrial wall. The right lower vein is not routinely imaged in a four-chamber view. Color Doppler imaging may help identify these venous structures.

TAPVR should be suspected in all cases of atrioventricular septal defects and in asplenia and polysplenia

syndromes. The prognosis is poor, with 75% dying within the first year after birth if no surgery is performed. Reconstruction of the pulmonary venous drainage into the left atrium has shown promising survival results.

Cardiosplenic Syndromes

Cardiosplenic syndromes are sporadic disorders characterized by a symmetric development of normally asymmetric organs or organ systems. The cardiosplenic syndromes are subdivided into asplenia and polysplenia syndromes. These two conditions are characterized by lack of the normal asymmetry of the visceral organs. The trunk tends to have two halves that are mirror images of one another. Generally speaking, asplenia is a condition of bilateral right-sidedness and polysplenia is bilateral left-sidedness.

In a fetus with asplenia, the following anomalies have been seen: the spleen is absent; the lungs are bilaterally trilobed with morphologic right bronchi on both sides; the liver is central; the stomach may be right, left, or central; the gut is malrotated; the superior vena cava is bilateral; the inferior vena cava lies to the right or left of the spine; and the aorta and cava are seen on the same side of the spine (instead of the aorta on the left and the cava on the right). Asplenia syndrome is twice as common in males.

There is a high association between asplenia and congenital heart disease. Total anomalous pulmonary venous return is seen in nearly all patients, atrioventricular septal defect in 85%, single ventricle in 51%, transposition of the great arteries in 58%, and pulmonary stenosis or atresia in 70%. In less than half of asplenic patients, dextrocardia is present.

Polysplenia syndrome is characterized by two or more spleens on both sides of the mesogastrium. Bilateral

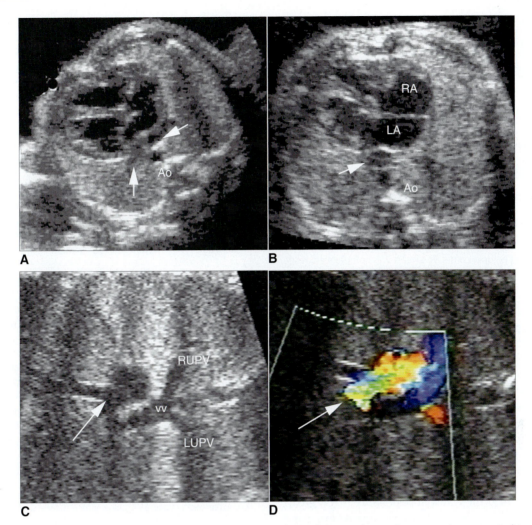

FIGURE 34-51 Total anomalous pulmonary venous return connection (TAPVR). Anomalous pulmonary veins connected to a confluence, which joined a vertical vein, ultimately draining into the inferior vena cava near the ductus venosus. **A,** Pulmonary vein connection *(arrows)* with the confluence that sits just in front of the descending aorta *(Ao)* behind the left atrium *(LA)* in **B** clearly demonstrates the confluence, the presence of which results in a gap between the posterior wall of the left atrium and the descending aorta, which normally is minimal. **C,** Pulmonary vein confluence then joins a vertical vein *(vv)* that ultimately connects below the diaphragm *(arrow)*. The left *(LUPV)* and right *(RUPV)* upper pulmonary vein connection to the confluence can be seen. **D,** Color Doppler confirms the direction of flow and presence of obstruction where the vertical vein connects with the inferior vena cava *(arrow)*.

morphologic left lungs and bronchi are found in 68% of patients. The liver and stomach are on the right or left, malrotation of the bowel is found in 80%, bilateral superior vena cava is seen in half the fetuses, and the inferior vena cava is absent in 70% (blood is drained by the azygos vein, which may be on the right or left).

Cardiac malformations are frequent, but not as common as with asplenia. The most common lesions found are TAPVR (70%), dextrocardia, atrial septal defect, AVSD, transposition of the great arteries, and double-outlet right ventricle.

The prognosis of this disease depends on the severity of the cardiac lesion. Surgical intervention has increased the survival rate.

◤ **Sonographic Findings.** The recognition of the cardiosplenic syndrome relies on the demonstration of both the abnormal relationship between the abdominal organs and the associated cardiac deformities. The abdominal situs must be determined clearly—with the stomach on the left, heart apex on the left, aorta on the left, and inferior vena on the right—to rule out a cardiosplenic syndrome.

Ectopic Cordis

Ectopia cordis is a heart lesion that results from an abnormal development of the primitive heart outside the embryonic disk in the early stage of development (Figure 34-52).

Associated anomalies include facial and skeletal deformities, ventral wall defects, and central nervous system malformations (meningocele and cephalocele). Cardiac anomalies include tetralogy of Fallot and transposition of the great arteries. The prognosis is poor for this fetus.

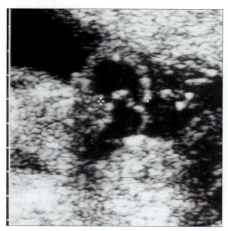

FIGURE 34-52 A fetus with pentalogy of Cantrell (multiple midline defects), including ectopia cordis. The heart was completely outside the thoracic cavity.

DYSRHYTHMIAS

The fetal heart undergoes multiple changes during the embryologic stages. One of these stages is the progression of the cardiac electrical system, which matures to cause a normal sinus rhythm in the cardiac cycle (Figure 34-53). It is not uncommon during the course of a fetal echocardiogram to see the normal fetal heart rate decelerate from 150 beats per minute to a bradycardia stage (under 55 beats per minute), or even to pause for a few seconds. This may happen if the baby is lying on the umbilical cord or if the transducer pressure is too great. The fetus should be given a recovery time to bring the heart rate to a normal sinus rhythm. This is usually done by changing the position of the mother or releasing the pressure from the transducer.

Other changes in rhythm patterns seen during fetal development may result from premature atrial and ventricular contractions, supraventricular tachycardia, tachycardia, or atrioventricular block (Table 34-2).

Ectopy

Premature Atrial and Ventricular Contractions

Electrical impulses generated outside the cardiac pacemaker (sinus node) can cause **premature atrial contractions (PACs)** or **premature ventricular contractions (PVCs)**. The sinus node is located along the lateral right atrial wall. It is not clearly understood why some patients develop these ectopic premature contractions. Some investigators have tried to link them to increased amounts of caffeine, alcohol, or smoking, but none of our patients with PACs has these associations. An increased redundancy of the flap of the foramen ovale has been noted in these patients. The flap is larger than seen in the normal fetus and appears to swing with a great excursion from the left atrium into the right atrial cavity, touching the right atrial node.

TABLE 34-2	Sonographic Pitfalls for Arrhythmias	
Heart Rate	**Rhythm**	**Features: Atrial to Ventricular Association**
40–60	Complete heart block	A-V dissociation
60–90	Atrial bigeminy	Every other atrial impulse blocked
80–110	Sinus bradycardia	Normal A-V conduction
105–185	Normal sinus rhythm	Normal A-V conduction
180–210	Sinus tachycardia	Normal A-V conduction
150–220	Ventricular tachycardia	A-V dissociation or 1:1 V-A conduction
180	SVT (ectopic)	1:1 A-V conduction, incessant
220–260	SVT (reentrant)	A-V conduction with sudden onset and cessation
150–600	Atrial flutter	1:1 A-V conduction or 2:1, 3:1, 4:1 A-V block
Any rate	Ectopy or blocked atrial PVCs	Frequent or occasional PACs conducted

A-V, Atrioventricular; *PACs,* premature atrial contractions; *PVCs,* premature ventricular contractions; *SVT,* supraventricular tachycardia.

The patient is usually referred for a fetal cardiac arrhythmia as heard on the routine obstetric examination by Doptone or auscultation. These techniques provide information about the ventricular rate only. To adequately assess the fetal rhythm, the ventricular and atrial rates must be analyzed simultaneously.

The atrium and ventricle may both experience extrasystoles and ectopic beats to give rise to complex echo patterns. The PACs may either be conducted to the ventricles or blocked, depending on the moment in which they occur in the cardiac cycle. Repeated PACs may lead to an increased or decreased ventricular rate. A blocked PAC must be differentiated from an atrioventricular block. This distinction relies on the demonstration of an atrial contraction that appears prematurely. PVCs are characterized by a PVC that is not preceded by an atrial contraction.

■ **Sonographic Findings.** The sonographer can help sort out the rhythm with M-mode or Doppler. To record the atrial and ventricular rates simultaneously, the four-chamber heart must be perpendicular to the transducer (Figure 34-54). The beam must dissect the ventricle and atria of the heart. It does not matter if the right or left side of the heart is more anterior. The best area to record

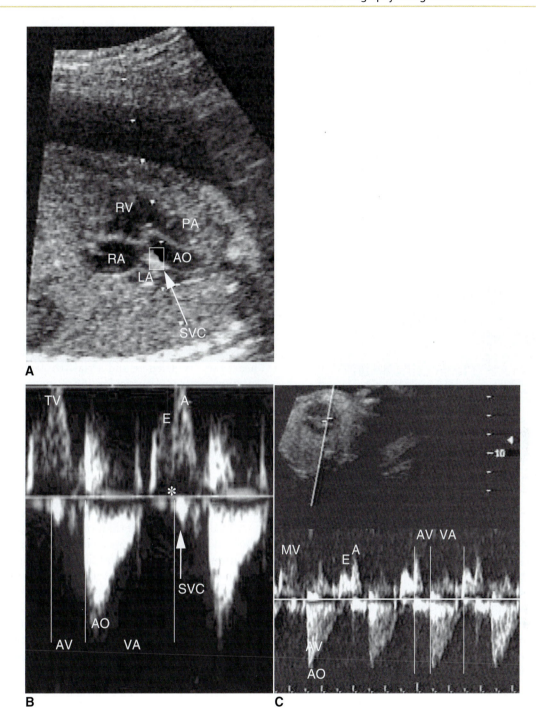

FIGURE 34-53 Doppler assessment of the normal fetal rhythm. **A** and **B,** Simultaneous pulsed Doppler recording of the ascending aorta *(A)* and superior vena cava *(SVC).* The Doppler sample volume *(–)* is placed between the two adjacent vessels. The time interval between the onsets of retrograde superior vena cava and antegrade flow, which corresponds to the atrioventricular *(AV)* conduction time, can be measured. The inflow through the tricuspid valve *(TV, E,* and A wave flow) is also demonstrated. **C,** Pulsed Doppler recording of the left ventricular inflow and outflow. The Doppler sample volume is positioned in the left ventricle to simultaneously demonstrate flow through the mitral valve *(MV)* and the aortic outflow *(AO).* The time interval between atrial (onset of A wave) and ventricular systole (onset of A) permits indirect assessment of atrioventricular conduction.

atrial motion is usually just superior to the atrioventricular junction along the lateral wall of the atria. The atrial pattern appears to move with a box type of motion. The ventricular rate is best recorded at the level of the atrioventricular valve and is seen to move as a smooth, uniform, well-defined pattern.

If the sonographer cannot obtain adequate images from the four-chamber view, the parasternal short-axis view may be used. The beam should be directed through the right atrial wall, aortic cusps, or the left atrial wall and aortic cusps. As the aorta moves in an anterior direction, the aortic cusps open in systole and

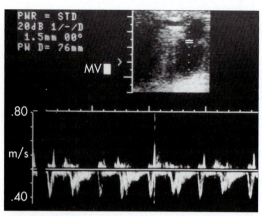

FIGURE 34-54 Fetus with premature atrial contractions. The fetus had normal cardiac anatomy.

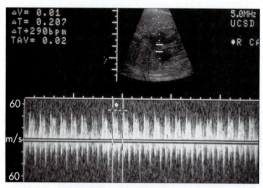

FIGURE 34-55 Fetus with supraventricular tachycardia showed normal conduction with a heart rate of more than 220 beats per minute.

close in diastole. Thus, the aortic leaflets may signify the ventricular systolic event, whereas the atrial wall signifies the atrial event.

The M-mode should be expanded to its full extent to clearly see the movement of the atrial and ventricular walls. Changes in the atrioventricular valve patterns are also noted in patients with arrhythmias. Doppler imaging of the atrioventricular valves demonstrates whether regurgitation is present during the disturbance in rhythm.

Patients with PACs and PVCs are assured that this development is a normal benign condition resulting from the immaturity of the electrical conduction system of the heart. This pattern is not associated with other cardiac anomalies.

Supraventricular Tachyarrhythmia

Supraventricular tachyarrhythmias include abnormal rhythms above 200 beats per minute with a conduction rate of 1:1 (Figure 34-55). These rhythm disturbances may be paroxysmal supraventricular tachycardia, paroxysmal atrial tachycardia, atrial flutter, or atrial fibrillation. In atrial flutter, the atrial rate is recorded at 300 to 460 beats per minute with a normal ventricular rate. Atrial fibrillation shows the atria to beat at more than

400 beats per minute, with a ventricular rate of 120 to 200 beats per minute.

Supraventricular tachycardia occurs by automaticity or reentry mechanisms. In cases of automatic induced tachyarrhythmias, an irritable ectopic focus discharges at a high frequency. The reentry mechanism consists of an electrical impulse reentering the atria, giving rise to repeated electrical activity. Reentry may occur at the level of the sinoatrial node, inside the atrium, at the atrioventricular node, and in the His-Purkinje system. Reentry may also occur along an anomalous atrioventricular connection, such as the Kent bundle in Wolff-Parkinson-White (WPW) syndrome.

Supraventricular tachycardia is the most frequent arrhythmia caused by atrioventricular nodal reentry, occurring in 1 in 25,000 births. Viral infections or hypoplasia of the sinoatrial tract may trigger supraventricular tachycardia.

Sonographic Findings. The finding of supraventricular tachycardia in a fetus is an emergency situation. The fetus should be scanned immediately to assess signs of heart rate, ventricular and atrial size, amount of regurgitation present, ventricular function, and presence of pericardial effusion and hydrops (Figure 34-56). With supraventricular tachycardia, the fetus develops suboptimal filling of the ventricles, decreased cardiac output, and right ventricular volume overload leading to subsequent congestive heart failure.

Other cardiac anomalies associated with supraventricular tachycardia are atrial septal defects, mitral valve disease, cardiac tumors, and WPW syndrome.

Atrial flutter and fibrillation often alternate and are thought to result from a mechanism similar to that found in supraventricular tachycardia. Atrial flutter and fibrillation have been described in patients with WPW syndrome, cardiomyopathies, and thyrotoxicosis.

The fetus with this arrhythmia is usually admitted to the hospital and medically treated with antiarrhythmic drugs to control the ventricular rate, with the goal of converting the rate into normal sinus rhythm. Fetal echocardiography may be clinically useful in monitoring these patients' recovery.

Atrioventricular Block

When the transmission of the electrical impulse from the atria to the ventricles is blocked, the condition is called an **atrioventricular block**. Normally the atria fill in ventricular diastole and empty in ventricular systole. Just before ventricular systole occurs, the pressure in the atria is at its peak. (This corresponds to the p wave on the ECG.) The QRS complex signifies the onset of ventricular systole, causing the pressure from the atria to open the atrioventricular valves so the left ventricle may fill. If this electrical process is blocked, the blood remains in the atria and does not cause the atrioventricular valves to open so blood can fill the ventricular cavities. This

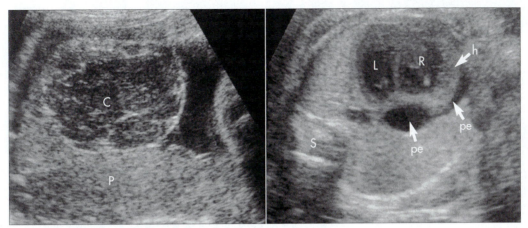

FIGURE 34-56 Pericardial effusion (*pe*) may be present if the arrhythmia is significant (i.e., supraventricular tachycardia). The fetus cannot withstand rapid changes in cardiac activity without developing signs of heart failure. *C*, Fetal cranium; *h*, heart; *L*, left ventricle; *P*, placenta; *R*, right ventricle; *S*, spine.

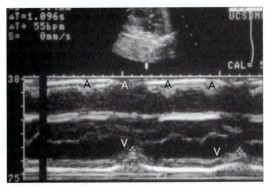

FIGURE 34-57 Mother with systemic lupus erythematosus presented at 20 weeks of gestation because of a "slow heart rate." The fetus was in 2:1 heart block with the atria beating twice as fast as the ventricle; every other beat was conducted. *A*, Atrium; *V*, ventricle.

condition may be attributed to immaturity of the conduction system, absence of connection to the atrioventricular node, or an abnormal anatomic position of the atrioventricular node. The fetus may have a first-, second-, or third-degree heart block.

The fetus with a third-degree atrioventricular block has been found to have associated structural anomalies, including corrected transposition, univentricular heart, cardiac tumors, and cardiomyopathies. Patients with a connective tissue disorder, such as lupus erythematosus, have also been found to develop heart block.

First- and second-degree atrioventricular blocks are not associated with any significant hemodynamic disturbance. A complete heart block may result in bradycardia,

leading to decreased cardiac output and congestive heart failure during fetal life.

Sonographic Findings. The fetal M-mode echocardiogram should be performed after the normal anatomic cardiac anatomy has been demonstrated (Figure 34-57). As described in the supraventricular tachycardia section, the four-chamber and parasternal short-axis views are best used to record atrial and ventricular events simultaneously.

First-degree heart block is not seen in the fetus, as the heart rate and rhythm are normal. The blockage of a normal atrial impulse can be diagnosed by demonstrating a normally timed atrial contraction that is not followed by a ventricular contraction.

Second- and third-degree heart blocks are defined by observing the relationship between the atrial and ventricular rates. In second-degree Mobitz type I block, only a few atrial impulses are not conducted; in Mobitz type II block, a submultiple of atrial impulses is transmitted. In complete heart block, atrial and ventricular rates are independent of each other, with the atrial rate slower. The fetus becomes symptomatic when the cardiac output is decreased and congestive heart failure develops.

REFERENCES

1. Callen PC: *Ultrasonography in obstetrics and gynecology*, ed 4, Philadelphia, 2000, WB Saunders.
2. Silverman NH, Schmidt KG: Ventricular volume overload in the human fetus: observations from fetal echocardiography, *J Am Soc Echocardiography* 3:20, 1990.

PART VI

Cerebrovascular

Extracranial Cerebrovascular Evaluation

Ann Willis and Mira L. Katz

The life of an individual is often dramatically affected by having a stroke. Not only is stroke a leading cause of adult disability in the United States, but approximately 143,000 of the 795,000 strokes that occur each year result in death.[23] Stroke is the third leading cause of death in the United States. Additionally, the direct (hospital, physician, rehabilitation, etc.) and indirect (lost productivity, etc.) costs associated with stroke in the United States tallied more than $65.5 billion for 2010.[23] Stroke is more prevalent among men, but women have a higher death rate. The rate of death by stroke is much higher in the African American population.

A stroke or "brain attack" is caused by an interruption of blood flow to the brain (ischemic stroke) or by a ruptured intracranial blood vessel (intracranial hemorrhage). Approximately 80% of all known strokes are ischemic, and the remaining 20% are hemorrhagic. Because extracranial carotid artery disease is responsible for more than 50% of all strokes, carotid ultrasound becomes an important imaging modality to identify disease that may be the potential cause of a stroke. This is important because prevention remains the best treatment for stroke.

STROKE RISK FACTORS, WARNING SIGNS, AND SYMPTOMS

Risk factors for stroke may be categorized into those that are not modifiable and those that are changeable or can be controlled. Nonmodifiable risk factors include age (risk of stroke dramatically increases with increasing age), sex (incidence of stroke is higher in males, although females generally have a more severe deficit), and race (African Americans have a higher stroke risk than other races). The modifiable or controllable risk factors include hypertension, atrial fibrillation and other cardiac diseases, diabetes mellitus, elevated cholesterol, smoking, and a history of a sedentary lifestyle.

The five warning signs of stroke are listed in Box 35-1. It is important to remember that symptoms of weakness or numbness of a leg or arm on one side of the body (**hemiparesis**) indicate disease in the contralateral carotid system. In other words, left body symptoms implicate the right carotid system and vice versa. Ocular symptoms, however, suggest disease in the carotid system on the ipsilateral (same) side. For example, transient blindness (**amaurosis fugax**) of the right eye suggests disease of the carotid system on the right side. Symptoms such as blurred vision, **dysarthria, ataxia, syncope, vertigo,** or overall weakness can be confusing as to which vascular system is involved. Bilateral-type symptoms such as these may be related to the vertebral system, especially if the carotid system proves to be clear. Patients are classified as asymptomatic (without symptoms) or symptomatic. Asymptomatic patients are usually referred for carotid duplex imaging because they are at high risk for stroke, or because of the presence of a cervical **bruit**. The classification of cerebrovascular symptoms includes the following: Stroke or **cerebrovascular accident (CVA)** is a permanent ischemic neurologic deficit; **reversible ischemic neurologic deficit (RIND)** is a neurologic deficit that resolves between 24 and 72 hours; **transient ischemic attack (TIA)** is an ischemic neurologic deficit that lasts less than 24 hours.

Other cerebrovascular (carotid and vertebral territory) symptoms include **aphasia**, dizziness, **dysphagia**, **diplopia**, and **hemianopsia**.

ANATOMY FOR EXTRACRANIAL CEREBROVASCULAR IMAGING

Aortic Arch

The ascending aorta originates from the left ventricle of the heart. The transverse aortic arch lies in the superior mediastinum and is formed as the aorta ascends and curves posteroinferiorly from right to left, above the left mainstem bronchus. It descends to the left of the trachea and esophagus. Three main arteries arise from the superior convexity of the arch in its normal configuration. The brachiocephalic trunk (innominate artery) is the first branch, the left common carotid artery the second, and the left subclavian artery the third branch in approximately 70% of cases.

The innominate artery divides into the right common carotid artery and the right subclavian artery, which gives rise to the right **vertebral artery**. The left common carotid artery originates slightly to the left of the innominate artery, followed by the left subclavian artery, which likewise gives rise to the left vertebral artery.

Anatomic variants of the major arch vessels occur frequently. The most commonly occurring variant (approximately 10%) is the left common carotid artery forming a common origin with or originating directly from the innominate artery. Less frequently, the left vertebral artery arises directly from the arch, the right subclavian artery originates from the arch distal to the left subclavian artery, the right common carotid artery originates directly from the arch, and a left innominate artery may exist, from which the left common carotid and the left subclavian originate.

Common Carotid Artery

Each **common carotid artery (CCA)** ascends through the superior mediastinum anterolaterally in the neck and lies medial to the jugular vein (Figure 35-1). The CCA usually measures between 6 and 8 mm in diameter. The left common carotid is usually longer than the right because it originates from the aortic arch. In the neck, the carotid artery, jugular vein, and vagus nerve are enclosed in connective tissue called the *carotid sheath*. The vagus nerve lies between and dorsal to the artery and vein. The CCA usually does not have branches, but occasionally it is the origin to the superior thyroid artery. The termination of the CCA is the carotid bifurcation, which is the origin of the internal carotid artery (ICA) and the external carotid artery (ECA). The CCA bifurcates in the vicinity of the superior border of the thyroid cartilage (approximately C4) in 70% of cases, and the level of the CCA bifurcations may be asymmetrical. The CCA bifurcation, however, has been described as low as T2 and as high as C1.

External Carotid Artery

The **external carotid artery (ECA)** originates at the mid-cervical level and is usually the smaller of the two terminal branches of the CCA. Initially, it lies anteromedial to the ICA, but as the ECA ascends, it courses posterolaterally. In approximately 15% of the population, the ECA originates lateral to the ICA. This anatomic variation occurs more frequently on the right (3:1). The ECA usually measures 3 to 4 mm in diameter.

Eight named branches of the ECA have been identified: the superior thyroid, ascending pharyngeal, lingual, facial, occipital, posterior auricular, and terminal branches, the superficial temporal, and the internal maxillary. The superior thyroid artery is the most commonly visualized branch of the ECA during carotid duplex imaging.

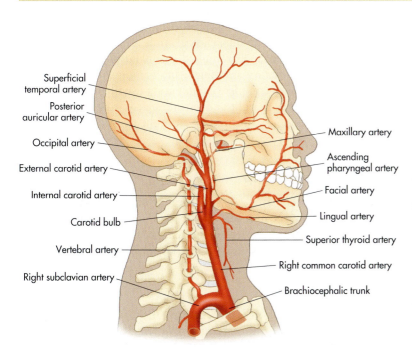

FIGURE 35-1 Anatomy of the extracranial carotid system. During carotid duplex imaging, the area of focus is the common carotid bifurcation because of its propensity for atherosclerotic plaque formation.

The abundant number of anastomoses between the branches of the ECA and the intracranial circulation underscores the clinical significance of the ECA as a **collateral pathway** for cerebral perfusion when significant disease is present in the ICA.

Internal Carotid Artery

The **internal carotid artery (ICA)** is usually the larger of the CCA terminal branches. The ICA is divided into four main segments: cervical, petrous, cavernous, and cerebral.

The cervical portion of the ICA is evaluated during carotid duplex imaging examinations. The cervical portion of the ICA begins at the CCA bifurcation and extends to the base of the skull. The ICA lies in the carotid sheath and runs deep to the sternocleidomastoid muscle. In the majority of individuals, the ICA lies posterolateral to the ECA and courses medially as it ascends in the neck. At its origin, the cervical ICA normally has a slight dilation, termed the carotid bulb. The carotid bulb may include the distal CCA, the proximal ICA, and the proximal ECA. The cervical ICA usually does not have branches and measures between 5 and 6 mm in diameter. The first branch of the ICA is located in the cavernous portion; it cannot be seen during a normal extracranial examination, but it can be an important collateral in cases of cervical ICA obstruction. With advancing age and progressive disease, the cervical ICA may become tortuous, coiled, or kinked (Figure 35-2).

Vertebral Artery

The vertebral arteries are large branches of the subclavian arteries. Atherosclerotic changes usually occur at

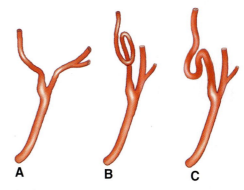

FIGURE 35-2 Morphologic variations in the internal carotid artery. **A,** Tortuosity: curving of the artery. **B,** Coiling: a redundant curve. **C,** Kinking: sharp and abrupt angulation.

the origin of the vertebral arteries. Occasionally, the vertebral artery arises directly from the aortic arch (4% of cases on the left side and rarely on the right side). The two vertebral arteries are asymmetrical in size in about 75% of cases, with the left vertebral artery being the dominant artery. The vertebral artery can be divided into four segments: extravertebral, intervertebral, horizontal, and intracranial.

The extravertebral segment is evaluated during the duplex imaging examination. This segment courses superiorly and medially from its subclavicular origin to enter the transverse foramen of the sixth cervical vertebra. The proximal segment of the vertebral artery is approximately 4 to 5 cm in length, and usually has no branches. The vertebral artery ascends within the transverse foramina of the upper cervical vertebrae (intervertebral segment), emerges from the transverse foramen of the atlas (horizontal segment), and becomes the intracranial portion of the vertebral artery as it pierces the spinal dura and arachnoid below the base of the skull at the foramen magnum. The two branches then combine to form the basilar artery.

TECHNICAL ASPECTS OF CAROTID DUPLEX IMAGING

The examination is explained and a medical history (risk factors, symptoms) obtained from the patient. Arm pressures may be recorded, and a difference of ≥20 mmHg pressure between arms suggests a proximal stenosis/occlusion of the subclavian or innominate artery on the side of the lower pressure. The presence of cervical bruits is documented by auscultation of the carotid arterial system. A bruit (noise) is caused by tissue vibration that is produced by blood flow turbulence. Not all stenosis in the carotid arteries will cause bruits, and a bruit may be identified from a normal artery, or the bruit may be transmitted (cardiac).

Suggested instrument setups for carotid duplex imaging are as follows:

1. Use a high-frequency (5-, 7- to 10-MHz) linear-array transducer.
2. The image orientation is usually such that the head is to the left of the monitor.
3. Although color is based on the direction of blood flow (toward or away) in relation to the transducer, red is usually assigned to arteries and blue to venous blood flow. Follow your institution's guidelines.
4. Keep the Doppler sample volume size small.
5. Use a 60-degree angle (or less) to the vessel wall. Make sure your angle is parallel to the vessel walls. Any error can have a large effect on true velocity readings.
6. The color and velocity scale (pulse repetition frequency [PRF]) should be adjusted throughout the examination to evaluate the changing velocity patterns.
7. The color and Doppler wall filter are set low.
8. The color "box" width affects frame rates (number of image frames per second), so the color display should be kept as small as possible.
9. The color, image, and Doppler gain should be adjusted throughout the examination as the signal strength changes.
10. Harmonics used in B-mode may help make hypoechoic plaque more visible.
11. If available, compound imaging will also make B-mode imaging technically better.
12. Beware of using time gain compensation (TGC) controls to make the vessels completely anechoic, as you may "erase" hypoechoic plaque or thrombus.

It is imperative that each institution develop a carotid imaging protocol that defines the standard examination (arteries to be evaluated, the numbers and locations of Doppler samples obtained from each artery, angle of insonation, etc.). This protocol must include information about the technique, clinical applications, indications for a complete and/or limited examination, interpretation criteria, quality assurance, and equipment maintenance. A standard complete examination usually includes evaluation of both right and left sides, acquiring both imaging and Doppler information from the carotid and vertebral arterial systems.

Patient Prep

Have the patient lie supine on an examination table. The patient's head is placed on a pillow and is turned slightly away from the side being scanned. The head of the bed can be raised slightly if the patient has trouble lying flat.

Procedure

The transducer is placed above the clavicle. Evaluate first in gray scale to determine the locations of the arteries, the CCA bifurcation, vessel tortuosity, and atherosclerotic plaque. This may be performed in a transverse or longitudinal view, depending on the preference of the operator. Longitudinal images are displayed with the distal segment (toward the head) of the artery on the left side of the monitor and the proximal artery on the right side of the monitor. Transverse images are usually displayed on the monitor as if the observer were looking toward the patient from his or her feet.

In a longitudinal view, the CCA is located and followed proximally as far as the clavicle will permit. The CCA can be distinguished from the internal jugular vein because the vein changes with respiration and compresses with pressure from the transducer (Figure 35-3). Although the origin of the right CCA is often located as it arises from the innominate artery, the left CCA originates from the arch and usually is not accessible to ultrasound imaging. The origin of the left CCA may be located in some cases by using a lower-frequency transducer with a smaller footprint angled inferiorly.

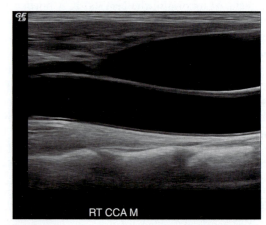

FIGURE 35-3 Normal common carotid artery *(CCA)* in gray scale. Internal jugular can be seen anterior to the CCA.

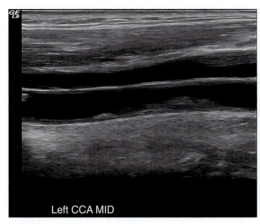

FIGURE 35-4 Hypoechoic plaque can be seen in the mid common carotid artery (CCA).

Slide the transducer up the neck, following the CCA to the level of the carotid bifurcation (thyroid cartilage). Document any plaque located in this vessel (Figure 35-4). The CCA bifurcation is a common site for the development of atherosclerotic disease. At the bifurcation, the ultrasound transducer is moved slightly anteriorly and posteriorly to image the origin of the ECA and ICA. The ICA and ECA are individually followed distally to the angle of the mandible. Multiple longitudinal views (anterior, lateral, and posterior to the sternocleidomastoid muscle) and transverse views are required to completely assess the cervical carotid arteries because of the eccentric shape of atherosclerotic plaque. Although the lateral approach provides the best visualization of the carotid system, the distal ICA is usually best visualized from a posterior approach. The transverse view provides the best cross-sectional view of the artery; therefore, any measurement of vessel diameter or plaque should be performed from this imaging plane.

The color Doppler and spectral Doppler interrogation of the carotid system is performed in the longitudinal plane using a 60-degree angle between the ultrasound beam and the vessel walls (placement of the Doppler sample volume parallel to the color jet has not undergone extensive validation testing and therefore should not be used). Use of a constant Doppler angle permits comparison of repeated studies in the same individual. Doppler angles greater than 60 degrees are not recommended because of an increase in measurement error. The sample volume should be small and placed in the center of the artery (or center stream). The Doppler sample volume is moved slowly throughout the length of the artery while searching for the highest velocity. "Spot" Doppler checks at specified locations will result in errors because areas of increased velocity may be missed. The color Doppler display will help to guide proper placement of the Doppler sample volume and is useful in locating sites of increased velocity (aliasing) suggesting disease. However, although color is helpful in locating an area of increased velocity, care must be taken

to evaluate that area for maximum velocity by slowly moving the sample volume in proximity to the color "jet" (change).

Doppler signals are recorded from the proximal, mid, and distal CCA; the origin of the ECA; the proximal, mid, and distal ICA; the origin of the vertebral artery; and, in some institutions, the subclavian artery bilaterally. In addition, Doppler signals are obtained from any area of stenosis. It is important to evaluate all Doppler signals bilaterally to correctly perform and interpret a carotid duplex imaging examination in an individual patient.

Common sources of technical error when performing carotid duplex imaging include the following: the transmitting frequency is too high for the vessel depth, the focal zone is not appropriately set to the depth of the vessel, the angle of the color box is too steep, the color gain setting is too low, and the color velocity scale (PRF) is set too high. Color and power Doppler imaging provide "roadmaps" that guide proper placement of the Doppler sample so that the artery is properly evaluated.

Normal Results

In the normal setting, the CCA spectral waveform will demonstrate a resistance pattern that is a combination of the low resistive ICA and the high resistive ECA (end-diastole above the zero baseline). The CCA Doppler signal will display a positive Doppler shift throughout the cardiac cycle. The normal CCA will have a continuous color pattern throughout the cardiac cycle. At peak systole, the color will fill the artery to the vessel walls and display an increased velocity (a lighter shade) in center stream. Doppler spectral waveforms should be evaluated from the proximal CCA, the midportion of the CCA, and the distal CCA (just proximal to the bifurcation). The CCA spectral Doppler waveform is important because it may indicate proximal disease or suggest distal disease. When calculating the ICA-to-CCA peak systolic ratio, the Doppler spectral waveform that is obtained from the straight portion (mid to distal) of the CCA is used. Investigators have shown that the velocity recorded from the CCA changes along its length.[20] Errors will occur if the spectral waveform obtained from the proximal tortuous CCA (increased velocity) or the distal CCA that may include the bulb (decreased velocity) is used in the calculation of the ratio.

Proper identification of the ICA and ECA is not a problem in most patients, but it is essential for performing accurate carotid duplex imaging. The most reliable method used to distinguish the ICA from the ECA is the Doppler signal (Figure 35-5). The ICA demonstrates blood flow velocity that is low resistive and above the zero baseline throughout the cardiac cycle. The shape of the waveform is smooth. The normal ICA will have a continuous color pattern throughout the cardiac cycle

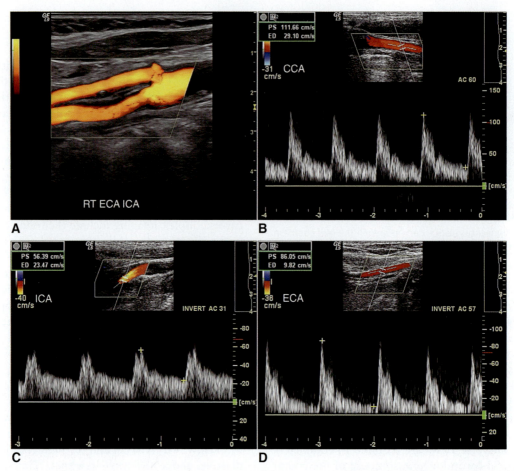

FIGURE 35-5 A, Doppler spectral waveforms from a normal extracranial carotid arterial system. **B** and **C,** Spectral waveforms from the common carotid artery *(CCA)* and the internal carotid artery *(ICA)* demonstrate low resistance. **D,** The external carotid artery *(ECA)* spectral waveform reflects a higher resistance.

caused by the low peripheral resistance of the brain. Because the carotid bulb usually includes the origin of the ICA, dilation of the proximal vessel produces a change in blood flow characteristics. Boundary layer separation, which is a normal flow disturbance, is detected as a transient reversal of blood flow along the posterior wall of the bulb. Boundary layer separation may be visualized in the color Doppler display and in the Doppler spectral waveform. Sample volumes for the ICA should start just distal to this area.

The ECA demonstrates a more pulsatile Doppler signal (high resistive, minimal diastolic flow) because it supplies blood to the skin and muscular bed of the scalp and face. The ECA usually has a faster slope to peak systole and blood flow velocity to or very close to zero in late diastole. The normal color flow pattern of the ECA will reflect the higher resistance of the scalp and face. The color pattern will decrease during diastole and may disappear at end-diastole. Additionally the ECA is smaller in diameter, usually originates anterior and medial at the carotid bifurcation, and has cervical branches. The superior thyroid artery is the ECA branch most visualized during a carotid duplex imaging examination.

The vertebral arteries are located by angling the transducer slightly laterally from a longitudinal view of the mid or proximal CCA. The vertebral artery lies deeper than the CCA. For the vertebral artery to be reliably identified, it should be followed distally, and periodic shadowing should be visualized from the transverse processes of the vertebrae (Figure 35-6). The vertebral artery is accompanied by the vertebral vein (Figure 35-7), and proper identification of the artery is made by the Doppler signal. Once the vertebral artery has been correctly identified, it should be followed as far proximally as possible. The use of color Doppler will greatly assist in locating the vertebral artery and its origin and in evaluating the direction of blood flow. Comparing the flow direction to the CCA will help confirm antegrade or retrograde flow. Decreasing the color velocity scale may be helpful in locating the vertebral artery. The color flow pattern in the vertebral artery will demonstrate continuous color throughout the cardiac cycle, and the blood flow velocity is low resistive and above the zero baseline throughout the cardiac cycle. The vertebral artery Doppler signal should be obtained near the origin of the vessel to identify any significant plaque formation.

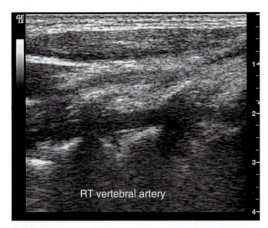

FIGURE 35-6 Normal vertebral artery seen in gray scale running between the transverse processes of the cervical spine.

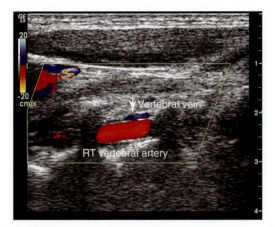

FIGURE 35-7 This is a color Doppler longitudinal view of the vertebral artery as it travels between the bony transverse processes. Note that the blood flow is in the correct direction *(head is to the left on the image)*. It is important to follow the vertebral artery proximally to obtain the Doppler signal near the origin of the artery. The vertebral vein can be seen just anterior to the artery.

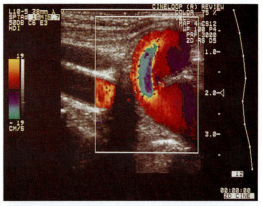

FIGURE 35-8 A complete loop in the proximal common carotid artery. Note the increased blood flow velocity (color Doppler aliasing) in the artery as it travels directly toward the transducer. This increased velocity may reflect the transducer-to-artery angle, rather than a true increase in blood flow velocity.

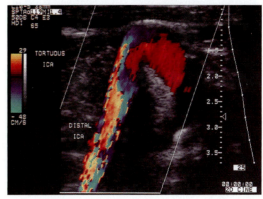

FIGURE 35-9 A distal internal carotid artery *(ICA)* dives deep away from the transducer. Doppler information from this artery cannot be taken 60 degrees to the vessel wall. It is important to note which angle was used during the examination, and to sweep the Doppler sample volume along the length of the vessel, noting any increases in velocity and poststenotic turbulence.

Tortuous Arteries. During a carotid duplex imaging examination, encountering tortuous arteries is very common (Figures 35-8 and 35-9). Normal blood flow disturbances occur because of the curves in the arteries. Usually, an increase in blood flow velocity is associated with a tortuous vessel. Correct placement of the Doppler sample volume and adjustment of the Doppler angle may be very difficult in some arteries. Often velocity is increased when scanning through a curve because of the acute Doppler angles relative to the changing blood flow direction, and not necessarily because of increased velocity of the blood flow. It is recommended that other evidence, such as poststenotic turbulence, be used to identify a stenosis in this setting. Additionally, whatever angle is used to evaluate the tortuous vessel should be documented and the same angle used for follow-up examinations in an individual patient.

Doppler Variations. Congestive heart failure (CHF) can have a profound effect on the Doppler signal. The velocity in the carotid system usually drops depending on the degree of CHF. This effect will be seen bilaterally. If it is seen on only one side, then obstruction should be considered as the reason for decreased flow. Patients on balloon pumps after surgery also exhibit unique flow (Figure 35-10).

Pathology

Atherosclerotic Disease. The location of any plaque visualized during the examination should be described, along with its length, surface characteristics (smooth vs. irregular), and echogenicity (homogeneous, heterogeneous, calcification). The extent of plaque may be measured in a longitudinal or transverse plane by subjectively tracing the border of the plaque using the software measurement packages included with most imaging systems. Measuring plaque, however, is not a reliable method for determining the percentage of narrowing. Although the

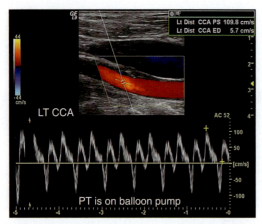

FIGURE 35-10 Common carotid artery *(CCA)* waveform with a patient on an intra-aortic balloon pump.

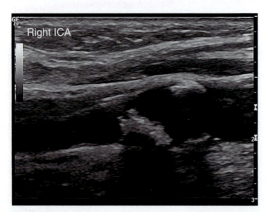

FIGURE 35-11 A longitudinal view of the internal carotid artery *(ICA)*. The plaque's surface is irregular.

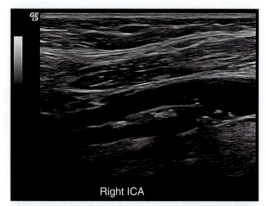

FIGURE 35-12 A calcified plaque near the origin of the internal carotid artery *(ICA)*. Calcified plaques cause a dropout deep to their location. This shadow can affect the gray scale and the color Doppler display.

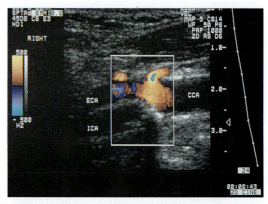

FIGURE 35-13 Occlusion of the internal carotid artery *(ICA)*. There is no color Doppler information, and a spectral Doppler waveform could not be located from the ICA. Blood flow is present in the external carotid artery *(ECA)*. The superior thyroid branch is visualized at the distal common carotid artery *(CCA)*.

surface of a plaque may be described as smooth or irregular (Figure 35-11), imaging is not a valid and reliable testing modality to identify plaque ulceration.[1,10,31] The echogenicity of plaque is usually described as homogeneous if it demonstrates a uniform level of echogenicity and texture throughout the plaque, and heterogeneous if the plaque has mixed areas of echogenicity and textures. This heterogeneity is important, as it may represent degenerative changes in the plaque or hemorrhage under the plaque that can result in plaque emboli. Calcification is very dense and is visualized as brightly echogenic areas in the plaque. A calcified plaque is usually visualized with an accompanying acoustic shadow that obscures imaging information deep to it (Figure 35-12). Multiple views of an artery from different scanning planes in most cases will minimize the shadowing associated with calcified plaque and will allow visualization and Doppler interrogation of the artery.

It is very important for patient management to differentiate between a high-grade stenosis and an occlusion of the ICA (Figure 35-13). An ICA occlusion is not amenable to surgical intervention. If an ICA is to be characterized as occluded, the artery should be evaluated with Doppler, color Doppler, and power Doppler to rule out the presence of trickle flow. In determining whether

the ICA is occluded, the color PRF should be decreased to document the presence of any slow-moving blood flow, and the color gain should be increased to enhance any blood flow that may be present. The ICA should be sampled at multiple sites with spectral Doppler. Increasing the sample volume size may be helpful when trying to locate the presence of any blood flow. Secondary ultrasound characteristics of an ICA occlusion include echogenic material filling the lumen, lack of arterial pulsations, reversed blood flow (color display) near the proximal origin of the occlusion, loss of diastolic blood flow in the ipsilateral CCA (Figure 35-14), increased blood flow velocity in the ipsilateral ECA, and increased velocity in the contralateral ICA. Occlusion of the ECA or CCA may also occur and should be documented during a carotid duplex imaging examination. At times, the CCA may be occluded and the ICA and ECA may remain patent. Usually, retrograde blood flow in the ECA supplies the ICA. In this imaging presentation, it is important to document the blood flow direction and the velocity in the ECA and the ICA.

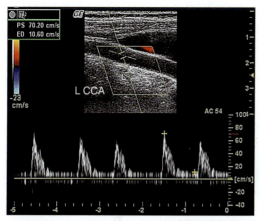

FIGURE 35-14 This common carotid artery *(CCA)* exhibits the high resistive waveform seen with distal internal carotid artery *(ICA)* occlusion. All the flow from the CCA is entering the external carotid artery *(ECA)*.

Aneurysms. Aneurysms of the cervical carotid system are rare. Most patients present with a pulsatile mass of the neck, and a bruit is often noted.

Sonographic Findings. In most cases, carotid duplex imaging demonstrates a tortuous CCA. In cases of aneurysms, however, the vessel diameter will be significantly increased. An aneurysm can be considered if the diameter of the vessel is 50% larger than the diameter just proximal to it. The abnormal blood flow pattern demonstrated within the aneurysm by color Doppler and by the Doppler signal depends on the size of the aneurysm.

Pseudoaneurysms. False aneurysms can occur in the presence of trauma, iatrogenically, or in association with pathologies that can weaken the arterial wall, such as dissections or arteritis. Patients will present with a pulsatile mass of the neck.

Sonographic Findings. A round, masslike lesion adjacent to the artery should be identified. This lesion may exhibit to-and-fro flow in color and spectral Doppler with connection to the artery by a neck. Sizes of the pseudoaneurysm and the neck connection can be variable depending on the cause and should be documented to help determine the choice of correction. Thrombosis may be seen in cases of spontaneous occlusion.

Dissection. Some of the common causes of a carotid artery dissection are blunt and penetrating trauma, acceleration-deceleration cervical injuries, and neck flexion. A carotid artery dissection can occur between any layers of the arterial wall. Thin-walled dissections may represent a tear between the intimal and medial layers, whereas thick-walled dissections may represent medial and adventitial layer separation (Figure 35-15). Dissections near the adventitial layer may result in a pseudoaneurysm. Flow between any of these walls is known as the *false lumen*. Dissections can be unilateral or bilateral. Evaluation of dissections is important

because they can cause complete obstruction in the carotid vessels, which can lead to an ischemic stroke.

Sonographic Findings. Different blood flow patterns in the two lumina should be documented with color Doppler and spectral Doppler waveforms. In some cases, the ICA has a gradual taper ending at the base of the skull, causing a decrease in peak systolic velocity with a high resistance pattern. Luminal narrowing of the vessel without visualization of plaque is characteristic of a dissection.

Fibromuscular Dysplasia. Fibromuscular dysplasia (FMD) is a nonatherosclerotic disease that usually affects the media of the arterial wall in medium-sized arteries. It predominantly occurs in the renal arteries and in the midsegment of the ICA, is bilateral in approximately 65% of cases, and occurs most often in females. FMD has been described as having a "string of pearls" appearance on arteriography. This pattern causes multiple arterial dilations separated by concentric stenosis.

Sonographic Findings. Color Doppler imaging may reveal turbulent blood flow patterns adjacent to the arterial wall, along with the absence of atherosclerotic plaque in the proximal and distal segments of the ICA. Diagnosis of this disease is usually made in conjunction with arteriography or computed tomography angiography (CTA) or magnetic resonance angiography (MRA) studies.

Carotid Body Tumors. Carotid body tumors are slow-growing neoplasms of the carotid body. The carotid body is a small (3- to 5-mm) chemoreceptor that lies within the adventitial layer on the posterior aspect of the carotid bifurcation. The carotid body assists in regulating heart rate, blood pressure, and respiration. The carotid body tumor is a relatively rare, hypervascular structure that usually lies between the ICA and ECA. Blood is supplied to most carotid body tumors via branches of the ECA.

Sonographic Findings. Carotid body tumors tend to be incidental findings on a carotid examination. The carotid body tumor usually lies between the ICA and ECA, may displace an artery from its normal location, and is supplied by branches of the ECA. Its hypervascularity is easily identified by color Doppler imaging (Figure 35-16).

Currently, the best carotid duplex imaging examinations will be achieved by proper attention to detail. Major areas of focus when performing carotid duplex imaging examinations are summarized in Box 35-2. Attention to these technical areas and interpretation details will ensure the best carotid duplex imaging results.

INTERPRETATION OF CAROTID DUPLEX IMAGING

Accurate interpretation of a carotid duplex imaging examination depends on the quality and the completeness of the evaluation. Often the patient's body habitus will affect the quality of the image, as will the sonographer's

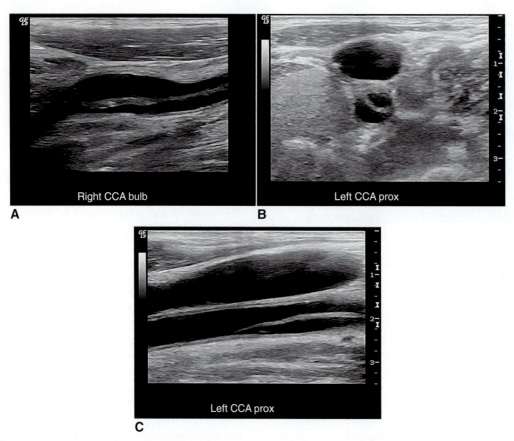

FIGURE 35-15 This is a 39-year-old female who presented to the ER with strokelike symptoms. Carotid sonography revealed bilateral common carotid artery *(CCA)* dissections due to uncontrolled hypertension *(HTN)*. **A,** The right CCA is near the bulb with a thick dissection. **B,** The left CCA is in transverse; true and false lumina are seen. **C,** Dissection is seen in the distal CCA on the left.

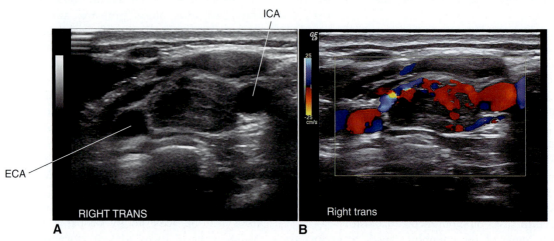

FIGURE 35-16 A, Transverse image of a carotid body tumor in gray scale. The internal carotid artery *(ICA)* and the external carotid artery *(ECA)* can be seen on each side of the tumor. **B,** Color flow in the tumor.

ability to search the entire carotid system with Doppler. The sonographer must be prepared to switch transducers if necessary to complete the carotid examination, and it is imperative to have a complete understanding of the equipment controls to optimize the image and Doppler information. Peak-systolic velocity, end-diastolic velocity, direction of blood flow, and shape of the Doppler spectral waveforms should be evaluated bilaterally.

Symmetry of the Doppler spectral waveforms should be noted. Abnormal waveform shape (increased or decreased pulsatility) may be an indicator of more proximal (innominate, subclavian) or distal (intracranial) disease. Blood flow reversal is uncommon; however, it may occur in patients with aortic valve regurgitation, arrhythmias, dissections, subclavian steals, or intra-aortic balloon pumps.

TABLE 35-1 | **Diagnostic Criteria for the Proximal Internal Carotid Artery***

Diameter Reduction	Peak Systolic Velocity	End-Diastolic Velocity
<50%	<125 cm/sec	N/A
50%–79%	≥125 cm/sec	N/A
80%–99%	>125 cm/sec	≥140 cm/sec
Occlusion	No signal	No signal

Courtesy Carotid Research Laboratory, University of Washington, 1991.
N/A, Not applicable.
*60-degree angle.

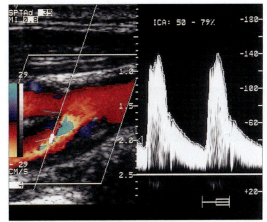

FIGURE 35-17 An example of a 50% to 79% diameter reduction of the internal carotid artery. The peak-systolic velocity is approximately 140 cm/sec, and the end-diastolic velocity is 35 cm/sec. The color Doppler information was used as a guide to sweep the Doppler sample volume through the area of increased velocity. Note that the Doppler signal was obtained with the sample volume parallel to the vessel walls, and not the color jet.

To determine the degree of stenosis present, complete Doppler evaluation of the carotid arterial system is necessary.[15] The Doppler spectral waveform should demonstrate elevated velocity through the narrowed segment, and color changes (aliasing) should be present. Poststenotic disturbances distal to the stenosis will be demonstrated by bidirectional turbulent blood flow patterns (spectral broadening). Additionally, a mottled color pattern will consist of aliasing and multiple directions of blood flow. The highest velocity obtained from an ICA stenosis is used to classify the degree of narrowing. Doppler signals obtained distal to the area of poststenotic flow disturbance may be normal or diminished, and the upstroke of the distal Doppler spectral waveform may be slowed. Multiple diagnostic criteria (peak-systolic velocity, end-diastolic velocity, ICA/CCA ratios) have been used to explain the varying degrees of narrowing of the ICA suggested by various investigators.[8,9,12,14,16,18,19,21,22,24,28] The most important recommendation is that each institution should establish its own diagnostic criteria by comparing carotid duplex imaging results versus conventional arteriography or magnetic resonance arteriography.

The information in Table 35-1 was put forth by the Carotid Research Laboratory at the University of Washington. These diagnostic criteria have been used successfully by many investigators to categorize disease from the origin of the ICA. These well-documented diagnostic criteria are a good starting point for any institution before it establishes its own diagnostic criteria (Figures 35-17 and 35-18). Internal carotid artery peak systolic velocities are normally approximately 60 to 80 cm/sec in older individuals and about 80 to 100 cm/sec in younger individuals.

Because the carotid endarterectomy trials (the North American Symptomatic Carotid Endarterectomy Trial [NASCET],[25] the Asymptomatic Carotid Atherosclerosis Study [ACAS],[13] and the European Carotid Surgery Trial [ECST])[29] used specific thresholds for surgical treatment, ultrasound criteria for ICA stenosis greater than 70% and greater than 60% were necessary to classify patients. Investigators have found that an ICA-CCA peak-to-systolic velocity (PSV) ratio is useful in grading ICA stenosis greater than 70% and greater than 60%. These ratios (Table 35-2) are calculated by using the highest PSV from the origin of the ICA divided by the highest PSV from the CCA (straight mid to distal segment). Again, many investigators have used different ICA-CCA ratios to document varying degrees of ICA narrowing.

In the presence of an ICA occlusion, the velocity in the contralateral ICA may be elevated. This may lead to overreading of the extent of disease in the patent ICA.[7,13,32] To avoid overestimation of the ICA stenosis contralateral to an ICA occlusion, new velocity criteria have been suggested.[13] The velocity criteria use a peak-systolic velocity greater than 140 cm/sec (instead of greater than 125 cm/sec) for a stenosis with a greater

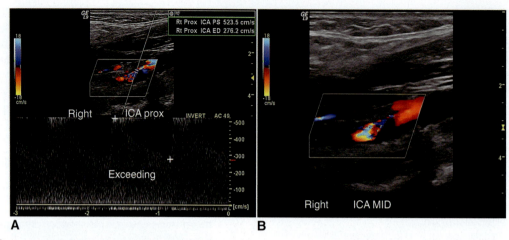

A   **B**

FIGURE 35-18 A, An example of a greater than 80% diameter reduction in stenosis of the internal carotid artery. The peak-systolic velocity is greater than 523 cm/sec, and the end-diastolic velocity is greater than 276 cm/sec. This waveform exceeded the Nyquist limit. **B,** Note the aliasing of the color Doppler near the origin of the internal carotid artery.

TABLE 35-2	ICA/CCA Peak-Systolic Velocity Ratios for the Proximal Internal Carotid Artery
Diameter Reduction	**Internal Carotid Artery/ Common Diameter Carotid Artery Peak Systolic Reduction Velocity Ratio**
70%–99%*	>4
60%–99%*	>3.2
>50%	>2.0

*Data from Moneta GL, Edwards JM, Papanicolaou G, et al: *J Vasc Surg* 21:989, 1995.

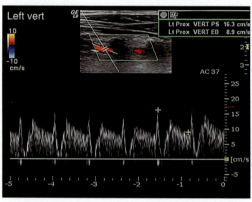

FIGURE 35-19 This left vertebra exhibits antegrade flow with a fast decline in flow velocity after the early systolic upstroke. This is what is known as the "bunny rabbit" sign. It represents an early indicator of subclavian steal syndrome.

than 50% diameter reduction. For a stenosis with greater than 80% diameter reduction of the lumen, the new criteria use an end-diastolic velocity of greater than 155 cm/sec (instead of greater than 140 cm/sec).

Evaluation of normal vertebral arteries produces wide variation in velocities. Absolute velocities are not useful in diagnosing stenosis. Poststenotic disturbances in the vertebral artery and dampening of the Doppler waveform may suggest a proximal obstruction. It is also important to evaluate the artery for the direction of blood flow and to look for any other changes in the waveform. A subclavian steal is present if reversal of vertebral artery blood flow direction occurs secondary to a significant obstruction proximal to the origin of the vertebral artery in the ipsilateral subclavian or innominate artery. Early signs of subclavian steal include a vertebral artery Doppler signal displaying an alternating (toward and away) pattern or antegrade flow with a fast decline in flow velocity after the early systolic upstroke. This gives the waveform the appearance of the "bunny rabbit" (Figure 35-19). If either pattern occurs in the vertebral artery, it may change to complete reversal of blood flow direction with arm exercise or after reactive hyperemia of the ipsilateral arm. This may be docu-

mented by monitoring the vertebral artery Doppler signal after release of a blood pressure cuff that has been inflated above systolic pressure on the ipsilateral arm for approximately 3 minutes.

The evaluation of normal subclavian arteries produces multiphasic high-resistance Doppler signals. The color flow pattern from the subclavian artery will reflect the high peripheral resistance. Blood flow will be toward the transducer in peak systole, away from the transducer in early diastole, and toward the transducer in late diastole. If a significant stenosis or occlusion of the proximal segment of this vessel occurs, the Doppler signal distal to the stenosis will be monophasic. A difference of blood pressure in the arms greater than 20 mmHg is usually associated with disease of the subclavian or innominate artery on the side with the lower blood pressure.

Other information important to include in the interpretation of a carotid duplex imaging examination is (1) the location of the stenosis, (2) the extent of the plaque and patency of the distal ICA, (3) the presence of tortuosity or kinking of the vessels, and (4) plaque characteristics (smooth vs. irregular surface, calcification). Additionally, the report should include any variation from the protocol, whether the quality of the examination was not optimal (e.g., body habitus), and any atypical Doppler waveforms noted.

At many institutions, carotid duplex imaging may be the only diagnostic imaging modality that is performed before a patient undergoes carotid endarterectomy. Careful imaging technique and the appropriate interpretation of results are essential in addressing several important questions. The questions that should be answered by a carotid duplex imaging examination are listed in Box 35-3.

Consistency of findings on gray scale, color Doppler, and Doppler spectral waveforms will limit errors in interpretation of carotid duplex imaging examinations. However, many pitfalls have been noted in the interpretation of these examinations. The more common errors encountered when interpreting carotid duplex imaging examinations are listed in Box 35-4. Proper technique is essential in performing accurate carotid duplex imaging examinations and minimizing errors in interpretation.

OTHER CLINICAL APPLICATIONS AND EMERGING TECHNIQUES

Intraoperative Use of Carotid Duplex Imaging

Assessment of the carotid endarterectomy site by duplex imaging for technical adequacy is an effective method to improve the results of the operation. Ultrasound transducers (10 MHz) designed for intraoperative use identify disturbed blood flow and anatomic abnormalities, such as residual plaque at the endarterectomy end point, thrombus, intimal flap, suture stenosis, platelet aggregation, and clamp or shunt trauma. Intraoperative carotid imaging is performed after the procedure, but before skin closure. The transducer is placed in a sterile sleeve, and imaging is performed on the exposed artery. It has been established that the detection of intraoperative peak systolic velocities greater than 150 cm/sec with the presence of an anatomic defect warrants correction because of its potential to progress.[5] Several investigators have reported that the use of routine intraoperative carotid duplex imaging has had a favorable impact on the stroke rate and the incidence of restenosis of the carotid artery.[2,5,11]

Carotid Duplex Imaging After Stent Placement or Endarterectomy

Carotid artery stenting is a technique that has been introduced as an alternative to carotid endarterectomy in selected patients.[6] The gray-scale image of a stent produces bright echoes (Figure 35-20). The velocity criteria established to identify disease in the native carotid arteries may not be sensitive in identifying a stenosis after carotid artery stent placement.[29] The stent is of a smaller diameter than the native vascular lumen, and the size difference or the lack of elasticity may cause an increase in velocity within the stent. Other anatomic configurations, such as the carotid bulb, may cause a significant diameter change between the native vessel and the stent, which may cause increased velocity within the stent. Duplex imaging, however, has been useful in detecting carotid artery stent occlusion. The performance of carotid duplex imaging following stent placement is in its infancy. As more experience is gained, diagnostic criteria will be developed and error in interpretation will be avoided in the future.

Carotid duplex imaging performed after carotid endarterectomy may reveal residual or recurrent stenosis in the ipsilateral ICA and disease progression in the contralateral ICA.[30] A follow-up duplex imaging examination should be performed approximately 1 to 3 months after a carotid endarterectomy. The time interval for follow-up after the initial postoperative study depends on the status of the artery after endarterectomy and the amount of disease present in the contralateral ICA. If a carotid patch is used, then imaging immediately after endarterectomy is difficult because the synthetic material often retains air, and information can be obtained only proximal and distal to the patch. The gas present in the synthetic material is usually reabsorbed within a few days and then can be evaluated.

If the operated carotid artery and the contralateral carotid artery demonstrate narrowing that is less than 50% diameter reduction, the patient is followed by carotid imaging annually. If the operated carotid artery or the contralateral nonoperated carotid artery demonstrates greater than 50% diameter reduction, the next postoperative scans are performed at 6-month intervals.

Also be aware of the occasional carotid bypass patients. These include carotid-to-carotid bypass for cases of severe proximal CCA stenosis, subclavian-to-ICA bypass for cases of complete CCA occlusion with still patent ICA, and proximal CCA-to-proximal ICA bypass (Figure 35-21) for cases of severe distal CCA stenosis. Bypasses are generally done in an emergency setting in patients with acute onset of stroke symptoms and no signs of collateral pathway flow.

Carotid Intima-Media Thickness

High-resolution gray-scale (B-mode) imaging is used to measure the intima-media thickness (IMT) of the carotid artery to detect early atherosclerotic changes. Carotid IMT is the distance between the lumen-intima interface and the media-adventitia interface. If monitored in a consistent method, IMT can be used as a marker of progression or regression of atherosclerotic disease.[3] Individuals with increased carotid IMT are more likely to suffer stroke and myocardial infarction than those with thinner walls.[4,26,27,33] Additionally, individuals with hypercholesterolemia have increased IMT compared with individuals with normal cholesterol levels.[17] To accurately measure carotid IMT, investigators must be experienced; must use an imaging protocol, modern equipment, and a high-frequency transducer (>7 MHz); and must acquire multiple samples from a longitudinal view (Figure 35-22). Some institutions consider 1 mm the upper limit of normal thickness.

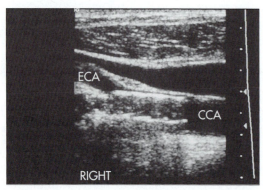

FIGURE 35-20 A longitudinal view of the carotid system. The bright echoes within the lumen are from the stent. The stent is placed in the distal common carotid artery *(CCA)* and extends into the bifurcation area near the origin of the external carotid artery *(ECA)*.

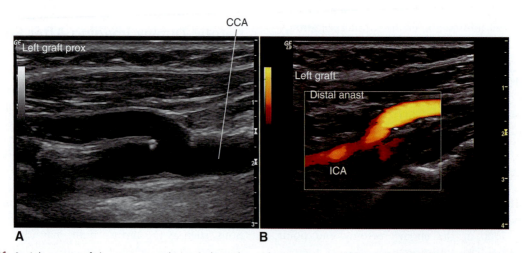

FIGURE 35-21 **A,** A bypass graft is anastomosed anteriorly to the mid common carotid artery *(CCA)*. **B,** Power Doppler demonstrates the flow from the graft into the proximal internal carotid artery *(ICA)*. A severe stenosis was present in the distal CCA that this graft was bypassing.

New Developments

Extended field of view, color Doppler, tissue harmonic imaging, echo-enhanced imaging, and B-flow imaging (Figures 35-23 and 35-24) are current developments in equipment capabilities that have improved the accuracy of carotid imaging. It is important to maintain state-of-the-art duplex imaging systems to provide accurate carotid evaluations for high-quality patient care.

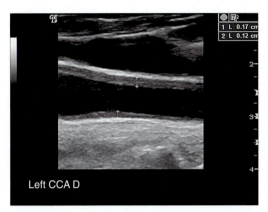

FIGURE 35-22 Intima-media thickness *(IMT)* see "crossbars" demonstrated on the anterior and posterior walls of the distal common carotid artery *(CCA)*. Both of these demonstrate abnormal thickness.

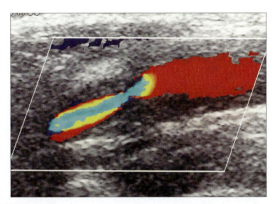

FIGURE 35-23 A color Doppler image of the origin of the internal carotid artery. Note the color Doppler aliasing, which suggests increased velocity associated with the plaque.

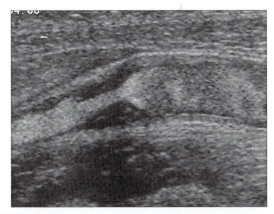

FIGURE 35-24 A B-flow image of the internal carotid artery shown in Figure 35-23. Note the improved visualization of the plaque versus the lumen near the origin of the vessel and the improved visualization of the distal vessel.

REFERENCES

1. Arnold JA, Modaresi KB, Thomas N, et al: Carotid plaque characterization by duplex scanning: observer error may undermine current clinical trials, *Stroke* 30:61-65, 1999.
2. Baker WH, Koustas G, Burke K, et al: Intraoperative duplex scanning and late carotid artery stenosis, *J Vasc Surg* 19:829-832, 1994.
3. Baldassarre D, Amato M, Bondioli A, et al: Carotid artery intima-media thickness measured by ultrasonography in normal clinical practice correlates well with atherosclerotic risk factors, *Stroke* 31:2426-2430, 2000.
4. Baldassarre D, Tremoli E, Amato M, et al: Reproducibility validation study comparing analog and digital imaging technologies for the measurement of intima-media thickness, *Stroke* 31:1104-1110, 2000.
5. Bandyk DF, Mills JL, Gahtan V, Esses GE: Intraoperative duplex scanning of arterial reconstructions: fate of repaired and unrepaired defects, *J Vasc Surg* 20:426-432, 1994.
6. Bowser AN, Bandyk DF, Evans A, et al: Outcome of carotid stent-assisted angioplasty versus open surgical repair of recurrent carotid stenosis, *J Vasc Surg* 38:432-438, 2003.
7. Busuttil SJ, Franklin DP, Youkey JR, Elmore JR: Carotid duplex overestimation of stenosis due to severe contralateral disease, *Am J Surg* 172:144-147, 1996.
8. Carpenter JP, Lexa FJ, Davis JT: Determination of duplex Doppler ultrasound criteria appropriate to the North American Symptomatic Carotid Endarterectomy Trial, *Stroke* 27:695-699, 1996.
9. Carpenter JP, Lexa FJ, Davis JT: Determination of sixty percent or greater carotid artery stenosis by duplex Doppler ultrasonography, *J Vasc Surg* 22:697-703, 1995.
10. Comerota AJ, Katz ML, White JV, Grosh JD: The preoperative diagnosis of the ulcerated carotid atheroma, *J Vasc Surg* 11:505-510, 1990.
11. Dykes JR 2nd, Bergamini TM, Dipski DA, et al: Intraoperative duplex scanning reduces both residual stenosis and postoperative morbidity of carotid endarterectomy, *Am Surg* 63:50-54, 1997.
12. Fillinger MF, Baker RJ Jr, Zwolak RM, et al: Carotid duplex criteria for a 60% or greater angiographic stenosis: variation according to equipment, *J Vasc Surg* 24:856-864, 1996.
13. Fujitani RM, Mills JL, Wang LM, Taylor SM: The effect of unilateral internal carotid artery occlusion upon contralateral duplex study: criteria for accurate interpretation, *J Vasc Surg* 16:459-467, 1992.
14. Grant EG, Duerinckx AJ, El Saden SM, et al: Ability to use duplex US to quantify internal carotid arterial stenoses: fact or fiction? *Radiology* 214:247-252, 2000.
15. Grant EG, Benson CB, Moneta GL, et al: Carotid artery stenosis: gray scale and Doppler US diagnosis. Society of Radiologists in Ultrasound Consensus Conference, *Radiology* 229:340-346, 2003.
16. Grant EG, Duerinckx AJ, El Saden SM, et al: Doppler sonographic parameters for detection of carotid stenosis: is there an optimum method for their selection? *AJR Am J Roentgenol* 172:1123-1129, 1999.
17. Hodis HN, Mack WJ, LaBree L, et al: The role of carotid arterial intima-media thickness in predicting clinical coronary events, *Ann Intern Med* 128:262-269, 1998.
18. Hood DB, Mattos MA, Mansour A, et al: Prospective evaluation of new duplex criteria to identify a 70% internal carotid stenosis, *J Vasc Surg* 23:254-261, 1996.

19. Kuntz KM, Polak JF, Whittemore AD, et al: Duplex ultrasound criteria for the identification of carotid stenosis should be laboratory specific, *Stroke* 28:597-602, 1997.

20. Lee VS, Hertzberg BS, Kliewer MA, Carroll BA: Assessment of stenosis: implications of variability of Doppler measurements in normal-appearing carotid arteries, *Radiology* 212:493-498, 1999.

21. Moneta GH, Edwards JM, Chitwood RW, et al: Correlation of North America Symptomatic Carotid Endarterectomy Trial (NASCET) angiographic definition of 70% to 99% internal carotid artery stenosis with duplex scanning, *J Vasc Surg* 17:152-159, 1995.

22. Moneta GH, Edwards JM, Papanicolaou G, et al: Screening for asymptomatic carotid internal carotid artery stenosis: duplex criteria for discriminating 60% to 99% stenosis, *J Vasc Surg* 21:989-994, 1995.

23. American Heart Association: *Heart disease and stroke statistics, 2005 update*, Dallas, 2005, American Heart Association.

24. Nehler MR, Moneta GL, Lee RW, et al: Improving selection of patients with less than 60% asymptomatic internal carotid artery stenosis for follow-up of carotid artery duplex scanning, *J Vasc Surg* 23:580-585, 1996.

25. North American Symptomatic Carotid Endarterectomy Trial Collaborators: Beneficial effect of carotid endarterectomy in symptomatic patients with high grade carotid stenosis, *N Engl J Med* 325:445-453, 1991.

26. O'Leary DH, Polak JF, Kronmal RA, et al: Thickening of the carotid wall: a marker for atherosclerosis in the elderly? Cardiovascular Health Study Collaborative Research Group, *Stroke* 27:224-231, 1996.

27. O'Leary DH, Polak JF: Intima-media thickness: a tool for atherosclerotic imaging and event prediction, *Am J Cardiol* 90:18L-21L, 2002.

28. Primozich JF: Color flow in the carotid evaluation, *J Vasc Tech* 15:112-122, 1991.

29. Randomized trial of endarterectomy for recently symptomatic carotid stenosis: final results of the MRC European Carotid Surgery Trial (ECST), *Lancet* 351:1379-1387, 1998.

30. Roth SM, Back MR, Bandyk MF, et al: A rational algorithm for duplex scan surveillance after carotid endarterectomy, *J Vasc Surg* 30:453-460, 1999.

31. Sitzer M, Müller W, Rademacher J, et al: Color-flow Doppler-assisted duplex imaging fails to detect ulceration in high-grade internal carotid artery stenosis, *J Vasc Surg* 23:461-465, 1996.

32. Spadone DP, Barkmeier LD, Hodgson KJ, et al: Contralateral internal carotid artery stenosis or occlusion: pitfall of correct ipsilateral classification—a study performed with color-flow imaging, *J Vasc Surg* 11:642-649, 1990.

33. Vemmos KN, Tsivgoulos G, Spengos K, et al: Common carotid artery intima-media thickness in patients with brain infarction and intracerebral haemorrhage, *Cerebrovasc Dis* 17:280-286, 2004.

Intracranial Cerebrovascular Evaluation

Ann Willis and Mira L. Katz

OBJECTIVES

On completion of this chapter, you should be able to:
- Distinguish normal from abnormal intracranial arterial anatomy
- Discuss the technical aspects of transcranial color Doppler imaging
- Describe the characteristics of the Doppler waveforms of arteries evaluated during a transcranial color Doppler examination

- List the clinical applications of transcranial color Doppler imaging and describe the diagnostic criteria associated with each
- Discuss common errors associated with performing and interpreting a transcranial color Doppler imaging examination

---

OUTLINE

Significant progress has been made in the noninvasive evaluation of cerebrovascular disease during the past 25 years, especially in the area of extracranial vasculature. Development of a noninvasive method to interrogate the intracranial arterial system lagged because of the attention focused on surgically correctable lesions of the carotid bifurcation and the difficulty in penetrating the skull with ultrasound. Technical sophistication has progressed and experience has been gained in the past decade to allow ultrasonic evaluation of the intracranial arterial system with the use of transcranial color Doppler (TCD) imaging.

The TCD technique was introduced in 1982 as a method to detect cerebral arterial vasospasm after subarachnoid hemorrhage. Since its introduction, TCD has been used for many different clinical applications (Box 36-1). A better understanding of intracranial arterial hemodynamics may be gained by using TCD in many different clinical settings.

Accurate interpretation of a patient's TCD examination is not possible without knowledge of the amount and location of atherosclerotic disease in the extracranial vasculature. Carotid and vertebral duplex imaging should be performed before the TCD examination because extensive extracranial disease may cause changes in the velocity profile or direction of blood flow in a patient's intracranial arterial system.

INTRACRANIAL ARTERIAL ANATOMY

Blood supply to the brain is provided by the carotid (anterior) and vertebral (posterior) arteries. Familiarity

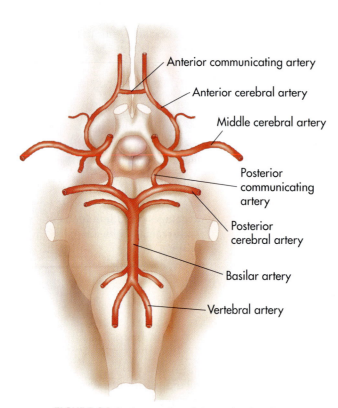

FIGURE 36-1 The arteries of the circle of Willis.

with the anatomy of the large intracranial arteries is requisite to performing accurate TCD imaging examinations.

This chapter concentrates on the intracranial arteries that make up the circle of Willis (Figure 36-1). The extracranial portion of the carotid and vertebral arteries is described in Chapter 35.

Internal Carotid Artery

The **internal carotid artery (ICA)** is divided into four main segments: (1) The cervical ICA originates at the common carotid bifurcation and ends as the artery enters the carotid canal of the temporal bone at the base of the skull; (2) the petrous section of the ICA begins as the ICA enters the carotid canal within the petrous portion of the bone and continues until it crosses over the cranial portion of the foramen lacerum and passes into the cavernous sinus; (3) the cavernous segment of the ICA runs from the foramen lacerum and cavernous sinus entrance to just medial of the anterior clinoid process; and (4) the supraclinoid portion of the ICA enters the intracranial space at the anterior clinoid and continues to its termination in the middle cerebral and anterior cerebral arteries. The portion of the ICA that forms two curves (S shape) is termed the *carotid siphon*. The segments of the ICA that are evaluated during a TCD examination are the terminal portion of the ICA just proximal to the origin of the middle cerebral artery and anterior cerebral artery and the carotid siphon. The internal carotid siphon may be the site of atherosclerotic disease in adults.

Ophthalmic Artery

The ophthalmic artery is the first branch of the ICA and is evaluated during TCD imaging. It courses anterolaterally and slightly downward through the optic foramen to supply the globe, orbit, and adjacent structures. The ophthalmic artery has three major groups of branches: the ocular branches, the orbital branches, and the extraorbital branches. The branches of the ophthalmic artery often play an important role in collateral pathways that form as a result of disease of the internal or external carotid arteries.

Middle Cerebral Artery

The **middle cerebral artery (MCA)** is the larger terminal branch of the ICA. From its origin, the MCA extends laterally and horizontally in the lateral cerebral fissure. The horizontal segment may course downward or upward. The MCA either bifurcates or trifurcates before the limen insulae (a small gyrus), where the branches turn upward into the Sylvian fissure, forming its genu ("knee"). The vessels course around the island of Reil, which is a triangular mound of cortex, and runs posterosuperiorly within the Sylvian fissure. Terminal branches of the MCA anastomose with terminal branches of the anterior cerebral and posterior cerebral arteries.

The middle cerebral artery is usually divided into four segments (M1 to M4). The M1 branch and the origin of the M2 branch are evaluated during TCD imaging. The main horizontal section from its origin to the limen insulae is the M1 segment. The M1 segment gives rise to numerous small lenticulostriate branches. The M2 segment is composed of the branches overlying the insular surface in the deep Sylvian fissure. The initial MCA bifurcation is the third most common site for congenital aneurysms, giving rise to approximately one fourth of all intracranial aneurysms. The anterior communicating and posterior communicating arteries are the first and second most common sites for aneurysm formation, respectively. The MCA may also be the site for arterial stenosis and occlusion.

Anterior Cerebral Artery

The **anterior cerebral artery (ACA)** is the smaller of the two terminal branches of the ICA. The ACA is a midline marker. From its origin, the ACA courses anteromedially over the optic chiasm and the optic nerve to the interhemispheric fissure (longitudinal cerebral fissure). The proximal horizontal segment of the ACA is known as the A1 segment and is connected to the contralateral A1 segment via the anterior communicating artery (ACoA). The A1 segment is evaluated during a TCD imaging examination. The contour of the A1 segment may take a horizontal course, ascend, or slightly descend. Complete absence of the A1 segment is unusual. An anomalous origin of the ACA is rare, but asymmetry between the two A1 segments is common. A direct correlation exists between size of the A1 segment and the size of the ACoA. A small or hypoplastic A1 is usually found in conjunction with a large ACoA because the contralateral A1 segment supplies most of the blood flow to both distal ACA territories. Individuals with anomalies of the A1 segment have a slightly higher incidence of ACoA aneurysms. The ACA is a rare site for stenosis or occlusion.

Distal to the ACoA, the ACA turns superiorly and runs side-by-side in the interhemispheric fissure. The ACA curves anterosuperiorly around the genu of the corpus callosum. The segment of the ACA from the ACoA to the distal ACA bifurcation (callosomarginal artery and pericallosal artery) is termed the *A2 segment*. The proximal portion of the A2 segments may be visualized during TCD imaging in some patients. The distal A2 segments anastomose with branches of the posterior cerebral arteries. A large medial striate artery, the recurrent artery of Heubner, is a major branch of the proximal A2 segment in approximately 80% of cases, but this artery can also originate from the distal A1 segment.

Anterior Communicating Artery

The **anterior communicating artery (ACoA)** is a short vessel that connects the anterior cerebral arteries (A1) at the interhemispheric fissure. The ACoA may be absent or may be a single, duplicated, or multichanneled system. The longer ACoAs are found to be curved, tortuous, or kinked. The ACoA often is the location for congenital anomalies. The ACoA frequently is a site for aneurysm formation and is the most common site for aneurysms associated with subarachnoid hemorrhage. The ACoA is

short in length; although it may be captured in the Doppler sample volume at midline, it cannot be visualized during TCD imaging.

Posterior Cerebral Artery

The **posterior cerebral arteries (PCAs)** originate from the terminal basilar artery and course anteriorly and laterally. The segment of the PCA from its origin to its junction with the posterior communicating artery (PCoA) is termed P1, the precommunicating portion. The P1 segment is evaluated during TCD imaging. Many perforating branches that supply the brain stem and thalamus originate from this segment. The portion of the vessel extending posteriorly from the PCoA to the posterior aspect of the midbrain is the P2 segment and may be visualized during transcranial imaging. The P3 and P4 segments of the PCA are not visualized during transcranial imaging. The proximal portion of the PCA is usually asymmetrical. In cases of "fetal" origin, the P1 segment is hypoplastic or smaller than the PCoA. It is uncommon for occlusive disease to be limited to the PCA, but if it does occur, the P2 segment is most commonly affected.

Posterior Communicating Artery

The **posterior communicating artery (PCoA)** courses posteriorly and medially from the ICA to join the posterior cerebral artery. The PCoA is variable in size and may angle upward or downward. Hypoplasia is the common PCoA anomaly. However, the PCoA can be large when the posterior cerebral artery is hypoplastic, which occurs in 15% to 25% of cases. This is termed a *fetal* origin of the posterior cerebral artery. The PCoA is usually a potential rather than an actual arterial conduit. The PCoA generally does not function as an important collateral pathway unless the patient has extensive extracranial occlusive disease bilaterally or lacks a patent anterior communicating artery. The PCoA may be evaluated during TCD imaging examinations.

Vertebral Artery

The **vertebral arteries** are large branches of the subclavian arteries. Atherosclerotic changes usually occur at the origin of the vertebral arteries. The two vertebral arteries are equal in size in approximately 25% of cases; in other words, asymmetry in size is common. The left vertebral artery is usually the dominant artery. The vertebral artery is divided into four segments: extravertebral, intervertebral, horizontal, and intracranial. During TCD examinations, the intracranial segment of the vertebral artery is evaluated. The intracranial portion begins as it pierces the dura and arachnoid immediately below the base of the skull at the foramen magnum. It continues anterior and medial to the anterior surface of the medulla and unites with the contralateral vertebral artery to form the basilar artery. Several major branches arise from this segment of the vertebral artery. The anterior spinal artery and the posterior inferior cerebellar artery (PICA) are sometimes visualized during TCD imaging. The PICA is the largest branch of the vertebral artery and commonly arises approximately 1 to 2 cm proximal to the confluence of the two vertebral arteries.

Basilar Artery

The **basilar artery (BA)** is formed by the union of the two vertebral arteries and is evaluated during TCD imaging. It is variable in its pathway, size, and length. It usually originates at the lower border of the pons, extends anteriorly and superiorly, and terminates by dividing into the paired posterior cerebral arteries. During its course, the basilar artery gives off several branches, including the anterior inferior cerebellar arteries, the internal auditory (labyrinthine) arteries, the pontine branches, and the superior cerebellar arteries just proximal to the posterior cerebral arteries. The basilar artery is often tortuous and may be duplicated or fenestrated.

Circle of Willis

The **circle of Willis** was first described in 1664 by Thomas Willis. The circle is composed of the A1 segments of the two ACAs, the ACoA, the two PCoAs, the two ICAs, and the P1 segment of the two PCAs. It is a polygon vascular ring at the base of the brain that permits communication between the right and left cerebral hemispheres (via the ACoA) and between the anterior and posterior systems (via the PCoAs). These communications are important when there is significant disease or occlusion of one of the major cervical arteries. Variations of the circle of Willis are common: A "classic" circle of Willis is found in only approximately 20% to 25% of cases. Significant hypoplasia and absence of the PCoA, ACoA, ACA (A1), and PCA (P1) are the most common variations.

TECHNICAL ASPECTS OF TRANSCRANIAL COLOR DOPPLER IMAGING

Color Doppler imaging is currently being used to investigate the intracranial arterial circulation. To obtain consistently reliable studies with TCD imaging, the operator must appreciate the importance of proper patient positioning, use the available anatomic landmarks that are important for accurate identification of the intracranial arteries, and be knowledgeable about proper use of the instrument's controls. The accuracy of the examination will be increased by using the gray-scale image and the color display to guide the TCD evaluation.

Instrumentation

Instrument controls and control settings vary depending on the manufacturer of the color Doppler imaging system. Therefore, it is important for the operator to be familiar with the particular imaging system being used. Hard copy records of the spectral waveforms may be made using any of the standard formats, but a videocassette recording has the advantage of documenting the audio signal, in addition to the spectral waveforms.

TCD imaging is performed with a phased-array imaging transducer. A 2-MHz transducer (imaging and Doppler) is ideal for this application, although transmitting frequencies as high as 2.5 MHz have been used with success. High-quality TCD imaging depends on proper adjustment of several instrument controls. It is important to optimize the gray-scale image, know how each color control will independently affect the image, and understand how the different controls affect each other. The patient's arterial hemodynamics and information that is relevant to the patient being evaluated may result in the adjustment of different controls.

Instrument controls to consider when adjusting the gray-scale image during TCD imaging are sector width, image depth, overall gain, time gain compensation (TGC), focal zone, frame rate, and dynamic range.

The color Doppler display is very important during TCD imaging. It is used as a guide for correct placement of the sample volume to obtain detailed hemodynamic information from the Doppler spectral waveforms. The color box is moved to the area of interest on the gray-scale image. During TCD imaging, the entire circle of Willis often can be captured within a small color box. If this is not done, to maintain a good frame rate, the color box should remain small and the anterior and posterior circulations evaluated separately by moving the position of the color box. Instrument controls to consider when adjusting the color Doppler display during TCD include color gain, scale (pulse repetition frequency [PRF]), wall filter, sensitivity (ensemble length), and persistence.

The real-time display of all Doppler shift frequencies over time is the Doppler spectral waveform. Time is recorded along the horizontal axis, and velocity (frequency) is recorded on the vertical axis. Velocity is recorded in centimeters per second (cm/sec). A positive Doppler shift (toward the transducer) is displayed above the baseline and a negative Doppler shift (away from the transducer) below the baseline. Accurate recording of the intracranial Doppler spectral waveform is critical, because this is the basis for interpretation of the TCD imaging examination. Instrument controls to consider when obtaining Doppler signals are sample volume size, gain, velocity scale (PRF), baseline, wall filter, and output. During TCD imaging, Doppler power should be increased for adequate penetration. However, this should be done at the lowest level necessary and applied for the shortest duration possible to obtain good clinical information. The ALARA (*as low as reasonably achievable*) principle should be applied during TCD imaging examinations.

Technique

The standard transtemporal, transorbital, suboccipital, and submandibular windows are used for TCD imaging (Figure 36-2). Interpretation criteria previously developed with the nonimaging TCD technique are used with TCD imaging. TCD imaging, however, permits identification of structural landmarks that assist in accurately locating the intracranial arteries. Anatomic landmarks that are helpful in locating the circle of Willis when the transtemporal approach is used are the petrous ridge of the temporal bone, sphenoid bone, cerebral falx, suprasellar cistern, and cerebral peduncles. When the suboccipital approach is performed, the foramen magnum and the occipital bone are used as anatomic landmarks to locate the vertebrobasilar system. The globe and optic nerve are helpful anatomic landmarks for locating the ophthalmic artery and the carotid siphon when the transorbital window is used.

Conventional color orientation for TCD examinations is set for shades of red indicating blood flow toward the transducer and shades of blue indicating flow away from the transducer. By keeping this color assignment constant, intracranial blood flow direction in the arteries can be readily recognized.

TCD evaluation of the intracranial arteries is performed with a large sample volume (5 to 10 mm) to obtain a good signal-to-noise ratio. Intracranial arterial velocities acquired with TCD imaging are also acquired assuming a zero-degree angle. Several investigators have evaluated the potential use of angle-adjusted (corrected) velocities during TCD imaging.[12,30,40] Angle-adjusted velocities are elevated compared with velocities taken assuming a zero-degree angle. Considering that an intracranial artery is tortuous and lies in different ultrasound planes, angle adjustment is possible only for a short segment of the artery.[13] Although the data for angle adjustment appear interesting, they have not been thoroughly evaluated, and it is recommended that routine TCD imaging be performed assuming a zero-degree angle.

Additionally, with the use of TCD imaging, many investigators are reporting TCD results using peak-systolic and end-diastolic velocities instead of the traditionally accepted mean velocities (time-averaged peak velocities). Each institution has to decide which velocity value to report and adjust diagnostic criteria accordingly.

Transtemporal Window. The **transtemporal window** approach is performed with the patient in the supine position with the head aligned straight with the body. The transducer is placed on the temporal bone cephalad to the zygomatic arch and anterior to the ear. A generous amount of acoustic gel is necessary to ensure good transducer-to-skin contact, especially in patients for whom angling the transducer to optimize the Doppler signal requires the footprint to be elevated from the skin's surface.

Finding this window can be difficult and at times frustrating because ultrasound penetration of the temporal bone is necessary. Other windows used during the TCD examination are usually less difficult to find because natural ostia allow easy intracranial penetration of the ultrasound beam. The transtemporal window varies in size and location with each patient and may vary in an individual from one side to the other. Attenuation of the Doppler signal occurs at the temporal bone interface, and its magnitude depends on the thickness of the bone. One study found that the power measured behind the skull was never greater than 35% of transmitted power, and the mean value of power loss was 80%.[15] The ability to penetrate the temporal bone is influenced by the patient's age, sex, and race. Hyperostosis of the skull is commonly found in older individuals, females, and African Americans. A transtemporal window is not located in approximately 10% to 30% of the population.

The transducer's orientation marker or light should be pointing in the anterior direction, with the transducer angled slightly superiorly. This orientation of the transducer produces an imaging plane that is a transverse oblique view. This view has the advantage of providing simultaneous visualization of the anterior and posterior intracranial circulation in many patients. The ipsilateral hemisphere is at the top and the contralateral hemisphere at the bottom of the monitor, with anterior being to the left side and posterior to the right side of the monitor. Although the contralateral hemisphere is visualized in many patients, each hemisphere should be separately studied through the ipsilateral ultrasound window to

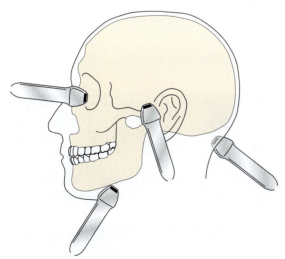

FIGURE 36-2 Placement of the ultrasound transducer for the four transcranial Doppler windows: transtemporal, transorbital, suboccipital, and submandibular approaches.

obtain the best artery-to-transducer angle. In patients with only a unilateral transtemporal window, however, evaluating the contralateral hemisphere is possible and may provide valuable information.

After the transtemporal window is located, identifying bony landmarks ensures position at the correct level within the skull to locate the circle of Willis. The reflective echo extending anteriorly is the lesser wing of the sphenoid bone, and the petrous ridge of the temporal bone extends posteriorly (Figures 36-3 and 36-4). The ipsilateral temporal lobe is at the top of the image.

Once the bony landmarks are identified, the color Doppler display is turned on (Figures 36-5 and 36-6). The terminal ICA (t-ICA) is visualized, and the direction of blood flow depends on the artery's anatomic configu-

ration. Blood flow is usually toward the transducer, and the mean velocity is normally 39 ± 9 cm/sec. At this anatomic location, mirror imaging artifact may be caused by the adjacent bone. The transducer is then angled anteriorly and superiorly so the MCA and ACA can be evaluated. The MCA courses adjacent to the sphenoid wing. The main trunk of the MCA is displayed in red because blood flow is normally toward the transducer. The mean velocity is normally 62 ± 12 cm/sec (Figure 36-7). The M2 branches are usually displayed in red but may appear blue as they curve and blood flows away from the transducer.

The ACA is displayed in shades of blue as it courses away from the transducer toward the midline. It may be necessary to angle the transducer slightly anteriorly and superiorly to visualize the ACA. The mean velocity is normally 50 ± 11 cm/sec. It may be necessary to decrease the color PRF to visualize this artery because of its lower velocity. The initial portion of the A2 segment often can be visualized and is displayed in blue extending in an anterior direction at midline.

The posterior circulation is visualized by angling the transducer slightly posteriorly and inferiorly, using the cerebral peduncles as an anatomic landmark. Normally

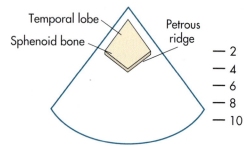

FIGURE 36-3 Schematic of the bony landmarks from the transtemporal approach.

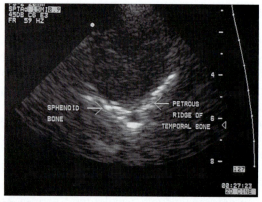

FIGURE 36-4 Image of the bony landmarks from the transtemporal approach.

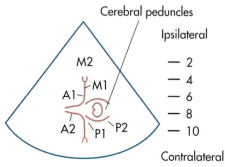

FIGURE 36-5 Schematic of the arteries in the circle of Willis from the transtemporal approach.

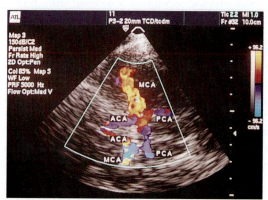

FIGURE 36-6 Color Doppler image of the intracranial arteries from the transtemporal approach. The ipsilateral hemisphere is at the top of the image, and the contralateral hemisphere at the bottom of the image. *ACA,* Anterior cerebral artery; *MCA,* middle cerebral artery; *PCA,* posterior cerebral artery.

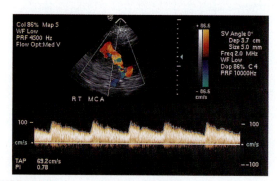

FIGURE 36-7 Doppler spectral waveform from the right *(RT)* middle cerebral artery *(MCA).* A zero-degree angle is used, and blood flow is toward the transducer.

the two cerebral peduncles are identical in size and shape and are of intermediate echogenicity. The PCA wraps around the cerebral peduncle. The color PRF may need to be decreased to visualize the PCAs because of lower blood flow velocity. The P1 segment is displayed in red because blood flow is normally toward the transducer. The normal mean velocity is 39 ± 10 cm/sec. Often the ipsilateral and contralateral P1 segments can be visualized at their origin as the basilar artery terminates. The ipsilateral P1 segment is seen in shades of red, and the contralateral P1 segment is displayed in shades of blue. The P2 segment may be displayed in red just distal to the origin of the PCoA but will be displayed in blue distally as it wraps around the cerebral peduncle. The color display of the P2 segment is variable because of the vessel's anatomic course and orientation to the transducer.

The ACoA is not visualized because it is short in length. However, the PCoA is longer in length and often is visualized connecting the anterior and posterior circulations in patients (Figure 36-8). The mean peak velocity in the PCoA is 36 ± 15 cm/sec, and the direction of blood flow may be toward or away from the transducer. The color PRF may need to be decreased to visualize the PCoA. Additionally, using power Doppler imaging may be helpful in locating the PCoA because this artery often courses parallel to the skin line.

Although the anterior and posterior circulations can be simultaneously visualized in many patients, the patient's anatomy often requires separate evaluation. Minor changes in the transducer's position on the surface of the skin or angle permit individual evaluation of either intracranial circulatory circulation.

The quality of the intracranial image depends on proper adjustment of many instrument controls. To obtain quality color Doppler images, increase the color gain to the appropriate level, maintain a small sector width and color box width to keep the highest possible frame rates, change the color PRF depending on the patient's hemodynamics or the particular intracranial artery being evaluated, and be aware of the color sensitivity and persistence settings. The color display is important because it assists in proper placement of the Doppler sample volume. The TCD examination is interpreted from the Doppler spectral waveform information. Doppler signals are obtained along the path of the artery using the color display as a road map. At each depth setting, it is important to adjust the sample volume and angle the transducer to optimize the Doppler signal. Additionally, it is important to remember that the color Doppler display is in two dimensions, and tortuous intracranial arteries frequently cannot be displayed along their length as a continuous color pathway.

Suboccipital Window. When the vertebrobasilar system is evaluated, the best results are obtained with the patient lying on his or her side with the head bowed slightly toward the chest. This position increases the gap between the cranium and the atlas. The orientation marker or light on the transducer should be pointing to the patient's right side. The transducer is placed on the posterior aspect of the neck inferior to the nuchal crest. The best images from this approach are acquired with the transducer slightly off midline, with the ultrasound beam directed toward the bridge of the patient's nose.

The large, circular, anechoic area seen from the **suboccipital window** is the foramen magnum, and the bright, echogenic reflection is from the occipital bone. Blood flow is normally away from the transducer in the vertebrobasilar system, and the color display appears as a blue Y. The right vertebral artery is displayed on the left side of the image, and the left vertebral artery is on the right side (Figure 36-9). The basilar artery is deep to the vertebral arteries (Figure 36-10). The mean velocity is 38 ± 10 cm/sec in the vertebral arteries and 41 ± 10 cm/sec in the basilar artery. Because the posterior circulation has lower velocities than the anterior circulation, the operator may need to decrease the color PRF to visualize the vertebrobasilar system.

TCD imaging allows visualization of the confluence of the vertebral arteries into the basilar artery. Attention to the color gain setting is critical when trying to measure the exact depth of the vertebral artery confluence. Additionally, branches of the vertebral arteries, especially the PICA, can often be visualized and are usually displayed in red as they curve and carry blood toward the transducer. Moving the transducer slightly inferiorly on the

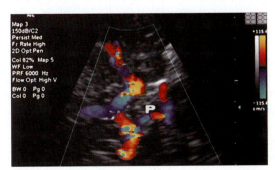

FIGURE 36-8 The posterior communicating artery (*P*) is visualized connecting the anterior and posterior intracranial arterial circulations.

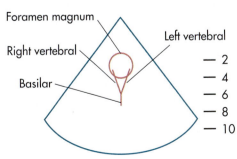

FIGURE 36-9 Schematic of the suboccipital approach during a transcranial Doppler imaging examination.

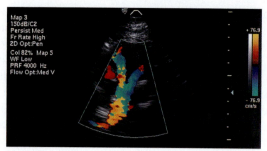

FIGURE 36-10 Color Doppler imaging from the suboccipital approach. Blood flow is away from the transducer and is displayed in blue. The right vertebral artery is on the left side of the image, and the left vertebral artery is displayed on the right side of the image. The basilar artery is deep to the vertebral arteries.

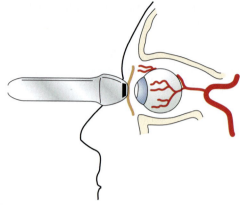

FIGURE 36-11 Schematic of the transorbital approach. The ophthalmic artery is a branch of the internal carotid artery.

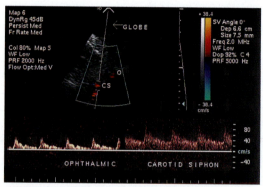

FIGURE 36-12 Color Doppler image of the transorbital approach. The ophthalmic Doppler spectral waveform demonstrates a high resistance signal, and the carotid siphon (*CS*) a low resistance signal. A mechanical index of 0.28 or less should be used when using the transorbital approach. *O*, Ophthalmic artery.

neck and angling superiorly often allows better visualization of the distal basilar artery. The terminal portion of the basilar artery as it bifurcates into the PCAs cannot be visualized from this TCD approach.

Transorbital Window. The **transorbital window** evaluation provides information about the ophthalmic artery and the carotid siphon. The U.S. Food and Drug Administration (FDA) has approved certain imaging transducers on various manufacturers' equipment for evaluation of the orbit. It is important for all operators to contact the appropriate ultrasound company to determine which transducer is approved for orbital imaging for their imaging system.

When imaging the orbit, it is important to decrease the power setting significantly before evaluating the orbit. Additionally, the examination time should be minimized. Although no observed bioeffects from ultrasound evaluation of the eye are known, the power settings raise concern for ocular damage. The current FDA maximum acoustic output allowable levels (derated) for ophthalmic imaging include a spatial peak temporal average intensity of 17 mW/cm^2 and a mechanical index of 0.28.

The examination is performed with the patient in the supine position and the transducer gently placed on the closed eyelid. A liberal amount of acoustic gel is important, and firm pressure on the eyelid is not necessary. The orientation marker on the imaging transducer should be pointed medially, toward the nose, when the right or left examination is performed. Evaluation of either eye produces an image with medial (nasal) on the left side and temporal on the right side of the monitor. A variation of this technique is to have the transducer's orientation marker directed to the patient's right side when evaluating either eye. This transducer orientation will produce an image with medial (nasal) on the monitor's left when examining the left eye and medial on the monitor's right side when evaluating the right eye. The globe is visualized at the top of the monitor.

The direction of blood flow in the carotid siphon depends on which segment (parasellar, genu, or supraclinoid) is insonated (Figure 36-11). Blood flow is bidirectional at the genu, toward the transducer in the parasellar portion, and away from the transducer in the supraclinoid segment. The mean velocity in the carotid siphon is 47 ± 14 cm/sec (Figure 36-12).

The **ophthalmic artery** is generally identified adjacent to the optic nerve. The color PRF should be decreased to visualize the ophthalmic artery. The ultrasound beam should be directed slightly medially along the anteroposterior plane. Blood flow is normally toward the transducer, with a mean velocity of 21 ± 5 cm/sec. The ophthalmic artery Doppler signal has a high pulsatility because this artery supplies blood to the globe and its structures.

Submandibular Window. The **submandibular window** approach is a continuation of the duplex imaging evaluation of the extracranial distal ICA. The transducer is placed at the angle of the mandible and is angled slightly medially and cephalad toward the carotid canal. The transducer's orientation marker or light is pointed in a superior direction. Distal ICA blood flow is away from the transducer and is displayed in shades of blue. Careful Doppler evaluation will distinguish the ICA's low resistance signal from the higher resistance signal from the extracranial artery (ECA). The mean velocity in the retromandibular portion of the ICA is normally 37 ± 9 cm/sec.

INTERPRETATION OF TRANSCRANIAL COLOR DOPPLER IMAGING

Standard interpretation criteria for TCD examinations have been reported in the literature. As the TCD examination evolved, however, it became apparent that important underlying physiologic variables may affect the intracranial velocities. Therefore, it is important to be aware of the factors that may affect intracranial hemodynamics and to interpret each case individually.

Proper identification of the intracranial vasculature is, of course, the first step in evaluating the TCD examination. Each TCD window provides access to specific arteries. Identification of the arteries is based on the following:

1. *Depth of the sample volume.* The sample volume depth is measured in millimeters (mm) and is the distance from the face of the ultrasound transducer to the middle of the Doppler sample volume. The sample volume length should be kept large (5 to 10 mm) to achieve the best signal-to-noise ratio. The depth ranges at which the intracranial arteries can be located from each TCD window are listed in Table 36-1. The depths of the arteries may vary with each individual, but in most adults, the artery in question will usually fall within these ranges. Midline is in the range of 70 to 80 mm in most adults.

2. *Angle of the transducer.* The angle of the transducer is important because different arteries can be insonated at the same depth from a TCD ultrasound window. The operator's position at the head of the patient will enable the best perception of the transducer-artery angle because it permits orientation of the ultrasound transducer to the body's axes and planes.

3. *Blood flow direction.* The normal direction of blood flow in the intracranial arteries relative to the ultrasound transducer is listed in Table 36-1. From the different approaches, Doppler spectral waveforms may demonstrate blood flow direction away from, toward, or in both directions (bidirectional). If the direction of blood flow is reversed from the established norm, it can be assumed that the artery is functioning as a collateral channel, or that there may be an anatomic variant.

4. *Spatial relationship.* Understanding the spatial relationship of one artery to another is helpful in properly identifying the intracranial arteries. Using the t-ICA bifurcation as a guide, the location of the intracranial arteries is determined with greater technical ease.

5. *Traceability of an artery.* The operator should be able to "trace" the anatomic route of the artery in stepwise fashion by increasing or decreasing the depth setting of the sample volume. The Doppler sample volume can be swept slowly along the path of the color Doppler display to correctly assess the entire length of the artery.

6. *Adjacent anatomic structures.* Using the anatomic structures visualized on gray scale as a guide to correctly identify the intracranial arteries is especially important. It is the major advantage of using imaging versus nonimaging TCD technique.

Normal Intracranial Arterial Velocities

The depths, mean velocities, and normal direction of blood flow relative to the ultrasound transducer for the intracranial arteries from each TCD window are listed in Table 36-1.

It is customary to assume a zero-degree angle (no angle correction) when performing TCD examinations. Different investigators have reported similar velocities for the same vessels, demonstrating good interobserver agreement. Mean velocities (time-averaged peak) are usually reported for TCD examinations because this parameter is less affected by changes in central cardiovascular factors (heart rate, peripheral resistance, etc.) than in systolic or diastolic values, thereby diminishing interindividual variation.

The **mean velocity** calculated during TCD imaging examinations is based on the time average of the outline velocity (maximum velocity envelope). The velocity envelope is a trace of the peak velocities as a function of

TABLE 36-1	Intracranial Arterial Identification Criteria		
Window/Artery	Depth mm	Mean Velocity cm/sec	Direction*
Transtemporal			
MCA	30–67	62 ± 12	Toward
ACA	60–80	50 ± 11	Away
t-ICA	55–67	39 ± 9	Toward
PCA	60–75	39 ± 10	Toward
PCoA	60–75	36 ± 15	Toward, away
Transorbital			
Ophthalmic	40–60	21 ± 5	Toward
ICA siphon	60–80	47 ± 14	Bi, away, toward
Suboccipital			
Vertebral	60–85	38 ± 10	Away
Basilar	>85	41 ± 10	Away
Submandibular			
ICA	35–80	37 ± 9	Away

*Relative to the ultrasound transducer.
ACA, Anterior cerebral artery; *Bi,* bidirectional; *ICA,* internal carotid artery; *t-ICA,* terminal internal carotid artery; *MCA,* middle cerebral artery; *PCA,* posterior cerebral artery; *PCoA,* posterior communicating artery.

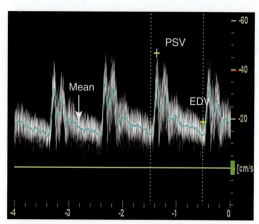

FIGURE 36-13 A Doppler spectral waveform from the middle cerebral artery. The cursors mark the peak-systolic velocity *(PSV)* and the end-diastolic velocity *(EDV)*. The mean velocity *(blue line)* is traced through each cycle of systole and diastole and is calculated by the machine.

time. The mean velocity can be estimated by positioning the horizontal cursor at the velocity where the area below the peak velocity and above the cursor are equal to the area below the cursor and above the peak velocity envelope in diastole (Figure 36-13).

Differences between intracranial arterial velocities are more important than the absolute values recorded from an individual. General observations of mean velocities in the intracranial arteries are as follows:

- Velocities are highest in the MCA.
- If ACA velocity is more than 25% greater than MCA velocity, the ACA may be hypoplastic or stenotic or may serve as a collateral vessel, or there may be an MCA distribution infarction.
- Velocities in the anterior circulation are higher than in the posterior circulation.

In the asymptomatic adult patient, side-to-side asymmetry should be minimal. The difference between sides has been reported to be less than 30%.[18,36] Small differences generally do not indicate an underlying pathologic condition. If a significant side-to-side difference is noted during the examination, try repeating the side with the lower velocities. Often by repeating the evaluation and modifying the transducer-to-artery angle, the side-to-side differences found on the initial examination can be reduced. If side-to-side differences occur, they should not be considered abnormal unless they exceed 30%. Additionally, asymmetries in the intracranial vertebral arteries make it difficult to interpret asymmetrical velocities from these arteries unless the differences are in a focal segment of the vessels.

The pulsatility index (PI) was first described in an attempt to quantify Doppler waveforms during evaluation of lower extremity arterial disease.[14] Most imaging systems automatically calculate the PI with each Doppler

display sweep, but it can be calculated from the following formula:

$$PI = \frac{\text{Systolic velocity} - \text{Diastolic velocity}}{\text{Mean velocity}}$$

When using the PI, the resistance that is encountered with each cardiac cycle is considered. For example, damped blood flow distal to an obstruction will have a decreased PI (diastolic velocity greater than 50% to 60% of peak systolic). Doppler signals obtained proximal to a high resistance (i.e., increased intracranial pressure), however, will have an increased PI (pulsatile spectral waveform). The PI in the MCA is normally in the range of 0.5 to 1.1.

Spectral broadening is observed in the Doppler waveforms obtained during TCD examinations. The Doppler sample volume size used during TCD imaging is usually larger than the intracranial arteries. In fact, the sample volume often includes the entire cross-sectional lumen of an intracranial artery and its small branches. Therefore, even though spectral broadening may be used as a diagnostic criterion for moderate degrees of stenosis in the extracranial carotid arteries, it is not helpful in refining the TCD interpretation.

Various technical factors, including the operator, can contribute to TCD measurement variability. Several studies have concentrated on interobserver and intraobserver variability.[25,36,39] The data provided by these studies indicate that day-to-day differences found by the same examiner usually do not exceed 20%. The size of the ultrasound window and the possibility of different angles of insonation may be the major sources of variability.

Physiologic Factors

Age. TCD velocities are affected by the age of the patient. Several investigators have found lower intracranial arterial velocities with increasing age.[3,17,19,20,31] The downward trend in intracranial arterial velocities may be multifactorial but primarily results from changes in cardiac output and corresponds to an age-related decrease in cerebral blood flow.

Sex. Penetration of the temporal bone with the ultrasound beam is more difficult in females than in males. However, once intracranial Doppler signals are obtained, there do not appear to be major differences in velocity readings due to the sex of the patient. Two studies, however, have demonstrated a slight increase (3% to 5%) in MCA velocities in females.[16,17] Possible explanations for these findings are that females have lower hematocrits, the intracranial arteries may be smaller in diameter, and women have higher hemispheric cerebral blood flow than men. The small differences documented in intracranial arterial velocities because of the sex of the patient need further investigation.

Hematocrit. Hematocrit (Hct) is the percentage of red blood cells by volume in whole blood and is a major determinant of blood viscosity. Blood viscosity is an important factor influencing intracranial arterial blood flow velocity. Intracranial arterial velocities increase in the presence of anemia (Hct <30%). If anemia is the cause of elevated velocities, then these changes should be detected from all of the intracranial arteries. Focal or localized velocity increases suggest a different cause.

Carbon Dioxide Reactivity. Changes in arterial carbon dioxide (CO_2) partial pressure (pCO_2) have an effect on cerebral blood flow and intracranial arterial velocities. An early study demonstrated angiographically that the diameters of the large basal arteries remain constant during changes in pCO_2.[19] Alteration of cerebral vascular resistance and changes in TCD signals result from changes at the level of the arteriolar channels. Hyperventilation (a deficiency of CO_2 in the blood known as *hypocapnia*) causes a decrease in the MCA mean velocity and an increase in the PI. Hypoventilation (an excess of CO_2 in the blood referred to as *hypercapnia*) causes an increase in MCA mean velocity and a decrease in PI. This information suggests that general changes in the intracranial arterial velocities caused by CO_2 reactivity must be taken into account when interpreting TCD data.

Heart Rate and Cardiac Output. Intracranial arterial velocities are also a reflection of an individual's heart rate. Most experienced TCD examiners caution against taking a reading if the patient is yawning, agitated, or experiencing pain, or if any other reason could be causing a change in the heart rate. Any cardiac arrhythmia will be reflected in the TCD recording. If there is a question concerning a change in the patient's heart rate, several display sweeps should be obtained before relying on the calculations. To compensate for extreme cases of bradycardia or tachycardia, the operator may need to adjust the instrument's Doppler display sweep time. Changes resulting from cardiac output not associated with hemodilution have little effect on the cerebral blood flow if autoregulation is intact. This suggests that TCD velocities should be relatively independent of small changes in cardiac output. Data on the relationship between cardiac output and intracranial arterial velocities are limited, and further investigation in this area is necessary.

Many parameters are involved in the accurate interpretation of TCD data. Each patient must be considered individually because of the variety of physiologic factors that affect intracranial arterial hemodynamics (Box 36-2). The parameters that affect the intracranial velocities can be categorized into those factors that are (1) proximal to the circle of Willis, (2) at the level of the circle of Willis, and (3) distal to the circle of Willis.

The most useful TCD results are derived by comparing velocities from different sample volume depths from the same artery and by comparing the velocities from different arteries within an individual. Bilateral symmetrical disease may be difficult to diagnose by TCD

BOX 36-2 | **Interpretation of Transcranial Color Doppler Imaging**

Proximal to the Circle of Willis
Patient's age
Amount and location of extracranial arterial obstruction
Hematocrit
Cardiac output

At the Level of the Circle of Willis
Vessel diameter
Blood viscosity
Turbulence

Distal to the Circle of Willis
Infarction
Intracranial arteriovenous malformations (AVMs)
Increased intracranial pressure
Change in partial pressure of carbon dioxide (pCO_2)

---

imaging. Correct identification of the intracranial arteries, knowledge of normal velocity ranges, familiarity with the technique's limitations, and an understanding of how cerebral hemodynamics may be affected by different physiologic parameters are essential for accurate interpretation of TCD examinations. It is imperative that each institution develop a TCD imaging protocol that defines the standard examination (arteries to be evaluated from each window, the number of Doppler samples from each artery, etc.). This protocol must include the technique, clinical applications, indications for a complete and/or limited examination, and interpretation criteria. A standard complete examination usually includes evaluation of the right and left sides, after acquiring Doppler information from the anterior and posterior intracranial arterial systems.

CLINICAL APPLICATIONS

Vasospasm

Cerebral vasospasm (vasoconstriction of the arteries) is a serious complication after subarachnoid hemorrhage (SAH) and is a significant cause of morbidity and mortality. The most common cause of SAH is leakage of blood from intracranial cerebral aneurysms into the subarachnoid space. Common sites for intracranial aneurysm formation are the ACoA, the MCA, and the PCoA. Early diagnosis and treatment reduce the devastating consequences of this disorder.

The hemodynamic effect of vasospasm produces an increase in blood flow velocity coupled with a pressure drop distal to the narrowed segment. Patients compensate for these changes and maintain cerebral blood flow through their collateral circulations and cerebral autoregulation. When intracranial pressure is increased or the vasomotor reserve has been exhausted, cerebral blood flow can be reduced to critical levels, resulting in isch-emia or infarction.

Examinations are usually performed bedside in the intensive care unit. Important technical features when studying the patient with vasospasm associated with SAH are as follows:

- The operator must be properly positioned at the patient's bedside to make appropriate adjustments in transducer angle and must be able to adjust the control settings on the equipment.
- Headphones are helpful because the high-velocity signals associated with vasospasm can be difficult to appreciate if there is extraneous background noise.
- The locations of the transtemporal window should be marked on the patient's skin, if possible, so that subsequent examinations can be performed from the same location, thereby ensuring the most reliable comparisons.
- If possible, repeat examinations should be performed by the same operator to eliminate interobserver variability.

In some patients, the surgical head dressing may need to be removed to access the transtemporal window. Sterile ultrasound gel is used if the transducer is placed near a wound. TCD recording is possible through a burr hole. However, the equipment's intensity levels should be decreased because the bone no longer causes attenuation of the Doppler signal. TCD imaging in this group of patients can be challenging because of variable patient cooperation, changing cardiovascular and cerebral hemodynamics, and less than optimal testing conditions. Clip artifacts may mask localized segments of increased velocity.

Vasospasm is unusual in the first 2 to 3 days after an SAH, so a TCD examination during this prespastic period serves as a valuable baseline. It allows monitoring of the rate at which vasospasm develops and provides a guide to future examinations because vessels in spasm are small and can be difficult to locate. The TCD examination should be performed daily or every other day for 2 weeks, and the highest velocity obtained from each artery should be recorded. Although a complete TCD examination is preferred, it is not always possible in these patients. Additionally, a cervical ICA signal is obtained at a depth of 45 to 60 mm (without angle adjustment) to calculate a hemispheric ratio. The frequency of follow-up studies will vary depending on the clinical symptoms and the degree of vasospasm. The pCO_2, Hct, and blood pressure should be recorded because these parameters may affect the intracranial arterial blood flow velocities. The time and the date of the examination are documented, and a graph plotting velocity versus time illustrates the time course of a patient's vasospasm. Following SAH, velocity increases

begin to occur about day 3, reach a maximum between days 7 and 12, and generally resolve at 2 to 3 weeks.

MCA mean velocities of 100 to 120 cm/sec correlate with mild vasospasm as demonstrated by arteriography. Moderate vasospasm is defined by velocities in the 120- to 200-cm/sec range (Figures 36-14 and 36-15), and severe vasospasm is characterized by velocities exceeding 200 cm/sec. Mean velocities greater than 200 cm/sec indicate that the patient is at risk of reduced cerebral blood flow (CBF). A rapid increase (greater than 25 cm/day) in velocity in the first few days after the hemorrhage is associated with a poor prognosis.

The MCA/ICA (distal extracranial ICA) mean velocity ratio may be used to determine vasospasm. This hemispheric ratio accounts for a possible increase in flow volume. The ratio increases with severe spasm resulting from increased MCA velocity, as well as with reduced blood flow volume in the ipsilateral extracranial ICA caused by an increase in cerebral vascular resistance. The normal range for the MCA/ICA ratio is 1.7 ± 0.4. An MCA/ICA ratio greater than 3 corresponds to MCA vasospasm, and a ratio greater than 6 demonstrates severe vasospasm.

The sensitivity for diagnosing vasospasm by TCD depends on the skill of the operator, the presence of a good transtemporal window, anatomic consistency, a good transducer-to-artery angle, the location and severity of the vasospasm, the presence of proximal hemodynamically significant lesions, physiologic parameters (increased intracranial pressure, blood pressure fluctuations, pCO_2 variations, Hct, etc.), the diagnostic criteria used, and the cooperation of the patient. The sensitivity of detecting vasospasm of the MCA has been reported to range from 39% to 94% and the specificity from 85% to 100%.[7,8,9,10,32] Data for detecting vasospasm in other intracranial arteries are limited but show lower sensitivity.[24,35] A negative TCD study does not exclude vasospasm. Sources of error are (1) a tortuous or aberrant artery, (2) distal branch vasospasm, (3) increased intracranial pressure, and (4) reduction in volume flow (with or without infarction).

Diagnosis of Intracranial Disease

The ability to detect intracranial arterial stenosis, occlusion, and aneurysm is a new and potentially important addition to the noninvasive cerebrovascular examination. However, to accurately assess the intracranial vasculature, one must be cognizant of the hemodynamic changes associated with intracranial (and extracranial) disease.

Stenosis. Intracranial arterial stenoses cause characteristic alterations in the Doppler signal (audio and spectral waveforms), including focal increases in velocity, local turbulence, and a poststenotic drop in velocity. These changes associated with a stenosis occur assuming that volume flow is maintained. Stenoses may also produce

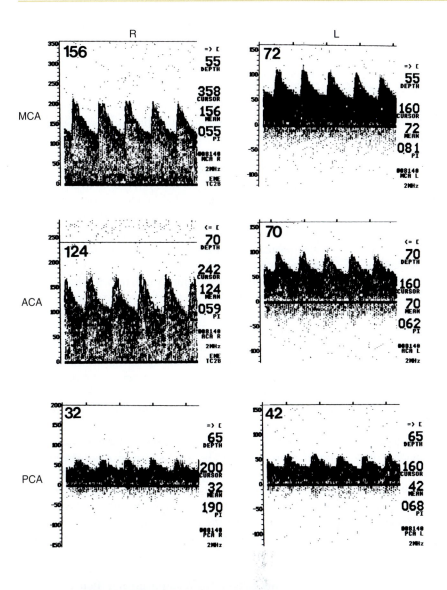

FIGURE 36-14 Doppler spectral waveforms from the middle cerebral artery *(MCA)*, anterior cerebral artery *(ACA)*, and posterior cerebral artery *(PCA)* bilaterally. Doppler spectral waveforms from the right *(R)* MCA and ACA demonstrate an increase in velocity, suggesting vasospasm in this 42-year-old patient. *L,* Left.

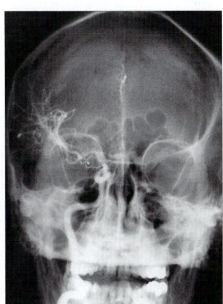

FIGURE 36-15 Corresponding arteriogram demonstrating vasospasm of the right middle cerebral and anterior cerebral arteries.

low-frequency enhancements around the baseline (bruit) or band-shaped enhancements symmetrical with and parallel to the baseline (musical murmur).

A stenosis greater than 60% in diameter reduction usually will be detected by TCD imaging. Absolute velocity criteria for the diagnosis of intracranial arterial stenoses are not reliable because of the many velocity alterations caused by nonvascular variables (age, Hct, etc.). Because absolute velocities are inaccurate, most investigators agree that a focal velocity increase of greater than or equal to 25% should raise suspicion of arterial narrowing. Intracranial stenoses are most commonly found in the MCA and the internal carotid siphon. The status of the cerebral tissue perfused can also have considerable impact on intracranial velocity profiles. Patients with central MCA stenosis without infarction demonstrate an increased MCA velocity. However, the same patient with a cerebral infarction has diminished MCA velocity because of decreased perfusion through the infarcted outflow bed.

Occlusion. TCD is limited in its ability to reliably identify intracranial arterial occlusion. The restriction to occlusion of the MCA is the result of inadequate transtemporal windows, anatomic variability, congenital aplasia, or severe hypoplasia of the other intracranial arteries.

MCA occlusion is suspected when an MCA Doppler signal is absent and high-quality Doppler signals are obtained from the uninvolved ipsilateral intracranial arteries (t-ICA, ACA, PCA). Locating the other ipsilateral arteries reveals that an adequate transtemporal window exists. An increase in the ipsilateral ACA velocity resulting from perfusion through leptomeningeal collaterals is considered corroborating evidence for an MCA occlusion.[21]

Information regarding the sensitivity and specificity of TCD in the diagnosis of intracranial stenoses and occlusion is limited.[5,10,18,22,37] The lack of reliable data is due to the overall low incidence of intracranial disease and the small number of patients who have quality intracranial arteriograms.

Aneurysm. Data are limited regarding TCD sensitivity in the diagnosis of intracranial aneurysms. Most investigators have found that detecting a patent intracranial aneurysm depends on the aneurysm's location and size, and sensitivity has been reported to range from 0% to 85%.[6,7,27,42] In one study, 26 of 37 intracranial aneurysms were identified using color power Doppler imaging.[43] In this exploratory study, investigators found the following features useful in identification of intracranial aneurysms: (1) rounded color areas projecting from an artery that appear noncontinuous at both ends with an artery; (2) color flow appearing in an unexpected area; (3) a color area that is wider than adjacent arteries; and (4) an area with greater expansion and contraction during the cardiac cycle compared with the adjacent artery. These ultrasound characteristics may be important in the identification of intracranial aneurysms; however, the importance of proper instrument control settings cannot be overemphasized. In one study, investigators reported the identification of ruptured intracranial aneurysms in patients with acute subarachnoid hemorrhage using three-dimensional power Doppler imaging.[28] As technology advances, TCD imaging may prove to be more useful for this clinical application in the future.

Collateral Pathways. The TCD examination reveals intracranial arterial collateral patterns in patients with extracranial arterial stenosis. An artery providing collateral circulation usually demonstrates an increased blood flow velocity. Unlike focal increases in velocity found in arterial stenosis, collateral pathways contain diffuse velocity increases throughout the length of the artery. Babikian and others have shown good correlation of TCD and arteriography in the identification of collateral patterns.[4]

The three main collateral pathways identified by TCD are (1) the ACoA, providing a channel from hemisphere to hemisphere; (2) the ophthalmic artery, providing a channel from the extracranial ECA to the intracranial ICA via the orbit; and (3) the PCoA, allowing blood flow between posterior and anterior circulation.

The most commonly found collateral pathway in response to significant extracranial disease is the ACoA. Ultrasound characteristics of this collateral pathway include (1) an increase in the contralateral ACA velocity; (2) a turbulent Doppler signal with increased velocity at midline (resulting from high-velocity blood flow through the small ACoA); and (3) reversal of blood flow direction in the ipsilateral ACA.

The ECA collateral pathway through the orbit is documented by reversed blood flow direction and a change in low-resistance Doppler signal in the ophthalmic artery carrying blood flow from the ECA to the ICA. Collateral perfusion from the posterior circulation to the anterior circulation via the PCoA is the third pattern and is found most often in patients with significant bilateral extracranial carotid artery disease.

Subclavian Steal. The **subclavian steal syndrome** is caused by a stenosis or occlusion of the left subclavian, innominate, or right subclavian artery proximal to the origin of the vertebral artery. Symptoms of this syndrome range from most commonly being asymptomatic[41] to having a variety of neurologic issues. A stenosis in this location may cause pressure in the upper extremity to be lower than normal. The production of a pressure gradient can cause reversal of flow in the vertebral artery, especially during exercise of the involved arm (Figure 36-16). If this occurs, the vertebral artery becomes a major collateral to the upper extremity. The "stealing" of blood from the basilar artery, via retrograde vertebral artery flow, causes the patient to experience neurologic symptoms of brain stem ischemia.

If a systolic pressure differential greater than 20 mmHg between arms is detected, a subclavian or innominate artery obstruction on the side of the lower pressure should be suspected. This physical finding is absent in rare instances and in cases of bilateral lesions.

If subclavian steal is suspected, a standard TCD examination should be performed, with special attention to the blood flow direction and the velocities in the vertebral and basilar arteries. Blood flow is normally away from the transducer (suboccipital approach) in the vertebrobasilar system. If flow is toward the transducer in a vertebral artery and the basilar artery, there is evidence of a steal. Often the reversed flow direction is found only in the vertebral artery, suggesting a possible vertebral-to-vertebral artery steal.

In the absence of blood flow reversal at rest, or when alternating blood flow is observed, the involved upper extremity should be stressed to reduce outflow resistance, thereby revealing the hemodynamics of a potentially latent steal. The baseline examination and the subsequent changes in spectral waveforms that occur after arm exercise or after occlusive hyperemia are

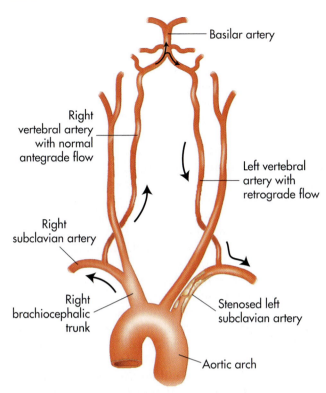

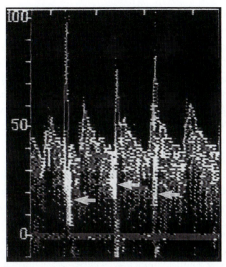

FIGURE 36-17 Emboli *(arrows)* recorded in the spectral Doppler waveform from a middle cerebral artery.

FIGURE 36-16 Subclavian steal. A narrowing of the left subclavian artery proximal to the vertebral artery causes a pressure drop that may cause reversal of blood flow direction in the left vertebral artery. This change in direction can be visualized in the extracranial or intracranial vertebral arteries.

recorded. To perform postocclusive reactive hyperemia, a blood pressure cuff is applied ipsilateral to the suspected stenosis/occlusion. The ipsilateral vertebral artery Doppler signal is located and monitored during inflation of the arm cuff. The blood pressure cuff is inflated above systolic pressure (greater than 20 mmHg above systolic) for approximately 3 minutes, and any changes in the Doppler signal are noted. Then the cuff is rapidly deflated, and changes in the vertebral artery blood flow direction and velocity are recorded. This procedure is repeated while monitoring the contralateral vertebral artery and the basilar artery. A 5- to 10-minute rest period is usually sufficient for the return of baseline arterial hemodynamics between evaluations. Resting basilar artery blood flow is rarely affected but may become abnormal if the contralateral feeding vertebral artery is also diseased.

Emboli Detection. Emboli detection has been reported during routine TCD testing in patients with carotid or cardiac disease. When monitoring the MCA for emboli, it is best to use the main trunk of the MCA (45 to 55 mm). A minimum of 15 to 20 minutes of monitoring is usually required, and a videotape recording is essential. The emboli rate is reported as the number of emboli per hour. Emboli cause an identifiable difference in the intensity of the returning Doppler signal

(Figure 36-17); therefore, proper Doppler gain setting is critical and should be reduced so that the emboli can be detected.

The Consensus Committee of the Ninth International Cerebral Hemodynamic Symposium has proposed minimal identification criteria for establishing microembolic signals.[3] An individual Doppler microembolic signal must have the following four features:

- The signal is transient, usually lasting less than 300 microseconds (μs).
- The amplitude of the signal is at least 3 decibels higher than the background blood flow signal.
- The signal is unidirectional within the Doppler spectral waveform.
- A microembolic signal is accompanied by a "snap," "chirp," or "moan" on the audio output.

In one study, bilateral MCAs were monitored for 20 minutes on each side.[26] No emboli were detected in 20 normal volunteers. However, emboli were detected in 24% (6/25) of symptomatic patients with a carotid stenosis (mean = 2.17 signals per 20 minutes), and in 38% (9/24) of patients with prosthetic cardiac valves (mechanical valves; mean = 17.6 signals per 20 minutes).

In another study, the MCA was monitored for 1 hour in 20 controls, 33 symptomatic patients, and 56 asymptomatic patients.[33] All patients had an extracranial ICA stenosis. No emboli were detected in the controls. However, emboli were observed in 16% (9/56) of asymptomatic patients and in 80% (27/33) of symptomatic patients.

Sixty-four asymptomatic patients were followed for a mean of 72 weeks.[34] Patients had a documented unilateral 70% to 99% stenosis of the extracranial ICA by carotid duplex imaging and did not have a history of atrial fibrillation or an artificial heart valve. The MCA was monitored for 1 hour. Thirteen percent (8/64) had two or more emboli per hour. This study demonstrated a significant association between two or more emboli per hour detected during a TCD examination and a subsequent neurologic event ($P = .005$). TCD imaging is currently being used to identify right-to-left shunts by detecting microbubbles.[2,11,38] To increase the sensitivity of detecting a patent foramen ovale, different patient positions have been recommended when TCD is used for this clinical application.

The detection of cerebral microemboli by TCD offers new information in the diagnosis and management of patients with cerebrovascular disease. Good interobserver agreement suggests that the detection of microemboli by TCD is sufficiently reproducible to be used in the clinical setting. Adding the potential advantage of microemboli detection to TCD monitoring must be balanced with known limitations.

Predicting Stroke in Sickle Cell Disease. TCD imaging is being used in the pediatric population, especially to screen children with sickle cell disease. Cerebral infarction in these patients is associated with an occlusion vasculopathy involving the terminal ICA, the MCA, and the ACA. Prevention of stroke may be feasible with chronic blood transfusion therapy if patients at risk can be identified.

The Stroke Prevention Trial in Sickle Cell Anemia (STOP) enrolled 130 children (ages 2 to 16) who were found to be at high risk for stroke on the basis of elevated (greater than 200 cm/sec) intracranial arterial mean velocities of the t-ICA or the MCA on two separate occasions.[1] The children were randomized to receive either standard supportive care or periodic blood transfusions. After 1 year, 10 children in the standard care group had a cerebral infarction compared with 1 child in the transfusion group. It is now recommended that children with sickle cell disease undergo screening with TCD. If the TCD examination is positive (greater than 200 cm/sec in MCA or t-ICA), the child is at high risk for developing a stroke. In addition, positive or negative TCD results have been shown to be highly correlated between family members.[23] Among children who had a sibling with a positive TCD examination, significant associations with elevated velocities were noted in siblings with sickle cell disease.[23] The clinical decision to start a child on chronic blood transfusion therapy should be made after careful consideration of the risks and benefits.

Technical adjustments for the evaluation of children by TCD imaging include using a smaller sample volume size (5 to 6 mm), applying different depth ranges for the intracranial arteries (these change with the age of the patient), and changing the PRF settings for the increase in intracranial arterial velocities (Figure 36-18).

Intracranial Venous Evaluation. TCD imaging has allowed investigators to begin to explore the intracranial venous system. Several instrument adjustments are important when evaluating intracranial venous blood flow. The ultrasound evaluation of normal intracranial veins produces low-amplitude, pulsatile Doppler signals. Therefore, color, Doppler PRF, and wall filter settings should be significantly reduced to ensure acquisition of high-quality intracranial venous Doppler signals.

Brain Death. TCD imaging can be used as a secondary test to confirm brain death. In a study of 40 patients, TCD was compared with the gold standard cerebral arteriography with 100% agreement on diagnosis.[29] The Doppler criterion for brain death is a brief forward systolic peak with either no diastolic flow or a slight reversal, or no flow at all seen in a patient with a previous examination that confirmed flow.

ADVANTAGES AND LIMITATIONS OF TRANSCRANIAL COLOR DOPPLER IMAGING

TCD imaging has several limitations (Box 36-3) and advantages when compared with the nonimaging TCD technique. Reducing the limitations and maximizing the advantages will ensure the most complete evaluation.

Proper TCD imaging technique requires that the operator has a sound understanding of color Doppler imaging principles. To obtain a quality study, this technique involves the proper use of more instrument controls than are used with the nonimaging technique. The distal basilar artery is difficult to visualize with the color Doppler display because of the larger beam width. However, the basilar artery can usually be followed distally by increasing the sample volume depth and

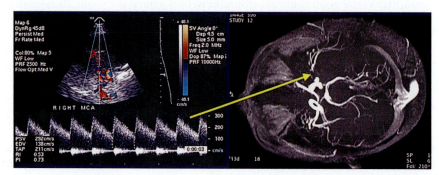

FIGURE 36-18 Transcranial color Doppler imaging examination and the corresponding magnetic resonance angiography in an 8-year-old patient with sickle cell disease. The mean velocity of the middle cerebral artery is greater than 200 cm/sec and corresponds to the intracranial arterial narrowing *(arrow)*.

- Operator inexperience
- Improper instrument control settings
- An uncooperative patient or patient movement
- Absent or poor transtemporal window
- Anatomic variations
- Arterial misidentification
- Distal branch disease
- Distal basilar artery
- Misinterpretation of collateral channels or vasospasm as a stenosis
- Displacement of arteries by an intracranial mass

BOX 36-4 | **Transcranial Color Doppler Imaging Guidelines**

- Obtain a patient history. Focus on medical history, risk factors, symptoms, and current medications.
- Obtain available laboratory values (hematocrit, intracranial pressure, blood pressure, heart rate, cardiac output).
- Know the status of the extracranial vessels.
- Be familiar with intracranial arterial anatomy, physiology, and pathology.
- Understand how each color control affects the image and how controls affect each other.
- Use the color/power Doppler display as a guide to obtain the Doppler spectral waveform information.
- Use a large Doppler sample volume (5 to 10 mm) and assume a zero-degree angle.
- Be aware of the Doppler spectral waveform configuration.
- Compare the Doppler spectral waveforms from the anterior and posterior circulations, and from left and right sides.
- Establish institutional diagnostic criteria for the various clinical applications.

continuing as with a nonimaging examination by using the Doppler signal. The larger beam width also hampers penetration of the temporal bone when the transtemporal ultrasound window is small.

The advantage of using transcranial color Doppler imaging is that anatomic landmarks guide the proper identification of the intracranial arteries. This instills confidence in the operator and leads to improved reliability. Those who are inexperienced with the TCD technique also find that the learning curve is shorter with the color Doppler imaging technique. Additionally, TCD imaging allows identification of the large M2 branches, accurate identification of contralateral arteries if a transtemporal window can be located only on one side, easy visualization of collateral pathways, ease in following tortuous vessels, and identification of the vertebral confluence in many patients. Imaging also provides a method to document the location from which the Doppler spectral waveform is derived, which becomes important with repeat examinations, in departments that include multiple operators and/or interpreters, and when quality improvement is desired.

Diagnostic Pitfalls

Sources of error in the TCD diagnosis of intracranial arterial disease are as follows:

- Misinterpreting collateral channels or vasospasm for stenosis. Vasospasm usually involves several arteries, and the velocities change with time.
- The technical limitations of evaluating distal branch disease (stenosis or occlusion)
- The misinterpretation of a tortuous or displaced MCA (by hematoma or tumor) diagnosed as occlusion
- Anatomic variability (location, asymmetry, tortuosity), especially in the vertebrobasilar system
- Technical difficulty in the evaluation of the distal basilar artery
- The location and size of cerebral aneurysms
- Poor-quality arteriography, leading to inaccurate correlations of TCD results

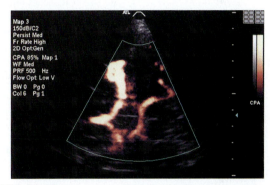

FIGURE 36-19 Color power Doppler imaging of the intracranial arteries. Power Doppler is helpful when trying to locate the small intracranial arteries.

TCD imaging offers new and important advantages to the TCD technique. By using the anatomic landmarks and proper instrument controls, a more accurate and reproducible evaluation of the intracranial arterial hemodynamics can be performed (Box 36-4). Hints to address common technical challenges associated with performing TCD examinations are located in Table 36-2. Color power imaging offers technical advantages in imaging small-caliber intracranial arteries, slower-moving blood flow, and intracranial arteries that course at unfavorable angles to the ultrasound beam (Figure 36-19). Future technology may offer improved visualization of the intracranial circulation by using power Doppler imaging, three-dimensional ultrasound imaging, and color Doppler imaging with contrast enhancement.

Currently, TCD imaging is being used to evaluate cerebral hematomas, differentiate between ischemic and hemorrhagic stroke, evaluate arteriovenous malformations, and evaluate the patient with an acute stroke.

TABLE 36-2	Transcranial Color Doppler Imaging: Technical Hints
Challenge	**Action**
No Doppler signal or color display Absent window, window not located, poor patient positioning, or an occluded intracranial artery	1. Undergo a systematic search for a better window. A TCD window may be located by repositioning the transducer on the skin, changing the angle of the transducer, changing the depth of the sample volume, or by changing the color control settings. 2. Check the equipment control settings to ensure that the maximum power is being used, especially when using the transtemporal window. Adjusting the color gain/PRF settings may also prove to be valuable when searching for a window. 3. Add more ultrasound gel to maintain good transducer-to-skin contact. 4. Use a lower MHz transducer (if available). 5. Reposition the patient to help in locating a Doppler signal, especially from the suboccipital window. 6. Use headphones (if available) to eliminate extraneous noise so that subtle Doppler signals may be detected.
Poor-quality Doppler signal Small or poor window, improper equipment control settings, poor technique, poor patient positioning, or intracranial pathology	1. Undergo a systematic search for a better window. A TCD window may be located by repositioning the transducer on the skin, changing the angle of the transducer, changing the depth of the sample volume, or changing the color control settings. 2. Check the equipment control settings to ensure that the maximum power is being used, especially when using the transtemporal window. Adjusting the color gain/PRF settings may also prove to be valuable when searching for a window. 3. Add more ultrasound gel to maintain good transducer-to-skin contact. 4. Use a lower MHz transducer (if available). 5. Reposition the patient to help in locating a Doppler signal, especially from the suboccipital window. 6. Use headphones (if available) to eliminate extraneous noise so that subtle Doppler signals may be detected. 7. Document any changes in blood flow velocity or spectral Doppler waveform shape that may indicate intracranial pathology (may be visualized).
Multiple Doppler signals Large sample volume size, anatomic variation, or overlapping vessel	1. Use a smaller sample volume size. 2. Search for a better window by repositioning the transducer on the skin or by changing the angle of the transducer.
Background noise in Doppler signal Improper gain settings or placement of sample volume	1. Adjust the gain setting so that the Doppler spectral waveform is optimized and the background noise is minimized. 2. Carefully adjust the angle of insonation to improve the signal-to-noise ratio. 3. Change the sample volume depth setting by a small increment to improve the quality of the signal.
Artifact in Doppler signal Patient movement, transducer movement, inadequate amount of ultrasound gel	1. Take the time to put the patient at ease or answer any questions to minimize patient movement. 2. Minimize transducer movement by properly adjusting the operator's position (arm resting on examination table). 3. Adjust the gain setting so that the Doppler spectral waveform is optimized and the background noise is minimized. 4. Carefully adjust the angle of insonation to improve the signal-to-noise ratio. 5. Change the sample volume depth setting by a small increment to improve the quality of the signal.
Aliasing of Doppler or color Doppler signal Detected frequency exceeding the Nyquist limit	1. Increase the PRF settings. 2. Decrease the zero baseline to increase the scale in one direction.
"I am lost" Not following examination protocol, patient movement, unusual window, anatomic variations, or intracranial pathology	1. Undergo a systematic search for a better window. A TCD window may be located by repositioning the transducer on the skin, changing the angle of the transducer, changing the depth of the sample volume, or changing the color control settings. If an unusual window is used, check the angle of the transducer. 2. Locate the anatomic landmarks from the specific window. 3. Locate the landmark t-ICA bifurcation signal and use it to locate the other arteries when using the transtemporal window. 4. Follow the examination protocol. 5. Remember that the patient's physiologic factors and any disease of the extracranial vessels may have an effect on the intracranial Doppler waveforms (velocity and configuration). 6. Take the time to put the patient at ease or answer any questions to minimize patient movement. 7. Remember the limitations of the technique.

PRF, Pulse repetition frequency; *TCD*, transcranial color Doppler; *t-ICA*, terminal internal carotid artery.

REFERENCES

1. Adams R, McKie VC, Hsu L, et al: Prevention of a first stroke by transfusions in children with sickle cell anemia and abnormal results on transcranial Doppler ultrasonography, *N Engl J Med* 339:5-11, 1998.
2. Anzola GP, Zavarize P, Morandi E, et al: Transcranial Doppler and risk of recurrence in patients with stroke and patent foramen ovale, *Eur J Neurol* 10:129-135, 2003.
3. Babikian V: Basic identification criteria of Doppler microembolic signals, *Stroke* 26:1123, 1995.
4. Babikian V, Sloan MA, Tegeler CH, et al: Transcranial Doppler validation pilot study, *J Neuroimaging* 3:242-249, 1993.
5. Baumgartner RW, Mattle HP, Schroth G: Assessment of ≥50% and <50% intracranial stenoses by transcranial color-coded duplex sonography, *Stroke* 30:87-92, 1999.
6. Baumgartner RW, Mattle HP, Kothbauer K, Schroth K: Transcranial color-coded duplex sonography in cerebral aneurysms, *Stroke* 25:2429-2434, 1994.
7. Becker GM, Greiner K, Kaune B, et al: Diagnosis and monitoring of subarachnoid hemorrhage by transcranial color-coded real-time sonography, *Neurosurgery* 28:814-820, 1991.
8. Burch CM, Wozniak MA, Sloan MA, et al: Detection of intracranial internal carotid artery and middle cerebral artery vasospasm following subarachnoid hemorrhage, *J Neuroimag* 6:8-15, 1996.
9. Compton JS, Redmond S, Symon L: Cerebral blood velocity in subarachnoid haemorrhage: a transcranial Doppler study, *J Neurol Neurosurg Psychiatr* 50:1499-1503, 1987.
10. deBray J-M, Joseph PA, Jeanvoine H, et al: Transcranial Doppler evaluation of middle cerebral artery stenosis, *J Ultrasound Med* 7:611-616, 1988.
11. Devuyst G, Piechowski-Józwiak B, Karapanayiotides T, et al: Controlled contrast transcranial Doppler and arterial blood gas analysis to quantify shunt through patent foramen ovale, *Stroke* 35:859-863, 2004.
12. Eicke BM, Tegeler CH, Dalley G, Myers LG: Angle correction in transcranial Doppler sonography, *J Neuroimag* 4:29-33, 1994.
13. Giller GA: Is angle correction correct? *J Neuroimag* 4:51-52, 1994.
14. Gosling RG, Dunbar G, King DH, et al: The quantitative analysis of occlusive peripheral arterial disease by a nonintrusive ultrasound technique, *Angiology* 22:52-55, 1971.
15. Grolimund P: Transmission of ultrasound through the temporal bone. In Aaslid R, editor: *Transcranial Doppler sonography*, New York, 1986, Springer-Verlag.
16. Halsey JH: Effect of emitted power on waveform intensity in transcranial Doppler, *Stroke* 21:1573-1578, 1990.
17. Halsey JH: Response: Letter to the editor, *Stroke* 22:533, 1991.
18. Hennerici M, Rautenberg W, Sitzer G, Schwartz A: Transcranial Doppler ultrasound for the assessment of intracranial arterial flow velocity, I. Examination technique and normal value, *Surg Neurol* 27:439-448, 1987.
19. Huber P, Handa J: Effect of contrast material, hypercapnia, hyperventilation, hypertonic glucose and papaverine on the diameter of the cerebral arteries: angiographic determination in man, *Invest Radiol* 2:17-32, 1967.
20. Kaps M, Seidel G, Bauer T, Behrmann B: Imaging of the intracranial vertebrobasilar system using color-coded ultrasound, *Stroke* 23:1577-1582, 1992.
21. Kaps M, Damian MS, Teschendorf U, Dorndorf W: Transcranial Doppler ultrasound findings in middle cerebral artery occlusion, *Stroke* 21:532-537, 1990.
22. Kirkham FJ, Neville BGR, Levin SD: Bedside diagnosis of stenosis of middle cerebral artery, *Lancet* 1:797, 1986 (letter).
23. Kwaitkowski JL, Hunter JV, Smith-Whitley K, et al: Transcranial Doppler ultrasonography in siblings with sickle cell disease, *Br J Haematol* 121:932-937, 2003.
24. Lennihan L, Petty GW, Fink ME, et al: Transcranial Doppler detection of anterior cerebral artery vasospasm, *J Neurol Neurosurg Psychiatr* 56:906-909, 1993.
25. Lippert H, Pabst R: *Arterial variations in man: classification and frequency*, New York, 1985, Springer-Verlag.
26. Markus HS, Droste DW, Brown MM: Detection of asymptomatic cerebral embolic signals with Doppler ultrasound, *Lancet* 343:1011-1012, 1994.
27. Martin PJ, Gaunt ME, Naylor AR: Intracranial aneurysms and arteriovenous malformations: transcranial colour-coded sonography as a diagnostic aid, *Ultrasound Med Biol* 20:689-698, 1994.
28. Perren F, Horn P, Kern R, et al: A rapid noninvasive method to visualize ruptured aneurysms in the emergency room: three-dimensional power Doppler imaging, *J Neurosurg* 100:619-622, 2004.
29. Poularas J, Karakitsos D, Kouraklis G, et al: Comparison between transcranial color Doppler ultrasonography and angiography in the confirmation of brain death. *Transplant Proc* 38:1213-1217, 2006.
30. Schoning M, Buchholz R, Walter J: Comparative study of transcranial color duplex sonography and transcranial Doppler sonography in adults, *J Neurosurg* 78:776, 1993.
31. Seibert JJ, Glasier CM, Kirby RS, et al: Transcranial Doppler, MRA, and MRI as a screening examination for cerebrovascular disease in patients with sickle cell anemia: an 8-year study, *Pediatr Radiol* 18:138-142, 1998.
32. Seidel G, Kaps M, Dorndor W: Transcranial color-coded duplex sonography of intracerebral hematomas in adults, *Stroke* 24:1519-1527, 1993.
33. Siebler M, Kleinschmidt A, Sitzer M, et al: Cerebral microembolism in symptomatic and asymptomatic high-grade internal carotid artery stenosis, *Neurology* 44:615-618, 1994.
34. Siebler M, Nachtmann A, Sitzer M, et al: Cerebral microembolism and the risk of ischemia in asymptomatic high-grade internal carotid artery stenosis, *Stroke* 26:2184-2186, 1995.
35. Sloan MA, Burch CM, Wozniak MA, et al: Transcranial Doppler detection of vertebrobasilar vasospasm following subarachnoid hemorrhage, *Stroke* 25:2187-2197, 1994.
36. Spencer MP, Whisler D: Transorbital Doppler diagnosis of intracranial arterial stenosis, *Stroke* 17:916-921, 1986.
37. Stolz E, Kaps M, Dorndorf W: Assessment of intracranial venous hemodynamics in normal individuals and patients with cerebral venous thrombosis, *Stroke* 30:70-75, 1999.
38. Telman G, Kouperberg E, Sprecher E, Yarnitsky D: The positions of the patients in the diagnosis of patient foramen ovale by transcranial Doppler, *J Neuroimaging* 13:356-358, 2003.
39. Totaro R, Marini C, Cannarsa C, Prencipe M: Reproducibility of transcranial Doppler sonography: a validation study, *Ultrasound Med Biol* 18:173-177, 1992.
40. Tsuchiya T, Yasaka M, Yamaguchi T, et al: Imaging of the basal cerebral arteries and measurement of blood velocity in adults by using transcranial real-time color flow Doppler sonography, *AJNR Am J Neuroradiol* 12:497-502, 1991.
41. Tummala RP, Ecker RD, and Levy EI: Variant of subclavian steal in the setting of ipsilateral common carotid artery occlusion: case report. *J Neuroimaging* 19:271-273, 2009.
42. Valdueza JM, Harms L, Doepp F, et al: Venous microembolic signals detected in patients with cerebral sinus thrombosis, *Stroke* 28:1607-1609, 1997.
43. Wardlaw JM, Cannon JC: Color transcranial "power" Doppler ultrasound of intracranial aneurysms, *J Neurosurg* 84:459-461, 1996.

Peripheral Arterial Evaluation

Ann Willis and Mira L. Katz

The noninvasive evaluation of patients with peripheral arterial disease has evolved greatly. With today's sophisticated technology, an anatomic and physiologic evaluation can be obtained both at rest and after exercise. Capabilities have advanced from simple oscillometric measurements to segmental pressures, pulse volume recordings, stress testing, and direct evaluation of arteries and bypass grafts by duplex imaging. Originally, the purpose of these tests was to offer objectivity in the diagnosis of arterial disease. Indications have been expanded, and currently the noninvasive evaluation is tailored to patients' specific needs, depending on the clinical presentation and the pathologic findings being evaluated.

The noninvasive arterial evaluation complements, but does not replace, a careful history and physical examination. Noninvasive testing is important because the clinical evaluation may not always detect underlying arterial occlusive disease, especially when concomitant neuropathy or osteoarthritis is present. A prospective study of 458 diabetic patients using noninvasive techniques detected lower extremity arterial disease in 31% (128/408) of patients who gave no history of claudication and in 21% (54/259) of patients with a normal physical examination.[25]

The noninvasive arterial examination is an important component in the evaluation of a patient with signs and symptoms of arterial occlusive disease. Although not required for diagnosis, noninvasive arterial testing is valuable to many patients and their doctors (Box 37-1).

Although indirect tests and peripheral arterial duplex imaging are discussed separately in this chapter, a combination of tests may be indicated, depending on the patient and the clinical presentation.

RISK FACTORS AND SYMPTOMS OF PERIPHERAL ARTERIAL DISEASE

Several risk factors have been associated with peripheral occlusive arterial disease, including increasing age, hypertension, diabetes mellitus, elevated cholesterol, tobacco smoking, documented atherosclerosis in the coronary or carotid system, and a family history of atherosclerosis.

Symptoms of lower extremity occlusive arterial disease include claudication and rest pain. Claudication is defined as walking-induced muscular discomfort of the calf, thigh, hip, or buttock due to ischemia. Most patients describe claudication as a cramping or aching in the muscles of their legs as they walk or exercise.

Claudication is relieved by resting for 2 to 5 minutes. Unless the disease is progressing, the distance most patients walk to the onset of symptoms is usually constant. Approximately 25% of patients with intermittent claudication will progress to rest pain within 5 years of onset of their claudication.

Ischemic rest pain points to critical ischemia of the distal limb when the patient is at rest. The patient usually complains of pain in the toes when lying down. The pain often awakens a patient who is sleeping. If the ischemia is severe, the patient may find relief by sitting with the affected limb in the dependent position during the day and night. This position permits gravity to assist in delivering blood flow to the foot.

Physical signs of peripheral occlusive arterial disease are elevation pallor and dependent rubor, ischemic ulcers, gangrene, bruits, and decreased peripheral pulses (femoral, popliteal, dorsalis pedis, posterior tibial, axillary, brachial, radial, and ulnar). Pulses are usually compared from side to side and are graded on a scale from 0 to 3+, with 0 = no pulse, 1+ = questionable pulse, 2+ = weak pulse, and 3+ = normal pulse.

ANATOMY ASSOCIATED WITH PERIPHERAL ARTERIAL TESTING

Lower Extremity

The descending aorta is the continuation of the aorta beyond the aortic arch. The descending aorta is divided into a thoracic section and an abdominal section. The thoracic section of the aorta terminates at the aortic opening in the diaphragm. The abdominal aorta begins at the level of the twelfth thoracic vertebra as it passes through the aortic hiatus of the diaphragm. The abdominal aorta terminates in the bifurcation of the right and left common iliac arteries (approximately at the level of the fourth lumbar vertebra) (Figure 37-1). Each of the common iliac arteries bifurcates into an internal iliac artery (hypogastric artery), which supplies the pelvis, and an external iliac artery, which continues distally to

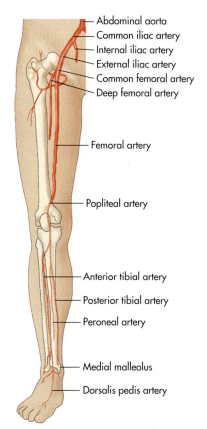

FIGURE 37-1 The arteries of the lower extremity.

- Abdominal aorta
- Common iliac artery
- Internal iliac artery
- External iliac artery
- Common femoral artery
- Deep femoral artery
- Femoral artery
- Popliteal artery
- Anterior tibial artery
- Posterior tibial artery
- Peroneal artery
- Medial malleolus
- Dorsalis pedis artery

supply the lower extremity. The external iliac artery terminates at the inguinal ligament, where it becomes the common femoral artery. The common femoral artery originates beneath the inguinal ligament and terminates by dividing into the femoral and profunda femoris arteries. The profunda femoris artery is posterior and lateral to the femoral artery. The profunda femoris (deep femoral) artery begins at the common femoral bifurcation and terminates in the lower third of the thigh. The profunda femoris artery supplies the muscles of the thigh and the hip joint. The femoral artery (FA) travels the length of the thigh, travels through Hunter's canal, and terminates at the opening of the adductor magnus muscle. The proximal FA is superficial and dives deep in the distal portion of the thigh. The popliteal artery begins at the opening of the adductor magnus muscle and travels behind the knee in the popliteal fossa. Major branches of the popliteal artery are the sural and genicular arteries. The popliteal artery terminates distally into the anterior tibial artery and the tibial-peroneal trunk.

The anterior tibial arteries take off at the popliteal and travel down the lateral calf in the anterior compartment to the level of the ankle. The dorsalis pedis artery is a continuation of the anterior tibial artery on the top of the foot. The arterial branches of the anterior tibial artery join branches of the posterior tibial artery to form the plantar arch. Arising off the plantar arch are the metatarsal arteries that divide into the digital branch arteries.

The **tibial-peroneal trunk** takes off after the anterior tibial artery and bifurcates into the posterior tibial artery and the peroneal artery. The posterior tibial artery travels down the medial calf in the posterior compartment and terminates between the ankle and the heel into the medial and lateral plantar arteries. The peroneal artery is located deep within the calf and travels near the medial aspect of the fibula. The peroneal artery terminates in the distal third of the calf, and its branches communicate with branches of the posterior and anterior tibial arteries.

Upper Extremity

The ascending aorta originates from the left ventricle of the heart. The transverse aortic arch lies in the superior mediastinum and is formed as the aorta ascends and curves posteroinferiorly from right to left, above the left mainstem bronchus. It descends to the left of the trachea and esophagus. Three main branches arise from the superior convexity of the arch in its normal configuration. The **innominate artery** (brachiocephalic trunk) is the first branch (divides into the right subclavian and the right common carotid artery); the left common carotid artery is the second; and the left subclavian artery is the third branch in approximately 70% of cases.

The **subclavian artery** originates at the inner border of the scalenus anterior muscle and travels beneath the clavicle to the outer border of the first rib, where it becomes the axillary artery (Figure 37-2). Major branches

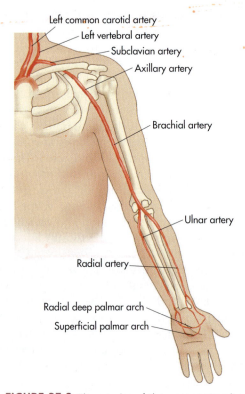

Left common carotid artery
Left vertebral artery
Subclavian artery
Axillary artery

Brachial artery

Ulnar artery

Radial artery

Radial deep palmar arch
Superficial palmar arch

FIGURE 37-2 The arteries of the upper extremity.

of the subclavian artery are the vertebral artery, thyrocervical trunk, costocervical trunk, internal mammary, and dorsal scapular.

The **axillary artery** is a continuation of the subclavian artery. It begins at the outer border of the first rib and terminates at the lower border of the tendon of the teres major muscle. The **brachial artery** is a continuation of the axillary artery. It originates at the lower margin of the tendon of the teres major muscle and usually terminates just below the antecubital fossa into the radial and ulnar arteries.

The **radial artery** begins at the brachial artery bifurcation. The radial artery travels down the forearm (thumb side) and terminates in the palm. The radial artery forms the deep palmar arch. The **ulnar artery** originates at the brachial artery bifurcation, is usually slightly larger than the radial artery, and travels down the forearm (small finger side) to the palm. The ulnar artery terminates and forms the superficial palmar arch. Both palmar arches supply blood to the digital arteries.

INDIRECT ARTERIAL TESTING

Segmental Doppler Pressures

Before the examination is begun, there should be a 15-minute rest period to allow the patient's blood pressure to stabilize and legs to recover from walking to the examination room. During this rest period, the patient's history can be obtained. The patient's history should document risk factors, current severity and location of symptoms, and previous history of arterial interventions, including arterial operations. Do not place cuffs on areas of graft placements.

Segmental pressures are obtained with the patient in the supine position. The legs should be at the same level as the heart because this position prevents hydrostatic pressure (gravity-induced) artifact. Blood pressure cuffs are placed bilaterally on the upper arm (brachial pressure), proximal thigh, low thigh (above the knee), calf (below the knee), and ankle just above the medial malleoli. Using a flow detector (continuous wave Doppler transducer) on the distal limb, each cuff is independently inflated about 20 to 30 mmHg above systolic pressure, then is slowly deflated. As the cuff pressure is lowered, the systolic pressure recorded at that cuff location is the pressure at which the audible arterial Doppler signal returns. Calf and ankle pressures are recorded using the Doppler signals from the dorsalis pedis and posterior tibial arteries. Proximal and low thigh pressures are recorded using the strongest distal Doppler signal. If no distal Doppler signals are noted (no measurable blood flow or occlusion of the distal vessels), thigh pressures are obtained by using the Doppler signal from the popliteal artery.

A continuous wave Doppler instrument is used when performing segmental limb pressures. An 8-MHz continuous wave transducer can be used for most patients. However, if the Doppler signal is attenuated because of depth, a 5-MHz transducer may be necessary to improve penetration. A generous amount of ultrasound gel should be used to ensure good transducer-to-skin contact. Use a transducer angle of 45 to 60 degrees. The pressure applied to the skin must maintain good contact but cannot be excessive, or it may obliterate the Doppler signal.

To obtain pressures comparable with direct intra-arterial measurements, the blood pressure cuff must have a width 20% greater than the diameter of the limb. When the width of the cuff is small compared with the girth of the limb, the pressure in the cuff may not be completely transmitted to the arteries, and measured pressures are often falsely elevated. In a normal person, pressure measurements increase from the ankle to the proximal thigh because of the relation between constant cuff width and the increase in limb girth. Blood pressure cuffs used for segmental pressure studies should have bladders that measure 12 × 40 cm, and cuffs with longer bladders (12 × 55 cm) may be used for proximal and distal thigh measurements.

Pressures may be falsely elevated in obese patients, and a proximal thigh pressure may be lower in extremely thin patients. The cuff-to-limb ratio should be kept in mind when the patient's legs are abnormally large or abnormally small.

Brachial pressures should be obtained in both arms. If a difference of ≥20 mmHg occurs between arms, an arterial obstruction (usually the subclavian artery) is suspected on the side with the lower systolic pressure. The proximal thigh pressure reading should be 30 mmHg greater than the brachial pressure because of the cuff size artifact rather than an actual increase in intra-arterial pressure. A proximal thigh pressure equal to or less than the brachial pressure suggests disease at or proximal to the level of the femoral artery. A pressure gradient of 20 mmHg between adjacent segments of the limb is abnormal and indicates intercurrent disease. Pressures measured at the same level of each leg should not differ by more than 20 mmHg. A significant pressure gradient (20 mmHg) between the proximal and distal thigh cuffs suggests disease of the femoral artery. Disease of the distal femoral artery, the popliteal artery, or both, is suspected if a significant pressure gradient is present from the low thigh to the calf. Disease of the tibial arteries is suspected if a 20-mmHg pressure gradient is present from the calf to the ankle.

When interpreting segmental pressures, it may be difficult to localize the disease when patients have multilevel disease. Proximal arterial obstruction or stenosis causing a significant pressure gradient may mask distal disease. Additionally, segmental pressure gradients cannot distinguish between a stenosis and an occlusion.

Because systemic pressures vary from person to person, and in the same patient from time to time, abso-

lute pressures are not used to categorize or follow patients. All pressures are divided by the highest brachial pressure and expressed as a ratio, and this pressure index (PI) is used to follow patients. The ad hoc committee on reporting standards for the Society for Vascular Surgery/International Society for Cardiovascular Surgery (North American chapter) concluded that an ankle-brachial index (ABI) change greater than 0.10 should be considered significant.[36] Another study demonstrated that an ABI must change by at least 0.15 before it can be considered significant.[1] Under constant conditions and with careful measurements, these values may be appropriate.

Modest variability in measuring ankle pressures is likely to be associated with normal patient or observer variability. The importance of body temperature in recording ABIs in claudicators has been demonstrated.[8] Variability in the ankle pressure index was documented as being higher after body cooling (0.79 ± 0.04) than during routine testing (0.69 ± 0.03) or after warming (0.65 ± 0.04).

Resting ABIs correlate with the degree of functional disability. The ABI has been found to be 1.11 ± 0.10 in the absence of arterial occlusion, 0.59 ± 0.15 in limbs with intermittent claudication, 0.26 ± 0.13 in limbs with ischemic rest pain, and 0.05 ± 0.08 in limbs with impending gangrene.[43]

ABIs are usually divided into four main categories (Table 37-1). Most patients' clinical symptoms and their ABIs fit into these four categories, but there tends to be some overlap between groups.

Lower extremity pressures may be artifactually elevated because of medial calcinosis, medial sclerosis, or both, with pressure indices exceeding 1.25. This affects the diabetic patient most commonly. When this occurs, toe pressures or pulse volume recordings are particularly valuable in evaluating the patient's ischemia because these tests are not affected by a noncompliant arterial wall.

Segmental pressure measurements of the lower extremity tend to underestimate the extent of the disease. Reasons for underestimation of the disease include (1) narrowing of the arterial lumen must be significant enough to cause a pressure change, (2) proximal disease may mask distal disease, and (3) calcified vessels may falsely elevate the pressures recorded. Indirect testing,

TABLE 37-1	Interpretation of Ankle-Brachial Pressure Index (ABI)
Clinical Presentation	**Ankle-Brachial Index**
Normal	>0.95
Claudication	0.50–0.95
Rest pain	0.21–0.49
Tissue loss	<0.21

however, provides information about the overall limb hemodynamics. These findings in combination with direct testing using duplex imaging will provide the best information in most patients.

Additionally, measuring penile blood pressure in persons who have proximal arterial disease may be necessary. A penile blood pressure cuff is placed at the base of the penis, and Doppler signals from the cavernosal arteries are used to obtain a pressure.

If arterial disease is severe, many of these patients will have sexual dysfunction. A normal potent male over the age of 40 years will have a penile-brachial pressure index of 0.75 or greater. A penile-brachial PI of less than 0.60 usually indicates some degree of impotence.

Other Extremity Testing

Arterial disease in the upper extremity does not occur as often as arterial disease in the lower extremity. Problems of the upper extremity may result from stenosis or obstruction of the large inflow arteries (innominate, subclavian). Plaque is not commonly seen in the arteries of the arms, but it can occur. Arterial embolization (cardiac origin) is another reason for upper extremity testing. Small emboli from atrial fibulation or aortic valve disease can cause ischemic reactions in the fingers and hands.

Thoracic outlet syndrome (TOS) (compression of neural and vascular structures by bone, ligament, or muscular obstacles) can cause ischemic reactions when the patient presents in certain positions. This is known as true TOS and can present with hand wasting (the affected hand is less muscular than the nonaffected hand). Vascular TOS can be related to impingement but also presents with some type of vascular stenosis, occlusion, or aneurysm. Symptoms resemble claudication in the legs, that is, cramping or pain in the muscles relieved by rest. To verify flow reduction, the patient is set up to record pulse volume waveforms using the fingers as testing sites. Photoplethysmographic (PPG) probes or pulse volume cuffs are placed on the index or middle finger and a normal waveform is obtained with the patient in an upright position and the arms at rest. The patient is then asked to perform a set of maneuvers while trying to assess the waveforms for changes related to impingement of the vascular structures. These maneuvers include the East position—arms in a "stick-them-up" manner with the chest poked out; the Adson maneuver—the arm extended back, hand externally rotated, and the patient looking back towards the hand; and the exaggerated military position—chest poked out with arms starting at the side then extended out to the sides and moved upward in 45-degree increments. The patient should also be tested in the position in which they experience symptoms. Any decrease or "flatlining" in the waveform indicates a flow-reducing position. Maneuvers may vary based on the patient's symptoms or the laboratory protocol. Testing can be

followed by a duplex study to look for any stenosis or occlusion.

Primary Raynaud's phenomenon is intermittent digital ischemia in response to cold or emotional stress. Patients present with color changes (white or blue) in the fingers or toes. Secondary Raynaud's phenomenon is caused by vascular occlusion or stenosis to the fingers or toes and can occur in response to cold or emotional stress. The key to treating this disease is to find the underlying cause of the symptoms, whether it is vascular blockage or just a vasospastic reaction. Segmental Doppler pressures and pulse volume recordings may be taken at the level of the upper arm, the forearm, the wrist, and the digits. If a difference of 20 mmHg or greater occurs between arms, an arterial obstruction (usually the subclavian artery) is suspected on the side with the lower systolic pressure. No more than a 10- to 15-mmHg difference should be observed between adjacent sites on the arm. Normal digital pressures will be within 20 mmHg of the brachial pressure. It is technically less challenging to use PPG as the end-point detector when taking digital pressures than to try to locate the digital arteries with a Doppler transducer. If the patient presents with normal pressures, a cold challenge can be performed. Attach PPGs to the fingers, and place the hand in a protective plastic bag. Pulse volumes are taken with the hand warmed and at rest. Then place the hand in cold water (if it is truly Raynaud's, this will not be well tolerated) for up to 1 minute. Assess the waveforms to see if there is any change in flow. Flow is considered abnormal if the waveform flatlines during the emersion or does not return to normal within 8 to 10 minutes.

Another test used to evaluate the hand is Allen's test. This test determines the flow in the superficial and deep palmar arch. Place PPGs on the thumb and the fifth digit of the hand to be examined. Record normal flow, then occlude the flow in the radial and ulnar arteries at the wrist with thumb pressure. Wait until both waveforms flatline, then release the radial artery and look for return of normal flow. If flow does not return to normal, then the palmar arch is not intact between the superficial and the deep system. If flow returns to normal, occlude both arteries again and repeat with the ulnar artery, while looking for the same results.

Toe Pressures

Toe pressures are a more accurate method of evaluating distal limb and foot perfusion in patients with falsely elevated segmental limb pressures. Toe pressures may also be used to determine if there is obstructive disease involving the pedal arch and digital arteries.

A digital cuff (2.5 × 9-cm bladder) is placed at the base of the big toe, and the pressure is obtained by using an audible Doppler signal from a digital artery, or by placing a PPG on the distal toe as an end-point detector. A toe pressure is considered normal if it is 50 mmHg or more than 64% of the brachial pressure, whichever is higher. The mean toe PI in patients with claudication and with rest pain is 0.35 ± 0.15 and 0.11 ± 0.10, respectively.

Pulse Volume Recordings

Pulse volume recordings measure changes in segmental limb volume with each cardiac cycle. The patient is examined in the supine position, and blood pressure cuffs are placed on the patient's arms, thighs, calves, ankles, and feet. Each cuff is inflated to a preset pressure (usually 65 mmHg) to maintain adequate contact between the cuff bladder and the limb. Accurate pulse volume tracings are possible only if the size of the blood pressure cuff (and of the bladder) is appropriate and if the cuff is correctly placed on the limb. The pulse volume waveforms are recorded on an analog chart recorder.

Pulse volume recordings are interpreted qualitatively and complement the systolic segmental pressure measurements. A normal pulse volume waveform is characterized by a rapid rise to a sharp peak during systole and a slower fall during diastole (Figure 37-3). The downslope of a normal pulse volume waveform contains a dicrotic notch that reflects the brief period of retrograde flow in the arteries during diastole.

Occlusive arterial disease causes changes in the amplitude and contour of the pulse volume waveform. Sequential changes in the waveform that occur with progressive occlusive arterial disease are that the dicrotic notch disappears, the upslope is slower, the peak is more rounded, and upslope and downslope times equalize (Figure 37-4). Recording of no pulse amplitude (a straight line) is pos-

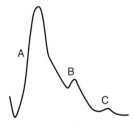

FIGURE 37-3 A normal pulse volume recording from the lower extremity. Note the rapid rise to a sharp peak during systole **(A)** and the slower fall during diastole **(C)**. The downslope of a normal pulse volume recording contains a dicrotic notch **(B)** that reflects the brief period of retrograde blood flow in the arteries during diastole.

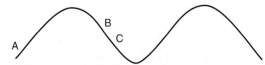

FIGURE 37-4 Arterial occlusive disease causes changes in the amplitude and contour of the pulse volume recording. The dicrotic notch disappears **(B)**, the upslope is slower **(A)**, the peak is more rounded, and the downslope time **(C)** equalizes to the upslope time.

sible in patients with severe occlusive arterial disease of the lower extremity.

The calf pulse volume waveform normally has greater amplitude than the thigh waveform because of cuff artifact. If the amplitude of the calf pulse volume waveform is equal to or smaller than that of the thigh waveform, femoral artery disease should be suspected.

Pulse volume recordings provide important information and are usually performed in addition to segmental pressure measurements. A discrepancy often occurs between pulse volume waveforms and segmental pressures when arteries cannot be compressed (systolic PI greater than 1.25). This frequently occurs when patients have diabetes mellitus. In this clinical presentation, pulse volume waveforms provide the only accurate information about the overall hemodynamics of the limb.

Arterial Stress Testing

In a normal individual without occlusive arterial disease, blood flow will increase with exercise because of a decrease in peripheral vascular resistance. This increase in blood flow demand will occur without a decrease in ankle systolic pressure. Some patients will have arterial lesions that are quiescent at rest (normal resting ABIs) but limit perfusion during exercise. They maintain their normal resting pressure by forming collaterals and by decreasing peripheral vascular resistance. These patients should be stressed with exercise or **reactive hyperemia** to further reduce peripheral resistance, thereby increasing the pressure gradient across the arterial segment and unmasking a hemodynamically significant lesion.

Contraindications to lower extremity arterial stress testing include symptomatic cardiac disease, severe pulmonary disease, severe hypertension, inability to walk on the treadmill, and cases of calcified vessels (unreliable pressure measurements; the use of pulse volume recordings may be helpful in some patients).

After the patient's brachial and ankle pressures are recorded at rest, the cuffs are left in place and exercise testing is performed on a treadmill at 1.5 to 2 mph on a 10% to 12% grade. Continuous electrocardiographic (ECG) monitoring during exercise testing is recommended. The patient walks for 5 minutes or until symptoms develop and pain forces the patient to stop. The patient is quickly returned to the supine position, and ankle pressures are recorded immediately and repeated every few minutes until the pressure returns to baseline. The time to onset of symptoms, the location and severity of the symptoms, and the total walking time are recorded and used to monitor changes in an individual patient over time.

The magnitude of the decrease in ankle pressure after exercise and the time required for the ankle pressure to return to baseline reflect the severity of the underlying arterial disease. In general, ankle pressures that fall after exercise and return to baseline within 5 minutes suggest single-segment occlusive disease. Multisegment arterial disease is usually associated with reduced ankle pressures that persist for longer than 10 minutes after exercise. When a patient stops walking because of symptoms associated with arterial disease, the ankle pressure is less than 60 mmHg. If ankle pressures are unchanged or improved after exercise, underlying arterial disease (even if present) can be excluded as a cause of the patient's symptoms.

An alternative method to stress the peripheral arterial circulation is reactive hyperemia. This testing is useful when patients cannot walk on the treadmill because of cardiac or other physical disabilities. This is not a well tolerated examination and should be used only in cases of extreme need. Resting ankle and arm pressures are recorded. A thigh cuff is inflated to a suprasystolic pressure for 3 to 5 minutes; this produces ischemia and vasodilation in the periphery. On release of the thigh cuff, ankle pressures are immediately recorded and measurements are repeated until they return to baseline. Normal individuals will experience up to a 30% decrease in ankle systolic pressure immediately after release of the thigh cuff. Patients with occlusive arterial disease will have a more pronounced effect after thigh cuff release and will take longer to return to baseline pressures.

Healing of Foot Ulcers and Amputations

Indirect arterial testing is helpful in predicting the likelihood of healing of skin lesions. This is especially helpful in diabetic patients, who often have foot ulcers and an abnormal physical examination. Ischemic skin lesions are not likely to heal if the ankle systolic pressure is below 55 mmHg (below 80 mmHg in diabetic patients), the toe pressure is below 30 mmHg, or the foot pulse volume recording fails to demonstrate pulsatile perfusion.

If a lower extremity amputation is required, segmental pressures and pulse volume recordings assist in selecting the appropriate amputation level. Pressure measurements have been reported as both helpful and misleading in predicting amputation site healing.[4,13,24,30,39] A below-knee amputation is likely to heal in patients with low thigh region or calf systolic pressures above 50 mmHg. In diabetic individuals, however, systolic pressures may be falsely elevated and amputation sites may fail to heal, even though pressure appears to be adequate.[25] Associated pulse volume recordings add valuable information for diabetic patients and those with calcified vessels.

Prediction of healing of forefoot and toe amputations is less precise. In general, a forefoot or toe amputation will not heal if the ankle pressure is less than 60 mmHg, or the toe pressure is less than 45 mmHg.

In summary, indirect methods of evaluation of the peripheral arterial system have provided much useful information over the past several decades. These techniques are limited, however, by failure to establish the exact disease location, by inability to detect disease that causes minor changes, by difficulties in differentiating the level and extent (stenosis vs. occlusion) of the disease, and by inability to accurately follow disease progression.

ARTERIAL DUPLEX IMAGING

Arterial duplex imaging provides direct anatomic and physiologic information, but it does not provide information regarding overall limb hemodynamics. Duplex imaging distinguishes between a stenosis and an occlusion, determines the length of the disease segment and the patency of the distal vessels, evaluates the results of intervention (angioplasty, stent placement), aids in diagnosis of aneurysm or pseudoaneurysm, and monitors patients' postoperative course with continuing bypass graft surveillance.

Color Doppler imaging provides a guide for accurate placement of the Doppler sample volume to obtain arterial Doppler spectral waveforms. Additionally, color Doppler imaging reduces the time required to perform an examination by visually identifying the blood flow disturbances on initial survey. When using color Doppler to guide the examination, however, properly adjusting the controls (e.g., pulse repetition frequency, color gain, frame rate) during the study is essential for an accurate examination.

The gray-scale image and color Doppler display are helpful in recognizing anatomic variations and in locating plaque and calcification, but are not accurate in determining the amount of arterial narrowing. The percent narrowing of an artery is determined from the Doppler spectral waveform information. A small Doppler sample volume is used for arterial imaging, and Doppler waveforms are obtained by maintaining a 60-degree angle to the vessel walls. If a 60-degree angle cannot be maintained, documentation of the angle used during the examination is important, especially in following the patient over time. It is best not to use an angle greater than 60 degrees because of the inherent error associated with using larger angles. The Doppler is swept through the color display to look for focal increases in velocity or blood flow disturbances. Representative Doppler signals are recorded from standard sites along the peripheral arteries. Additionally, if an area of narrowing is noted, Doppler signals proximal to the area, at the narrowing, and distal to the narrowing will provide the complete documentation necessary for an accurate interpretation.

It is imperative that each institution develop an arterial imaging protocol that defines the standard examination (arteries to be evaluated, the location of Doppler samples, etc.). This protocol must include information about the technique, clinical applications, indications for a complete and/or limited examination, and interpretation criteria. A standard complete examination for arterial occlusive disease usually includes acquiring both imaging and Doppler information from the entire extremity.

Lower Extremity

Peripheral arterial imaging begins at the level of the aortic bifurcation. Visualization of the proximal arteries is improved if patients do not take anything by mouth the morning of the examination. It is best to use a low-frequency transducer (2.0 to 3.5 MHz) for the proximal segment of the examination. The aortic bifurcation is best seen with the patient turned to the left side and with the transducer placed just in front of the right iliac crest in a longitudinal plane. The distal aorta and the origin of both common iliac arteries can usually be visualized. Doppler signals should be obtained from all three vessels at this location.

The patient should be placed in a lateral decubitus position (side being evaluated up) to evaluate the internal and external iliac arteries with the transducer placed between the iliac crest and the umbilicus. Doppler waveforms should be obtained from the internal and external iliac arteries, noting direction of blood flow and velocity. If difficulty is encountered in locating the iliac arteries from this approach, the arteries may be located by identifying the femoral arteries at the groin level and following the arteries proximally.

The patient should return to the supine position, and a higher-frequency, linear array transducer (5 to 10 MHz) should be used for evaluation of the arteries of the lower extremity. The common femoral artery is located at the level of the groin. The artery lies lateral to the common femoral vein. Imaging should be performed in the longitudinal plane, and a Doppler signal should be obtained from this artery. The vessel should be followed distally on the leg to the origin of the femoral and profunda femoris (deep femoral) arteries. Doppler signals should be obtained from the origin of both the femoral artery and the deep femoral artery. The femoral artery is followed distally as it courses down the medial aspect of the thigh. Doppler signals should be obtained along its pathway and at areas of questionable narrowing. The distal portion of the femoral artery may be easier to evaluate from the distal posterior thigh. This artery is followed distally in the limb and becomes the popliteal artery. The popliteal artery should be followed through the popliteal fossa. The popliteal artery lies deep to the vein, and a Doppler spectral waveform should be obtained from this vessel.

Following the distal popliteal artery in a longitudinal plane, the origin of the anterior tibial artery can usually be visualized diving deep on the monitor. The anterior tibial artery can be followed for only a short distance from this approach. The remainder of the vessel can be located distally by placing the transducer on the lateral calf and following to the level of the ankle. The tibial-peroneal trunk extends into the calf from the popliteal artery. The posterior tibial and peroneal arteries are usually visualized by placing the transducer on the medial calf. The peroneal artery lies deep and runs parallel to the posterior tibial artery. These vessels are located above the malleolus and are followed proximally.

The dorsalis pedis artery is found on top of the foot between the navicular and intermediate cuneiform bones. It is extremely superficial, so depth must be set at its minimum. Place the probe sagittally between the extensor longus tendons on top of the foot to see this artery. Finding the pulse of this artery can also help in locating with color Doppler (Figure 37-5).

Penile Evaluation

Arterial duplex imaging of the penile arteries can be used as a follow-up to penile pressure studies to assess erectile dysfunction. A high-frequency (7 to 10 MHz) linear probe should be utilized. Scanning on the dorsal side of the penis, flow should be evaluated in the **cavernosal arteries** and veins that run through the **corpus cavernosum**. These arteries are the main source of blood to fill this tissue during an erection. In the flaccid state, the flow in these arteries should be high resistive. As an erection occurs, the flow becomes low resistive, and venous drainage should cease. When the erection reaches a plateau, peak-to-systolic velocity (PSV) should be ≥35 cm/sec and venous flow should be ≤5 cm/sec (high resistive again). Any flow less than 35 cm/sec is considered erectile dysfunction related to arterial inflow disease. If inflow is normal but venous flow exceeds 5 cm/sec, then the dysfunction is related to venous disease. Or you may have a combination of both. These studies may require a pharmacologic injection for the patient to obtain an erection for your study. Prostaglandin E and papaverine, the most common drugs for this reaction, are injected directly into the corpus cavernosum.

Upper Extremity

Arteries of the upper extremity may also be evaluated with arterial duplex imaging. A low-frequency transducer should be used to evaluate the proximal vessels. The subclavian artery is evaluated from a supraclavicular

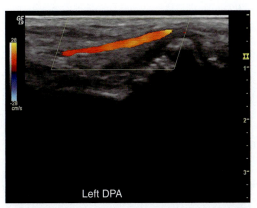

FIGURE 37-5 Normal dorsalis pedis artery (DPA) in the foot with color Doppler.

and infraclavicular approach. Segments of the subclavian artery may not be visualized because of shadowing from the clavicle. A Doppler signal should be obtained from the subclavian artery (Figure 37-6). The axillary artery may be evaluated from an infraclavicular approach or from the axilla.

The arteries in the arm should be evaluated with a higher-frequency linear-array transducer. The brachial artery should be followed along the length of the upper arm. The brachial artery divides into the radial and ulnar arteries near the antecubital fossa. The radial and ulnar arteries are visualized in a longitudinal plane along the length of the forearm. These vessels are superficial and may become very small at the wrist level.

Changes in arterial blood flow to the arms may be related to intermittent compression of the proximal arteries (thoracic outlet syndrome). The patient should be sitting with arms relaxed and alongside the body. Arterial Doppler signals should be recorded in the proximal brachial artery at rest and can be monitored during positional maneuvers.

Interpretation

Arterial duplex imaging examination of the lower extremities focuses on answering a number of important questions (Box 37-2). The duplex imaging criteria for normal arterial evaluation of the lower extremity have been established.[17] In normal vessels, the arterial Doppler signal is triphasic from the abdominal aorta to the tibial arteries at the ankle (Figure 37-7). This characteristic waveform has a high-velocity forward flow component during systole (ventricular contraction), followed by a brief reversal of flow in early diastole (because of peripheral resistance), and a final low-velocity forward flow phase in late diastole (elastic recoil of the vessel wall). Peak-systolic velocity gradually decreases from the proximal to the distal arteries. The peak velocity in the abdominal aorta is 100 cm/sec, and the velocity gradually decreases to 70 cm/sec in the popliteal artery.

Criteria have been developed for duplex imaging used to detect abnormal arterial segments.[20] A triphasic waveform with an increase in peak velocity of 30% to 100% relative to the adjacent proximal segment indicates disease, defined as a stenosis with a narrowing of less than 50% of the diameter of the artery. A 50% to 99% diameter reduction stenosis produces a monophasic waveform with extensive spectral broadening (caused by turbulence) and a peak-systolic velocity of more than 100% relative to the adjacent proximal segment; reduced systolic velocity is present distal to the stenosis (Figures 37-8 through 37-11). Three major changes in the spectral Doppler arterial waveform that occur because of a significant stenosis are (1) an increase in peak-systolic velocities (greater than 100%), (2) marked spectral broadening caused by turbulence, and (3) loss of reversal of blood flow during diastole. The color Doppler display

---

BOX 37-2 | Essential Questions to be Answered for Arterial Duplex Imaging

- Is disease present in the lower extremity?
- Is the disease a stenosis, an occlusion, an arteriovenous fistula, an aneurysm, or a pseudoaneurysm?
- What is the location of the narrowing? What is its length and severity?
- What is the location of the occlusion? What is the length of the occlusion? Are collaterals identified near the occlusion?
- Is there adequate inflow into the leg?
- Is an outflow vessel identified?
- Is an adequate superficial vein identified that may be used as an arterial conduit?
- Is an arteriovenous fistula identified? What is the location of the fistula?
- Is a patent arterial aneurysm identified? What is the location of the aneurysm and its dimensions?
- Is a pseudoaneurysm identified? What are its location and dimensions? Is the neck of the pseudoaneurysm identified? What is the vessel of origin?

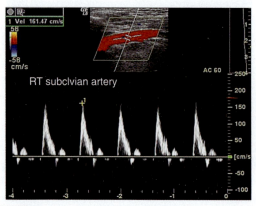

FIGURE 37-6 Normal triphasic waveform in the subclavian artery.

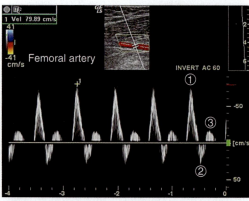

FIGURE 37-7 A normal color Doppler image and spectral Doppler waveform from a superficial femoral artery. The triphasic Doppler signal demonstrates a fast upstroke to peak systole **(1)**, reversal of blood flow during early diastole **(2)**, and a forward flow component during late diastole **(3)**.

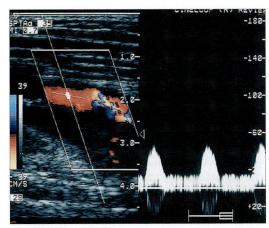

FIGURE 37-8 Color Doppler imaging in a patient who presented with claudication. A 40-mm Hg drop in pressure occurred from the upper to the lower thigh. The Doppler signal is proximal to the narrowed segment. Peak-systolic velocity is approximately 55 cm/sec, and the waveform shape is abnormal.

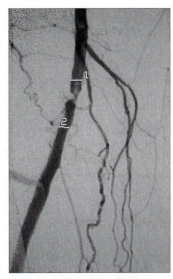

FIGURE 37-11 Corresponding arteriogram demonstrates narrowing of the superficial femoral artery.

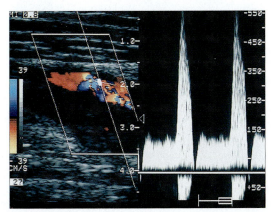

FIGURE 37-9 An area of increased velocity (color aliasing) was noted in the distal superficial femoral artery. At the site of narrowing, the peak-systolic velocity increases to greater than 450 cm/sec.

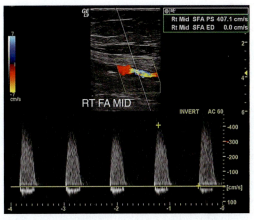

FIGURE 37-12 Severe stenosis seen in the femoral artery. Spectral Doppler is displaying a velocity of 407 cm/sec.

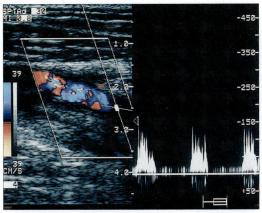

FIGURE 37-10 Distal to the segment of arterial narrowing, the Doppler spectral waveform is turbulent and the peak-systolic velocity is approximately 150 cm/sec.

also provides information that identifies the presence of significant arterial narrowing. Color aliasing, color persistence (continuous signal), and color bruit (tissue vibration caused by severe blood flow disturbance) indicate the presence of a blood flow abnormality (Figure 37-12).

No color Doppler or Doppler spectral waveform will be obtained in areas of occlusion. Damped proximal arterial Doppler spectral waveforms are obtained, and these demonstrate low velocity with little or no diastolic blood flow. The color Doppler display may reveal collaterals near the occluded segment. Power Doppler imaging improves visualization of areas of tight stenosis, especially in vessels running parallel to the skin line.

To define its accuracy, duplex imaging has been compared with lower extremity arteriography.[19,21,28,41] These studies demonstrate a sensitivity of 77% to 92% and a specificity of 92% to 98% for correctly categorizing a stenosis as greater or less than 50% diameter reduction. These reports evaluated the capabilities of duplex imaging in the proximal vessels, but limited information is available regarding its sensitivity in the calf arteries.[16]

All studies reported high negative predictive values (87% to 98%), indicating that significant occlusive arterial disease can be excluded in patients with normal duplex imaging examinations. Limitations of the lower extremity arterial duplex imaging examination are listed in Box 37-3.

Aneurysms and Pseudoaneurysms. Arterial duplex imaging has also become valuable for evaluating patients with aneurysms and pseudoaneurysms of the extremity. Duplex imaging distinguishes between aneurysms (Figure 37-13), pseudoaneurysms (Figure 37-14), perigraft fluid collections (Figure 37-15), and hematomas. Information about size, location, site of communication, and presence of luminal thrombus is easily obtained in most cases.

Evaluation of arterial aneurysms by duplex imaging is considered an accurate method in determining size, position, patency, and associated arterial blood flow dynamics. Aneurysms may be located in the distal abdominal aorta and the iliac, common femoral, and popliteal arteries. To accurately measure the size (length and width) of an aneurysm, the artery should be evaluated in both longitudinal and transverse imaging planes.

A **pseudoaneurysm** is a perivascular collection (hematoma) that communicates with an artery or a graft and contains pulsating blood entering the collection. A track (neck) of variable length connects the native vessel to the collection. Pseudoaneurysms may occur as a result of trauma, at vascular anastomoses, in angioaccess grafts, or at puncture sites (usually following cardiac catheterization).

A pseudoaneurysm may be unilocular or multilocular and may partially contain thrombus. Pseudoaneurysms occur in variable sizes, and the size of the pseudoaneurysm changes during each cardiac cycle. Although spontaneous thrombosis of pseudoaneurysms has been reported in the literature,[18,22,32] fatal spontaneous hemorrhage of pseudoaneurysms has also occurred.[26] The risk of rupture is present in those pseudoaneurysms measuring greater than 3 cm.

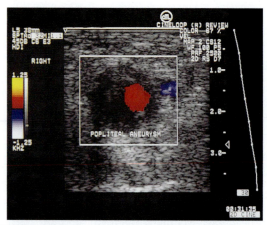

FIGURE 37-13 A popliteal artery aneurysm. The red represents the blood flow within the aneurysm. Blood flow within the popliteal vein is displayed in blue.

BOX 37-3	**Limitations of the Lower Extremity Arterial Duplex Imaging Examination**

- Nonvisualization of the iliac system because of bowel gas or obesity
- Shadowing because of calcification
- Imaging of the popliteal trifurcation
- Difficulty evaluating lesions distal to tight stenoses because of low velocities in these segments

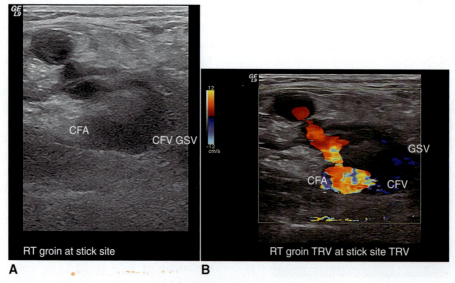

FIGURE 37-14 A bilobed pseudoaneurysm in a 49-year-old female is seen extending from the common femoral artery *(CFA)* post heart catheterization. **A,** Gray scale of the double-lobed pseudo. **B,** Color flow within the double lobes extending from the neck attached to the common femoral artery. *CFA,* Common femoral artery; *CFV,* common femoral vein; *GSV,* greater saphenous vein.

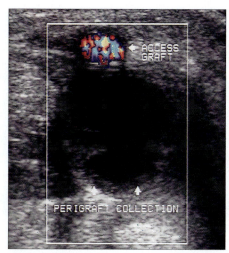

FIGURE 37-15 Color Doppler image of a patent access graft with adjacent perigraft collection.

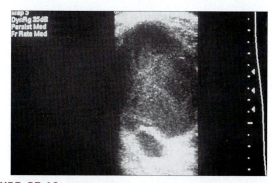

FIGURE 37-16 A large pseudoaneurysm from an axillofemoral bypass graft. The swirling of blood is visualized in gray scale.

■ **Sonographic Findings.** Swirling blood within the collection is often visualized in gray-scale imaging (Figure 37-16). The use of color Doppler imaging helps to identify the neck of the pseudoaneurysm. Identification of the neck of the pseudoaneurysm is important when ultrasound-guided compression therapy is attempted, and color Doppler imaging permits identification of the vessel of origin, which is important when planning surgical interventions.

A spectral Doppler waveform obtained from the neck of a pseudoaneurysm displays a to-and-fro (bidirectional) pattern. During systole, blood flows from the native artery into the pseudoaneurysm; during diastole, blood flow returns to the native artery. Additionally, the size (length, width, and depth) of the pseudoaneurysm should be measured. Some pseudoaneurysms are very large, and it is difficult to capture the entire area in one image for measurement. The sensitivity and specificity in the identification of pseudoaneurysms range from 94% to 100%.

Compression Therapy. Compression therapy of the pseudoaneurysm may be attempted if the neck of the pseudoaneurysm has been clearly identified during arterial duplex imaging. The neck of the pseudoaneurysm is

the area that is compressed when pressure is placed on the skin by the ultrasound transducer. The goal is to stop blood flow into the pseudoaneurysm by occluding the neck. It is extremely important not to occlude blood flow in the native artery, so distal blood flow should be monitored during compression therapy.

A considerable amount of time and upper body strength are necessary to perform ultrasound compression therapy of pseudoaneurysms for an extended period. Compression cycles of 15 to 20 minutes are usually performed, with progress evaluated between cycles. In most cases, it will take at least 30 to 60 minutes to achieve a successful thrombosis of the pseudoaneurysm. Most investigators suggest bed rest (6 to 24 hours) after a successful compression procedure and reexamination of the area the next day. Recurrence rates have been reported for ultrasound compression, and a second attempt to compress the pseudoaneurysm may be warranted.[15]

Success rates of ultrasound compression of pseudoaneurysms have varied from 70% to 86%.[9,12] Success varies depending on the size and age of the pseudoaneurysm, and whether the patient is on anticoagulation therapy. Failure to thrombose a pseudoaneurysm occurs more often in large pseudoaneurysms, when the pseudoaneurysm has been present for a prolonged period, and when the patient has been given anticoagulants. Additionally, some patients cannot tolerate the pain associated with the compression technique. Complications of ultrasound compression therapy for pseudoaneurysms have included occlusion of the native artery, development of deep vein thrombosis, and rupture of the pseudoaneurysm.

As an alternative to ultrasound compression therapy, some investigators have performed ultrasound-guided thrombin injection of pseudoaneurysms.[7,23,31,33,35,38,42] As the thrombin is injected, results are continuously monitored with color Doppler imaging. Thrombin injection is stopped when blood flow is no longer documented (visualized color Doppler). In addition, distal pulses and other signs of arterial disease are closely monitored. Follow-up imaging can be repeated immediately and within 24 hours. Successful treatment occurs in approximately 97% of reported patients. Complications of this technique are few (about .05% to 1.3% of cases) and include thrombosis of the feeding artery.[40] Investigators use this technique in uncomplicated pseudoaneurysms and suggest that complicated pseudoaneurysms (arteriovenous fistula [AVF], rapid expansion, infection, hemorrhage, etc.) should be managed surgically. Important issues associated with the successful repair of pseudoaneurysms using this technique are the size, location, and size of the neck; the thrombin dose; and the number of injections.

Transluminal Angioplasty. Lower extremity arterial duplex imaging is important in the evaluation and follow-up of patients who may be candidates for percutaneous intervention. Because duplex imaging can identify the extent and location of the arterial disease, it may eliminate the need for an arteriogram in patients who are considered candidates for balloon angioplasty but not operative reconstruction.

One study compared color Doppler imaging and arteriography in 84 lower extremities in 61 patients being evaluated for angioplasty.[11] Differentiation between a normal and a diseased artery was possible, with a sensitivity of 83% and a specificity of 96%. For identifying stenosis greater than 50% diameter reduction, sensitivity was 87% and specificity was 99%. In the detection of occluded arterial segments, sensitivity and specificity were 81% and 99%, respectively. In this group of patients, color Doppler imaging accurately provided information in 48/51 (94%) of arterial occlusions, including four extremities for which the original arteriogram overestimated the length of the occlusion.

A study used color Doppler imaging to evaluate 62 patients with limiting claudication.[10] Twenty-six patients were believed to be suitable candidates for percutaneous balloon angioplasty and underwent arteriography. Duplex imaging and arteriography agreed in 97% (62/64) of femoral and popliteal segments and in 97% (93/96) of tibial and peroneal arteries.

One hundred ten patients who had lower extremity arterial duplex imaging before arteriography were evaluated.[14] Fifty patients were selected for transluminal balloon angioplasty on the basis of the duplex imaging examination. Three of the 50 patients did not have angioplasty performed because of the lesion's location or extent. The authors concluded that duplex imaging allowed accurate prediction of which arterial lesions can be treated by transluminal balloon angioplasty. The authors therefore recommended duplex imaging as a screening test. This is now replaced by CT angioplasty.

Duplex imaging allows accurate identification of the location, length, and severity of arterial lesions, which is important in planning the best type of intervention. Duplex imaging is also ideal in the follow-up examination of patients after intervention for lower extremity arterial disease (Figure 37-17). Although pressure measurements can be valuable when observing these patients, they cannot distinguish between restenosis of the angioplasty site and progression of proximal or distal disease, or both. Duplex imaging can identify recurrent stenosis before occlusion and, if indicated, allows for a repeat angioplasty.

Bypass Graft Surveillance. The patency of bypass grafts can be significantly prolonged if developing graft lesions are corrected before graft thrombosis. Therefore, all lower extremity bypass grafts should be monitored for technical adequacy, hemodynamic function, and development of postimplantation lesions (Figures 37-18 and 37-19). Graft abnormalities, such as myointimal stenosis, retained valve cusps, arteriovenous fistulas, degenerative aneurysmal formation, and low flow states, can be detected with arterial duplex imaging, even if no

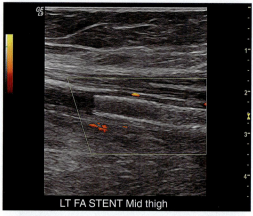

FIGURE 37-17 An occluded femoral artery stent 2 days post placement in a 79-year-old female.

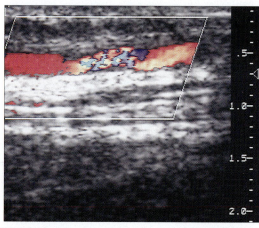

FIGURE 37-18 A color Doppler image of an in situ bypass graft. An area of increased blood flow velocity (color change) is seen within the graft.

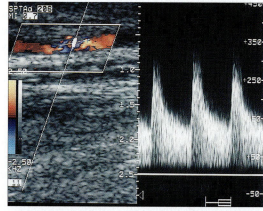

FIGURE 37-19 Doppler spectral waveform from the area of narrowing in the in situ bypass graft demonstrates an increase in peak-systolic velocity to approximately 300 cm/sec.

changes in ankle pressure are obvious.[5,27] A graft surveillance program should identify bypass grafts at risk for thrombosis, provide information on the mechanism of failure (Figure 37-20), and, with appropriate intervention, reduce the incidence of unexpected graft failure.

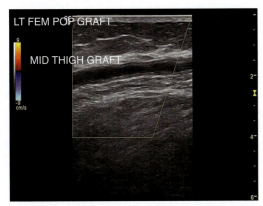

FIGURE 37-20 An occluded fem-pop bypass graft in a patient with increasing claudication.

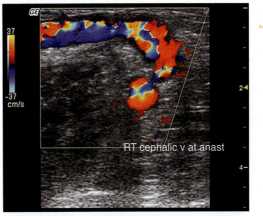

FIGURE 37-21 A dialysis fistula created between the cephalic vein and the brachial artery in color Doppler.

Surveillance programs by arterial duplex imaging have resulted in assisted primary patency rates of 82% to 92% at 5 years compared with 60% to 70% patency for bypasses followed clinically, and 30% to 50% patency rates after secondary procedures to salvage thrombosed vein grafts.[2,3,36]

To accurately evaluate bypass grafts with arterial duplex imaging, it is important to know the location and type of graft before beginning the study. The technique is similar to the color Doppler imaging of native arteries. The entire length of the bypass graft should be evaluated with color Doppler and Doppler signals. Additionally, the inflow and outflow vessels should be evaluated and close attention paid to the proximal and distal anastomoses.

The timing of bypass graft surveillance will vary with each surgeon. Some authors suggest performing an examination after the operation before the patient is discharged from the hospital. This baseline duplex examination permits identification of bypass grafts with residual graft defects. If the baseline postoperative duplex evaluation is considered normal, follow-up examinations are performed at 4- to 6-week, 3-month, and 3- to 6-month intervals for the first postoperative year. During the second postoperative year, evaluations are performed at 18 and 24 months and then on an annual basis. If graft surveillance detects a stenosis, more frequent evaluations may be performed to follow the patient, or the decision to intervene may be indicated.

A change from the triphasic Doppler signal to a monophasic waveform with a decrease in peak-systolic velocity to below 45 cm/sec is diagnostic of a lesion placing the graft at risk. Additionally, repair of graft stenosis is recommended with peak systolic velocities greater than 300 cm/sec or a peak systolic ratio greater than 3.5.[36]

A wide range of peak velocities may be identified in normal grafts.[6] The peak-systolic velocity in a bypass graft is due to the size of the graft and the outflow resistance. A low velocity in a bypass graft may relate to a large graft diameter, poor arterial inflow, and small vessel runoff. A significant decrease in peak-systolic velocity within a graft on serial duplex imaging may be a better indicator of pending graft failure.

Other investigators suggest using a velocity ratio to determine graft stenosis. Doubling of the velocity ratio has been noted to indicate a significant graft stenosis.[34] The velocity ratio is calculated by dividing the peak-systolic velocity at the site of the flow disturbance by the peak-systolic velocity in the adjacent proximal segment. A velocity ratio greater than 2.0 was associated with a sensitivity of 95% and a specificity of 100% for detection of stenosis greater than 50% diameter reduction.

Arterial duplex imaging plays an important role in the follow-up of patients with lower extremity arterial bypass grafts. Identification of arterial lesions during the preocclusive phase is critical for prolonging the patency of the graft.

Dialysis Access Grafts. The evaluation of dialysis access grafts is an area of increasing interest. Dialysis grafts (autogenous or synthetic) are typically placed in the forearm. The Brescia-Cimino arteriovenous fistula is a direct connection of the radial artery and the cephalic vein. Other direct connections include cephalic vein to brachial artery (Figure 37-21), basilic vein to brachial artery, and basilic vein to ulnar artery. The other type of dialysis access uses a synthetic graft interposed between the artery and the vein (straight or loop graft). These can be placed in the lower or upper arm or in the upper leg. They are usually easily identifiable under the surface of the skin and produce a thrill when palpated. The most common problems associated with these grafts are caused by venous outflow obstruction, venous anastomotic stenosis, pseudoaneurysm, hematoma (Figure 37-22), perigraft fluid collection, or arterial anastomotic stenosis (Figure 37-23). Patients are referred for evaluation and mapping of the veins before access placement, or because of inadequate dialysis, suspicion of a steal, a stenosis, thrombosis, or a pseudoaneurysm. The ultrasound examination should include recording of Doppler velocity signals from throughout the native arterial system, the graft, and the venous outflow system, paying close attention to each anastomosis. This evaluation should include checking for stenosis and thrombosis within the graft and the native circulation. Typically, access grafts will demonstrate an increased velocity that has continuous forward diastolic flow and notable spectral broadening. These velocities will be slightly lower moving toward the venous limb of the graft. Peak sys-tolic velocities are usually in the range of 200 cm/sec or higher (Figure 37-24). Decreases in peak velocities between 100 cm/sec and 200 cm/sec are suspicious for the development of a problem (usually an outflow stenosis). Lack of Doppler signals and intraluminal echoes provides evidence for occlusion of the graft. Using an ultrasound surveillance program for the early detection and treatment of problems associated with hemodialysis access grafts has demonstrated that the patency of access grafts can be significantly prolonged if developing graft lesions are corrected before graft thrombosis.[29,37]

GUIDELINES FOR EVALUATION

Peripheral arterial testing provides valuable information by addressing specific questions at the patient's original visit and during follow-up studies (Table 37-2).

Performing high-quality and complete examinations is essential to the diagnostic value of these tests. The best peripheral arterial evaluation will be achieved by proper attention to detail. Major areas of focus when performing a peripheral arterial evaluation are summarized in Box 37-4. Attention to these technical areas and interpretation details will ensure the best peripheral arterial evaluation.

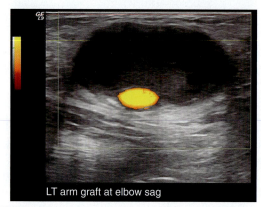

FIGURE 37-22 A hematoma seen post dialysis. Flow is seen in the graft posterior to the hematoma. The patient presented with a palpable mass.

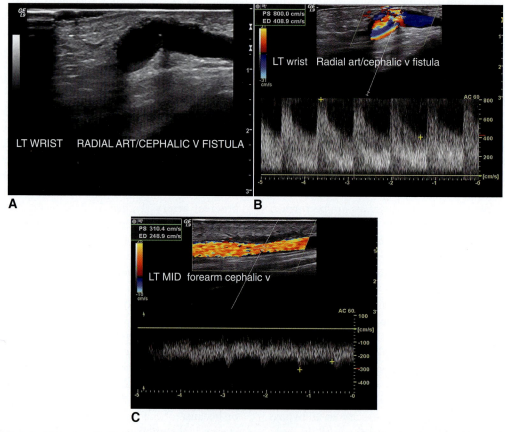

FIGURE 37-23 Brescia-Cimino graft. **A,** Gray-scale image of the radial artery and cephalic vein connection. **B,** Color and spectral Doppler of a stenosis at the anastomosis of the artery and vein. Flow is 800 cm/sec. **C,** Distal flow in the cephalic vein reveals a normal flow velocity of 310 cm/sec.

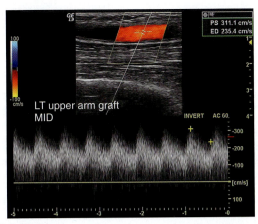

FIGURE 37-24 Normal flow of 311 cm/sec through a synthetic graft. Flow velocities through these grafts are normally high.

| BOX 37-4 | **Arterial Evaluation Guidelines** |

- Take a patient history.
- Be familiar with arterial anatomy, physiology, and pathology.
- When measuring ankle pressures, always use the highest brachial pressure when calculating an ankle-brachial index.
- When performing arterial duplex imaging, optimize the gray-scale image.
- Understand how each color control affects the image and how the controls affect each other.
- Use a longitudinal imaging plane to obtain color Doppler information, and use it as a guide to obtain the spectral Doppler waveforms.
- Use a small Doppler sample volume size and a 60-degree angle.
- Be aware of the Doppler spectral waveform velocity and its configuration.
- Establish institutional diagnostic criteria.

TABLE 37-2	**Evaluation Guidelines Based on Clinical Presentation**	
Clinical Presentation	**Questions**	**Noninvasive Test**
Initial visit	Is disease present? How severe is the process? What segments are involved?	Resting segmental pressures, pulse volume tracings, exercise testing (select patients)
Focal problems	Is pulsatile mass an aneurysm or a pseudoaneurysm? What is the size/location of the aneurysm?	Duplex imaging
Before angioplasty	What is the location of the lesion? Is it a stenosis or an occlusion? What is the length of the disease segment? What is the status of the runoff vessels?	Duplex imaging
After angioplasty	Was the angioplasty successful? What is the degree of improvement?	Pressure measurements and duplex imaging
Bypass graft	Is the bypass graft patent? What is the degree of improvement? Is the graft at risk for failure?	Pressure measurements and duplex imaging

---

REFERENCES

1. Baker JD, Dix D: Variability of Doppler ankle pressures with arterial occlusive disease: an evaluation of ankle index and brachial-ankle pressure gradient, *Surgery* 89:134-137, 1981.
2. Bandyk DF, Mills JL, Gahtan V, Esses GE: Intraoperative duplex scanning of arterial reconstructions: fate of repaired and unrepaired defects, *J Vasc Surg* 20:426-432, 1994.
3. Bandyk DF, Cato RF, Towne JB: A low flow velocity predicts failure of femoropopliteal and femorotibial bypass grafts, *Surgery* 98:799-809, 1985.
4. Barnes RW, Shanik GD, Slaymaker EE: An index of healing in below-knee amputation: leg blood pressure by Doppler ultrasound, *Surgery* 79:13-20, 1976.
5. Barnes RW, Thompson BW, MacDonald DM, et al: Serial noninvasive studies do not herald postoperative failure of femoropopliteal or femorotibial bypass grafts, *Ann Surg* 210:486-493, 1989.
6. Belkin M, Raffery KB, Mackey WC: A prospective study of the determinants of vein graft flow velocity: implications for graft surveillance, *J Vasc Surg* 17:259-265, 1994.
7. Brophy DP, Sheiman RG, Amatulle P, Akbari CM: Iatrogenic femoral pseudoaneurysms: thrombin injection after failed US-guided compression, *Radiology* 214:278-282, 2000.
8. Carter SA, Tate RB: The effect of body heating and cooling on the ankle and toe systolic pressures in arterial disease, *J Vasc Surg* 16:148-153, 1992.
9. Coley BD, Roberts AC, Fellmeth BD, et al: Postangiographic femoral artery pseudoaneurysm: further experience with US-guided compression repair, *Radiology* 194:307-311, 1995.
10. Collier P, Wilcox G, Brooks D, et al: Improved patient selection for angioplasty utilizing color Doppler imaging, *Am J Surg* 160:171-174, 1990.
11. Cossman DV, Ellison JE, Wagner WH, et al: Comparison of contrast arteriography to arterial mapping with color flow duplex imaging in the lower extremities, *J Vasc Surg* 10:552-558, 1989.
12. Cox GS, Young JR, Gray BR, et al: Ultrasound-guided compression repair of postcatheterization pseudoaneurysms: results of treatment in one hundred cases, *J Vasc Surg* 19:683-686, 1994.
13. Dean SM, Olin JW, Piedmonte M, et al: Ultrasound-guided compression closure of postcatheterization pseudoaneurysms during concurrent anticoagulation: a review of seventy-seven patients, *J Vasc Surg* 23:28-34, 1996.
14. Edwards JM, Coldwell DM, Goldman ML, Strandness DE Jr: The role of duplex scanning in the selection of patients for transluminal angioplasty, *J Vasc Surg* 13:69-74, 1991.

15. Feld R, Patton GM, Carabasi RA, et al: Treatment of iatrogenic femoral artery injuries with ultrasound-guided compression, *J Vasc Surg* 16:832-840, 1992.

16. Hatsukami TS, Primozich JF, Zierler RE, et al: Color Doppler imaging of infrainguinal arterial occlusive disease, *J Vasc Surg* 16:527-531, 1992.

17. Jager KA, Ricketts HJ, Strandness DE: Duplex scanning for the evaluation of lower limb arterial disease. In Bernstein EF, editor: *Noninvasive diagnostic techniques in vascular disease*, ed 3, St Louis, 1985, Mosby.

18. Johns JP, Pupa LE, Bailey SR: Spontaneous thrombosis of iatrogenic femoral artery pseudoaneurysms: documentation with color Doppler and two-dimensional ultrasonography, *J Vasc Surg* 14:24-29, 1991.

19. Keagy BA, Pharr WF, Thomas D, Bowes DE: Comparison of reactive hyperemia and treadmill tests in the evaluation of peripheral arterial disease, *Am J Surg* 142:158-161, 1981.

20. Kohler TR, Nance DR, Cramer MM, et al: Duplex scanning for diagnosis of aortoiliac and femoropopliteal disease: a prospective study, *Circulation* 76:1074-1080, 1987.

21. Kohler TR, Andros G, Porter JM, et al: Can duplex scanning replace arteriography for lower extremity arterial disease? *Ann Vasc Surg* 4:280-287, 1990.

22. Kotval PS, Khoury A, Shah PM, Babu SC: Doppler sonographic demonstration of the progressive spontaneous thrombosis of pseudoaneurysms, *J Ultrasound Med* 9:185-190, 1990.

23. Liau CS, Ho FM, Chen MF, Lee YT: Treatment of iatrogenic femoral artery pseudoaneurysm with percutaneous thrombin injection, *J Vasc Surg* 26:18-23, 1997.

24. Malone JM, Anderson GG, Lalka SG, et al: Prospective comparison of noninvasive techniques for amputation level selection, *Am J Surg* 154:179-184, 1987.

25. Marinelli MR, Beach KW, Glass MJ, et al: Noninvasive testing vs. clinical evaluation of arterial disease: a prospective study, *JAMA* 241:2031-2034, 1979.

26. McCann RL, Schwartz LB, Pieper KS: Vascular complications of cardiac catheterization, *J Vasc Surg* 14:375-381, 1991.

27. Mills JL, Harris EJ, Taylor LM Jr, et al: The importance of routine surveillance of distal bypass grafts with duplex scanning: a study of 379 reversed vein grafts, *J Vasc Surg* 12:379-386, 1990.

28. Moneta GL, Strandness DE: Peripheral arterial duplex scanning, *J Clin Ultasound* 15:645-651, 1987.

29. Neyra NR, Ikizler TA, May RE, et al: Change in access blood flow over time predicts vascular access thrombosis, *Kidney Int* 54:1714-1719, 1998.

30. Nichols GG, Myers JL, DeMuth WE: The role of vascular laboratory criteria in the selection of patients for lower extremity amputation, *Ann Surg* 195:469-473, 1982.

31. Partap VA, Cassoff J: Ultrasound-guided percutaneous thrombin injection for treatment of femoral pseudoaneurysms: technical note, *Can Assoc Radiol J* 50:182-184, 1999.

32. Paulson EK, Hertzberg BS, Paine SS, Carroll BA: Femoral artery pseudoaneurysms: value of color Doppler sonography in predicting which ones will thrombose without treatment, *Am J Radiol* 159:1077-1081, 1992.

33. Pezzullo JA, Dupuy DE, Cronan JJ: Percutaneous injection of thrombin for the treatment of pseudoaneurysms after catheterization: an alternative to sonographically guided compression, *AJR* 175:1035-1040, 2000.

34. Polak JF, Donaldson MC, Dobkin GR, et al: Early detection of saphenous vein arterial bypass graft stenosis by color-assisted duplex sonography: a prospective study, *Am J Radiol* 154:857-861, 1990.

35. Reeder SB, Widlus DM, Lazinger M: Low-dose thrombin injection to treat iatrogenic femoral artery pseudoaneurysms, *AJR Am J Roentgenol* 177:595-598, 2001.

36. Roth SM, Bandyk DF: Duplex imaging of lower extremity bypasses, angioplasties, and stents, *Semin Vasc Surg* 12:275-284, 1999.

37. Safa AA, Valji K, Roberts AC, et al: Detection and treatment of dysfunctional hemodialysis access grafts: effect of a surveillance program on graft patency and the incidence of thrombosis, *Radiology* 199:653-657, 1996.

38. Taylor BS, Rhee RY, Muluk S, et al: Thrombin injection versus compression of femoral artery pseudoaneurysms, *J Vasc Surg* 30:1052-1059, 1999.

39. Wagner WH, Keagy BA, Kotb MM, et al: Noninvasive determination of healing of major lower extremity amputation: the continued role of clinical judgment, *J Vasc Surg* 8:703-710, 1988.

40. Webber GW, Jang J, Gustavson S, Olin JW. Contemporary management of postcatheterization pseudoaneurysms, *Circulation* 115:2666-2674, 2007.

41. Whelan JF, Barry MH, Moir JD: Color-flow Doppler ultrasonography: comparison with peripheral arteriography for the investigation of peripheral vascular disease, *J Clin Ultrasound* 20:369-374, 1992.

42. Wixon CL, Philpott JM, Bogey WM Jr, Powell CS: Duplex-directed thrombin injection as a method to treat femoral artery pseudoaneurysms, *J Am Coll Surg* 187:464-466, 1998.

43. Yao JST: Haemodynamic studies in peripheral arterial disease, *Br J Surg* 57:761-766, 1970.

Peripheral Venous Evaluation

Mira L. Katz and Ann Willis

Venous disease may be categorized as an acute or a chronic process. Deep vein thrombosis (DVT), the acute process, may be located in the lower and/or upper extremities. The chronic process, post-thrombotic syndrome, is a complication that can follow DVT. It is responsible for patient morbidity caused by leg swelling, pain, hyperpigmentation, and venous ulceration. Although the exact incidence or prevalence of DVT in the United States is unknown because many episodes are not clinically detected, it has been estimated that DVT affects more than 600,000 individuals annually.[10] Almost 1 in 20 individuals will develop DVT over their lifetime.[15] Historically, upper extremity DVT was considered an uncommon clinical event that was usually caused by compression at the thoracic inlet ("effort thrombosis"). The incidence of upper extremity DVT is on the rise, however, because of the increasing use of central venous lines.

A potentially lethal complication of acute DVT is pulmonary embolism (PE). The number of fatal PEs in the United States has caused 300,000 deaths per year.[7] Nonfatal pulmonary embolism has been estimated to occur three times more often than fatal PE.

The symptoms and signs of DVT are common and may have several possible causes (e.g., musculoskeletal disorders, ruptured Baker's cyst, cellulitis). Because the clinical diagnosis of DVT is unreliable, noninvasive methods to diagnose DVT were developed. Venous duplex imaging has emerged as a valuable diagnostic test because it is more accurate than other noninvasive techniques (nonimaging Doppler, impedance plethysmography), and unlike with venography, no risks are associated with this technique. The ability to correctly diagnose DVT is critical to patient management. Treatment of DVT with anticoagulants has reduced the occurrence of PE, relieved symptoms, and prevented extension of DVT. Additionally, it is critical to correctly identify patients without DVT, so that patients are not exposed unnecessarily to the risks associated with anticoagulant therapy.

RISK FACTORS AND SYMPTOMS OF VENOUS DISEASE

In response to a wide variety of stimuli, elements within the blood alter themselves to form a thrombus or blood clot. In 1856, Rudolph Virchow presented classic concepts on the causes of clot formation within the intact venous system.[22] The three factors associated with thrombus formation—Virchow's triad—include (1) a hypercoagulable state, (2) venous stasis (blood pools in the veins), and (3) vein wall injury (endothelium of the vein is damaged, exposing the subendothelium to blood and triggering platelet adhesion and aggregation, which promotes blood coagulation). The interplay of these three factors creates the most likely setting for the development of deep venous thrombosis.

The risk factors for DVT are listed in Box 38-1. An individual with an increasing number of risk factors is at greater risk of developing DVT.

Deep vein thrombosis and **pulmonary embolism (PE)** may be symptomatic or asymptomatic. Severe forms of lower extremity DVT include phlegmasia alba dolens (swollen, painful white leg) and phlegmasia cerulea dolens (swollen, painful cyanotic leg). Both of these affect arterial inflow and are limb threatening. Symptoms commonly associated with DVT and PE are listed in Box 38-2.

The chronic venous process, post-thrombotic syndrome, is caused by increased ambulatory venous pressure. Increased ambulatory venous pressure may result from venous obstruction and/or incompetent venous valves. DVT tends to accumulate around the valve leaflets. Over time, this can damage the leaflets, causing them to become incompetent. Transmission of venous hypertension to the capillaries over time may result in damage to the capillaries and may produce edema (Figure 38-1), stasis dermatitis (redness, itching, flaking skin), hyperpigmentation, and ulceration.

Additionally, varicose veins may occur. **Varicose veins** are dilated, elongated, tortuous superficial veins. Primary varicose veins are congenital, are an inherent weakness of the venous walls, and occur without coexisting deep venous disease. Secondary varicose veins occur secondary to pathology (DVT, absence of valves) of the deep venous system. Ultrasound-guided sclerotherapy is being used for the treatment of varicose veins. With sclerotherapy, a substance is injected into the veins, causing them to shrink and eventually disappear. Ultrasound guidance can help the physician find vessels under the skin surface that are not readily apparent.

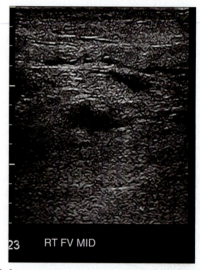

23   RT FV MID

FIGURE 38-1 Edema is seen in the tissue anterior to a chronic deep venous thrombosis *(DVT)*.

BOX 38-1	Risk Factors for Deep Vein Thrombosis

- Age (greater than 40 years old)
- Malignancy (cancer)
- Previous deep venous thrombosis or pulmonary embolism
- Immobilization (bed rest, paralysis of legs, extended travel)
- Fracture of the pelvis, hip, or long bones
- Myocardial infarction, stroke
- Congestive heart or respiratory failure
- Pregnancy and postpartum
- Oral contraceptives and hormone replacement therapy
- Extensive dissection at major surgery (especially orthopedic surgery)
- Trauma (multiple)
- Hereditary factors (antithrombin deficiency, protein C and protein S deficiencies)
- Obesity
- Central venous lines, pacemakers
- Intravenous drug abuse

BOX 38-2	Symptoms and Signs Associated With Deep Vein Thrombosis and Pulmonary Embolism

Deep Vein Thrombosis
- Persistent calf, leg, or arm swelling
- Pain or tenderness of the leg (usually the posterior calf) or arm-shoulder region
- Venous distention
- Increased temperature and redness
- Superficial venous dilation
- Homan's sign (calf discomfort on passive dorsiflexion)

Superficial Venous Thrombosis
- Local erythema
- Tenderness or pain
- Palpable subcutaneous "cord"

Pulmonary Embolus
- Dyspnea (shortness of breath)
- Chest pain
- Hemoptysis (spitting up blood)
- Sweats
- Cough

ANATOMY FOR VENOUS DUPLEX IMAGING

The peripheral veins return deoxygenated blood back to the heart. The venous systems of the lower and upper extremities consist of superficial, deep, and perforating (communicating) veins. Perforating veins provide a channel between superficial and deep veins. Venous blood flow is normally from the superficial veins to the deep veins.

A unique feature of the venous system is the venous valve. **Valves** are folds of the intima, the innermost layer of the vein wall. Venous valves are bicuspid, are more numerous in the distal leg, and often are located near a vein confluence. Venous valves are important in maintaining unidirectional blood flow from the peripheral veins to the central veins. They also help fight against the effects of hydrostatic pressure, which is essentially gravity when standing upright. At the level of the right atrium, this pressure equals 0 mmHg, and when standing upright, the pressure increases because of gravity as you travel toward the periphery in the lower segment of the body. No venous valves are present in the inferior vena cava, superior vena cava, innominate veins, or soleal sinuses.

Lower Extremity

Deep Veins. In the lower extremity, the primary route of drainage is via the deep veins of the leg (Figure 38-2). The lower extremity deep veins have corresponding arteries. The **anterior tibial veins** drain blood from the dorsum of the foot (dorsalis pedis veins) and the anterior compartment of the calf. The anterior tibial veins originate near the tibia at the ankle, lie anterior to the interosseous membrane as they ascend the lower leg, and move toward the fibula. They join at a variable level and pattern with the posterior tibial veins to become the **popliteal vein.**

The **posterior tibial veins** originate from the plantar (superficial and deep) veins of the foot. They run from the medial malleolus along the medial calf with the posterior tibial artery. The posterior tibial veins drain blood from the posterior compartment of the lower leg. They often unite as a single vein and receive the combined **peroneal veins** (tibial-peroneal trunk) before uniting with the anterior tibial veins to become the popliteal vein.

The peroneal veins course along the peroneal artery near the fibula. They lie deep to the soleus and gastrocnemius muscles and parallel the path of the posterior tibial veins. The peroneal veins drain blood from the lateral compartment of the lower leg. They unite as a single vein before joining the posterior tibial veins.

Lying within the deep muscular compartment of the calf are the soleal sinuses and the gastrocnemius (sural) veins. The **soleal sinuses** are large venous reservoirs that

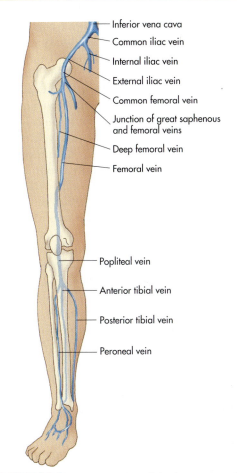

FIGURE 38-2 The deep veins of the lower extremity.

Inferior vena cava
Common iliac vein
Internal iliac vein
External iliac vein
Common femoral vein
Junction of great saphenous and femoral veins
Deep femoral vein
Femoral vein
Popliteal vein
Anterior tibial vein
Posterior tibial vein
Peroneal vein

lie in the soleus muscle and empty into the posterior tibial or peroneal veins. The gastrocnemius veins are paired, accompany an artery, and lie in the medial and lateral gastrocnemius muscles. The gastrocnemius veins terminate in the popliteal vein.

The popliteal vein accompanies the popliteal artery. The popliteal vein originates from the confluence of the anterior tibial veins with the posterior and peroneal veins (tibial-peroneal trunk). A duplicated popliteal vein occurs in approximately 30% to 35% of the population. The popliteal vein lies superficial to the artery. In the lower popliteal fossa, the popliteal vein lies medial to the artery. The vein passes to the lateral side of the artery as it ascends through the popliteal space.

The **femoral vein (FV)**, which is the companion of the femoral artery, is a deep vein that originates at the hiatus of the adductor magnus muscle in the distal thigh and ascends through the adductor (Hunter's) canal. The vein courses deep to the artery and terminates in Scarpa's (femoral) triangle. The femoral vein is duplicated in 20% to 30% of limbs. These have been commonly known as the *superficial femoral vein and artery.* Anatomists have always referred to this set as just the *femoral artery* and *femoral vein.* Adding the word *superficial* has caused confusion for physicians who may not treat DVT found in this vein, because they assume from the name *superficial femoral vein,* that it is not part of the deep system. An international interdisciplinary committee of physicians met in 2002 to discuss issues regarding terminology of the lower extremity veins. Committee members came to the agreement that only the terms *femoral vein* and *femoral artery* should be used. Their findings have been published in many vascular and surgical journals.[3]

The deep femoral (profunda femoris) vein travels with the profunda femoris artery, which unites with the femoral vein to form the common femoral vein. The confluence of the profunda femoris vein and the femoral vein is distal in the leg to the bifurcation of the common femoral artery. The deep femoral vein drains the deep muscles of the proximal thigh.

The **common femoral vein (CFV)** lies in Scarpa's triangle medial to the common femoral artery. The common femoral vein is formed by the confluence of the profunda femoris and the femoral vein and receives the greater saphenous vein. The common femoral vein terminates at the level of the inguinal ligament and becomes the external iliac vein.

The **external iliac vein** is a single vein that travels with the artery, beginning at the level of the inguinal ligament. It is joined with the internal iliac vein to become the common iliac vein. The internal iliac vein is a single vein that travels with the internal iliac artery. The internal iliac vein drains the pelvis.

The **common iliac vein** is formed by the confluence of internal and external iliac veins. The right common iliac vein is shorter than the left, is oriented vertically, and ascends posterior and then lateral to its companion artery. The left common iliac vein is longer than the right and is oriented obliquely. It lies to the medial side of the left common iliac artery, and while it ascends, the vein crosses beneath the right iliac artery, where it joins the right common iliac vein. This anatomic feature of the left common iliac vein crossing beneath the right iliac artery causes mild compression of the vein and has been cited as the reason for a slightly greater number of left-side deep vein thromboses. This is known as May-Thurner syndrome. DVT that cannot be explained by any other means may be the result of May-Thurner syndrome. If narrowing of the left iliac vein can be identified, stenting may be necessary to keep the vein widely patent.

The union of the right and left common iliac veins forms the inferior vena cava, which lies to the right of the aorta.

Superficial Veins. The superficial veins of the leg lie beneath the skin and between the two layers of superficial fascia. The greater (long) saphenous vein originates on the dorsum of the foot and ascends anterior to the medial malleolus and along the anteromedial side of the calf and thigh (Figure 38-3). The **greater saphenous vein (GSV)** ends as it joins the common femoral vein (saphenofemoral junction) in the proximal thigh. The greater saphenous vein is the longest vein in the body, has

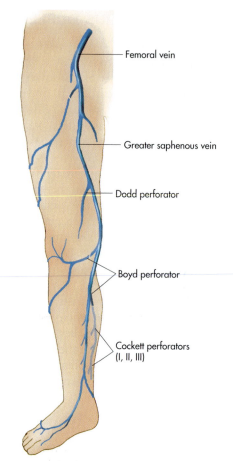

FIGURE 38-3 The greater saphenous vein is a superficial vein. It courses along the medial thigh and calf. Many perforators join the greater saphenous vein.

approximately 10 to 20 valves, and receives many tributaries.

The lesser (short) saphenous vein originates on the dorsum of the foot, ascends posterior to the lateral malleolus, and runs along the midline of the posterior calf (Figure 38-4). The **lesser saphenous vein** terminates when it joins the popliteal vein. The level of entry of the lesser saphenous vein into the popliteal vein is variable; it has even been visualized to enter the femoral vein in the mid thigh. The lesser saphenous vein has approximately 6 to 12 valves and receives many tributaries.

The **posterior arch vein** is a main tributary of the greater saphenous vein in the lower leg. This vein arises posterior to the medial malleolus and terminates in the greater saphenous vein below the knee. It communicates with the deep vein through multiple perforators in the gaiter (region above the medial malleolus) area of the leg.

The **perforating veins** connect the superficial and deep venous systems. Perforating veins penetrate the deep fascia and contain valves that permit unidirectional blood flow from the superficial to the deep veins. Many named perforators (Cockett's, Boyd's, Dodd's, Hunterian) are present in the lower extremity.

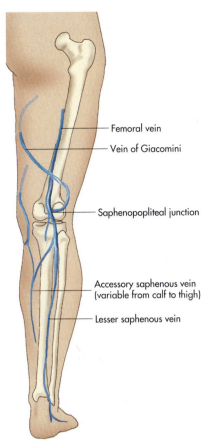

FIGURE 38-4 The lesser saphenous vein is a superficial vein that courses along the posterior calf. The lesser saphenous vein usually enters the popliteal vein.

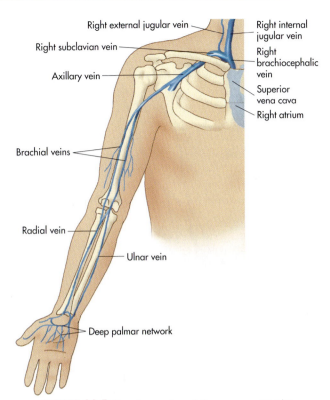

FIGURE 38-5 The deep veins of the upper extremity.

Upper Extremity

Deep Veins. The deep veins (superficial and deep palmar venous arches) draining the hand form the paired radial and ulnar veins (Figure 38-5). The radial veins accompany the radial artery, and the ulnar veins accompany the ulnar artery in the forearm. Near the antecubital fossa, the radial and ulnar veins join to form the brachial veins. The brachial veins are paired veins that travel with the brachial artery in the upper arm.

The **axillary vein** is a single vein. It begins where the basilic vein joins the brachial veins in the upper arm and terminates beneath the clavicle at the outer border of the first rib. The axillary vein receives the cephalic vein near its termination.

The **subclavian vein** is a continuation of the axillary vein. It extends from the outer border of the first rib to the inner end of the clavicle, where it joins the internal jugular vein to form the innominate vein. The subclavian vein lies beneath the clavicle and is inferior and anterior to the subclavian artery.

Right and left innominate (brachiocephalic) veins are present. On the right side, the innominate vein courses almost vertically downward, joining the left innominate vein just below the first rib to form the superior vena cava. It lies superficial and to the right of the innominate

artery. The right innominate vein receives the right vertebral, internal mammary, and inferior thyroid veins. The left innominate vein is longer than the right vein. It courses from the left to the right side of the chest beneath the sternum and at a slight downward angle to join the right innominate vein to form the superior vena cava. It receives the left vertebral, internal mammary, inferior thyroid, and left superior intercostal veins.

Superficial Veins. In the upper extremity, the superficial venous system is the primary route of drainage (Figure 38-6). The superficial veins lie beneath the skin and between the two layers of superficial fascia and outside the deep investing fascia.

The **cephalic vein** begins on the thumb side of the dorsum of the hand. It courses along the outer border of the biceps muscle and the deltopectoral groove, penetrates the deep fascia at variable levels, and joins the axillary vein just below the clavicle.

The **basilic vein** originates on the small finger side of the dorsum of the hand. The basilic vein is large, courses medially along the inner side of the biceps muscle, pierces the deep fascia, and enters the brachial veins in the upper arm, which then become the axillary vein.

TECHNICAL ASPECTS OF VENOUS DUPLEX IMAGING

Lower Extremity

Imaging Examination. The venous duplex imaging examination is explained to the patient. A history taken

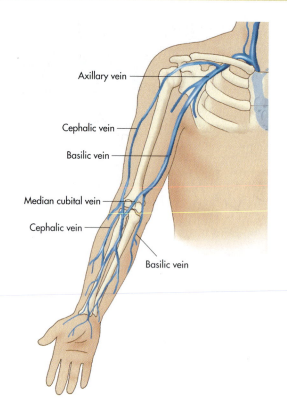

Axillary vein

Cephalic vein

Basilic vein

Median cubital vein

Cephalic vein

Basilic vein

FIGURE 38-6 The superficial veins of the upper extremity.

from the patient focuses on risk factors, signs, and symptoms (if present) of venous disease. If the patient is symptomatic, this helps in locating the area of pain and in measuring limb swelling at the calf level.

Patients are evaluated in the supine position on a hospital bed or on an examination table. The bed or table should be placed in reverse Trendelenburg's (head elevated) position, which promotes venous distention and optimizes visualization of the veins. The leg being evaluated is externally rotated, and the knee slightly flexed.

Ultrasound gel is placed on the leg along the anatomic route of the veins to ensure good transducer-to-skin contact. The transverse view is used to locate the veins and to perform the examination. The transverse view is mandatory for an accurate examination and interpretation when evaluating the veins in the lower extremity. The transverse view allows visualization of multiple venous segments and of the entire lumen (lumina) of the vein(s) during compression maneuvers.

The venous duplex examination begins by locating the CFV at the level of the inguinal crease. The vein is usually large at this location and easy to locate compared with the smaller veins located distally in the leg. Veins can be distinguished from arteries by the characteristics listed in Box 38-3. In general, compared with the common femoral artery, the common femoral vein will collapse with light to moderate transducer pressure on the skin and usually will change in size with respiration. If the artery is deformed by the compression maneuver, then

the operator knows that adequate pressure has been applied to compress the vein.

After locating the vein, follow it as far proximally as possible. The distal external iliac vein is usually the most proximal vein imaged. The mid and proximal external iliac and common iliac veins lie deep in the pelvis and are often obscured by the overlying bowel.

To evaluate the proximal iliac veins, a low-frequency sector transducer will usually provide the best images. During this portion of the examination, it is not possible to perform accurate compression testing of the veins. The iliac veins are evaluated in a longitudinal view using color Doppler as a guide. Usually, blue is the color assigned to venous blood flow. Follow your institution's protocol for color assignment. Careful attention to color control settings is critical, and evaluation of venous Doppler signals is essential for performing an accurate examination of the veins at this level.

After examination of the proximal veins, a higher-frequency (5 to 7.5 MHz) linear-array transducer is placed at the inguinal crease in a transverse imaging plane. The transducer's orientation marker should be toward the patient's right side (transducer orientation may vary by institutional protocol). Using the transducer, pressure is applied to the skin to evaluate the compressibility of the vein. During each compression maneuver, the vein is observed to confirm that the vein walls "touch" each other (coapt), demonstrating the absence of intraluminal material. The lumen of the vein should reopen with release of the transducer's pressure on the skin. The amount of transducer pressure necessary to compress the vein varies with its location and the patient's body habitus. The veins are followed transversely distally along the length of the thigh, and transducer pressure is applied to the leg approximately every width of the transducer's footprint. Do not lift the transducer's footprint off the skin. You want to visualize the entire length of each vessel evaluated. Following this technique along the pathway of the venous system will provide the best results when performing venous duplex imaging.

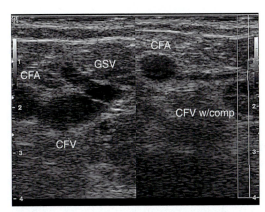

FIGURE 38-7 Normal common femoral vein *(CFV)* with *(left)* and without compression *(right)* at the level of the greater saphenous vein *(GSV)*. *CFA*, Common femoral artery.

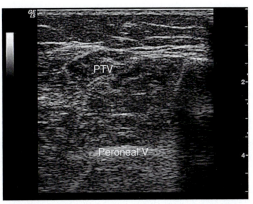

FIGURE 38-8 Transverse image of the posterior tibial veins *(PTVs)* and peroneal veins in the lower calf. The peroneals can be seen just anterior to the fibula.

At the level of the inguinal ligament, the common femoral vein is located and evaluated for compressibility. The transducer is moved distally on the limb, and the proximal GSV is compressed at the saphenofemoral junction (Figure 38-7). If superficial thrombophlebitis is suspected, the GSV should be followed along its entire length. The GSV lies beneath the skin and may be compressed by the weight of the transducer on the skin. If the saphenous vein is not visualized, reduce the pressure on the transducer to make sure that the vein is not inadvertently being compressed. This problem can be avoided by adding more gel to the leg to maintain contact and by not using any transducer pressure on the skin. The proximal greater saphenous vein is important to evaluate during venous duplex imaging because it is often the site of a clot that propagates and extends into the deep system. While the transducer is moved distally on the leg from the common femoral vein, the origin of the FV and the **deep femoral vein (DFV)** will be visualized. The origins of the two veins are evaluated with transducer pressure applied to the skin. The compressibility of the origin of the DFV varies with patients but can usually be evaluated with color Doppler for patency. When the vein is followed in the distal thigh, it will course deep and may be difficult to follow. The femoral vein is followed along its length in the thigh. The FV usually lies deep to the femoral artery. The FV can be difficult to coapt at the level of the adductor canal in the distal thigh because of the surrounding tissue. The distal FV may be imaged and compressed from the medial distal thigh by compressing the vein inward toward the femur.

The popliteal vein is evaluated from a posterior approach with the patient's knee rotated externally (frog-legged), with the patient supine or in the decubitus position, or with the patient in the prone position with the foot elevated on a pillow to eliminate extrinsic compression of the vein. The popliteal vein should be followed proximally to the distal FV and distally to the proximal calf veins. While the popliteal vein is followed along its length, it is evaluated in a transverse plane with the venous imaging compression technique. The popliteal vein usually lies superficial to the popliteal artery. Although venous aneurysms are rare vascular anomalies, popliteal venous aneurysms do occur and may be visualized during venous duplex imaging examinations.

The paired calf veins (posterior tibial and peroneal) are evaluated in the same manner (transverse view) along their length. The posterior tibial and peroneal veins are usually visualized by placing the transducer in a transverse imaging plane along the medial calf. The posterior tibial veins are located near the medial malleolus and are followed proximally in the calf. The peroneal veins lie deep and travel near the fibula (Figure 38-8). The posterior tibial and peroneal veins run parallel to their corresponding artery and can usually be visualized in the same imaging plane. In the upper calf, the two posterior tibial veins form a common trunk with the two peroneal veins (tibial-peroneal trunk). The anterior tibial veins are not usually evaluated, only if symptoms are focal in the anterior tibial region.[1] They are small and are located in the proximal calf by placing the transducer on the lateral calf in a transverse imaging plane. The anterior tibial veins travel with the anterior tibial artery. The anterior tibial veins are located medial to the fibula in the proximal calf, travel just superior to the interosseous membrane, and gradually move in the direction of the tibia in the distal calf.

In addition to the paired calf veins, two sets of muscular calf veins may be visualized: the gastrocnemius and soleus calf veins. The paired gastrocnemius veins accompany an artery and can be visualized in the proximal calf as they enter the popliteal vein. The **gastrocnemius veins** lie in the muscles and are easily compressed with transducer pressure on the skin. The soleal sinuses lie deeper in the calf muscle and empty into the posterior tibial or peroneal veins. Additionally, the lesser saphenous vein runs along the posterior calf, lies just beneath the skin, is easily compressed by transducer pressure on the skin, and usually enters the popliteal vein.

Doppler. Evaluation of the lower extremity veins by Doppler is performed during the imaging examination. Doppler signals should be obtained from the longitudinal imaging plane. Angle correction of the Doppler signal is not necessary during venous duplex imaging because the actual peak velocity does not provide any clinical information. The pattern of the venous Doppler signal is what is clinically relevant. The Doppler scale should be reduced to visualize the low-velocity venous Doppler signals. Additionally, the Doppler sample volume may be increased to include the entire diameter of the lumen.

Following are the characteristics of a normal venous Doppler signal from a lower extremity:

- *Spontaneous:* **Spontaneous** flow means flow is present without augmentation maneuvers (usually not found in calf veins).
- *Respiratory phasicity:* **Respiratory phasicity** means that blood flow velocity changes with respiration (usually not found in calf veins). In the lower extremity, on inspiration the diaphragm descends and causes intra-abdominal pressure to rise, compressing the vena cava and impeding venous outflow from the legs. With expiration, the diaphragm rises, intra-abdominal pressure decreases, and venous blood flow from the legs increases toward the vena cava.
- *Augmentation:* Blood flow velocity increases with distal limb compression or with the release of proximal limb compression.

Venous Doppler signals should be obtained from the common femoral vein and the popliteal vein. The signal from the common femoral vein helps to identify proximal obstruction (loss of phasicity), and the popliteal venous Doppler signal provides information about possible calf vein thrombosis (absent or decreased **augmentation**). During a unilateral venous imaging examination, the contralateral femoral venous Doppler signal should be documented. Venous Doppler signals may be obtained from other veins according to each institution's protocol.

Upper Extremity

Imaging Examination. The examination is explained to the patient. A history taken from the patient focuses on risk factors, signs, and symptoms (if present) of venous disease. Additionally, documentation of the history or presence of a line placed in the veins is critical.

Unless contraindicated, the patient is evaluated in the supine position. The arm is positioned at the side of the patient. The head should be turned away from the side being examined. The internal jugular vein (IJV) is evaluated along its route in the neck in a transverse plane. The IJV can usually be compressed with transducer pressure on the skin. If the IJV cannot be compressed, and if the lumen is echo free, the use of color Doppler or spectral Doppler may be helpful. In this situation, the IJV will usually compress when the patient's head is raised. Evaluate the IJV carefully for intraluminal echoes. Often after indwelling lines or catheters are removed, partial thrombus may be noted in the IJV. If an indwelling line or catheter is in place, special attention should be paid to imaging this area carefully (Figure 38-9). Compressive ultrasound technique will be limited. A clot is often visualized near the line or by its tip. The subclavian and **innominate veins** are evaluated from a supraclavicular approach. A low-frequency transducer with a small footprint will improve visualization of the central veins. Mirror imaging artifacts may occur when evaluating the central veins because of the clavicle. Normal Doppler signals from the central veins are pulsatile (right side of heart) with a phasic respiratory variation superimposed on the venous velocity pattern (Figure 38-10). The superior vena cava may be visualized from a supraclavicular or a suprasternal approach, depending on the patient.

Next, from an infraclavicular approach, the subclavian and axillary veins are evaluated in a transverse plane, and the compression technique can be attempted. Shadowing from the clavicle is a problem with this approach, and it may take multiple views to fully visualize the subclavian vein. The patient's arm is repositioned to allow access to the axilla. A low-frequency (5 to 7.5 MHz) linear-array transducer is used to evaluate the veins in the arm. A higher-frequency (7.5 to 10 MHz)

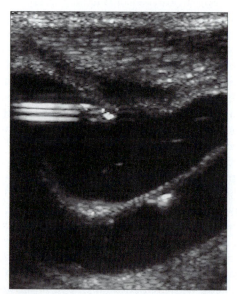

FIGURE 38-9 A longitudinal view of the internal jugular vein and the common carotid artery. The internal jugular vein lies superficial to the artery. The indwelling line produces bright echoes within the venous lumen. The tip of the line is against the vessel's wall. When imaging a patient who has an indwelling line, careful attention must be paid to the area surrounding the line.

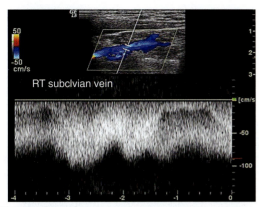

FIGURE 38-10 Normal phasic flow seen in the subclavian vein.

linear-array transducer may be used to evaluate the more superficial veins, depending on the patient. The axillary vein travels with the axillary artery and receives the cephalic vein. The axillary vein is followed distally on the arm to the confluence of the basilic vein. Distally on the arm, the axillary vein becomes the brachial vein after the entrance of the basilic vein. The brachial veins travel with the brachial artery, and the veins tend to be small.

Near the antecubital fossa, the radial and ulnar veins can be visualized as they travel with their respective arteries along the length of the forearm. Although they are often small in diameter, they can usually be evaluated without too much difficulty. The forearm veins should compress with transducer pressure on the skin. The radial and ulnar veins can usually be followed to the wrist level.

The cephalic and basilic veins are the superficial veins in the upper extremity. The cephalic vein is a superficial vein and is not accompanied by an artery. This vein travels along the lateral aspect of the biceps muscle and may be followed from the axillary vein to the level of the wrist. The basilic vein is a superficial vein, is usually large, and does not travel with an artery; it travels along the medial side of the arm and enters the brachial vein.

Doppler. Evaluation of upper extremity veins by Doppler imaging is a critical part of the venous imaging examination. Color Doppler is very helpful in locating the central veins and in identifying filling defects from a clot. Doppler signals should be obtained from the longitudinal plane. Angle correction of the Doppler signal is not necessary during venous duplex imaging because the actual peak velocity does not provide any clinical information. Additionally, the Doppler sample volume may be increased to include the entire lumen of the vein, and the Doppler scale should be reduced to visualize low-velocity venous Doppler signals. The pattern of the venous Doppler spectral waveform is what is important and extremely critical in examination of the views of the upper extremity.

Following are the characteristics of a normal venous Doppler signal from an upper extremity:

- *Spontaneous:* Flow is present without augmentation maneuvers.
- *Pulsatility:* Pulsatile signals should be present in the jugular, subclavian, innominate, and superior vena cava because of retrograde transmission of right atrial pressure.
- *Respiratory phasicity:* Blood flow velocity changes with respiration. In the upper extremity (central veins), the venous Doppler signal will increase with inspiration and decrease with expiration.
- *Augmentation:* Blood flow velocity increases with distal limb compression or with release of proximal limb compression (limited in the upper extremity examination).

Venous Doppler signals should be obtained from the superior vena cava and jugular, innominate, subclavian, and axillary veins. Brachial, radial, ulnar, cephalic, and basilic veins may be evaluated with Doppler when symptoms indicate distal arm or hand DVT. Protocols will vary by institution. When evaluating the upper extremity, it is helpful to compare Doppler signals from the right and left sides. During a unilateral venous imaging examination, the contralateral internal jugular or subclavian venous Doppler signal should be documented. Lack of pulsatility in the central veins suggests venous obstruction.

General tips when performing venous duplex imaging are listed in Table 38-1. The best quality and most reliable examination will be obtained by careful attention to venous anatomy and imaging technique.

INTERPRETATION OF VENOUS DUPLEX IMAGING

It is imperative that each institution develop a venous imaging protocol that defines the standard examination (veins to be evaluated during a lower and upper extremity examination, locations for Doppler signal documentation). This protocol must include the technique, clinical applications, indications for a complete and/or limited examination, and interpretation criteria. The interpretation criteria for venous duplex imaging (Table 38-2) are based on three components: The patent vein is free of echogenic material, compresses fully with transducer pressure on the skin (Figures 38-11 and 38-12), and exhibits a normal (Figure 38-13) venous Doppler signal. Congestive heart failure (CHF) can cause extremely pulsatile signals, and bilateral comparison is necessary to confirm this as the cause (Figure 38-14).

Consistency of findings on gray-scale imaging, by compression technique, and with color Doppler and/or the venous Doppler spectral waveform will limit errors when interpreting venous duplex imaging examinations.

However, many pitfalls are involved in the interpretation of these examinations. Proper technique is essential

TABLE 38-1	Venous Duplex Imaging Tips
Challenge	**Action**
Nonvisualization of veins	Veins may collapse easily with pressure from the transducer. If a vein cannot be visualized, lessen pressure applied to the transducer. Release of the transducer's pressure on the skin allows the vein to be visualized from the correct anatomic position.
Veins do not compress	If a vein segment appears patent but does not compress, transducer pressure may be applied from a different site on the skin or by repositioning the patient. Often an adjacent bone or tendon prevents compression of the vein.
Pressure assessment	Adequate pressure has been applied to compress a vein if the adjacent artery is compressed by the compression maneuver.
Imaging in a longitudinal plane	Multiple veins or vein segments are common and may be missed if imaging only in a longitudinal plane.
Imaging limitations	Obesity, extensive edema, leg wounds, calcified arteries, anatomic structures (clavicle), and casts may limit the venous duplex imaging study or affect the quality of the examination. Use transducers of different frequency, and use different imaging planes, to improve visualization of the veins.
Color Doppler limitations	Color Doppler may obscure a nonoccluding thrombus. When evaluating the vein in the longitudinal plane, visualization of a nonoccluding thrombus depends on the angle of the imaging plane and accurate setting of the instrument controls.
Venous Doppler	Angle correction is not necessary during venous duplex imaging. The actual peak velocity is not critical. The pattern of the Doppler spectral waveform is what is important during venous imaging. Doppler signals are taken in the longitudinal plane, and the sample volume may be increased to the size of the diameter of the vein.
Upper extremities	During upper extremity imaging, use color Doppler to help locate the central veins; the central veins should have a pulsatile and phasic signal; compare Doppler signals from the right and left sides; be aware of mirror imaging artifact caused by the clavicle.

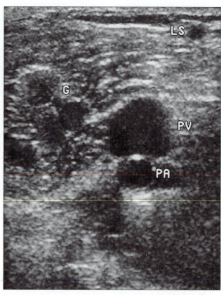

FIGURE 38-11 Transverse view at the popliteal fossa without transducer pressure. The popliteal vein *(PV)* lies superficial to the popliteal artery *(PA)*. The lesser saphenous *(LS)* vein lies just below the skin line. A set of paired gastrocnemius *(G)* veins are located on either side of the accompanying artery.

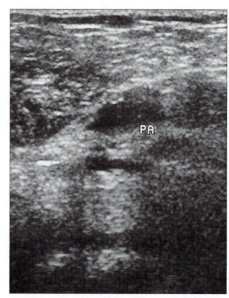

FIGURE 38-12 Transverse view at the popliteal fossa with transducer pressure on the skin. The vein walls collapse, suggesting no evidence of venous thrombosis in the lesser saphenous, popliteal, or gastrocnemius veins. The popliteal artery *(PA)* is visualized and does not collapse.

for providing accurate venous duplex imaging examinations and minimizing errors in interpretation.

If inconsistent findings are obtained when performing a venous duplex imaging examination, several technical and equipment adjustments should be considered before the final interpretation (Table 38-3).

It is important to remember that the most significant diagnostic criterion during venous imaging is how the vein responds to transducer pressure. To check whether adequate pressure was used during the examination,

TABLE 38-2	Interpretation Criteria of Venous Duplex Imaging	
Gray Scale/Compression	Doppler Signal	Color Doppler
Normal		
No intraluminal echoes Vein compresses	Normal. Phasic, augments with distal compression (pulsatile for upper extremities)	Color fills lumen
Abnormal: Nonocclusive		
Vein lumen partially filled with echoes Vein partially compresses	May be normal or abnormal	Defect in color as it is displayed around thrombus; may appear normal if thrombus is small or if instrument controls are not adjusted properly
Abnormal: Occlusive		
Vein filled with intraluminal echoes Vein does not compress	Abnormal. Absence of Doppler signal, a continuous signal, absent or reduced phasicity, and the lack of pulsatility in the central veins of the upper extremity	Absence of color

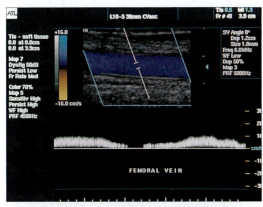

FIGURE 38-13 Normal venous Doppler signal of the femoral vein. Note that color fills the lumen of the vein when a low-color pulse repetition frequency is used. The venous spectral Doppler waveform demonstrates low velocity and the phasic characteristic of a normal venous Doppler signal.

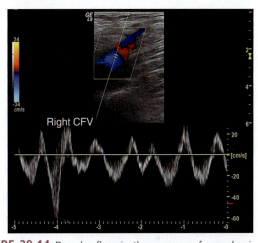

FIGURE 38-14 Doppler flow in the common femoral vein (CFV) in a patient with congestive heart failure. Notice the extreme pulsatility. Augmentation is seen within the erratic flow.

TABLE 38-3	Technical Adjustments for Venous Duplex Imaging
Challenge	Action
Vein does not compress; lumen is echo-free	**Technique:** Move the transducer on the skin to attempt compression from a different approach. Use the correct transverse plane, and check for adequate pressure. **Patient Position:** Repositioning the patient's extremity often results in ability to compress the vein. **Anatomy:** At times, the depth of the vessel and the surrounding tissue will make vein compression impossible.
Vein compresses; lumen is filled with echoes	**Equipment:** Gain settings too high **Technique:** Use the correct transverse plane to make sure that there is complete compression of the venous lumen.

look at the effects of compression on the artery. Adequate pressure was used if the artery is deformed during the compression maneuver.

If the vein does not compress and the lumen is echo-free, try repositioning the extremity. If the vein still does not compress, remember that visualization of the thrombus is variable. At times, the thrombus is very echogenic and may blend into the surrounding tissue (Figure 38-15); at other times, the clot is anechoic. A vein may not compress because the clot is present in the lumen but is not visualized with gray-scale imaging. Additionally, trying to determine the age of the thrombus by the degree of its echogenicity is unreliable (Figure 38-16).

A free-floating clot may be visualized moving freely within the lumen during venous duplex imaging (Figure 38-17). When this phenomenon occurs, the compression technique is not performed at that level on the limb. Compression should be limited for the rest of the examination, and color Doppler can be used to confirm patency.

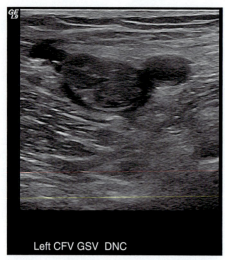

FIGURE 38-15 The common femoral artery *(CFA)* and vein *(CFV)* are visualized in a transverse view with transducer pressure on the skin. The vein walls do not coapt, and echogenic material fills the lumen of the vein, suggesting thrombosis.

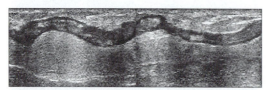

FIGURE 38-16 A longitudinal view of the basilic vein demonstrates venous thrombosis of mixed echogenicity.

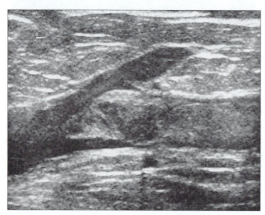

FIGURE 38-17 A longitudinal view of the femoral vein. A free-floating clot is visualized within the lumen of the vein. Blood flows around the tip of the thrombus. Distally in the vein *(right side of the image)*, the clot attaches to the vein walls.

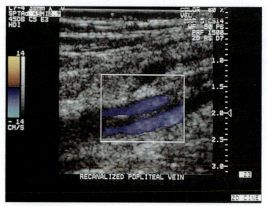

FIGURE 38-18 Longitudinal view of the popliteal vein demonstrating recanalization of the venous thrombosis. The color Doppler display demonstrates blood flow channels.

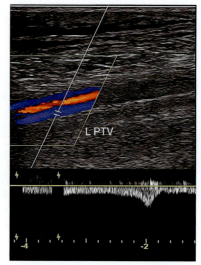

FIGURE 38-19 A longitudinal view at the level of the lower calf. The post tibial and peroneal veins are clearly seen in color.

In follow-up studies, the resolution of a clot varies dramatically from patient to patient. Complete resolution of an extensive clot may occur at 3 months, 6 months, or 1 year, or it may never occur in an individual patient. Recanalization of veins occurs often, and blood flowing through small channels can be documented on color Doppler imaging (Figure 38-18).

In a review of more than 30 studies, the results of venous duplex imaging compared with venography demonstrated good sensitivity for the detection of DVT.[5] In symptomatic patients, the sensitivity for proximal DVT ranges from 89% to 100%. The specificity for DVT is greater than 90%. Additionally, good results have been reported for proximal disease in the asymptomatic high-risk patient. Sensitivity in these patients ranges from 63% to 100%, and specificity is greater than 90%. It is important to note that the distribution and magnitude of DVT may vary, depending on the type of patient. Screening of high-risk patients has revealed an increase in the number of nonoccluding thrombi compared with symptomatic patients.[6]

Evaluation of the calf veins is becoming easier with the advent of newer technology. The size and number of the veins can be evaluated with better sensitivity than in the past few years. Reports in the literature describe a sensitivity of greater than 80% for detecting DVT in the calf veins. This is due to better resolution obtained with the use of state-of-the-art imaging systems and color Doppler imaging in most patients (Figure 38-19).

COMBINED DIAGNOSTIC APPROACH

A newer and somewhat controversial approach to the diagnostic evaluation of DVT has been to use a combined approach of ultrasound imaging, D-dimer assays, and a detailed clinical risk assessment score.[2,4,21,23,24] The assays measure D-dimer, which is a fibrin-specific degradation product that detects cross-linked fibrin resulting from endogenous fibrinolysis. The precise role of using D-dimer assays in conjunction with venous ultrasound has not been clearly established. The D-dimer assays have not been standardized, and results are variable depending on thrombus size, location, and interpretation of results. Algorithms for diagnosing DVT using a clinical risk assessment score, venous imaging of the entire leg, and D-dimer testing have been proposed, and they will probably be more widely used in the future in an attempt to limit costs and improve efficiency in the diagnosis of DVT.

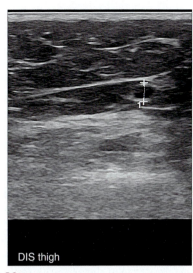

FIGURE 38-20 Transverse image of the greater saphenous vein in the mid thigh with measurements.

VEIN MAPPING

The purpose of superficial vein mapping is to determine the vein's suitability for use as a bypass conduit and to identify its anatomic route. Vein mapping is usually performed before lower extremity arterial bypass or coronary bypass operations. Accurate mapping of the location of the veins is important when the surgeon plans an in situ bypass graft of the lower extremity or harvests the vein. Preoperative vein mapping avoids exposing inadequate veins; this, in turn, decreases operative time and the possibility of wound complications from unnecessary incisions.

A high-frequency linear-array (7 to 10 MHz) transducer provides the best resolution for evaluating the superficial veins of the lower (greater and lesser saphenous veins) and upper extremities (cephalic and basilic veins). Light transducer pressure on the skin is critical because the superficial veins lie below the skin line and are easily compressed with minimal pressure from the transducer. The patient should be in the supine position. The bed may be placed in reverse Trendelenburg's position to promote venous distention if necessary.

Imaging begins at the groin level in a transverse plane. The common femoral vein should be located and followed distally on the limb. The saphenofemoral junction is usually located a few centimeters distally on the leg from the inguinal ligament. The greater saphenous vein travels along the anteromedial side of the thigh and calf, has many branches, and usually has valves. The anatomy of the greater saphenous vein is variable, and a double system for short segments of the vein is common. The vessel should be measured in the transverse plane at different locations while traveling down the leg (Figure 38-20). Vascular surgeons can use vessels that measure 2 to 2.5 mm or larger.[9,16] Institutional protocol should include acceptable vessel diameters.

If an adequate greater saphenous vein is not located in either leg, the lesser saphenous vein should be evaluated bilaterally. The lesser saphenous vein extends from posterior to the lateral malleolus and terminates at variable levels of the popliteal vein; it has branches and usually has valves. If the superficial veins on the lower extremity are not adequate, the superficial veins on the arms may be evaluated for their suitability. If the arm veins are difficult to visualize, try using a tourniquet on the upper arm to promote venous dilation.

Confirm the patency of the vein along its length by using the compression technique. The size of the vein and the presence of thickened walls, calcification, recanalization, and stenotic valves should be documented. If the physician requests it, mark the vein's path and its branches on the skin using an indelible marker. When marking the skin, make sure that the vein is centered in the ultrasound image. With some type of small but blunt-ended object (ball point pen, pen cap, etc.), press the skin just hard enough to leave a small mark. Wipe away the gel, and begin "connecting your dots" with the indelible marker.

VENOUS REFLUX TESTING

The purpose of venous reflux testing is to identify the presence and the location of incompetent venous valves. Patients who suffer from chronic venous insufficiency may benefit from this type of study. Symptoms include chronic leg swelling, induration (hard, firm, almost leather-like appearance of the skin around the ankles), and possibly ulcers. Repair of valves is now possible to help those who experience chronic symptoms. The venous reflux examination is explained to the patient. A history taken from the patient focuses on risk factors, signs, and symptoms of venous disease, especially any history of DVT. If the patient has not had one recently, a complete lower extremity DVT study should be done before this test is performed to rule out any existing pathology. Evaluation of venous reflux by duplex imaging is performed using a low-frequency (5 MHz) linear-array imaging transducer. This examination is performed with the patient standing and holding onto a frame for support, and with full body weight placed on the opposite leg. Although venous valves may be visualized at different locations in many individuals, the gray-scale image is not used for determining valvular incompetence. The absence or presence of venous reflux is measured from the venous spectral Doppler waveform.

A longitudinal view of the saphenofemoral junction is located. The Doppler sample volume size is adjusted to the vein's width. The Doppler sample volume is positioned in the femoral vein distal to the saphenofemoral junction, and distal limb compression is performed. In the presence of incompetent valves, sudden release of distal compression produces retrograde blood flow (reflux), which is recorded and measured on the spectral Doppler waveform display (Figure 38-21). The valves are considered incompetent if retrograde blood flow is present and lasts longer than 1 second. Absence of retrograde blood flow indicates competent valves. The examination is repeated with the sample volume located in the greater saphenous vein distal to the saphenofemoral junction. The popliteal and lesser saphenous veins are selectively evaluated in a similar manner, with the imaging transducer located over the popliteal fossa. Depending on the patient, any vein, including the perforators, may be evaluated for venous reflux.

Duplex imaging provides the ability to quantify reflux in the individual (deep, superficial, perforating) veins of the thigh and calf. It is technically difficult to operate the imaging system, hold the transducer on the patient's leg, and compress the patient's distal limb to test for venous reflux. Two examiners are necessary to ensure proper testing, or a distal automatic cuff compression-release device must be used. A cuff compression-release device is used on the leg distal to the imaging transducer and ensures standard compression pressure and timing of the release.

Performing a complete venous duplex imaging examination for reflux takes approximately 30 minutes per extremity. With the addition of color Doppler imaging, identification of the veins with reflux is immediate, and individual vein Doppler sample volume placement is not necessary. Although using color Doppler to test for venous reflux may reduce examination time and technical difficulty, appropriate color control settings are essential for an accurate diagnosis. The venous duplex imaging examination for venous reflux provides accurate information about the individual veins. It does not provide information about the limb's overall venous hemodynamics.

CONTROVERSIES IN VENOUS DUPLEX IMAGING

Complete Versus Limited Examination

Why examine the entire leg in a symptomatic patient? The standard technique for venous duplex imaging of the lower extremity in symptomatic patients has been to evaluate the veins from the level of the inguinal ligament to and including the calf veins. Limited venous ultrasound of the lower extremity has been defined multiple ways in the literature. Investigators have described a limited examination as an evaluation limited to the common femoral and popliteal veins, imaging limited to the full length of the femoral and popliteal veins, imaging limited to the common femoral vein, and imaging limited to the popliteal vein. It has been suggested that a "two-point" venous duplex examination in symptomatic patients would detect a clot in a high percentage of cases and would significantly reduce examination time.[13] The abbreviated study employs compression of the veins at the level of the common femoral and popliteal veins.

In a prospective study of 53 symptomatic patients (56 limbs), the results of a limited examination were compared with those from the routine venous imaging examination.[13] The limited examination preceded the routine examination. During the limited examination, the CFV from the inguinal ligament to the deep femoral (profunda) takeoff and the popliteal vein above and below the knee to the level of its trifurcation were visualized. Limited venous evaluations were performed in transverse and longitudinal views.

Of the 56 cases, 7 (12%) demonstrated deep vein thrombosis on limited and routine venous examinations. Both techniques failed to visualize an isolated iliac vein clot that was depicted by computed tomography (CT) scan. The average time for the limited examination was 8.3 minutes; for the routine examination, the average time was 18.0 minutes.

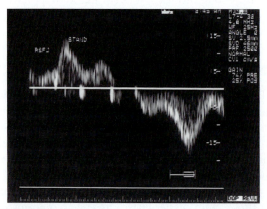

FIGURE 38-21 The Doppler spectral waveform obtained during a venous reflux test. Reversal of blood flow that lasts longer than 1 second is obtained with release of distal compression, suggesting venous reflux.

In another study, investigators performed 755 venous duplex imaging examinations in 721 symptomatic patients (1024 limbs).[8] Acute DVT was visualized in one or more veins in 131 (17.4%) of 755 examinations. DVT was limited to a single vein in 28 (21.4%) of 131 examinations in which DVT was detected. Isolated thrombus in the CFV was noted in 8 examinations (6.1%), in the SFV in 6 examinations (4.6%), and in the popliteal vein in 14 examinations (10.7%). Investigators concluded that DVT limited to a single vein occurs frequently, and that adoption of an abbreviated venous duplex imaging examination may be potentially dangerous for patients.

It is currently recommended that the routine venous duplex imaging examination should be performed in most cases. The abbreviated or limited venous duplex examination may have a role in the symptomatic, critically ill patient or in symptomatic patients with limited mobility. The limited venous duplex examination should not be performed when screening patients at high risk for DVT.

Unilateral Versus Bilateral

Why examine the asymptomatic leg in a patient with unilateral symptoms? Traditionally, only the symptomatic limb was evaluated in a patient when the accepted diagnostic test for DVT was venography. However, it was customary to study both lower extremities when vascular laboratories were using nonimaging Doppler and plethysmographic techniques that relied on comparison of venous hemodynamics from one limb versus the other for an accurate interpretation.

In a prospective bilateral venous duplex imaging study of the proximal veins in patients with unilateral symptoms, the diagnosis of DVT was made in 37 (18%) of 206 patients.[17] No patient was found to have thrombosis in the asymptomatic limb. Investigators suggest that unilateral imaging will not subject the patient to any risks but will improve cost-effectiveness.

Another study retrospectively reviewed bilateral venous duplex imaging examinations in symptomatic patients.[20] Two hundred forty-eight of 1694 patients had acute DVT. No case of acute DVT occurred in the asymptomatic limb if the symptomatic limb was normal. Investigators recommend that patients with unilateral symptoms should undergo unilateral venous duplex imaging because treatment in these patients would not have been altered, and unilateral imaging improves cost efficiency.

In a prospective study of patients referred for venous duplex imaging, DVT was present in 121 of 488 (25%) patients.[12] A total of 245 patients had unilateral signs and symptoms of DVT. Deep venous thrombosis was present in 65 of the 245 patients with unilateral signs and symptoms. If only the symptomatic leg was evaluated, 3 patients with DVT of the contralateral asymptomatic limb would have been missed. Additionally, 18 patients with unilateral symptoms were found to have DVT bilaterally. In these 18 patients, the diagnosis of DVT would have been made, but the extent of disease would not have been appreciated. This may affect the patient in the future if follow-up venous imaging is performed for new signs and symptoms. Investigators concluded that bilateral venous duplex imaging should be performed on all patients with unilateral symptoms.

Currently, it is recommended to image the contralateral asymptomatic extremity if DVT is visualized in the symptomatic extremity. This procedure will document the patency of the femoral vein (access for percutaneous placement of vena caval filters) and the presence of any DVT that may prove to be helpful in follow-up studies. If DVT is not detected in the symptomatic limb, then DVT in the asymptomatic, contralateral limb occurs in approximately 1% of patients with unilateral symptoms. A protocol for this clinical situation should be established by each institution.

Bilateral Symptoms

Why perform venous duplex imaging in patients with bilateral leg symptoms? It has been suggested in the literature that patients with symptoms of bilateral edema of the lower extremity may have cardiac disease as the dominant cause of their leg swelling. Other causes of bilateral lower extremity symptoms may include peripheral arterial disease, venous stasis, trauma, or venous thrombosis.

In a study of 488 patients evaluated with venous duplex imaging, 149 had bilateral signs and symptoms of DVT.[12] Of the 149 patients, 35 (23%) were found to have proximal DVT by venous duplex imaging. Ten patients had unilateral DVT, and 25 patients had bilateral DVT. Investigators concluded that bilateral venous duplex imaging should be performed in patients with bilateral signs and symptoms of DVT.

In a prospective study of 500 symptomatic patients referred for venous duplex imaging, 50 patients had bilateral symptoms.[18] No DVT was diagnosed in the 50 patients with bilateral symptoms, although the overall detection rate of DVT was 17.4% in this patient population. On the basis of the patient's medical history, a possible alternative cause for the patient's symptoms was found in 34 of the 50 patients. Alternative causes for symptoms included cardiac disease in 18 patients, peripheral arterial disease in 6 patients, and superficial thrombophlebitis or cellulitis in 12 patients. The remaining 16 patients had no history that could explain the development of bilateral symptoms. Investigators suggested that DVT in the patient with bilateral symptoms is rare, and that venous duplex imaging should not be performed if the patient's medical history indicates a more likely alternative cause.

Calf Vein Imaging

Why examine the calf veins in patients at high risk for developing DVT or in patients suspected of having DVT? This controversy centers on three distinct points. It is thought that calf veins can be difficult to image in many patients. Physicians often do not treat an isolated calf clot, and patients with calf clot are unlikely to have signs or symptoms of pulmonary embolism. Additionally, patients can be followed serially with venous duplex imaging for propagation of the clot, which occurs in approximately 20% of cases.

Critical for direct evaluation of the calf veins are knowledge of venous anatomy and the use of proper technique. Improvements in gray-scale resolution and in color Doppler capability have made possible the identification of calf veins. Evaluation of the calf veins adds approximately 10 minutes to the examination of the lower extremity. Evaluation of the calf veins for DVT provides the clinician with the option to initiate treatment. Additionally, imaging of the calf veins documents calf clot; this may provide an explanation for a patient's symptoms or important information on the high-risk patient being screened for DVT.

Assessment of Pulmonary Embolus

Why examine the lower extremities with venous duplex imaging if the patient has signs and symptoms of a pulmonary embolus? Clinicians not wishing to order pulmonary arteriography have determined that if venous duplex imaging detects DVT in patients suspected of PE, then anticoagulation therapy may be initiated.[14] Because most pulmonary emboli originate from the lower extremity, using venous duplex imaging to clarify an indeterminate lung scan may also help to confirm clinically suspected PE. However, it has been shown that approximately half of patients with pulmonary embolism documented by pulmonary arteriography do not have clots in their legs.[11] Therefore, a negative venous duplex imaging study of the legs does not exclude the diagnosis of PE, and further workup in these patients is necessary. Venous duplex imaging should not be used as the first or only diagnostic test for the diagnosis of pulmonary embolus.

OTHER PATHOLOGY

A **Baker's cyst** is a common fluid collection that can be found in the popliteal fossa. It is a collection of synovial fluid that is associated with the knee joint. This excess fluid can be related to any type of arthritis, more commonly, osteoarthritis and rheumatoid arthritis, or to trauma such as cartilage tears. Baker's cysts can be unilateral or bilateral. Symptoms mimic DVT symptoms with swelling and tightness behind the knee or severe pain in the upper calf in cases of cyst rupture and dis-

section into the upper calf muscles. The keys to this pathology are to prove a widely patent popliteal vein to rule out DVT; evaluate the popliteal artery to rule out an aneurysm; and visualize the fluid collection separate from these structures (Figure 38-22). These cysts tend to take a crescent shape and can be anechoic or complex as the result of hemorrhage or infection (Figure 38-23). The use of color Doppler can confirm lack of flow within the structure.[19]

Abscesses, cellulitis, and hematomas can cause focal areas of redness and swelling that may mimic symptoms of DVT. Proving that there is no DVT in the deep venous system is the first goal in these cases; evaluating the focal area is secondary. Small fluid collections within the tissue or muscle planes may be seen with these types of tissues (Figure 38-24).

Lymph nodes in the groin in the common femoral or external iliac veins can sometimes be confused with DVT. Visualizing these structures in transverse and sagittal excludes them from venous pathology. Enlarged lymph nodes should be documented when seen (Figure 38-25). Color may be seen flowing in from the hilum. Nodes can be enlarged as the result of infection or as an early sign of lymphoma.

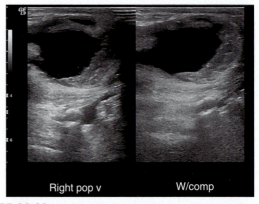

FIGURE 38-22 Dual-screen image of a patent, then compressed popliteal vein, sitting posterior to a large Baker's cyst. The object of this image is to clear the popliteal vein of deep vein thrombosis.

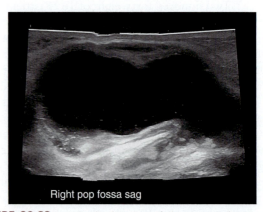

FIGURE 38-23 Longitudinal image of the same Baker's cyst for evaluation.

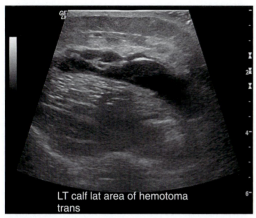

FIGURE 38-24 Large hematoma in the calf of an older female post traumatic fall. Examination was ordered to rule out deep vein thrombosis.

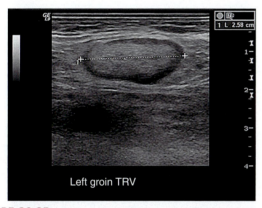

FIGURE 38-25 Large lymph node seen in the groin of an elderly gentleman with an elevated white blood cell count. These cases have been confused with deep vein thrombosis in the common femoral vein.

IMAGING GUIDELINES

Producing high-quality and complete venous duplex examinations is essential if the examination is to have diagnostic value. The best examinations are achieved by proper attention to detail. Technical areas and interpretation details that will ensure the best venous duplex imaging results are listed in Box 38-4.

REFERENCES

1. AbuRahma AF, Bergan JJ: *Noninvasive vascular diagnosis: a practical guide*, ed 2, New York, 2007, Springer Publishing
2. Anderson DR, Kovacs MJ, Kovacs G, et al: Combined use of clinical assessment and D-dimer to improve the management of patients presenting to the emergency department with suspected deep vein thrombosis (the EDITED study), *J Thromb Haemost* 1:645-651, 2003.
3. Caggiati A, Bergan J, Gloviczki P, et al: Nomenclature of the veins of the lower limbs: an international interdisciplinary consensus statement, *Journal of Vascular Surgery* 36:416-422, 2002.
4. Caprini JA, Glase CJ, Anderson CB, et al: Laboratory markers in the diagnosis of venous thromboembolism, *Circulation* 109:I4-I8, 2004.

5. Comerota AJ, Katz ML, Hashemi HA: Venous duplex imaging for the diagnosis of acute deep venous thrombosis, *Haemostasis* 23:61-71, 1993.
6. Comerota AJ, Katz ML, Grossi RJ, et al: The comparative value of noninvasive testing for diagnosis and surveillance of deep vein thrombosis, *J Vasc Surg* 7:40-49, 1988.
7. Dalen JE, Paraskos JA, Ockene IS, et al: Venous thromboembolism: scope of the problem, *Chest* 89:370S-373S, 1986.
8. Frederick MG, Hertzberg BS, Kliewer MA, et al: Can the US examination for lower extremity deep vein thrombosis be abbreviated? A prospective study of 755 examinations, *Radiology* 199:45-47, 1996.
9. Hobson RE, Wilson FJ, Dekker M: *Vascular surgery, principles and practice*, ed 3, New York, 2004, McGraw-Hill.
10. Kahn SR: The clinical diagnosis of deep venous thrombosis: integrating incidence, risk factors, and symptoms and signs, *Arch Intern Med* 158:2315-2323, 1998.
11. Killewich LA, Nunnelee JD, Auer AI: Value of lower extremity venous duplex examination in the diagnosis of pulmonary embolism, *J Vasc Surg* 17:934-939, 1993.
12. Naidich JB, Torre JR, Pellerito JS, et al: Suspected deep venous thrombosis: is US of both legs necessary? *Radiology* 200:429-431, 1996.
13. Pezzullo JA, Parkins AB, Cronan JJ: Symptomatic deep vein thrombosis: diagnosis with limited compression US, *Radiology* 198:67-72, 1996.
14. Rosen MP, Sheiman RG, Weintraub J, McArdle C: Compression sonography in patients with indeterminate or low probability lung scans: lack of usefulness in the absence of both symptoms of deep vein thrombosis and thromboembolic risk factors, *AJR Am J Roentgenol* 166:285-289, 1996.
15. Schreiber D: Deep venous thrombosis and thrombophlebitis, Updated July 10, 2008. Available at: http://emedicine.medscape.com/article/758140-overview
16. Seeger JM, Schmidt JH, Flynn TC: Preoperative saphenous and cephalic vein mapping as an adjunct to reconstructive arterial surgery, *Ann Surg* 205:733-739, 1987.
17. Sheiman RG, McArdle CR: Bilateral lower extremity US in the patient with unilateral symptoms of deep vein thrombosis: assessment of need, *Radiology* 194:171-175, 1995.
18. Sheiman RG, Weintraub JL, McArdle CR: Bilateral lower extremity US in the patient with bilateral symptoms of deep vein thrombosis: assessment of need, *Radiology* 196:379-381, 1995.
19. Shiver SA, Blaivas M: Acute lower extremity pain in an adult patient secondary to bilateral popliteal cysts, *J Emerg Med* 34:315-318, 2008.
20. Strothman G, Blebea J, Fowl RJ, Rosenthal G: Contralateral duplex scanning for deep venous thrombosis is unnecessary in patients with symptoms, *J Vasc Surg* 22:543-547, 1995.
21. Tick LW, Ton E, van Voorthuizen T, et al: Practical diagnostic management of patients with clinically suspected deep vein

thrombosis by clinical probability test, compression ultrasonography, and D-dimer test, *Am J Med* 113:630-635, 2002.

22. Virchow R: Neuer fall von todlicher emboli der lungenarterie, *Virchows Arch Pathol Anat* 10:225-231, 1856.

23. Wells PS, Anderson DR, Rodger M, et al: Evaluation of D-Dimer in the diagnosis of suspected deep-vein thrombosis, *N Engl J Med* 349:1227-1235, 2003.

24. Zierler BK: Ultrasonography and diagnosis of venous thromboembolism, *Circulation* 109:I9-I14, 2004.

PART VII

Gynecology

Normal Anatomy and Physiology of the Female Pelvis

Candace Goldstein and Sandra L. Hagen-Ansert

Understanding the anatomy and physiology of the female genital organs is important for understanding the pathophysiology of the female pelvis. Many pelvic landmarks, ligaments, and muscular structures within the pelvis are important to know to differentiate normal reproductive organs from muscular and vascular structures. This chapter presents a discussion of the normal anatomy and physiology of the female genital organs. The sonographically significant muscular structures and pelvic ligaments will also be discussed because a basic understanding of these structures is essential for performing an adequate pelvic ultrasound examination.

Two approaches are used to evaluate the female pelvis sonographically: transabdominal and transvaginal. A transabdominal approach requires a full urinary bladder for use as an acoustic window and typically necessitates the use of a 3.5- to 5-MHz transducer for adequate penetration. A transvaginal examination performed with an empty bladder allows the use of a higher-frequency transducer, typically 7.5 to 10 MHz. It is generally recommended that a complete pelvic examination should consist of a transabdominal scan followed by a transvaginal examination. The transabdominal scan offers a wider field of view for a general screening of the pelvic anatomy. The transvaginal examination will usually offer a more detailed study but is limited in its field of view and depth of penetration. The approach used will depend on the patient's age and sexual status. Transvaginal examinations are typically contraindicated in minors who are not sexually active. Transvaginal examinations are not contraindicated for the non–sexually active adult female who has had a previous gynecologic exam or has used tampons and consents to the procedure.

When using a transabdominal scanning technique, a distended urinary bladder is optimal. An adequately filled bladder will tilt the uterus posteriorly and push the bowel up and out of the pelvic cavity into the lower abdominal cavity, making visualization of the uterine fundus and adnexa easier. An overly distended bladder, on the other hand, will often push the uterus too far posteriorly, making the pelvic structures difficult to see. An overdistended bladder may also cause compression and distortion of the pelvic organs. If the bladder appears overly distended, throwing the pelvic structures too deep, it may be necessary to have the patient partially or fully void. Because over-distention can alter the true lie of the pelvic organs, it is advised to look at the pelvis from a variety of windows—full, empty, and transvaginally—before making a final assessment.

When transvaginal ultrasound is used to evaluate the pelvic structures, the patient should empty her bladder completely before the transvaginal transducer is inserted into the vaginal canal. With the urinary bladder empty, the uterus and iliac vessels become the primary landmarks used to evaluate and image the pelvic organs.

PELVIC LANDMARKS

External Landmarks

The external genitalia in the female, also known as the *vulva* or the *pudendum,* consist of the mons pubis, labia majora, labia minora, clitoris, urethral opening, and vestibule of the vagina (Figure 39-1). (The vagina itself is the part of the female genitalia that forms a canal from the orifice through the vestibule to the uterine cervix. It is behind the bladder and in front of the rectum.) These external structures are important to recognize when using translabial and transvaginal scanning techniques. The mons pubis is a pad of fatty tissue and thick skin that overlies the symphysis pubis and is covered by pubic hair after puberty. The labia are folds of skin at the

opening of the vagina, with labia majora being the thicker external folds and labia minora the thin folds of skin between the labia majora. The clitoris is located anterior to the urethra and is usually partially hidden between the labia majora. Posterior to the clitoris, the urethral opening and vestibule of the vagina can normally be identified between the labia minora. The most posterior orifice is the anus.

The Bony Pelvis

The bony pelvis consists of four bones: two innominate (coxal) bones, the sacrum, and the coccyx. The innominate bones make up the anterior and lateral margins of the bony pelvis, whereas the sacrum and coccyx form the posterior wall. Anatomically, the pelvis is divided into two continuous compartments (true and false pelves) by an oblique plane that passes through the pelvic brim. This plane of division passes from the superior border of the sacrum to the superior margin of the pubic symphysis and corresponds to the **iliopectineal line** (Figure 39-2). The **false pelvis,** also known as the greater or major pelvis, is located above the brim. The false pelvis communicates with the abdominal cavity superiorly and with the pelvic cavity inferiorly. The **true pelvis,** also known as the lesser or minor pelvis, is the area below the pelvic brim.

The Pelvic Cavity and Perineum

The true pelvis, situated inferior to the caudal portion of the parietal peritoneum, is considered the pelvic cavity

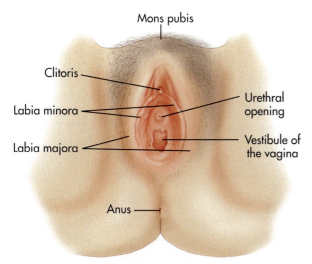

FIGURE 39-1 External genitalia as viewed in the lithotomy position.

Mons pubis
Clitoris
Labia minora
Labia majora
Urethral opening
Vestibule of the vagina
Anus

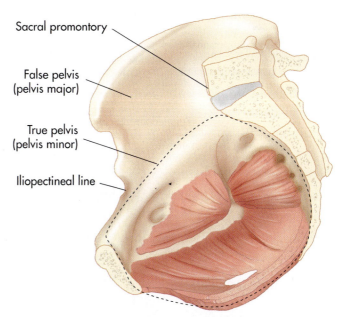

Sacral promontory
False pelvis (pelvis major)
True pelvis (pelvis minor)
Iliopectineal line

FIGURE 39-2 Sagittal plane through the lateral pelvis. The true pelvis is the most inferior portion of the body cavity. It is separated from the false pelvis by the pelvic brim, which corresponds with the iliopectineal line and the sacral promontory.

(Figure 39-3 and Box 39-1). The posterior wall of the pelvic cavity is formed by the sacrum and coccyx, whereas the margins of the posterolateral wall are formed by the piriformis and **coccygeus muscles** (see Figure 39-6). The anterolateral walls of the pelvic cavity are formed by the hip bones and the obturator internus muscles, which rim the ischium and pubis (see Figure 39-10). The lower margin of the pelvic cavity, the pelvic floor, is formed by the **levator ani** and coccygeus muscles and is known as the pelvic diaphragm. The area below the pelvic floor is the perineum.

MUSCLES OF THE PELVIS

The sonographer must be able to identify several primary muscle groups in the pelvis. These muscles serve as

landmarks that may be used to help differentiate the reproductive organs and should be recognized sonographically to prevent misidentifying the muscles as a mass (Box 39-2). Pelvic muscles vary in shape, but typically appear hypoechoic with characteristic hyperechoic **striations** when viewed in their long axis. The pelvic muscles are easiest to locate and identify sonographically if classified by region. The major pelvic muscles can be differentiated as muscles of the abdominal wall, those running through the false pelvis, and those found within the true pelvis.

The Abdominal Wall

The muscles of the anterior abdominal wall extend superiorly from the xiphoid process to the symphysis pubis inferiorly. These muscles include the paired rectus abdominis muscles anteriorly and the external oblique, internal oblique, and transversus abdominis muscles anterolaterally (Figure 39-4). These muscles are described in greater depth in Chapter 7.

Muscles of the False Pelvis

Muscles of the false pelvis include the psoas major and iliacus muscles. The **psoas major muscles** originate at the transverse process of the lumbar vertebrae and descend inferiorly through the false pelvis on the pelvic sidewalls.

> **BOX 39-1** | **Pelvic Cavity**
>
> - Posterior: occupied by rectum, colon, and ileum
> - Anterior: occupied by bladder, ureters, ovaries, fallopian tubes, uterus, and vagina

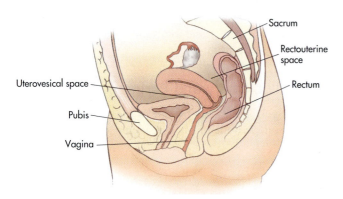

FIGURE 39-3 Sagittal plane through the female pelvis. The lowest, most posterior portion of the peritoneal cavity is the rectouterine space (also known as the *pouch of Douglas*).

> **BOX 39-2** | **Pelvic Muscles**
>
> - Psoas major: pelvic sidewall
> - Iliacus: pelvic sidewall
> - Piriformis: posterolateral wall
> - Obturator internus: anterolateral pelvic sidewall
> - Levator ani: pelvic floor (diaphragm)
> - Coccygeus: posterior pelvic floor (diaphragm)

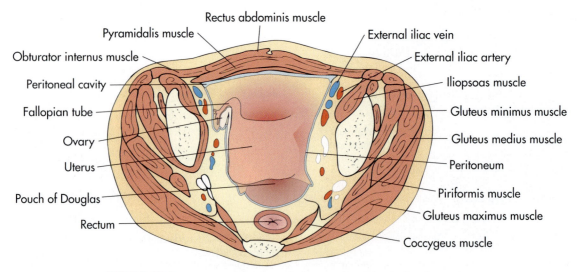

FIGURE 39-4 Transverse plane through the anterior abdominal wall muscles.

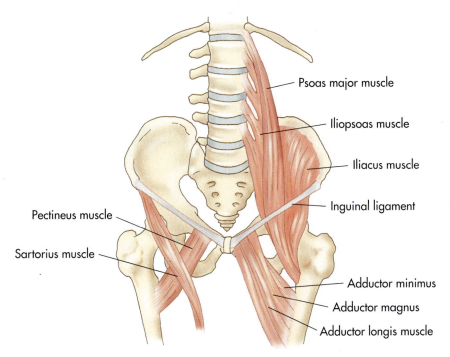

FIGURE 39-5 Anterior diagram of the psoas major muscle extending from the abdominal cavity into the false pelvis. The iliacus muscle joins the psoas muscle to form the iliopsoas muscle along the sidewall of the false pelvis.

In the false pelvis, they join with the **iliacus muscles** to form the iliopsoas muscles. The iliopsoas muscles pass anterior to the hip and insert into the lesser trochanters on the posterior aspect of the femurs (Figure 39-5). Note that the iliopsoas muscles pass outside the pelvic bones and do not enter the true pelvis.

Muscles of the True Pelvis

The muscles found within the true pelvis include the piriformis muscles, obturator internus muscles, and muscles of the pelvic diaphragm. The **piriformis muscles** are flat, triangular muscles that arise from the anterior sacrum and pass through the greater sciatic notch on the posterior aspect of the innominate bone to insert into the superior aspect of the greater trochanter of the femur (Figures 39-6 and 39-7). The **obturator internus muscles** are triangular sheets of muscle that arise from the antero-lateral pelvic wall and surround the obturator foramen. They pass out of the pelvic cavity through the lesser sciatic foramen, where they insert into the superior aspect of the greater trochanter of the femur (see Figures 39-6 and 39-7). The pelvic diaphragm is formed by the levator ani and coccygeus muscles and makes up the floor of the true pelvis (Figure 39-8). The levator ani is a group of three muscles that extend across the pelvic floor like a hammock. This group of muscles consists of the pubococcygeus muscles, the iliococcygeus muscles, and the puborectalis muscles. The pubococcygeus muscles are the most anterior and medial of the three levator ani muscles. They extend from the pubic bones anteriorly to the coccyx posteriorly and surround the urethra, vagina, and rectum. The iliococcygeus muscles extend from the anterolateral pelvic wall to the coccyx

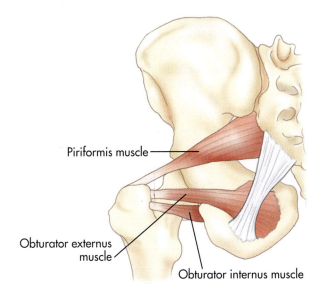

FIGURE 39-6 Posterior view of the piriformis and obturator internus muscles.

posteriorly. The puborectalis muscles arise from the lower part of the pubic symphysis and surround the lower part of the rectum, forming a sling. The levator ani, in addition to forming the floor of the pelvis, has an important role in rectal and urinary continence.

BLADDER AND URETERS

The urinary bladder is located in the anterior portion of the pelvic cavity, posterior to the pubic symphysis (see Figure 39-2 and Box 39-3). The function of the bladder is to collect and store urine until it empties through the urethra. When the bladder is empty or only slightly filled,

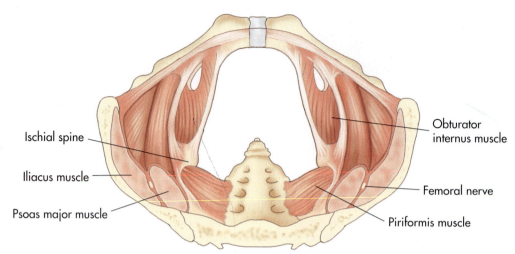

FIGURE 39-7 Pelvic cavity viewed from above. The piriformis and obturator internus muscles pass out from the pelvis through the sciatic foramina to attach to the greater tuberosity of the femur.

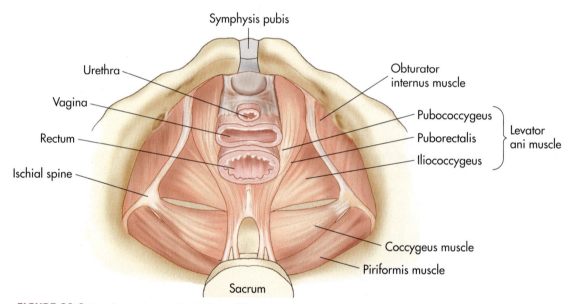

FIGURE 39-8 The floor of the pelvis is formed by the coccygeus and levator ani muscles (*as viewed from above*).

BOX 39-3   Bladder

- Apex: located posterior to pubic bones
- Base: anterior to vagina, superior surface related to uterus
- Neck: rests on upper surface of urogenital diaphragm; inferolateral surfaces relate to retropubic fat, obturator internus, levator ani muscles, and pubic bone

BOX 39-4   Ureters

- Cross the pelvic inlet anterior to bifurcation of common iliac arteries
- Run anterior to internal iliac arteries and posterior to the ovaries
- Run anteriorly and medially under the base of the broad ligament, where they are crossed by the uterine artery
- Run anterior and lateral to the upper vagina to enter the posteroinferior bladder

it remains entirely within the true pelvis; as it becomes distended, it rises up behind the lower anterior abdominal wall and pushes the peritoneum away from the wall.

The ureters are the two tubes that carry urine from the kidneys to the urinary bladder (Box 39-4). As the ureters descend inferiorly from the kidneys, they run anteriorly and medially, passing anterior to the psoas major muscles, behind the peritoneum, and along the lateral aspect of the cervix and upper portion of the vagina, where they enter the bladder at the trigone. As the ureters descend from the retroperitoneal cavity, they pass anterior to the internal iliac arteries and posterior to the ovaries and uterine arteries. The ureters are not normally visualized sonographically (unless obstructed) but may be identified by the visualization of "ureteral jets" in the posteroinferior portion of the urinary bladder as it fills. The ureteral jets are identified by a swirling of urine, which is easily identified with color Doppler. The urinary bladder and ureters are discussed in detail in Chapter 14. Pregnancy, uterine fibroids, ovarian masses, or distal ureteral calculi can lead to compression and dilation of the ureters, resulting in hydronephrosis.

VAGINA

The vagina is a collapsed muscular tube that extends from the external genitalia to the cervix of the uterus. It lies posterior to the urinary bladder and urethra, and anterior to the rectum and anus (Figure 39-9). It is normally directed upward and backward, forming a 90-degree angle with the uterine cervix. It measures approximately 9 cm in length and is longest along its posterior wall (Box 39-5). The vaginal canal is a potential space in which the anterior and posterior walls usually touch. It is the passageway for the products of menstruation and is easily distended during sexual intercourse and childbirth. The vagina has a mucous membrane lining its muscular walls. This membrane receives secretions from the vaginal wall, the mucous glands of the cervix (around ovulation), and the vestibular glands of the vagina (during sexual excitement).

The uterine cervix protrudes into the upper portion of the vaginal canal, forming four archlike recesses called *fornices*. The posterior vaginal wall attaches higher on the cervix, and the fornices are blind pockets formed by the inner surface of the vaginal walls and the outer surface of the cervix. It is a continuous ring-shaped space with the posterior fornix running deeper than its anterior counterpart. This design eases the use of the transvaginal probe and concomitant visualization of the cervix and uterus (Figure 39-10).

UTERUS

Normal Anatomy

The uterus and vagina are derived from the embryonic müllerian (paramesonephric) ducts as they elongate, fuse, and form a lumen between the 7th and 12th weeks of embryonic development. The uterus is pear-shaped and is the largest organ in the normal female pelvis when the urinary bladder is empty (Box 39-6). The average menarcheal uterus measures approximately 6 to 8 cm in length and 3 to 5 cm in anteroposterior and transverse dimensions. The size of the uterus varies with age and parity (Box 39-7 and Table 39-1).

The uterus consists of a fundus, body, and cervix (Figure 39-11). The fundus is the widest and most

---

BOX 39-5	Vagina

- Extends upward and backward from the vulva
- Upper half lies above pelvic floor.
- Lower half lies within perineum.
- Area of vaginal lumen surrounding the cervix is divided into four fornices.
- Arterial supply is from vaginal and uterine arteries; drains into the internal iliac vein.

BOX 39-6	Uterus

- Hollow, pear-shaped organ
- Divided into fundus, body, and cervix
- Usually anteflexed and anteverted
- Covered with peritoneum except anteriorly below the os, where peritoneum is reflected onto bladder
- Supported by levator ani muscles, cardinal ligaments, and utero-sacral ligaments
- Round ligaments hold uterus in anteverted position.

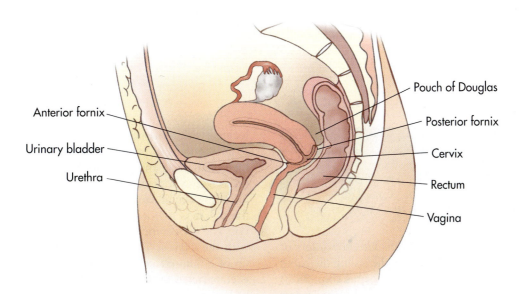

FIGURE 39-9 Lateral view of the pelvis demonstrating the relationship of the anterior and posterior fornices to the cervix and vagina.

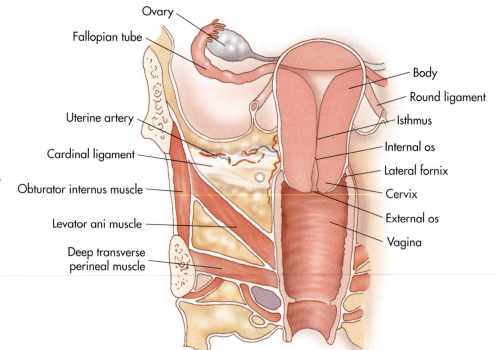

FIGURE 39-10 Coronal view of the vagina, cervix, and uterus.

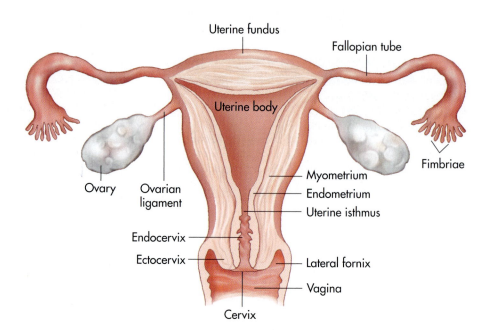

FIGURE 39-11 Normal female pelvic anatomy.

BOX 39-7	Uterine Size

- Premenarcheal: 1.0 to 3.0 cm long by 0.5 to 1.0 cm wide
- Menarcheal: 6.0 to 8.0 cm long by 3.0 to 5.0 cm wide
- With multiparity: increases in size by 1.0 to 2.0 cm
- Postmenopausal: 3.5 to 5.5 cm long by 2.0 to 3.0 cm wide

superior portion of the uterus. At the lateral borders of the fundus are the cornua, where the fallopian tubes enter the uterine cavity. The body or corpus (Box 39-8) lies between the fundus and the cervix and is the largest portion of the uterus. The uterine cavity is centrally located within the pelvis and is a potential space for fluid to accumulate, allowing for dynamic changes during the menstrual cycle and pregnancy. The cervix (Box 39-9) is the lower cylindrical portion of the uterus that projects into the vaginal canal (see Figure 39-11). The surface of the cervix is divided into an exocervix and an endocervix. The exocervix is a squamous epithelium continuous with the vagina. The surface of the endocervix is made up of columnar cells, which excrete mucus. The cervix is constricted at its upper end by the internal os and at its lower end by the external os. The isthmus is the outer transition point between the body of the uterus and

TABLE 39-1	Uterine Size				
	Length, cm	Width, cm	AP, cm	Volume, mL	Cervix/Corpus Ratio
Adult (nulliparous)	6–8	3–5	3–5	30–40	1:2
Adult (parous)	8–10	5–6	5–6	60–80	1:2
Postmenopausal	3–5	2–3	2–3	14–17	1:1

From Standring S, editor: *Gray's anatomy*, New York, 2009, Churchill Livingstone.

BOX 39-8 | Body of the Uterus

- Posterior to the vesicouterine pouch and the superior surface of the bladder
- Anterior to the rectouterine pouch (of Douglas), the ilium, and the colon
- Medial to the broad ligaments and uterine vessels
- Uterine cavity is funnel shaped in coronal plane; "slitlike" in sagittal plane

BOX 39-9 | Cervix

- Projects into vaginal canal
- Endocervix: cervical canal; communicates with uterine cavity by the internal os; the vagina by the external os
- Exocervix: continuous with the vagina

BOX 39-10 | Layers of the Uterus

- Perimetrium: serous outer layer of the uterus; serosa
- Myometrium: muscular middle layer of the uterus composed of thick, smooth muscle supported by connective tissue
- Endometrium: inner mucous membrane, glandular portion of the uterine body

BOX 39-11 | Uterine Ligaments

- Broad: lateral aspect of uterus to pelvic sidewall
- Mesovarium: posterior fold of the broad ligament; encloses the ovary
- Mesosalpinx: upper fold of the broad ligament; encloses the fallopian tube
- Round: fundus to anterior pelvic sidewalls; hold uterus forward
- Cardinal: extend across the pelvic floor laterally; firmly support the cervix
- Uterosacral: extend from uterine isthmus downward, alongside the rectum to the sacrum; firmly support the cervix
- Suspensory: extend from lateral aspect of ovary to the pelvic sidewall
- Ovarian: extend medially from the ovary to the uterine cornua

---

the cervix. This is the point where the uterus bends anteriorly (anteversion) or posteriorly (retroversion) with an empty bladder.

The uterine wall consists of three histologic layers: the serosa or **perimetrium,** the myometrium, and the endometrium (see Figure 35-11). The external layer, the serosa, reflects on the anterior surface of the uterus at the isthmus. The muscular middle layer, the myometrium, is the thickest layer of the uterus and is primarily smooth muscle that is longitudinal and circular (Box 39-10). The mucous membrane, glandular tissue lining the uterine cavity is the endometrium.

Endometrium

The endometrium consists primarily of two layers: the superficial functional layer (zona functionalis) and the deep basal layer (zona basalis). The functional layer is a superficial layer of glands and stroma (supporting tissue) that sheds with **menses.** The basal layer is a thin layer of

the blind ends of endometrial glands that regenerates new endometrium after menses. The endometrium changes dynamically in response to the cyclic hormonal flux of ovulation and varies in sonographic appearance and histologic structure, depending on the patient's menstrual status and the period of life in which it is studied.

Uterine Ligaments

The uterus is supported in its midline position by paired broad ligaments, round ligaments, uterosacral ligaments, and cardinal ligaments (Figure 39-12 and Box 39-11). The **broad ligaments** are a double fold of peritoneum that drapes over the fallopian tubes, uterus, and ovaries (Figure 39-13). They extend from the lateral sides of the uterus to the sidewalls of the pelvis. The broad ligaments provide a small amount of support for the uterus and contain the uterine blood vessels and nerves. The upper fold of the broad ligament, known as the **mesosalpinx,** encloses the fallopian tube as it extends from the cornua of the uterus. The posterior portion of the broad ligament that is drawn out to enclose the ovary is the **mesovarium.**

The **round ligaments** are fibrous cords that occur in front of and below the fallopian tubes between the layers of broad ligament. These two cords commence on each side of the superior aspect of the uterus, course upward and lateral to the inguinal canal, insert into the labia majora, and help to hold the uterine fundus and body in a forward position. The cervix is the only portion of the

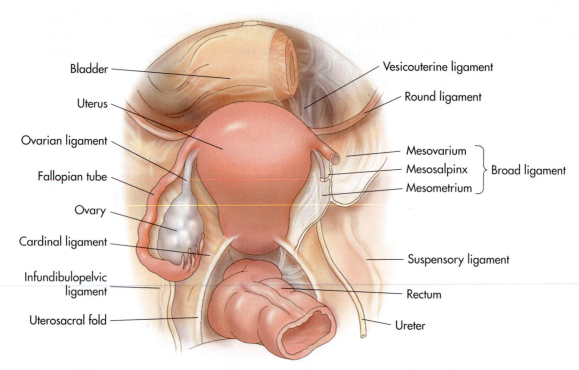

FIGURE 39-12 View of the pelvic cavity from above, looking inferiorly, showing the attachment of the round ligament and broad ligament to the uterus.

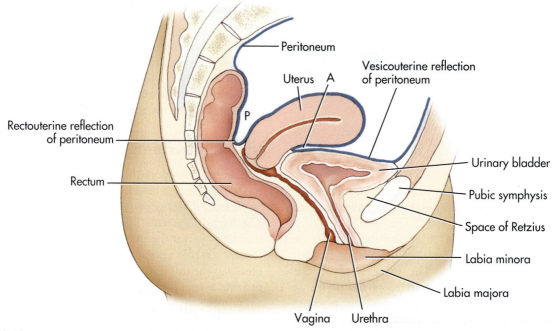

FIGURE 39-13 The peritoneum drapes over the uterine fundus and body to divide the pelvis into anterior (A) and posterior (P) sections. The peritoneum extends laterally from the uterus, forming the broad ligaments and creating the mesosalpinx as it folds over the fallopian tubes. The mesovarium is another fold of the peritoneum, which forms posterior to the broad ligament as it folds over the ovary.

uterus that is firmly supported. It is fixed in position by the **cardinal** and **uterosacral ligaments.** The cardinal ligaments are a continuation of the broad ligaments that extend across the pelvic floor laterally. The uterosacral ligaments originate at the lateral uterine isthmus and extend downward along the sides of the rectum to the third and fourth bones of the sacrum.

Positions of the Uterus

The position of the uterus is variable. The average uterine position is considered to be anteverted and anteflexed. The uterine position is described as **anteverted** when the cervical canal forms a 90-degree or smaller angle with the vaginal canal and as **anteflexed** when the body and fundus of the uterus are curved forward upon the cervix (Figure 39-14 and Box 39-12). In the nulliparous female, the round ligaments help to hold the uterus in an anteverted, anteflexed position. In multiparous females, the entire uterus may tip backward rather than forward and is described as a **retroverted** position. The term *retroverted* is used to describe the uterine position when the cervical canal forms an angle less than 90 degrees with the vaginal canal. The uterine fundus or body may also curve backward upon the cervix, and this position is described as **retroflexed.** It is not uncommon to see a uterus that has variations of version and flexion. For example, a common variation from the average uterine position is retroverted and retroflexed. Another variation from the normal uterine position is for the entire uterus

to tilt to the right (dextro) or to the left (levo) of midline. Abnormal dropping of the uterus (uterine prolapse) occurs if the uterine ligaments and pelvic floor muscles are weak, allowing the uterus to protrude into the vagina. It is also important to recognize that filling of the bladder will affect uterine position. A full urinary bladder will tip the average anteverted, anteflexed uterus backward.

FALLOPIAN TUBES

The fallopian tubes, or oviducts, are coiled, muscular tubes that open into the peritoneal cavity at their lateral end. They are approximately 10 to 12 cm in length and 1 to 4 mm in diameter (Box 39-13). The fallopian tubes lie superior to the utero-ovarian ligaments, round

BOX 39-12	Uterine Positions

- Anteversion: most common position; fundus and body bent forward toward the cervix (degree of anteversion is dependent on bladder distention)
- Dextroversion or levoversion: normal variant in absence of pelvic masses
- Retroversion: entire uterus tilted posteriorly
- Retroflexion: fundus and body bent backward toward the cervix

BOX 39-13	Fallopian Tubes

- Infundibulum: funnel-shaped lateral tube that projects beyond the broad ligament to overlie the ovaries; "free edge" of the funnel has fimbriae (fingerlike projectors draped over the ovary)
- Ampulla: widest part of the tube, where fertilization occurs
- Isthmus: hardest part; lies just lateral to the uterus
- Interstitial portion: pierces the uterine wall at the cornua
- Length: 12 cm; blood is supplied by ovarian arteries and veins

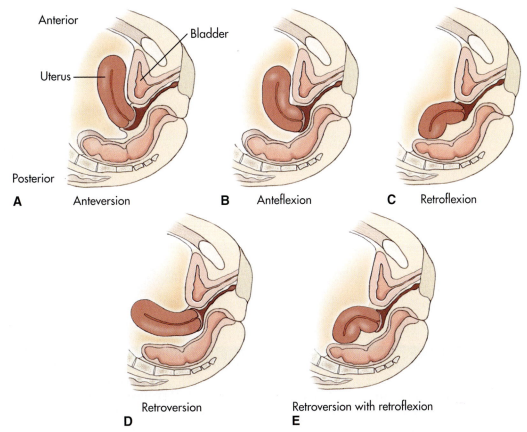

FIGURE 39-14 The uterus may be found in one of several positions: **A,** Anteversion (entire uterus tipped forward). **B,** Anteflexion (body and fundus folded anteriorly toward the cervix). **C,** Retroflexion (body and fundus folded posteriorly upon the cervix). **D,** Retroversion (entire uterus tilted backward). **E,** Retroversion with retroflexion (entire uterus tilted backward with fundus and body folded posteriorly upon the cervix).

ligaments, and tubo-ovarian blood vessels. They are contained in the upper margin of the broad ligament and extend from the cornua of the uterus laterally, where they curve over the ovary.

The fallopian tubes are divided into four anatomic portions (Figure 39-15): infundibulum (lateral segment), ampulla (middle segment), isthmus (medial segment), and interstitial portion (segment that passes through the uterine cornua). The interstitial portion is the narrowest segment of the fallopian tube. The tube widens as it extends laterally, with the infundibulum being the wide, trumpet-shaped, lateral portion. The infundibulum is often referred to as the fimbriated end of the fallopian tube because it contains fringelike extensions, called *fimbriae*, which move over the ovary, directing the ovum into the fallopian tube after ovulation. The ampulla is the longest and most coiled portion of the fallopian tube and is the area in which fertilization of the ovum most often occurs because it is the most distensible region of the tube. The innermost region of the fallopian tube, with its mucosal layer, runs directly into the mucosal layer of the uterus (the endometrium). The continuous nature of the endometrium and the endocervical canal can act as a pathway for organisms, infection, and hemorrhage, because it is the most distensible.

The normal fallopian tubes are difficult to distinguish sonographically from surrounding ligaments and vessels. Doppler interrogation may help differentiate prominent blood vessels from the fallopian tubes.

OVARIES

Position and Size of the Ovaries

The ovaries are almond-shaped structures, measuring approximately 3 cm long in a menarcheal female (Table 39-2 and Box 39-14). They usually lie posterior to the uterus at the level of the cornua. They are suspended from the posterior aspect of the broad ligament in a fold of peritoneum called the mesovarium. The ovaries are usually located medial to the external iliac vessels and anterior to the internal iliac vessels and ureter (Box 39-15). The ovarian arteries have a double supply of blood. The primary blood supply to the ovaries is from the ovarian arteries, which arise from the lateral aspect of the abdominal aorta, below the renal arteries. The

BOX 39-14	Ovaries

- Almond-shaped
- Attached at posterior aspect of the broad ligament by mesovarium
- Lie in ovarian fossa
- Fossa is bounded by external iliac vessels, ureter, and obturator nerve
- Dual blood supply; receives blood from ovarian artery and uterine artery
- Blood drained by ovarian vein into inferior vena cava on the right and into renal vein on the left

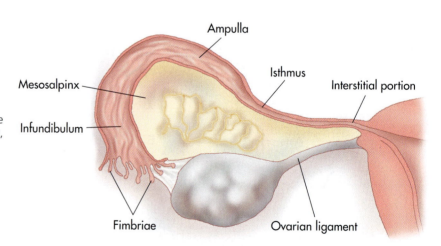

FIGURE 39-15 Diagram of the fallopian tube showing the fimbriae, infundibulum, ampulla, isthmus, and interstitial portions.

TABLE 39-2	Normal Ovarian Volume by Menstrual Status		
Group	Mean Volume, cm³	Standard Deviation	No. of Ovaries Evaluated	95% Confidence Interval, cm³*
Premenarcheal	3.0	2.3	32	0.2–9.1
Menstruating	9.8	5.8	866	2.5–21.9
Postmenopausal	5.8	3.6	100	1.2–14.1

From Cohen HL, Tice HM, Mandel FS: *Radiology* 177:189, 1990.
*Calculated on the basis of cube root values, then transformed back to cubic centimeters.

ovarian artery anastomoses with the uterine artery, providing additional blood to the ovary (Box 39-16).

Normal Anatomy

The ovaries consist of an outer layer or cortex, which surrounds the central medulla. The cortex consists primarily of follicles in varying stages of development and is covered by a layer of dense connective tissue, the tunica albuginea. The tunica albuginea is surrounded by a single, thin layer of cells known as the *germinal epithelium.* The central medulla is composed of connective tissue containing blood, nerves, lymphatic vessels, and some smooth muscle at the region of the hilum.

The ovaries produce the reproductive cell, the **ovum,** and two known hormones: **estrogen,** secreted by the follicles, and **progesterone,** secreted by the **corpus luteum.** These steroidal hormones are responsible for producing and maintaining secondary gender characteristics and for preparing the uterus for implantation of a fertilized ovum; they are also responsible for development of mammary glands in the female.

Ovarian Ligaments

The ovaries are supported medially by the **ovarian ligaments,** originating bilaterally at the cornua of the uterus, and laterally by the **suspensory (infundibulopelvic) ligament,** extending from the infundibulum of the fallopian

tube and ovary to the sidewall of the pelvis. The ovary is also attached to the posterior aspect of the broad ligament via the mesovarium (see Figure 39-15).

PELVIC VASCULATURE

The common iliac arteries course anterior and medial to the psoas muscles, providing blood to the pelvic cavity and lower extremities. The common iliac arteries normally bifurcate into the external and internal iliac (hypogastric) arteries at the level of the superior margin of the sacrum (Figure 39-16; see Box 39-16). The external iliac arteries course along the pelvic brim and continue inferiorly as the common femoral arteries, supplying blood to the lower extremities. The internal iliac arteries extend into the pelvic cavity, along the posterior wall, and provide multiple branches that perfuse the pelvic structures to include the urinary bladder, uterus, vagina, and rectum. The ovarian veins follow a slightly different course, as the left ovarian vein drains into the left renal vein, whereas the right ovarian vein drains directly into the inferior vena cava (IVC).

Blood is supplied to the uterus by the uterine artery, which arises from the anterior branch of the internal iliac artery (Figure 39-17). From the internal iliac artery, the uterine artery crosses above and anterior to the ureter, extending medially in the base of the broad ligament to the uterus at the level of the cervix. The uterine artery is tortuous and spirals up the sides of the uterus within the broad ligament to the cornua, where it courses laterally to anastomose with the ovarian artery. The uterine artery gives off many branches that perforate the serosa and carry blood to the myometrium (Figure 39-18). These branches anastomose extensively anteriorly and posteriorly within the myometrium, forming arcuate (arclike) vessels that encircle the uterus. The arcuate vessels can often be identified sonographically as anechoic tubular structures in the outer third of the myometrium.

Blood is supplied to the endometrium by the radial arteries, which "radiate" from the arcuate arteries within the myometrium. The radial arteries extend through the myometrium to the base of the endometrium, where straight and spiral arteries branch off the radial arteries to supply the zona basalis of the endometrium. The spiral arteries will lengthen during regeneration of the endometrium after menses to traverse the endometrium and supply the zona functionalis. Blood from the spiral arteries is shed during menses. The pelvic vessels supply blood to the functional layer of the endometrium.

PHYSIOLOGY

The Menstrual Cycle

A female's reproductive years begin around 11 to 13 years of age at the onset of menses (menstruation) and end around age 50, when menses ceases. The average

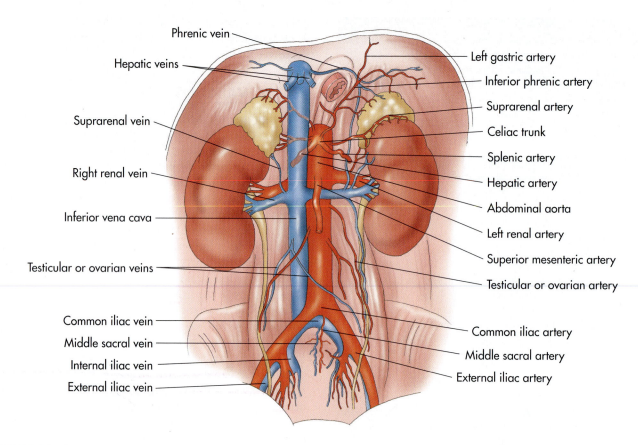

FIGURE 39-16 Blood is supplied to the pelvic cavity by the external and internal iliac arteries; the iliac veins drain the pelvis. The ureter enters the pelvis and courses anterior to the internal iliac artery to empty into the posterior base of the bladder.

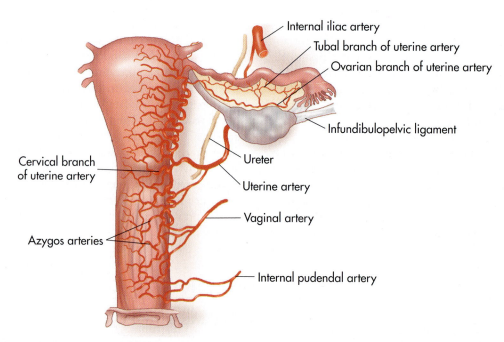

FIGURE 39-17 Blood is supplied to the uterus and vagina by the uterine artery (arising from the internal iliac artery) and the vaginal artery (arising from the uterine artery). The ovaries receive blood from branches of the uterine artery and from the ovarian arteries arising from the abdominal aorta.

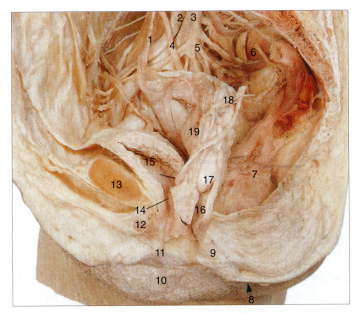

FIGURE 39-18 Female pelvic vessels and viscera (seen on the right side in a sagittal section) after removal of most of the peritoneum.

1. Ovarian vessels	10. Labium majora
2. External iliac artery	11. Labium minora
3. External iliac vein	12. Clitoris
4. Ureter	13. Pubic symphysis
5. Internal iliac vessels and branches	14. Urethra
6. Piriformis	15. Bladder
7. Rectum	16. Vagina
8. Anus	17. Cervix of uterus
9. Perineal body	18. Left uterine artery
	19. Body of uterus

BOX 39-17 | The Menstrual Cycle

Menstruation
- Days 1 to 14

Proliferative Phase
- Days 5 to 14
- Corresponds to the follicular phase of ovarian cycle
- Thin endometrium
- Estrogen level increases as ovarian follicles develop.
- Increasing estrogen levels cause uterine lining to regenerate and thicken
- Ovulation occurs on day 14

Secretory Phase
- Days 15 to 28
- Corresponds to the luteal phase of ovarian cycle
- Ruptured follicle becomes corpus luteum
- Corpus luteum secretes progesterone
- Endometrium thickens
- If no pregnancy, estrogen and progesterone decrease

menstrual cycle is approximately 28 days in length, beginning with the first day of menstrual bleeding (Box 39-17). The length of the menstrual cycle can, however, vary considerably from one woman to another.

Menstrual status is described using the terms *premenarche*, *menarche*, and *menopause*. **Premenarche** is the physiologic status of prepuberty, the time before the onset of menses. **Menarche** is the state after reaching puberty in which menses occurs normally every 28 days. **Menopause** refers to the cessation of menses. The menstrual cycle is regulated by the hypothalamus and is dependent upon the cyclic release of estrogen and progesterone from the ovaries.

Follicular Development and Ovulation

During the menarcheal years, an ovum is released once a month by one of the two ovaries. This process is known as ovulation. Ovulation normally occurs midcycle on about day 14 of a 28-day cycle. It is speculated that ovum release alternates between the two ovaries: one month from the right, the next month from the left. All ova begin development during embryonic life and remain in suspended animation within a preantral follicle as an immature **oocyte** until the onset of menarche.

Each female ovary contains approximately 200,000 oocytes at the time of birth. Some of these oocytes will mature and be released from the ovaries during ovulation, whereas others will degenerate.

The process of ovulation is regulated by the hypothalamus within the brain. When a young girl reaches puberty, the hypothalamus begins the pulsatile release of the **gonadotropin-releasing hormones (GnRHs)**, which stimulate the anterior pituitary gland to secrete varying levels of **gonadotropins** (primarily **follicle-stimulating hormone [FSH]** and **luteinizing hormone [LH]**).

Secretion of FSH by the anterior pituitary gland causes the ovarian follicles to develop during the first half of the menstrual cycle. This phase of the ovulatory cycle, known as the *follicular phase*, begins with the first day of menstrual bleeding and continues until ovulation on day 14 (Figure 39-19). As the ovarian follicles grow, they fill with fluid and secrete increasing amounts of estrogen. Although typically five to eight preantral follicles will begin to develop, only one usually reaches maturity each month. This mature follicle is known as a *graafian follicle* and typically measures 2 cm right before ovulation. As the estrogen level in the blood rises with follicle development, the pituitary gland is inhibited from further production of FSH and begins to secrete LH. The luteinizing hormone level will typically increase rapidly 24 to 36 hours before ovulation in a process known as *the LH surge*. This surge is often used as a predictor for timing ovulation for conception. LH level usually reaches its peak 10 to 12 hours before ovulation. It is the LH surge, accompanied by a smaller FSH surge, that triggers ovulation on about day 14.

Ovulation is the explosive release of an ovum from the ruptured graafian follicle. Rupture of the follicle is associated with small amounts of fluid in the posterior cul-de-sac midcycle. Some women can tell when they're ovulating

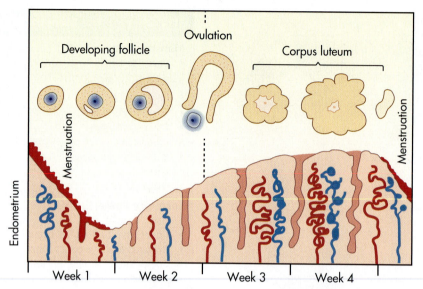

FIGURE 39-19 The average menstrual cycle is approximately 28 days, beginning with the first day of bleeding. As the menstrual lining is shed, the pituitary gland begins to secrete follicle-stimulating hormone (FSH), which causes five to eight preantral ovarian follicles to develop. As the ovarian follicles grow, they fill with fluid and secrete increasing amounts of estrogen. This estrogen stimulates the superficial layer of the endometrium to regenerate and grow. As the estrogen level in the blood rises, the pituitary gland is inhibited from further production of FSH and begins to secrete luteinizing hormone (LH). The LH surges 24 to 36 hours before ovulation and is accompanied by a smaller FSH surge that triggers ovulation on about day 14. Ovulation occurs as the follicle ruptures, releasing the mature ovum. After ovulation, the cells lining the ruptured ovarian follicle begin to multiply and create the corpus luteum. The corpus luteum immediately begins to secrete progesterone. Progesterone causes the spiral arteries and endometrial glands to enlarge as the endometrium prepares for implantation should conception occur. Without conception, the corpus luteum degenerates 9 to 11 days after ovulation, causing progesterone levels to decline. Declining progesterone levels cause the spiral arterioles to constrict, resulting in decreasing blood flow to the endometrium with ischemia and shedding of the zona functionalis. As menstruation occurs, the menstrual cycle begins again.

because at midcycle they have pain, typically a dull ache on either side of the lower abdomen lasting a few hours. The term "mittelschmerz," from the German word meaning *middle pain,* is often used to describe this sensation. After ovulation, the ovary enters the luteal phase. This phase begins with ovulation and is about 14 days in length. It is interesting to note that the luteal phase does not usually vary in length. When a menstrual cycle is shorter or longer than 28 days, it is the follicular phase that is altered. Menstruation almost always occurs 14 days after ovulation. During the luteal phase, the cells in the lining of the ruptured ovarian follicle begin to multiply and create the corpus luteum, or yellow body. This process, known as *luteinization,* is stimulated by the LH surge. The corpus luteum immediately begins to secrete progesterone. Nine to 11 days after ovulation, the corpus luteum degenerates, causing progesterone levels to decline. As progesterone levels decline, menstruation occurs and the cycle begins again. Should conception and implantation occur, the human chorionic gonadotropin (hCG) produced by the zygote causes the corpus luteum to persist, and it will continue to secrete progesterone for 3 more months until the placenta takes over. (Box 39-17) summarizes the phases of the menstrual cycle.

Endometrial Changes

Varying levels of estrogen and progesterone throughout the course of the menstrual cycle induce characteristic changes in the endometrium. These changes correlate with ovulatory cycles of the ovary. The typical endometrial cycle is identified and described in three phases, beginning with the menstrual phase (see Figure 39-19). The menstrual phase lasts approximately 1 to 5 days and begins with declining progesterone levels, causing the spiral arterioles to constrict. This causes decreased blood flow to the endometrium, resulting in ischemia and shedding of the zona functionalis. These first 5 days coincide with the follicular phase of the ovarian cycle. As the follicles produce estrogen, the estrogen stimulates the superficial layer of the endometrium to regenerate and grow. This phase of endometrial regeneration, called the *proliferative phase,* will last until luteinization of the graafian follicle around ovulation. With ovulation and luteinization of the graafian follicle, the progesterone secreted by the ovary causes the spiral arteries and endometrial glands to enlarge. This will prepare the endometrium for implantation, should conception occur. The endometrial phase after ovulation, referred to as the *secretory phase,* extends from approximately day 15 to the onset of menses (day 28). The secretory phase of the endometrial cycle corresponds to the luteal phase of the ovarian cycle.

The sonographic appearance of the endometrium changes dramatically among the three phases of the endometrial cycle and should be correlated with the patient's menstrual status (Figure 39-20). During menses, it is not uncommon to see varying levels of fluid and

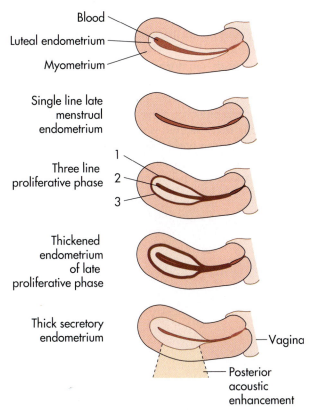

FIGURE 39-20 Cyclic changes in the endometrium. The menstrual cycle begins with approximately 5 days of bleeding. During menses, varying levels of fluid and debris may be seen within the uterine cavity. The thickness of the endometrium decreases with menstruation, becoming a thin echogenic line during the early proliferative phase. As regeneration ensues, the endometrium thickens and appears hypoechoic with a "three-line" sign. The outer echogenic line surrounding the hypoechoic functionalis represents the zona basalis, whereas the central echogenic line represents the uterine cavity. As ovulation nears, the endometrium becomes isoechoic with the myometrium. The secretory phase occurs after ovulation, when the endometrium reaches its thickest dimension and becomes hyperechoic.

debris within the uterine cavity; likewise, the thickness of the endometrium will decrease with menstruation, becoming a thin echogenic line during the early proliferative phase. As regeneration of the endometrium occurs during the proliferative phase, the endometrium will thicken to an average of 4 to 8 mm in the proliferative phase, when measured as a double layer from anterior to posterior. The endometrium characteristically appears hypoechoic with the appearance of the "three-line" sign. The three echogenic lines seen in the proliferative endometrium represent the zona basalis anteriorly and posteriorly, with the central line representing the uterine cavity. Right before ovulation, the endometrium averages 6 to 10 mm and becomes isoechoic with the myometrium. After ovulation, during the secretory phase, the endometrium reaches its thickest dimension, averaging 7 to 14 mm, and becomes echogenic, blurring the "three-line" appearance. The endometrium in anovulatory patients (e.g., those on the birth control pill, postmeno-

pausal patients) will usually appear as a thin, echogenic line. Postmenopausal patients who are not on hormone replacement therapy (HRT) should have an endometrial thickness of less than 5 mm. Postmenopausal patients on HRT or taking tamoxifen (a drug used as adjuvant palliative therapy to help in the prevention of breast cancer) may demonstrate normal endometrial thicknesses of up to 8 mm.

Abnormal Menstrual Cycles

Several terms are used to describe abnormal menstrual cycles and should be familiar to the sonographer. The term **menorrhagia** is used to describe abnormally heavy or long periods and is often associated with uterine fibroids, intrauterine contraceptive devices (IUDs), or hormonal imbalances. Persistent menorrhagia can lead to anemia. The term **oligomenorrhea** describes abnormally short or light periods and is often associated with polycystic ovary syndrome (PCOS). Oligomenorrhea can also be caused by emotional and physical stress, chronic illnesses, tumors that secrete estrogen, poor nutrition and eating disorders, such as anorexia nervosa, and heavy exercise. **Polymenorrhea** is when the menstrual cycle occurs at intervals of less than 21 days.

Many patients complain of **dysmenorrhea** or painful periods. Dysmenorrhea is often associated with endometriosis.

The term **amenorrhea** refers to the absence of menstruation. Amenorrhea is considered primary when menarche is delayed beyond 18 years of age, and secondary when cessation of uterine bleeding occurs in women who have previously menstruated. Amenorrhea may be due to a congenital vaginal or cervical stenosis or may result from infection, trauma, ovarian dysfunction, or other endocrine disturbances that affect ovarian function, such as pituitary disease.

PELVIC RECESSES AND BOWEL

The peritoneal cavity contains two potential spaces formed by the caudal portion of the parietal peritoneum (Box 39-18). These potential spaces are sonographically significant in that fluid may accumulate or pathology may be present in these locations. The **vesicouterine recess (pouch)**, or anterior cul-de-sac, is located anterior to the fundus of the uterus between the urinary bladder and the uterus, whereas the **rectouterine recess (pouch)**, or posterior cul-de-sac, is located posterior to the uterus between the uterus and the rectum. The rectouterine pouch is often referred to as the *pouch of Douglas* and is normally the most inferior and most posterior region of the peritoneal cavity. One additional area that is sonographically significant is the retropubic space (also called the **space of Retzius**). It can be identified between the anterior bladder wall and the pubic symphysis. This space normally contains subcutaneous fat, but a hematoma or abscess in this location may displace the urinary bladder posteriorly.

It is normal to observe a small accumulation of free fluid throughout the menstrual cycle in the posterior cul-de-sac (see Figure 39-3). The greatest quantity of free fluid in the cul-de-sac normally occurs immediately following ovulation when the mature follicle ruptures. A small amount of fluid in the posterior cul-de-sac is considered normal; however, there is no sonographic means of confirming that the fluid is related to ovulation. Hemorrhage or infection within the fluid may be related to a ruptured cyst, ascites, a ruptured corpus luteum cyst, ectopic pregnancy, or pelvic inflammatory disease.

The Sonographic and Doppler Evaluation of the Female Pelvis

Candace Goldstein, Sandra L. Hagen-Ansert, and Barbara J. Vander Werff

OBJECTIVES

On completion of this chapter, you should be able to:
- Demonstrate how to take a patient history specific to a pelvic ultrasound examination
- Discuss the indications and contraindications for transabdominal and transvaginal scans
- Name the important muscles in the pelvic cavity
- Describe the scan orientation for transabdominal and transvaginal ultrasonography
- Describe both the sonographic technique for evaluating the uterus and adnexal area and their sonographic appearances
- Discuss quantitative Doppler measurements

OUTLINE

Ultrasonography is an important diagnostic tool for the evaluation of pelvic anatomy and pathology both in adult and in pediatric populations. The noninvasive nature of sonography, its high-resolution imaging capabilities, and its ability to separate fluid from soft tissue structures in multiple imaging planes have proved clinically useful.

In the pediatric population, transabdominal ultrasound is used in a variety of clinical circumstances, including the evaluation of ambiguous genitalia, pelvic masses, and disorders of puberty. It is also used to further evaluate pelvic or lower abdominal pain that may result from appendicitis.

The size, location, contour, vascularity, and physiologic state of pelvic organs are easily obtained using both transabdominal and transvaginal ultrasound. The information obtained complements the clinical evaluation and aids the process of forming differential considerations.

Color and spectral Doppler have evolved to play a role in assessing normal and pathologic blood flow. Sonohysterography can provide more detailed evaluation of the endometrium. Sonography also plays an important role in guiding interventional procedures.

The role of the sonographer is to gather the clinical history, identify the referring physician's indications for the study (working diagnosis), review the previous imaging results, and tailor the ultrasound exam to each patient. Critical thinking by the sonographer produces valid, reliable, and reproducible results that are the basis of an effective diagnostic medical sonographic practice.

PATIENT PREPARATION AND HISTORY

A complete history is critical in order to tailor the ultrasound exam and correlate ultrasound findings with the proper differential consideration. It is useful for the sonographer to use a routine patient questionnaire requesting the following information: date of last menstrual period, gravidity, parity, physiologic menstrual status, hormone regimen, symptoms, history of cancer, family history of cancer, past pelvic surgeries, laboratory tests, previous Pap or biopsy results, and pelvic examination findings. A review of previous examinations (ultrasound, CT, MRI, PET) should be done before the start of the ultrasound exam to determine if a mass was previously present and to assess if there has been any change in size or internal characteristics.

The patient's menstrual status is described by using the terms *premenarche*, *menarche*, and *menopause*. **Premenarche** is the physiologic status of prepuberty, the time before the onset of menses. **Menarche** is the state after reaching puberty in which menses occur normally every 21 to 28 days. Perimenopause, or premenopause, is a transitional stage of 2 to 10 years before complete cessation of the menstrual cycle. This is the stage of gradually declining estrogen during which menstrual cycles may become shorter, longer, or irregular. **Menopause** is when menses have ceased permanently, generally agreed to be defined as 1 year without menses.

After the clinical history has been taken, the sonographer should carefully explain the examination to the patient. If both the transabdominal (TA) and transvaginal (TV) examinations are going to be performed, the patient should be instructed that the pelvic ultrasound examination will be performed in two parts. The first is the transabdominal approach, in which the transducer is carefully scanned across her lower abdomen after warm gel has been applied, and the second is the transvaginal approach, which is an internal ultrasound and similar to a pelvic examination. The sonographer should tell the patient that she will be allowed to empty her bladder completely after the first part of the examination is completed. After receiving a brief explanation of the entire ultrasound examination, the patient is placed in the supine position. Ideally the scanning should be performed on a gynecologic ultrasound examination table, which can be modified for the TV examination.

By understanding all of the patient's clinical history and by talking and listening to the patient, the sonographer can gain a perspective as to what questions the ultrasound examination needs to answer and can tailor a plan of how to accomplish this. Once the scanning begins, the sonographer adds the information gained to develop a clinical and diagnostic image for each patient.

PERFORMANCE STANDARDS FOR THE ULTRASOUND EXAM

Four major organizations have determined standards for the pelvic ultrasound examination: the Society of Diagnostic Medical Sonography, the American Institute of Ultrasound in Medicine, the American College of Obstetrics & Gynecology, and the American College of Radiology. These organizations can be investigated by visiting their websites. This chapter uses the standards set by the American College of Radiology (ACR) as its primary example. The ACR Standard for the Performance of Ultrasound Examination of the Female Pelvis outlines the following guidelines when performing a pelvic ultrasound examination:

1. Ultrasound examination of the pelvis should be performed only when there is a valid medical reason.
2. The lowest possible ultrasonic exposure settings should be used to gather the necessary information. The American Institute of Ultrasound in Medicine (AIUM) Bioeffects Committee identified ultrasound intensity (free-field spatial peak, temporal average [SPTA]) of 100 mW/cm² as the intensity below which no significant biologic effects in mammalian tissues exposed in vivo have been confirmed.
3. All relevant structures (anatomy and pathology) should be identified by the transabdominal and the transvaginal approach; in most cases both techniques are utilized unless contraindicated.
4. Alternatively a transperineal, also known as translabial, approach can be useful in patients who are not candidates for transvaginal scanning. Such patients might include those with suspected rupture of membranes in pregnancy or uterine prolapse.

The ACR also sets standards for personnel, protocols, documentation, equipment, quality control, and quality improvement.

SONOGRAPHIC TECHNIQUE

The female pelvis is routinely evaluated with at least one of two ultrasound techniques: transabdominal (TA) and transvaginal (TV) (Box 40-1). The TA examination is performed from the anterior abdominal wall using a curvilinear, or sector, transducer with frequencies of up to 5 MHz. TA scans typically use the distended urinary bladder as a "sonic" window to identify the uterus and **adnexa** as an overview of the other pelvic structures. If the protocol is to do a TA study in conjunction with a TV study, not all institutions begin with the urinary bladder fully distended. Even when the urinary bladder is only partially distended or is empty, a TA scan may still help as an overview to the pelvic structures.

The TV examination is performed with the patient's bladder empty, using higher transducer frequencies of 7.5 MHz or more. These higher frequencies have better near-field focusing and resolution, which permit greater detail and characterization of the uterus and adnexa.

Transabdominal and transvaginal sonography are complementary techniques, and both are used extensively in evaluation of the female pelvis. Anatomy and pathology should be identified in at least two orthogonal planes, usually *sagittal* and *axial* or *coronal* and *transverse*, using both techniques (Figure 40-1).

BOX 40-1 | Pelvic Ultrasound Examination

Uterus
- Vagina and uterus serve as anatomic landmarks
- Document the following:
  Uterine size, shape, and orientation
  Endometrium
  Myometrium
  Cervix
- Vagina serves as a landmark for the cervix and lower uterine segment
- Uterine length measured in the long axis from the fundus to the cervix
- Anteroposterior depth of the uterus measured in the long axis from its anterior to posterior walls, perpendicular to the length
- Width measured from the transaxial or coronal view
- Cervical diameters (length and width) can be obtained (usually performed in pregnancy)
- Endometrium analyzed for thickness and echogenicity
- Myometrium and cervix evaluated for contour changes, echogenicity, and masses

Adnexa (Ovaries and Fallopian Tubes)
- Ovaries should be identified anterior to the internal iliac (hypogastric) vessels
- Document the following:
  Size, shape, contour, and echogenicity
  Position relative to the uterus
- Ovarian size determined by measuring the length of the long axis with the anteroposterior dimension measured perpendicular to the length
- Ovarian width measured in the transaxial or coronal view
- Ovarian volume may be calculated

Cul-de-sac
- Evaluate cul-de-sac for the presence of free fluid or a mass
- If a mass is detected, document its size, position, shape, echographic pattern (cystic, solid, or complex) and its relationship to the ovaries and uterus
- Differentiate normal loops of bowel from a mass

When a mass is found on sonography, the following features should be characterized:

- Location (uterine or extrauterine)
- Size
- External contour (well-defined, ill-defined, or irregular borders)
- Internal consistency (cystic, complex, predominantly cystic, complex, predominantly solid, or solid)

Ultrasound scanning equipment usually has built-in "presets" to optimize visualization techniques. These can be fine-tuned, and each ultrasound lab can develop its own unique techniques. Included are the use of harmonic imaging (clean-up on the anterior noise in fluid-filled structures), compound scanning (improved echo texture), and a variety of penetration and resolution capabilities. Sonographers need to be aware of these techniques and their capabilities to improve diagnostic imaging and avoid artifacts that can lead to an inaccurate diagnosis.

Transabdominal (TA) Ultrasonography

The transabdominal approach visualizes the entire pelvis and gives a global overview. The transabdominal technique may be limited in patients who are obese and unable to fill their urinary bladders, older patients who are unable to fill due to incontinence issues, or in patients with a **retroverted** uterus. This technique gives a less optimal characterization of adnexal masses because of its distance from the transducer and interference from the bowel.

For an initial study of the female pelvis, it is recommended that a TA study be made, especially if the patient has not had a previous ultrasound. The TA exam is performed with a distended urinary bladder. Instruction should be given to the patient to drink at least 32 oz of fluid 1 hour before examination time and not to empty her bladder before the scheduled appointment. The full bladder displaces the bowel and any gas it contains from the field of view and "flattens" the anteflexed uterus slightly so it is more perpendicular to the transducer angle. The distended bladder also becomes an acoustic window to view pelvic anatomy and pathology and serves as a "cystic" reference. The bladder is considered optimally full when it covers the fundus of the normal-sized uterus (Figure 40-2). Overdistention of the bladder may compromise the sonographic evaluation and compress, distort, and displace anatomy (Figure 40-3). When this occurs, imaging may be repeated after the patient partially empties the bladder.

In most average-size patients, the anatomic survey is usually performed with a transducer frequency range of 3.5 to 5 MHz. If the ovaries lie anteriorly, the use of a higher-frequency transducer may be preferable. If the patient is obese, the lower-frequency transducer may be used. The TA examination is best initiated by identifying the urinary bladder and evaluating its walls and lumen. It is important to definitely identify the urinary bladder to rule out the possibility of a midline cystic, complex mass, or free fluid, which can inadvertently be mistaken for the bladder. The patient may even feel that she has a full bladder if a large mass is pushing against the urinary bladder. The bladder shape may be helpful because a well-distended bladder typically has a triangular or elongated shape on midline scans. If there is any question as to whether a cystic structure in the pelvis represents the bladder, it can be confirmed by having the patient void or by checking for ureteral jets entering the bladder.

The uterus should then be identified in its long axis. This may not be in a true anatomic **sagittal plane** because the uterus can normally deviate toward either the right or the left. A somewhat oblique angulation through the distended bladder may be necessary to visualize the entire uterus and cervix. Anatomic orientation is correct for longitudinal scans (Figure 40-4) when the left side of the screen represents cephalic anatomy (toward the

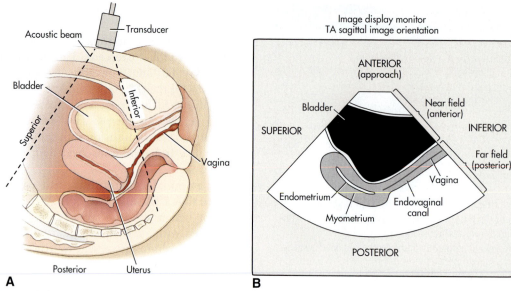

A

B

FIGURE 40-1 Sagittal plane/transabdominal approach illustrates how transabdominal pelvic sonography may be performed from an anterior approach using the fully distended urinary bladder as the acoustic window.

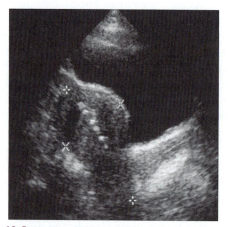

FIGURE 40-2 Sagittal image of the distended urinary bladder covering the fundus of the uterus. The endometrial cavity is seen as bright linear reflectors. The cervix is seen posterior to the angle of the bladder; the vagina is the tubular structure posterior to the bladder.

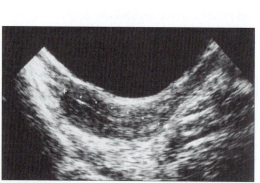

FIGURE 40-3 Sagittal image of an overdistended bladder compressing the uterine cavity.

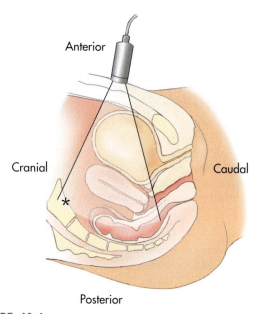

FIGURE 40-4 Longitudinal plane is oriented with the patient's head toward the left of the image and the feet to the right.

patient's head) and the right side of the screen represents caudal anatomy (toward the patient's feet). Once the long axis has been established, parallel sagittal scans are then obtained to the right and left to evaluate the uterine margins and the adnexa. The adnexal area may be imaged by scanning obliquely from the contralateral side and scanning through the fluid-filled bladder. In many instances, the adnexal area can be visualized by scanning directly over the adnexal area. Gentle pressure with the transducer on the pelvic area may be necessary to bring the area of interest within the focal zone. The iliac vessels can be used as a landmark to identify the lateral adnexal borders.

By again identifying the true sagittal plane of the uterus and cervix, and then rotating the transducer 90 degrees, the axial or axial-coronal (transverse) images can be obtained. Again, angulation from the contralateral side or direct visualization may help to image the adnexa. Anatomic correlation is correct for axial scans when the left side of the screen correlates with the right side of the patient (Figure 40-5). Applying gentle pressure on the transducer or placing the free hand on the abdomen helps move overlying bowel gas to bring the area of interest within the focal zone. The ovaries tend to travel cephalad with increasing bladder disten-

tion and may come to lie superior to the uterine fundus. When this occurs, it may be necessary to have the patient empty her bladder before the exam can be completed.

Documentation and scanning techniques should be methodical and become routine for viewing by both the sonographer and the physician. A routine protocol consists of longitudinal and transverse scans of the uterus (to include the **myometrium** and **endometrium**), cervix, rectouterine recess (cul-de-sac), right adnexa, and left adnexa (Box 40-2; Figures 40-6 to 40-8). Measurements of normal structures and pathology are made in the length, width, and depth dimensions. Additional information may be obtained by the Doppler evaluation of all pelvic anatomy and pathology.

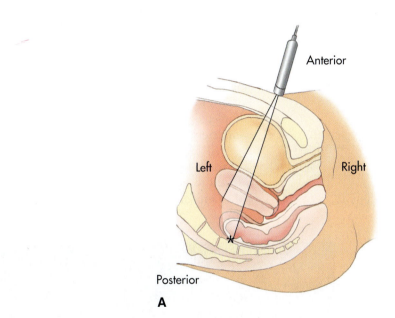

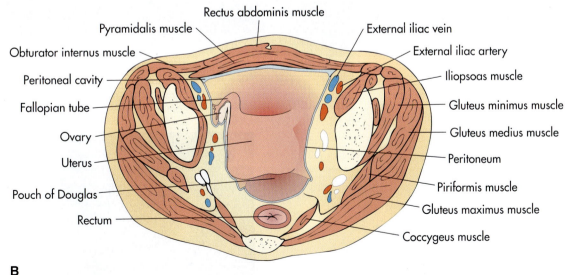

FIGURE 40-5 A, Transverse plane is 90 degrees to the longitudinal plane. The right of the patient is located on the left side of the image. **B,** Cross section of the female pelvis just below the junction of the sacrum and coccyx. The anterior inferior spine of the ilium and the greater sciatic notch are shown. The uterine artery and vein and the ureter are shown dissected beyond the uterine wall. The bladder is anterior to the uterus. The ovaries are cut through their midsections at this level.

If pathology is present, documentation of the right upper quadrant (Morison's pouch and subphrenic area) and bilateral renal areas must be obtained. The evaluation of these areas demonstrates the presence or absence of free fluid, hydronephrosis (either renal in origin or as a secondary result of a pelvic mass), or anatomic variants related to pelvic findings.

BOX 40-2 | Transabdominal Pelvic Ultrasound Protocol

Survey the pelvic area before images are recorded.

Longitudinal
Midline. Distended urinary bladder, uterus, endometrium, cervix, vagina (Figure 40-6)
Measure length of uterus from the fundus to the cervix
Angle right of midline. Bladder, uterus, area of right ovary (Figure 40-7, *A*)
Angle left of midline. Bladder, uterus, area of left ovary (Figure 40-7, *B*)
Look at both right and left adnexal areas in true pelvis (iliacus muscle is lateral border)

Transverse
Low. Distended urinary bladder, vagina, cervix
Mid. Bladder, body of uterus, endometrium; look for ovaries (Figure 40-8)
High. Fundus of uterus, endometrium; look for ovaries lateral to cornu of uterus

It is important to have adequate bladder filling for all TA exams. The examination routinely begins with a TA exam to look for large masses, fluid collections, or any obvious abnormalities. The survey of the pelvis is made to identify the uterus and ovaries. Then scan both the right and left flanks, and document the sagittal and transverse the liver–right kidney interface and the spleen–left kidney interface. The patient is then instructed to void and the TV scan is performed.

Transvaginal Ultrasonography

The inclusion of the transvaginal (TV) transducer in standard gynecologic sonography protocols has vastly improved the effectiveness of the pelvic exam. This exam allows the sonographer and physician a better visual survey by shortening the distance from the transducer to the ovaries, uterus, and adnexal regions. The resolution of pelvic structures has improved and the ability to zoom in on smaller objects has been enhanced. This advance in technology brings with it more frequent detection of small tissue differences.

Patient Instructions. After the transabdominal study is completed, the patient is asked to empty her bladder completely. If the bladder is very full from all the fluids ingested before the examination, the patient may void and think the bladder is "empty" because it had been difficult to hold so much urine during the transabdominal examination. Ask the patient to wait a few seconds

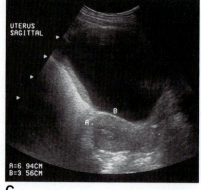

FIGURE 40-6 A, Sagittal midline image of the pelvic cavity demonstrates the urinary bladder *(B)*, uterus *(u)*, cervix *(cx)*, and vagina *(V)*. **B,** The image is magnified to better view the myometrium and endometrial canal within the uterus. **C,** Measurements of the length *(A)* and anteroposterior *(B)* dimensions of the uterus are shown.

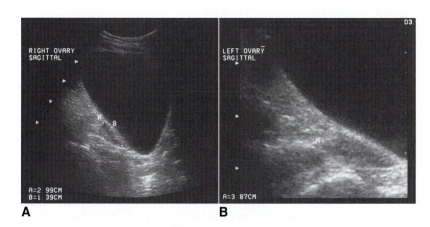

FIGURE 40-7 A, Sagittal image to the right of midline shows the bladder with the right ovary posterior. The ovarian length (A) and depth (B) are measured. **B,** Sagittal image to the left of midline shows the left ovary posterior to the urinary bladder. The length (A) is measured.

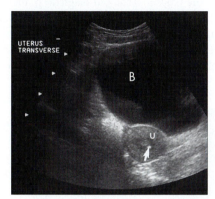

FIGURE 40-8 Transverse image of the bladder (B) with the uterus (u) posterior. The endometrial cavity (arrow) is seen in the center of the uterine cavity.

after her bladder has been emptied and try to void again; this technique is usually successful in completely emptying the bladder. If the bladder is not completely empty, reverberation artifacts may obscure crucial structures, and problem areas may be pushed too far away from the transducer. This is also an opportune time to reiterate the transvaginal procedure, obtain a verbal consent, and answer any questions the patient may have.

An adequate explanation of the procedure is essential. Many patients are apprehensive at any mention of an "internal" examination, and the referring physician may not have explained the possibility of having one. It is important to explain why it is necessary to perform the transvaginal exam and to stress that the examination is a simple, usually painless procedure and that only part of the probe is inserted. Many labs require a verbal or written consent from the patient and examiner for the transvaginal examination. If the examiner is a male, it is essential to have a female staff member in the room during the examination to act as a chaperone.

Transvaginal sonography is performed using transducer frequencies of 7.5 MHz or more. These higher frequencies have better near-field resolution, which often permits greater detail of the uterus and adnexal anatomy. The primary disadvantage of high-frequency transvaginal ultrasound is the limited field of view and penetration

(8 to 10 cm) because of the high frequency of the transducer and limited movement of the probe within the vagina. TV is often the preferred method of evaluation because it provides optimal visualization of the pelvic organs and should always be performed in women with suspected endometrial disorders, a strong family history of ovarian cancer, or a suspected pelvic mass. Contraindications include patient refusal, lack of patient tolerance (usually secondary to intense pelvic pain), and age, both premenarchal and menopausal. It is not recommended that a transvaginal examination be performed in patients who have never been sexually active, have an intact hymen, or have a narrow vaginal canal. If a patient experiences discomfort with an attempted insertion of the transducer, the examination should be discontinued.

Probe Preparation. The TV transducer is prepared with coupling gel on the transducer face and then covered with a sterile probe cover. Currently most institutions are using latex-free probe covers to prevent allergic reactions in latex-sensitive patients. Instruct the patient that only a short portion of the end of the transducer is introduced into the vaginal canal, because the length of the probe can be intimidating. After the protective sheath has been put on, any air bubbles should be eliminated to prevent artifacts. A sterile external lubricant is then applied to the outside of the probe cover. This provides lubrication for insertion of the probe and is especially important in older women. If the examination is performed on an infertility patient, the use of water to lubricate the transducer is preferred because water does not have a negative effect on sperm mobility.

Examination Technique. After the patient has completely voided, she is asked to undress from the waist down, given a gown, and covered with a sheet. The patient position should be supine, knees gently flexed, and hips elevated slightly on a pillow or folded sheets and feet flat on the table, approximately shoulder length apart. The head and shoulders are slightly elevated with a pillow. A slightly reversed Trendelenburg's position may be helpful in lowering the pelvic organs to enhance visualization and detect free intraperitoneal fluid that gravitates to the posterior cul-de-sac. Current ultrasound scanning tables allow the lower section to be dropped with stirrups added to provide for ease of patient positioning. It is important that the patient's buttocks be at the end of the table with the patient's heels in the stirrups. This elevation is necessary to provide adequate mobility of the transducer handle. Being able to easily position the patient, cart, ultrasound equipment, and sonographer chair enhances the ergonomic position and reduces musculoskeletal stress on the sonographer. The height adjustment of the scanning table may permit the sonographer to sit or stand during the TV exam. The use of a chair with arms to rest on takes the strain off the examiner's shoulder and elbow.

Scan Orientation. The most accepted method of orientation used during transvaginal scanning is such that the left side of the screen corresponds to the cephalic and right side of the patient, whereas the right side of the screen corresponds to the caudal and left side of the patient (Figures 40-9 to 40-11). This method of orienta-

tion is the same one for radiography and conventional ultrasound. Residual fluid in the bladder is a helpful orientation landmark and should always appear in the right upper corner of the screen in the sagittal plane. For an **anteverted** uterus, the cervix would be seen on the right side of the screen, whereas the fundus of the uterus is found on the left side of the screen. In the case of a retroverted uterus, the cervix would be seen on the left with the fundus on the right.

Scanning Planes. When inserting the transducer in the sagittal plane, the flat part of the transducer is along the top surface of the handle so that the beam is projected in the midline anteroposterior aspect of the body. From the sagittal plane, the transducer is limited in motion because of the vagina. True parasagittal planes are never obtained, but angulation from this central point is considered sagittal imaging (Figure 40-12, *A*). As in the TA examination, oblique angulation is often necessary to visualize the entire uterus and cervix. It is often necessary

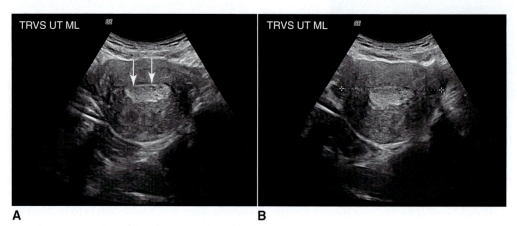

FIGURE 40-9 A, Transvaginal coronal image of the uterus. Note the echogenic central echo pattern of the endometrium *(arrows).* **B.** The maximum dimension of the uterine width is measured. Here it is 6.46 cm.

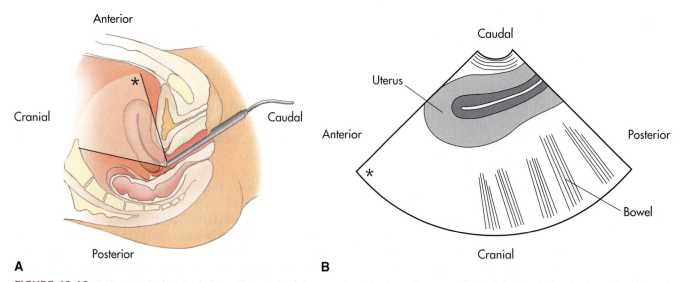

FIGURE 40-10 A, Transvaginal sagittal plane. The notch of the transducer is along the top surface of the handle so the beam is projected in the midline anteroposterior aspect of the body. **B,** The bladder is emptied, so only the uterine cavity and endometrial canal are seen.

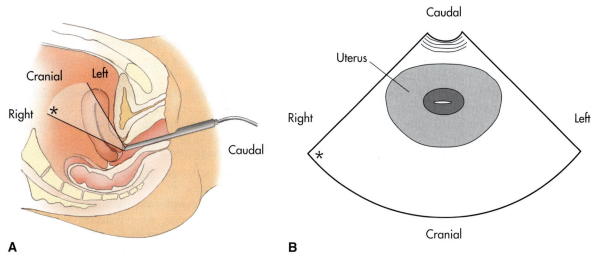

FIGURE 40-11 **A,** Transvaginal coronal plane. The notch of the transducer is rotated toward the sonographer so the beam may image the uterus in a coronal view. **B,** Coronal view of the uterus with the endometrial canal centrally located.

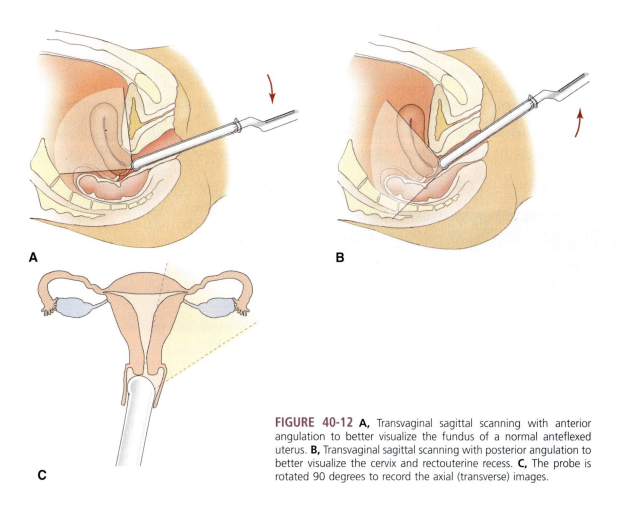

FIGURE 40-12 **A,** Transvaginal sagittal scanning with anterior angulation to better visualize the fundus of a normal anteflexed uterus. **B,** Transvaginal sagittal scanning with posterior angulation to better visualize the cervix and rectouterine recess. **C,** The probe is rotated 90 degrees to record the axial (transverse) images.

to advance the transducer slightly, angling anterior to visualize the fundus, and then withdraw slightly, away from the external os, while angling posterior to see the cervix and rectouterine recess (Figure 40-12, *B*). The uterus is surveyed by scanning from the midline to the right and left. Angulation and tilting of the transducer directs the sound beam to visualize the adnexa in

an oblique sagittal plane. Applying manual external pressure (either by the sonographer or the patient) to the outer abdominal wall may help displace the bowel and bring the ovaries into the focal zone, helping to visualize and delineate the borders of the ovaries.

When the transducer is rotated 90 degrees from the sagittal plane, image orientation represents the **coronal** plane (Figure 40-12, C). Rotating the transducer 360 degrees is possible. If the uterus is retroverted, better resolution may be obtained by inverting the transducer 180 degrees. The image should be inverted to properly document the retroverted uterus. It may also help to rotate the transducer 180 degrees in the coronal plane to better image the left ovary. The sonographer should check the orientation to guarantee that the left side of the screen represents the right side of the patient and again invert the image as necessary.

A helpful technique for locating the ovary is to first obtain a coronal image of the uterine fundus and then to angle the probe out to the **cornua** and ovarian ligament. Once this region is identified, the ovary can usually be identified by slowly sweeping the beam anteriorly and posteriorly.

By sweeping from the cervix through the lower, mid, and fundal portions of the uterus, the entire organ can be evaluated and measurements can be taken. For an anteverted uterus, the sweep will be posterior to anterior. A retroverted uterus will be anterior to posterior.

Scan Technique. The orientation of the transvaginal probe is controlled by probe rotation and angulation. The probe can be rotated up to 90 degrees, angled or pointed in any direction, and inserted or withdrawn to allow structures to be placed in the focal zone of the transducer rotation (Box 40-3; Figures 40-13 to 40-16). Varying the depth of the transducer may optimize the

imaging of a structure in that field of view. Movement of the transducer is centered around the **introitus.** Any tilting movement of the transducer handle produces reciprocal motion at the probe tip. Rotation of the probe along its long axis provides 360-degree longitudinal visualization of the pelvis. Pushing or pulling the probe can bring the tip close to a region of interest and provide a method of indirect palpation, allowing evaluation of focal tenderness or fixation.

The insertion of the transducer into the vagina should be done in real time as the sonographer watches the anatomy, because real time appears to ensure proper orientation. The probe may be inserted or guided by the patient, sonographer, or physician. It should not be inserted beyond the external cervical os. To maintain patient dignity and privacy, the patient should be properly draped at all times, and all practitioners who will be observing the examination should be present from the beginning of the examination.

Scan Protocol. Before recording any images, a complete pelvic survey should be performed. This survey is performed by slowly sweeping the beam in a sagittal plane from the midline through both adnexa to the lateral pelvic sidewalls. The probe is then rotated to the coronal plane, and the beam swept from the cervix to the fundus of the uterus. The survey will orient the sonographer to the relative positions of the uterus and ovaries and identify any obvious masses. After the survey, standard views are obtained. These include the following:

- *Sagittal plane.* Cervix, endocervical canal, posterior cul-de-sac, uterus (midline, right, and left), endometrium, right ovary and adnexa, and left ovary and adnexa.
- *Coronal plane.* Vagina, cervix and posterior cul-de-sac, uterine corpus and endometrium, uterine fundus and endometrium, right ovary and adnexa, and left ovary and adnexa.

Length, width, and axial measurements of the uterus and ovaries should be documented. The thickness of the endometrium should be measured in the sagittal plane (Figure 40-17). By sweeping side to side through the endometrium, the thickest portion can be identified and any areas of focal irregularity can be evaluated. It may be helpful either to zoom or to decrease the field of view to obtain an accurate measurement. Do not include any internal fluid in the endometrium measurement. Additional views of pathology or areas indicated should be obtained and measured in three dimensions.

Obtaining the standard images indicates that the entire organ and regions imaged have been carefully assessed in real time in two orthogonal planes. Any pathology or variant of normal must be assessed and appropriate images recorded. Color flow Doppler, power Doppler, and pulsed Doppler are added to the examination, depending on the clinical situation and pathology demonstrated on gray scale.

BOX 40-3	Transvaginal Scanning Pelvic Protocol

Survey the pelvic area before images are made.

Sagittal: Uterus
Image the uterus from cervix to fundus, endometrial cavity: measure the long axis (Figure 40-13, *A*).
Angle slowly to right of uterus (Figure 40-13, *B*).
Angle slowly to left of uterus (Figure 40-13, *C*).
Pull probe out slightly to image cervix (Figure 40-13, *D*).

Coronal: Uterus
Rotate transducer 90 degrees; image uterine fundus, body, and cervix with endometrial canal (Figure 40-14, *A-E*).
Look for free fluid surrounding uterine cavity.

Sagittal: Ovaries
Follow the fundus of the uterus to the area of the cornu to image the ovaries; the internal iliac vessels serve as their posterior border (Figures 40-15, *A*, and 40-16, *A*). Color imaging may be used to separate vascular structures from the ovary (Figures 40-15, *C* and 40-16, *C*). Look for follicles surrounding the periphery of the ovary.
Measure long axis.

Coronal: Ovaries
Rotate transducer 90 degrees once sagittal plane of ovary is obtained (Figures 40-15, *B* and 40-16, *B*).
Measure width and depth (Figure 40-15, *B*).

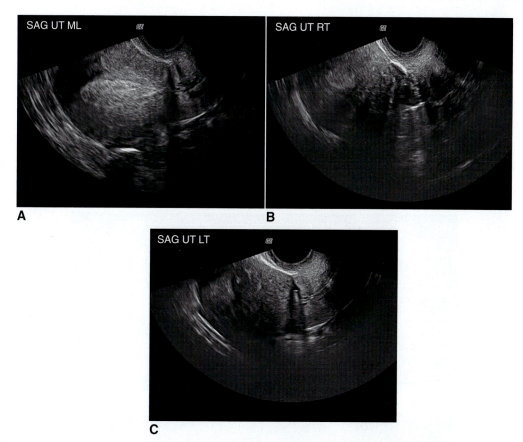

FIGURE 40-13 **A,** The uterus is imaged from the cervix to the fundus, showing the endometrial stripe; measure the long axis of the uterus. **B,** The probe should be angled slowly to the right and left side of the uterus. **C,** The probe is then angled slightly to the left of the uterus. Withdraw the probe slightly to image the cervix.

Translabial (transperineal) sonography provides an alternative technique to transvaginal scanning in the event that TV is contraindicated. The most common scenarios would be premature rupture of membranes (PROM), in which one would want to avoid contact with prolapsed membranes, cervical incompetence, and uterine prolapse. A 3.5- to 5-MHz sector transducer is covered with a sterile probe cover and placed at the vaginal introitus and oriented in the direction of the vagina. Partial bladder filling may assist visualization of the cervix. Transperineal sonography is technically more challenging. Rectal gas and the pubic symphysis may obscure visualization and the identification of anatomic landmarks. These limitations can be overcome by elevation of the hips (as in transvaginal scanning), better application of the transducer on the perineum, or changes in the orientation of the probe. The transvaginal probe may also be placed at the vaginal introitus or slightly inserted within. This can assist in imaging the lower cervical area and distal vagina. If the transvaginal transducer is already well within the vaginal vault, withdraw the transducer to visualize the lower cervix.

Disinfecting Technique. The use of an intracavitary device requires the prevention of cross contamination between patients. After completing the TV exam, the sterile probe cover should be removed. This can be done easily with the gloved scanning hand by sliding the probe cover off into the glove, removing the glove, and disposing of both into the waste container. The transducer should then be wiped clean with the facility disinfectant (be sure to read the vendor's recommendation for cleaning transducers) and dried with a towel. The transducer should then be soaked in a disinfectant between uses for at least the minimum recommended amount of time from the equipment manufacturer (10 to 20 minutes). Disinfection for extended times can cause damage or degradation to the transducer face. Most disinfectants are now nonglutaraldehyde based (e.g., Cidex OPA) and care should be taken when handling these caustic and toxic chemicals. Staff members must wear gloves, and some manufacturers recommend the use of safety goggles. There are various safety "stations" that are commercially available and that contain the required venting for this toxic chemical. Emergency eyewash stations should be available onsite. After the transducer has been soaked in a Cidex-type of solution (high-grade disinfectant), it is important to rinse the transducer with water and dry it before applying the coupling gel and protective nonlatex sheath. It is advisable to contact the probe manufacturer if the manual does not provide information regarding the type of disinfectant and immersion time limit.

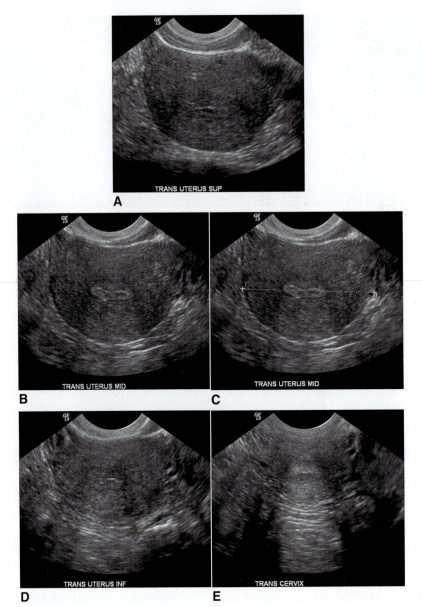

FIGURE 40-14 A, Rotate the probe 90 degrees; image the uterine fundus, body, and cervix with the endometrial stripe. This is the fundus of the uterus. **B,** The probe is angled caudally to image the miduterine cavity. **C,** The width of the uterus is measured. **D,** The probe is angled slightly more caudal to image the lower uterine segment. **E,** The probe is withdrawn slightly to image the cervix.

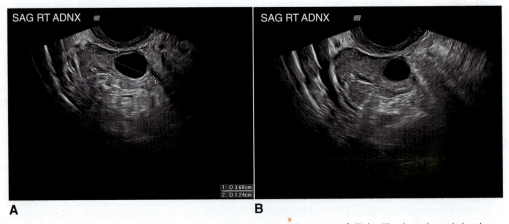

FIGURE 40-15 A and **B,** Long axis of the right ovary well demarcated by a large follicle. The length and depth are measured.

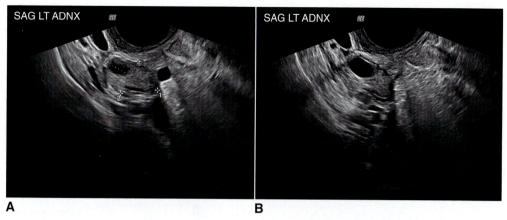

FIGURE 40-16 A and **B** Long axis of the left ovary again, well demarcated by follicles. The length is measured.

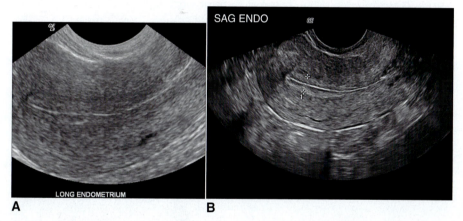

FIGURE 40-17 A, Sagittal image of the endometrial canal within the uterus. **B,** Measurement of the endometrial canal is made from leading edge to leading edge.

SONOGRAPHIC EVALUATION OF THE PELVIS

Bony Pelvis

Ultrasound is essentially absorbed by bone. The shadow is produced because no sound is returned to the transducer because it is virtually all absorbed. The bony pelvis resembles a ring or funnel in shape. Anteriorly, the pubic symphysis is formed by the articulation of the pubic bones with each other. The transabdominal study is begun just superior or cephalad to this midline landmark. Posteriorly, the sacroiliac joint on either side forms the connection between the os ilium and the sacrum. Sonographically, the sacrum may appear as a bright line with an overlying bowel shadow. This is more apparent in infants, children, and thin patients.

Muscles of the Pelvis

The filled urinary bladder displaces the bowel and acts as an acoustic window for evaluating three major groups of muscles (Figure 40-18). Pelvic muscles may be mistaken for ovaries, fluid collections, or masses. A sym-

metric bilateral arrangement indicates that they are muscles. The rectus abdominis muscles insert on the pubic rami and are paired parasagittal straps in the abdominal wall; they appear as hypoechoic structures with echogenic striations. The rectus sheath separates the sonographic appearance of the rectus abdominis muscle from surrounding fat and bowel as a bright linear echogenic reflector (Figure 40-19).

Obturator Internus Muscles. In the lesser or true pelvis, the urinary bladder, reproductive organs, levator ani, and obturator internus muscles can be identified. Sonographically, sections of the obturator internus muscle are seen at the posterior lateral corners of the bladder at the level of the vagina and cervix. This muscle is hypoechoic, ovoid, and surrounded by the obturator fascia, which serves as a tendinous attachment for the levator ani muscle (Figure 40-20).

Pelvic Floor Muscles. The levator ani muscle is best visualized sonographically in a transverse plane with caudal angulation at the most inferior aspect of the bladder. It is a hypoechoic, hammock-shaped area that is medial, caudal, and posterior to the obturator internus (Figure 40-21). The two other muscles of the lesser pelvis, the coccygeus and piriformis, are located deep,

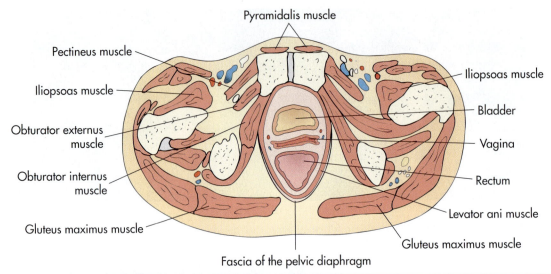

Pyramidalis muscle

Pectineus muscle

Iliopsoas muscle

Obturator externus muscle

Obturator internus muscle

Gluteus maximus muscle

Fascia of the pelvic diaphragm

Iliopsoas muscle

Bladder

Vagina

Rectum

Levator ani muscle

Gluteus maximus muscle

FIGURE 40-18 The bladder serves as an acoustic window to image the muscles of the pelvis.

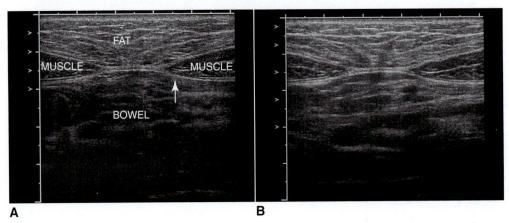

A

B

FIGURE 40-19 **A** and **B.** The rectus abdominis muscle is visualized with a 14-MHz linear transducer. The rectus sheath *(arrow)* separates the muscle from surrounding fat and bowel.

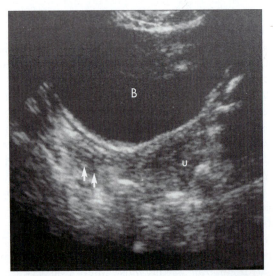

FIGURE 40-20 The obturator internus muscle *(arrows)* is visualized with the transabdominal sector transducer as hypoechoic-ovoid muscles lateral to the bladder *(B).* Angle the transducer through a distended bladder from the contralateral side to demonstrate these muscles. *u,* Uterus.

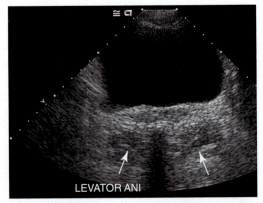

LEVATOR ANI

FIGURE 40-21 The levator ani muscle *(arrows)* is visualized with the transabdominal sector transducer as hypoechoic, hammock-shaped muscles medial, caudal, and posterior to the obturator internus. Angle from the most superior aspect of the urinary bladder caudally to demonstrate these muscles.

cranially, and posteriorly. They are not routinely visualized on ultrasound examination and are not distinguished from other surrounding muscles. The piriformis muscles are located on either side of the midline posterior to the upper half of the uterine body and fundus. This is the most common muscle to be mistaken for the ovary.

Iliopsoas Muscles. The iliopsoas muscles can be seen in the greater pelvis. The iliopsoas muscle is a combination of the iliacus muscle and the psoas major. The psoas major originates bilaterally at the paravertebral lumbar region and courses caudally. The iliacus muscle is contiguous with and arises posterior to the psoas major at the level of the superior two thirds of the iliac fossa. Together, they form the iliopsoas muscle, which continues in the caudal direction, coursing anterolaterally to its insertion on the lesser trochanter of the femur.

The sonographic appearance of this muscle varies greatly depending on its development. On ultrasound examination, the iliopsoas muscle is discretely marginated and hypoechoic (Figure 40-22). The bright echogenic line representing the interposed fascial sheath can often determine the separation of the iliacus and psoas muscles. Both longitudinal and transverse images may be obtained through the urinary bladder midline with lateral angulation. Transvaginally, the positions of these muscles are deep and beyond the field of view.

Pelvic Vascularity

Pelvic vascularity can easily be evaluated using real-time and Doppler imaging. The use of color Doppler techniques (color flow, power, and pulsed) permits the vessel to be localized, allows the sample gate to be placed exactly in the area of interest, and reduces examination time. The quantitative waveform is displayed and analyzed in one of the following indices:

S/D ratio (or A/B ratio) (A equals peak systolic and B equals end diastolic)
Pourcelot resistive index (RI) (A–B/A)
Pulsatility index (PI) (A–B/mean)

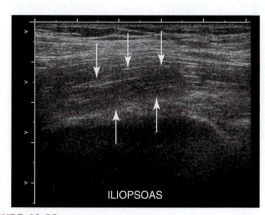

FIGURE 40-22 Sagittal image of the iliopsoas muscle (*arrows*).

Because the Doppler velocities are assessed as ratios, the waveform values are angle independent. (Remember that to obtain accurate Doppler velocities, it is critical to have the Doppler as parallel to the flow as possible; however, when ratios are determined, the difference in flow between systole and diastole is assessed and therefore the angle is not as critical.)

Imaging with transabdominal and transvaginal ultrasound, the internal iliac vessels can almost always be visualized and used as a landmark for the lateral pelvic wall and ovary. This vessel is commonly seen lateral and deep to the ovary (see Figure 39-17). The internal iliac vessel has classic characteristic blood flow, demonstrating parabolic flow with an even distribution of velocities throughout the waveform. The pulsatility and slow movement of blood flow can often be appreciated on gray-scale imaging. It is important to differentiate the vessels from an ovarian cyst because of its proximity to the ovary. If uncertain, the sonographer can use Doppler technique or rotate on the structure to elongate a vessel into a tube.

The arteries may be noted anterior to the veins in the pelvis. To assess the uterine vessels, the sonographer interrogates just lateral to the cervix and lower uterine segment at the level of the **internal os.** Uterine flow in the nonpregnant female usually shows a resistive pattern with a resistive index (RI) of 0.88 in the proliferative phase, decreasing slightly beginning the day before ovulation.

The vagina has two sources of blood. The anterior surface of the vagina and cervix is supplied with blood from a branch off the uterine artery before it reaches the uterus. The posterior surface of the vagina is supplied with blood from a branch off the internal iliac vessel (see Figure 39-17).

The ovary receives its blood supply from the aorta. The ovarian arteries also have a tortuous course from the lateral posterior border of the ovary to anastomose, with the uterine artery in the broad ligament adjacent to the cornual area (see Figure 39-17). This is considered the ovarian branch of the uterine artery, which is the most consistent and successful area for assessing ovarian Doppler flow. The blood flow of the functional ovary varies with the menstrual cycle. The changes in resistive index (RI) are thought to be a result of hormone-mediated changes in vessel wall compliance, allowing increased blood flow to the ovary in the late follicular and early luteal phases. A low-velocity, highly resistive flow pattern is shown during the follicular phase of the menstrual cycle. At ovulation, the maximal velocity increases and the RI decreases. The RI reaches 0.44 ± 0.004, and 4 to 5 days later it rises slightly before menstruation. The nonresistive flow pattern during ovulation probably results from the neovascularization of the follicle and subsequent corpus luteum. A normal pregnancy causes persistent low-resistive corpus luteum flow throughout the first trimester.

Uterus

The uterine muscle consists of three layers, and the outer serosa of the uterus is not visualized sonographically. The middle layer is the myometrium of the uterus. This layer should have a homogeneous echotexture with smooth-walled borders. Any areas of increased or decreased echotexture should be noted and measured. The inner layer is the endometrium. This layer is thin, compact, and relatively hypovascular. The endometrium is hypoechoic and surrounds the relatively echogenic endometrial stripe, creating a subendometrial halo. The thin outer layer is separated from the intermediate layer by the arcuate vessels.

The normal **arcuate vessels** are often seen in the periphery of the uterus and should not be mistaken for pathology (Figure 40-23). The radial arteries arise as multiple branches from the arcuate arteries and travel centrally to supply the rich capillary network in the deeper layers of the myometrium and the endometrium. Before entering the endometrium, the radial arteries give rise to the straight and spiral arteries of the endometrium (Figure 40-24). These vessels are most often demon-strated between 1 and 3 weeks after the onset of the last menses. Just before the onset of menses and during menses, these vessels are less apparent. The vasodilating actions of estrogens on the uterus during midcycle and the vasoconstricting hormonal influences during the late luteal phase before menses explain the normal dynamic changes of these vessels. Calcifications may be seen in the arcuate arteries in postmenopausal women and appear as peripheral linear echoes with shadowing. This is a normal aging process that may be accelerated in diabetic patients. Echogenic foci in the inner layer of the myometrium, which are usually nonshadowing, are thought to represent dystrophic calcification related to previous instrumentation. Although they are of no clinical significance, they should be distinguished from calcified leiomyomas. Uterine perfusion (the vascular blood flow within the myometrium) can be assessed by Doppler sonography of the uterine arteries. The Doppler waveform usually shows a high-velocity, high-resistance pattern.

The body of the uterus is separated from the cervix by the isthmus at the level of the internal os and is identified by the narrowing of the canal. Tissue echogenicity surrounding the cervical canal should appear homogeneous. One can frequently visualize cervical inclusion cysts, known as nabothian cysts, near the endocervical canal. These are generally less than 1 to 2 cm wide and are anechoic smooth-walled structures with acoustic enhancement posteriorly; they are of no clinical significance and generally are not measured (Figure 40-25).

The cervix is fixed in the midline, but the uterine body is mobile and may lie obliquely on either side of the midline. Flexion refers to the axis of the uterine body relative to the cervix, whereas version refers to the axis of the cervix relative to the vagina. The uterus is usually anteverted and anteflexed. The uterus may also be retroflexed when the body is tilted posteriorly or retroverted when the entire uterus is tilted backward (Figure 40-26).

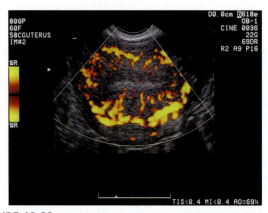

FIGURE 40-23 Transvaginal coronal view of the uterus with color Doppler that outlines the vascularity of the uterine cavity. The arcuate arteries are in the periphery of the uterine myometrium.

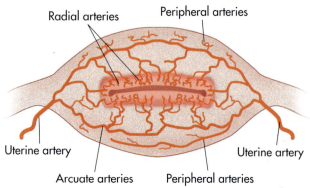

FIGURE 40-24 The blood is supplied to the uterus from the uterine artery, which bifurcates into the arcuate artery, radial arteries, and peripheral arteries. These vessels are tortuous and have many anastomotic sites.

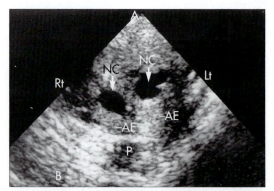

FIGURE 40-25 Transvaginal coronal view of the cervix with nabothian cysts. Naboth's cysts are often multiple and demonstrated in the coronal plane. *A,* Anterior; *AE,* acoustic enhancement; *B,* bowel; *Lt,* left side of patient; *NC,* Naboth's cyst; *P,* posterior; *Rt,* right side of patient.

The fundus of a retroverted or retroflexed uterus is difficult to assess by transabdominal sonography. It may appear hypoechoic because it is situated a distance from the transducer and may mimic a mass in the rectouterine space. This can be confused for a fibroid. Transvaginal sonography is close to the posteriorly located fundus and is much better for assessing the retroverted or retroflexed uterus. As discussed earlier, it is necessary to use all three motions of the transvaginal transducer to optimize the image. The true "lie" of the uterus is seen transvaginally with an empty bladder.

The transabdominal technique is the best way to measure the cervical-fundal dimension of the uterus in the longitudinal plane. Oblique angulation may be necessary to elongate and measure the entire length of the longitudinal plane of the uterus. Its length is always measured from the distal end of the fundus to the distal end of the cervix (Figure 40-27). Either transabdominal or transvaginal scanning technique may be used to measure the width and anteroposterior dimensions of the uterus (Figure 40-28). Because of the proximity of the uterus to the broad ligament and surrounding vessels, it may be difficult to delineate the lateral borders of the uterus. Color Doppler technique or changing postprocessing controls may help delineate these borders.

The size and shape of the normal uterus varies throughout life and is related to age, hormonal status, and **parity**. Neonatally the uterus is pear-shaped secondary to maternal hormonal stimulation (Figure 40-29). Prepubertally the cervix occupies two thirds of the uterine length and the uterus is about 1 to 3 cm in length and 0.5 to 1 cm in width and diameter (Figure 40-30). The nulliparous cervix occupies one third of the uterine length and is about 6 to 8 cm in length and 3 to 5 cm in width and diameter; add 2 cm for multiparous dimensions. The postmenopausal cervix occupies two thirds of the uterine length. The uterus is about 3 to 5 cm in length and 2 to 3 cm in width and diameter.

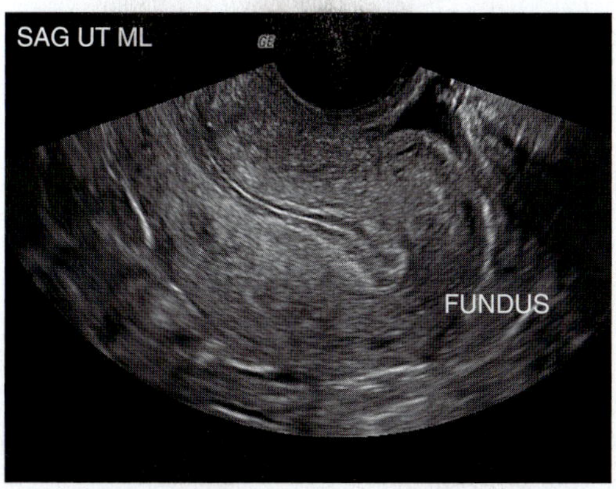

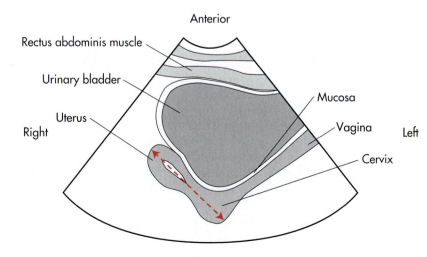

FIGURE 40-26 Transvaginal sagittal image of the retroflexed uterus.

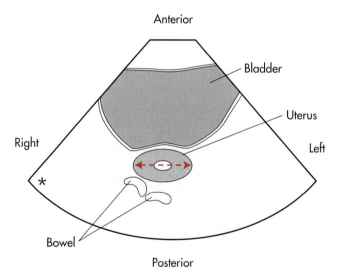

FIGURE 40-28 The width of the uterus is measured on the transverse image at the widest diameter of the body.

FIGURE 40-27 The length of the uterus is measured on the longitudinal image from the fundus to the cervix.

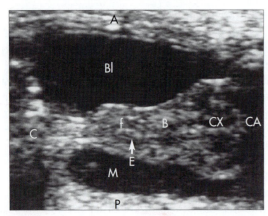

FIGURE 40-29 Transabdominal sagittal scan of a 1-day-old neonatal uterus. The cervix occupies two thirds of the entire uterine length secondary to maternal hormonal stimulation. *A,* Anterior; *B,* body of uterus; *Bl,* bladder; *C,* cephalic; *CA,* caudal; *CX,* cervix of uterus; *E,* endometrial canal; *f,* fundus of uterus; *M,* meconium; *P,* posterior.

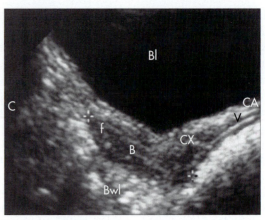

FIGURE 40-30 Transabdominal sagittal scan of a 6-year-old prepubertal uterus. The cervix occupies two thirds of the entire uterine length, but loses the pear shape of a neonatal uterus. *B,* Body of uterus; *Bl,* bladder; *Bwl,* bowel; *C,* cephalic; *CA,* caudal; *CX,* cervix of uterus; *f,* fundus of uterus; *V,* vagina.

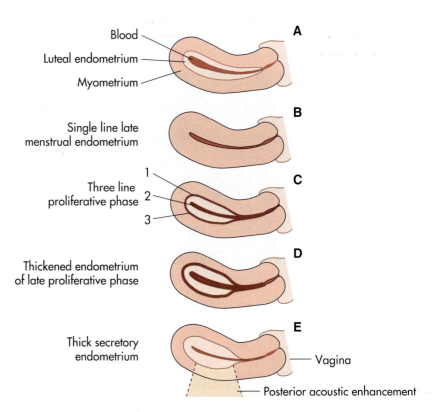

FIGURE 40-31 Endometrial changes through a normal menstrual cycle. **A,** Endometrium (days 1 to 4) of early menses. The hypoechoic central cavity represents blood and tissue. This is surrounded by a hyperechoic endometrial echo. **B,** Endometrium (days 3 to 7) as menses progress. The hypoechoic area that represented blood is sloughed. **C,** Proliferative phase (days 5 to 9) endometrium presents as the three-line sign. The thin endometrial center cavity is surrounded by a hypoechoic halo (the functionalis). The thin surrounding echogenic layer represents the basalis. **D,** The endometrium of the late proliferative phase (days 10 to 14) increases in thickness and echogenicity, representing the basalis. **E,** The secretory endometrium is at its greatest thickness and echogenicity with posterior acoustic enhancement.

Endometrium

Sonographic images of the endometrium disclose a characteristic appearance at each phase of the menstrual cycle. To optimally visualize and discern the endometrium, transvaginal scanning is performed.

The sonographic appearance of the endometrial canal is seen as a thin echogenic line as a result of specular reflections from the interface between the opposing surfaces of the endometrium. The endometrium consists of a superficial functional layer and a deep basal layer.

During **menstruation** (days 1 to 4), the endometrial canal appears as a hypoechoic central line representing blood and tissue and reaching 4 to 8 mm, including the basal layer. This is surrounded by a hyperechoic basal endometrial echo. If menstrual flow is heavy, the entire endometrial cavity can appear anechoic (Figure 40-31). During this phase of early menses, acoustic enhancement posterior to the endometrium may appear. As menses progress (days 3 to 7), the hypoechoic echo that represented blood disappears and the endometrial stripe is a discrete thin hyperechoic line, which is usually only 2 to 3 mm.

In the **early proliferative phase** (days 5 to 9), the endometrial canal appears as a single thin stripe. The functionalis layer is seen as a hyperechoic halo encompassing it. The basalis layer of the endometrium represents the thin surrounding hyperechoic outermost echo. This complex creates the three-line sign (Figure 40-32). Early in the proliferative phase (days 5 to 9), the endometrial complex is thin, measuring 6 mm, and becomes thicker, 10 mm, from days 10 to 14 before ovulation. The thin surrounding hyperechoic layer of endometrium represents the innermost layer of the myometrium and is not included in the measurement. In the **late proliferative phase** (days 10 to 14), ovulation occurs.

During the **secretory (luteal) phase** (days 15 to 28), the endometrium is at its greatest thickness and echogenicity with posterior enhancement (Figure 40-33). The posterior enhancement is thought to be attributable to the increased vascularity of the endometrium. The functionalis layer becomes isoechoic with the basalis layer. The endometrial complex measures 7 to 14 mm during the secretory phase (Figure 40-34).

The endometrial thickness is measured from the highly reflective interface of the basalis layer of the endometrium and myometrium in the sagittal view. This sonographic measurement includes both the anterior and posterior layers of the endometrium (Figure 40-35). The surrounding hypoechoic area represents the innermost layer of myometrium and is not included in the measurement (Figure 40-36). Similarly, fluid presenting within the endometrial cavity should not be included in the measurement of the endometrial complex (Figure 40-37). With the use of electronic calipers and transvaginal scanning, measurements of endometrial thickness have been found to be within 1 mm of measurements from pathology examinations.

In all stages of a female's life, the normal measurement of the endometrium varies depending on hormonal status. In an infant, the endometrium may appear thick and echogenic because of maternal hormonal stimulation. In the childbearing ages, the endometrium varies between 4 and 14 mm. During menopause the endometrium becomes atrophic because it is no longer hormonally stimulated. Sonographically, the postmenopausal

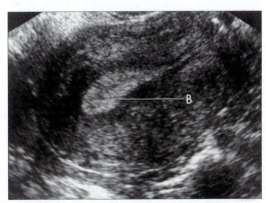

FIGURE 40-34 Transvaginal scan of the endometrium during late proliferative (early secretory) phase (see Figure 40-31 correlation). *B,* Basalis.

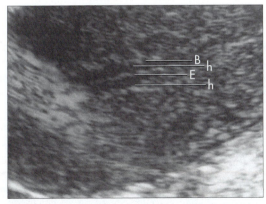

FIGURE 40-32 Transvaginal scan of the endometrium during menses (see Figure 40-31 correlation). *Bld,* Blood and tissue; *E,* endometrial echo.

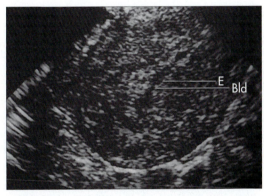

FIGURE 40-33 Transvaginal scan of the endometrium during proliferatice phase (see Figure 40-31 correlation). *B,* Echogenic basalis; *E,* endometrial echo; *h,* halo (functionalis).

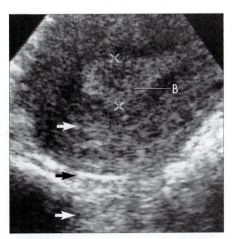

FIGURE 40-35 Transcaginal scan of the endometrium during the secretory phase (see Figure 40-31 correlation). The basalis (*B*) is at its greatest thickness and echogenictiy with posterior acoustic enhancement (*arrows*).

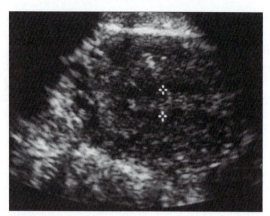

FIGURE 40-36 Transvaginal sagittal uterus. The endometrial measurement includes both the anterior and posterior layers of the endometrium. The hypoechoic area surrounding the endometrium is not included.

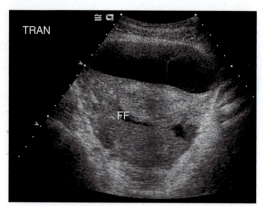

FIGURE 40-38 Transvaginal transverse view of free fluid (*FF*) in the cul-de-sac with the partially filled bladder anterior.

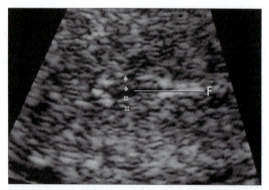

FIGURE 40-37 Transvaginal sagittal uterus. Fluid that is within the endometrial cavity is excluded from the measurement. Measure the anterior and posterior layers separately and add together. *F,* Fluid.

endometrial complex is seen as a thin echogenic line measuring less than 8 mm unless the patient takes hormone therapy. The literature varies for postmenopausal values of the nonhormonally stimulated endometrium. The generally accepted range is between 4 and 10 mm. Patients with postmenopausal bleeding and an endometrial double-layer thickness greater than 5 mm should have further evaluation.

Fallopian Tubes

The normal fallopian tube can be difficult to identify by transabdominal or transvaginal sonography unless it is surrounded by or filled with fluid (dilated). Developmental abnormalities are rare. The normal fallopian tube is a tubular structure of approximately 8 to 10 mm in width and running posterolateral from the uterus to near the ovaries. It is divided into intramural, isthmic, infundibular, and ampullary portions. In the transverse view transabdominally, or the coronal view transvaginally, the fallopian tube region can be followed laterally from either side of the cornua at the fundal level of the uterus to the ovaries. The high resolution of transvaginal scan-

ning allows improved visualization of the fallopian tube. It is not unusual to visualize the region of the proximal tube and surrounding ligaments. If the tubes are distended with or surrounded by a sufficient amount of fluid, they can be easily outlined by the contrasting fluid. The patient is placed in reverse Trendelenburg's position to use any fluid in the peritoneum as a contrast agent (Figures 40-38 and 40-39).

Ovaries

The sonographic approach to evaluate the ovary is often initially performed transabdominally. The transabdominal approach is especially important when the ovary is in an obscure location (i.e., high in the pelvis) so as to determine a general location to interrogate transvaginally. Transabdominal evaluation is also necessary to evaluate a large adnexal mass and determine its origin. The ovary is very mobile and can move considerably in the pelvis, depending on bladder volume and whether women have had a previous pregnancy. Uterine location influences the position of the ovaries. The ovaries are elliptical in shape, with the long axis usually oriented vertically. Transvaginal scanning is superior for characterizing the ovary and its contents and for visualizing ovaries that are not visible transabdominally.

Typically the ovary is located just lateral to the uterus and anteromedial to the internal iliac vessels, which can be used as a landmark to localize the ovary. Transvaginally, the ovaries are easiest to locate in the coronal plane lateral to the cornua. However, it is not uncommon to find the ovaries located above the uterus or posterior in the rectouterine cul-de-sac area.

Sonographically, the normal ovary appears as an ovoid medium-level echogenic structure; follicular cysts may be seen peripherally in the cortex. The appearance of the ovary changes with age and the menstrual cycle. During the proliferative phase, many follicles develop and increase in size until about day 8 or 9 of the menstrual cycle. This is caused by stimulation of follicle-stimulating hormone (FSH) and luteinizing hormone

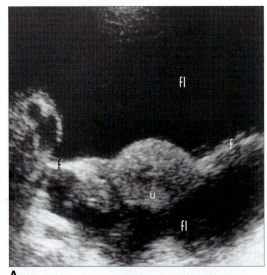

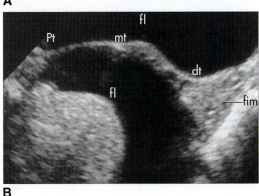

FIGURE 40-39 A, Transabdominal transverse scan of uterus and fallopian tubes. *f,* Fallopian tube; *fl,* free-fluid. *u,* uterus. **B,** Transvaginal coronal scan of fallopian tube surrounded by free fluid within peritoneum. *dt,* Distal tube; *fim,* fimbriae; *fl,* free fluid; *mt,* mid (ampulla) tube; *Pt,* proximal (isthmus) tube.

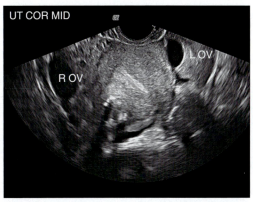

FIGURE 40-40 Transvaginal image of the prominent ovaries with multiple follicles allows the visualization of the ovaries with sonography. The bladder is partially filled. The uterus separates the two ovaries.

(LH). At that time one follicle becomes dominant and increases in size to about 2 to 2.5 cm at the time of ovulation. The other follicles become atretic. If the fluid is not reabsorbed in the nondominant follicles, a follicular cyst develops.

Following ovulation, the corpus luteum develops and, if fertilization has not occurred, involutes before menstruation. Sonographically, these cysts are unilocular, anechoic structures with well-defined thin walls and posterior acoustic enhancement. Corpus luteum cysts may have a thicker wall and a peripheral rim of color around the wall on color Doppler.

The best sonographic marker for the ovary is identification of a follicular cyst, which has the classic appearance of being thin-walled and anechoic with through-transmission posteriorly. The normal range in diameter of a mature graafian follicle is 1.8 to 2.4 cm. These cysts may be present in normal premenarchal, menstruating, and menopausal ovaries (Figure 40-40).

The ovary is measured in the sagittal or longitudinal plane at its longest length and anteroposterior dimension

(see Figures 40-15 and 40-16). In transverse or coronal scans, the width is measured at the widest point. With the use of color Doppler technique, a vessel and a cyst can easily be distinguished. Because of the variability in shape, ovarian volume is considered the best method for determining ovarian size. The volume of the ovary is calculated using the formula for a prolate ellipse: 0.523 = length × thickness × width. The mean volume for a premenarchal ovary is 3 cm³, with an upper limit of 8 cm³; for a normal menstruating ovary, 9.8 cm³, with an upper limit of 21.9 cm³; and for a postmenopausal ovary, 5.8 cm³, with an upper limit of 8 cm³.

Because of its smaller size and lack of follicles, the postmenopausal ovary may be difficult to see on ultrasound. Scanning must be done slowly to look for peristalsis, so that stationary loops of the bowel are not mistaken for the ovary. Changes in imaging parameters (e.g., decreased frame averaging) may also help. The absence of a uterus following hysterectomy may also make it more difficult to visualize the ovaries. A difference in size of one ovary greater than twice the volume of the contralateral ovary should also be considered abnormal. Small anechoic cysts (less than 3 cm in diameter) may be seen in some postmenopausal ovaries. These may disappear or change in size over time. Surgery is generally recommended for postmenopausal women who have cysts greater than 5 cm and for those who have cysts containing septations or solid nodules.

Occasionally, echogenic ovarian foci are seen in the normal ovary. These are usually tiny (1 to 3 mm) and are nonshadowing foci, which can be peripheral or diffuse. They are thought to represent inclusion cysts and associated calcifications. These are insignificant findings and do not need further follow-up. Focal calcifications may occasionally be seen and are thought to be a stromal reaction to previous hemorrhage or infection. The calcifications are suggested for follow-up to rule out an early neoplasm.

The ovarian arteries arise from the aorta laterally, slightly inferior to the renal arteries. After giving off branches to the ovary, they continue to anastomose with the branches of the uterine artery. The ovarian veins leave the ovarian hilum and communicate with the uterine plexus of veins. The right ovarian vein drains into the inferior vena cava, and the left ovarian vein drains directly into the left renal vein.

Rectouterine Recess and Bowel

The rectouterine recess (posterior cul-de-sac) is the most posterior and inferior reflection of the peritoneal cavity. It is located between the rectum and uterus and is also known as the pouch of Douglas. The posterior cul-de-sac is frequently the initial site for intraperitoneal fluid collection. In asymptomatic women, small amounts of fluid can normally be seen in the cul-de-sac during all phases of the menstrual cycle. Possible causes include follicular rupture and retrograde menstruation. Pathologic fluid collections may be seen in association with ascites, blood from ruptured ectopic pregnancy or hemorrhagic cyst, or pus resulting from an infection. Transvaginal scanning is better at demonstrating echoes within the fluid and helping to identify the type of fluid along with the clinical indications.

Gas- and fluid-filled bowel loops are poorly defined, echo-free mobile structures that usually demonstrate peristalsis under observation. Solid material in the bowel is hyperechoic and may produce shadowing, as does gas (Figure 40-41). An empty bowel can look like an irregular bull's-eye with a thin, sharp, hypoechoic outline on a cross section. When rectal gas obscures the cul-de-sac and it is necessary to differentiate a mass from bowel, a saline or water enema may delineate the rectosigmoid, posterior uterus, and cul-de-sac in a transabdominal view.

Fluid-filled small bowel loops can appear cystic, but they are easily identified by their swirling activity demonstrated on real-time imaging. Fluid may accumulate in the small bowel with rapid oral hydration. The movements of bowel outlining the ovary often aid a transvaginal search for ovaries. Immobile, dilated, or distorted bowel should be further investigated.

Sonohysterography

Sonohysterography, also known as *saline infused sonography (SIS)* or *hysterosonography,* involves the instillation of sterile saline solution into the endometrial cavity. This technique is used to further evaluate the endometrium when it exceeds the normal thickness or shows focal areas of thickening and polyps are suspected. The patient is prepared in the same manner as for a pelvic examination. The physician inserts a sterile speculum, and the cervix is cleansed with an antiseptic solution. A very small catheter (5 to 7 French) filled with saline solution or contrast medium (Albunex) is inserted into the uterine cavity to the level of the uterine fundus. The catheter should be prefilled with saline before insertion to minimize air artifact. The speculum is removed with the catheter in place, and the transvaginal transducer is inserted into the vagina. A hysterosalpingography catheter may have a balloon to prevent retrograde leakage of saline into the vagina. Use fluid to inflate the balloon to minimize air artifact in the lower uterine segment. The balloon should be placed as close to the internal os as possible. The tip of the catheter may be localized on ultrasound, and then 10 to 15 ml of sterile normal saline is injected to distend the endometrial cavity while under continuous sonographic evaluation.

The uterus is surveyed with ultrasound in sagittal and coronal planes to delineate the entire endometrial cavity (Figure 40-42). Appropriate images are recorded or cine clips may be recorded in the sagittal and coronal planes. This technique is clinically useful to outline the endometrial cavity to determine the presence of polyps, tumors, or hyperplasia. In addition, the cornu of the uterus may be demonstrated with the interstitial area of the fallopian

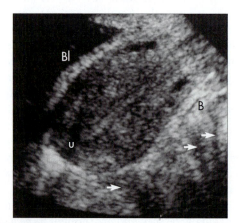

FIGURE 40-41 Transvaginal sagittal uterus *(u)*. *B,* Bowel. Peristalsis is often observed in the cul-de-sac. Solid material in bowel is hyperechoic and produces shadows posteriorly *(arrows)*. The bladder *(Bl)* is always oriented in the upper left corner.

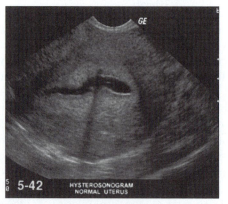

FIGURE 40-42 Transvaginal hysterosonogram of the uterus with a small amount of saline solution injected into the endometrial cavity.

tube. The examination is contraindicated in patients with pelvic inflammatory disease.

The procedure is usually performed on premenopausal women between days 6 and 10, or soon after the cessation of bleeding in women with irregular cycles. Postmenopausal women who are not on sequential hormone replacement can have the procedure performed at any time. In most cases, there is no special patient preparation. Prophylactic antibiotic can be given for women with chronic pelvic inflammatory disease and women with a history of mitral valve prolapse or other cardiac disorders.

Three-Dimensional Ultrasound

Three-dimensional ultrasound (3D ultrasound) is now an accepted additional technology in ultrasound that allows imaging from volume sonographic data rather than conventional planar data. Volume data are generally obtained by acquiring many slices of conventional ultrasound data, identifying the location of the slices in space, and reconstructing them into a volume. That data (voxels) can then be viewed as a 3D object and displayed using a variety of formats to rotate and view the images from different angles for optimal visualization of anatomy and pathology (Figure 40-43). An additional approach to acquiring volume data is to use multidimensional arrays. Display of 3D data has improved greatly. Currently the most common methods include multiplanar display of perpendicular slices through the volume and volume rendering. The display can be optimized to emphasize soft tissue or be changed to optimize vessels. Volume editing can be performed to eliminate or mask structures that obscure the areas of interest. Archived volume data may be further reviewed after the patient exam has been completed, permitting the reviewer to "rescan" the patient in the computer workstation.

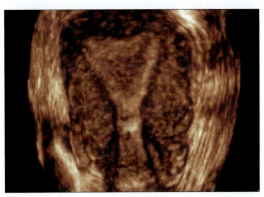

FIGURE 40-43 Three-dimensional reconstruction of the uterus showing a coronal image of the endometrium.

Volumes often require significant storage media and currently may be stored on magnetic optical disks, CD-ROMs, or hard drives or transferred to computer networks with Internet capabilities.

The current AIUM guidelines regarding 3D sonography state that because it is still a developing technology, its role is that of an adjunct to, not a replacement for, two-dimensional ultrasound. Continued work will likely show that the most promise for 3D ultrasound in the pelvis is its ability to provide unique planes for improved evaluation of organs, tubal morphology, tumor invasion, accurate volume estimation, and guidance for invasive procedures. Sonohysterography also benefits from volume scanning. The exact location of a polyp, fibroid, or adhesion is readily identified.

As the 3D technology becomes available in many more clinical sites, additional benefits will be identified. Four-dimensional ultrasound data are another new technology that allows 3D imaging in a real-time mode versus computerized imaging postcapture. These technologies are exciting areas in development along with efforts to improve resolution and application.

Pathology of the Uterus

Candace Goldstein and Sandra L. Hagen-Ansert

Sonography is traditionally applied in the female pelvis to delineate the size, texture, vascularity, and structure of pelvic anatomy. The examination may also supply information on the morphology of malfunctioning organs that seem normal on pelvic examination. Small, nonpalpable submucosal myomas or polyps may cause abnormal bleeding. The localization of intrauterine contraceptive devices (IUCDs) may be assessed by pelvic ultrasound examination. The homogeneity of the myometrium is assessed, and the thickness of the endometrial cavity is measured, in addition to the length and width of the uterus and cervix. Both transabdominal and transvaginal sonography are important in these evaluations. Transabdominal imaging furnishes a survey of anatomy, whereas transvaginal imaging provides better characterization of internal architecture of the vagina, cervix, and uterus. Color and spectral Doppler sonography can also play a role in assessing normal and pathologic blood flow, as well as identify vessels separate from fluid-filled structures. Newer techniques include sonohysterography, a process in which a small catheter, placed under ultrasound guidance, introduces sterile saline into the endometrial canal to provide a detailed evaluation of an intracavitary, endometrial, or submucosal lesion. Additionally, three-dimensional (3D) ultrasound now provides us with coronal representation of the uterus. Other imaging modalities used to evaluate pelvic anatomy and pathology include magnetic resonance imaging (MRI) and computed tomography (CT). These two modalities are particularly useful in the staging of malignant disease.

PATHOLOGY OF THE VAGINA AND CERVIX

The Vagina

The vagina runs anterior and caudal from the cervix, between the bladder and rectum (Figure 41-1). Occasionally, sonography is used to characterize a vaginal

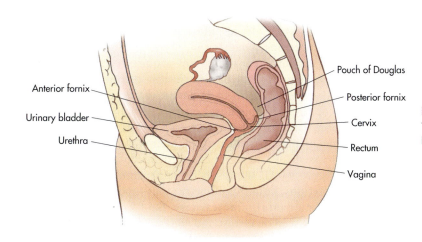

FIGURE 41-1 Lateral view of the pelvis demonstrating the relationship of the pelvic organs to the bladder and pouch of Douglas.

mass, such as a **Gartner's duct cyst.** These are the most common cystic lesions of the vagina and usually are found incidentally during sonographic examination. The most common congenital abnormality of the female genital tract is an imperforate hymen that results in obstruction. Obstruction of the uterus or the vagina may result in an accumulation of fluid (hydrometra), blood (hematometra), or pus (pyometra).

Solid masses of the vagina are rare. As with carcinoma of the cervix, sonography is not used for diagnosis of carcinoma of the vagina, but it may play a role in staging. When found, the lesion is usually vaginal adenocarcinoma and rhabdomyosarcoma. The lesions appear as a solid mass, occasionally with areas of necrosis. Translabial scanning may be used to best evaluate the vaginal area.

The Vaginal Cuff

A vaginal cuff is seen in hysterectomy patients after surgery. The upper size limit of a normal vaginal cuff is 2.1 cm. If the cuff is larger than this or contains a well-defined mass or areas of high echogenicity, it should be regarded with suspicion for malignancy, especially in the patient who has a previous history of cancer. Nodular areas in the vaginal cuff may be due to postirradiation fibrosis.

Rectouterine Recess

The rectouterine recess (posterior cul-de-sac) is the most posterior and inferior reflection of the peritoneal cavity (see Figure 41-1). It is located between the rectum and uterus and is also called the pouch of Douglas. Because of its location, it is frequently the site of intraperitoneal fluid collections. As little as 5 ml of fluid has been detected by transvaginal sonography. Fluid in the cul-de-sac is a normal finding in asymptomatic women and can be seen during all phases of the menstrual cycle. Pathologic fluid collections may be associated with ascites,

BOX 41-1	Nabothian Cysts

- Benign cysts in cervix
- Chronic inflammatory retention cysts
- Asymptomatic

blood resulting from a ruptured **ectopic pregnancy,** hemorrhagic cyst, or pus resulting from an infection. Pelvic abscesses and hematomas can also occur in the cul-de-sac. Sonographic characteristics help to differentiate these findings.

Cervix

Benign Conditions. Transvaginal sonography should be used to obtain high-quality images of the cervical area. The cervix lies posterior to the bladder between the lower uterine segment and the vaginal canal (see Figure 41-1). The cervical canal extends from the internal os, where it joins the uterine cavity, to the external os, which projects into the vaginal vault. It is a cylindrical portion of the uterus that enters the vagina and measures 2 to 4 cm in length. Transvaginal scanning of the cervix is performed after the patient empties her bladder. The transducer is inserted into the vagina with the patient supine, knees gently flexed, and hips elevated on a pillow. After the uterine cavity has been examined, the probe should be slowly pulled back slightly to image the internal and external cervical os. In the sagittal view, the handle of the transducer is slowly moved upward or back to better image the cervix (see Chapter 40). With gentle rotation and angulation of the transducer, coronal images are also obtained.

The most common finding is the presence of **nabothian cysts** (Box 41-1), which result from chronic cervicitis and are seen frequently in middle-aged women. This cyst results from an obstructed dilated transcervical gland and is also called epithelial inclusion cyst.

On sonographic evaluation, these lesions appear along the cervical canal as discrete, round, fluid-filled anechoic structures, usually measuring less than 2 cm; they may be multiple (Figure 41-2). Occasionally, nabothian cysts may have internal echoes that may be caused by hemorrhage or infection.

Cervical polyps may present clinically with irregular bleeding. This benign condition arises from the hyperplastic protrusion of the epithelium of the endocervix or **ectocervix**. Chronic inflammation is the most likely factor. The polyps may be pedunculated, projecting out of the cervix, or broad-based, and ultrasound may or may not see cervical polyps, depending on their location. Women in their late middle age are more likely to develop polyps.

A small percentage of leiomyomas (myoma tumors) occur in the cervix (Figure 41-3). When the myomas are small, the patient is asymptomatic, but as the mass enlarges, bladder or bowel obstruction may result. The myoma may be pedunculated (Figure 41-4) and prolapse into the vaginal canal. Sonography may assist in

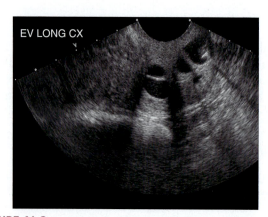

FIGURE 41-2 Transvaginal sagittal image of the cervix shows multiple very small nabothian cysts just inferior to the endometrial cavity in the center of the cervix with increased through-transmission beyond. The areas of shadowing represent poor contact or air bubbles between the transducer and the vaginal wall.

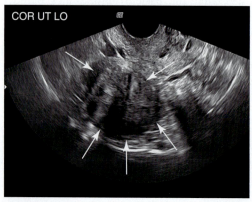

FIGURE 41-3 Transavaginal coronal view of the cervix reveals a cervical myoma (*arrows*).

determining the location of the stalk and the thickness of the stalk. Fluid infusion with sonohysterography enhances this visualization.

Cervical stenosis is an acquired condition with obstruction of the cervical canal at the internal or external os resulting from radiation therapy, previous cone biopsy, postmenopausal cervical atrophy, chronic infection, laser or cryosurgery, or cervical carcinoma. The menopausal patient may be asymptomatic even though the stenosis can produce a distended, fluid-filled uterus (Figure 41-5), the result of an accumulation of uterine secretions, fluid (hydrometra), pus (pyometra), or blood (hematometra). Intracavitary fluid collections can be readily seen on ultrasound and may be an indirect indicator of cervical stenosis. Premenopausal patients may experience abnormal bleeding, oligomenorrhea or amenorrhea, cramping, **dysmenorrhea**, or infertility.

Cervical Carcinoma. **Squamous cell carcinoma** is the most common type of cervical cancer. Precursors to this disease are the cervical dysplasias classified as mild, moderate, or severe. When the full thickness of the epithelium is composed of undifferentiated neoplastic cells, the lesion is referred to as carcinoma in situ. The detection of these abnormalities is attributed to screening with Papanicolaou (PAP) smears because most of the early lesions are asymptomatic. Advanced cervical cancer is usually evident clinically (Box 41-2 and Figure 41-6). Sonography may demonstrate a solid retrovesical mass, which may be indistinguishable from a cervical myoma. Transvaginal and translabial ultrasound may demonstrate bladder, ureteral, vaginal or rectal involvement and may be used in staging cervical cancer. CT and MRI are preferable, however, because they are superior methods for staging and evaluating lymphatic spread. Areas of increased echogenicity or hypoechoic areas with an irregular outline signify changes compatible with cervical carcinoma (Figure 41-7). Multiple cystic areas within a solid cervical mass are a rare cervical neoplasm arising from the endocervical glands termed *adenoma malignum* or *minimal deviation adenocarcinoma*. Ultrasound is also helpful in guiding biopsies of the cervix and vagina.

Translabial or transperineal sonography may be used instead of or with the transvaginal approach to help define the cervical area. A 5.0- to 7.5-MHz sector or curvilinear transducer is covered with a sterile probe cover and applied to the vestibule of the vagina in the sagittal plane. Partial bladder filling may assist visualization of the cervical area. Rotation of the transducer

---

BOX 41-2 | **Cervical Carcinoma**

- Affects women of menstrual age
- Clinical findings: Vaginal discharge or bleeding
- Sonographic findings: Retrovesical mass, obstruction of ureters, invasion of bladder

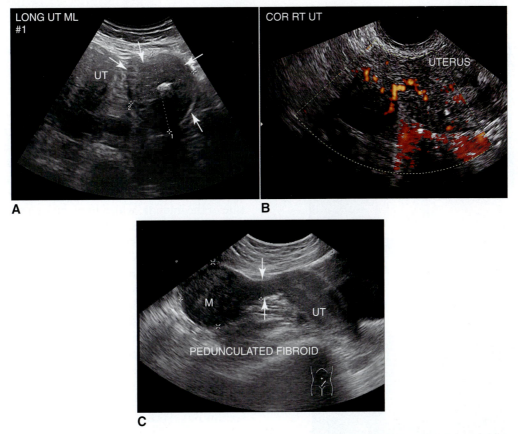

FIGURE 41-4 **A,** Transavaginal view of the uterus *(UT)* with a 5.5-cm hypoechoic myoma *(mass outlined by calipers and arrows).* **B,** Increased vascularity is noted in the cervical myoma. **C,** Large pedunculated fibroid is shown extending from the fundus of the uterus by a pedicle *(arrows).*

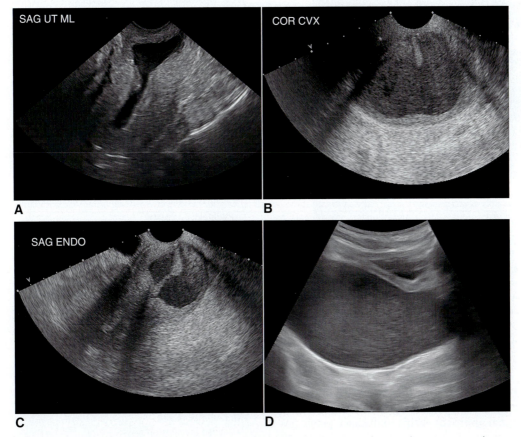

FIGURE 41-5 **A–C,** A 63-year-old asymptomatic woman on cyclic hormone replacement therapy demonstrates a large endometrial fluid collection. She underwent dilation for cervical stenosis, and bloody fluid was drained. **D,** Hematometrocolpos presents as a moderately echogenic collection in the cervical area.

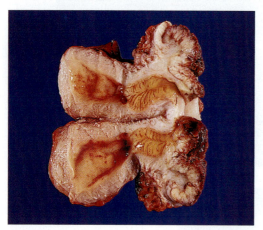

FIGURE 41-6 Gross pathologic findings of cervical squamous cell carcinoma.

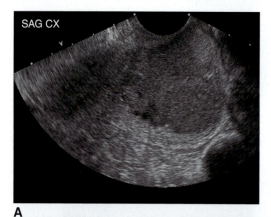

A

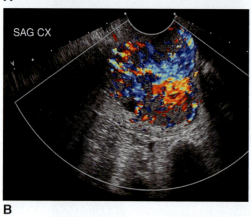

B

FIGURE 41-7 A, Transvaginal images of the lower uterine segment. The cervical area is enlarged and hypoechoic with decreased through-transmission. **B,** Color Doppler demonstrates increased vascularity in the mass. The patient was found to have cervical carcinoma at surgery.

obliquely in a counterclockwise direction shows the coronal images and defines the second plane for visualization. Positioning the patient with the hips elevated, as in the transvaginal approach, helps to displace pelvic gas and identify anatomy. Limitations can be overcome by elevation of the hips, better application of the transducer to the perineum, or changes in the orientation of the probe.

PATHOLOGY OF THE UTERUS

The uterus lies in the true pelvis between the urinary bladder anteriorly and the rectosigmoid colon posteriorly (see Figure 41-1). Uterine position is variable and changes with the degrees of bladder and rectal distention. The body of the uterus may lie obliquely on either side of the midline, which may mimic a mass on physical exam. Flexion refers to the axis of the uterine body relative to the cervix. Version refers to the axis of the cervix relative to the vagina. The uterus is usually anteverted and anteflexed. It may also be retroflexed (when the body tilts posteriorly) or retroverted (when the uterine fundus tilts backward) (Figure 41-8). Transvaginal sonography has proven to be excellent for assessing the retroverted or retroflexed uterus because the transducer is close to the posteriorly located fundus. The size and shape of the normal uterus are related to age, hormonal status, and parity.

Common differential considerations for the uterus are seen in Box 41-3.

BOX 41-3	Differential Considerations for the Uterus

Enlarged Uterus
Pregnancy
Postpartum
Leiomyoma
Adenomyosis
Bicornuate or didelphic uterus

Uterine Tumor
Leiomyoma
Carcinoma

Thickened Endometrium
Early intrauterine pregnancy
Endometrial hyperplasia
Retained products of conception or incomplete abortion
Trophoblastic disease
Endometritis
Adhesions
Polyps
Inflammatory disease
Endometrial carcinoma

Endometrial Fluid
Endometritis
Retained products of conception
Pelvic inflammatory disease
Cervical obstruction

Endometrial Shadowing
Gas (abscess)
Intrauterine device
Calcified myomas or vessels
Retained products of conception

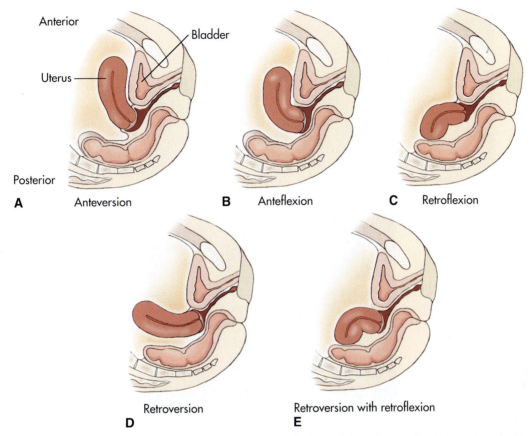

FIGURE 41-8 Variations in uterine position. **A,** Anteversion. **B,** Anteflexion. **C,** Retroflexion. **D,** Retroversion. **E,** Retroversion with retroflexion.

Normal Variations of the Uterus

Ultrasound is the first clinical exam ordered to evaluate the enlarged uterus. There are common variations of uterine morphology, the bicornuate or "two-horned uterus" and the didelphic uterus, that can be visualized with great specificity with sonography. These developmental variations are discussed in detail in the pediatric chapter. A detailed exam can reveal the endometrium in each horn, identify pathology, or document pregnancy (Figure 41-9).

Leiomyomas

Leiomyomas, commonly called myomas, are the most common gynecologic tumors, occurring in approximately 20% to 30% (or greater depending on the reference source) of women over the age of 30 years. They are more common in African American women.

Myoma tumors are composed of spindle-shaped, smooth muscle cells arranged in a whorl-like pattern with variable amounts of fibrous connective tissue, which can degenerate into a number of different histologic subtypes (Figure 41-10). The tumors consist of nodules of myometrial tissue and are usually multiple. The myoma is encapsulated (Figure 41-11) with a pseudocapsule and separates easily from the surrounding myometrium. With atrophy and vascular compromise as a result of outgrowing their blood supply, fibrotic changes and degeneration of the myomas can occur. Liquefaction, necrosis, hemorrhage, and ultimate calcification may take place. Hyalinization (development of an albuminoid mass in a cell or tissue) occurs most often, making the myomas appear more lucent or hypoechoic than the myometrium. Ten percent of myomas contain calcification, and a similar number have areas of hemorrhage. Other myomas contain tissue that has undergone necrosis and liquefaction and become myxoid in texture.

Myomas are estrogen dependent and may increase in size during pregnancy, although about half of all myomas show little change during pregnancy. Myomas identified in the first trimester are associated with an elevated risk of pregnancy loss, and this risk is higher in patients with multiple myomas. They rarely develop in postmenopausal women, and most stabilize or decrease in size following menopause because of a lack of estrogen stimulation. They may increase in size in postmenopausal patients who are undergoing hormone replacement therapy. Tamoxifen has also been reported to cause growth in leiomyomas. A rapid increase in myoma size, especially in a postmenopausal patient, should raise the level of concern for a neoplasm.

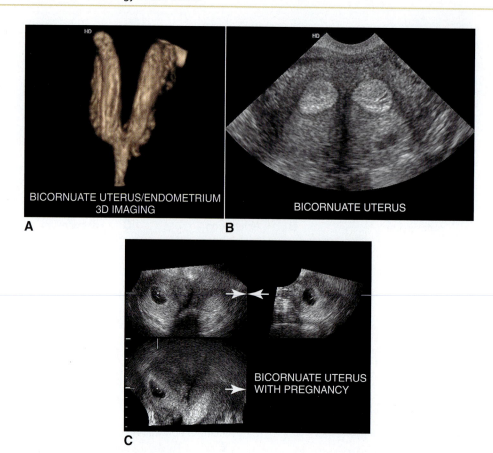

FIGURE 41-9 Bicornuate uterus. **A,** 3D reconstruction of a bicornuate uterus that clearly demonstrates the two uterine horns and echogenic endometrium. **B,** Transvaginal image of the bicornuate uterus. **C,** Patient with a known bicornuate uterus presents with a gestational sac in one horn.

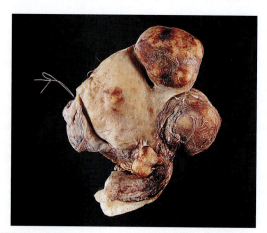

FIGURE 41-10 Gross pathologic findings of the uterine cavity with multiple subserosal myoma tumors arising from its walls.

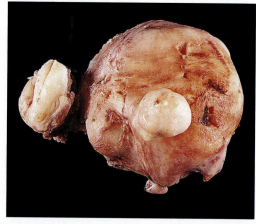

FIGURE 41-11 Gross pathologic findings of the uterus with the encapsulated leiomyoma in the submucosal area.

Clinically, myomas cause uterine irregularity and enlargement with the sensation of pelvic pressure and sometimes pain. Patterns of irregular bleeding, menometrorrhagia, or heavy menstrual bleeding (menorrhagia) are the primary clinical problems. Myomas may contribute to infertility by distorting the fallopian tube or endometrial cavity; if located in the lower uterine segment or cervix, the tumor may interfere with normal vaginal

delivery. Because of the increased estrogen during pregnancy, the tumor may grow and bleed within, causing pain. Box 41-4 summarizes the characteristics of leiomyomas.

Leiomyomas can affect any portion of the uterine wall; however, the tumor may also be uncommonly found in the lower uterine segment, the cervix, and in the broad ligament. Leiomyomas are either **submucosal**

- Most common pelvic tumor
- Smooth muscle cell composition
- Fibrosis occurs after atrophic or degenerative changes
- Degeneration occurs when myomas outgrow their blood supply; calcification
- May be pedunculated
- Clinical findings: Enlarged uterus, profuse and prolonged bleeding, pain

| BOX 41-5 | **Uterine Locations of Leiomyomas** |

Submucosal

Disruption into endometrial cavity—heavy bleeding; infertility

Intramural

Within myometrium—may enlarge to cause pressure on adjacent organs; infertility or recurrent pregnancy loss

Subserosal

Arise from myometrium, project exophytically—may enlarge to cause pressure on adjacent organs

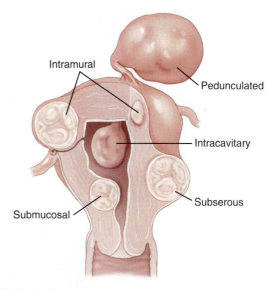

FIGURE 41-13 Various locations of fibroid tumors found within the uterine cavity.

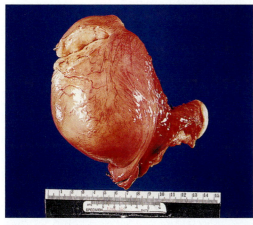

FIGURE 41-12 Gross pathologic findings of a pedunculated subserosal myoma of the uterus.

(displacing or distorting the endometrial cavity with subsequent irregular or heavy menstrual bleeding), **intramural** (confined to the myometrium, the most common type), or **subserosal** (projecting from the peritoneal surface of the uterus). Sometimes subserosal leiomyomas become pedunculated and appear as extrauterine masses (Box 41-5 and Figure 41-12).

The signs and symptoms of leiomyomas depend on their size and location (Figure 41-13). Submucosal myomas may erode into the endometrial cavity and cause irregular or heavy bleeding, which may lead to anemia. Fertility may be affected by submucosal or intramural myomas, which may impede sperm flow, prevent adequate implantation, or cause recurrent miscarriages. It is particularly important to diagnose submucosal leiomyomas because they are a well-established cause of dysfunctional uterine bleeding, infertility, and spontaneous abortion. Small submucosal leiomyomas may be removed hysteroscopically.

Uncommonly, a pedunculated subserosal lesion develops a long stalk and is migratory; it can implant into the blood supply of the broad ligament, omentum, or the bowel mesentery. Transvaginal sonography is often helpful in showing the uterine origin of the mass and identifying the stalk. Occasionally a pedunculated myoma becomes adherent to surrounding structures and develops an auxiliary blood supply.

Sonographic Findings. Leiomyomas have variable sonographic appearances. The earliest sonographic finding of myomas is the demonstration of uterine enlargement or irregular uterine wall contour with a heterogeneous myometrial texture pattern. The sonographer should also look for contour distortion along the interface between the uterus and the bladder (Figure 41-14). The myoma alters the normal homogeneous myometrium. Discrete myomas usually are hypoechoic but can be hyperechoic if they contain dense fibrous tissue. Bright clusters of echoes occur with calcific deposits and produce typical distal acoustic shadowing (Figure 41-15). Some myomas demonstrate an area of acoustic attenuation without a discrete mass, making it impossible to estimate size. The attenuation is thought to be caused by dense fibrosis within the substance of the tumor. The ultrasound technique and gain controls often must be manipulated to provide increased penetration, or a lower frequency may be necessary to fully evaluate the uterus. If extensive calcification is present, the uterus and adnexa may be difficult to image because of shadowing. In such cases, transvaginal imaging is helpful in visualizing the ovaries. Myomas as small as 0.5 cm can be detected by transvaginal sonography and their relationship to the endometrial cavity defined precisely.

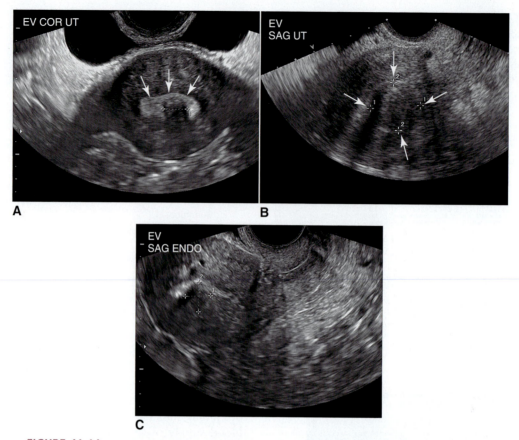

FIGURE 41-14 **A–C,** Transvaginal views of the uterus reveal subtle submucosal myomas *(arrows).*

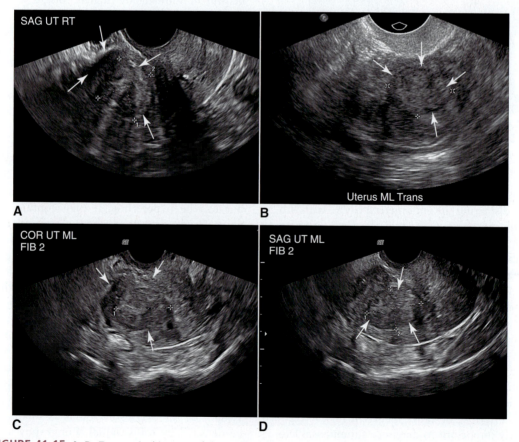

FIGURE 41-15 **A–D,** Transvaginal images of the uterine cavity with a moderate size intramural myoma *(arrows).*

Larger myomas cause heterogeneous uterine enlargement and may be better outlined by transabdominal sonography.

The sonographic study should include measurement of the uterus in three dimensions: (1) cervix to fundus, (2) widest anteroposterior diameter, and (3) widest transverse diameter at fundus diameter (Figure 41-16). The texture of the myoma (calcific, complex, or anechoic), size, and location are described. Individual myomas are measured if they are discrete. The shape of the endometrial complex and its thickness are also described;

alterations in the endometrial border will be evident if a myoma is present (Figure 41-17). This is especially important in women with a history of abnormal bleeding. Myomas can be associated with endometrial infection or cancer. Blood debris and polyps can artifactually widen the endometrium; therefore, definitive diagnosis of the cause of abnormal bleeding might require an endometrial biopsy or sonohysterography.

Cystic degeneration of myomas causes lucencies that are well visualized with transvaginal sonography. Cystic degeneration can occur during pregnancy and cause

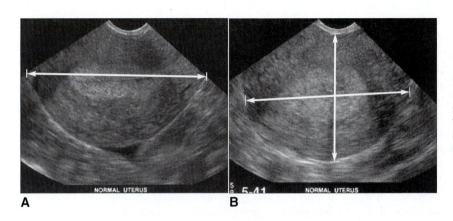

FIGURE 41-16 Transvaginal images of the uterus for measurement. **A,** Sagittal image should measure the uterus at the longest point from the fundus to the cervix. **B,** Coronal image at the level of the fundus measures the antero-posterior dimension and the width of the uterus.

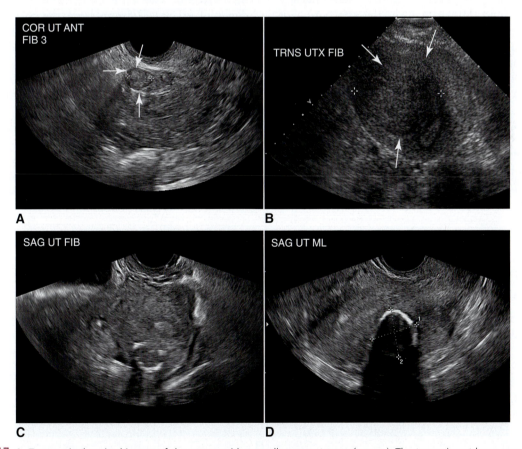

FIGURE 41-17 A, Transvaginal sagittal image of the uterus with a small myoma tumor *(arrows)*. The tumor is not large enough to displace the endometrium. **B,** This myomatous tumor *(arrows)* is displacing the endometrium posteriorly. **C,** Moderate size myoma with calcification. **D,** Calcified rim of the fibroid with complete shadowing posterior.

pain. Doppler should be used to assess the vascularity of myomas as a possible predictor of growth. Sonography shows thin vessels with low-velocity flow within myomas. In cases of cystic degeneration, these vessels with low-velocity flow are not seen (Figure 41-18). Giant leiomyomas with multiple cystic spaces resulting from edema have also been described.

Although ultrasound is used to identify myomas in women with abnormal bleeding, uterine enlargement, or infertility, MRI, with its tissue differentiation characteristics, can be more sensitive for evaluating the exact location, size, and number of myomas.

Treatment of Myomas. The decision to treat or not treat myomas depends on the clinical state of the patient. In the case of infertility and a submucosal myoma, surgery by myomectomy is generally the treatment of choice. In cases of menorrhagia, women now have several choices. The least invasive treatment is hormonal suppression to stop bleeding. Several newer techniques are also now available. Endometrial ablation uses radiofrequency, microwaves, freezing, or heating ablative technology to ablate or remove the endometrium and any small surrounding myomas. Uterine artery embolization (UAE) is another method to obstruct blood flow to large myomas. Small plastic particles are injected into the blood supply to the myoma to terminate flow. The myoma eventually becomes necrotic. High-intensity focused ultrasound (HIFU) involves the application of "therapeutic" sonic waves to the uterus and myoma. The myoma is ablated by heating the tissue and causing tissue death. Currently, only MRI-guided HIFU is approved in the United States. Ultrasound-guided HIFU is approved and in use in several European countries, Russia, and China.

Uterine Calcifications

Myomas are the most common cause of uterine calcifications. A less common cause is arcuate artery calcification in the periphery of the uterus. These calcifications are thought to occur as a consequence of calcific sclerosis within these vessels and can indicate underlying disease, such as diabetes mellitus, hypertension, and chronic renal failure. Such calcifications have been termed *Monckebergs's arteriosclerosis* and appear in arteries throughout the body.

Sonographic Findings. Calcifications may occur as focal areas of increased echogenicity with shadowing or as a peripheral echogenic rim (Figure 41-19).

Adenomyosis

Adenomyosis is a benign disease, commonly diffuse, with global infiltration of the endometrium, which sonographically presents as a bulky enlarged uterus without focal mass. Adenomyosis is the ectopic occurrence of endometrial tissue within the myometrium and is more common in the posterior aspect. On occasion, adenomyosis may be focal with discrete masses or be identified with adenomyomas in the wall of the uterus. The exact cause is unknown, but the most commonly accepted theory suggests that a compromise of the natural barrier between the endometrium and myometrium occurs, commonly from uterine surgery, allowing the growth of ectopic endometrial bands and stroma within the uterine myometrium. The tissue penetration usually reaches a depth of at least 2.5 mm from the basal layer of the endometrium. Adenomyosis may arise from multiple pregnancies and deliveries with subsequent uterine shrinking. Elevated estrogen levels may also promote the growth of myometrial islands of endometrial tissue.

Adenomyosis is often classified into diffuse and focal forms. The more common form is diffuse adenomyosis. It represents a reactive hypertrophy of the myometrial muscle, which produces uterine enlargement, but usually not to the extent seen with leiomyomas. Focal adenomyosis is sometimes called *adenomyoma*, referring to isolated implants that typically cause reactive

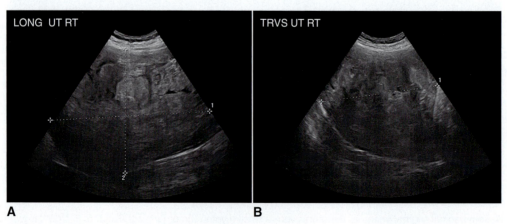

LONG UT RT   TRVS UT RT

A   B

FIGURE 41-18 A and B, Transvaginal sagittal image of the uterus in a pregnant woman with a large myoma. No flow within the myoma was observed on color Doppler imaging.

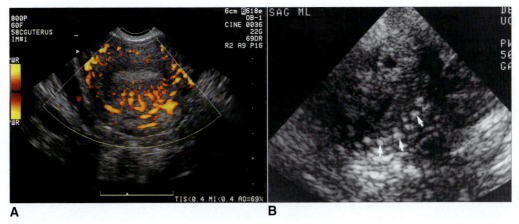

FIGURE 41-19 A, Color Doppler image of normal arcuate artery flow within the periphery of the uterus. **B,** Transvaginal sagittal view of the uterus demonstrates multiple echogenic foci in the region of the arcuate vessels. These are consistent with arcuate artery calcifications *(arrows)*.

hypertrophy of the surrounding myometrium and produce diffuse uterine enlargement. Less common than the diffuse form, focal adenomyosis (adenomyoma) lacks a hypoechoic border that is seen with fibroids, not endometriosis. Adenomyosis can be appropriately managed with hormone therapy.

Clinically, both adenomyosis and endometriosis are identical with respect to structure and function, but they are usually regarded as separate and distinct processes. Patients with adenomyosis are often multiparous and older than patients with endometriosis. The patient presents with heavy, painful abnormal menses, and, on physical examination, the uterus is found to range from normal to three times normal size and is globular in contour, boggy, and somewhat tender.

An estimated 60% of women with adenomyosis experience abnormal uterine bleeding (hypermenorrhea), prolonged/profuse uterine bleeding (menorrhagia), or irregular, acyclic bleeding (**metrorrhea**). Approximately 25% of patients with adenomyosis also suffer from pelvic pain during menstruation (dysmenorrhea). Currently, only 10% to 20% of adenomyosis cases are correctly diagnosed before surgery. This low rate is thought to exist because many adenomyosis patients are asymptomatic in the absence of other uterine pathology, and its presence may be overshadowed by associated pathology, such as leiomyomas, endometriosis, or endometrial polyps.

Sonographic Findings. Sonographically, the diagnosis of adenomyosis may be difficult. The most common presentation of extensive adenomyosis is diffuse uterine enlargement, thickening of the posterior myometrium, indistinct border between the endometrium and myometrium (the involved area being slightly more anechoic than normal myometrium) (Figure 41-20), and myometrial cysts. Typically, adenomyosis involves the inner two thirds of the myometrium, where a slight decrease in echo content of the involved areas may be observed.

Hemorrhage in the islands of endometrial tissue appears as small hypoechoic myometrial cysts. This has previously been described as a *swiss cheese* or *honeycomb* pattern. Lesions of this size are at the limit of ultrasound resolution. The fluid nature of these lesions produces increased posterior acoustic enhancement rather than the degree of attenuation that is normally seen posterior to the uterus. Further evaluation using signal processing (preprocessing and postprocessing) is helpful to better distinguish the contour and border differentiation of any coexisting pathology, such as leiomyomas. Doppler studies have also proven helpful in differentiating uterine pathology, as color flow studies of uterine masses show that myomas and sarcomas typically demonstrate a feeding artery, but adenomyosis rarely demonstrates feeding arteries.

Calcifications resulting from prior instrumentation are seen along the inner myometrium and cervix (Figure 41-21). Localized adenomyomas may be seen by transvaginal sonography as inhomogeneous, circumscribed areas in the myometrium, having indistinct margins and containing anechoic lacunae. They may be difficult to distinguish from leiomyomas, as these two conditions frequently occur together.

Adenomyosis is not always reliably diagnosed by ultrasonography, and caution is advised because these findings are similar in appearance to uterine myomas, muscular hypertrophy, myometrial contractions, endometritis, endometrial carcinoma, and the presence of increased endometrial secretions.

Localized adenomyomas may be seen by transvaginal sonography as inhomogeneous, circumscribed areas in the myometrium, having indistinct margins and containing anechoic cavities. These can be difficult to distinguish from leiomyomas. The presence of myomas has been shown to limit the ability to diagnose the severity of adenomyosis. Although not reliably diagnosed by ultrasonography, adenomyosis is well characterized by MRI,

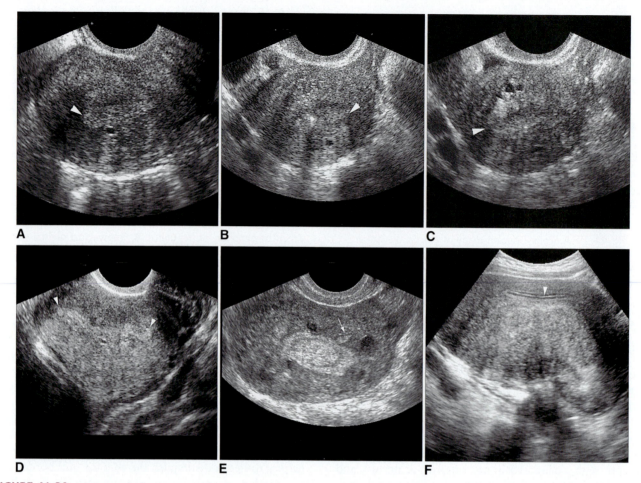

FIGURE 41-20 Adenomyosis on transvaginal scans—spectrum of appearances. **A,** Subendometrial cyst *(arrowhead).* **B,** Cysts with heterogeneity in both anterior and posterior myometrium. **C,** Cysts with heterogeneity in anterior myometrium. **D,** Myometrial heterogeneity with ill-defined endometrial borders *(arrowheads).* **E,** Multiple subendometrial cysts and echogenic nodule *(arrow).* **F,** Large area of myometrial heterogeneity producing a focal mass effect and displacing endometrium *(arrowhead).* This may mimic a fibroid.

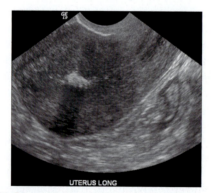

FIGURE 41-21 Transvaginal image of the uterine cavity with a bright echogenic echo in the endometrium. Shadowing is present beyond the calcification.

which currently is thought by many to be the best technique for the presurgical diagnosis of adenomyosis. The MRI hallmark is the appearance of diffuse or focal widening of the junctional zone or the appearance of an indistinctly bordered myometrial mass (Figure 41-22).

Arteriovenous Malformations

Uterine arteriovenous malformations (AVMs) consist of a vascular plexus of arteries and veins without an intervening capillary network. They are rare, usually involving the myometrium and rarely the endometrium. They can be congenital, but most are teratogenic (acquired) resulting from pelvic trauma, surgery, and gestational trophoblastic neoplasia. Clinically, women of childbearing years have metrorrhagia with blood loss and anemia. Diagnosis is critical because dilation and **curettage** may lead to catastrophic hemorrhaging.

▶ **Sonographic Findings.** Sonographically, serpiginous, anechoic structures are seen within the pelvis. Uterine AVMs may appear as subtle myometrial inhomogeneity, tubular spaces within the myometrium, intramural uterine mass, endometrial or cervical mass, or sometimes as prominent parametrial vessels. Color Doppler is diagnostic to show blood flow within the anechoic structures (Figure 41-23). There may be a florid colored mosaic pattern with apparent flow reversals and areas of color aliasing. Spectral Doppler shows high-velocity,

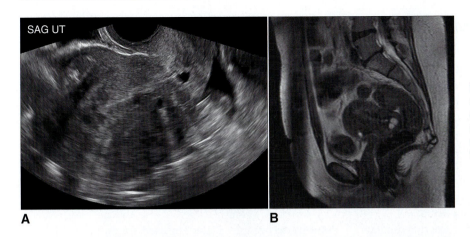

FIGURE 41-22 Adenomyosis. **A,** Transvaginal view of the uterus demonstrates an enlarged heterogeneous uterus. **B,** MRI shows an enlarged uterus with heterogeneous decreased signal intensity throughout the myometrium.

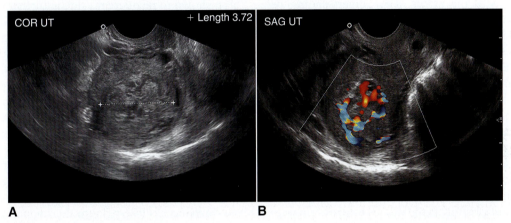

FIGURE 41-23 Uterine arteriovenous malformation. **A,** Transvaginal images show a textural inhomogeneity in the uterine fundus. **B,** Color Doppler image shows a floridly colored mosaic pattern with apparent flow reversals and areas of color aliasing.

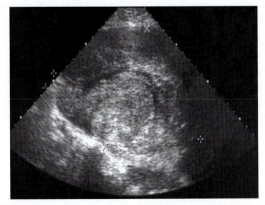

FIGURE 41-24 A 61-year-old woman with lower abdominal "fullness" and frequency of urination. Transvaginal ultrasound showed a large heterogeneous mass in the uterus. A large leiomyosarcoma was found at surgery.

BOX 41-6	Leiomyosarcoma

- Rare, solid tumor arising from the myometrium or endometrium
- Commonly in fundus of uterus
- Most common in women 40 to 60 years of age
- Rapid growth
- Sarcoma botryoides: Very rare condition in children characterized by grapelike clusters of tumor mass

---

low-resistance arterial flow coupled with high-velocity venous flow, with an arterial component. Treatment and confirmation include angiography with embolic therapy.

Uterine Leiomyosarcoma

Leiomyosarcoma is rare, accounting for 1% of all uterine malignancies (Figure 41-24). The tumors originate from the myometrium or the endometrial lining, are highly aggressive, and have a poor prognosis. Benign leiomyomas and leiomyosarcomas may occur in the same patient, though the two are genetically distinct and different structures (Box 41-6). The most common presentation is abnormal vaginal bleeding, pelvic pain, and an enlarged uterus. Occasionally patients are asymptomatic.

Sonographic Findings. Leiomyosarcoma may resemble myomas or endometrial carcinoma with features of solid or mixed-solid and cystic texture. Clinically, the rapid enlargement of a solid uterine mass in the perimenopausal or postmenopausal patient raises concern about the development of a malignancy.

PATHOLOGY OF THE ENDOMETRIUM

The endometrial canal is the landmark for the identification of the long axis of the uterus. The echogenicity of the endometrial tissue is compared with the homogeneous, medium-level echogenicity of the middle layer of the myometrium. A hypoechoic layer of inner myometrium surrounds the endometrium. Progressive thickening and increased reflectivity of the endometrium occurs in the majority of patients until it is shed during menstruation. In the immediate preovulatory and postovulatory periods (approximately 2 days), an additional inner hypoechoic layer appears secondary to edema.

The endometrium should be measured perpendicular to the long axis of the uterus. The calipers should be placed at the maximum anterior to posterior diameter of the outer borders. The hypoechoic halo surrounding the endometrium should not be included in the measurement because this represents the inner compact layer of myometrium. Fluid, if present, should not be included in endometrial measurements (Table 41-1). Additionally, the 2009 AIUM pelvic sonography guidelines recommend a 3D reconstruction of the uterus and endometrium whenever possible.

Improved resolution with transvaginal sonography is better able to image and see subtle abnormalities within the endometrium. Knowledge of the normal sonographic appearance of the endometrium allows for earlier recognition of the pathologic conditions where the endometrium is thickened, irregular, or poorly defined. An abnormally thick endometrium results from a variety of conditions, including early intrauterine pregnancy, gestational trophoblastic disease, endometrial hyperplasia, secretory endometrium, estrogen replacement therapy, polyps, or endometrial carcinoma. Many endometrial pathologies—such as hyperplasia, polyps, and carcinoma—can cause abnormal bleeding, especially in the postmenopausal patient.

Disorders of the endometrium may also occur in menopausal patients with breast cancer who are receiving tamoxifen therapy. This is a partial estrogen receptor antagonist used in postmenopausal women with estrogen receptor positive breast cancer. The effects on the uterus include epithelial metaplasia, hyperplasia, and even carcinoma. In these patients, transvaginal scanning may show thickened, irregular cystic endometrium. These patients frequently have biannual serial ultrasound exams of their uterus and endometrium. A biopsy is performed in suspicious cases. New medications have been developed that purport to have less effect on the endometrium. These include Aromasin, Femara, Raloxifen, and Evista.

Sonohysterography

Sonohysterography (saline-infused sonography, SIS) has been shown to be of great value in further evaluating the abnormally thickened endometrium. By distending the endometrial cavity with saline, the examiner can distinguish endometrial growths and abnormalities. After performing routine transvaginal exam to orient the sonographer to the patient's anatomy and pathology, the doctor should explain the procedure to the patient and obtain consent. A sterile speculum is inserted into the vagina, and the cervix is cleansed with an antiseptic solution. A hysterosalpingography catheter is inserted into the uterine cavity beyond the cervical os. The catheter is prefilled with sterile saline before insertion to minimize air artifact. The speculum is removed and the transvaginal transducer is inserted into the vagina. The catheter is identified in the endometrial cavity by locating the saline-filled balloon, and the saline is slowly injected through the catheter under sonographic visualization. The uterus is scanned systematically in sagittal and coronal planes to delineate the entire endometrial cavity. Appropriate images are obtained under the direction of the physician performing the procedure. A sweep of the fluid-filled endometrium in both planes can be captured on cine clips to further document the presence of any pathology.

In premenopausal women, the procedure is performed in the midmenstrual cycle, usually between days 6 to 10. This will prevent the possibility of disrupting an early pregnancy and prevent blood clots artifactually filling some of the endometrial cavity. For women with irregular cycles, the procedure is performed soon after the cessation of bleeding, if possible. In postmenopausal women, the procedure can be performed at any time or shortly after the monthly bleeding period if they are on sequential hormone replacement therapy. The procedure is *not* performed in women with acute pelvic inflammatory disease. In most cases there is no special patient preparation. Prophylactic antibiotics are given to women with chronic pelvic inflammatory disease and to women with a history of mitral valve prolapse or other cardiac disorders.

◢ **Sonographic Findings.** Sonographically, after the saline is injected, the endometrial canal fills with saline and the borders are clearly identified (Figure 41-25). Any projections or filling defects can be delineated and

TABLE 41-1	Endometrial Thickness Related to Phases of Menstrual Cycle	
Phase of Menstrual Cycle	**Endometrial Thickness* (mm)**
Menstrual	2-3
Early proliferative	4-6
Periovulatory	6-8
Secretory	8-15

Data from Goldberg BB, Kurtz AB: *Ultrasound measurements*, St. Louis, 1990, Mosby.
*Measured as full thickness, anteroposterior (AP), from outer border to outer border of hypoechoic interface.

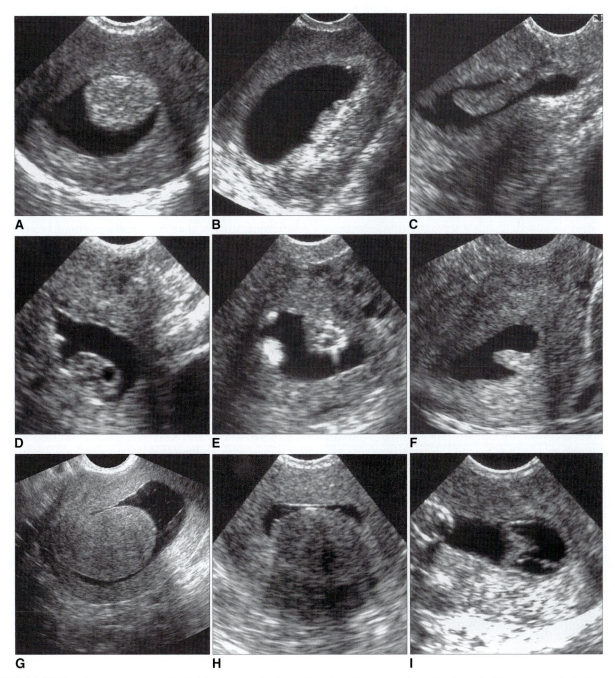

FIGURE 41-25 Sonohysterograms. **A,** Well-defined, round echogenic polyp. **B,** Carpet of small polyps. **C,** Polyp on a stalk. **D,** Polyp with cystic areas. **E,** Small polyp. **F,** Small polyp. **G,** Hypoechoic submucosal fibroid. **H,** Hypoechoic attenuating submucosal fibroid. **I,** Endometrial adhesions. Note bridging bands of tissue within the fluid-filled endometrial canal.

confirmed in the sagittal and coronal planes. By using color Doppler, a vascular pedicle can be identified in polyps. The clinician carefully removes the catheter while injecting a small amount of the saline to help distinguish the cervical area.

Endometrial Hyperplasia

Endometrial hyperplasia (Box 41-7) is the most common cause of abnormal uterine bleeding in both

BOX 41-7	Endometrial Hyperplasia

- Follows prolonged endogenous or exogenous estrogenic stimulation
- May be precursor of endometrial cancer
- Sonographic findings: Abnormal thickening of endometrium

premenopausal and postmenopausal women. Hyperplasia develops from unopposed estrogen stimulation. It appears as thickening of the endometrium. In premenopausal women, if the endometrium measures more than 14 mm (double thickness), hyperplasia is suggested. The optimal time period for this assessment in a woman still having menses is day 6 through day 10, after bleeding and before the endometrium is again stimulated. In asymptomatic postmenopausal women, 8 mm (double thickness) is the upper limit of normal. However, women on sequential estrogen and progesterone replacement regimens may have endometrial thickness up to 15 mm during the estrogen phase; the thickness decreases after progesterone is added. Ideally a woman using sequential hormones should be studied at the beginning or end of her hormone cycle, when the endometrium is theoretically at its thinnest. Common hormonal regimens in menopausal women are listed in Box 41-8. Hyperplasia is less common during the reproductive years, but it may occur with persistent anovulatory cycles, with polycystic ovarian disease, and in obese women with increased production of endogenous estrogens. Hyperplasia may also be seen in women with estrogen-producing tumors, such as granulose cell tumors and thecomas of the ovary.

Because hyperplasia has a nonspecific sonographic appearance, an endometrial biopsy is necessary for diagnosis. Sonohysterography can also be performed to evaluate the internal structure of the endometrial canal.

Most women with postmenopausal uterine bleeding are experiencing endometrial atrophy. On transvaginal sonography, an atrophic endometrium is thin, measuring less than 5 mm. If the postmenopausal patient has irregular bleeding and a thickened endometrium, this may warrant a sonohysterography procedure or an endometrial biopsy. Ultrasound is used to help the clinician triage which patients are candidates for biopsy. Clinicians may use the endometrial measurement alone (for example, greater than 5 to 8 mm without bleeding), or they may use symptoms as their criteria (for example, less than 5 to 8 mm with bleeding),

Sonographic Findings. The endometrium is usually diffusely thick and echogenic with well-defined margins (Figures 41-26 and 41-27). Focal or asymmetrical thickening can occur. Small cysts representing dilated cystic glands may be seen within the endometrium. Although cystic changes within a thickened endometrium are more frequently witnessed in benign conditions, they can also be observed in endometrial carcinoma.

Endometrial Polyps

Patients with **endometrial polyps** can be asymptomatic, or they may present with uterine bleeding. Histologically, polyps are overgrowths of endometrial tissue covered by epithelium. They contain a variable number of glands, stroma, and blood vessels. Approximately 20% of endometrial polyps are multiple. They may be pedunculated, broad based, or have a thin stalk. They typically cause diffuse or focal endometrial thickening and are more frequently seen in perimenopausal and postmenopausal women. In menstruating women, they may be associated with menometrorrhagia or infertility. In postmenopausal women, especially those being investigated for bleeding, the major differential considerations are hyperplasia, submucosal myomas, or, less commonly, endometrial carcinoma.

BOX 41-8	**Common Hormonal Regimens in Menopausal Women**

1. No hormones.
2. Unopposed estrogen (usually Premarin). If uterus is present, unopposed estrogen is associated with increased risk for endometrial hyperplasia or carcinoma.
3. Continuous/combined estrogen and progesterone (Premarin and Provera). This combination produces endometrial atrophy after 3 to 6 months. Usually there is no risk of endometrial cancer; however, women may have "breakthrough" bleeding during the month or annoying progesterone side effects (i.e., irritability, depression, bloating, and breast tenderness).
4. Sequential estrogen and progesterone (Premarin first half then Provera second half of month). Women have predictable withdrawal bleeding at end of each month.

In the United States, regimens 2 and 4 are most commonly used.

Beneficial Effects
Estrogen
Alleviates menopausal symptoms (hot flashes, night sweats, painful intercourse)
Reduces risk of osteoporosis, vertebral and hip fractures
Reduces risk of heart attacks, strokes

Progesterone
Produces endometrial atrophy; reduces risk of endometrial hyperplasia/cancer

Negative Effects
Estrogen
Increases risk of endometrial hyperplasia/cancer

Progesterone
Increases risk of breast cancer
Irritability, depression, breast tenderness in some women

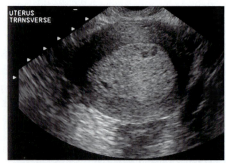

FIGURE 41-26 Transvaginal coronal image of the uterus with a very prominent endometrium measuring more than 23 mm. On biopsy the patient had endometrial hyperplasia.

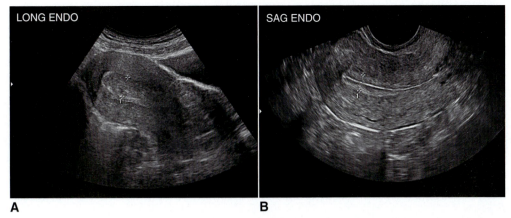

FIGURE 41-27 Normal variation in endometrial thickness from cyclic hormone replacement in a 62-year-old woman. **A,** Day 9, three-layer endometrium, 10-mm thick. **B,** Day 3, 4-mm thick endometrium. Women taking sequential hormones should be examined after the progesterone phase of the cycle, when the endometrium is theoretically at its thinnest.

Sonographic Findings. Sonographically, polyps appear toward the end of the luteal phase and are represented by a hypoechoic or isoechoic region within the hyperechoic endometrium. They initially may appear as nonspecific echogenic endometrial thickening. The polyp may be diffuse or focal and may also appear as a round echogenic mass within the endometrial cavity (Figure 41-28). Cystic areas representing histologically dilated glands may be seen within a polyp. A feeding artery in the pedicle may be identified with color Doppler, especially with the newer systems that have sensitive power Doppler or high-definition flow. Individual polyps are better visualized when outlined by intracavitary fluid. Sonohysterography is a valuable technique when transvaginal sonography is unable to differentiate an endometrial polyp from a submucosal leiomyoma. Color Doppler sonohysterography can be particularly useful in discriminating polyps from submucosal myomas based on the presentation of feeding vessels. Polyps present most often with one primary feeding vessel, whereas myomas typically have multiple microvessels arising from the inner myometrium.

Endometritis

Endometrial thickening or fluid may indicate endometritis (Box 41-9). **Endometritis** is an infection within the endometrium of the uterus. It occurs most often in association with pelvic inflammatory disease (PID), in the postpartum state, or following instrumentation of the uterus. In patients with pelvic infection, the uterus is the conduit for infectious spread to the tubes and adnexa. Postpartum patients may develop endometritis after prolonged labor, vaginitis, premature rupture of the membranes, or retained products of conception. Clinically, the patient has intense pelvic pain.

Sonographic Findings. Sonographically, the endometrium appears prominent, irregular, or both, with a small amount of endometrial fluid (Figures 41-29 and 41-30).

BOX 41-9 | Endometritis

- Inflammation of the endometrium
- Clinical findings: Low back pain and fever; lower abdominal pain; dysmenorrhea; menorrhagia; sterility; constipation
- Sonographic findings: Endometrium appears prominent or irregular; pus may be seen in the cul-de-sac; enlarged ovaries with multiple cysts secondary to periovarian inflammation; dilated fallopian tubes

---

Pus may be demonstrated in the cul-de-sac as echogenic particles or debris. Enlarged ovaries with multiple cysts and indistinct margins may be seen secondary to periovarian inflammation. Dilation of the fallopian tube shows fluid-filled tubular shapes in a folded configuration and well-defined echogenic walls. A thickened tubal wall (5 mm or more) indicates acute disease. These should be distinguished from a fluid-filled bowel by gentle compression on the pelvic wall to look for peristalsis or movement in the bowel lumen.

As the infection worsens, periovarian adhesions may form and fuse the inflamed tube and ovary, called the tubo-ovarian complex. Further progression results in a tubo-ovarian abscess that appears as a complex multiloculated mass with septations, irregular shaggy margins, and scattered internal echoes. There can be posterior enhancement and a fluid-debris level. Gas bubbles are present in rare cases; however, these also are observed in normal postpartum patients. In the immediate postpartum period, the presence of retained tissue is difficult to distinguish from inflammatory debris or blood clots. The sonographic appearance can be similar to that of other adnexal masses, so clinical correlation is important. Sonography can also be useful in following the response to antibiotic therapy or in guided transvaginal aspirations and drainage. If the aspirate is purulent, catheter drainage is used. In chronic PID, fibrosis and adhesions may make identification of pelvic organs difficult. Torsion

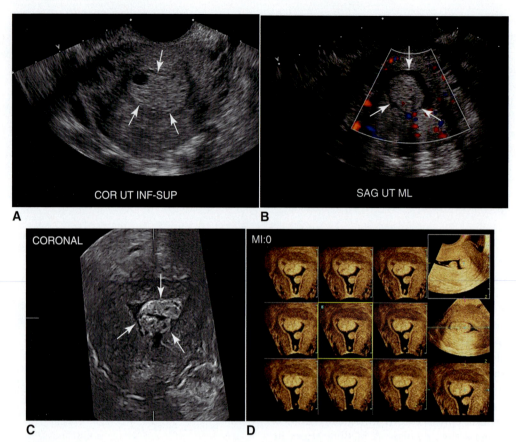

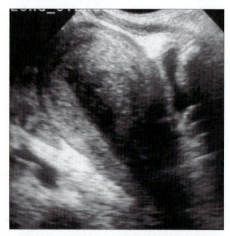

FIGURE 41-28 A and **B,** Transvaginal image of endometrial polyp shows a focal thickening within the endometrial cavity *(arrows)*. **C,** 3D reconstruction of the polyp. **D,** Multiplane reconstruction of the endometrial polyp.

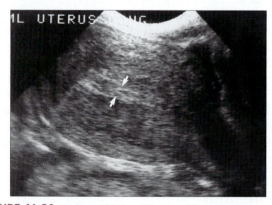

FIGURE 41-30 Endometritis in a 31-year-old woman. A transvaginal sagittal view of the uterus 3 days postpartum demonstrates a slightly irregular endometrium *(arrows)*.

FIGURE 41-29 The enlarged uterus with an edematous complex endometrium in a patient who presented 10 days postoperatively with intense pelvic pain. She was diagnosed with endometritis.

of the tube is uncommon, but it occurs in association with chronic hydrosalpinx.

Synechiae

Intrauterine synechiae (endometrial adhesions, Asherman's syndrome) are found in women with posttraumatic or postsurgical histories, including uterine curettage. Synechiae can cause infertility or recurrent pregnancy loss.

Sonographic Findings. Ultrasonography may demonstrate bright echoes within the endometrial cavity in this condition. The diagnosis is difficult unless fluid is distending the endometrial cavity. This is best identified during the secretory phase when the endometrium is more hyperechoic. Synechiae are more easily observed in the gravid uterus, where they appear as a hyperechoic band traversing the uterus from anterior to posterior.

Sonohysterography is an excellent technique for demonstrating adhesions and should be performed in cases of suspected adhesions. Adhesions appear as bridging bands of tissue that distort the cavity or as thin, undulating membranes that connect from one side of the uterus to the other. Thick, broad-based adhesions may prevent distention of the uterine cavity. Adhesions can be divided under hysteroscopy.

Endometrial Carcinoma

Endometrial carcinoma is the most common gynecologic malignancy in North America, and its incidence has been rising. Most endometrial malignancies are adenocarcinomas occurring in postmenopausal patients. The most common clinical presentation is uterine bleeding, although only 10% of women with postmenopausal bleeding will have endometrial carcinoma. There is a strong association with replacement estrogen therapy. In the premenopausal woman, anovulatory cycles and obesity are also considered risk factors. The earliest change of endometrial carcinoma is a thickened endometrium. An abnormally thick endometrium is also associated with endometrial hypertrophy and polyps.

Recent studies of patients with postmenopausal bleeding show that an endometrial thickness (double layer) of less than 5 mm reliably excludes significant endometrial abnormality.[1–4] At present, most investigators believe biopsies should be performed for all symptomatic patients. In the future, however, transvaginal ultrasonography may be used to follow symptomatic patients with normal endometrial thickness for whom biopsy is contraindicated or who do not wish to undergo an invasive procedure.

Although increased endometrial thickness is an early finding in endometrial carcinoma, enlargement with lobular contour of the uterus and mixed echogenicity are correlated with more advanced stages of the disease. The risk of malignancy increases with the presence of a large endometrial fluid collection or clinical symptoms, such as abdominal pain or bleeding.

Sonographic Findings. Transvaginal examination is helpful in screening for early changes of endometrial hyperplasia or carcinoma by accurately measuring endometrial thickness. Sonographically, a thickened endometrium (greater than 4 to 5 mm, and this value varies institution to institution) must be considered cancer until proven otherwise (Figure 41-31). Demonstration of myometrial invasion is clear evidence for endometrial carcinoma. Transvaginal ultrasonography demonstrates myometrial invasion as thickening and irregularity of the central endometrial interface with echogenic or hypoechoic patterns combined with infiltration of hyperdense structures in the myometrium (Box 41-10). Cystic changes within the endometrium are more commonly seen in endometrial atrophy, hyperplasia, and polyps, but can also be seen with carcinoma. Endometrial masses containing numerous vascular branches with color imaging should also raise the level of suspicion for carcinoma.

Endometrial carcinoma may obstruct the endometrial canal, resulting in **hydrometra** or **hematometra.** The level of myometrial invasion (superficial versus deep) also can be detected by transvaginal ultrasonography, although contrast-enhanced MRI is more sensitive. Intactness of the subendometrial halo (the inner layer of myometrium) usually indicates superficial invasion, whereas obliteration of the halo is indicative of deep invasion. Magnetic resonance imaging is also valuable in evaluating extrauterine extension and involvement of lymph nodes.

Tamoxifen, a nonsteroidal antiestrogen compound, is widely used for adjuvant therapy in premenopausal and postmenopausal women with breast cancer and has secondary effects on the endometrium. Various new

---

BOX 41-10 | Endometrial Carcinoma

- Associated with estrogen stimulation
- Clinical findings: Postmenopausal bleeding
- Sonographic findings: Prominent endometrial complex; enlarged uterus with irregular areas of low-level echoes

---

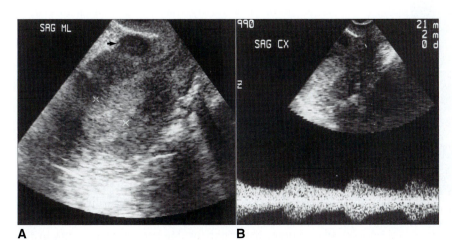

A   B

FIGURE 41-31 Endometrial carcinoma in a 52-year-old woman. **A,** Sagittal view of the uterus demonstrates a 2-cm-thick endometrium. A small myoma *(arrow)* is also present. **B,** Doppler examination of the uterine artery shows abnormal increased diastolic flow (resistive index, 0.5).

medications have been developed for the postmenopausal woman, including Aromasin, Evista, and Femara. An increased risk of endometrial carcinoma, hyperplasia, and polyps has been reported in patients on tamoxifen therapy. On sonography, tamoxifen-related endometrial changes are nonspecific and similar to those described in hyperplasia, polyps, and carcinoma. Because it may be difficult to distinguish the endometrial-myometrial border in many of these patients, sonohysterography is valuable.

Sonography may be helpful in staging carcinoma and in distinguishing between tumors limited to the uterus (stages I and II) and those with extrauterine extension (stages III and IV). Both MRI and CT are useful in staging by demonstrating lymphadenopathy and distant disease (stages III or IV). Endometrial biopsy is usually required for a definite diagnosis.

Doppler Evaluation. The role of color and spectral Doppler in the diagnosis of endometrial carcinoma is controversial. Doppler ultrasonography of the uterine artery may help distinguish between benign and malignant endometrial thickening. Pulsed Doppler is used to evaluate the resistive index (RI = peak systolic –end diastolic/peak systolic) or pulsatility index (PI = peak systolic – end diastolic/mean). The technique of this examination is discussed in Chapter 40. Low-resistance flow (RI < 0.4) has been found in patients with endometrial carcinoma and high-resistance flow (RI > 0.5) in normal or benign endometria. If a pulsatility index is used, the cutoff is 1. Intratumoral neovascularity is a more sensitive marker of endometrial carcinoma than resistive index alone.

Small Endometrial Fluid Collections

Small endometrial fluid collections also occur with ectopic pregnancy, endometritis, degenerating myomas, and recent abortion (Figure 41-32).

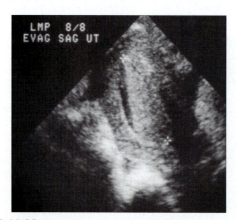 **Sonographic Findings.** Transvaginal sonography, with its improved resolution, sometimes shows tiny endometrial fluid collections not seen on transabdominal

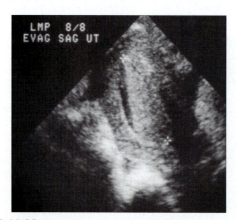

FIGURE 41-32 Transvaginal image in a 23-year-old woman after a dilation and curettage demonstrates a central fluid collection with a fluid debris level representing a hematometra.

scans. These small endometrial fluid collections (less than 2 ml) are common in women during the menstrual phase of the cycle. They are seen in postmenopausal women, especially during the menstrual phase in women taking sequential hormones. In a uterus with a fluid collection, the anteroposterior diameter of the fluid should be subtracted from the endometrial measurement for a true assessment of endometrial thickness.

Large Endometrial Fluid Collections

Large endometrial fluid collections should be regarded with suspicion. Obstruction of the cervical os results in the accumulation of secretions, blood, or both in the uterus. Before menstruation, the accumulation of secretions is referred to as hydrometrocolpos. Following menstruation, hematometrocolpos results from the presence of retained menstrual blood. The obstruction may be congenital, imperforate hymen (most common), vaginal septum, vaginal atresia, or a rudimentary uterine horn. Hydrometra and hematometra may also be acquired as a result of cervical stenosis from endometrial or cervical tumors or from postirradiation fibrosis. They may also be caused by uterine, cervical, tubal, or ovarian carcinoma. Hyperplasia and polyps also cause endometrial fluid collections, so these collections also indicate increased risk of endometrial carcinoma. However, large amounts of endometrial fluid also are associated with benign conditions, such as congenital anomalies or cervical stenosis from prior instrumentation or childbirth.

The patient typically complains of abdominal pain and has an enlarged abdominal mass. She may or may not have vaginal bleeding. The presence of fever suggests infection of the blood collection. Lab results show an elevated white blood count. In simple hematometra, the uterine cavity returns to normal promptly after dilation and curettage. **Pyometra** is more likely to occur with uterine cancer. Abnormal development of the vagina or uterus may result in a cystic uterine or vaginal collection of mucus in children. When menstruation begins, the collection consists of blood.

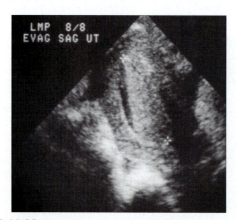 **Sonographic Findings.** The sonographic picture of large endometrial cavity fluid collections is that of a centrally cystic, round, moderately enlarged uterus. This may contain echogenic material if pus or blood is present (Figure 41-33).

INTRAUTERINE CONTRACEPTIVE DEVICES

Lost Intrauterine Device

Intrauterine contraceptive devices (IUCDs) are devices placed in the uterine cavity during menses for the purpose of birth control. Proper placement is verified by weekly digital palpation of the string in the cervix, performed by the patient. If the patient does not feel the string in the cervix, the IUCD may have been expelled or more likely the string has fallen off or retracted into the uterus. A pregnancy test is performed. If it is negative, the gynecologist explores the uterine cavity with a sterile hooked probe. If no string is found or if the pregnancy test is positive, an ultrasound examination is performed. Sonography can demonstrate malposition, perforation, and incomplete removal of the IUCD. Eccentric position of an IUCD from midline suggests myometrial penetration. If the IUCD is not observed during sonography, a radiograph should be done. The IUCD may be difficult to see with coexisting intrauterine abnormalities, such as blood clots or an incomplete abortion. In the first trimester, the IUCD can usually be removed safely under ultrasound guidance. After the first trimester, an IUCD is very difficult to visualize. Patients with IUCDs are at increased risk for ectopic pregnancy and pelvic inflammatory disease. In these women, tubo-ovarian abscess (TOA) may be unilateral; more commonly, though, it is bilateral.

▶ **Sonographic Findings.** Transabdominal and transvaginal scanning demonstrate the IUCD. The sonographic appearance of an IUCD varies according to the components of the device. The most commonly used

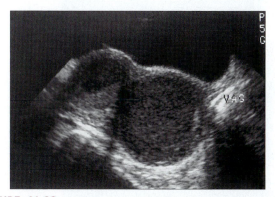

FIGURE 41-33 Large endometrial fluid collection. TV image of obstructed right horn of a bicornuate uterus. This elderly woman was placed on cyclic hormone replacement therapy. She underwent dilation for cervical stenosis; bloody fluid was drained.

IUCDs are currently the Paraguard, a T-shaped flexible plastic wrapped in copper, and the Mirena, a T-shaped flexible plastic that releases low amounts of progestin to act as an additional measure to prevent pregnancy. Traditionally, the metal-containing devices appear as highly echogenic linear structures in the endometrial cavity within the uterine body. Do not confuse them with the normal, central endometrial echoes. The newer plastic polymer hormone-releasing Mirena appears only mildly echogenic and may be difficult to appreciate when visualizing for the first time. For this reason it is important to ask the patient what type of IUCD she has. An analysis of in vivo and in vitro transabdominal images of the many types of IUCDs previously used in the United States found that the shafts of all of them appeared as a double line. This is because of entrance-exit reflections of sound waves when scanned perpendicular to the uterine cavity with high-resolution equipment. Posterior shadowing occurs when the ultrasound beam is entirely interrupted. This requires that the scanning plane be placed perpendicular to the IUCD. The development of 3D scanning has greatly enhanced our ability to fully demonstrate IUCD position by displaying the coronal plane. This acquisition is highly recommended for all IUCD localization exams.

The Copper 7 is shaped like a 7, with a copper wire spiraled around the vertical shaft. The Tatum T and Progestasert are T-shaped (Figures 41-34 and 41-35), and the Lippes loop is serpentine. Occasionally a thick midcycle endometrium obscures the bright IUCD echo when transabdominal ultrasonography is used. If no intrauterine IUCD is identified on ultrasound examination and the pregnancy test is negative, a thin metal probe is inserted into the uterine cavity to mark it, and abdominal x-ray films are obtained to search for the IUCD in an extrauterine location. Perforation of the uterus by an IUCD almost always occurs at the time of insertion. The displaced IUCD may not be suspected until an abscess or painful bowel involvement occurs. If the IUCD is displaced caudally in the lower uterine

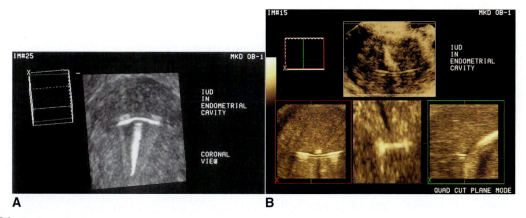

A   **B**

FIGURE 41-34 A, Three-dimensional reconstruction of a safety coil intrauterine contraceptive device located within the uterine cavity. **B,** X, Y, and Z axes of the IUCD.

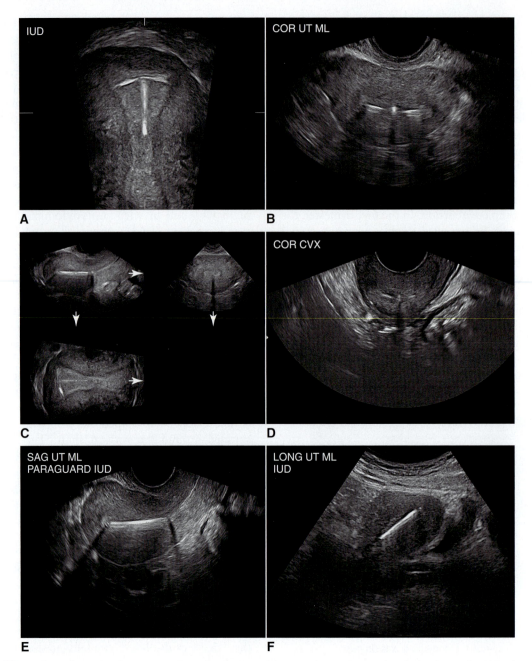

FIGURE 41-35 A, Three-dimensional reconstruction of a Paraguard intrauterine contraceptive device located within the uterine cavity. **B–F,** The Paraguard IUCD should be easily identified by the echogenic linear stripe within the endometrial cavity.

segment, approaching the cervix, this should be reported to the clinician. The IUCD may not be effective in this location and may be at risk for being expelled.

When a pregnancy is present, either transabdominal or transvaginal ultrasound examination demonstrates both gestational age and the location of the IUCD. Occasionally a string is visible in the external os of a pregnant uterus. Approximately 50% of pregnancies abort on extraction of the IUCD. With transvaginal scanning, the location of the IUCD can be detected relative to the sac, and it may be possible to predict which pregnancy will be disrupted. Intrauterine contraceptive devices are always external to fetal membranes.

REFERENCES

1. Carlson JA Jr, et al: Clinical and pathologic correlation of endometrial cavity fluid detected by ultrasound in the postmenopausal patient, *Obstet Gynecol* 77:119, 1991.
2. Goldstein SR, et al: Endometrial assessment by vaginal ultrasonography before endometrial sampling in patients with postmenopausal bleeding, *Am J Obstet Gynecol* 163:119, 1990.
3. Karlsson B, Granberg S, Wikland M, et al: Endovaginal ultrasonography of the endometrium in women with postmenopausal bleeding: a Nordic multicenter study, *Am J Obstet Gynecol* 172:1488-1494, 1995.
4. Varner RE, et al: Endovaginal sonography of the endometrium in postmenopausal women, *Obstet Gynecol* 78:195, 1991.

Pathology of the Ovaries

Candace Goldstein, Sandra L. Hagen-Ansert, and Barbara J. Vander Werff

OBJECTIVES

On completion of this chapter, you should be able to:
- Describe the effects of hormones on the ovarian cycle
- Define the characteristics of the simple ovarian cyst and a functional ovarian cyst
- Discuss the sonographic findings of the common cystic and complex ovarian masses, common solid ovarian masses, ovarian neoplasms, and a dermoid tumor

- List the characteristics of the ovarian syndromes discussed in this chapter
- Discuss the benign pelvic masses found in neonates and adolescent girls
- Differentiate between mucinous and serous types of tumors
- Define the Doppler parameters used in ovarian torsion

OUTLINE

Anatomy of the Ovaries
  Normal Sonographic
    Appearance
Sonographic Evaluation of the
  Ovaries
  Simple Cystic Masses
  Complex Masses
  Solid Tumors
  Doppler of the Ovary
Benign Adnexal Cysts
  Functional Ovarian Cysts
  Ovarian Syndromes
  Other Benign Ovarian Cysts

Endometriosis
Ovarian Torsion
Sonographic Evaluation of Ovarian
  Neoplasms
Ovarian Carcinoma
  Doppler Findings in Ovarian
    Cancer
Epithelial Tumors
  Mucinous Cystadenoma
  Mucinous Cystadenocarcinoma
  Serous Cystadenoma
  Serous Cystadenocarcinoma
  Other Epithelial Tumors

Germ Cell Tumors
  Teratoma
  Immature and Mature Teratomas
  Dysgerminoma
  Endodermal Sinus Tumor
Stromal Tumors
  Fibroma and Thecoma
  Granulosa
  Sertoli-Leydig Cell Tumor
  Arrhenoblastoma
  Metastatic Disease
Carcinoma of the Fallopian Tube
Other Pelvic Masses

Sonography is clinically useful to characterize adnexal masses, evaluate abnormal bleeding, assess infertility, monitor follicular growth, perform endovaginal needle aspiration and biopsy, and screen for ovarian carcinoma. Both transabdominal and transvaginal sonography are important in these evaluations. Transabdominal imaging furnishes a global survey of anatomy, whereas transvaginal imaging provides better characterization of internal architecture of the ovary, vascular anatomy, and adnexal area. It is important to note that information from the clinical pelvic examination is required for optimal interpretation of the sonographic studies, thus necessitating good communication between the referring physician and the sonologist.

A woman will ovulate nearly 400 times in her reproductive life, and a quarter of a million follicles will be stimulated to varying degrees during this time. It is not surprising that an organ as dynamic as the ovary can

form more than 100 different types of tumors, both benign and malignant. These masses are described on the sonographic examination as primarily cystic, complex, or predominantly solid. However, the final diagnosis is left to the pathologist upon surgical excision. Precise diagnosis on the basis of sonography alone is highly predictive, although not conclusive until the surgery. The primary role of sonography is to indicate the need for surgical or medical intervention.

ANATOMY OF THE OVARIES

The ovaries are paired, almond-shaped structures situated one on each side of the uterus close to the lateral pelvic wall (Figure 42-1). The ovaries can vary in position and are influenced by the uterine location and the ligament attachments. In the anteflexed midline uterus, the ovaries are usually identified laterally or

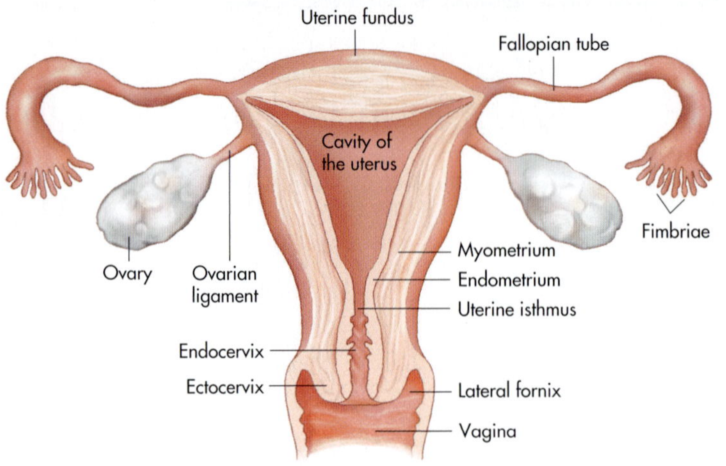

FIGURE 42-1 Normal anatomy of the female pelvis. Note the relationship of the ovaries to the lateral walls of the uterus and the position of the fallopian tubes to the ovaries.

posterolaterally. When the uterus lies to one side of the midline, the ipsilateral ovary often lies superior to the uterine fundus. In a retroverted uterus, the ovaries tend to be lateral and superior, near the uterine fundus. When the uterus is enlarged, the ovaries tend to be displaced more superiorly and laterally. Following hysterectomy, the ovaries tend to be located more medially and directly superior to the vaginal cuff. They can be located high in the pelvis or in the cul-de-sac. Superiorly or extremely laterally placed ovaries may not be visualized by the transvaginal approach because they are out of the field of view. Ovaries are ellipsoid in shape, with their cranio-caudad axes paralleling the internal iliac vessels, which lie posterior and serve as a reference point.

Normal Sonographic Appearance

The normal ovary has a homogeneous echotexture, which may exhibit a central, more echogenic medulla. Small anechoic or cystic follicles may be seen peripherally in the cortex (Figure 42-2). The appearance of the ovary varies with age and the menstrual cycle (Figure 42-3). During the reproductive years, three phases are recognized sonographically during each menstrual cycle. During the early proliferative phase, many follicles develop and increase in size until about day 8 or 9 of the menstrual cycle. This is due to stimulation by both follicle-stimulating hormone (FSH) and luteinizing hormone (LH). At that time one follicle becomes dominant, reaching up to 2 to 2.5 cm at the time of ovulation. The cumulus oophorus may occasionally be detected as an eccentrically located, cystlike, 1-mm internal mural protrusion. Although visualization of the cumulus indicates a mature follicle and imminent ovulation, no reproducible sonographic sign is reliable. The other follicles become atretic. A **follicular cyst** develops if the fluid in the nondominant follicles is not reabsorbed. Usually the dominant follicle disappears immediately after rupture at ovulation. Occasionally the follicle decreases in size and develops a wall that appears crenulated (scalloped).

Fluid in the cul-de-sac commonly occurs after ovulation and peaks in the early luteal phase. Following ovulation in the luteal phase, a mature corpus luteum develops and may be identified sonographically as a small hypoechoic or isoechoic structure peripherally within the ovary. It may appear irregular with echogenic crenulated walls and contain low-level echoes. Less frequent appearances include a typical "ring" color Doppler pattern around the wall of an isoechoic corpus luteum. In the absence of fertilization, the corpus luteum begins to undergo involutional changes on postovulatory days 8 or 9, and disappears shortly before or with the onset of menstruation.

Multiple small, punctate, echogenic foci are commonly seen in the normal ovary. These foci are reported to be a common finding with transvaginal examination. They are generally very small (1 to 2 mm) and located in the periphery. The foci are nonshadowing and can be multiple. A possible source of these foci of specular reflections is from the walls of tiny unresolved cysts below the spatial resolution of ultrasound. More central punctate echogenic foci are thought to represent stromal reaction to previous hemorrhage or infection. Since they do not indicate significant underlying disease, no follow-up is necessary.

Following menopause, the ovary atrophies and the follicles disappear with increasing age. For this reason, the postmenopausal ovary may be difficult to visualize sonographically because of the smaller size and lack of discrete follicles. A stationary loop of the bowel may mimic a small shrunken ovary, so scanning must be done slowly to look for peristalsis in the bowel. After a hysterectomy, the ovaries can be difficult to visualize with ultrasound. The use of both transabdominal and transvaginal approaches increases the chance of visualization.

Because of the variability in ovarian shape and size, the volume measurement is the best method for determining overall ovarian size. The volume measurement is based on the prolate ellipse formula ($0.523 \times$ length $\times$

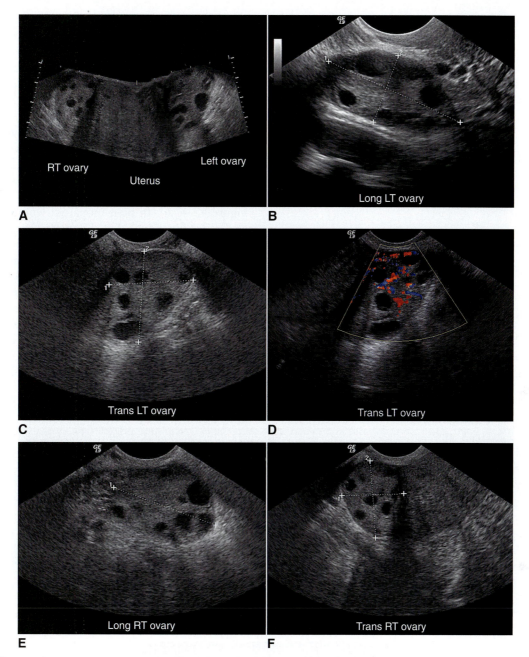

FIGURE 42-2 Normal transvaginal image of the ovaries with multiple follicles. **A,** Both ovaries are well seen with multiple follicles. **B,** Long left ovary. **C,** Transverse left ovary. **D,** Normal color Doppler of the ovary. **E,** Long right ovary. **F,** Transverse right ovary.

width × height). In the adult menstruating female, a normal ovary may have a volume as large as 22 cc,[3] with a mean ovarian volume of 9.8 ± 5.8 cc. An ovarian volume of more than 8 cc is definitely considered abnormal for the postmenopausal patient. An ovarian volume more than double that of the opposite side should also be considered abnormal, regardless of the actual size. Three-dimensional (3D) ultrasound may provide the most accurate method of ovarian volume measurement by allowing accurate determination of the ovarian long axis and objective calculation of stromal and cystic volume components. Further development in this technology will define future applications.

SONOGRAPHIC EVALUATION OF THE OVARIES

Simple Cystic Masses

An ovary's function is to mature oocytes until ovulation under the influence of luteinizing hormone and follicle-stimulating hormone from the pituitary. At the same time, the ovary synthesizes **androgens** (male hormones) and converts them to **estrogens** (female hormones). Finally, it produces progesterone after ovulation to sustain early pregnancy until the placenta can do so at 10 to 12 weeks of gestation.

Usually only one follicle enlarges from 3 mm to approximately 24 mm over about 10 days in the mid- and late-follicular phases of the cycle. This is followed by ovulation. The resulting corpus luteum or an abnormal unruptured follicle can persist as a simple or complex cystic structure from 1 to 10 cm in size. These so-called functional cysts may produce discomfort or delayed menses but can be observed to regress within 8 weeks with serial ultrasound studies. If a cyst greater than 6 cm persists more than 8 weeks, surgical intervention may be considered.

Ultrasound-guided needle aspiration has become another option for reducing recurrent **simple ovarian cysts** in carefully selected cases. The majority of ovarian masses are simple cysts, most of which are benign. Sonographic criteria for a simple cyst include a thin smooth wall, anechoic contents, and acoustic enhancement (Figure 42-4, *A*). In premenopausal women, these cysts usually are functional. The differential considerations of simple adnexal cysts include functional cyst, paraovarian cyst, cystadenoma, cystic teratoma, endometrioma, and rarely tubo-ovarian abscess (TOA) (Box 42-1).

Small anechoic cysts may be seen in postmenopausal ovaries. They can disappear or change in size over time. Serial sonographic studies can monitor the size and document any changes. Surgery is generally recommended for postmenopausal cysts greater than 5 cm and for those containing internal septations or solid nodules.

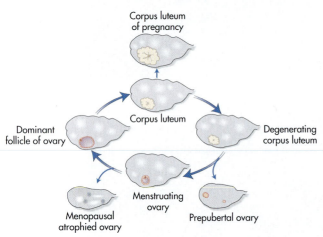

FIGURE 42-3 Diagram of cyclic changes of the normal ovary.

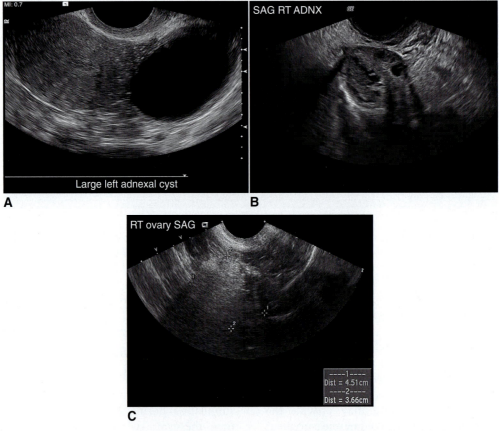

FIGURE 42-4 A, Simple ovarian cyst. The cyst is well defined and anechoic, with increased through-transmission. **B,** Complex ovarian cyst. Transvaginal sagittal image of a simple cyst that has hemorrhaged; this mass had resolved spontaneously when the patient was rescanned 2 weeks later. The borders of the mass are well defined; there are low-level internal echoes within the mass. On real-time imaging, swirling of these echoes could be seen. **C,** Solid mass. Transvaginal sagittal image of a large, solid ovarian mass in a 56-year-old woman. The mass has irregular borders with a heterogeneous texture and decreased through-transmission. This was a dermoid tumor.

BOX 42-1	Common Cystic or Homogeneous Ovarian Masses

- Follicular cyst
- Corpus luteum cyst of pregnancy
- Cystic teratoma
- Paraovarian cyst
- Hydrosalpinx
- Endometrioma (low-level echoes)
- Hemorrhagic cyst

BOX 42-2	Common Complex Masses

- Cystadenoma
- Dermoid cyst
- Tubo-ovarian abscess
- Ectopic pregnancy
- Granulosa cell tumor

BOX 42-3	Common Solid Masses

- Solid teratoma
- Adenocarcinoma
- Arrhenoblastoma
- Fibroma
- Dysgerminoma
- Torsion

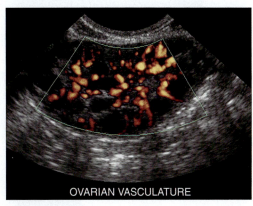

OVARIAN VASCULATURE

FIGURE 42-5 Color or power Doppler is useful to distinguish cystic structures from vessels.

Complex Masses

Any simple cyst that hemorrhages as it involutes may appear as a complex mass (Box 42-2). In patients of reproductive age, the classic differential considerations of a complex adnexal mass are ectopic pregnancy, endometriosis, and pelvic inflammatory disease (PID) (Figure 42-4, B). Dermoids and other benign tumors can appear in a similar fashion.

Solid Tumors

Mixed solid to cystic ovarian masses are typical of all the epithelial ovarian tumors; the most common are the serous types: **cystadenoma** and **cystadenocarcinoma** (Figure 42-4, C). During the peak fertile years, only 1 in 15 is malignant; this ratio becomes 1 in 3 after age 40.

The more sonographically complex the tumor, the more likely it is to be malignant, especially if associated with ascites. The epithelium of serous tumors is tubal in type, and there may be one or multiple cysts. One fourth of them are bilateral, and most occur in women over age 40. They are large and often fill the pelvic cavity.

The differential considerations of a solid-appearing adnexal mass include pedunculated fibroid, dermoid, fibroma, thecoma, granulosa cell tumor, Brenner tumor, and metastasis. Tubo-ovarian abscess, ovarian torsion, hemorrhagic cysts, and ectopic pregnancy also may appear solid. Solid adnexal masses are often difficult to diagnose because normal ovarian size varies widely. However, as previously noted, an ovary that has a volume double that of the opposite side is generally considered abnormal. When a solid mass is found, care should be taken to identify a connection with the uterus to differentiate an ovarian lesion from a pedunculated fibroid (Box 42-3). The use of color Doppler can be helpful, as color can be used to identify a vascular pedicle between the uterus and the mass, as can often be identified with pedunculation.

Doppler of the Ovary

When any abnormality of the ovary is detected, Doppler examination should be performed. In the case of a suspected cystic lesion, color Doppler is helpful in differentiating a potential cyst from adjacent vascular structures (Figure 42-5). Color also can be used to localize flow to further determine flow velocity with pulsed Doppler, which can be obtained on all ovarian masses. Pulsed Doppler interrogation of the adnexal branch of the uterine artery, the ovarian artery, or intratumoral flow is performed to determine the resistive index or pulsatility index (Figure 42-6). Patients with normal menstrual cycles are best scanned in the first 10 days of the cycle to avoid confusion with normal changes in intraovarian blood flow, because high diastolic flow occurs in the luteal phase (Figure 42-7).

A debate in the literature exists regarding the value of a resistive index (RI) in distinguishing between benign and malignant adnexal masses. The largest study in the literature uses a cutoff of greater than 0.4 as a normal RI in a nonfunctioning ovary.[7] Other investigators employ a pulsatility index of greater than 1 as normal.[1,5] Intratumoral vessels, low-resistance flow, and absence of a normal diastolic notch in the Doppler waveform are signs that may be worrisome for malignancy. In addition, abnormal waveforms can be seen in inflammatory masses, metabolically active masses (including ectopic pregnancy), and corpus luteum cysts. The most

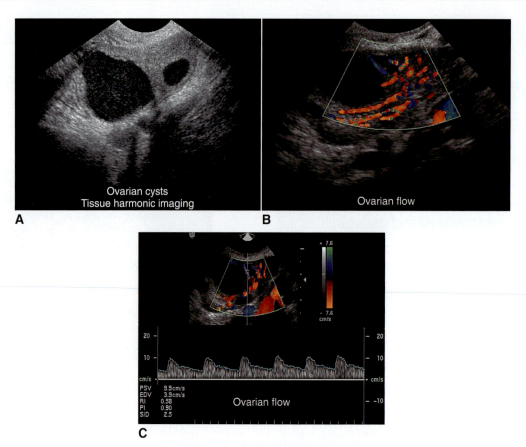

FIGURE 42-6 A, Simple cyst. Coronal view of the right ovary in an asymptomatic 52-year-old woman demonstrates a simple cyst. **B** and **C,** Ovarian artery Doppler shows a normal flow pattern with low diastolic flow.

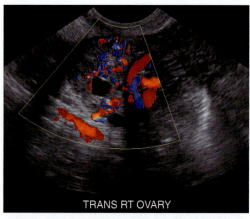

FIGURE 42-7 Transvaginal color Doppler view of the right adnexa in a woman during the hyperstimulation phase. Note the prominent flow to the ovary during this phase of treatment for infertility.

significant problem in the use of an RI is that it is not a sensitive indicator of malignancy. One study found a low RI in only 25% of malignant lesions.[8]

The color Doppler central distribution of the small arteries within an ovarian mass may be an important factor in malignancy. Two pulsed Doppler indices have been analyzed, comparing the relative amount of diastolic to systolic components of their arterial waveforms.

The **pulsatility index (PI)** is calculated as peak-systolic velocity minus end-diastolic velocity divided by the mean velocity. The **resistive index (RI)** is the peak-systolic velocity minus the end-diastolic velocity divided by the peak-systolic velocity. Although these indices have different cutoff values, increased diastolic flow suggests neovascularity and the likelihood of malignancy. The cutoff value for the PI is 1 and the value for the RI is 0.4, with malignancy considered more likely below and benign disease more likely above these values. Inflammatory masses, active endocrine tumors, and trophoblastic disease (ectopic pregnancies) may give low indices, thus mimicking cancer.

A mass showing a complete absence or minimal diastolic flow (very elevated RI and PI values) is usually benign. A diastolic notch in early diastole may also be a sign of benign disease. This finding is not often noted and its absence has no diagnostic value.

The PI and RI values may vary considerably in the fertile patient during the menstrual cycle, and this can complicate the pulsed Doppler analysis. In the first 7 days, the flow to the ovaries has the greatest resistance with the lowest diastolic flow and the indices are at their highest. Later in each cycle, the diastolic flow increases, particularly to the dominant ovary, and may lower the indices sufficiently to falsely suggest a malignant process.

A Doppler study can be performed at any time during the cycle. If the indices are in the benign range, they do not need to be repeated. However, if a suspicious mass is present and the indices suggest possible malignancy and are expected to affect management, a repeat study should be performed to confirm the abnormal indices in the first week of another cycle.

BENIGN ADNEXAL CYSTS

Functional Ovarian Cysts

Functional cysts result from the normal function of the ovary. They are the most common cause of ovarian enlargement in young women. Functional cysts include follicular, corpus luteum, hemorrhagic, and theca-lutein cysts. Hormonal therapy is sometimes administered to suppress a cyst. Most cysts measure less than 5 cm in diameter and regress during the subsequent menstrual cycle. A follow-up sonographic examination in 6 weeks usually documents change in size.

Follicular Cysts. A follicular cyst forms when a mature follicle fails to ovulate or involute postovulation (Box 42-4). These cysts are usually unilateral, asymptomatic, and less than 2 cm in size, but they can be as large as 20 cm in diameter. They regress spontaneously and are frequently detected incidentally on sonographic examinations.

Corpus Luteum Cysts. **Corpus luteum cysts** result from failure of resorption or from excess bleeding into the corpus luteum. These cysts usually are less than 4 cm in diameter and are unilateral. They are prone to hemorrhage and rupture. The presenting feature is often pain. If the ovum is fertilized, the corpus luteum continues as the corpus luteal cyst of pregnancy during the first trimester of pregnancy, when maximum size is reached by 10 weeks, and resolution occurring by 12 to 16 weeks (Box 42-5).

Sonographic Findings. Because of the hemorrhagic nature of these cysts, they usually appear as complex masses with central blood clot and echogenic septations (Figure 42-8). This appearance is difficult to distinguish from ectopic pregnancy and endometriosis. They may exhibit posterior acoustic enhancement, depending on the content.

Duplex Doppler reveals prominent diastolic flow in corpus luteum cysts. This low-velocity waveform is present throughout the luteal phase of the cycle. They may also have a peripheral rim of color around the wall of color Doppler, sometimes termed the "ring of fire."

BOX 42-4	Follicular Cysts

- Occur when a dominant follicle does not succeed in ovulating and remains active though immature
- Usually unilateral
- Thin-walled, translucent, watery fluid; may project above or within surface of the ovary
- May grow 1 to 8 cm
- Usually disappear spontaneously by resorption or rupture
- Clinical findings: Asymptomatic to dull, adnexal pressure and pain, abnormal ovarian function, torsion of the ovary resulting in severe pain
- Sonographic findings: Simple cyst

BOX 42-5	Corpus Luteum Cysts

- Result from hemorrhage within a persistently mature corpus luteum
- Filled with blood and cystic fluid
- May grow 1 to 10 cm in size
- May accompany intrauterine pregnancy (IUP)
- Clinical findings: Irregular menstrual cycle, pain, mimic ectopic pregnancy, rupture
- Sonographic findings: "Cystic" type of lesion; may have internal echoes secondary to hemorrhage and increased color

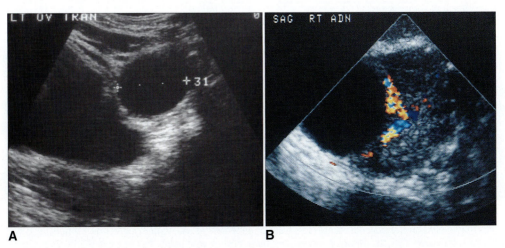

A **B**

FIGURE 42-8 Hemorrhagic corpus luteum cyst. Transabdominal **(A)** and transvaginal **(B)** views of the right adnexa demonstrate a 3.5-cm cystic mass with internal echoes. The acoustic enhancement posterior to this mass confirms its cystic nature.

Hemorrhagic Cysts. Internal hemorrhage may occur in follicular cysts or more commonly in corpus luteal cysts. The patient may present with an acute onset of pelvic pain.

◤ **Sonographic Findings.** The sonographic picture is variable depending on the amount of hemorrhage, clot formation, and time passed since hemorrhage (Figure 42-9). The internal characteristics are better visualized by transvaginal scanning, but transabdominal scanning should also be performed for a global view. An acute hemorrhagic cyst is usually hyperechoic and may mimic a solid mass. It usually has a smooth posterior wall and shows posterior acoustic enhancement indicating its cystic component. Diffuse low-level echoes may be seen but are more commonly seen in endometriomas. As time goes on, the internal pattern becomes more complex.

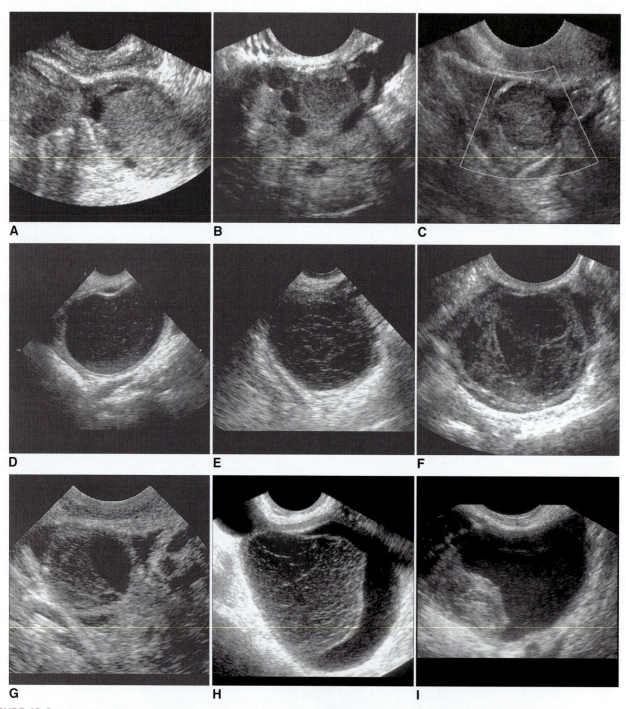

FIGURE 42-9 Hemorrhagic cysts on transvaginal scans—spectrum of appearances. **A,** Acute hyperechoic hemorrhagic cyst. **B,** Acute hemorrhagic cyst mimicking a solid lesion. **C,** Color Doppler shows peripheral ring of vascularity, but not vascularity within the cyst. **D,** Large cyst containing multiple internal low-level echoes. **E,** Reticular pattern of internal echoes and septations within cyst. **F,** Reticular pattern. **G-I,** Variations in clot retraction. The clot in **I** suggests a solid mass. Lack of color Doppler signal supports its benign nature.

The clotted blood becomes more echogenic and may show a fluid level. Echogenic free intraperitoneal fluid in the cul-de-sac can help confirm the diagnosis of a ruptured or leaking hemorrhagic cyst. This may mimic a ruptured ectopic pregnancy, so it is critical to know if the patient has a positive pregnancy test.

Theca-Lutein Cysts. Theca-lutein cysts are the largest of the functional cysts and appear as very large, bilateral, multiloculated cystic masses. They are associated with high levels of human chorionic gonadotropin (hCG). They are seen most frequently in association with gestational trophoblastic disease (30%). Similar cysts occur in normal pregnancies, especially multiple gestations, and in some patients being treated with infertility drugs, particularly Pergonal (Box 42-6). These cysts may undergo hemorrhage, rupture, and torsion (Figure 42-10).

Ovarian Syndromes

Ovarian Hyperstimulation Syndrome. Ovarian hyperstimulation syndrome (OHS) is a frequent iatrogenic complication of ovulation induction. This hyperstimulation can result in mild, moderate, and severe forms. In the mild form, the patient presents with pelvic discomfort but no significant weight gain. The ovaries are enlarged but measure less than 5 cm in diameter (Figure 42-11). With severe hyperstimulation, the patient

has severe pelvic pain, abdominal distention, and notably enlarged ovaries, measuring greater than 10 cm in diameter. There can also be associated ascites, pleural effusions, and numerous large, thin-walled cysts throughout the periphery of the ovary. When treated, this condition usually resolves within 2 to 3 weeks.

Polycystic Ovarian Syndrome. Polycystic ovarian syndrome (PCOS), which includes Stein-Leventhal syndrome (infertility, oligomenorrhea, hirsutism, and obesity), is an endocrine disorder associated with chronic anovulation (Box 42-7). An imbalance of LH and FSH results in abnormal estrogen and androgen production. The serum LH level is high and the FSH level is low. An elevated LH/FSH ratio is characteristic. Pathologically, the ovaries are rounded, usually two to five times normal size, with an increased number of follicles. Clinically, PCOS encompasses a spectrum of findings from hyperandrogenism in lean, normally menstruating women to obese women with severe hirsutism and oligomenorrhea or amenorrhea, as originally described by Stein and Leventhal. Manifestations of unopposed estrogenic hyperplasia and endometrial carcinoma occur in a significant proportion of patients, so long-term follow-up is recommended. PCOS is a common cause of infertility and a higher-than-usual rate of early pregnancy loss.

Sonographic Findings. On sonography, the ovaries appear normal or enlarged with echogenic stroma (Figure 42-12). Multiple small follicles are seen, often bilaterally, in the size range of 5 to 8 mm. The reported number of immature follicles varies in the literature from 11 to less than 15. The ovaries have a more rounded shape, with the follicles usually located peripherally, commonly referred to as the "string of pearls." Small cysts of variable size can also occupy both the subcapsular and stromal parts of the ovary. It is the multitude of these small cysts that contributes to the enlarged size of the ovary. Transvaginal sonography is more sensitive for detecting these small follicles than is transabdominal scanning. The diagnosis of PCOS is usually made biochemically, but sonography is useful. Serial studies show the follicles persist because ovulation does not occur.

Ovarian Remnant Syndrome. Infrequently, a cystic mass may be seen in a patient who has a history of bilateral oophorectomy. This usually results in a technically difficult surgery (because of adhesions), in which a

---

BOX 42-6	Theca-Lutein Cysts

- Large, bilateral, multiloculated cysts
- Associated with high levels of human chorionic gonadotropin
- Seen in 30% of patients with trophoblastic disease
- Clinical findings: Nausea and vomiting
- Sonographic findings: Multilocular cysts in both ovaries

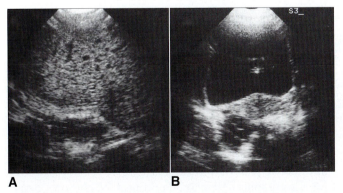

A   B

FIGURE 42-10 A, A patient in her 15th week of pregnancy came to the clinician with size larger than dates. The ultrasound examination showed an enlarged uterus completely filled with grapelike clusters. **B,** Evaluation of both ovaries demonstrated enlargement with multiple septations, suggesting the presence of bilateral theca-lutein cysts with the molar pregnancy.

BOX 42-7	Polycystic Ovarian Syndrome

- Includes Stein-Leventhal syndrome
- Bilaterally enlarged polycystic ovaries
- Occurs in late teens through twenties
- May have endocrine imbalance
- Spectrum of ultrasound appearances
- Clinical findings: Amenorrhea, obesity, infertility, hirsutism
- Sonographic findings: Multiple tiny cysts around the periphery of the ovary; ovary may be normal size or enlarged

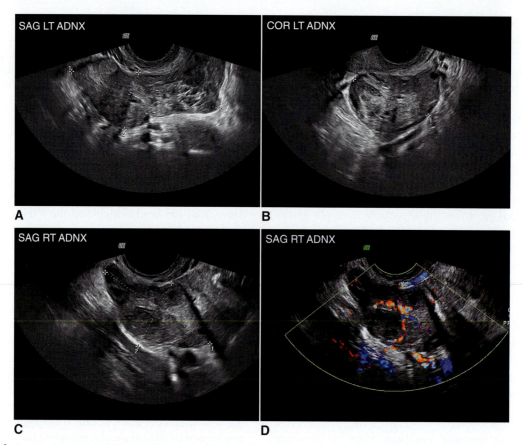

FIGURE 42-11 Ovarian hyperstimulation. **A,** Transvaginal image showing a notably enlarged and round ovary with multiple complicated cysts. **B,** Coronal image of the left ovary. **C,** Sagittal image of the prominent right ovary. **D,** Increased vascularity of the hyperstimulated ovary on the right.

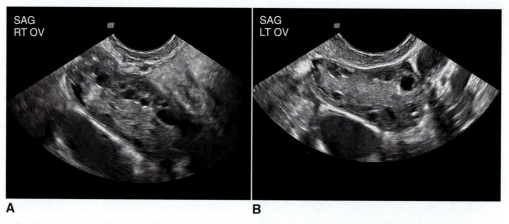

FIGURE 42-12 Polycystic ovarian syndrome. **A,** The right ovary is enlarged with prominent follicles around the periphery of the outer margin. **B,** The left ovary is likewise enlarged with the "string of pearls" enlarged follicles.

small amount of residual ovarian tissue has been unintentionally left behind. The residual ovarian tissue can become functional and produce cysts with a thin rim of ovarian tissue in the wall.

Other Benign Ovarian Cysts

Peritoneal Inclusion Cysts. Peritoneal inclusion cysts are lined with mesothelial cells and are formed when adhesions trap peritoneal fluid around the ovaries, resulting in a large adnexal mass. Clinically, most patients have pelvic pain or a pelvic mass.

Sonographic Findings. Peritoneal inclusion cysts (benign cystic mesothelioma) are multiloculated cystic adnexal masses. The diagnosis must include the presence of an intact ovary either within or on the margin of the cyst. The fluid may contain echoes as a result of hemorrhage or proteinaceous fluid (Figure 42-13).

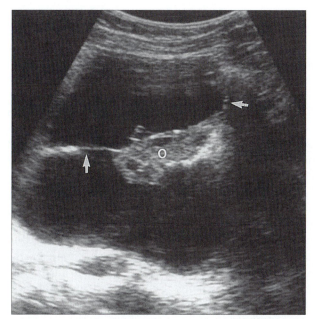

FIGURE 42-13 Peritoneal inclusion cyst. Transabdominal scan shows multiple fluid-filled cystic areas with linear septations *(arrows)* representing adhesions attached to normal ovary *(O)*.

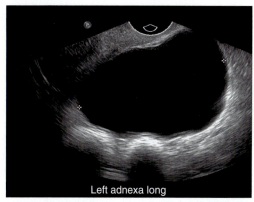

Left adnexa long

FIGURE 42-14 Paraovarian cyst. Transvaginal image of the paraovarian cyst that completely fills the adnexal region.

BOX 42-8 | **Paraovarian Cysts**

- Usually simple
- Can bleed or torse
- Wolffian duct remnants
- Ten percent of all adnexal masses
- Located in broad ligament
- Clinical findings: Asymptomatic
- Sonographic findings: Simple cyst adjacent to ovary

Predominantly these occur in premenopausal women with a history of abdominal surgery. The cyst may also occur in patients with a history of trauma, pelvic inflammatory disease, or endometriosis. The risk of recurrence after surgical resection is 30% to 50%. Do not confuse this condition with hydrosalpinx, which appears as a tubular or ovoid cystic structure with visible folds, where the ovary lies outside of the cystic structure.

Paraovarian Cysts. Paraovarian cysts account for approximately 10% of adnexal masses (Box 42-8). They arise from the broad ligament and usually are of mesothelial or paramesonephric origin. They may occur at any age but are more common in the third and fourth decades of life. A specific diagnosis of a paraovarian cyst is possible only by demonstrating a normal ipsilateral ovary close to, but separate from, the cyst. The cyst may undergo hemorrhage, torsion, or rupture similar to other cystic masses.

Sonographic Findings. Paraovarian cysts have thin, deformable walls that are not surrounded by ovarian stroma. They are difficult to distinguish from ovarian cysts and may contain small nodular areas and occasionally have septations. Paraovarian cysts vary in size and

can become large enough to extend into the upper abdomen. Paraovarian cysts can arise anywhere in the adnexal structures, and if they fill the pelvis, their point of origin may not be clear (Figure 42-14). Their size does not change with the hormonal cycle.

Fluid Collections in Adhesions. Fluid collections in adhesions can create cystic structures of odd shapes throughout the abdomen. Omental cysts tend to be higher in the abdomen, and urachal cysts are midline in the anterior abdominal wall peritoneum above the bladder. Any tumor may have cystic elements, and the sonographer should demonstrate if the tumor is a simple cyst or a complex mass.

Benign Cysts in Fetuses and Adolescents. Small simple cysts (1 to 7 mm) normally occur in fetuses and newborn girls because of stimulation by maternal hormones. In premenarchal girls, small follicles (less than 9 mm) are common. Larger cysts also are seen in otherwise healthy premenarchal girls. These may be followed closely if they are regressing, as long as the child's growth and development appear normal. Occasionally, ovarian cysts produce symptoms of precocious puberty in young girls. These may arise spontaneously or in association with other hormonal derangements.

Simple Cysts in Postmenopausal Women. Palpable ovaries in postmenopausal women are of concern. However, the cause of ovarian enlargement is often a simple adnexal cyst. In postmenopausal women, small (up to 3 cm) simple cysts of the ovaries are seen in approximately 15% of patients. These cysts commonly change in size and often disappear completely.

A large majority of ovarian malignancies are epithelial in origin and most are cystic. In the past, the occurrence of any ovarian cyst in a postmenopausal woman was considered abnormal and an indication for surgery. However, several retrospective studies have evaluated simple ovarian cysts and concluded that simple cystic lesions of the ovary, especially cysts less than 5 cm in diameter, are not likely to be malignant. It has therefore been recommended that if the resistive index is normal (greater than 0.4), these simple adnexal cysts should be followed sonographically rather than surgically removed.

ENDOMETRIOSIS

Endometriosis is a common condition in which functioning endometrial tissue is present outside the uterus. The ectopic tissue can be found almost anywhere in the pelvis, including the ovary, fallopian tube, broad ligament, the external surface of the uterus, and scattered over the peritoneum, cul-de-sac, and even the bladder. The endometrial tissue cyclically bleeds and proliferates. In the diffuse form, this leads to disorganization of the pelvic anatomy with an appearance similar to pelvic inflammatory disease (PID) or chronic ectopic pregnancy. Two forms of endometriosis have been described: diffuse and localized (endometrioma). The diffuse form is more common and consists of endometrial plantings within the peritoneum and is rarely diagnosed by sonography. The localized form consists of a discrete mass called an *endometrioma,* or *chocolate cyst,* and can frequently be found in multiple sites. The patient with an endometrioma is usually asymptomatic.

There are two possible explanations for endometriosis. The first is that the chronic reflux of menstrual fluid through the tubes and into the pelvis may, in some women, produce implantation and proliferation of endometrial cells with cyclic bleeding. The second theory involves the evolution of endometrial activity in susceptible cells that retain the embryonic capacity to differentiate in response to chronic irritation (for example, by menstrual fluid) or to hormonal stimulation. The resulting tissue bleeds and proliferates in response to cyclic hormones, producing pain, scarring, and distortion of adherent pelvic organs and endometrium-lined collections of blood known as endometriomas in the ovary. These may become moderately enlarged and create a surgical emergency by rupturing or by causing the ovary to twist on the vessels that supply it (torsion). Further discussion of endometriosis may be found in Chapter 43.

▶ **Sonographic Findings.** Endometriosis may appear as bilateral or unilateral ovarian cysts with patterns ranging from anechoic to solid, depending on the amount of blood and its organization (Figure 42-15). The ovaries are typically adherent to the posterior surface of the uterus or stuck in the cul-de-sac and may be intimately

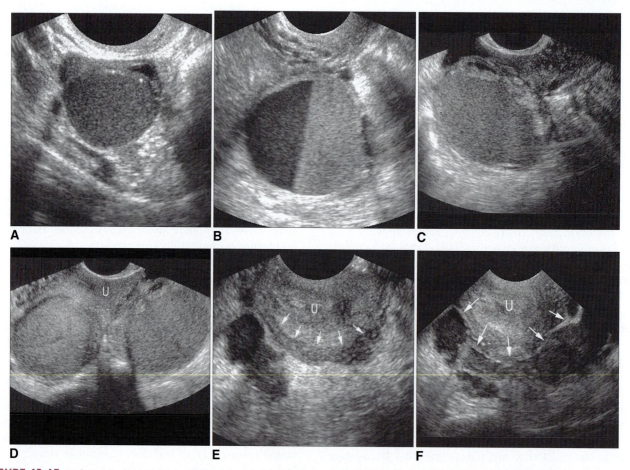

FIGURE 42-15 Endometriosis—spectrum of appearances. Transvaginal scans. Images **A** to **D** show uniform low-level echoes within a cystic ovarian mass. **A,** Typical peripheral echogenic foci. **B,** A fluid-filled level. **C,** Avascular marginal echogenic nodules. **D,** Bilateral disease. **E,** Endometriotic plaque on the posterior surface of the uterus *(arrows)* filling the pouch of Douglas **(F)** *(arrows). U,* Uterus.

associated with the rectosigmoid colon and difficult to define. Obscured organ borders and multiple irregular cystic masses also suggest either disseminating cancer or pelvic infection, and the clinical picture and serial sonographic studies determine when and if exploratory surgery is indicated.

The endometrioma is a well-defined unilocular or multilocular, predominantly cystic mass containing diffuse homogeneous, low-level internal echoes (Figure 42-16). It is better characterized on transvaginal scanning. Occasionally a fluid-fluid level can be seen. Small linear hyperechoic foci may be present in the wall and are thought to be cholesterol deposits accumulating in the cyst wall. Clinical symptoms help to differentiate endometriosis from a hemorrhagic ovarian cyst, ovarian neoplasm, or tubo-ovarian abscess.

OVARIAN TORSION

Torsion of the ovary is caused by partial or complete rotation of the ovarian pedicle on its axis. Torsion usually occurs in childhood and adolescence and is common in association with adnexal masses. **Ovarian torsion** produces an enlarged edematous ovary, usually greater than 4 cm in diameter. The classically described appearance is of multiple tiny follicles around a hypoechoic mass, but the most common presentation is that of a completely solid adnexal mass. Free fluid often is present in the pelvis. Doppler examination usually reveals absent blood flow to the torsed ovary (Box 42-9). Occasionally, however, blood flow can be detected to torsed ovaries. This is thought to be the result of the dual blood supply of the ovary or because of venous thrombosis, leading to symptoms before arterial thrombosis occurs.

Ovarian torsion is an unusual but serious problem because it accounts for 3% of gynecologic operative emergencies. Ovarian torsion is an acute abdominal condition requiring prompt diagnosis and surgical intervention. The ovarian pedicle partially or completely rotates on its axis, compromising the lymphatic and venous drainage. This causes edema and eventual loss of arterial perfusion with subsequent infarct. Torsion typically involves not only the ovary but also frequently the fallopian tube. It may also be seen in women during the

---

BOX 42-9 | Ovarian Torsion

- Usually associated with a mass
- Hypoechoic, enlarged ovary, with or without peripheral follicles
- Absent blood flow on Doppler examination
- Free fluid in cul-de-sac
- Surgical emergency

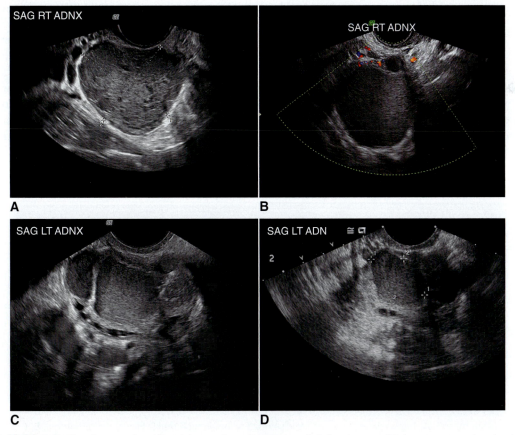

A   B

C   D

FIGURE 42-16   A-D, On ultrasound, endometriomas demonstrate a well-defined mass with homogeneous low-level echoes.

fertile years and even occurs during pregnancy in 20% of the cases. Torsion may present at any time in female life, from childhood to the postmenopausal period. Occasionally the lead point is an ovarian mass. Once torsion has occurred, there is a 10% increased incidence of torsion occurring in the contralateral adnexa. Torsion of a normal ovary usually occurs in children and younger females with mobile adnexa, preexisting ovarian cyst or mass, or pregnancy.

Clinically, acute severe unilateral pain is typically the presenting symptom in patients with torsion. Intermittent pain may precede the acute pain by weeks. These symptoms can be mimicked by many other pelvic or lower abdominal processes, and therefore quite frequently torsion is part of a differential diagnostic list. The patient may also have fever, nausea, and vomiting. More than 50% of patients feel a palpable mass. The right ovary is three times more likely to torse than the left.

🔖 **Sonographic Findings.** As a general rule, ovarian torsion is unlikely when the ovary is normal in size and texture with sonography. The torsed ovary is typically enlarged and heterogeneous in appearance, owing to edema, hemorrhage, or necrosis (Figure 42-17). There is often a lead mass, but in some cases this mass is not appreciated because it is mixed in with the necrosis and hemorrhage of the torsed mass. Torsed masses are often large (greater than 4 cm in diameter), vary in appearance from cystic to solid, and vary in echogenicity from relatively anechoic to markedly hyperechoic. A palpable mass may be present. Torsion occurs more frequently on the right side, and the pain may mimic acute appendicitis.

The differentiation of torsion from other adnexal masses is often not possible unless there is clinical suspicion. The sonographic picture varies, depending on the duration and degree of vascular compromise. The ovary is enlarged and may have multiple cortical follicles. Free fluid in the cul-de-sac is a common finding. Color and spectral Doppler may show absent flow in the affected ovary. However, Doppler findings may vary on the degree and chronicity of the torsion and whether or not there is an associated adnexal mass. If torsion is intermittent, a "hyperemic" increased diastolic flow during the times when torsion is not present may be seen. This could be related to the dual ovarian arterial blood supply from the ovarian artery and ovarian branches of the uterine artery. Different appearances include target, ellipsoid, or tubular structures with internal heterogeneous echoes. Doppler may show the presence of circular, coiled twisted vessels, known as the *whirlpool sign*. The presence of arterial or venous flow or both does not exclude the diagnosis of torsion. Comparison with the appearance of morphology and flow patterns in the contralateral ovary helps in the evaluation.

SONOGRAPHIC EVALUATION OF OVARIAN NEOPLASMS

Sonographic screening finds adnexal cysts in 1% to 15% of postmenopausal women. Only 3% of ovarian cysts less than 5 cm are malignant. Therefore, it is recommended that a cyst greater than 5 cm be surgically removed. In the postmenopausal woman, the ovaries are enlarged; if a mass is seen, it may be mixed texture to solid with papillae within. Well-defined anechoic lesions are more likely to be benign, whereas lesions with irregular walls, thick irregular septations, mural nodules, and solid echogenic elements favor malignancy. Doppler examination shows a low-resistive pattern. Extension beyond the ovary into the omentum or peritoneum and liver metastases should be evaluated. Malignant ascites may also be present. Unilocular or thinly septated cysts are more likely to be benign. Multilocular, thickly septated masses and masses with solid nodules are more likely to be malignant. In advanced stages, peritoneal carcinomatosis with malignant ascites and peritoneal implants can be seen.

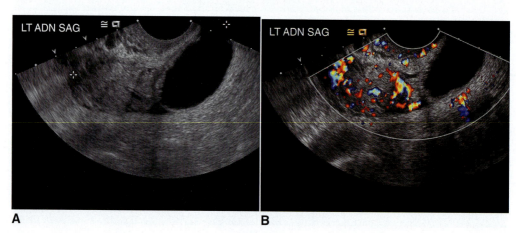

A   **B**

FIGURE 42-17 Ovarian torsion. **A,** Transvaginal images of the distended fallopian tube that is filled with hematoma. **B,** Color Doppler shows increased flow surrounding the inflamed tubal torsion.

Any change in ovarian echogenicity or volume of more than 20 ml should be considered suspicious. In postmenopausal women, the ovaries become atrophic and often do not have follicles. Thus, the ovary can be difficult to identify. Only women receiving hormone replacement therapy continue to have normal-sized ovaries. Abnormal ovaries suggestive of malignancy are defined as enlarged echogenic ovaries (more than twice the size of normal ovaries or greater than two standard deviations above the norm [for the woman's age]).

Although ultrasound is able to identify masses and subtle changes in ovaries, it is not often able to distinguish benign from malignant. Doppler imaging has been studied to determine whether it can detect the neovascularity of malignant masses. Pulsed Doppler imaging is then performed to analyze the vascular component. When evaluating the soft tissue from the margins of the abnormal ovary or mass, care must be taken so that the sample volume does not obtain flow patterns from adjacent normal structures.

OVARIAN CARCINOMA

Ovarian cancer is often detected by a combination of physical examination and laboratory and imaging findings. Every year **ovarian carcinoma** kills more women than cancer of the uterine cervix and body combined and is the fourth leading cause of cancer death. The American Cancer Society estimates that there were 22,000 new cases of ovarian cancer in the United States in 2009 and that about 15,000 women die from this disease annually. Approximately 1 in 70 women develop the disease. Ovarian carcinoma is the leading cause of death from gynecologic malignancy (25%) in the United States. Sixty percent of the ovarian malignancies occur in women between 40 and 60 years of age. About 80% of cases involve women over 60 years of age, with the risk of cancer increasing with age. New chemotherapeutic and surgical techniques have done little to decrease mortality, so continued efforts are being directed at developing methods of early diagnosis. The 5-year survival rate is 50% (stages I through IV). If the cancer is found early (stage I), the survival greatly improves to 93%; however, less than 20% of all ovarian cancer is found at this stage.

Ovarian malignancy is a "silent" cancer. Because of its relative absence of symptoms early in the disease, ovarian cancer commonly is not detected until advanced, either having spread beyond the capsule but still within the pelvis (stage II) or into the abdomen (stage III). At the time of initial detection, 50% of women present with stage III spread. The adnexal finding on physical examination is variable, ranging from almost "normal" to slightly enlarged firm irregular ovaries to pelvic masses. In advanced disease, ascites and omental masses may be palpated. The blood chemistry test CA 125 is helpful in some patients but has been disappointing as a screening test because of its inability to detect many cases of ovarian cancer. It has many false-positive and false-negative results, and elevated levels are found in only 50% of patients with stage III ovarian cancer. If a baseline level is known, however, such as for patients who have undergone resection of primary ovarian cancer, then an elevated follow-up level has greater significance.

Ovarian cancer can present as either a complex, cystic, or solid mass, but it is more likely predominantly cystic; as many as 20% are bilateral. Differential diagnoses include endometriosis, hemorrhagic ovarian cyst, ovarian torsion, PID, and benign ovarian neoplasms (e.g., serous cystadenoma, mucinous cystadenoma, dermoid, fibroma, and thecoma). An exophytic fibroid or a nongynecologic mass may also appear in the adnexa and resemble an ovarian neoplasm. The likelihood of malignancy is increased by the greater the amount of solid tissue in a complex ovarian mass and the presence of complex ascites.

The size of the ovarian mass, age of the patient, and ultrasound characteristics of the mass relate directly to its potential for being malignant. Masses less than 5 cm in their longest axis are much more likely to be benign, whereas masses larger than 10 cm are much more likely to be malignant. Increasing patient age also correlates with an increased incidence of malignancy. The primary clinical problem with this disease is the asymptomatic and undetectable nature of the cancer in the earliest stages. Often the patient will seek medical attention after ascites has initiated abdominal distention. The 5-year survival rate for stage IV ovarian cancer is 5%; stage I tumors diagnosed early and confined to the capsule show a survival rate of 90% at 5 years.

The incidence of ovarian cancer is greatly increased in women who have had breast and colon cancer. This appears primarily related to genetic mutations in the BRCA1 and BRCA2 genes and less commonly in the MSH2 and MLH1 genes.

The strongest risk factor is a family history of ovarian or breast cancer. Women with carcinoma of the breast have increased risk of developing ovarian cancer, and women with ovarian cancer are three to four times more likely to develop breast cancer. Other risk factors include increasing age, nulliparity, infertility, uninterrupted ovulation, and late menopause. About 3% to 5% of women with a family history of ovarian cancer will have a hereditary ovarian cancer syndrome. The three main hereditary syndromes associated with ovarian cancer are the breast-ovarian, nonpolyposis colorectal, and site-specific ovarian cancer syndrome. They have an earlier age of onset than do other ovarian cancers.

Clinical symptoms include vague abdominal pain, swelling, indigestion, frequent urination, constipation, and weight change (ascites). Over 70% of the women first seen by their doctors are in advanced stages of the disease. Although the median age of diagnosis is 63 years, the peak age ranges between 55 and 59 years, although it may also affect women in their forties.

Ovarian cancer arises primarily from epithelial tumors (60% to 70%), including serous cystadenocarcinoma (50%), endometrioid tumor similar to endometrial adenocarcinoma (15% to 30%), mucinous cystadenocarcinoma (15%), clear cell carcinoma (5%), Brenner tumor (2.5%), and undifferentiated tumor (less than 5%).[4] Germ cell tumors contribute 15% to 30% of the malignancies and are more common in girls and young women (age 4 to 27 years); they include mature teratoma, dysgerminoma, immature teratoma, transdermal sinus tumor, malignant mixed germ cell tumor, choriocarcinoma, and embryonal carcinoma. Metastases (5% to 10%) and stromal tumors (5%) are the remaining tumors that contribute to ovarian cancer.

On laparotomy, the cancer is classified into one of the following stages:

Stage I: Limited to ovary
  a. Limited to one ovary
  b. Limited to two ovaries
  c. Positive peritoneal lavage (ascites)
Stage II: Limited to pelvis
  a. Involvement of the uterus/fallopian tubes
  b. Extension to other pelvic tissues
  c. Positive peritoneal lavage (ascites)
Stage III: Limited to abdomen-intraabdominal extension outside pelvis/retroperitoneal nodes/extension to small bowel/omentum
Stage IV: Hematogenous disease (liver parenchyma)/spread beyond abdomen

The treatment for ovarian carcinoma includes surgery and chemotherapy initially, followed by a second laparotomy in 6 months and follow-up CA 125 blood tests and computed tomography (CT) scans.

The CA 125 test is a serum marker for ovarian cancer; it is elevated in more than 80% of epithelial ovarian cancers. It has not been found effective as a screening tool because only 50% of stage I malignant ovarian tumors have CA 125 levels higher than 35 U/ml, and the method has a high false-positive rate that is attributed to nonmalignant gynecologic disease. It is also insensitive to mucinous and germ-cell tumors. Levels of CA 125 may be elevated in benign conditions, such as endometriosis, pelvic inflammatory disease, uterine fibroids, pregnancy, and in other types of cancer not arising from the ovaries.

Sonographic Findings. Sonographically, ovarian cancer usually presents with an adnexal mass (Figure 42-18). Although sonography can detect morphologic characteristics of the tumor, it cannot (with the exception of dermoid cysts) histologically distinguish benign from malignant tumors. In general, well-defined, smooth bordered anechoic lesions are more likely to be benign. Lesions with irregular walls, thick, irregular septations, mural nodules, and solid echogenic elements are frequently malignant. Mixed cystic and solid masses are the most frequent presentation of the common epithelial

tumors of the ovary. Ascites, extension to adjacent organs, peritoneal implants, lymphadenopathy, and hepatic metastases support the diagnosis of malignant disease (Figure 42-19).

Doppler Findings in Ovarian Cancer

Abnormal tumor vascularity and abnormal RI or PI are also worrisome for malignancy. The results of the many studies using Doppler are quite variable. It is difficult to compare studies because of many factors, such as the lack of standardization of equipment, technical settings and techniques, and differences in various patient populations. Absence of flow within a lesion usually indicates a benign lesion. This is based on the premise that malignant masses, because of internal neovascularization, will have high diastolic flow, which can be seen on spectral Doppler waveforms. Malignant tumor growth is dependent on angiogenesis with the development of abnormal tumor vessels. This leads to decreased vascular resistance and higher diastolic flow velocity.

Contrast imaging in ultrasound will enable us to image the anatomic area better and give the physician more confidence in determining whether an exam is abnormal or normal. It might allow us to distinguish between benign and malignant lesions. Vascular contrast agents consist of surfactant coated or encapsulated gas microbubbles less than 10 U/m in diameter. These agents are injected into the bloodstream via a peripheral vein and then circulate through the body. The vascular contrast agent Echovist, used to diagnose ovarian malignancies, shows increased brightness of power Doppler signal and the amount of recognizable vascular areas after contrast administration. The contrast agent enhancement was significantly higher in malignant than benign adnexal masses. There was also an increase in the number of recognizable vessels after contrast agent administration. Contrast agent uptake times were significantly shorter in malignant than benign tumors. For differentiation of benign from malignant tumors, the kinetic properties of the contrast agent, such as uptake and washout times, have significant potential in diagnosis.

EPITHELIAL TUMORS

Gynecologic tumors that arise from the surface epithelium and cover the ovary and the underlying stroma are termed **surface epithelial-stromal tumors**. This group accounts for 65% to 75% of all ovarian neoplasms and 80% to 90% of all ovarian malignancies. The two most common types are serous and mucinous tumors. Serous tumors are the most common and constitute 30% of all ovarian neoplasms. Mucinous tumors account for 20% to 25% of ovarian neoplasms. The benign or low-malignancy potential form is termed *adenoma* and the malignant form is termed *adenocarcinoma*. The prefix *cyst* is added if the lesion is cystic, and *fibroma* is added

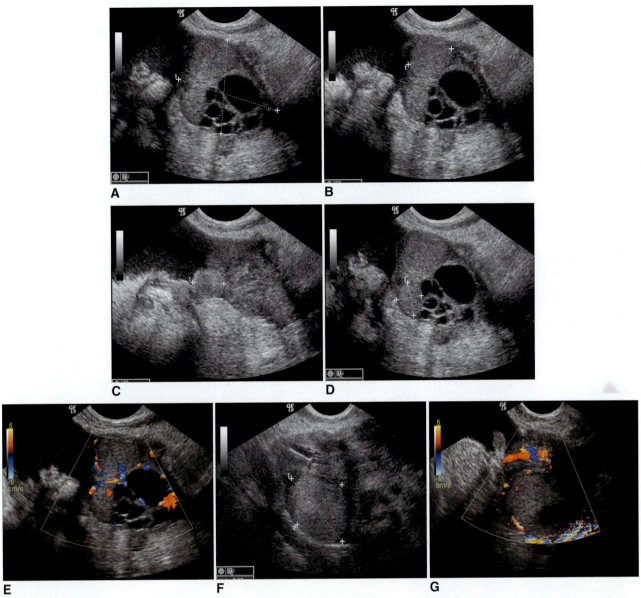

FIGURE 42-18 Ovarian carcinoma with bilateral metastases. **A,** Transverse left adnexa shows large complex mass. **B,** Transverse left adnexa. **C,** Transverse left adnexa shows nodule superior to uterine fundus. **D,** Transverse left adnexa shows uterus, mass, ovaries, and vascular structures. **E,** Color Doppler of increased vascular flow. **F,** Right transverse of large mass. **G,** Increased vascularity demonstrated with color Doppler.

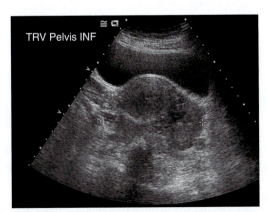

FIGURE 42-19 Ovarian carcinoma. A large, solid mass was found adjacent to the uterus in the right adnexa in this 49-year-old woman whose presenting symptom was a palpable mass. Complications of advanced stages of ovarian carcinoma led to malignant ascites.

if the tumor is more than 50% fibrous. Mucinous tumors are less frequently bilateral than are the serous type.

Some investigators believe that benign-appearing tumors (which are anechoic, thin walled, have no septation, and are acoustically enhanced) can be aspirated safely.[2,6]

Metastatic spread is primarily intraperitoneal, although direct extension to surrounding structures and lymphatics is not uncommon. Hematogenous spread usually occurs late in the course of the disease.

  Sonographic Findings. Serous and mucinous tumors vary greatly in size but can be very large. They often fill the pelvis and extend into the abdomen. In general, serous tumors are smaller than mucinous tumors (Figure 42-20).

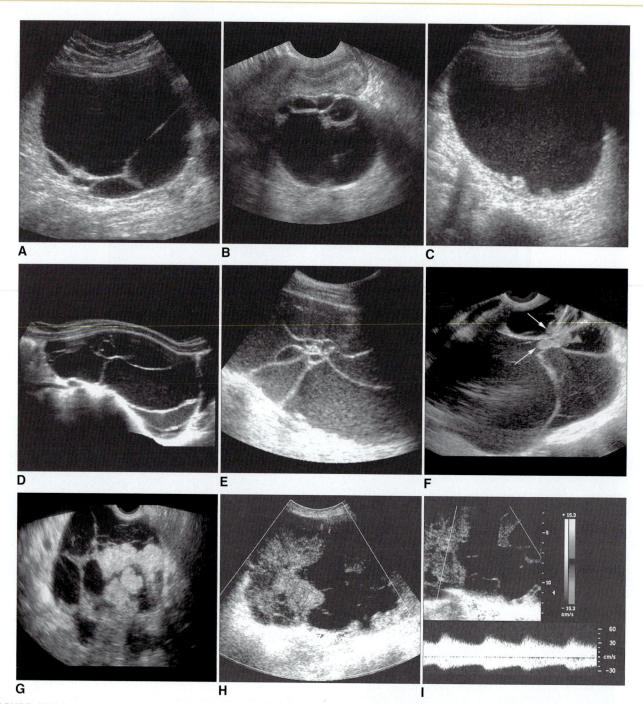

FIGURE 42-20 Epithelial ovarian neoplasms—spectrum of appearances. **A, B,** and **C** show serous cystadenomas. In **A,** septations within a cystic mass are fairly thin. In **B,** septations are thicker, and in **C,** there are low-level echogenic particles and small mural nodules. **D** and **E** are mucinous cystadenomas, and **F** is a mucinous cystadenocarcinoma. Large size and septations are characteristic; septal nodularity is marked in **F** *(arrows)*. **G, H,** and **I** are images in a single patient with a serous cystadenocarcinoma. Extensive nodularity shows vascularity confirming the morphologic suspicion of a malignant mass. There is high diastolic flow resulting in a low resistive index.

Mucinous Cystadenoma

Mucinous cystadenoma is a type of epithelial tumor that is lined by the mucinous elements of the endocervix and bowel. It constitutes 20% to 25% of all benign ovarian neoplasms. When benign, it is a mucinous cystadenoma; when malignant, it is a cystadenocarcinoma. This type of tumor is usually found in a woman between the ages of 13 and 45 years. A reported 80% to 85% of mucinous tumors are benign. These tumors can be large, measuring 15 to 30 cm in diameter, and weigh more than 100 pounds. They can fill the entire pelvis and abdomen. The tumor is usually benign and unilateral (5% bilateral) (Box 42-10).

▶ **Sonographic Findings.** In 75% of patients with mucinous tumors, ultrasound examination shows simple or

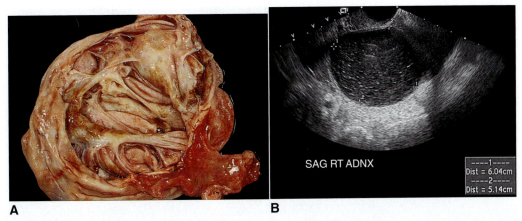

A   **B**

FIGURE 42-21 Mucinous cystadenoma. **A,** Gross pathology of a mucinous cystadenoma of the intestinal type. **B,** A 37-year-old woman presented with pelvic pressure and fullness. A large pelvic mass was found on pelvic examination. The sonogram shows a large homogeneous cystic-appearing mass with smooth borders.

BOX 42-10	Mucinous Cystadenoma

- Unusually large (15 to 30 cm)
- Most common cystic tumor
- Usually unilateral
- Cyst filled with sticky, gelatin-like material
- Multilocular cystic spaces
- Benign type more common than malignant
- Clinical findings: Pressure, pain, increased abdominal girth
- Sonographic findings: Simple or septate thin-walled multilocular cysts

BOX 42-11	Mucinous Cystadenocarcinoma

- Bilateral
- May occur in menopausal women (10%)
- Large, likely to rupture—ascites
- Clinical findings: Pelvic pressure, pain when ruptured
- Sonographic findings: Ascites appears as hypoechoic fluid with bright punctate echoes; thick, irregular walls and septations

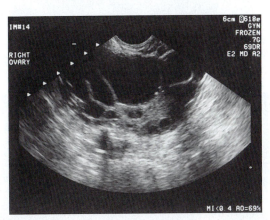

FIGURE 42-22 Mucinous cystadenocarcinoma. A large septated mass with thick, irregular walls was found in this 33-year-old woman.

septate thin-walled multilocular cysts (Figure 42-21). They often contain internal echoes with compartments differing in echogenicity caused by the mucoid material in the dependent portions.

Mucinous Cystadenocarcinoma

Mucinous cystadenocarcinoma most frequently occurs in women 40 to 70 years old and accounts for 5% to 10% of all primary malignant ovarian neoplasms; 15% to 20% are bilateral when malignant (Box 42-11); 10% occur in menopausal women. These tumors can also become very large and are more likely than the benign form to rupture. If the tumor ruptures, it is associated with pseudomyxoma peritoneum. This causes loculated ascites with mass effect.

  Sonographic Findings. On examination, malignant cysts tend to have thick, irregular walls and septations with papillary projections and echogenic material (Figures 42-22 and 42-23). They generally have a sonographic appearance similar to that of serous cystadenocarcinomas.

Penetration of the tumor capsule or rupture may lead to the mucoid ascites that appears as hypoechoic fluid with bright punctate echoes. This condition, known as pseudomyxoma peritonei, can be seen in mucinous cystadenomas and cystadenocarcinomas or mucinous tumors of the appendix and colon. It may contain multiple septations and low-level echogenic material that fills much of the pelvis and abdomen.

Serous Cystadenoma

Serous cystadenoma is the second most common benign tumor of the ovary (after the dermoid cyst) and represents 20% to 25% of all benign ovarian neoplasms (Figure 42-24). This tumor is usually unilateral (20% are bilateral) (Box 42-12).

  Sonographic Findings. Serous tumors are usually unilocular or multilocular with thin septations (Figure 42-25). They are smaller than the mucinous cysts (up to

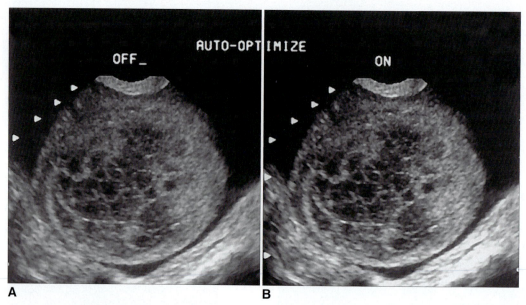

FIGURE 42-23 Mucinous cystadenocarcinoma. Adjustments in equipment features with auto optimization may help the sonographer to better determine the thickness of the septations within the large ovarian mass.

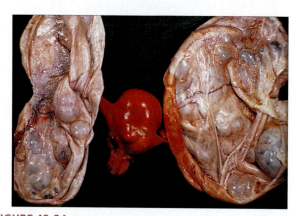

FIGURE 42-24 Serous cystadenoma. Gross pathology of the lesion that demonstrates the multiple small cystic areas within the mass.

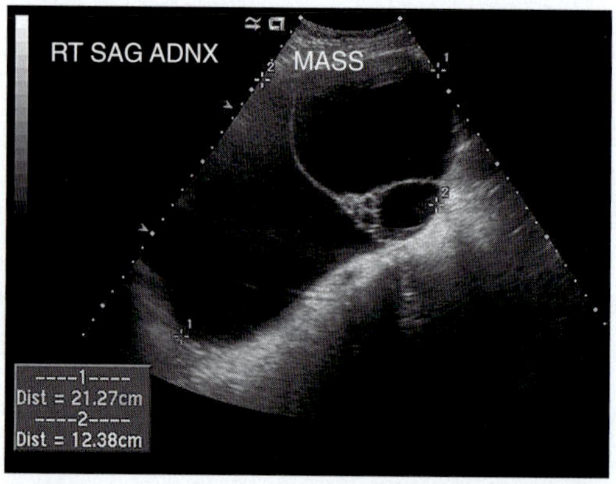

FIGURE 42-25 Serous cystadenoma. Multilocular mass with septations is seen in this ovarian mass posterior to the bladder.

BOX 42-12 | **Serous Cystadenoma**

- Usually unilateral
- Smaller than mucinous cysts
- Multilocular cysts with septations
- Clinical findings: Pelvic pressure, bloating
- Sonographic findings: Multilocular cyst—may have nodule

BOX 42-13 | **Serous Cystadenocarcinoma**

- External papillary mass adhesions and infection lead to bilateral involvement
- Loss of capsular definition and tumor fixation; calcifications
- Peritoneal implants; ascites; metastases to omentum, lymph nodes, liver, and lungs
- Clinical findings: Pelvic fullness, bloating
- Sonographic findings: Cystic structure with septations or papillary projections; internal and external papillomas usually present

---

20 cm); borders are irregular with a loss of capsular definition. Multilocular cysts contain a small amount of solid tissue in chambers of varying size with occasional internal septum or mural nodules.

Serous Cystadenocarcinoma

Serous cystadenocarcinoma constitutes 60% to 80% of all ovarian carcinomas. More than half of these tumors are bilateral.

Sonographic Findings. Serous cystadenocarcinomas are smaller than mucinous cysts, but they still may be quite large, with irregular borders and a loss of capsular definition (Box 42-13). The tumor may be accompanied by bilateral ovarian enlargement. Multilocular cysts contain chambers of varying size with septated, internal papillary projections. Calcifications may be present.

Solid elements or bilateral tumors suggest malignancy (Figure 42-26). Ascites forms secondary to peritoneal surface implantation and is frequently seen. The tumor may spread to the lymph nodes (e.g., periaortic, mediastinal, and supraclavicular).

Other Epithelial Tumors

Less common varieties of epithelial tumors are endometrioid, clear cell, Brenner (transitional cell), and undifferentiated carcinoma. Endometrioid tumors are nearly all malignant and are the second most common epithelial malignancy. Approximately 25% to 30% are bilateral and occur most frequently postmenopausal; peak age ranges from 50 to 60 years. Clear cell tumors are considered to be of müllerian duct origin and a variant of the endometrioid carcinoma. Clear cell tumors are nearly always malignant and are bilateral about 20% of the time. Peak age ranges from 50 to 70 years. Transitional cell tumor, also known as *Brenner tumor,* is uncommon. The Brenner tumor is found in 1.5% to 2.5% of patients; peak age ranges from 40 to 70 years. It is nearly always benign and 6% to 7% are bilateral; 30% are associated with cystic neoplasms in the ipsilateral ovary.

Sonographic Findings. These types of epithelial tumors cannot be distinguished sonographically; however, they are more frequently found unilaterally. They are usually small and present as a nonspecific, complex, predominantly cystic mass. Occasionally the tumor may contain hemorrhage or necrosis. The Brenner tumors are hypoechoic, solid masses that may contain calcifications in the outer wall. They are composed of dense fibrous stroma and appear similar to ovarian fibromas and thecomas.

GERM CELL TUMORS

Germ cell tumors are derived from the primitive germ cells of the embryonic gonad. They account for 15% to 20% of ovarian neoplasms, with approximately 95% being benign cystic teratomas. Besides teratomas, germ cell tumors include dysgerminoma, embryonal cell carcinoma, choriocarcinoma, and transdermal sinus tumor. These types are rare and occur mainly in adolescents and are the most common ovarian malignancy in this age group. Germ cell tumors often occur as mixed tumors with elements of two or three varieties of germ cell tumors. They are associated with elevated alpha-fetoprotein (AFP) and hCG levels.

Clinical symptoms include pelvic or abdominal pain and a palpable mass (average diameter is 15 cm). The germ cell tumor is usually unilateral; 40% of tumors will calcify. The tumor ranges in texture from homogeneously solid (3%), predominantly solid (85%), to predominantly cystic (12%).

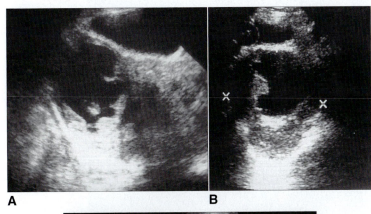

A   B

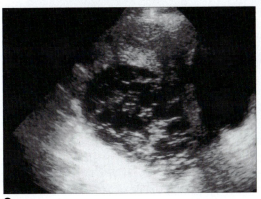

C

FIGURE 42-26 Serous cystadenocarcinoma. **A** and **B,** A 14-cm mass was found in a 62-year-old woman. This mass had papillary projections within. **C,** In another patient, the ovarian mass showed multiple thick septations within. Massive ascites was seen throughout the pelvic cavity.

Teratoma

Dermoid Tumors. Dermoid tumors are the most common ovarian neoplasm, constituting 20% of ovarian tumors. Up to 15% are bilateral. About 80% occur in women of childbearing age, but they may occur at any age. They are composed of well-differentiated derivatives of the three germ layers: ectoderm, mesoderm, and endoderm. In 10% of cases, the tumor is diagnosed during pregnancy. A rare dermoid that is composed of thyroid tissue is termed a *stroma ovarii* (thyroid tissue) and may produce insuppressible thyrotoxicosis. Malignant degeneration into squamous cell carcinoma is uncommon (2%) in teratomas, usually in older women.

Sonographic Findings. Dermoids have a spectrum of sonographic appearances, depending on which elements (ectoderm, mesoderm, or transderm) are present. Teeth, bones, and fat can be seen on plain films (Box 42-14). Clinical findings include abdominal mass or pain secondary to torsion or hemorrhage.

Sonography may demonstrate one of several patterns: (1) a completely cystic mass, (2) a cystic mass with a very echogenic nodule along the mural wall representing a "dermoid plug," (3) a fat-fluid level, (4) high-amplitude echoes with shadowing (e.g., teeth or bone), or (5) a complex mass with internal septations (Figures 42-27 and 42-28). Echogenic dermoids are often confused with bowel, as the mass may have characteristics similar to those of complex bowel tissue with shadowing posterior. If a palpable pelvic mass is present that is not identified on sonography, an echogenic dermoid must be considered and further imaging is usually performed. Indentation on the bladder wall will be a clue that a pelvic mass is present. The calcification within the pelvic cavity is also shown on the radiograph.

The term "tip-of-the-iceberg" refers to a mixture of matted hair and sebum producing ill-defined acoustic shadowing that obscures the posterior wall of the lesion.

BOX 42-14	Dermoid Tumors

- Size ranges from small to 40 cm
- Unilateral, round to oval mass
- Contains fatty, sebaceous material, hair, cartilage, bone, teeth
- Clinical findings: Asymptomatic to abdominal pain, enlargement and pressure; pedunculated, subject to torsion
- Sonographic findings: Cystic/complex/solid mass, echogenic components; acoustic shadowing

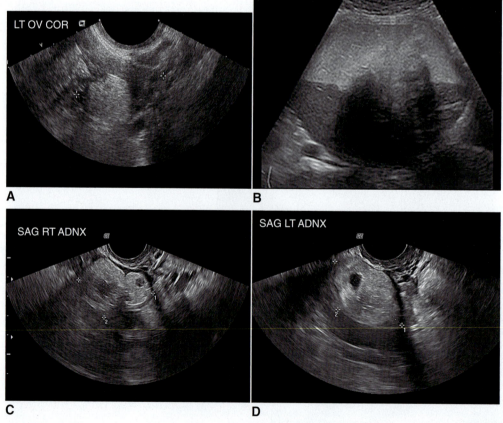

FIGURE 42-27 Dermoid tumor. Spectrum of appearances on sonography. **A,** Complex dermoid with an echogenic mural nodule. **B,** Solid dermoid with calcification and shadowing. **C,** Calcification and shadowing are shown in this complex dermoid tumor. **D,** Complex pattern of a dermoid tumor.

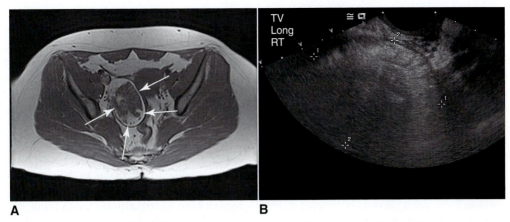

FIGURE 42-28 A, MRI of a young female with a calcified dermoid tumor shown within the pelvic cavity *(arrows)*. **B,** Transvaginal image of the large calcified dermoid tumor in the right pelvic cavity.

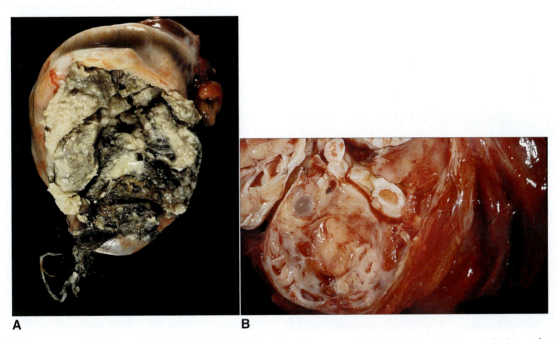

FIGURE 42-29 A, Gross pathology of the dermoid cyst filled with sebaceous material and hair. **B,** Gross pathology of an immature teratoma.

The "dermoid mesh" refers to multiple linear hyperechoic interfaces floating within the cyst and represent hair.

Acute hemorrhage into an ovarian cyst or an endometrioma may be so echogenic that it resembles a dermoid or a dermoid plug. Posterior sound enhancement is usually seen where a dermoid plug usually causes attenuation. Other pitfalls include a pedunculated fibroid or an appendicolith in a perforated appendix.

Immature and Mature Teratomas

Immature teratomas are uncommon and occur in girls and young women 10 to 20 years of age. These are rapidly growing, solid malignant tumors with many tiny cysts. Alpha-fetoprotein is elevated in 50% of patients. The tumor is unilateral and small in size, although it may grow to a larger dimension (Figure 42-29).

Sonographic Findings. On examination, the texture of immature teratomas ranges from cystic to complex; the teratoma usually is solid with internal echoes. Calcifications are commonly seen.

Dysgerminoma

Dysgerminoma is a rare malignant germ cell tumor that is bilateral in 15% of cases. The mass constitutes 1% to 2% of primary ovarian neoplasms and 3% to 5% of ovarian malignancies. An entirely solid ovarian mass in a woman less than 30 years of age is usually a dysgerminoma. The dysgerminoma and the serous cystadenoma are the two most common ovarian neoplasms seen in pregnancy (Figure 42-30).

Sonographic Findings. Dysgerminoma is a hyperechoic solid mass with areas of hemorrhage and necrosis on ultrasound examination. It may show a speckled pattern of calcifications. In a postmenopausal patient, a fibroma or thecoma is most likely.

Endodermal Sinus Tumor

Endodermal sinus tumors are rare rapidly growing tumors also called *yolk sac tumors*. The lesion usually occurs in women under 20 years of age and is almost always unilateral. Increased serum AFP may be seen. Endodermal sinus tumor has a poor prognosis and is the second most common malignant ovarian germ cell neoplasm after dysgerminoma. The sonographic appearance is similar to that of the dysgerminoma.

STROMAL TUMORS

Sex-cord stromal tumors typically are solid adnexal masses that arise from the sex cords of the embryonic gonadal or ovarian stroma. This category includes granulosa cell tumor, thecoma, fibroma, and Sertoli-Leydig cell tumors (androblastoma). This group accounts for 5% to 10% of all ovarian neoplasms and 2% of all ovarian malignancies. Thecomas and fibromas are the most common of these. They are benign solid hypoechoic adnexal masses that occur in middle-aged women.

Sonographic Findings. Stromal tumors are often so hypoechoic as to appear cystic, but there is lack of through-transmission.

Fibroma and Thecoma

Both fibroma and thecoma tumors arise from the ovarian stroma and are pathologically similar (Figure 42-31). Tumors with an abundance of thecal cells are called thecomas, and those with an abundance of fibrous tissue are called fibromas. Thecomas are usually benign and unilateral, comprising 1% of all ovarian neoplasms, and 70% occur in postmenopausal women. They frequently show signs of estrogen production.

Fibromas comprise 4% of ovarian neoplasms. Unlike thecomas, they are rarely associated with estrogen production. Clinical signs include lack of symptoms if the tumor is small; if large, increasing pressure and pain are apparent. Ascites has been reported in up to 50% of patients with fibromas larger than 5 cm in diameter. Associated ascites along with pleural effusion, referred to as **Meigs' syndrome**, occurs in 1% to 3% of patients with fibroma, but it is not specific, as it can occur with other ovarian neoplasms as well. The tumor is found in postmenopausal women. Fibromas occurring with basal cell nevus syndrome are commonly bilateral and calcified and occur in women with a mean age of 30 years.

Sonographic Findings. Fibromas are usually unilateral (90%) and range from small to melon size, with a

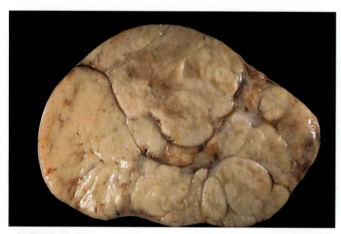

FIGURE 42-30 Gross pathology of a dysgerminoma shows a large lobulated tumor.

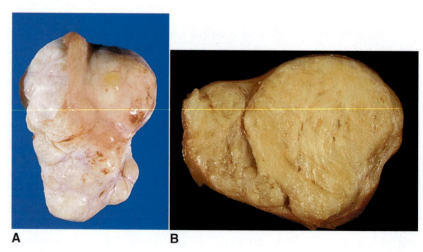

FIGURE 42-31 A, Gross pathology of a fibroma. **B,** Gross pathology of a thecoma.

A   B

variable sonographic appearance. A hypoechoic mass with posterior attenuation is seen from the homogeneous fibrous tissue. The larger tumors are pedunculated and prone to torsion, edema, and cystic degeneration (Figure 42-32).

Granulosa

A granulosa is a feminizing neoplasm composed of cells resembling the Graafian follicle. It is the most common hormone-active estrogenic tumor of the ovary but is rarely found (1% to 3%). It is more common after menopause (50%) but is also seen in the reproductive ages (45%) and in adolescence (5%). Clinical symptoms of estrogen production may include precocious puberty or vaginal bleeding and full breasts. Pain, pressure, and fullness may also be present. The tumor may twist on itself to cause torsion or rupture, leading to Meigs' syndrome. Malignant transformation is rare, but when it occurs, the lesion spreads via the lymphatics and bloodstream.

Sonographic Findings. On examination, adult granulose cell tumors have a variable appearance. A mass without torsion is similar to an endometrioma or cystadenoma, with low-level homogeneous echoes (Figure 42-33); if torsion occurs, a multilocular cyst containing blood or fluid is seen. The solid masses may have an echogenicity similar to that of uterine fibroids. The size may range up to 40 cm in diameter; the mass is usually unilateral. Endometrial glandular hyperplasia may be apparent. Metastases are uncommon and appear as peritoneal-based masses.

Sertoli-Leydig Cell Tumor

Sertoli-Leydig cell tumors (also called *androblastomas*) are rare. They generally occur in women under 30 years and constitute less than 0.5% of ovarian neoplasms. Almost all are unilateral, and malignancy occurs in 10% to 20% of these tumors. Clinically, symptoms of virilization occur in about 30% of patients. Occasionally, these tumors may be associated with estrogen production.

Sonographic Findings. Sonographically, the tumor usually appears as a solid hypoechoic mass.

Arrhenoblastoma

Arrhenoblastoma is a masculinizing ovarian tumor that occurs in females 15 to 65 years of age, with a peak incidence at 25 to 45 years. Clinical features are the same as for other pelvic masses, with the addition of amenorrhea and infertility. This mass may undergo malignant transformation in 22% of patients.

Sonographic Findings. The tumor is a solid mass with cystic components; it is lobulated and well encapsulated. In 95% of patients the mass is unilateral, and the size ranges from 2 to 30 cm.

Metastatic Disease

The ovaries are more involved with metastatic disease than any other pelvic organ, and these metastases often mimic the appearance of advanced stage II to III primary ovarian cancer. Approximately 5% to 10% of ovarian neoplasms are metastatic in origin. Metastatic cancer can arise from the breast, upper gastrointestinal tract, and other pelvic organs by direct extension or lymphatic spread. Krukenberg tumors are "drop" metastases to the ovaries from the gastrointestinal tract, primarily from the stomach, but also from the biliary tract, gallbladder, and pancreas (Figure 42-34). These masses are typically solid. Cystic metastatic masses appear to result more commonly from rectosigmoid colon cancers. Regardless of the site of origin, when there are metastases to the ovaries these malignancies are often widespread, with metastasis to the peritoneum (including ascites) and to

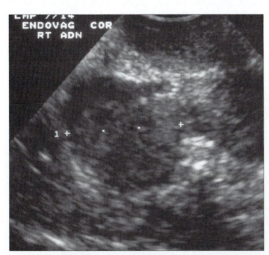

FIGURE 42-32 Fibroma. A 65-year-old woman presented with fullness in her abdomen. A homogeneous, well-defined mass was found in the right ovary. At surgery, an endometrioid cyst adenofibroma was removed.

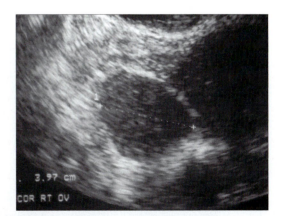

FIGURE 42-33 Granulosa. A 46-year-old woman was found to have a grapefruit-size mass on pelvic examination. The ultrasound image showed a well-defined, homogeneous mass in the right ovary, which was surgically removed.

the mesentery. The ovary is a common site of metastasis from carcinoma of the bowel (Krukenberg's tumor), breast, and endometrium and from melanoma and lymphoma.

   Sonographic Findings. Metastatic disease to the ovaries frequently is bilateral and is often associated with ascites (Figure 42-35). Metastases are usually completely solid or solid with a "moth-eaten" cystic pattern that occurs when they become necrotic. Lymphoma involving the ovary is usually diffuse and disseminated and is also frequently bilateral. Sonographically, the mass appears as a solid hypoechoic tumor similar to lymphoma elsewhere in the body.

CARCINOMA OF THE FALLOPIAN TUBE

Carcinoma of the fallopian tube is the least common (less than 1%) of all gynecologic malignancies. Adenocarcinoma is the most common histologic finding. It occurs most frequently in postmenopausal women with pain, vaginal bleeding, and a pelvic mass. The tumor usually involves the distal end, but it may involve the entire length of the tube.

   Sonographic Findings. Sonographically, carcinoma of the fallopian tube appears as a sausage-shaped, complex mass, with cystic and solid components often with papillary projections. The clinical and sonographic findings are similar to those of ovarian carcinoma.

OTHER PELVIC MASSES

Not all pelvic masses are gynecologic in origin. Pelvic kidneys, omental cysts, distended impacted feces in the rectosigmoid colon, a distended bladder, hydroureters, colonic cancer or masses, diverticular abscesses, and retroperitoneal masses can all be identified by ultrasound examination. In addition, the use of ultrasound in detecting an ectopic pregnancy has been well documented (Figure 42-36). The location, size, consistency, and source of adnexal masses can be defined by a flexible combination of transvaginal and transabdominal scanning. It is of key importance to try to distinguish solid ovarian masses from pedunculated myomas by identifying the uterine connection and searching for an ovary. Any fluid present in the pelvis can be used to outline dependent portions of the pelvic organs by tilting the

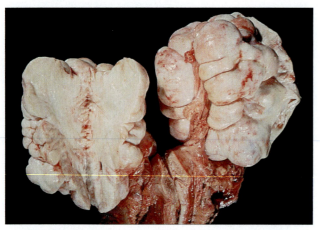

FIGURE 42-34 Gross pathology of a Krukenberg tumor.

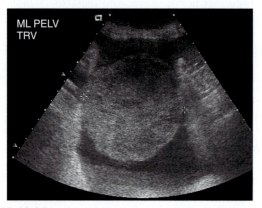

FIGURE 42-35 Transvaginal image of the solid Krukenberg tumor in this patient with pancreatic carcinoma.

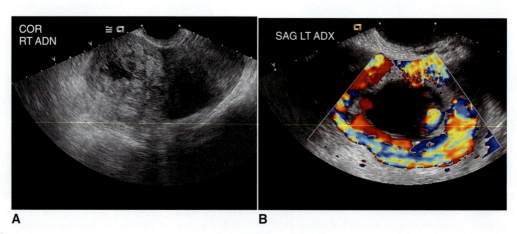

A   **B**

FIGURE 42-36 Ectopic pregnancy. **A,** Transvaginal coronal image showing the empty uterus in a patient who presented with vaginal bleeding and elevated hCG levels. **B,** Increased color Doppler flow surrounding the ectopic pregnancy "ring of fire."

patient, using a transvaginal approach, or both. Large palpable tumors rising out of the pelvis are best viewed with transabdominal technique.

Sonography is useful in defining symptomatic or palpable masses, as described previously. It allows the surgeon to observe functional-appearing cysts without resorting to immediate surgery and to plan a strategy for surgical exploration and treatment when necessary. Obvious signs of malignancy, such as sonolucent liver metastases or nodular peritoneum outlined by ascites, assist in the preoperative assessment. With current equipment, excellent resolution is available, and the experienced sonographer may frequently identify the tumor by its texture if the clinical context is understood. However, histologic diagnosis is the job of the pathologist.

REFERENCES

1. Bourne T, et al: Endovaginal colour flow imaging: a possible new screening technique for ovarian cancer, *Br Med J* 299:1367, 1989.

2. Bret PM, et al: Endovaginal US-guided aspiration of ovarian cysts and solid pelvic masses, *Radiology* 185:377, 1992.

3. Cohen HL, et al: Ovarian cysts are common in premenarchal girls: a sonographic study of 101 children 2-12 years old, *Am J Roentgenol* 159:89, 1992.

4. Dahnert W: *Radiology review manual*, ed 3, Baltimore, 1996, Williams & Wilkins.

5. Fleischer AC, Kepple DM, Vasquez J: Conventional and color Doppler endovaginal sonography in gynecologic infertility, *Radiol Clin North Am* 30:693, 1992.

6. Granberg S, et al: Comparison of endovaginal ultrasound and cytological evaluation of cystic ovarian tumors, *J Ultrasound Med* 10:9, 1991.

7. Kurjak A, et al: Evaluation of adnexal masses with endovaginal color ultrasound, *J Ultrasound Med* 10:295, 1991.

8. Levine D, et al: Sonography of adnexal masses: poor sensitivity of resistive index for identifying malignant lesions, *Am J Roentgenol* 162:1355, 1994.

Pathology of the Adnexa

Candace Goldstein, Sandra L. Hagen-Ansert, and Barbara J. Vander Werff

OBJECTIVES

On completion of this chapter, you should be able to:
- List the causes of and risk factors for pelvic inflammatory disease
- Describe the sonographic findings of salpingitis, pyosalpinx, tubo-ovarian abscess, endometrioma, and adenomyosis
- List the locations of endometrial implants in the body
- Discuss the development of endometritis in the postpartum patient
- Discuss the role of ultrasound in pelvic inflammatory disease

OUTLINE

Pelvic Inflammatory Disease
  Salpingitis, Hydrosalpinx, and
    Pyosalpinx

Tubo-ovarian Abscess (TOA)
  Peritonitis
Endometritis

Endometriosis and Endometrioma
Interventional Ultrasound
Postoperative Uses of Ultrasound

Pelvic inflammatory disease (PID) and endometriosis are diffuse disease processes of the female pelvic cavity. Most commonly, PID is caused by sexually transmitted diseases, including gonorrhea and chlamydia. Although uncommon, PID can also be caused by a ruptured appendix and peritonitis. PID and endometriosis have very different clinical presentations and pathologies. However, early in the disease the clinical presentation of both endometriosis and PID is nonspecific and may mimic functional bowel disease.

PID is an inclusive term that refers to all pelvic infections (e.g., endometritis, salpingitis, hydrosalpinx, pyosalpinx, **periovarian inflammation, tubo-ovarian complex,** and tubo-ovarian abscess). The infection usually occurs bilaterally and may be found in the endometrium (**endometritis**), the uterine wall (**myometritis**), the uterine serosa and broad ligaments (**parametritis**), the ovary (**oophoritis**), and the most common location, the oviducts (**salpingitis**) (Figure 43-1). Sonography has limited value during acute PID or at early onset when inflammatory changes have not yet begun to manifest. In cases of chronic PID, ultrasound can identify dilated fallopian tubes (hydrosalpinx or pyosalpinx), abscess, and complex intraperitoneal fluid.

Endometriosis is the presence of endometrial glands or stroma in abnormal locations. It occurs most commonly in two forms: **adenomyosis** of the uterus and endometriosis of the adnexa. In most cases, endometriosis is diagnosed clinically and is not detectable by sonography. When identified sonographically, it presents as an adnexal mass or masses (endometriomas) of variable echogenicity, shape, and size.

PELVIC INFLAMMATORY DISEASE

The occurrence of pelvic inflammatory disease (PID) is becoming more common. PID occurs in 11% of young women during reproductive age, with a peak incidence at 20 to 24 years, affecting 750,000 American women each year. The increased incidence in younger populations may be due to the immaturity of the cervix and consequent higher risk of sexually transmitted infections. Risk factors include early sexual contact, multiple sexual partners, history of sexually transmitted disease, previous history of PID, use of an intrauterine contraceptive device (IUCD), and douching (douching may push bacteria into the upper genital tract). Although sexually transmitted diseases such as gonorrhea and chlamydia are the most common forms of infection, other routes of infection are possible, such as direct extension from appendiceal, diverticular, or postsurgical abscess collections that have ruptured into the pelvis, the string from an IUCD, or puerperal and postabortion complications. Other types of invasive instrumentation procedures in

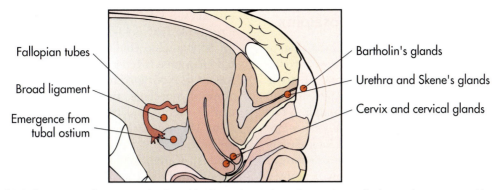

FIGURE 43-1 Pelvic inflammatory disease may be found in the endometrium, the uterine wall, the uterine serosa and broad ligaments, the ovary, and the fallopian tubes.

BOX 43-1	Pelvic Inflammatory Disease

- Inflammatory disease (acute or chronic); infection spreads to pelvis
- Large, palpable, bilateral complex mass; ovary may be seen separate from mass
- Free fluid in cul-de-sac
- Doppler image shows increased vascularity and diastolic flow
- Associated with infertility and endometritis

BOX 43-2	Sonographic Findings of Pelvic Inflammatory Disease

- Endometritis: Thickening or fluid in the endometrium
- Periovarian inflammation: Enlarged ovaries with multiple cysts, indistinct margins
- Salpingitis: Nodular thickening, irregularity of tube with diverticula
- Pyosalpinx or hydrosalpinx: Fluid-filled irregular fallopian tube with or without echoes
- Tubo-ovarian abscess: Complex mass with septations, irregular margins, and internal echoes; usually in cul-de-sac

---

the pelvic cavity may leave the route more open to bacterial invasion. PID is usually found as a bilateral collection of fluid and pus within the pelvic cavity, except when it is caused by direct extension of an adjacent inflammatory process, in which case it is most commonly unilateral (Box 43-1).

Infrequently, particularly in patients with PID resulting from gonorrhea, a pelvic infection may travel upward through the right flank, causing a perihepatic inflammation. The pain may mimic liver, gallbladder, or right renal pain. Perihepatic inflammation can be detected sonographically by scanning along the liver margin and identifying a hypoechoic rim between the liver and the adjacent ribs. This perihepatic inflammation is called the Fitz-Hugh-Curtis syndrome.

Sexually transmitted PID is spread via the mucosa of the pelvic organs through the cervix into the uterine endometrium (endometritis) and out the fallopian tubes (acute salpingitis) to the area of the ovaries and peritoneum. As the tube becomes obstructed, it fills with pus (pyosalpinx). In the setting of extensive PID, the margins of the ovaries and other pelvic structures can become difficult to distinguish from each other.

The bacterial infection may arise from *Chlamydia trachomatis* and *Neisseria gonorrhea*. Other bacteria that have been found in PID patients include aerobes (*Streptococcus* sp., *Escherichia coli*, *Haemophilus influenzae*), anaerobes (*Bacteroides*, *Peptostreptococcus*, and *Peptococcus*), *Mycobacterium tuberculosis*, *Actinomycetes* sp. in IUCD users, and herpesvirus hominis type 1.

If the pregnancy test result is positive in a woman with previously treated PID, a careful evaluation of the adnexa is indicated, even if a normal intrauterine pregnancy is detected. From the previous fallopian tube damage, the incidence of an ectopic pregnancy is significantly increased. The possibility of a rare heterotopic pregnancy (a concomitant intrauterine and extrauterine pregnancy) increases in this patient.

Clinically, patients may present with intense pelvic pain and tenderness described as dull and aching, with constant vaginal discharge. Other symptoms include fever, pain in the right upper abdomen, painful intercourse, and irregular menstrual bleeding. A history of infertility may also be present. Lab tests may show an elevated white blood cell count (WBC) in PID, particularly when caused by a chlamydial infection. The patient may be asymptomatic or the disease may produce only minor symptoms, even though it can seriously damage the reproductive organs. A palpable mass may be present on clinical examination. Current criteria of the Centers for Disease Control and Prevention (CDC) for diagnosing PID include pelvic or lower abdominal pain and one or more of the following: cervical motion tenderness, uterine tenderness, or adnexal tenderness.

The sonographic findings may be normal early in the course of the disease (Box 43-2). As the disease progresses or becomes chronic, a variety of findings may occur. Differential considerations may include hematoma, dermoid cyst, ovarian neoplasm, and endometriosis.

Salpingitis, Hydrosalpinx, and Pyosalpinx

Salpingitis is inflammation of a fallopian tube (Figure 43-2). This condition may be acute, subacute, or chronic. Clinical signs may range from asymptomatic to pelvic fullness or discomfort, or a low-grade fever. An obstructed tube filled with serous secretions is a **hydrosalpinx**; this can occur as a result of PID, endometriosis, or postoperative adhesions. The sonographer should look closely at the fundal uterus to search for prominent or enlarged fallopian tubes. The dilated tube may show a pointed beak at the swollen end of the tube near the isthmus where the tube enters the uterus. If the dilated tube becomes infected, it is called **pyosalpinx.** The likelihood of recurrent infection and ectopic pregnancy increases significantly. Infected or hemorrhagic pelvic fluid may also be present. Infection can obscure normal tissue planes, making anatomy unclear. Severe pain requires gentle use of ultrasound probes in acute PID, and in some cases a full bladder for transabdominal study is intolerable (Table 43-1).

◤ **Sonographic Findings.** Sonographically, the normal fallopian tube is generally not visualized unless fluid surrounds it. If outlined by ascitic fluid, it is a thin, less than 5-mm hypoechoic tissue band originating from the uterine fundus and can be imaged in an axial-coronal view. The sonographer can try to follow the dilated fallopian tube as it enters the cornu of the uterus (at the fundus). Careful oblique angulations of the transducer are necessary to trace the pathway of the tube. If fluid, pus, or products of conception fill the tube, detection is easier. If the lumen is outlined and shows irregularity and multiple diverticula, a pathologic state is probable.

If distinct tubular structures are instead seen, hydrosalpinx (dilated tubes) is diagnosed. Hydrosalpinx has variable presentations, from subtle dilated tubular structures to massive tortuous cystic areas. Although both tubes may be damaged, they may be asymmetric in size, with only the more dilated tube appreciated sonographically. Although contrast-enhanced salpingography is the definitive test, ultrasound appears accurate in identifying this process, particularly when performed transvaginally. Hydrosalpinx may present as echogenic fluid or fluid-debris levels (Figure 43-3), indicating infection (pyosalpinx).

Severe and chronic pyosalpinx often contain thick, echogenic mucoid pus, which does not transmit sound as well as serous fluid or blood. A pyosalpinx may appear as a complex mass. A transvaginal exam is particularly useful for identifying the tubular nature and folds of the dilated tube, thus avoiding the mistaken diagnosis of a mass. Careful coronal scanning and rotation of the probe will help the sonographer to discern a dilated tube from an adnexal cyst.

Acute salpingitis is evident as a thick-walled nodular hyperemic tube (Figure 43-4). The dilated tubes usually surround the ovaries like two lunar crescents encircling

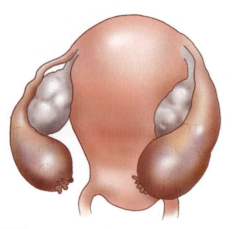

FIGURE 43-2 Salpingitis is an inflammation of the fallopian tubes that causes nodular dilation. This infection may be unilateral or bilateral.

TABLE 43-1	Salpingitis, Hydrosalpinx, and Pyosalpinx		
	Description	**Clinical Findings**	**Sonographic Findings**
Salpingitis	Inflammation of fallopian tube Acute, subacute, or chronic	Asymptomatic to pelvic fullness or discomfort Low-grade fever	Dilated tube Tortuous
Hydrosalpinx	Obstructed tube filled with serous secretions Occurs secondary to PID, endometriosis, or postoperative adhesions	Asymptomatic to pelvic fullness or discomfort Low-grade fever	Walls become thin secondary to dilation Appearance of multicystic or fusiform mass Follow dilated tubes from fundus of uterus Look for pointed "beak" at swollen end of tube near isthmus Bilateral Ampullary portion more dilated than interstitial part of tube
Pyosalpinx	Retained pus in oviduct with inflammation	Asymptomatic to pelvic fullness or discomfort Low-grade fever	May appear as complex mass Pus within dilated tube very thick Transmission and echogenic–poor sound

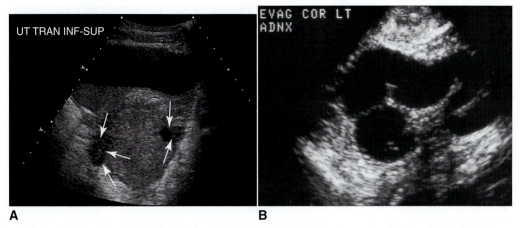

FIGURE 43-3 A, Transvaginal coronal image of the very dilated fallopian tube (*arrows*). **B,** When swollen with fluid, the tube bends and curls in the adnexal area.

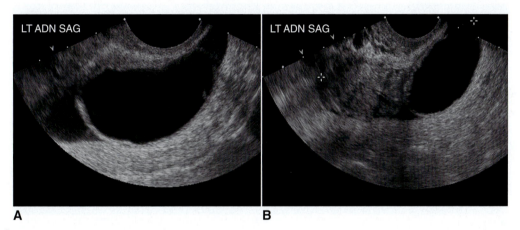

FIGURE 43-4 A and **B,** Transvaginal sagittal images of a patient with acute salpingitis. The tube is very dilated with echogenic debris.

the posterior surface of the uterus and filling the cul-de-sac.

The sonographer should be sure not to confuse the dilated tube with a dilated ureter or prominent vessel. Occasionally, prominent blood vessels may be present in the adnexa. Although these may initially be misinterpreted as a hydrosalpinx, color or pulsed Doppler imaging will show blood flow in an adnexal blood vessel and no flow in a hydrosalpinx. Evaluation of the kidneys for possible hydronephrosis and trying to trace the dilated ureter to the bladder should help. The ovaries may be difficult to delineate because of surrounding tissue, edema, and pus. In addition to hydrosalpinx or pyosalpinx, sonographic findings of PID include fluid in the cul-de-sac (Figure 43-5), mild uterine enlargement, and endometrial fluid or thickening. Transabdominal and transvaginal sonography can reveal the presence of pelvic intraperitoneal fluid in the cul-de-sac. Pelvic fluid may frequently have internal echoes, septations, and fluid levels, a sign that the fluid is not simple but rather may be infected or hemorrhagic (Figure 43-6).

Any simple cyst that hemorrhages may appear as a complex mass. In patients of reproductive age, the classic differential diagnosis of a complex adnexal mass is hemorrhagic cyst, ectopic pregnancy, endometrioma, and PID. Dermoids and other benign tumors can appear in a similar fashion.

Tubo-ovarian Abscess (TOA)

The adhesive, edematous, and inflamed serosa may further adhere to the ovary and/or other peritoneal surfaces, which distorts anatomy. As the infection worsens, periovarian adhesions may form. The ovary cannot be separated from the inflamed dilated tube and is called the tubo-ovarian complex. In trying to determine if an adnexal mass is separate from the ovary, gentle pushing with the transvaginal transducer can be used to identify separate or contiguous movement. Periovarian adhesions fuse the inflamed ovary and tube, and the ovary cannot be separated from the tube. This causes a further loculation of pus known as a **tubo-ovarian abscess (TOA)**. This may be unilateral abscess or bilateral and appears as a complex mass in the posterior cul-de-sac.

The tubo-ovarian complex or abscess usually responds well to antibiotic treatment without the need for surgical

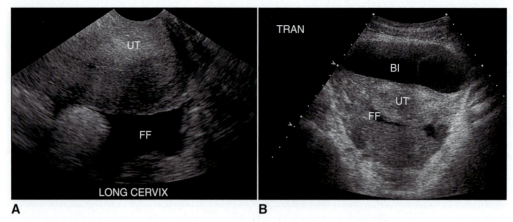

FIGURE 43-5 Free fluid. **A,** Sagittal and **B,** transverse views of the uterus *(UT)* in an asymptomatic, postmenopausal female demonstrate a small free fluid collection *(FF)* posterior to the uterus. *BI,* bladder.

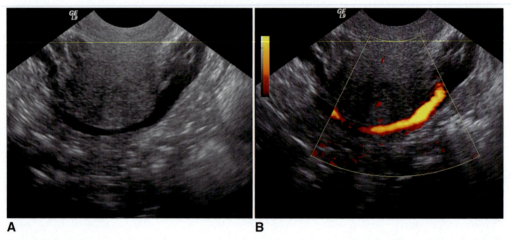

FIGURE 43-6 A, Transvaginal transverse image of the uterus with sonolucent structure posterior. **B,** Power Doppler shows the structure to be vascular in origin, not free fluid.

drainage. Serial ultrasound images during treatment allow observation of resolution and can indicate which patients need prolonged intravenous antibiotics and which patients may benefit more from removal of the involved tissue. Sonographic guidance can be used to assist in percutaneous or transvaginal drainage, for culture and sensitivity or complete drainage, and thus hasten recovery.

Sonographic Findings. A pelvic abscess is usually a complex mass in the cul-de-sac that distorts pelvic anatomy (Figure 43-7). It can involve the ovary alone or the fallopian tube and ovary as a tubo-ovarian abscess. The TOA appears as a complex multiloculated mass with variable septations, irregular margins, and scattered internal echoes. The ovaries are often difficult to recognize as separate from the mass because of surrounding tissue, edema, and pus (Figure 43-8). As noted, TOAs usually are bilateral, but they may be unilateral if an IUCD is present or if there is direct extension from an abdominal abscess. There is usually posterior acoustic enhancement. Occasionally a fluid-debris level or gas may be seen within the mass. Gas within the abscess may

appear as hyperechoic, punctate echoes that exhibit a comet tail shadowing effect. Drainage of the collection of pus may be done with interventional sonography (Figure 43-9). Recognizable ovarian tissue may be identified within the inflammatory mass by transvaginal sonography.

The sonographic appearance may be indistinguishable from other adnexal masses, and clinical correlation is necessary for the correct diagnosis. The transvaginal approach is helpful in assessing the extent of the disease. Dilated tubes, periovarian inflammatory change, and the internal characteristics of tubo-ovarian abscesses are better defined with transvaginal scanning.

Peritonitis

Peritonitis is the inflammation of the peritoneum, the serous membrane lining the abdominal cavity and covering the viscera. This inflammation is caused by infectious organisms that gain access by way of rupture or perforation of the viscera or associated structures; via the female genital tract; by piercing the abdominal wall; via the

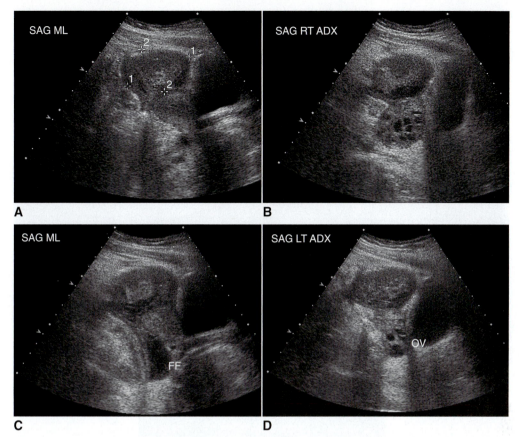

FIGURE 43-7 **A,** Transabdominal midline sagittal image of the bladder *(B)*, uterus *(UT)*, and complex mass *(M)* that is displacing the uterus anteriorly. **B,** The scan over the right adnexal area shows the uterus *(UT)* with the right ovary posterior *(OV)*. The bladder *(B)* is seen inferiorly. **C,** The scan over the midline of the pelvis demonstrates the mass *(M)* posterior to the uterus *(UT)*. Free fluid *(FF)* is seen adjacent to the complex mass. **D,** The scan over the left adnexal area shows the left ovary *(OV)* and uterus *(UT)*.

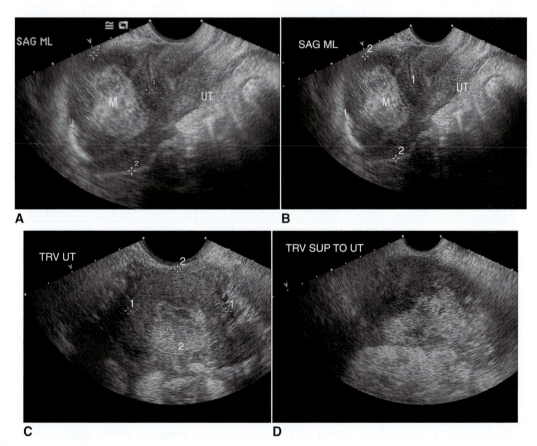

FIGURE 43-8 **A,** Transvaginal sagittal midline image of the uterus *(UT)* with a large complex echogenic mass *(M)* adjacent to the uterine cavity. **B,** The complex mass *(M)* is clearly separate from the uterus *(UT)*. **C,** Transvaginal image of the uterus. **D,** Transvaginal image superior to the uterine fundus shows the complex mass.

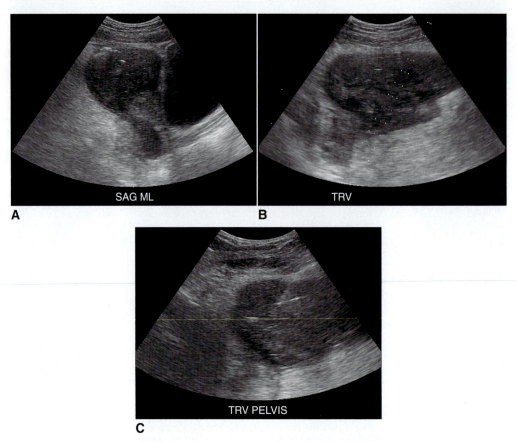

FIGURE 43-9 A, TA sagittal midline image of the pelvis shows the distended urinary bladder *(B)*, the complex mass *(M)* anterior to the uterus *(UT)*. **B,** TA transverse image over the complex mass. **C,** A drainage catheter is inserted into the mass *(arrows)*.

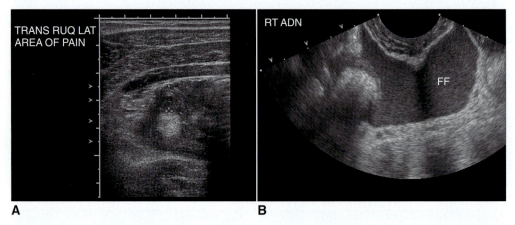

FIGURE 43-10 A, Transvaginal sagittal image in a 24-year-old female who had acute pelvic pain. A complex mass was observed in the right adnexa secondary to a ruptured appendix (marked by calipers in **A**). **B,** Free fluid collection was noted in the right adnexal area *(FF)*.

bloodstream or lymphatic vessels; via surgical incisions; or by failure to practice antiseptic techniques during surgery. If the infectious process spreads to involve the bladder, ureter, bowel, and adnexal area, it becomes pelvic peritonitis.

Sonographic Findings. If the abscess collection has gas-forming bubbles within, it may be difficult to delineate well with sonography because the beam is reflected from the area of interest. The sonographer should look for loculated areas of fluid within the pelvis, the

paracolic gutters, and mesenteric reflections (Figure 43-10). Evaluation of the space between the right kidney and liver and the left kidney and spleen should also include a check for fluid.

ENDOMETRITIS

Endometritis, infection of the endometrium, can be divided into obstetric and nonobstetric cases. Nonobstetric infection is associated with either PID or gynecologic instrumentation. Endometritis can be acute or chronic. Obstetric cases occur in the immediate postpartum period. Endometritis is the most common cause of fever in the postpartum patient. Postpartum fever is considered a temperature >101° F (38° C) on any 2 of the first 10 days postpartum (excluding the initial 24-hour period). Although good data on postpartum infections are lacking, a 2001 study by Yokoe and colleagues found that 5.5% of vaginal deliveries and 7.4% of cesarean sections incurred a postpartum infection. Endometritis accounted for almost 50% of the infections after cesarean delivery (3.4% of C-sections). Clinical presentation includes fever, uterine/adnexal tenderness, and bleeding.

Sonographic Findings. On sonography the endometrium may appear thick; contain fluid, air or clot; or appear normal (Figure 43-11). The endometrium is considered normal in size up to 20 mm. A measurement of greater than 20 mm should raise the suspicion of endometritis, hemorrhage, or retained products of conception (POCs). The risk for endometritis goes up with premature rupture of membranes, retained clot or products of conception (POCs), and prolonged labor.

ENDOMETRIOSIS AND ENDOMETRIOMA

Endometriosis is one of the most common gynecologic diseases. It is defined as the presence of functioning endometrial tissue in abnormal locations. The ectopic tissue can be found almost anywhere in the body including the ovaries, fallopian tubes, broad ligaments, the external surface of the uterus, and scattered over the peritoneum, bowel, or bladder, especially in the dependent parts of the pelvis or cul-de-sac (Figure 43-12). The incidence of endometriosis is found in up to 15% of premenopausal women. It affects women in their third to fourth decade of life and is dependent on normal hormonal stimulation. Clinical findings include severe dysmenorrhea, chronic pelvic pain from peritoneal adhesions and bleeding, or dyspareunia (Table 43-2).

The cause may arise from peritoneal seeding from retrograde travel of endometrial cells through fallopian

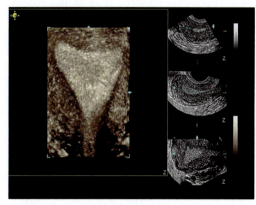

FIGURE 43-11 Transvaginal multislice image of the endometrial cavity.

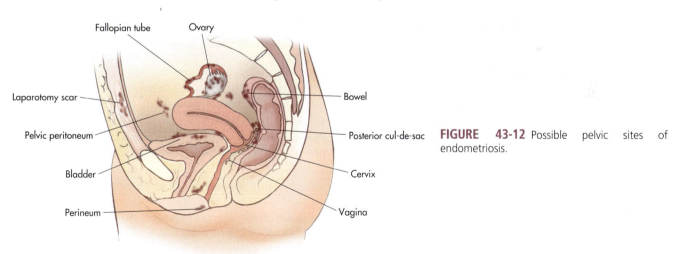

FIGURE 43-12 Possible pelvic sites of endometriosis.

TABLE 43-2	Endometriosis	
Description	**Clinical Findings**	**Sonographic Findings**
Presence of functional ectopic endometrial glands and stroma outside the uterine cavity.	Not distinctive
Complaints of dysmenorrhea with pelvic pain
Premenstrual dyspareunia
Sacral backache during menses
Infertility	Bilateral or unilateral ovarian cysts
Cysts are anechoic to solid, depending on amount of blood
Ovaries adherent to posterior uterus or in cul-de-sac; difficult to define
Obscured organ borders
Focal mass is endometrioma ("chocolate cyst") with low-intensity echoes and acoustic enhancement

tubes (perhaps through the contractions of the uterus associated with the menstrual cycle), metaplastic transformation of peritoneal epithelium into endometrial tissue, or through traumatic spread from uterine surgery or amniocentesis.

Endometriosis has two forms: internal and external. Internal endometriosis occurs within the uterus (adenomyosis). External endometriosis is outside the uterus and may be found in the pouch of Douglas; surface of the ovary, fallopian tube, and uterus broad ligaments; or rectovaginal septum.

The more common form of endometriosis is the external, or indirect, form. The disease process for the external form varies in extent from small foci to widespread sheets of tissue to focal discrete masses. The endometrial tissue in endometriosis cyclically bleeds and proliferates as stimulated by changes in hormonal influence. Though the true prevalence of endometriosis is unknown (as most cases are asymptomatic), it is estimated that 5.5 million women in North America are currently affected.

The second less common form of endometriosis, known as the internal, or direct form, is called adenomyosis. Endometrial cells begin to grow into the uterine body, invading the junctional zone and the myometrium. The clinical symptoms of adenomyosis are heavy menstrual bleeding, painful menses, and uterine enlargement. Adenomyosis is most common in women who have had uterine surgery, including cesarean section and myomectomy. Sonographically, the uterus may appear bulbous, there may be myometrial "cysts," and the border between the endometrium and myometrium becomes indistinct. This "blurred border" appearance is more common in the posterior aspect of the uterus. MRI is more specific than ultrasound in making this distinction.

Endometriosis can be either diffuse or localized. The diffuse form is most common and is rarely diagnosed by sonography because the implants are so small. The diffuse form leads to disorganization of the pelvic anatomy with an appearance similar to PID or chronic ectopic pregnancy. The localized form, on the other hand, consists of a discrete mass called an **endometrioma**, or "chocolate cyst." Endometriomas are usually asymptomatic and can frequently be multiple and have a unique sonographic appearance. They may become moderately enlarged and create a surgical emergency by rupturing or by causing the ovary to twist on the vessels that supply it and cause torsion.

Two possible explanations for the cause of endometriosis are presented. The first is that the chronic retrograde flow of menstrual fluid through the tubes and into the pelvis may produce implantation and proliferation of endometrial cells with cyclic bleeding. This is the "transtubal migration" theory. The second theory involves the evaluation of endometrial activity in susceptible cells that retain the embryonic capacity to differentiate in response to hormonal stimulation. The resulting tissue bleeds and proliferates with the resultant production of pain, scarring, and endometrium-lined collections of blood known as endometriomas.

Endometriosis may occur in any menstruating female. Clinical symptoms include painful periods (dysmenorrhea) or painful intercourse (dyspareunia); lower abdominal, pelvic, and back pain; irregular bleeding; and infertility secondary to adhesions and fibrosis. Differential diagnosis would include hemorrhagic ovarian cyst, TOA, cystic ovarian neoplasm, solid ovarian tumor, or ectopic pregnancy. Clinically, most women with an acute hemorrhagic cyst or abscess present with acute pelvic pain, whereas women with an endometrioma are asymptomatic or have more chronic discomfort associated with their menses.

Symptoms depend on the location and extent of the disease, but there is no direct relationship between the extent of disease and severity of symptoms. Patients can be asymptomatic if the condition is confined to the ovaries, or they can suffer severe pain if it is widespread. Although typically associated with infertility, endometriosis may be identified in a pregnant patient, by evidence of an endometrioma.

Sonographic Findings. Diffuse endometriosis, the more common form, is rarely detected sonographically unless a focal mass, an endometrioma, is present. Endometriomas may appear as bilateral or unilateral ovarian masses with patterns ranging from anechoic (rare) to solid, depending on the amount of blood and its state of organization (Figure 43-13). The ovaries typically adhere to the posterior surface of the uterus or are stuck in the cul-de-sac and may be difficult to define. Obscured organ borders and multiple irregular cystic masses are also suggestive of either disseminating cancer or pelvic infection.

An endometrioma often appears as a well-defined, predominantly cystic mass with transabdominal ultrasound, but, with transvaginal ultrasound, uniform internal echoes are usually evident. The most common presentation is termed a "chocolate cyst" because of the presence of low level echoes (secondary to internal bleeding and organization) and acoustic enhancement. The echogenicity of endometriomas can vary from cystic to solid, and their size varies widely from less than 1 cm to more than 10 cm in diameter. The masses are the result of multiple episodes of bleeding. Fluid-fluid levels and internal septations are frequently noted. Some endometriomas are multiloculated, often with varied internal echo patterns and interconnecting loculations. Endometriomas may be multiple and present in both adnexa. Endometriomas can have a similar appearance to inflammation (abscess), trophoblastic tissue (ectopic pregnancy), and dermoids.

Other appearances include an enlarged multicystic ovary with a thick wall and internal septations or a cyst with fluid-debris levels (because of different degrees of organization of the hemorrhage). Small linear hyperechoic foci may be present in the wall of the cyst and are

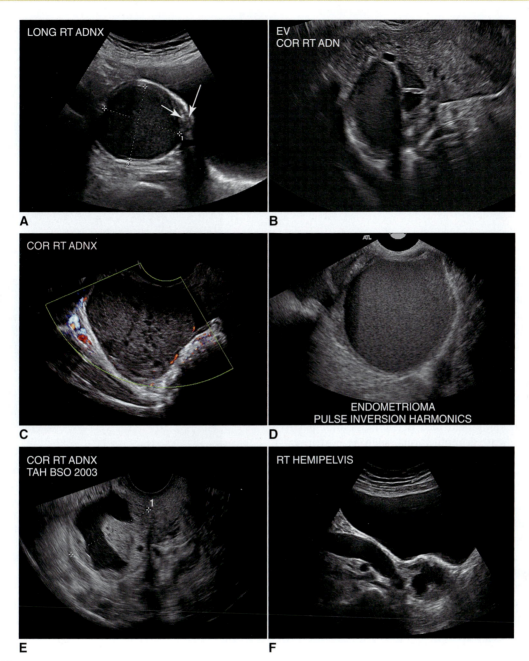

FIGURE 43-13 A, Transvaginal sagittal view of the uterus demonstrates endometrial calcification *(arrows)* with shadowing in a 34-year-old female with pelvic fullness. **B,** The transvaginal coronal image shows a complex mass in the right adnexal area. **C,** Color Doppler imaging shows increased flow in the pelvic vessels surrounding the endometrioma. **D,** A different patient with a large endometrioma that is completely filled with low-level homogeneous echoes ("chocolate cyst"). Transvaginal coronal image **(E)** and sagittal TA image **(F)** of the right adnexa in a patient with a dilated right hydroureter.

thought to be caused by cholesterol deposits accumulating in the cyst wall. Endometriomas may also demonstrate microcalcification. Ovarian abscesses or hemorrhagic ovarian cysts may demonstrate sonographic appearances similar to endometriomas; however, the clinical picture is usually different.

INTERVENTIONAL ULTRASOUND

Ultrasound-guided percutaneous biopsy and abscess drainage have become valuable diagnostic and

therapeutic procedures (see Chapter 19). Interventional biopsy has also decreased patient costs by obviating the need for surgery and a lengthy hospital stay. Contraindications to needle biopsy include uncorrectable coagulopathy, lack of a safe biopsy route, and an uncooperative patient. A patient's bleeding history can be evaluated with a platelet count, INR, prothrombin time, and partial thromboplastin time. Evaluation of the patient's use of aspirin, Coumadin, or heparin should also be used to screen for an increased risk of bleeding. If these values are abnormal, the procedure should be delayed if deemed necessary after consulting with the patient's doctor. Transabdominal or transvaginal guidance is used for aspiration of benign-appearing cysts. Transvaginal drainage is helpful in TOAs; other pelvic abscesses, such as appendicitis and diverticulitis; and drainage of postoperative fluid collections (Figure 43-14). Transrectal drainage can be used for deep pelvic abscesses. Transvaginal sonography is also used in obtaining biopsies for benign and malignant solid pelvic masses and to drain recurrent malignant collections. Biopsy kits can be used with the transvaginal transducers to allow direct visualization of the region of interest.

Ultrasonically, guided needle drainage of abscesses and stable hematomas, either through the abdominal wall or the vagina, is diagnostic and therapeutic. Recurrent tumor masses may be biopsied in a similar fashion. The transvaginal ultrasound and needle guide make entering the anterior or posterior cul-de-sacs safer and easier for pelvic fluid aspiration, biopsies, or radiation needle placement.

POSTOPERATIVE USES OF ULTRASOUND

Pain and the development of a pelvic mass after pelvic surgery can indicate complications, such as postoperative bleeding, hematomas, or abscess formation Postoperative ultrasound can be used to distinguish a distended bladder from an abnormal fluid collection at the operative site. The ability to palpate specific structures with the transvaginal probe and avoid the abdominal wound is valuable in determining the site of pain in a postoperative pelvis. Resolving hematomas often appear to be of a solid consistency and can be followed as they recede.

An expert combination of transvaginal and transabdominal techniques is essential as new gynecologic applications of ultrasound continue to be found for screening, diagnosis, and therapy of pelvic pathology in a female patient. The inclusion of translabial and

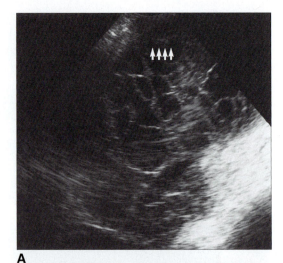

A

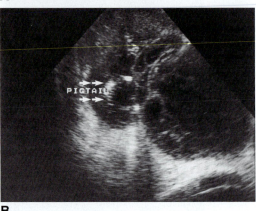

B

FIGURE 43-14 Hematometra in a 23-year-old woman 4 weeks after a dilation and curettage. **A,** Transabdominal longitudinal view of the uterus demonstrates a central fluid collection with a fluid debris level *(arrows).* **B,** Transvaginal image in the same patient again demonstrates the pigtail catheter *(arrows).* The fluid is monitored by ultrasound guidance.

the perineal approaches to gynecologic imaging allows another field of view for the sonographer to evaluate the pelvic structures. Three-dimensional imaging will surely add additional understanding of ovarian pathologies.

The Role of Ultrasound in Evaluating Female Infertility

Carol Mitchell, Barbara Trampe, and Dan Lebovic

OBJECTIVES

On completion of this chapter, you should be able to:
- Define *infertility* and list its treatment options
- List the female pelvic organs to be imaged in an infertility workup
- State anatomic variations or pathologies that need to be defined when imaging an infertility patient
- List complications that may occur because of infertility treatments

OUTLINE

Ultrasound has come to play an important role in the management and guidance of treatment for the infertile patient. By definition, infertility is the inability to conceive within 12 months with regular coitus (or within 6 months for those 35 years or older). It is estimated that infertility affects one in seven couples in America. Approximately 40% of the cases of infertility are attributable to the female, 40% to the male, and the remaining 20% are combined male/female or unexplained factors.[3] Traditionally, infertility has been divided into cervical, endometrial/uterine, tubal, ovulatory, peritoneal, and male factor causes.[3] Male factor causes of infertility are an inadequate number of sperm and decreased motility of sperm, obstruction of the spermatic ducts or vas deferens, and scrotal varicoceles. This chapter focuses on female factors, including discussion of cervical, uterine/endometrial, tubal, ovulatory, and peritoneal causes of infertility.

As reproductive technologies continue to advance, it is important for the sonographer to be aware of the different treatment plans and the role that ultrasound plays in evaluating the infertile patient because many of these patients will come to the ultrasound lab very knowledgeable about their procedures. The sonographer should be compassionate toward each patient's situation.

EVALUATING THE CERVIX

The role of the cervix in fertility is to provide a nonhostile environment to harbor sperm. The cervix does this with glands that secrete mucus and crypts that hold the sperm. Ultrasound can be used to evaluate the cervical length during pregnancy to assess for cervical incompetence. However, in the nongravid uterus, both the length of and any opening in the cervix are difficult to assess. Hysterosalpingography (HSG) can be used to evaluate the internal os diameter. A diameter less than 1 mm by HSG may indicate cervical stenosis.

EVALUATING THE UTERUS

When evaluating the uterus of the infertility patient, the sonographer has two main objectives: (1) to assess the structural anatomy and (2) to assess the endometrium. Assessing for structural anatomy refers to evaluating the uterine shape (i.e., unicolis, bicornuate, congenital malformations) (Figure 44-1) and evaluating echogenicity. Is the uterus uniform in echogenicity? Are there any masses suggestive of fibroids that may impede implantation of the fertilized egg (Figure 44-2)? When assessing the endometrium, the sonographer wants to evaluate the

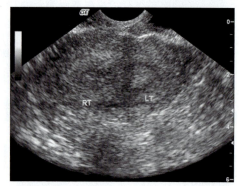

FIGURE 44-1 A bicornuate uterus. *RT*, right. *LT*, left.

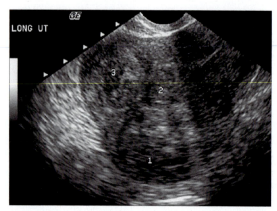

FIGURE 44-2 Longitudinal transvaginal image of the uterus with multiple fibroids.

thickness and echogenicity characteristics as well as any intracavitary lesions.

Congenital Uterine Anomalies

It is estimated that congenital uterine anomalies occur in 1% of women.[2] Congenital uterine anomalies are the result of defects in müllerian duct development, fusion, or resorption and are associated with renal anomalies. Although there are seven classes used to describe uterine anomalies, this chapter discusses only those that ultrasound is best suited to evaluate. The congenital anomalies most easily assessed with ultrasound are a septate or bicornuate uterus and uterus didelphys. Although these three entities are difficult to accurately confirm with ultrasound, ultrasound is good at depicting the two endometrial interfaces in the transverse plane. This finding should alert the sonographer to further evaluate the pelvic anatomy for two versus one cervix and vagina. Didelphys uterus is not usually associated with fertility problems, but bicornuate uterus is associated with a low incidence of fertility complications.

A uterine anomaly that is associated with a high incidence of infertility is the septate uterus. This congenital anomaly presents with two uterine cavities and a single fundus. In this case, the septum causes a problem for

implantation. If the pregnancy implants along the septum, the pregnancy may be at an increased risk of failure because of inadequate blood supply from the septum. For these patients, the septum can be removed hysteroscopically to improve implantation and fertility success, so this is an important diagnosis to make.

On ultrasound, the septate uterus appears as two endometrial cavities without a fundal notch compared with the bicornuate and didelphys uterus, which have two endometrial cavities, a wide uterine body, and a fundal notch (see Figure 44-1). The septate uterus should not be confused with a uterine cavity filled with myomatous tumors, as shown in Figure 44-2.

The T-shaped uterus is another uterine anomaly to evaluate. This congenital anomaly is caused by exposure to diethylstilbestrol (DES) in utero. DES was a medication given to women to treat for threatened abortion from 1950 to 1970. The T-shaped uterus also is at risk for cervical incompetence, and there is no treatment known for this type of congenital anomaly. Because many uteruses imaged will not fit completely into one of these categories, the anatomy needs to be described as thoroughly as possible and may not be given a label immediately. Magnetic resonance imaging (MRI) and HSG are other imaging methods that are better suited to evaluating the wide range of uterine anomalies.

Recently, three-dimensional ultrasound imaging has provided the ability to view the coronal plane. The coronal plane has afforded a diagnostic opportunity that two-dimensional imaging was unable to obtain. Figure 44-3 demonstrates the standard two-dimensional images of a septate uterus as well as the three-dimensional coronal plane. Note that in the coronal plane, the diagnosis of septate uterus becomes apparent.

EVALUATING THE ENDOMETRIUM

The endometrium can be measured throughout the menstrual cycle to look for appropriate changes. The thickness encompasses the thickness of both anterior and posterior endometrial layers in the sagittal plane. During the first half of the menstrual cycle, the mucosa begins to proliferate because of increasing estrogen levels. On ultrasound exam, the proliferative endometrial phase is seen as a triple line sign consisting of the hypoechoic mucosa and the echogenic interface where they meet in the central plane of the uterus (Figure 44-4). After ovulation, progesterone is secreted by the corpus luteum. This secretion of progesterone begins the secretory phase of the endometrial cycle. During the secretory phase, the endometrium becomes thickened and very echogenic as a result of stromal edema, and there is loss of the triple line sign (Figure 44-5). A thickness of at least 6 mm appears to represent a central threshold for achieving pregnancy. If not enough progesterone is produced in the luteal phase, the endometrial lining may be thinner than expected on ultrasound evaluation. This lack of

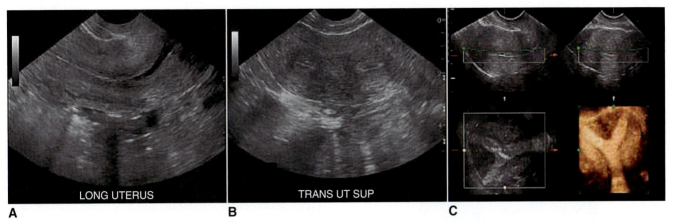

A   **B**   **C**

FIGURE 44-3 A, Longitudinal image of the uterus. **B,** Transverse image of the uterus. **C,** Three-dimensional reconstruction of the same patient demonstrating a septate uterus.

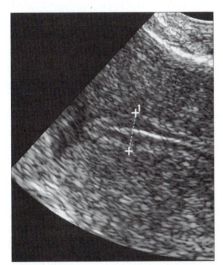

FIGURE   44-4 Longitudinal   image   of   the   proliferative endometrium.

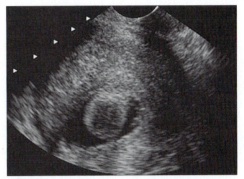

FIGURE 44-6 Submucosal fibroid with saline infusion sonography (SIS).

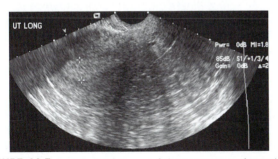

FIGURE 44-5 Longitudinal image of the secretory endometrium.

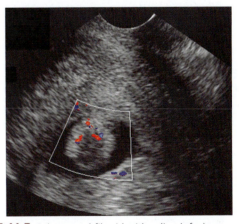

FIGURE 44-7 Submucosal fibroid with saline infusion sonography (SIS) and color Doppler showing circumferential flow.

progesterone production is known as "luteal phase deficiency" and may be associated with infertility and early pregnancy loss. The endometrial appearance has particular importance for planning for infertility treatment with embryo transfer.

Other things that can make the endometrium appear irregular or more echogenic than normal are submucosal fibroids, polyps, and adhesions. Saline infusion sonogra-

phy (SIS) can be used in these situations to further delineate the anatomic structure of the endometrium. SIS can demonstrate fibroids and polyps by outlining the endometrial cavity. Fibroids tend to have a broad base and are more isoechoic to the uterine myometrium. They also tend to have circumferential flow around them (Figures 44-6 and 44-7). Polyps tend to have a uniform hyperechoic appearance, a narrow base attachment to the endometrium (a stalk), and a vascular pedicle feeding

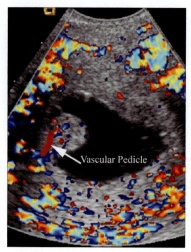

FIGURE 44-8 A polyp with SIS. Note the color Doppler demonstrating the vascular pedicle.

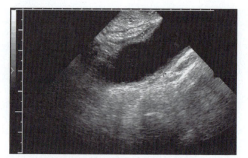

FIGURE 44-10 A hydrosalpinx.

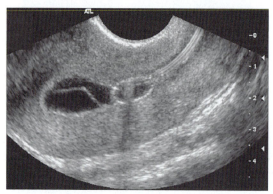

FIGURE 44-9 Uterine synechia with SIS.

them (Figure 44-8). Fibroids and polyps can potentially impede implantation, and therefore if found they can be removed to enhance fertility. SIS can also be used to evaluate the uterine cavity for synechiae, which are scars from uterine trauma (Figure 44-9). Synechiae are typically seen on ultrasound as linear strands of tissue extending from one wall of the uterine cavity to the other.

EVALUATING THE FALLOPIAN TUBES

The fallopian tubes can be examined by ultrasound for hydrosalpinx and to assess patency. A hydrosalpinx is a fallopian tube containing fluid (Figure 44-10). On ultrasound, this appears as multiple cystic tubular structures in the adnexa. Hydrosalpinx is associated with a 50% reduction in pregnancy rate and a doubling of the spontaneous miscarriage rate. Removal of such damaged tubes can dramatically improve in vitro fertilization (IVF) success. Tubal patency is assessed by injecting saline into the tube and looking for spillage of fluid into the cul-de-sac or by using contrast to evaluate for spillage. Before performing a saline or contrast study of the

fallopian tubes, it is recommended that the sonographer perform a transvaginal ultrasound to assess pelvic anatomy. The transvaginal exam allows the sonographer to see where the ovaries are in relation to the uterus and to assess for mobility of the tube and ovary. This is done by using probe pressure and hand palpation of the lower abdomen. After performing the transvaginal ultrasound, an SIS is recommended in order to evaluate the structure of the endometrial cavity. Because of the expense of contrast imaging, most centers prefer to start with a saline injection for evaluation of a tube patency, and then if it is indeterminate, to move on to air instillation or contrast imaging. To perform a saline infusion assessment of the fallopian tube, ideally a catheter is placed in the cervical canal. At this point the balloon tip of the catheter is inflated with the minimal amount of saline required to maintain its location. Afterward, and with the vaginal transducer in place, 10 to 30 cc of sterile saline is injected to assess for patency. If saline is inconclusive, air can be injected to induce echogenic bubbles. The approximate position of the fallopian tube is going to be between the ovary and the cornu. The sonographer is looking for spillage of saline or air around the ovary or into the posterior cul-de-sac. If this is seen, patency is inferred. If no spillage is noted and the patient complains of pain during injection, it may be because the tube is blocked. Obstruction of the fallopian tube can be caused by adhesions.

Before the use of ultrasound to assess for patency, there were two nonsurgical methods: the Rubin's test and hysterosalpingography (HSG). The Rubin's test involves insufflation of the fallopian tube with carbon dioxide gas, and HSG involves inserting a catheter through the cervix and then injecting contrast medium to assess the uterine cavity and fallopian tube anatomy under fluoroscopic imaging. A surgical method used to evaluate the fallopian tubes is laparoscopic chromopertubation.

EVALUATING THE OVARIES

During the ovarian follicular phase, there are several antral follicles on the ovary that are less than 5 mm in diameter (Figure 44-11). A follicle is selected to develop into a dominant follicle in response to follicle-stimulating

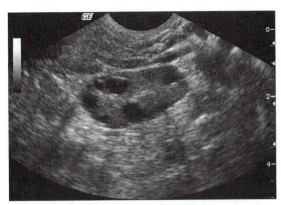

FIGURE 44-11 Ovarian follicular phase.

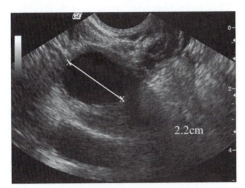

2.2cm

FIGURE 44-12 Dominant follicle.

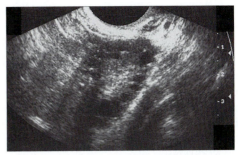

FIGURE 44-13 A polycystic ovary and the "string of pearls" sign.

Sonographic Findings. Polycystic ovary syndrome typically presents as a round ovary with multiple small immature follicles on the periphery. Usually these follicles are 2 to 9 mm in diameter. This sonographic finding has been described as the "string of pearls" sign (Figure 44-13), with the periphery of the ovary representing the neck and the multiple small cysts around the outside representing a string of pearls. The second is a normal-appearing ovary. When evaluating for PCOS, transvaginal sonography is the preferred method and is more sensitive for detecting this syndrome.

PERITONEAL FACTORS

Peritoneal factors may be the cause for as many as 25% of infertility cases. Peritoneal factors are adhesions and endometriosis. Adhesions are bands of scar tissue that can obstruct the fimbriated end of the fallopian tube. Sometimes fluid will collect in between these adhesions, resulting in a peritoneal inclusion cyst. Endometriosis is caused by the ectopic placement of endometrial tissue outside the uterus. The most common site of endometriosis is the ovaries, and often there is additional peritoneal disease. The gold standard for evaluating pelvic adhesions and endometriosis is laparoscopy.

Endometriosis involving the ovary can lead to the formation of endometriomas, which are blood-filled cysts with endometrial tissue lining the cyst wall. They range in size from smaller than 1 cm to larger than 10 cm, on rare occasion. Endometriomas typically have a characteristic sonographic appearance with homogeneous low-amplitude internal echoes.

TREATMENT OPTIONS

Ovarian Induction Therapy

Ovarian induction therapy refers to a treatment in which ovarian stimulation is achieved in a controlled setting. The first step in this process is to obtain a baseline transvaginal ultrasound of the ovaries to rule out an ovarian cyst and assess for the presence of a dominant follicle. If a cyst measuring greater than 15 mm is detected, it could represent persistent follicular activity that could interfere

hormone (FSH). The dominant follicle will grow at a rate of approximately 1 to 3 mm/day until it reaches an average diameter of 22 mm (Figure 44-12). Once reaching a mean diameter of 22 mm, the dominant follicle will rupture. Rupture may be associated with an increase or decrease in size. Sonographic findings associated with ovulation are echoes within the fluid left behind (corpus luteum cyst) or free fluid in the peritoneal cavity. However, the best predictor of ovulation is the serum p4 level of at least 3 ng/mm. At this time, luteinizing hormone (LH) rises just before ovulation and can also be found in the patient's urine.

One condition that can inhibit the release of FSH and LH is polycystic ovary syndrome (PCOS). PCOS often occurs with the diagnostic triad of (1) oligoovulation, (2) hyperandrogenism, and (3) polycystic ovaries. With PCOS, follicles begin to grow but do not develop normally. In this syndrome, the immature follicles continue to produce estrogen and androgen. This production of estrogen and androgen inhibits the pituitary gland's function and prevents normal ovulation. This is due to the pituitary gland producing more LH than FSH, which causes the follicles to remain in an arrested state of development, leading to no mature ova being released. Women with PCOS may often present with irregular bleeding and a thickened endometrium as a result of the chronic elevation of estrogen. Because of the chronic elevations of androgens, some women may have hirsutism.

with response to ovarian stimulation medication. The presence of follicular activity may be further evaluated by correlating the sonographic findings with serum estradiol levels. If serum estradiol is elevated and a large ovarian cyst is present, then oral contraceptives may be indicated to suppress follicular activity before starting ovarian stimulation therapy. This is an optimal time to assess for intracavitary masses (polyp, fibroid), because the lining of the uterus is usually at its thinnest during this early proliferative phase.

Ovarian induction therapy is usually accomplished by administering clomiphene citrate (Clomid) or human menopausal **gonadotropins**. The administration of these medications is expected to result in the enlargement of multiple follicles compared with a single dominant follicle in a naturally occurring menstrual cycle. Once therapy has started, ultrasound is used to monitor the number and size of follicles in days 8 to 14 (follicular phase) of the menstrual cycle. When evaluating the number and size of follicles, the sonographer needs to count and measure all follicles greater than 1 cm in longitudinal and transverse planes (Figure 44-14). The optimal mean measurement of a mature follicle is between 16 and 20 mm. During this time, ultrasound can be correlated with the serum estradiol levels to determine if the follicular growth corresponds with adequate Estradiol (E2) production. Correct measurement of the follicles is important because **human chorionic gonadotropin (hCG)**, a substitute for LH, may need to be given intramuscularly to trigger ovulation.

One method of evaluating ovarian reserve (decrease in quantity and quality of the ovarian follicle pool) is a sonographic antral follicle count (AFC). During the early follicular phase of the menstrual cycle, the numbers of follicles sized 2 to 6 mm from both ovaries are added to give a total AFC. High AFC values generally represent an abundance of antral follicles and thus predict a vigorous response to hormonal induction, whereas low AFC values (<5) predict lower pregnancy rates.

Monitoring the Endometrium

The endometrium is also evaluated during ovarian stimulation by assessing the thickness and echogenicity pattern of the endometrial cavity. A normal endometrial response associated with ovarian stimulation is an increasing thickness from 2 to 3 mm to 12 to 14 mm. To measure the endometrial thickness, the sonographer should image the uterus transvaginally and in the longitudinal/sagittal plane. Calipers should measure from the anterior endometrial interface to the posterior endometrial interface (Figure 44-15). This is referred to as the "double-layer" thickness. Also important to evaluate is the echogenicity pattern. A normal pattern is trilaminar. This would be similar to the echographic pattern of the periovulatory endometrium. A thin endometrium (less than 6 mm in diameter) and an abnormal echographic pattern have been associated with decreased fertility.

In Vitro Fertilization and Embryo Transfer

In vitro fertilization (IVF) is a method of fertilizing the human oocyte outside the body. Mature oocytes are collected and mixed in a dish with a sample of sperm. The resulting embryos are then placed back into the uterus. The treatment plan for IVF consists of ovarian monitoring, needle aspiration of oocytes, incubation of oocytes, fertilization, and transferring the embryos into the uterus. The ovarian monitoring is performed as described in the ovarian induction therapy section, with one difference: instead of evaluating for two optimal follicles, four follicles are identified before triggering evaluation. Oocyte retrieval is accomplished by transvaginal ultrasound guidance.

Transvaginal sonography is used as a guide to locate the ovaries when the ovaries are more posterior in location, such as in the cul-de-sac. The transvaginal transducer is covered with a protective sheath (e.g., transducer

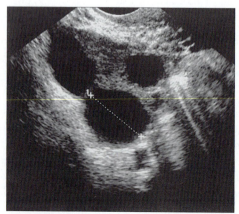

FIGURE 44-14 Enlargement of multiple ovarian follicles.

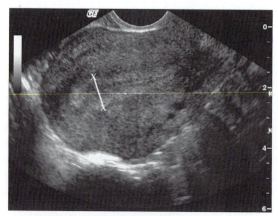

FIGURE 44-15 Endometrial measurement.

cover) and the needle guide is attached. Sterile gel should be placed in the tip of the protective sheath. If using an ultrasound machine with needle guide software, the sonographer turns on the needle guide function. This function shows where the needle will go in relationship to the image. Once the transducer is prepared, it is inserted into the vagina and the ovary imaged. A 30-cm, 18-gauge needle is placed in the guide and introduced transvaginally following the outlined needle path, and under ultrasound imaging one will see the needle tip go into the desired follicle. Some centers prefer using a scored needle tip, which is more easily seen on ultrasound. Once the needle tip is in the follicle, the fluid in the follicle is aspirated with the intention that the oocyte is within this aspirate. Occasionally the ovum may be stuck to a wall; some clinicians may use a buffer solution injected into the follicle to flush out the cavity. The solution is then reaspirated to maximize the potential for ovum retrieval.

Once the oocytes are retrieved, they are fertilized in a dish and incubated for a few days before **embryo transfer** into the uterus. Embryo transfer is done by ultrasound guidance. Ultrasound is first used to map the endometrial cavity. This can be done by using the trace function on the ultrasound machine and tracing the endometrial interface from cervix to the apex of the fundus to determine the length of the uterine cavity. Optimal placement of the embryos is considered to be within 2 cm of the apex of the fundus, so it is important for the clinician to know the length of the uterine cavity to ensure proper placement of the embryos. After the endometrium is mapped, using transabdominal ultrasound guidance, a catheter is inserted through the cervix and placed within 2 cm of the fundus of the uterine cavity. The embryos are then slowly released, and a transfer air bubble is visible on ultrasound after the embryos are released from the catheter. After embryo transfer, the catheter is checked under a stereomicroscope to ensure that all embryos are transferred.

Intrauterine Insemination

Intrauterine insemination is a technique used to treat male factor infertility. With intrauterine insemination, a catheter containing sperm is placed into the uterine fundus. The sperm preparation may be from a donor, and this is referred to as artificial insemination using donor sperm or therapeutic donor insemination (TDI). Sometimes ultrasound is used to guide this procedure.

COMPLICATIONS ASSOCIATED WITH ASSISTED REPRODUCTIVE TECHNOLOGY

Complications associated with **assisted reproductive technology (ART)** include **ovarian hyperstimulation syndrome (OHSS)**, multiple gestations, and ectopic pregnancy. OHSS is a syndrome that presents sonographically as enlarged ovaries with multiple cysts, abdominal ascites, and pleural effusions. This syndrome is often seen in patients who have undergone ovulation induction after administration of follicle-stimulating hormone or a GnRH analogue followed by hCG. This syndrome is more common in patients with a history of polycystic ovary syndrome and can be graded based on patient symptoms. In mild cases of OHSS, patients complain of lower abdominal pain and back pain. On ultrasound exam, a mild case of OHSS will demonstrate enlarged ovaries (5 to 10 cm) with multiple cysts. More severe cases of OHSS will present with leg edema, ascites, pleural effusions, hypotension, and polycythemia. Sonographic findings in severe OHSS cases will demonstrate enlarged ovaries with multiple cysts, ascites, and pleural effusions (Figure 44-16).

Patients who undergo in vitro fertilization are at an increased risk for having multiple gestations. It is estimated that about 30% of in vitro fertilization pregnancies result in a multiple gestation. The concern with multiple gestations is that if there are three or more fetuses, there is an increased risk of fetal or neonatal morbidity and mortality. Therefore, pregnancies that have three or more fetuses are often counseled about fetal reduction options. Fetal reduction is performed by injecting potassium chloride into the fetal chest/heart.

Patients who undergo assisted reproductive technologies are at an increased risk for ectopic pregnancy. An ectopic pregnancy is a pregnancy that is implanted outside of the uterus. These patients are also at risk for having a heterotopic pregnancy. A heterotopic pregnancy is an ectopic pregnancy coexisting with an intrauterine pregnancy (Figures 44-17 and 44-18). This used to be a rare occurrence (1:4000). However, with the advancement in ART, the estimated occurrence is 1:100 in this patient population.[1] The incidence of a heterotopic pregnancy with an intrauterine multiple gestation is 1:10,000, but in the ART patient subgroup, this risk may increase to 1:100.[1] In this patient population, when an

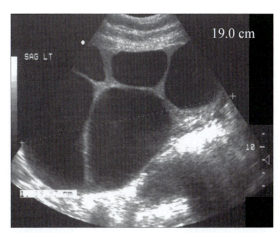

FIGURE 44-16 An enlarged ovary with multiple cysts in a patient with OHSS.

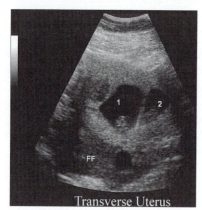

FIGURE 44-17 An intrauterine twin pregnancy. *FF*, free fluid.

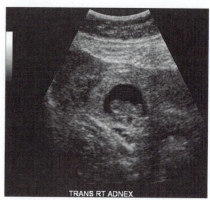

FIGURE 44-18 A live heterotopic pregnancy in the same patient shown in Figure 44-17.

intrauterine pregnancy is visualized, it is important to carefully image the adnexa, not just for ovarian pathology but also to evaluate for a heterotopic pregnancy.

REFERENCES

1. Barnhart KT: Ectopic pregnancy, *N Engl J Med* 361(4):379-387, 2009.
2. Buttram VC: The American Fertility Society classification of adnexal adhesions, distal tubal occlusion, tubal occlusion secondary to tubal ligation, tubal pregnancies, Mullerian anomalies and intrauterine adhesions, *Fertil Steril* 49:944-955, 1988.
3. Thurmond AS: Imaging of female infertility, *Radiol Clin N Am* 41:757-767, 2003.

PART VIII

Obstetrics

The Role of Sonography in Obstetrics

Jean Lea Spitz

OBJECTIVES

On completion of this chapter, you should be able to:
- Discuss indications for obstetric sonography
- Analyze the differences among standard, specialized, and limited obstetric sonography examinations
- List maternal risk factors that increase the chances of producing a fetus with congenital anomalies
- Recount important questions to ask the patient before beginning the obstetric sonography examination
- Describe the biologic effects of diagnostic medical ultrasound energy and related patient safety
- Describe the steps of the first-, second-, and third-trimester sonography protocols
- List fetal anatomy visualization required as part of the standard second-trimester examination
- Discuss the use of sonography as a diagnostic and screening test

OUTLINE

Sonography is the primary tool for evaluating the developing fetus during pregnancy. Obstetric sonography allows the clinician to assess the development, growth, and well-being of the fetus. When an abnormal condition is recognized prenatally, obstetric management may be altered to provide optimal care for the fetus and mother. The visualization of pregnancy with sonography has revolutionized obstetrics. Conditions that were previously detected only at delivery are now diagnosed early in pregnancy and monitored with sonography. Prenatal diagnosis has led to prenatal treatments performed under ultrasound visualization. Sharing of sonographic images and diagnostic results facilitates prenatal parental education and counseling. Although obstetric sonography is popular in many aspects of our culture, including books, television, and family gatherings, its value lies in its medical use.

The sonographer performing fetal studies must understand both sonographic and obstetric principles to accurately and thoroughly compile pertinent information and to provide an optimal sonographic assessment of the fetus. Fetal sonography should be performed only when there is a valid medical reason and using the lowest possible ultrasound energy exposure settings to gain the necessary diagnostic information. The sonographer has a responsibility to obstetric patients and clinicians to provide competent, safe, and appropriate examinations.

Practice guidelines produced by the American College of Radiology (ACR), the American Institute of Ultrasound in Medicine (AIUM), and the American College of Obstetricians and Gynecologists (ACOG) recommend specific components of a standard obstetric sonography examination. Sonographers must strive during each examination to meet the recommended requirements. In addition, components may be altered or added to serve the interests of the patient or the referring clinician. It is often the responsibility of the sonographer, under the general direction of a physician, to apply knowledge, competence, and critical thinking to determine and perform appropriate examination components based on the specific indication for the study and the clinical history of the mother.

In accordance with recommended guidelines, the sonographer should establish a systematic scanning protocol that encompasses all criteria indicated in the guidelines. An organized approach to scanning ensures completeness and reduces the risk of missing a detectable obstetric or fetal concern.

This chapter describes the medical indications for obstetric sonography examinations and the types of obstetric examinations performed; reviews practice guidelines as outlined by ACR, AIUM, and ACOG; reviews the safety of ultrasound in obstetrics; and describes maternal risk factors and history that may alter examination protocols.

INDICATIONS FOR OBSTETRIC SONOGRAPHY

The sonographer needs to be aware of the indications for obstetric sonography and to understand the medical complications associated with each indication. Recommended indications for obstetric sonography examinations are incorporated into diagnosis codes and billing codes. The National Institute of Child Health and Human Development in the National Institutes of Health Consensus Report on Safety of Ultrasound first defined these indications in 1984. Current practice guidelines include indications for first-trimester obstetric sonography and second- and third-trimester obstetric sonography that were adapted from the 1984 list. These indications are listed in Boxes 45-1 and 45-2. Additional explanation for these indications is provided in the following paragraphs.

1. Estimation of **gestational (menstrual) age** for patients with uncertain clinical dates or verification of dates for patients who are to undergo scheduled elective repeat cesarean delivery, indicated induction of labor, or elective termination of pregnancy. Sonographic confirmation of dating permits proper timing of cesarean delivery or labor induction to avoid premature delivery.

2. Evaluation of fetal growth, for example, when the patient has an identified cause for uteroplacental insufficiency, such as severe preeclampsia, chronic hypertension, chronic renal disease, or severe diabetes mellitus, or for other medical complications of pregnancy in which fetal malnutrition (e.g., **intrauterine growth restriction [IUGR]**, or **macrosomia**) is suspected. Measuring fetal growth by sonography at 2- to 4-week intervals permits assessment of the impact of a complicating condition of the fetus and guides pregnancy management.

3. Vaginal bleeding of undetermined cause in pregnancy. Sonography often allows determination of the source of bleeding and the status of the fetus.

4. Serial evaluation of cervical length in pregnant women with increased risk for recurrent preterm birth or primary preterm birth.

BOX 45-1 Indications for First-Trimester Sonography

- To confirm the presence of an intrauterine pregnancy
- To evaluate a suspected ectopic pregnancy
- To define the cause of vaginal bleeding
- To evaluate pelvic pain
- To estimate gestational (menstrual) age
- To diagnose or evaluate multiple pregnancy
- To confirm cardiac activity
- As an adjunct to chorionic villous sampling, embryo transfer, or localization and removal of an intrauterine device
- To assess for certain fetal anomalies, such as anencephaly, in patients at high risk
- To evaluate maternal pelvic or adnexal masses or uterine abnormalities
- To screen for fetal aneuploidy
- To evaluate suspected hydatidiform mole

BOX 45-2 Indications for Second- and Third-Trimester Sonography

- Evaluation of gestational age
- Evaluation of fetal growth
- Evaluation of vaginal bleeding
- Evaluation of cervical insufficiency
- Evaluation of abdominal and pelvic pain
- Determination of fetal presentation
- Evaluation of suspected multiple gestation
- Adjunct to amniocentesis or other procedure
- Significant discrepancy between uterine size and clinical dates
- Evaluation of pelvic mass
- Examination of suspected hydatidiform mole
- Adjunct to cervical cerclage placement
- Evaluation of suspected ectopic pregnancy
- Evaluation of suspected fetal death
- Evaluation of suspected uterine abnormality
- Evaluation of fetal well-being
- Evaluation of suspected amniotic fluid abnormalities
- Evaluation of suspected placental abruption
- Adjunct to external cephalic version
- Evaluation for premature rupture of membranes and/or premature labor
- Evaluation for abnormal biochemical markers
- Follow-up evaluation of a fetal anomaly
- Follow-up evaluation of placental location for suspected placenta previa
- Evaluation of those with a history of previous congenital anomaly
- Evaluation of fetal condition in late registrants for prenatal care
- Assessment of findings that may increase the risk of aneuploidy
- Screening for fetal anomalies

5. Evaluation of abdominal or pelvic pain in pregnancy that may be associated with ectopic pregnancy, **abruptio placentae,** or maternal appendicitis, renal calculi, pelvic mass, or other conditions.

6. Determination of fetal presentation when the presenting part cannot be adequately determined in labor, or the fetal presentation is variable in late pregnancy. Accurate knowledge of presentation guides management of delivery.

7. Suspected multiple gestation based on detection of more than one fetal heartbeat pattern, fundal height larger than expected for dates, or prior use of fertility drugs. Pregnancy management may be altered in multiple gestation.

8. Adjunct to **amniocentesis.** Sonography permits guidance of the needle to avoid the **placenta** and fetus, to increase the chance of obtaining amniotic fluid, and to decrease the chance of pregnancy loss.

9. Significant discrepancy between uterine size and clinical dates. Sonography permits accurate dating and detection of such conditions as **oligohydramnios** and **polyhydramnios,** along with multiple gestation, IUGR, and anomalies.

10. Evaluation of pelvic mass. Sonography can detect the location and nature of the mass and can aid in diagnosis.

11. **Hydatidiform mole** suspected on the basis of clinical signs of hypertension, proteinuria, or the presence of ovarian cysts felt on pelvic examination or failure to detect fetal heart tones with a Doppler ultrasound device after 12 weeks. Sonography permits accurate diagnosis and differentiation of this neoplasm from fetal death.

12. Adjunct to cervical **cerclage** placement. Sonography aids in timing and proper placement of the cerclage for patients with **incompetent cervix.**

13. Suspected ectopic pregnancy, or pregnancy that occurs after tuboplasty or prior ectopic gestation. Sonography is a valuable diagnostic aid for this complication.

14. Evaluation of suspected fetal death. Rapid diagnosis enhances optimal management.

15. Suspected uterine abnormality (e.g., clinically significant leiomyomas; congenital structural abnormalities, such as bicornuate uterus or uteri didelphys). Serial surveillance of fetal growth and state enhances fetal outcome.

16. Evaluation of fetal well-being. Biophysical evaluation for fetal well-being after 28 weeks' gestation may include assessment of amniotic fluid, fetal tone, body movements, breathing movements, and heart rate patterns.

17. Evaluation of suspected amniotic fluid abnormalities such as suspected polyhydramnios or oligohydramnios. Confirmation of the diagnosis and identification of the cause of the condition in certain pregnancies are necessary.

18. Suspected abruptio placentae. Confirmation of diagnosis and extent of abruption assists in clinical management.

19. Adjunct to external version from breech to vertex presentation. The visualization provided by sonography facilitates performance of this procedure.

20. Estimation of fetal weight and presentation in premature rupture of the membranes or premature labor. Information provided by sonography guides management decisions on timing and method of delivery.

21. Evaluation following maternal serum biochemical marker results. Elevated **maternal serum alpha-fetoprotein (MSAFP)** increases the risk for open defects such as neural tube defects. Other biochemical markers in the first trimester or **quad screen** biochemistry in the second trimester may indicate increased risk for certain obstetric or fetal conditions.

22. Follow-up observation of identified fetal anomaly. Sonographic assessment of progression or lack of change may assist in clinical management.

23. Follow-up evaluation of placenta location for suspected **placenta previa.**

24. Evaluation for those with a history of previous congenital anomaly. Detection of recurrence may be facilitated, or psychological benefit to patients may result from reassurance of no recurrence.

25. Evaluation of fetal condition in late registrants for prenatal care. Assessment of gestational age and fetal size assists in pregnancy management decisions for this group.

26. Assessment of findings that may increase the risk of **aneuploidy.**

27. Screening for fetal anomalies.

TYPES OF OBSTETRIC SONOGRAPHY EXAMINATIONS

The three practice guidelines define the major types of sonographic examinations performed in the second and third trimesters of pregnancy, using the terms "limited," "standard," and "specialized." In practice, the examinations may also be referred to by the CPT (current procedure terminology) code most commonly used for billing of the examinations. The major types of obstetric sonography examinations are listed in Box 45-3 and are described in the following sections.

The standard obstetric sonography examination (CPT code 76805) is typically performed during the second trimester around 18 weeks' gestational age. The standard examination includes an evaluation of gestational age by fetal biometry, fetal number, placental position, cardiac activity, amniotic fluid volume, and fetal anatomic survey, including all of the elements specified in the guidelines. The standard examination may include the maternal cervix and adnexa as well when clinically appropriate and technically feasible.

The limited obstetric sonography examination (CPT code 76815) is used when the answer to a specific clinical question such as presentation of the fetus, placental location, cervical length, amniotic fluid volume, or verification of fetal heart motion is required. A limited examination is done when a previous standard obstetric examination has been recorded.

A repeat obstetric sonography examination (CPT code 76816) is similar to a standard obstetric examination and typically includes biometry to evaluate fetal growth, and reevaluation of anatomy that may or may not have been well visualized on the standard examination. The repeat obstetric examination is done when a previous standard obstetric examination has been recorded and the second examination is ordered for the same indication.

The specialty obstetric sonography examination (CPT code 76811) is also known as a targeted sonogram. It is typically done when an anomaly is suspected based on maternal history, biochemistry, or the results of a previous obstetric sonogram. The specialty obstetric sonography examination includes all components of the standard examination plus a more in-depth view of fetal anatomy. The specialty examination typically includes additional views of the fetal heart and may include color Doppler views of the heart. The specialty examination may include additional views of the extremities and a focus on areas of anomalous or expected findings associated with the patient history. The specialty obstetric sonography examination is typically performed in referral centers with specific expertise in high-risk obstetrics.

The first-trimester examination (CPT code 76801) is performed before 13 weeks and 6 days' gestation. The examination includes the uterus, the **cervix,** and the maternal adnexa, as well as the gestational sac and embryo. The pregnancy is dated based on embryonic size, and fetal heart motion is documented if these findings are present. Uterine anomalies and pelvic masses associated with pregnancy are more easily seen in first-trimester examinations. The chorionicity and amnionicity of multiple gestations should be documented at this time as well.

The first-trimester risk assessment examination (CPT code 76813) is also known as the **nuchal translucency**

examination. This examination is performed only when women choose first-trimester screening tests for aneuploidy. The examination includes measurement of fetal crown-rump length and measurement of nuchal translucency using standard criteria. In some centers, the examination may also include visualization of the fetal nasal bone and other risk assessment parameters. Sonographers who perform these examinations must demonstrate competence in the standardized measurement of nuchal translucency and must participate in an ongoing quality-monitoring program.

Additional CPT codes are used for transvaginal obstetric examinations, multiple gestations, fetal echocardiography, three-dimensional (3D)/four-dimensional (4D) examinations, biophysical profiles, and invasive procedures. Sonographers performing obstetric sonography must know the components required for each type of examination. Health care compliance regulations require that the billing or CPT code must match the examination performed.

PATIENT HISTORY

The sonographer should ask the patient several important questions before beginning the obstetric sonography evaluation. Both open-ended questions such as "Do you have concerns?" and closed questions such as "When was your last normal period?" are used in gathering important patient information.

Gravidity and Parity

Key obstetric history of the patient is summarized using gravidity (G) and parity (P). The sonographer should recognize this clinical description of the pregnant patient. **Gravidity** is the number of pregnancies, including the present one. **Parity** is reported using a numeric system that describes all possible pregnancy outcomes. The letter "P" followed by four numbers in sequence, P0000, is commonly used. The numbers represent, in order, full-term deliveries, premature births and stillborns, early pregnancy loss or termination, and living children. For instance, a G4P2103 describes a patient undergoing her fourth pregnancy. She has had two full-term deliveries, one premature birth, no early pregnancy losses, and three living children.

Clinical Dates

The sonographer first tries to determine the clinical dates of the pregnancy. It is important to document the clinical date reported by the patient and the date determined by the earliest sonographic examination. An accurate clinical date facilitates correlation of obstetric measurements with the expected gestational age.

The first date of the last normal menstrual period (LMP or LNMP) is the standard way to date a pregnancy in the United States. Human pregnancy lasts 266 days plus or minus 10 days. If conception occurs on day 14 from the LNMP, the pregnancy duration from LNMP is 280 days or 40 weeks. Pregnancy is divided into **trimesters** of approximately 13 weeks. A pregnant woman is in the first trimester until 13 weeks 6 days' gestational age (GA), and in the second trimester from 14 weeks to 26 weeks 6 days' GA. The third trimester begins at 27 weeks' GA and lasts until term.

In reality, the assessment of gestational age is often not precise. Many women have irregular periods, conceive within 3 months of coming off birth control pills when ovulation is irregular, or do not record dates. Even with a known menstrual date, conception may occur from day 6 to day 27, which is a difference of 3 weeks in gestational age as determined by sonography. Physicians may use clinical parameters such as uterine size and growth or ovulation indications to estimate pregnancy dates. Gestational age provides an estimate of how long a patient has been pregnant, but the exact date that labor will begin cannot be determined owing to the variable length of human pregnancy.

The sonographer first asks the patient the first day of her last menstrual period. If the patient does not remember the date of her LNMP, the sonographer may ask for the expected date of delivery (EDD). The sonographer should also ask if previous sonographic examinations were performed before 20 weeks and the estimated date of delivery determined by the earliest sonographic examination. By recording this information, the sonographer can provide an estimation of the clinical dates and their accuracy.

Dates established by sonography performed in the first or second trimester typically take precedence over menstrual dates when the discrepancy is greater than 7 days in the first trimester or greater than 10 days in the second trimester. Sonography may be considered to confirm menstrual dates if there is gestational age agreement within a week by crown-rump length or within 10 days by second-trimester fetal biometry. The pregnancy should not be dated by sonographic measurements in the third trimester, and dates should not be changed after they have been calculated from an early examination. It is ultimately the responsibility of the obstetrician who is following the pregnancy to determine the clinical gestational age.

Nägele's Rule

The EDD may be calculated using Nägele's rule (Box 45-4). According to this method, the EDD is derived by subtracting 3 months from the LNMP and adding 7 days. For example, an LNMP of 10/17 would result in an EDC of 7/24 (10/17 – 3 months = 7/17 – 7 days = 7/24). A sonographer familiar with this rule may determine EDD or LNMP when the patient verbally reports only one. Commercial date wheels simplify this method to

BOX 45-4	Nägele's Rule
EDD = LNMP – 3 months + 7 days	
LMP = EDD – 3 months + 7 days	

EDD, Estimated date of delivery; *LNMP,* last normal menstrual period.

determine the due date and to assign fetal age at the time of the sonography study.

Maternal Risk Factors

It is important for sonographers to ask if the patient has latex allergies. Many sonography laboratories use only latex-free materials to prevent allergic reactions. It is also important to ask if the patient has experienced supine hypotension (i.e., difficulty lying on her back during pregnancy) and to caution the patient to report any sense of warmth, dizziness, or syncope experienced during the sonography examination.

The sonographer needs to know if the patient is currently taking any medication or has experienced clinical problems with the pregnancy, such as bleeding, decreased fetal movement, or pelvic pain. If the patient has had problems with previous pregnancies, such as incompetent cervix, fibroids, fetal macrosomia or growth restriction, or congenital or chromosomal fetal anomalies, this information must be documented. Finally, the sonographer needs to know if the patient has maternal risk factors for anomalies that may have an impact on the examination or interpretation.

Factors that may affect the risk of producing a fetus with congenital anomalies include increased maternal age, first- or second-trimester maternal serum biochemistry values, first-trimester increased nuchal translucency, maternal disease (e.g., diabetes mellitus, systemic lupus erythematosus), and a pregnant uterine cavity that is too small or too large for dates. Other risk factors include a previous child born with a chromosomal disorder or exposure to a known teratogenic drug or infectious agent known to cause birth defects. Some anomalies are caused by a reduced or increased number of fetal chromosomes. These anomalies, the most common of which is Down syndrome, trisomy 21, are called aneuploidies. Other anomalies are thought to have both genetic and environmental causes. For example, neural tube defects have a genetic component but are influenced by the maternal environment, especially by a lack of adequate folic acid before pregnancy and during the early embryonic period. Assessment of maternal risk may include discussion of both genetic and family history; environmental triggers, such as maternal disease and nutrition; and available testing. Genetic counselors are trained to assist patients in determining risks before or during pregnancy. With adequate counseling and environmental factor control, some anomalies may be prevented.

THE SAFETY OF ULTRASOUND

U.S. government census bureau prenatal statistics estimate that approximately 65% of all pregnant women in the United States are examined with sonography. Ultrasound imaging has been used in pregnancy since the 1950s without apparent side effects. The first studies conducted to determine the safety of ultrasound in pregnancy were small and were hampered by imprecise dosimetry and poorly matched control groups. Physicists and researchers have made tremendous strides in defining the variables of importance in terms of bioeffects and the types of tissue interactions and damage that may occur. Using human epidemiology studies, animal experiments, and in vitro studies of tissue and cells, scientists continue to study the safety of ultrasound, but challenges remain. Existing human studies are not large enough to document small increases in normally occurring anomalies that may occur as the result of sonography. Similarly, it is difficult to determine potential long-term effects of prenatal ultrasound imaging. Animal experiments and therapeutic applications document that high-intensity ultrasound may modify biologic structures and functions. Studies in pregnancy with animals and humans have suggested possibilities of growth differences (reduction in animals), increased nonright-handedness, and delayed speech.

The major biologic effects of ultrasound are believed to be thermal (a rise in temperature) and mechanical forces, including cavitation (production and collapse of gas-filled bubbles). Sonographers can minimize thermal effects by not staying in one spot, especially over fetal bone, for long periods of time and by extending the focus of the beam as deeply into the body as is reasonable to obtain adequate images. Cavitation is dependent on the presence of preexisting gas within the tissue. Sonographers who work with newborns may choose to be cautious of long examinations through newborn lungs filled with gas.

The AIUM has a committee of scientists, clinicians, sonographers, and engineers who regularly review and summarize information regarding bioeffects. The AIUM statement on Prudent Use and Clinical Safety adopted in 2007 is as follows:

Diagnostic ultrasound has been in use since the late 1950s. Given its known benefits and recognized efficacy for medical diagnosis, including use during human pregnancy, the American Institute of Ultrasound in Medicine herein addresses the clinical safety of such use: No independently confirmed adverse effects caused by exposure from present diagnostic ultrasound instruments have been reported in human patients in the absence of contrast agents. Biological effects (such as localized pulmonary bleeding) have been reported in mammalian systems at diagnostically relevant exposures but the clinical significance of such effects is not known. Ultrasound should be used by qualified health professionals to provide medical benefit to the patient.

In summary, it is important to remember the following:

1. There are theoretical effects of ultrasound energy on the fetus; potential biologic effects have not been documented.
2. The energy produced by ultrasound equipment today is higher than that produced by earlier equipment. Doppler imaging produces higher energy. The history of safety with energy at the level in use today is not long.
3. Studies on ultrasound bioeffects are not definitive, and continued research is essential.
4. Sonographers have a responsibility to be knowledgeable regarding ultrasound bioeffects and to use the least amount of energy necessary to obtain the clinical information needed.

It is the responsibility of sonographers to integrate their knowledge of bioeffects into their scanning.

In March 2008, the AIUM adopted a statement on the *As Low As Reasonably Achievable (ALARA) principle*, which states the following:

The potential benefits and risks of each examination should be considered. The ALARA (As Low As Reasonably Achievable) principle should be observed when adjusting controls that affect the acoustical output and by considering transducer dwell times.

THE SAFETY OF DOPPLER FOR THE OBSTETRIC PATIENT

Doppler ultrasound provides a noninvasive method to assess the physiology and pathophysiology of fetal and maternal circulations when such examinations are required for diagnosis. In most cases, pulsed wave Doppler rather than continuous wave Doppler is used in the fetus. Doppler may be used to detect flow in the maternal vessels, the fetal vessels (umbilical artery and vein, aorta and inferior vena cava, renal arteries, and cerebral vessels), the fetal **ductus venosus,** the fetal heart, and the placenta. Doppler interrogation is an important part of fetal echocardiography examinations and aids in the diagnosis of fetal heart defects. Specific applications of Doppler in obstetrics are presented in the respective chapters.

Recently, several authors have demonstrated the feasibility of examining the fetal heart during the first trimester. Doppler is performed at a higher energy level because these are difficult examinations that may require prolonged dwell times, and because the embryo at this stage is small and receives total body insonation.

Therefore, the use of Doppler ultrasound during the first trimester has generated some controversy.

The benefits of Doppler imaging most likely outweigh the risks when specific indications require Doppler interrogation. Fetal sonography with or without Doppler should be performed only when there is a valid medical reason, and the lowest possible ultrasonic exposure settings should be used to obtain the necessary diagnostic information.

GUIDELINES FOR FIRST-TRIMESTER AND STANDARD SECOND- AND THIRD-TRIMESTER OBSTETRIC SONOGRAPHY EXAMINATIONS

In the late 1980s, in response to concerns about variability in quality and practices, obstetric examination guidelines were introduced by three professional organizations. AIUM published obstetric standards in 1985, which were revised in 1991, 2003, and 2007. ACOG first published standards in 1988, and the current version of ACOG standards (*ACOG Practice Bulletin Number 101: Ultrasonography in Pregnancy*) was published in February 2009. The ACR first adopted standards in 1990, with revisions following in 1995 and 2007. These three professional societies collaborate on the clinical aspects of their statements and include identical wording related to classification and specifications for examinations. Portions of their statements, including information related to physician qualifications, procedure documentation, quality control, background, and clinical recommendations, differ between organizations.

The purpose of the current guidelines is to provide practitioners with information regarding the criteria for a complete examination. These guidelines are often cited as a legal standard, although this use was not intended. Although it is not possible to detect all fetal anomalies with sonography, adherence to practice guidelines and referral of any suspicious studies for further evaluation will optimize the possibilities of detection.

It is important that all sonographers strive to consistently meet or exceed minimum standards during every obstetric sonographic examination. Quality standards include not only the components of the examination protocol but also the qualifications of personnel performing the examination, documentation, equipment specifications, fetal safety, quality control, infection control, and patient education concerns.

Although no mechanism exists to absolutely ensure technical competence, the standard of practice for personnel in sonography is national board certification. The purpose of certification or registry is to assure the public that the person performing sonography has the necessary knowledge, skills, and experience to provide this service.

Documentation standards require that a permanent record be maintained that includes the measurements and anatomic findings. Images should be labeled with the patient's name, date, and image orientation if appropriate. A written report of the examination must be maintained in the patient records. Fetal echocardiography is often stored in a real-time format for future reference and review. A written report by the physician should outline the findings of the study. The availability of real-time sonography equipment with transabdominal and transvaginal transducers is essential to confirm fetal life and to permit the sonographer to view fetal anatomy and movements, and to obtain the biometric parameters used to determine fetal age and growth.

Transducer frequency selection and equipment settings should balance optimal imaging resolution and penetration. The lowest possible exposure setting should be used according to the ALARA principle. Policies and procedures related to patient information, infection control, quality control, and safety should be developed and implemented in every laboratory. Policies typically address personnel and patient safety and may address musculoskeletal injury concerns for the sonographer. A monitor mounted on the wall for patient viewing provides ergonomic protection for the sonographer in obstetric laboratories.

First Trimester

Indications for first-trimester sonography are shown in Box 45-1. A transabdominal or transvaginal transducer may be used for examination of the first-trimester embryo and fetus. If a transabdominal examination is not definitive, a transvaginal or transperineal examination is required. A transabdominal examination may provide an overview of the entire pelvic cavity and enable the sonographer to image the uterus from the **cervix** to the fundus, evaluate the ovaries and adnexal areas for abnormal collections of fluid or a mass, and look for the presence of free fluid. The transvaginal transducer provides a more limited view of the pelvic cavity but allows excellent visualization of the **embryo, yolk sac, amnion, chorion,** and **gestational sac.**

Sample Protocol

1. The uterus and adnexa should be evaluated for the presence of a gestational sac.
   - If a gestational sac is seen, its location (intrauterine or extrauterine) should be noted.
   - The gestational sac should be recorded when the embryo is not identified during the **zygote** or implantation stage of pregnancy. Caution must be used in diagnosing a gestational sac without the presence of a yolk sac or embryo because intrauterine fluid collections may appear similar.
   - The presence or absence of a yolk sac and an embryo should be noted.
   - The crown-rump length is the most accurate measurement of gestational age during the first

trimester and should be recorded when an embryo is present.

- The earliest structure seen within the gestational sac is the yolk sac (the yolk sac will indicate the presence of an intrauterine pregnancy).
- The embryo is seen at 4 weeks (menstrual age) as an echogenic curved structure adjacent to the yolk sac.
- Blood tests (human chorionic gonadotropin [hCG] levels) should be positive at 7 to 10 days' **embryonic age (conception age).**
- The placenta is seen as a thickened density (trophoblastic reaction) along part of the margin of the gestational sac.
- The bowel herniates out from the fetal abdomen at 8 to 11 weeks, then returns to the abdominal cavity.

2. Presence or absence of cardiac activity should be reported.
- Cardiac motion is usually seen when the embryo is 5 mm or greater in length.
- The fetal heart rate is much faster than the mother's heart rate. The fetal heart rate changes according to fetal development stages; early in embryologic development, the heart rate is slow (90 beats per minute). The rate may go up to 180 beats per minute in the middle of the first trimester, before returning to 120 to 160 beats per minute throughout the remainder of the pregnancy.

3. Fetal number should be documented.
- Count only the embryo and yolk sac to determine multiple pregnancies. The membrane structure and the number of amniotic and chorionic membranes should be documented in all multiple pregnancies. The chorionicity is most reliably documented during the first trimester.

4. Evaluation of the uterus, adnexal structures, and cul-de-sac should be performed.
- It is important to document the texture of the ovaries and the presence of **corpus luteum** or other adnexal masses; look for inhomogeneous uterine texture that may represent leiomyomatous growth that may be stimulated by the hormonal changes of pregnancy.

Second and Third Trimesters

The indications for second- and third-trimester sonography are shown in Box 45-2. Guidelines for the second- and third-trimester ultrasound examination, which include a biometric and anatomic survey of the fetus, suggest the following:

1. Fetal cardiac motion, fetal number, presentation, and activity should be documented.
- In multiple gestations, the following individual studies should be performed on each fetus: amnionicity, chorionicity, comparison of fetal sizes, estimation of amniotic fluid (increased, decreased, or normal) on each side of the membrane, and fetal gender (when visualized).

2. A qualitative or semiquantitative estimate of the volume of amniotic fluid should be reported. Abnormal fluid amounts should be described.
- In early pregnancy, amniotic fluid is produced by the placenta; the fetal kidneys begin to produce urine, which contributes to the production and replacement of amniotic fluid as the fetus swallows and urinates. The fluid increases in volume until the 34th week of gestation.
- Experienced observers may subjectively estimate amniotic fluid volume. Semiquantitative methods, including the four-quadrant amniotic fluid index (AFI), the single deepest pocket, and the two-diameter pocket, may be used.
- Excessive fluid is termed *hydramnios (polyhydramnios);* too little fluid is called *oligohydramnios.*

3. Placental localization, appearance, and relationship to the internal cervical os should be recorded. The **umbilical cord** should be imaged, and the number of vessels should be evaluated when possible.
- The maternal bladder must be adequately filled to reveal the cervical os in the **lower uterine segment.** The sonographer should document that the lower end of the placenta is away from the cervical os to rule out placenta previa.
- An overdistended maternal urinary bladder or a contraction in the lower uterine cavity can give a false impression of placenta previa.
- Placental location in early pregnancy may not correlate well with its location at the time of delivery.
- Transvaginal or transperineal imaging may be necessary to document cervical length when it appears shortened or if there is a history of regular uterine contractions. The value of routine cervical length measurements in low-risk pregnancy has not been established.

4. Gestational (menstrual) age should be assessed by sonographic biometry. Crown-rump length measured during the first trimester is the most accurate method to assess gestational age. During the second and third trimesters, multiple sonographic parameters can be used to estimate gestational age. The variability of these measurements increases as the pregnancy progresses. If the clinical gestational age and sonographic parameters demonstrate significant discrepancies, the possibility of fetal growth abnormalities, such as macrosomia or IUGR, is suggested. Biometric parameters that may be used include the following:
- Biparietal diameter (BPD) is measured in an axial plane that includes the thalamus and the cavum septi pellucidi. The cerebellar hemispheres should not be visible in the image where the BPD is measured. The biparietal measurement is taken from the outer edge to the inner edge of the skull. The head may normally be more rounded

(brachycephaly) or elongated (dolichocephaly), which will make measurement of the head circumference more accurate than measurement of the BPD.

- Head circumference is measured at the same level as BPD, around the outer perimeter of the calvarium. Head circumference is not affected by head shape.
- Femur length, that is, the length of the femoral diaphysis, is reliably measured after the 14th week of gestation. The most accurate measurements are taken when the femoral shaft is perpendicular to the acoustic beam.
- Abdominal circumference is measured on a transverse view at the level of the junction of the umbilical vein and the portal sinus. Circumference should be measured at the skin line on a true transverse view of the fetal abdomen, where the portal sinus, fetal stomach, and umbilical vein are visible. Abdominal circumference is used to estimate fetal weight.
- Fetal weight may be estimated by using the abdominal circumference measurement in mathematical formulations along with other sonographic parameters. The best fetal weight estimates may yield significant errors. Interval growth may be determined by sonographic measurements taken 2 to 4 weeks apart.

5. Evaluation of maternal anatomy, including uterine, adnexal, and cervical evaluations, should be performed to document the presence, location, and size of uterine or adnexal masses, which may complicate obstetric management. Normal maternal ovaries may not be imaged during the second and third trimesters.

6. Fetal anatomy may be adequately assessed after 18 weeks' gestation. Anatomy may be difficult to image because of fetal movement, size, or position; maternal scars; or increased wall thickness. When anatomy is not seen because of technical limitations, the sonographer should note the reason. A follow-up examination may be ordered.

The guidelines recommend that the following anatomy should be documented during a standard obstetric sonography examination. More detailed studies may be performed if the anatomy appears questionable or abnormal. Documentation and images of the required anatomy should be retained. Anatomic areas to be assessed are listed in Box 45-5 and include the following:

1. Head and neck
   - Cerebellum
   - Choroid plexus
   - Cisterna magna
   - Lateral cerebral ventricles
   - Midline falx
   - Cavum septi pellucidi
   - Upper lip

BOX 45-5 Essential or Minimal Elements of a Standard Examination of Fetal Anatomy

- Head, face, and neck*
  - Cerebellum
  - Choroid plexus
  - Cisterna magna
  - Lateral cerebral ventricles
  - Midline falx
  - Cavum septi pellucidi
  - Upper lip
- Chest/Heart: The basic cardiac examination includes a four-chamber view of the fetal heart. If technically feasible, views of the outflow tracts should be attempted as part of the cardiac screening examination.
- Abdomen
  - Stomach (presence, size, and situs)
  - Kidneys
  - Bladder
  - Umbilical cord insertion site into the fetal abdomen
  - Umbilical cord vessel number
- Spine—cervical, thoracic, lumbar, and sacral spine
- Extremities—legs and arms (presence or absence)
- Gender—medically indicated in low-risk pregnancies only for the evaluation of multiple gestations

*Measurement of the nuchal fold may be helpful during a specific age interval to suggest increased risk of aneuploidy.

2. Chest
   - Four-chamber view of the fetal heart
   - If technically feasible, an extended basic cardiac examination that includes both outflow tracts may be attempted.
3. Abdomen
   - Stomach (presence, size, and situs)
   - Kidneys
   - Bladder
   - Umbilical cord insertion into the fetal abdomen
   - Umbilical cord; number of vessels
4. Spine
   - Cervical, thoracic, lumbar, and sacral spine
5. Extremities
   - Presence or absence of arms and legs
6. Gender
   - Medically indicated in low-risk pregnancies only for assessment of multiple pregnancies

DIAGNOSTIC AND SCREENING ASPECTS OF OBSTETRIC SONOGRAPHY EXAMINATIONS

Obstetric sonography examinations are both diagnostic and screening tests. Diagnostic tests can give definitive information about a clinical question or the presence or absence of a finding. Obstetric sonography examinations are typically diagnostic with respect to fetal heart motion, fetal number, fetal biometry, fetal presentation, location of the placenta, presence of a maternal pelvic or adnexal mass, and major disruptions of fetal anatomy such as **anencephaly.**

Obstetric sonography may also diagnose other fetal problems, but, in general, it is considered a screening test for detection of fetal anomalies. A screening test does not provide a definitive diagnosis but indicates whether the patient or pregnancy is at greater or lesser risk. In other words, an obstetric sonography examination with normal findings may reduce the risk of that fetus having an anomaly but does provide certainty that the fetus is not affected.

The sensitivity of routine sonography in detecting fetal anomalies has been analyzed in multiple studies. It is generally agreed that sensitivity depends on many factors, including maternal habitus, the expertise of the sonographers and physicians responsible for the study, the risk level of the patient, the number and timing of sonography examinations, and the type of anomaly. Sensitivity tends to be higher for defects of the central nervous system and urinary system, and lower for defects of the heart and great vessels. Sensitivity is higher in tertiary care centers and with specialty obstetric examinations. Maternal obesity is known to have an impact on sonographic visualization of anatomy. In one review of 36 studies involving more than 900,000 fetuses, overall sensitivity for the detection of fetal anomalies by obstetric sonography was 40.4%, and the range was 13.3% to 82.4%.

It is important that patients be counseled about the limitations of obstetric sonography. This counseling should inform patients that screening examinations do not detect all anomalies, that false-positive findings are possible, and that the sensitivity of sonography is not certain in any situation.

Clinical Ethics for Obstetric Sonography

Jean Lea Spitz

Ethical codes are important regulators in health care. Patient trust is built on the expectation that health care professionals will follow established ethical principles and guidelines. Medical ethics promotes excellence and protects patients by encouraging practitioners to reflect on, communicate, and demonstrate optimal care.

Sonographers have ethical responsibilities to their patients and colleagues. The principles of nonmaleficence, beneficence, autonomy, respect for persons, veracity and integrity, and justice must be implemented in the sonography laboratory to ensure ethical practice. Sonographers who regularly participate in ethical discussions and discourse within their environment may best meet these requirements. The Society of Diagnostic Medical Sonography (SDMS) has adopted a code of ethics for sonographers. This code includes elements consistent with principles of nonmaleficence, beneficence, autonomy, veracity, justice, and confidentiality.

MORALITY AND ETHICS DEFINED

Ethics is defined as systematic reflection on and analysis of morality. **Morality** concerns right and wrong conduct (what we ought or ought not to do) and good and bad character (the kinds of persons we should become and the virtues we should cultivate in doing so). Morality reflects duties and values. Freedom and autonomy are integral to morality because they allow values to be expressed. All aspects of morality, duties, values, and rights are of importance in the clinical ethics of sonography practice.

In a pluralistic, multicultural society such as the United States, moral beliefs and behaviors vary widely. Morality is learned through personal experiences and family traditions, and from normative behavior within communities, ethnic and racial groups, or geographic regions. Religions disagree about conduct and character, and religious ethics provides an inadequate foundation for professional ethics in a culturally diverse society. National identity and history also contribute to beliefs, as do the laws of the states and the federal government. These many sources of moral beliefs can sometimes cause conflict. Health care providers with good intentions may disagree among themselves or with patients on moral directions. When these disagreements are discussed and analyzed, a collaborative and ethical resolution of the conflict can be achieved. It is this type of discussion, reflection, and discourse on morality that constitutes ethics.

Whereas morality has to do with the protection of cherished values, ethics is a discipline of study that seeks to articulate clear, consistent, coherent, and practical guidelines for conduct and character. Ethics tries to answer the key question, "What is good?" To be applicable to a medical context like sonography, ethics must transcend moral pluralism by offering an approach with minimal ties to any substantive prior belief about moral conduct and character. This is what philosophical ethics attempts to do because it requires only a commitment to the results of rational discourse in which all substantive commitments about what morality ought to be are open to question. Every such substantive moral claim requires intellectual justification in the form of rigorous ethical analysis and argument. Philosophical ethics therefore properly serves as the foundation for medical ethics, especially in an international context.

HISTORY OF MEDICAL ETHICS

Medical ethics has evolved since the beginning of civilization, when health care knowledge was shared orally and healers exemplified a community's moral code. Prince Hammurabi of Babylon recorded the responsibilities of health care providers in 1727 BC, and early Hindu writers at about the same time cautioned healers to treat patients with respect, gentleness, and dignity. Fundamental principles of Western medical ethics were first recorded in ancient Greece in about the 5th century BC. Hippocrates cautioned his students, *"primum non nocere,"* which famously means, "First, do no harm." In ethics, this is known as the *ethical principle of nonmaleficence.* Hippocrates' teachings emphasize choosing treatment based on knowledge that would best benefit patients, treating patients as one would treat family members, upholding confidentiality, and practicing personal piety.

Ethical norms, elements, and principles were refined through the centuries. Thomas Percival (1740–1805) wrote a treatise that substantially changed medical ethics. Previously, a patient was someone who paid for treatment, but Percival redefined *patient* as anyone needing care. He also foresaw a team approach in health care and public health. Percival emphasized patient care provided by all professionals and ordered competitive or professional interests as secondary to the needs of the patient.

Modern medical ethics was codified after the Nuremberg trials, which judged the atrocities done in medical experimentation by Nazi doctors. The judges in the Nuremberg trial issued a verdict that included a section on permissible human experimentation. That section, which became known as the Nuremberg code, was incorporated into regulatory policy in the United States. The same protections were adopted internationally and published within the Helsinki report in 1964. The Nuremberg code emphasized individual rights and autonomy and has become a key element of modern ethics.

Basic principles of medical ethics have been incorporated into research regulations, professional codes, and clinical practices throughout the world. The ethical codes of different professional groups may differ slightly in definition and emphasis, but the basic principles of autonomy, justice, beneficence, nonmaleficence, integrity, and respect for persons are universal.

The *Code of Ethics for the Profession of Diagnostic Medical Sonography* has been adopted and is maintained by the SDMS.

PRINCIPLES OF MEDICAL ETHICS

Nonmaleficence

The principle of **nonmaleficence** directs the sonographer to not cause harm. Application of the principle of nonmaleficence requires the sonographer to obtain appropriate education and clinical skills to ensure competence in performing each required examination. Ensuring an appropriate level of competence imposes a rigorous standard of education and continuing education. Two problems result when obstetric sonographers do not maintain a baseline level of competence in the techniques and interpretation of sonographic imaging: (1) They may cause unnecessary harm to the pregnant woman or fetal patient, for example, from mistaken impressions of fetal anomalies that in turn lead to unnecessary anxiety or testing; and (2) they may undermine the **informed consent** process regarding the management of pregnancy by reporting in an incomplete or inaccurate manner to the physician, who in turn reports misinformation to the pregnant woman.

Sonographers need to be accountable for and participate in regular assessment and review of protocols, equipment, procedures, and results to ensure that patients are not harmed by outdated procedures or poorly functioning equipment. Appropriate oversight and approval of protocols by research or hospital committees contribute to patient safety. Protocols and diagnostic criteria should be established by peer review. Sonographers may contribute to the safety of patients by sharing with others and publishing peer-reviewed information about mistakes made or lessons learned.

The sonographer must practice emergency procedures and strive to ensure patient safety in all procedures and circumstances. Sonographers must refrain from substance abuse or any activity that may alter their judgment or ability to provide safe and effective patient care.

Because ultrasound energy poses a theoretical risk to the fetus, the principle of nonmaleficence requires sonographers to perform only medically indicated examinations and to perform all examinations in keeping with ALARA, an energy exposure that is as low as reasonably achievable, to obtain the desired results. Sonographers should not perform obstetric ultrasound examinations for entertainment purposes.

Sonographers need to read the current medical literature to stay abreast of new developments related to patient safety. Sonographers should not perform ultrasound examination without medical benefit.

Beneficence

Protections for patients and subjects based on the ethical principle of nonmaleficence only partially explain what is in the patients' interests because medicine, and therefore sonography, seeks to benefit patients, not simply to avoid harming them. The use of obstetric ultrasound, like other medical interventions, must be justified by the goal of seeking the greater balance of clinical "goods" over "harms," not simply avoiding harm to the patient at all cost. This ethical principle is called **beneficence** and is a more comprehensive basis for ethics in sonography than is nonmaleficence.

Goods and harms are to be defined and balanced from a rigorous clinical perspective. The goods that obstetric sonography should seek for patients include preventing early or premature death (not preventing death at all costs); preventing and managing disease, injury, and handicapping conditions; and alleviating unnecessary pain and suffering. Pain and suffering are unnecessary and therefore represent clinical harms to be avoided when they do not contribute to seeking the good of the beneficence-based clinical judgment. *Pain* is a physiologic phenomenon involving central nervous system processing of tissue damage. *Suffering* is a psychological phenomenon involving blocked intentions, plans, and projects. Pain often causes suffering, but one can suffer without being in pain.

The principle of beneficence obligates the obstetric sonographer to seek the greatest benefit in the care of pregnant patients. Beneficence encourages sonographers to go beyond the minimum standard protocol and to seek additional images and information if achievable and in the best interests of patients. Beneficence requires sonographers to focus on small comforts for the patient, respecting their privacy and including their family upon request. Kindness and attention to small details minimize suffering caused by frustration or anger. Beneficence, like nonmaleficence, requires competency, knowledge, and excellent sonographic skills to ensure that the patient and the fetus receive the greatest benefit from the examination.

Fetal interests in sonography are understood exclusively in terms of beneficence. This principle explains the moral (as distinct from legal) status of the fetus as a patient and generates ethical obligations owed by physicians and sonographers to the fetus. In the technical language of beneficence, the sonographer has beneficence-based obligations to the fetal patient to protect and promote fetal interests and those of the child it will become, as these are understood from a rigorous clinical perspective. The clinical good to be sought for the fetal patient includes prevention of premature death, disease, handicapping conditions, and unnecessary future pain and suffering. It is appropriate therefore to refer to fetuses as patients, except when a patient elects to terminate her pregnancy.

In clinical practice, beneficence may have to be balanced against other ethical principles. A health professional's duty of beneficence may suggest one course of action and the patient may choose another. In these cases, beneficence must be balanced by respect for a person's autonomy. The principles of veracity and integrity on occasion may conflict with beneficence when truth-telling will cause undue stress and complications. The principle of justice or fair distribution of benefits may conflict with beneficence for individual patients who need extra resources. Fortunately in most situations, it is in the patients' best interests to respect their autonomy, to tell the truth, and to distribute benefits justly.

Autonomy

In the 21st century, **autonomy,** or the right to self-determination, has become a key ethical principle. **Respect for persons** incorporates both respect for the autonomy of individuals and the requirement to protect those with diminished autonomy. Patients, including pregnant women, have their own perspective on their interests, which should be respected as much as the clinician's perspective on patients' interests. A patient's perspective on her interests is shaped by wide-ranging and sometimes idiosyncratic values and beliefs. *Autonomy* refers to a person's capacity to formulate, express, and carry out value-based preferences. The ethical principle of respect for autonomy obligates the sonographer to acknowledge the integrity of a patient's values and beliefs and of her value-based preferences; to avoid interfering with the expression or implementation of these preferences; and, when necessary, to assist in their expression and implementation. This principle generates the autonomy-based obligations of the sonographer.

Informed consent is an autonomy-based right. Each health professional has autonomy-based obligations regarding the informed consent process. This process must include discourse about what sonography examinations can and cannot detect, the sensitivity and frequency of false-negatives and false-positives of the sonography techniques employed, and the difficult and sometimes uncertain interpretation of sonographic images. In the face of medical uncertainty about the clinical good and harm of routine ultrasound, it is obligatory to inform pregnant patients about that uncertainty and to give them the opportunity to make their own choices about how that uncertainty should be managed. In routine examinations, it is also important to inform the woman of the possibility of confronting an anomaly that will lead her to decide whether to terminate the pregnancy or take it to term.

As the protocols and options for gaining medical information regarding potential fetal anomalies increase and risk assessment becomes more individualized, requirements are increased for patient education that is sufficient for informed choice. Genetic counselors, patient educators, sonographers, and physicians often work together to counsel women regarding their options and choices.

The sonographer respects the patient's autonomy by providing a detailed explanation of the examination, including appropriate choices such as the right to view the screen or to learn the gender of the fetus. Respect for maternal autonomy dictates responding frankly to requests from the pregnant woman for information about the gender of the fetus. As part of the disclosure process, the pregnant woman should be made aware of the uncertainties of ultrasound gender identification. The sonographer can use his or her own experience to help the pregnant woman understand these uncertainties. A second choice that may be presented during obstetric examinations is the choice to view the images. This choice concerns the phenomenon of apparent bonding of pregnant women and their families to the fetus as a result of seeing the sonographic images. Such bonding often enriches pregnancies that will be taken to term, but at other times can complicate decisions to terminate a pregnancy.

A current ethical issue is the nonmedical use of sonography for the videotaping or photography of "baby pictures." There is nothing intrinsically wrong with the practice if it is a side product of a legitimate ultrasound examination. However, when videotaping or photography is performed to generate revenue, this practice trivializes medical sonography and may result in harm because problems that could be diagnosed may be missed. It is the responsibility of sonographers to ensure that women have the information necessary to make informed choices.

It is an autonomy-enhancing strategy for a woman to be allowed to insert a vaginal probe herself to make the experience more comfortable and less threatening. It is also a sonographer's obligation to respect a patient's right to refuse a procedure.

Maternal interests are protected and promoted by both autonomy-based and beneficence-based obligations of the sonographer to the pregnant woman. Fetuses are incapable of having their own perspective on their interests because the immaturity of their central nervous system renders them incapable of having the requisite values or beliefs. Thus there can be no autonomy-based obligations to the fetus. The pregnant woman also has beneficence-based obligations to the fetal patient when the pregnancy will be taken to term. She is expected to protect and promote the fetal patient's interests and those of the child it will become. When a pregnant woman elects to have an abortion, however, these obligations do not exist. A sonographer with moral objections to abortion should keep two things in mind: First, the moral judgment and decision of the pregnant woman to end her pregnancy should not be criticized or commented on in any way; her autonomy demands respect as shown by the sonographer and the physician being neutral to her judgment and decision. Second, the sonographer is free to follow his or her conscience and to withdraw from further involvement with patients who elect abortion. Physicians should as a matter of office policy respect this important matter of individual conscience on the part of the sonographer.

Veracity and Integrity

Telling the truth is an ethical practice that most sonographers have been taught from a young age. Yet, the vast majority of us on occasion will tell "white lies" in kindness or to escape unwanted consequences. The universal acceptance and even cultural preference in some countries for white lies is evidence of the difficulty involved in adhering to the principle of veracity. **Veracity** means truthfulness. **Integrity** means adherence to moral and ethical principles. Integrity is related to the word *integrate*, meaning "to bring together." In terms of honesty, integrity means that there is no difference between what you think, what you say, and what you do: They all come together in ethical behavior.

In medical care, patients properly rely for their protection on the personal and professional integrity of their clinicians. A crucial aspect of that integrity on the part of physicians is willingness to refer to specialists when the limits of their own knowledge are being approached. Integrity should also be one of the fundamental virtues of sonographers and thus a standard for judging professional character. Similar to other virtues, such as self-sacrifice and compassion, integrity directs sonographers to focus primarily on the patient's interests as a way to blunt mere self-interest. Sonographers must avoid conflicts of interest and situations that exploit others, create unreasonable expectations, or misrepresent information.

Veracity with respect to abilities and limitations is absolutely essential among sonographers. If a practitioner asks a sonographer to perform an examination that he or she is not competent to do, it is essential for the sonographer to be truthful about his or her limitations to protect the patient. A sonographer asked by a patient or a colleague must accurately represent his or her level of competence, education, and credentials.

Premature disclosure of the results of an abnormal sonographic examination raises significant clinical ethical issues for sonographers. Sonographers are justified in disclosing findings of normal anatomy directly to the pregnant woman. When images reveal abnormal findings, sonographers must not act "dumb" or tell the patient that they do not know what they are seeing. Veracity is upheld by telling the patient in a nonalarming way the procedure for diagnosis, that "multiple eyes need to look at some of the images," and that the physician will determine the results. Disclosure of, and discussion about, abnormal findings by sonographers is inappropriate because it is not in the best interest of the patient. If the disclosure and the discussion are to respect and enhance maternal autonomy and avoid unnecessary psychological harm to the pregnant woman, the discussion should occur in a setting where the alternatives and choices available to manage the pregnancy are presented. Sonographers cannot by training or by experience claim the clinical competence to engage in such discussions. Physicians can and therefore should.

Sonographers must strive to supply patients and colleagues with complete and accurate information. The sonographer's integrity is an essential safeguard for the patient's autonomy. At times, the sonographer will need to become an advocate, even a vigorous advocate, for disclosure of information to a patient. In such cases, sonographers must address their concerns not to the patient but to the practitioner involved. Failure to make patient disclosures undermines professional integrity and the moral authority of health care professionals. When the sonographer disagrees with the clinical judgment of his or her supervising physician, professional communication and discussion of the matter need to occur. The best interests of the health care team and the patient are enhanced by such conversations.

Justice

Justice is the ethical principle that requires fair distribution of benefits and burdens; an injustice occurs when a benefit to which a person is entitled is withheld, or when a burden is unfairly imposed. Justice means simply that sonographers must strive to treat all patients equally. In practical terms, justice requires that translators be used when necessary to ensure adequate and appropriate communication with all patients. Sonographers should strive to ensure that disabled patients have access to reasonable accommodations and pathways, and that obese patients have comfortable chairs, gowns, and stretchers. Children, adults, and geriatric patients need to feel equally welcome and cared for within the sonography laboratory.

Justice is served when protocols are standardized. Men and women with similar symptoms should receive similar tests and interventions. If a group is denied services or is asked to assume an undue burden to obtain care provided to others, justice is not being served.

Justice and autonomy are the ethical principles that determine the timing of obstetric sonography examinations. The information obtained from a sonogram enhances women's choices. It is an injustice to provide this information to some women and not to others. It is for this reason that recommendations are made that all women be offered risk assessment for anomalies during the first trimester. Sonography results, such as risk for an abnormality, are relevant to the woman's decision about whether she will seek an abortion. In pregnancies that will be taken to term, sonography enhances a pregnant woman's autonomy. The timing of the information is also relevant if anomalies are detected and she does not choose abortion, as she may begin to prepare herself for the decisions that she will confront later regarding management of the anomalies in the intrapartum and postpartum periods. Providing requested information early in pregnancy permits a pregnant woman ample time to deal with psychological and practical issues before she must confront decisions.

The principle of justice implies that health care professionals should act in accordance with the best interest of the community. As health care costs increase, insurance costs skyrocket, and bankruptcy becomes associated with chronic illness, the societal aspects of medical justice are receiving more attention. The traditional focus of medical ethics is the individual patient. In some cases, however, the costs and benefits of treating one patient may place an undue burden on others. An individual ethical focus may be in conflict with a society focus when an individual uses a disproportionate amount of health care without paying for it. This forces others to pay for the service—a burden that society accepts if the service is considered essential. However, as the benefit of the service decreases, as in experimental protocols, or as the cost of the service increases, the conflict grows. If the resources used are not replaced, others may be deprived of similar services. The solution to such conflicts is not clear politically, socially, or ethically. What is clear, however, is that the community aspect of justice will receive more attention in the future. Sonographers can support community interests by performing only medically indicated procedures prescribed by a clinician.

CONFIDENTIALITY OF FINDINGS

Confidentiality concerns the obligation of caregivers to protect clinical information about patients from unauthorized access. The obligation of confidentiality derives from the principles of beneficence (patients will be more forthcoming) and respect for autonomy (patients' privacy rights are protected). Others, including the pregnant woman's spouse and/or sex partner and family, should be understood as third parties to the patient–sonographer relationship. Diagnostic information about a woman's pregnancy is confidential. It can be justifiably disclosed to third parties *only* with the pregnant woman's *explicit permission*. Federal regulations, including the Health Insurance Portability and Accountability Act (HIPAA), determine acceptable conditions for releasing confidential information. To prevent awkward situations, sonographers and their supervising physicians should establish policies and procedures that reflect the ethics of confidentiality.

The ethics of confidentiality when the pregnant woman is younger than the age of 18 years should be the same as when the patient is 18 years of age and older. The law, however, may complicate matters because pregnancy does not emancipate a minor in every jurisdiction, and different jurisdictions give different levels of protection to the privacy of the physician–patient relationship when the patient is younger than 18 years of age.

ACKNOWLEDGMENTS

The author would like to acknowledge the work of Frank A. Chervenak and Laurence B. McCullough on the sixth edition of this book.

The Normal First Trimester

Jean Lea Spitz

First-trimester obstetric sonography is an increasingly important component of prenatal care. These examinations may diagnose conditions that require intervention, and even in "normal" intrauterine pregnancies, they provide patients and clinicians with information that influences management. Information about multiple pregnancies, uterine anomalies, and pelvic masses that is readily visualized during the first trimester may be more difficult to obtain later.

Aspects of prenatal fetal diagnosis are shifting from second trimester to first trimester. First-trimester aneuploidy screening protocols have higher detection rates than second-trimester tests. The current standard of care suggests offering aneuploidy screening during the first trimester to all obstetric patients, and where available offering diagnostic genetic testing through **chorionic villi sampling (CVS)** between 11 and 13 weeks. Fetal anatomy has not been routinely assessed until the second trimester, but recent studies have demonstrated the possibility of achieving similar rates of anomaly detection earlier. In the morbidly obese gravida, assessment of fetal anatomy through transvaginal sonography in the late first trimester is reported to be an improvement over second-trimester scanning.

Although the ability to image the first-trimester pregnancy with ultrasound may seem routine, the potential for false-positive and false-negative diagnoses for any given pathology is substantial. Extreme care should be taken when evaluating the first-trimester pregnancy sonographically.

OVERVIEW OF THE FIRST TRIMESTER

A Note on Terminology

It is especially important to have a clear understanding of terminology when discussing embryology. Embryologists state time in *conceptual age,* also known as *embryologic age,* with conception as the first day of pregnancy. Clinicians and sonographers use *gestational age,* also known as *menstrual age,* to date the pregnancy, with the first day of the last menstrual period as the beginning of gestation. Thus the gestational age would add 2 weeks onto the conceptual age. For 12 days after conception,

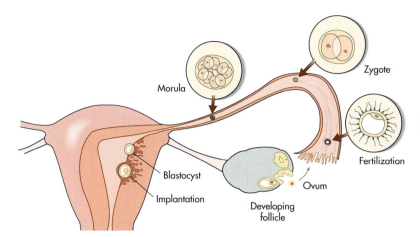

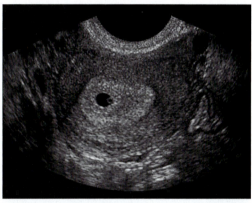

FIGURE 47-1 Diagram illustrates the zygote stage from conception through implantation.

during the implantation process, the conceptus is called a **zygote.** From the time of implantation until the end of the 10th week menstrual age, the conceptus is called an embryo. After the first 10 weeks, the embryo is called a fetus.

Normal Pregnancy Progression

Except when specifically noted, dates in this chapter reflect menstrual age rather than embryologic age (conceptual age). The gestational age (also known as menstrual age) is calculated by adding 2 weeks (14 days) to the conceptual age. Menstrual age refers to the length of time calculated from the first day of the LMP to the point at which the pregnancy is being assessed. During a 28-day menstrual cycle, a mature ovum is typically released at day 14. The ovum is swept into the distal fallopian tube via fimbriae; fertilization occurs within this region 1 to 2 days after ovulation. Meanwhile, the follicle that released the mature ovum hemorrhages and collapses to form the corpus luteum, which begins to secrete progesterone and estrogen (Figure 47-1).

The fertilized conceptus that is now referred to as a zygote undergoes rapid cellular division to form the 16-cell morula. Further cell proliferation brings the morula to the blastocyst stage. The blastocyst contains trophoblastic cells and the "inner cell mass," which forms the embryo. The trophoblastic cells begin to secrete **human chorionic gonadotropin (hCG)** that is absorbed within the tubes and stimulates maternal pregnancy responses.

hCG causes the uterine endometrium to convert to decidua, a glycogen-rich mucosa that nourishes the early pregnancy. The blastocyst typically enters the uterus 4 to 5 days after fertilization. Implantation into the uterine decidua is completed within 12 days post fertilization. During implantation, proteolytic enzymes produced by the trophoblasts "eat into" decidual tissue, creating spaces for trophoblastic cell proliferation. Blood pools known as *lacunae* that form as maternal capillaries erode nourish the proliferating trophoblastic cells. A primitive blood exchange network between mother and conceptus

FIGURE 47-2 The thickened decidua, the gestational sac (chorionic cavity), and the secondary yolk sac are seen in this transverse image of an early first-trimester 5-week intrauterine gestation.

is formed, and the lacunae and trophoblastic cells develop into a mature placental/maternal circulation complex that will sustain the pregnancy. By the end of the implantation process, the zygote has buried itself within one wall of the uterus. The implantation process sometimes results in light vaginal bleeding about the same time as the expected menstrual period.

When implantation is complete, the trophoblast has formed primary villi, which initially encircle the early gestational sac. Within the conceptus, the inner cell mass matures into the bilaminar embryonic disk, the future embryo, and the primary yolk sac. At approximately 23 days' menstrual age, the **primary yolk sac** is pinched off by the extraembryonic coelom, forming the **secondary yolk sac.** The secondary yolk sac is the yolk sac seen sonographically throughout the first trimester (Figure 47-2). The amniotic and chorionic cavities also develop and evolve during this period of gestation.

The embryonic phase occurs from week 4 through week 10. It is during this phase that all major internal and external structures begin to develop (Table 43-1). The cardiovascular system undergoes rapid development, with the initial heartbeat occurring at between $5\frac{1}{2}$ and 6 weeks. The embryo's appearance changes from a flat, disklike configuration to a C-shaped

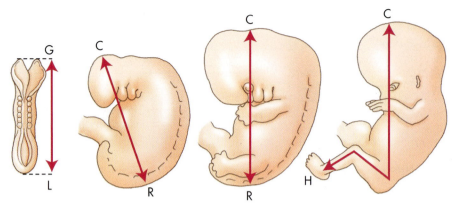

FIGURE 47-3 The relationship of neural tube development to crown-rump length in the first trimester. Note the size of the embryo's head relative to the body.

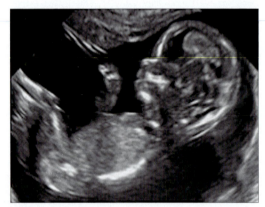

FIGURE 47-4 At the beginning of the fetal period in the late first trimester, the embryo's head measures almost half of the crown-rump length. Notice the ossification of the frontal bones, vertebrae, long bones, and fingers.

structure, and it develops a human-like appearance (Figure 47-3). During this period of embryogenesis, the **crown-rump length (CRL)** develops rapidly, measuring 35 mm by the end of the 10th week.

The last 2 weeks of the first trimester (weeks 11 and 12) constitute the beginning of the fetal period. During the fetal period growth of the organs and structures formed during the embryonic period continues. At this stage, the fetal head is disproportionately larger than the rest of the fetus, constituting one half of the CRL (Figure 47-4). As the fetus grows, body growth accelerates, and this proportionality becomes less pronounced. Fetal anatomy is fully developed in the late first trimester, and the goal of sonography at this stage includes anomaly detection.

MATERNAL SERUM BIOCHEMISTRY IN EARLY PREGNANCY

Maternal serum biochemistry values can be very useful in evaluation of the early pregnancy. A direct relationship exists in early pregnancy between the sonographic findings and quantitative serum hCG levels. Gestational sac size and hCG levels increase proportionately until 10 menstrual weeks, at which time the gestational sac is approximately 45 mm mean sac diameter (**MSD**), and an embryo should be easily detected by transabdominal or transvaginal sonography.

Because the quantitative hCG levels correlate with gestational sac size in normal pregnancies, the sonographer or clinician may use the objective biochemistry measurement to establish whether the pregnancy is normal or abnormal when the embryo is too small to be imaged with ultrasound. Discriminatory hCG level for detecting an intrauterine sac varies somewhat from laboratory to laboratory according to the standard against which the hCG is calibrated. However, when the hCG level and the sonographic findings are combined, accuracy is improved to rule in an intrauterine pregnancy or an ectopic pregnancy. A normal gestational sac can be consistently demonstrated when the hCG level is 1800 mIU/ml (Second International Standard) or greater when transabdominal sonography is used. This detection threshold is significantly reduced by transvaginal sonography and may be as low as 500 mIU/ml. Many laboratories use hCG levels of 1000 to 2000 mIU/ml as the number that indicates a pregnancy should be visible with sonography (Table 47-2). The sonographer must be aware that when the hCG value is at this level and the gestational sac is not seen within the uterus, an ectopic pregnancy may be considered.

Ectopic pregnancies demonstrate a lower hCG level than intrauterine pregnancies perhaps owing to limited absorption outside the uterus. The rate of rise or increase in hCG during early pregnancy may help detect ectopic pregnancies. The normal intrauterine pregnancy at less than 7 weeks demonstrates doubling of quantitative maternal serum hCG levels every 3.5 days, or an increase of 66% in hCG levels within 48 hours. If this normal rate of increase is not seen, there is a greater chance that the pregnancy is ectopic. However, some ectopic pregnancies will show a normal rate of increase, and some normal pregnancies will show a reduced rate.

Abnormal pregnancies demonstrate a low hCG level relative to gestational sac development, and it has been shown that hCG levels fall before spontaneous expulsion of nonviable gestations. Sonographers need to obtain quantitative hCG levels whenever possible before first-trimester obstetric exams are performed and must correlate hCG levels with the gestational sac appearance. This is particularly important when vaginal bleeding or pelvic pain is present, or when an ectopic pregnancy is suspected.

At 9 to 10 weeks, hCG levels plateau and subsequently decline while gestation continues. In pregnancies where the fetus is trisomy 21, the hCG levels plateau later and fall much more slowly. Levels of hCG are increased in these pregnancies as compared with normal pregnancies, and the difference increases as gestation advances. Consequently, increased hCG levels can be used as a screening marker for Down syndrome during the first and second trimesters. Increased hCG is not a strong marker and does not have sufficient sensitivity to be used by itself in screening for Down syndrome. It is combined with other independent markers to enhance detection. hCG is a component of first-trimester risk assessment and a component of triple-screen and quad-screen testing performed during the second trimester. The sensitivity of hCG for Down syndrome assessment is improved by measurement of the free beta subunit. Both total hCG and free beta hCG are used for aneuploidy screening in the United States.

Pregnancy-associated plasma protein–A (PAPP-A), also known as pappalysin-1, is an insulin-like growth factor produced by trophoblastic (placental) cells during pregnancy. It is involved in proliferative growth processes such as bone and tissue formation. Maternal serum PAPP-A increases with advancing gestation. In trisomy 21–affected pregnancies, PAPP-A levels are initially lower than in normal pregnancies, but the difference decreases with increasing gestational age. Decreased values of maternal serum PAPP-A may be a marker for Down syndrome during the first trimester but are not useful in the second trimester. Currently, PAPP-A analysis at 9 to 11 weeks' gestational age is the strongest biochemical marker for Down syndrome. PAPP-A is not sensitive enough to be used by itself, however, and is combined with hCG levels for serum biochemistry screening or with hCG and sonographic markers for combined screening. Recent studies project an association between PAPP-A levels in early pregnancy and pregnancy pathology such as preterm labor and preeclampsia.

SONOGRAPHIC TECHNIQUE AND EVALUATION OF THE FIRST TRIMESTER

First-trimester obstetric sonography has evolved rapidly during the past decade with the development of **transvaginal (TV) transducers,** which allow the gravid uterus and adnexa to be visualized with improved resolution by allowing higher frequencies (5 to 8 MHz) and transducer placement closer to anatomic structures when compared with transabdominal scanning. With transvaginal transducers, the pelvic anatomy is imaged in both sagittal and coronal/semicoronal planes. Such coronal imaging of the pelvis is unique within sonography, and the images should not be misconstrued as transverse sections (Figure 47-5).

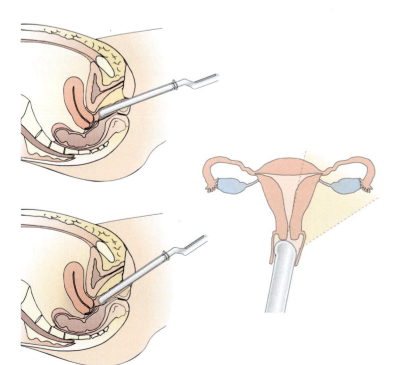

FIGURE 47-5 Schematic demonstrating transvaginal transducer techniques of sagittal and coronal/semicoronal anatomic planes.

Although transvaginal sonography has gained overall acceptance within the medical community because of its improved image quality, transabdominal (TA) and transperineal sonography should not be overlooked. The transabdominal approach allows visualization of a larger field of anatomy, which is important when specific anatomic relationships are in question. For instance, the size, extent, and anatomic relationships of a large pelvic mass with surrounding structures can be determined only with transabdominal techniques.

The transperineal approach can be used to visualize the cervix.

Three-dimensional sonography has been performed in the first trimester, but its clinical value during this stage of pregnancy has not been established.

The value of pulsed Doppler analysis of early gestation in some situations has been reported. Pulsed Doppler should be performed in early pregnancy only when there are clear benefits.

Indications for first-trimester obstetric sonography that have been outlined by professional organizations, including the American College of Radiology (ACR), the American Institute of Ultrasound in Medicine (AIUM), and the American College of Obstetricians and Gynecologists (ACOG) (see Box 45-1), and sample protocols for these examinations are recorded in Chapter 45. The major components of a routine first-trimester examination include the following:

- The uterus and adnexa are evaluated for the presence of a gestational sac.
- Sonographic measurements of the embryo and/or sac are recorded.
- The presence or absence of cardiac activity is documented.
- Fetal number is documented and chorionicity is assessed in multiple pregnancies.
- The uterus, adnexal structures, and cul-de-sac are evaluated.

Visualization of Early Gestation

During the 5th week of embryonic development, the intrauterine pregnancy (**IUP**) can be visualized sonographically. It appears as a 1- to 2-mm sac with an echogenic ring having a sonolucent center. The anechoic center represents the chorionic cavity. The circumferential echogenic rim seen surrounding the gestational sac represents trophoblastic tissue and the associated decidual reaction. The echogenic ring around the gestational sac can be divided embryologically into several components. The portion on the myometrial or burrowing side of the conceptus is known as the **decidua basalis**. The villi covering the developing embryo are referred to as the **decidua capsularis** (Figure 47-6). The interface between the decidua capsularis and the echogenic, highly vascularized decidua on the opposite wall of the endometrial cavity forms the **double decidual sac sign,** which has been reported to be a reliable sign of an early intrauterine gestation. The gestational sac is eccentrically placed in relation to the endometrial cavity, secondary to its implantation. Typically, a fundal location is noted (Figure 47-7).

The normal sonographic features of a gestational sac include a round or oval shape; a fundal position in the uterus, or an eccentrically placed position in the middle portion of the uterus; smooth contours; and a decidual wall thickness greater than 3 mm (Figure 47-8). Implantation in the lower uterine segment may be associated with placenta accreta or placenta previa.

A yolk sac should be seen when the MSD is greater than 12 mm. An embryo should be seen when the MSD is greater than 18 mm (Box 47-1). Once the gestational sac is sonographically imaged, rapid growth and development occur. The gestational sac size grows at a predictable rate of 1 mm/day in early pregnancy.

Often the first intragestational sac anatomy seen is the sonographic yolk sac (secondary yolk sac), which is routinely visualized at between 5 and 5½ weeks' gestation.

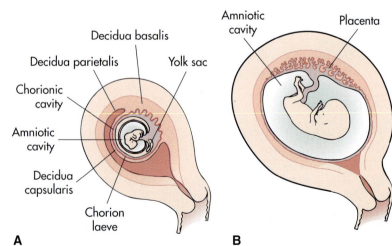

FIGURE 47-6 Schema showing the relation of the fetal membranes and the wall of the uterus. **A,** End of the second month. Note the yolk sac in the chorionic cavity between the amnion and chorion. At the abembryonic pole, the villi have disappeared (chorion laeve). **B,** End of the third month. The amnion and chorion have fused and the uterine cavity is obliterated by fusion of the chorion laeve and the decidua parietalis.

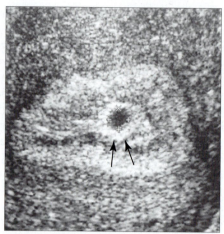

FIGURE 47-7 The early gestational sac is seen embedded in the decidual basalis on one side of the endometrial cavity. The arrows are pointing to the decidua capsularis.

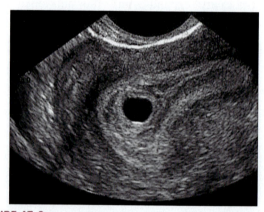

FIGURE 47-8 A normal gestational sac is seen in a fundal location on this longitudinal uterine scan.

BOX 47-1	Sonographic Features of a Normal Gestational Sac

- **Shape:** round or oval
- **Position:** fundal or middle portion of uterus; a center position relative to endometrium (double decidual sac or intradecidua finding)
- **Contour:** smooth
- **Wall (trophoblastic reaction):** echogenic
- **Internal landmarks:** yolk sac present when gestational sac is larger than 12 mm; embryo present when gestational sac is larger than 18 mm
- **Growth:** 1 mm/day (range, 0.7 mm to 1.5 mm/day)

From Nyberg DA, Hill LM: Normal early intrauterine pregnancy: sonographic development and hCG correlation. In Nyberg DA, et al, editors, *Endovaginal ultrasound*, St Louis, 1992, Mosby.

The yolk sac is seen before the beating embryonic heart, because embryonic heart motion begins at approximately 5½ weeks. The yolk sac may be used as a landmark to image the embryo, given the connection between yolk sac and embryo.

At this point in gestation, rapid embryonic development increases gestational sac size, leading to better defined visualization of gestational structures. Between 5½ and 6 weeks' gestation, the amniotic cavity and membrane, chorionic cavity, yolk sac, and embryo should be seen.

Yolk Sac. The yolk sac is the earliest intragestational sac anatomy seen. The yolk sac is normally seen from 5 weeks' gestation. The secondary or sonographic yolk sac has essential functions in embryonic development, including (1) provision of nutrients to the developing embryo, (2) **hematopoiesis,** and (3) development of embryonic endoderm, which forms the primitive gut.

Initially, the yolk sac is attached to the embryo via the yolk stalk, but with amniotic cavity expansion, the yolk sac, which lies between the amniotic and chorionic membranes, detaches from the yolk stalk at approximately 8 weeks' gestation (Figure 47-9).

Visualization of the yolk sac predicts a viable pregnancy in more than 90% of cases. Conversely, failure to visualize the yolk sac, with a minimum of 12 mm MSD, using transvaginal sonography, should provoke suspicion of abnormal pregnancy. Transabdominal studies have shown that the yolk sac should be seen within MSDs of 10 to 15 mm and should always be visualized with an MSD of 20 mm (Figure 47-10).

The growth rate of the yolk sac has been reported to be approximately 0.1 mm/ml of growth of the MSD when the MSD measures less than 15 mm, and 0.03 mm/ml of growth of the MSD through the first trimester. The normal diameter of the yolk sac should not exceed 6 mm. Enlarged yolk sacs may have ominous outcomes (Figure 47-11).

The number of yolk sacs is consistent with the number of amnion membranes. In twin pregnancies, one yolk sac signifies a monochorionic, monoamniotic pregnancy, whereas two yolk sacs signifies a diamniotic, monochorionic or a diamniotic, dichorionic pregnancy. Double

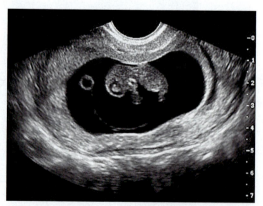

FIGURE 47-9 The yolk sac located between the chorion and amnion moves away from the embryo as the amniotic cavity increases in size. This is illustrated in this view of a 7.5- to 8-week pregnancy.

yolk sacs have been reported in singleton pregnancies without effect.

Typically, the yolk sac resorbs and is no longer seen sonographically by 12 weeks. Persistent yolk sac does occur. A persistent yolk sac may be visualized at the placental umbilical cord insertion, where the amniotic and chorionic membranes are fused.

Embryo. At the beginning of the 5th week, the bilaminar embryonic disk undergoes gastrulation and is converted into the trilaminar (three germ layer) embryonic disk. It is at this point that organogenesis begins.

The early embryo often is not identified until heart motion is detected at approximately 5½ weeks, when the CRL is approximately 3 mm. The embryonic heartbeat must be seen in a viable embryo when the CRL is greater than 4 mm. At this stage, the embryo is seen between the secondary yolk sac and the immediate gestational sac wall. Because the amniotic cavity is still relatively small, it appears that no space lies between the

yolk sac and embryo (Figure 47-12). As pregnancy progresses, the amniotic cavity grows in size, and the corresponding space between the embryo and the yolk sac, which is located outside the amniotic sac, increases (see Figure 47-9).

Between the 5th and 6th weeks' gestation, identification of the amniotic membrane may not be possible using transabdominal techniques. Using transvaginal transducers, the amniotic membrane that separates the **amniotic** and **chorionic cavities** is routinely seen after 5½ weeks. Although with normal gain settings the chorionic cavity (extraembryonic coelom) may appear sonolucent, increased overall gain settings may fill the fluid with low-level echoes. This appearance corresponds to increased density of the chorionic cavity fluid in relation to the amniotic fluid (Figure 47-13). The chorionic cavity is the initial dumping ground for embryonic waste. Later the placenta takes over the process of waste removal, the amniotic cavity expands, and the chorionic cavity

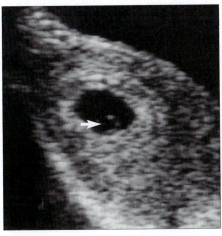

FIGURE 47-10 An approximate 6-week gestational sac with normal-appearing secondary or sonographic yolk sac *(arrow).*

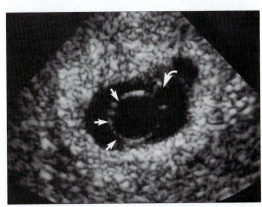

FIGURE 47-11 An enlarged yolk sac, measuring approximately 9 mm *(arrows).* Also note the enlarged, or hydropic, amniotic sac *(curved arrow).* Although embryonic heart motion was initially detected, follow-up studies diagnosed embryonic demise at 8½ weeks' gestation.

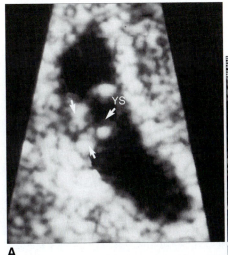

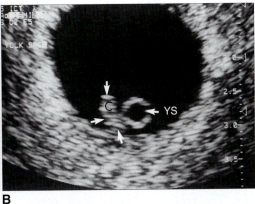

A   **B**

FIGURE 47-12 A, A 5½-week embryo. Note the straight, disklike appearance *(arrows).* **B,** A 6.2-week gestation is seen at the beginning stages of embryonic "curling." *C,* Embryonic cranium. *YS,* Yolk sac.

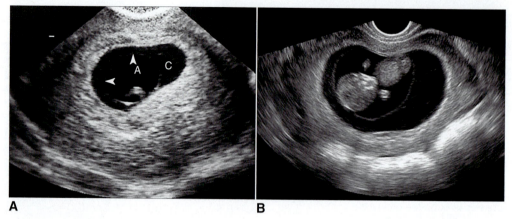

FIGURE 47-13 The fluid in the extraembryonic coelom between the chorion and the amnion has low-level echoes and greater density when compared with the amniotic fluid. *A,* Amniotic cavity *(arrows). C,* Chorionic cavity. **B,** The same fluid differences are seen at approximately 9 weeks' gestation.

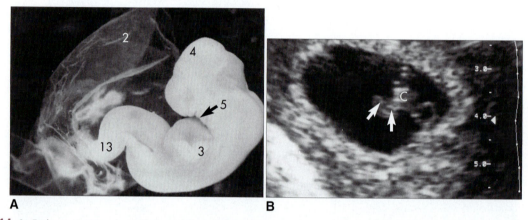

FIGURE 47-14 A, Embryo at approximately 6 weeks' gestation, demonstrating early limb buds *(3)* and embryonic tail *(13). 2,* Amnion; *4,* cranium; *5,* heart. **B,** Corresponding sonogram of a 6-week gestation, demonstrating embryonic tail *(arrows). C,* Embryonic cranium.

decreases in size. Fusion of the membranes, that is, chorioamniotic fusion, occurs at approximately 14 to 15 weeks.

At the beginning of the 6th week of gestation, the trilaminar embryonic disk folds into a C-shaped embryo (Figure 47-14). While embryonic folding continues, the embryonic head, caudal portions, and lateral folds form, resulting in constriction or narrowing between embryo and yolk sac, creating the **yolk stalk.** During embryonic folding, the dorsal aspect of the yolk sac is incorporated into the embryo, developing the foregut, midgut, and hindgut and forming the entire gastrointestinal tract, liver, biliary tract, and pancreas. The yolk stalk, connecting stalk, and allantois are brought together by the expanding amnion, which covers the three structures forming the umbilical cord (Figure 47-15).

Visualization of the Embryo: 6 to 10 Weeks' Gestational Age

The time between 4 and 10 weeks' gestation is often considered the **embryonic period.** A distinct pattern of

development occurs through the embryonic and fetal periods and is outlined in Tables 47-1 to 47-3. The appearance of the embryo changes so rapidly and is so characteristic during the first trimester that the experienced sonographer or sonologist can often date the pregnancy by observation.

Embryonic Cranium and Spine. The spine, which develops from ectoderm, initially evolves from the primitive neural tube, which closes about the 6th week of gestation. The developing spine may be visualized sonographically as parallel echogenic lines at 6 weeks' gestation (Figure 47-16).

Although the embryonic cranium undergoes dramatic changes from the 6th to 10th week of gestation (Figure 47-17), specific anatomy can be visualized sonographically. The cranial neural folds and closure of the neuropore are completed by 7 weeks, forming a cranial vault that is recognizable sonographically (Figure 47-18). At 7 weeks, the brain may appear to have a single fluid-filled vesicle (Figure 47-19).

By 8 weeks, three primary vesicles are seen within the fetal brain: the prosencephalon, the mesencephalon, and

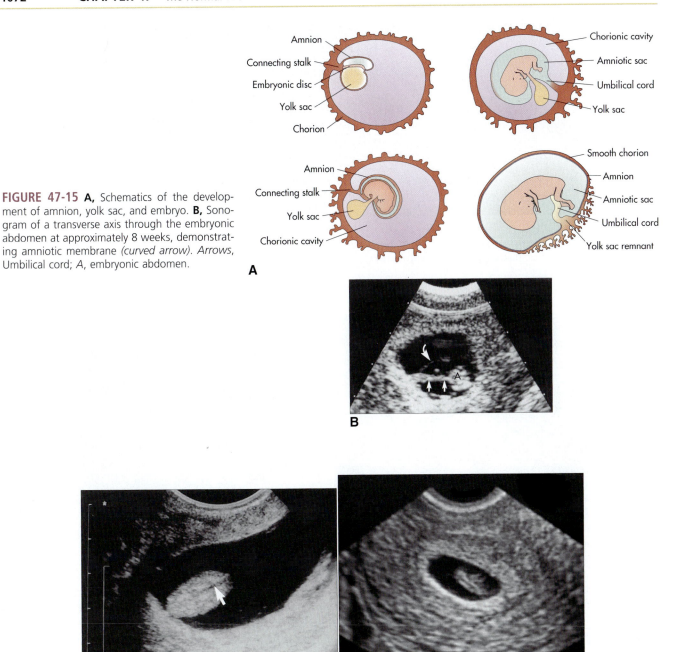

FIGURE 47-15 A, Schematics of the development of amnion, yolk sac, and embryo. **B,** Sonogram of a transverse axis through the embryonic abdomen at approximately 8 weeks, demonstrating amniotic membrane *(curved arrow). Arrows,* Umbilical cord; *A,* embryonic abdomen.

FIGURE 47-16 A, Sonogram of an 8-week embryo demonstrating parallel echogenic lines with the sonolucent center representing spine *(arrow).* **B,** Similar image demonstrating early spinal formation.

the rhombencephalon (Figure 47-20). The rhombencephalon divides into two segments: the cephalic portion or metencephalon, and the caudal component or myelencephalon. Once the rhombencephalon divides with its corresponding flexure, the cystic rhomboid fossa forms. The cystic rhomboid fossa can be imaged sonographically routinely from the 8th to the 10th week of gestation (Figure 47-21). This cystic structure, seen within the posterior aspect of the embryonic cranium, should not be confused with pathology, such as Dandy-Walker malformation.

By 9 weeks, the midline falx has formed and the echogenic choroid plexus tissue is seen in the lateral ventricles. The echogenic choroid plexus, which fills the lateral cerebral ventricles, is prominent. Sonolucent cerebrospinal fluid can be demarcated around the choroid plexus. The lateral ventricles completely fill the cerebral vault at this time in gestation. Although the cerebral hemispheres may be seen at around 9 weeks' gestation, the hemispheric brain tissue is relatively small compared with the rest of the brain. Cerebral brain tissue develops rapidly at the beginning of the second trimester. The

TABLE 47-1	Normal Embryonic Development
Menstrual Age	**Embryonic Observations**
Week 5	Prominent neural folds and neural groove are recognizable.
Day 36	Heart begins to beat.
Week 6	Anterior and posterior neuropores close and neural tube forms.
Day 41	Upper and lower limb buds are present.
Day 42	Crown-rump length is 4.0 mm.
Day 46	Paddle-shaped hand plates are present. Lens pits and optic cups have formed.
Day 48	Cerebral vesicles are distinct.
Day 50	Oral and nasal cavities are confluent.
Day 52	Upper lip is formed.
Day 54	Digital rays are distinct.
Day 56	Crown-rump length is 16.0 mm.
Week 9	Cardiac ventricular septum is closed. Truncus arteriosus divides into aorta and pulmonary trunk. Kidney collecting tubules develop.
Day 58	Eyelids develop.
Day 64	Upper limbs bend at elbows. Fingers are distinct.
Week 10	Glomeruli form in metanephros.
Day 73	Genitalia show some female characteristics but are still easily confused with male genitalia.
Day 80	Face has human appearance.
Day 82	Genitalia have male and female characteristics but still are not fully formed.
Day 84	Crown-rump length is 55 mm.
Month 7	Ossification is complete throughout vertebral column.
Month 8	Ossification centers appear in distal femoral epiphysis.

From Neiman HL: Sonoembryology. In Nyberg DA, et al, editors: *Transvaginal ultrasound*, St Louis, 1990, Mosby.

TABLE 47-2	Beta–Human Chorionic Gonadotropin (hCG) Levels During Pregnancy
Menstrual Weeks	**hCG Levels, mIU/ml**
3	0–5
4	5–426
5	18–7340
6	1080–56,500
7–8	7650–229,000
10–12	25,700–288,000

Note: hCG rates will likely decrease after the first trimester when the placenta takes over.
Note: Even if levels are rising, failure of the levels to double every few days is not a good sign and the pregnancy will likely end in miscarriage. If the test is low or borderline, a repeat test will be ordered in a few days.

TABLE 47-3	Appearance of Embryonic Structures
Menstrual Week of Appearance	**Structure**
4–5	Gestational sac
5	Yolk sac
5.5–6	Fetal heartbeat
6	Fetal pole
7	Single ventricle
7.5	Spine
7.5	Lower limbs
8	Upper limbs
9	Falx
9	Body movements
9.2	Limb movements
9.5	Midgut herniation
9.5	Choroid plexus
9.5	Hindbrain
12	Fingers
12	Jaw
12.5	Toes

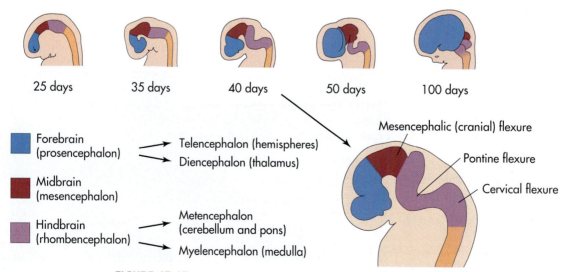

25 days   35 days   40 days   50 days   100 days

Forebrain (prosencephalon) → Telencephalon (hemispheres)
→ Diencephalon (thalamus)

Midbrain (mesencephalon)

Hindbrain (rhombencephalon) → Metencephalon (cerebellum and pons)
→ Myelencephalon (medulla)

Mesencephalic (cranial) flexure
Pontine flexure
Cervical flexure

FIGURE 47-17 Schematic of the embryonic development of the brain.

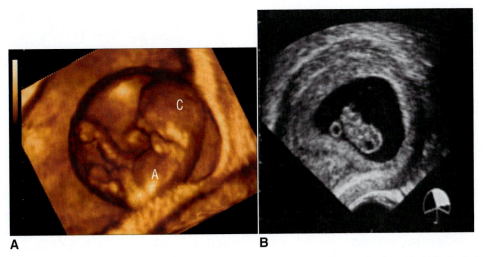

FIGURE 47-18 A, Three-dimensional sonogram demonstrating a 7- to 7½-week gestation. Note the morphologic distinction between the embryonic cranium *(C)* and the embryonic abdomen *(A)*. **B,** Two-dimensional sonogram showing the same gestational age.

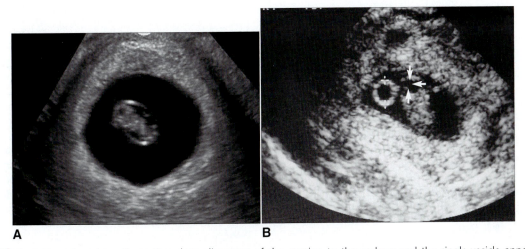

FIGURE 47-19 A, A 7-week embryo illustrating close alignment of the amnion to the embryo and the single-vesicle appearance of the fetal brain. **B,** Sonogram of a 7-week gestation demonstrating the single-vesicle appearance within the fetal cranium *(arrows)*. Note yolk sac between calipers.

FIGURE 47-20 A, An embryo at 7.5 to 8 weeks' gestation demonstrating the three-vesicle appearance of the fetal brain. The cystic vesicles represent the prosencephalon, the mesencephalon, and the rhombencephalon. *4V,* fourth ventricle. *UC,* Umbilical cord. **B,** Notice the three vesicles, including the rhombencephalon *(arrow)*. Arrow is pointing to the yolk sac.

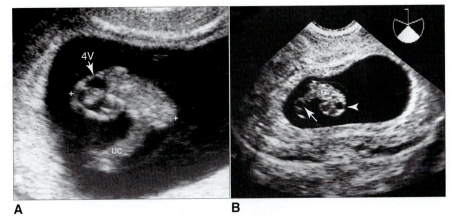

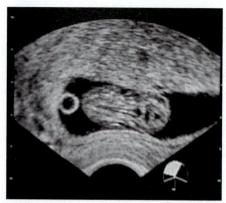

FIGURE 47-21 The cystic rhomboid fossa is seen in this image of an 8-week fetus.

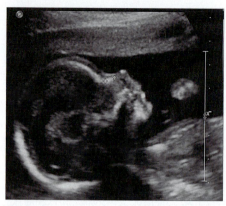

FIGURE 47-23 Fetal knuckles can be seen in this image of a first-trimester embryo.

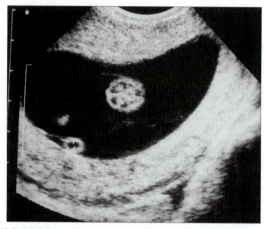

FIGURE 47-22 Axial plane sonogram of a 10-week embryo demonstrating cerebral falx and choroid plexus. Note that the lateral ventricles and the choroid plexus occupy the entire cranial vault at this gestational age.

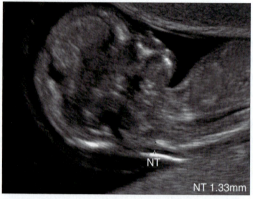

FIGURE 47-24 Calcification of the bony palate can be seen in this embryo at approximately 11 weeks' gestational age.

cerebral falx and midline may also be seen in axial views of the embryonic brain (Figure 47-22).

At 10 weeks, further evolution of the cerebellum, medulla, and medulla oblongata encloses the rhomboid fossa to form the primitive fourth ventricle and part of the cerebral aqueduct of Sylvius. The cerebellum is fused, and the brain structure is completed shortly thereafter.

Limb Development. The limb buds are embryologically recognizable during the 6th week of gestation, as is the embryonic tail, which is not unlike that of a tadpole (see Figure 47-14). The upper limbs form first, followed by the lower limbs. The hands and feet develop later in the first trimester and are completely formed by the end of the 10th week of gestation. Sonographically, limb buds may be detected from the 7th week on; however, the limbs are not routinely identified until calcification of the long bones begins at 10 weeks. Fingers and toes have been identified using transvaginal sonography at 10 weeks (Figure 47-23).

Skeletal Ossification. Calcification of the clavicle begins at approximately 8 weeks, followed by ossifica-

tion of the mandible, palate, vertebral column, and neural arches. Frontal cranial bones begin to calcify at 9 weeks, followed by long bones. Palate fusion occurs late in the first trimester. Sonographically, the embryonic face typically cannot be seen with diagnostic detail. By the 9th week, the maxilla and the mandible are noted as brightly echogenic structures; further bony palate development may be visualized from the 10th week (Figure 47-24).

Physiologic Herniation of Bowel. The anterior abdominal wall is developed by 6 weeks' gestation from the fusion of four ectomesodermal body folds. Simultaneously, the primitive gut is formed as a result of incorporation of the dorsal yolk sac into the embryo. The midgut, derived from the primitive gut, develops and forms the majority of the small bowel, cecum, ascending colon, and proximal transverse colon. Because the midgut is in direct communication with the yolk sac, amniotic cavity expansion pulls the yolk sac away from the embryo, forming the yolk stalk.

As amniotic expansion occurs, the midgut elongates faster than the embryo is growing, causing the midgut to herniate into the base of the umbilical cord. Until approximately 10 weeks' gestation, the midgut loop continues to grow and rotate before it descends into the fetal abdomen at about the 11th week.

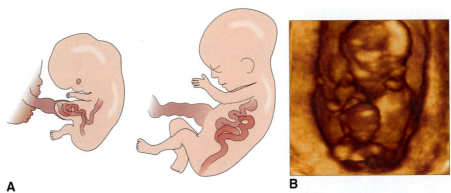

A   **B**

FIGURE 47-25 **A,** Schematic demonstrating normal gut migration. The bowel normally migrates into the base of the umbilical cord between 8 and 12 menstrual weeks (6 to 10 embryonic weeks). The bowel returns to the abdominal cavity by 12 menstrual weeks. **B,** Sonogram of a 10-week gestation demonstrating echogenic "mass" at the base of the umbilical cord. Note that no echogenic material is present within the embryonic abdomen.

Sonographically, this transition of the bowel within the base of the umbilical cord can readily be visualized. The small bowel appears as an echogenic mass within the base of the umbilical cord; little echogenic bowel is seen within the embryonic or fetal abdomen. After 12 weeks' gestation, the echogenic umbilical cord mass is no longer visualized, and echogenic bowel is seen within the fetal abdomen. It is important that this normal embryologic event not be confused with pathologic processes, such as omphalocele or gastroschisis (Figure 47-25).

Embryonic Heart. The heart is the first organ to function within the embryo. The embryonic heart starts beating at approximately 35 days (5 to 5½ weeks), when the endocardial heart tubes fuse to form a single heart tube. Complex embryonic evolution occurs so that by the end of the 8th week of gestation, the heart has reached its adult configuration.

Embryonic cardiac activity should always be seen by 46 menstrual days, or when the CRL is greater than 4 mm. Embryonic cardiac rates vary with gestational age. Rates of 90 to 115 beats per minute at 6 weeks increase to rates of 140 to 160 beats per minute at 9 weeks, with rates of approximately 140 beats per minute through the remainder of the late first and second trimesters (Table 47-4). Documenting a fetal heartbeat of more than 100 beats per minute allows discrimination from the maternal heartbeat.

Although with present technology detailed morphologic anatomy of the first-trimester heart may not always be seen, the situs of the heart is apparent by 9 weeks and should be documented.

DETERMINATION OF GESTATIONAL AGE

It is widely accepted that the most accurate pregnancy dating is obtained via first-trimester sonography. Two parameters for sonographic gestational dating may be used: (1) CRL and (2) gestational sac size.

TABLE 47-4	First-Trimester Fetal Heart Rates
Gestational Age, Weeks	Mean Fetal Heart Rate, Approximate beats/min
5	92–109
6	112–136
7	112–140
8	126–160
9	126–150
10	126–150
11	120–150
12	125–160

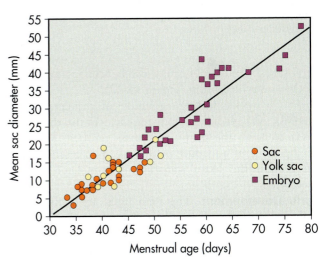

FIGURE 47-26 Graph correlating growth of gestational sac, yolk sac size, and embryo length in relation to mean sac diameter and menstrual days.

Gestational Sac Size

Mean gestational sac size correlates closely with menstrual age during early pregnancy (Figure 47-26). As a rule, the gestational sac size remains accurate through the first 8 weeks of gestation. Sonographically, the

gestational sac size or MSD is determined by calculating the average sum of the length, width, and height of the gestational sac. These measurements are obtained in both sagittal and coronal/semicoronal sonographic planes. When measuring the MSD, the sonographer should measure only the gestational sac fluid space, not including the echogenic decidua (Figure 47-27).

To calculate MSD, the following formula should be used:

$$\text{Length (mm)} + \text{Width (mm)} + \text{Height (mm)}/3 = \text{MSD}$$

$$\text{MSD (mm)} + 30 = \text{Menstrual age (days)}$$

$$\text{Menstrual age (days) divided by } 7 = \text{Menstrual age (weeks)}$$

It is important to note that precise standard deviations for gestational sac size have not been determined, although linear regression analysis demonstrates excellent correlation of MSD and menstrual age.

Crown-Rump Length

Determination of first-trimester gestational dates by direct measurement of the embryo using the CRL was first reported in 1975. This produced gestational dating standard deviations of plus or minus 5 to 7 days, by far the most accurate dating parameters within obstetric biometry. Hadlock and others reevaluated CRL data using modern equipment and determined gestational age standard deviation to be plus or minus 8% throughout the first trimester—essentially unchanged from the original data (Figure 47-28).

CRL measurements can be obtained as early as 5½ weeks using transvaginal sonography. Visualization of embryonic heart motion is a marker signifying the beginning of CRL measurements.

CRLs are considered the most accurate method for dating through 12 weeks' gestation. At this time, the fetus begins to "curl" into the fetal position, making measurement of length more difficult (Figure 47-29).

From 13 weeks on, second-trimester biometric measurements, such as biparietal diameter and femur length, are used for pregnancy dating.

FIRST-TRIMESTER ANATOMY VISUALIZATION

A growing body of literature has reported on the visualization of fetal anatomic structures using transvaginal and transabdominal techniques between 11 and 14 weeks' gestation. Timor-Tritsch found that trained sonographers could successfully visualize 37 anatomic structures in 64% to 99% of patients. Souka found that noncardiac anatomy was seen successfully in 84% of patients with a CRL of 45 to 54 mm and in 96% of patients with a CRL greater than 65 mm. Many studies have documented successful visualization of the four-chamber view of the fetal heart and outflow tracts at between 11 and 14 weeks.

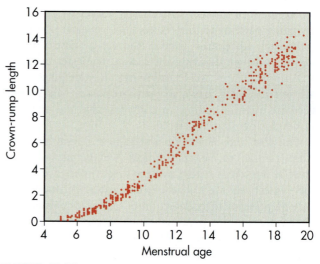

FIGURE 47-28 Graph demonstrating crown-rump length versus menstrual age.

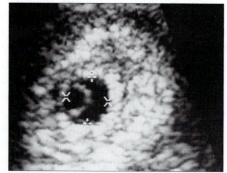

FIGURE 47-27 Sagittal sonogram of an approximate 6-week gestational sac demonstrating caliper placement for appropriate mean sac diameter measurement. Coronal images would also be taken for a third dimension.

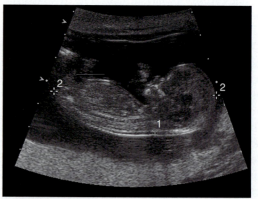

FIGURE 47-29 Sonogram demonstrating crown-rump length measurement on a 10-week embryo.

Reports have described early detection of anomalies, including urinary tract and skeletal anomalies, heart defects, omphaloceles, gastroschisis, and major anomalies of the central nervous system (CNS). Several studies have reported detection rates of fetal structural anomalies similar to rates obtained in the second trimester. These studies, however, vary significantly with regard to the populations screened, gestational age at the time of examination, the anatomy visualized, and the experience of the sonographer.

It is unclear how a first-trimester anatomy survey might be used. Limitations have been recognized, for example, some CNS anomalies—particularly those involving the corpus callosum, the posterior fossa, and the cerebellum—may not be apparent until the second trimester. Similarly, some heart defects such as hypoplastic left heart syndrome and valvular disorders, although structurally present in the first trimester, may not be detectable until the second trimester.

Some authors have suggested two anatomy surveys, adding a first-trimester anatomy survey at the time of nuchal translucency measurement. Others have studied replacement of the second-trimester survey by randomly assigning patients to first- or second-trimester scans and comparing detection rates. Adding a first-trimester survey and then delaying the second-trimester anatomy scan until after 20 weeks, allowing more detailed views of the fetal heart, has also been proposed. Many practices are already adding an early transvaginal anatomy survey for obese gravidas.

The cost and benefit of first-trimester fetal anatomy scans remain to be determined. Significant questions must be answered before routine first-trimester anatomy surveys can be used. The current literature documents the potential for early detection of fetal structural anomalies; however, this potential alone increases the responsibility of the sonographer to visualize and record structures whenever possible.

FIRST-TRIMESTER RISK ASSESSMENT

Women may choose before birth to seek information regarding chromosomal anomalies in the fetus that they are carrying. There are many reasons to seek this information. Prior knowledge provides the opportunity to connect with support groups, to learn about resources and treatments, to choose a delivery hospital that can meet special medical needs, perhaps to find out about special needs adoptions, to choose further testing such as fetal echocardiography, or to choose pregnancy termination.

Women may choose not to seek this information, participate in noninvasive screening tests to determine the level of individual risk, or have an invasive and definitive diagnostic test. There is not a right or wrong choice; the choice is up to the individual woman and her family.

Invasive obstetric techniques allow definitive diagnosis of chromosomal anomalies, including trisomy 21. CVS may be performed between 10 and 14 weeks. Amniocentesis may be performed at 16 weeks. With both techniques, cells from the conceptus are obtained, cultured, and analyzed for chromosomal number and distribution. These diagnostic techniques are definitive but invasive and carry a risk of fetal loss of approximately 1 loss per 300 procedures when done by experienced physicians.

Because chromosomal anomalies are relatively rare, performing invasive procedures on every woman who wants additional information may lead to an unacceptable procedure-related loss of normal fetuses. Offering noninvasive screening tests initially directs women at higher risk toward invasive testing.

Screening for aneuploidy initially focused on maternal age alone. Because the risk for Down syndrome at age 35 is 1:200 (approximately the same as the reported amniocentesis-related risk in the 1980s), women over the age of 35 were offered amniocentesis. Younger women have many more babies than older women, however, and although their risk is lower, 75% to 80% of Down syndrome babies in the United States are born to women younger than 35 years of age.

Second-trimester biochemical screening tests were developed to help determine which women were at greater risk. The triple screen includes measurement of hCG, estriol, and alpha-fetoprotein. The quad screen involves measurement of hCG, estriol, alpha-fetoprotein, and inhibin. These second-trimester tests are used along with age to assess a woman's individual risk.

When CVS became available, there was an incentive to move prenatal screening and diagnosis of aneuploidy into the first trimester. Performing these tests in the first trimester provides earlier reassurance for more than 95% of patients and earlier diagnosis for affected pregnancies. The results can be obtained before the pregnancy is visible, and when termination is chosen, it is seven times safer when performed in the first trimester. First-trimester testing also allows more time for counseling and additional options for testing.

The standard for first-trimester risk assessment is the combined test using maternal age, the nuchal translucency measurement, and biochemistry analyses of hCG and PAPP-A. The combined first-trimester test has a higher detection rate (at the same false-positive rate) than maternal age alone, triple screen, or quad screen (Figure 47-30). It is important to note that none of the first-trimester markers should be used alone for risk assessment. The combination of multiple markers is required. Risk assessment markers are incorporated into examinations when women choose to have aneuploidy screening tests, and when the combination test, including serum biochemistry and nuchal translucency, is performed.

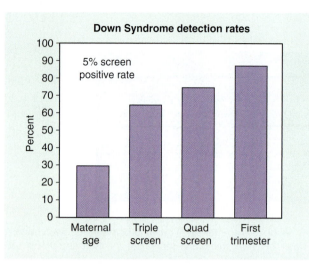

FIGURE 47-30 Down syndrome detection rates based on maternal age alone, second-trimester triple screen, second-trimester quad screen, and the combined first-trimester risk assessment.

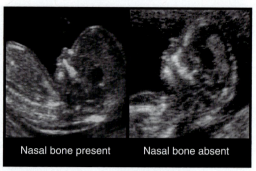

FIGURE 47-32 The presence or absence of the nasal bone in the late first trimester is assessed for aneuploidy risk.

BOX 47-2	Nuchal Translucency (NT) Measurement Criteria

- The margins of the NT edges are clear.
- The fetus is in a midsagittal plane.
- The fetus occupies the majority of the image.
- The fetal head is in a neutral position.
- The fetus is observed away from the amnion.
- (+) calipers are used.
- Horizontal crossbars are placed correctly on the inner surface of the border of the lucency.
- Calipers are placed perpendicular to the long axis of the fetus.
- The measurement is taken at the widest NT space.

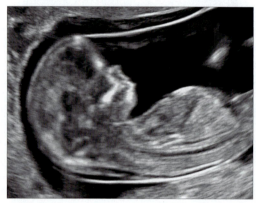

FIGURE 47-31 The fluid-filled space known as the nuchal translucency (NT) is seen in this image of an 11-week embryo. The boundary of the NT is seen separate from the amnion.

First-Trimester Risk Assessment Sonography Techniques

Nuchal Translucency Measurements. The normal first-trimester fetus has a small pocket of fluid along its back that is known as the nuchal translucency (NT) (Figure 47-31). Measurement of the NT is a component of first-trimester risk assessment. The NT must be measured in a standardized way (Box 47-2), and measurement techniques need to be monitored and continually assessed to ensure that accurate risks based on these measurements are given to women and their families.

To participate in NT measurements and first-trimester risk assessment, sonographers and sonologists must demonstrate competency to measure the NT. The Maternal Fetal Medicine Foundation Nuchal Translucency Quality Review program (http://www.ntqr.org) and the Fetal Medicine Foundation USA (http://

www.fetalmedicineusa.com) provide credentialing and ongoing quality monitoring in the United States.

Nasal Bone. Absence of the fetal nasal bone in late first-trimester sonography is associated with trisomy 21. Nasal bone imaging is a useful adjunct to NT and serum biochemistry (Figure 47-32). Many laboratories will incorporate the presence or absence of the fetal nasal bone into their risk algorithm and will provide to women a risk adjusted for nasal bone. A small nose and midface hypoplasia are well-known components of the Down syndrome phenotype. It is important to note these characteristics and to look for the fetal nasal bone in both first- and second-trimester examinations.

Tricuspid Regurgitation. Studies have linked the early presence of tricuspid regurgitation (TR) to increased risk for aneuploidy. Because tricuspid flow analysis requires interrogation of a very small fetus with pulsed Doppler, it is recommended that tricuspid flow be used to further define risk for women who are borderline or high risk by other techniques. Ongoing research is needed to determine the appropriate use of TR in a low-risk population.

Additional Risk Assessment Techniques. Risk assessment strategies, including measurement of facial angles and Doppler assessment of the ductus venosus, are incorporated into first-trimester risk assessment protocols in some centers. Risk assessment is an active area of research, and new measurements and techniques may be

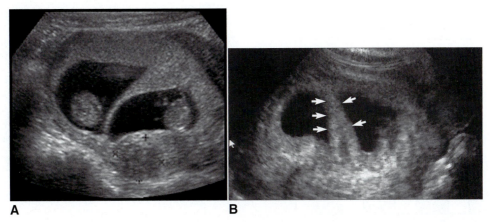

FIGURE 47-33 A, A dichorionic pregnancy. Notice the thick wall and the V shape of placental tissue growing between the two chorionic membranes. **B,** Sonogram showing a dichorionic-diamniotic pregnancy. Note the thick membrane separating the two gestational sacs *(arrows).*

available. Ongoing research is looking at fetal nucleic acid in the maternal blood system. If these particles can be captured from maternal blood noninvasively for analysis, then genetic diagnosis will be more widely available during pregnancy.

MULTIPLE GESTATIONS

The sonographic diagnosis of multiple gestations within the first trimester is valuable information for the obstetrician. A multiple-gestation pregnancy is, by definition, high risk, with significant increases in morbidity and mortality rates in relation to singleton pregnancies. Overall, twin gestations have a seven to ten times greater mortality rate than singletons. Risk increases when the twins are monozygotic and share membrane components.

Using transvaginal sonography, multiple gestations can be readily diagnosed at very early gestational ages, between 5½ and 6½ weeks. Sonographic identification of multiple gestational sacs with incorporated yolk sacs, amniotic membranes, and, ideally, embryos with cardiac motion allows definitive diagnosis.

The first trimester is the ideal time to determine membrane structures of multiple pregnancies. It is extremely important to identify and document chorionicity and amnionicity in twin pregnancies imaged during the first trimester.

Dizygotic twin pregnancies, which account for 70% of all twins, are by definition **dichorionic** and **diamniotic.** Sonographically, dichorionic and diamniotic twins appear as two separate gestational sacs with individual trophoblastic tissue, which allows the appearance of a thick dividing membrane. As pregnancy progresses, this membrane becomes thinner secondary to the diminished space between the two sacs, so this diagnosis may be

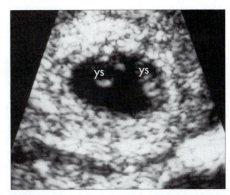

FIGURE 47-34 A sonogram demonstrating a monochorionic-diamniotic pregnancy. There is only one thick-walled structure and one chorionic sac, so the pregnancy is monochorionic. The amnions are not seen, but the presence of two yolk sacs *(ys)* indicates that this is a diamniotic pregnancy.

more difficult later in gestation. In a dichorionic-diamniotic pregnancy, each sac has an individual yolk sac, amniotic membrane, and embryo (Figure 47-33).

Monochorionic-diamniotic twins appear to be contained within a single gestational/chorionic sac; two amnions, two yolk sacs, and two embryos are identified (Figure 47-34). The amnion membranes may be difficult to observe within the chorionic sac. **Monoamniotic-monochorionic** twin gestation is a crucial diagnosis to make. This type of twinning has a mortality rate of approximately 50%. Sonographic visualization would include one gestational sac containing one yolk sac, one amniotic membrane, and two embryos within a single amniotic cavity.

First-trimester NT measurements in multiple pregnancies may contribute to risk assessment. Differences in NT measurements between normal twins may be an early sign of twin-to-twin transfusion syndrome.

First-Trimester Complications

Candace Goldstein and Sandra L. Hagen-Ansert

The first trimester consists of a series of complex, sequential events that make up the early stage of embryonic development. Interruption in development may lead to complications in the embryonic period. Approximately 15% of clinically recognized pregnancies are spontaneously miscarried. The loss rate may be even higher for early pregnancies that are not clinically recognized. The most common presentation for complications is vaginal spotting or frank bleeding, which occurs in nearly 25% of patients during the early stage of pregnancy. In many cases, bleeding is inconsequential, resulting from implantation of the conceptus into the decidualized endometrium. However, if bleeding is accompanied by severe pain, uterine contractions, or a dilated cervix, the pregnancy is unlikely to progress. Patients benefit from early transvaginal examination to carefully investigate the uterine cavity for the presence of an embryo, a fetal heartbeat, a yolk sac, or retained products of conception.

A threatened abortion covers a wide range of conditions based on the stage of development and the sonographic appearance of the products of conception. *Threatened abortion* is a term used for pregnancies of fewer than 20 weeks when the patient has a viable embryo, documented fetal heartbeat, and vaginal bleeding. The diagnosis of *threatened abortion* is made when

the cervix is long and closed in a patient with vaginal bleeding. At least 50% of pregnant women with these complications will go on to spontaneously lose or "abort" the pregnancy. Specific terminology has been adopted to describe the complications of these pregnancies. *Embryonic demise* is used when there is clear evidence of a nonviable embryo. *Blighted ovum,* or *anembryonic pregnancy,* is used to describe a uterus containing a gestational sac but no visible embryo.

Other conditions that may present clinically as a threatened abortion are ectopic pregnancy and gestational trophoblastic disease. Knowledge of the quantitative level of serum human chorionic gonadotropin (hCG) is necessary to make this diagnosis and should be correlated with the sonographic appearance.

FIRST-TRIMESTER BLEEDING AND SONOGRAPHIC APPEARANCES

Placental Hematomas and Subchorionic Hemorrhage

The embryonic placenta, or frondosum, may become detached, resulting in the formation of a hematoma, which typically causes vaginal bleeding. Most of these hemorrhages are contiguous with a placental edge. Although no risk factors have been associated with first-trimester placental separation, it has been reported to have a 50% or greater fetal loss rate. Although the prognosis seems to depend on the size of the hematoma, no specific volumes have been correlated in the first trimester with fetal outcomes. That said, improved outcomes do seem to be consistent with smaller hematomas.

Sonographically, placental hematomas may be difficult to distinguish from subchorionic hemorrhages. Placental hematomas do not cause symptoms, bleeding, or spotting because they are within the chorionic sac and have no communication with the endometrium.

Subchorionic Hemorrhage. The most common occurrence of bleeding in the first trimester is from subchorionic hemorrhage. These low-pressure bleeds result from the process of implantation of the fertilized ovum into the endometrial cavity and myometrial wall. The hemorrhage is found between the myometrium and the margins of the gestational sac and may or may not be associated with the placenta. This finding can help distinguish a subchorionic hemorrhage from abruptio placentae, which generally occurs in the second trimester and may present as a lucency posterior to the placenta. Clinical findings may include bleeding, spotting, or uterine cramping. If the hemorrhage becomes large enough, this can lead to **spontaneous pregnancy loss (SPL).**

Sonographic Findings. The appearance of bleeding varies with the stage of its organization. An early bleed may appear slightly echogenic as the red blood cells actively fill the area of hemorrhage. With time, the hemorrhage becomes more anechoic and may be seen between the uterine wall and the fetal membrane (Figure 48-1). Color flow Doppler will demonstrate the avascular nature of the hemorrhage. Patients may present with active vaginal bleeding, and the subchorionic bleed is easily seen by ultrasound adjacent to the gestational sac. Other patients may have no bleeding yet have a subchorionic lucency that can be seen with imaging. Patients may be symptomatic with a large subchorionic bleed, or asymptomatic with a small subchorionic bleed, perhaps only seen with transvaginal imaging.

Absent Intrauterine Sac

Sonography is routinely used to evaluate for the presence or absence of an intrauterine gestational sac. If the patient presents with a positive pregnancy test, the uterus appears normal but the endometrial complex shows no sign of a gestational sac; the differential diagnosis would include a very early intrauterine pregnancy, a nondeveloping pregnancy, or possible ectopic pregnancy.

Characteristics for the sonographic diagnosis of an absent intrauterine sac include an empty uterus with no evidence of an endometrial fluid collection (early gestational sac), absence of adnexal masses or free fluid, and positive beta-hCG levels. Clinical findings may be characterized by bleeding and cramping. Correlation between the serum beta-hCG level and uterine findings can be used to confirm whether the sonographic indications of a first-trimester pregnancy have been met. Recall that the gestational sac is identified sonographically at 4.5 weeks' gestation. The sac grows approximately 1 mm per day in the first trimester. The yolk sac should be visualized transvaginally when the gestational sac reaches 8 mm in size, and the embryo should be visualized when the mean sac diameter (MSD) is greater than 16 mm. The normal embryo grows at a rate of 1 mm per day. Cardiac activity is visible by 5.5 to 6.5 weeks (Table 48-1). Failure to observe these developmental markers suggests an abnormal pregnancy.

In the case of pregnancy loss (complete abortion), serial hCG levels demonstrate successive decline. Caution should be taken when a positive pregnancy test and an empty uterus are seen, given the possibility that an early normal intrauterine pregnancy between 3 and 5 weeks' gestation may be present. Consequently, serial hCG levels should always be obtained and followed for appropriate rise or decline.

If the endometrium is abnormally thick or irregularly echogenic, the differential diagnosis includes intrauterine blood, retained products of conception after an incomplete spontaneous abortion, a decidual reaction associated with an ectopic pregnancy, or decidual changes resulting from an early but not yet visible intrauterine pregnancy. **Incomplete spontaneous abortion** may show several sonographic findings, ranging from an intact gestational sac with a nonviable embryo to a collapsed gestational sac that is grossly misshapen (Figure 48-2).

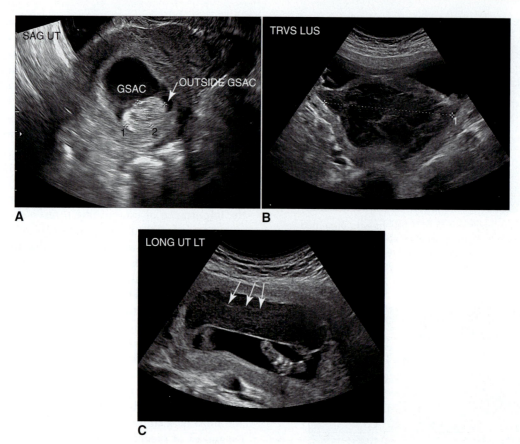

FIGURE 48-1 Subchorionic hemorrhages are shown at **(A)** 8 weeks' gestation, **(B)** 14 weeks' gestation, and **(C)** 16 weeks' gestation. Note the separation of the anterior placenta from the uterine wall *(arrows)*. GSAC, Gestational sac.

TABLE 48-1	Sonographic Findings for Abnormal Pregnancy in the First Trimester
Condition	**Sonographic Findings**
Embryonic bradycardia	<60 beats per minute
Embryonic tachycardia	>170 beats per minute
Complete abortion	– Empty uterus – No adnexal mass – No free fluid in pelvis – Positive hCG levels with rapid decline
Incomplete abortion	Variable findings: – Intact gestational sac with nonviable embryo to collapsed sac – Thickened endometrium >8 mm – Retained embryonic parts
Anembryonic pregnancy	– Large (>18 mm), empty gestational sac with failure to develop – No yolk sac, amnion, or embryo
Molar pregnancy – Hyperemesis – Increased hCG levels – Bleeding – Preeclampsia	– Uterus larger than dates – "Snowstorm" of multiple tiny clusters of grapelike echoes within the uterine cavity – Theca lutein cysts may be present

hCG, Human chorionic gonadotropin.

Women who are clinically undergoing a spontaneous abortion or who have had an elective termination often require follow-up sonography to determine whether retained products of conception are present. Sonographic signs of retained products may be subtle; a thickened endometrium greater than 8 mm and increased vascularization of the endometrial complex with color Doppler are strongly predictive. The presence of visible embryonic parts, a gestational sac, or an embryonic disk is obvious evidence of retained products of conception

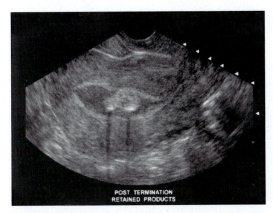

FIGURE 48-2 Transvaginal scan of a patient who presented with fever, pain, and bleeding secondary to an abortion 2 days previously. The endometrial cavity is distended, with retained products of conception casting small shadows into the myometrial cavity.

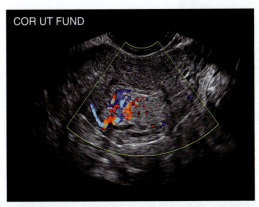

FIGURE 48-3 Transvaginal coronal color Doppler image demonstrates an increased flow velocity throughout the molar tissue. This patient had a positive pregnancy test and was experiencing vaginal bleeding.

(Figure 48-3). It sometimes can be difficult to distinguish retained products of conception from blood clots. Quantitative hCG levels, which do not decline normally, a thickened endometrium, and increased vascular flow will provide discriminating evidence for retained products.

Gestational Sac Without an Embryo or Yolk Sac

A gestational sac without an embryo or yolk sac on sonography may represent one of three conditions: (1) a normal early intrauterine pregnancy of less than 5 weeks, (2) an abnormal intrauterine pregnancy, or (3) a pseudogestational sac in a patient with an ectopic pregnancy.

Criteria for Abnormal Sac

The gestational sac should be imaged consistently by both transabdominal and transvaginal sonography when its mean diameter is 5 mm, which corresponds to a ges-

tational age of 4 to 5 weeks. Transvaginal sonography may demonstrate the sac as early as 4 weeks, when it measures 2 to 3 mm. Measuring the gestational sac at this early stage provides a baseline for monitoring appropriate interval growth. Caution should be used in evaluating these early stages of pregnancy to allow for the possibility that someone may have inaccurate dates for their last menstrual period. Sequential scanning can document appropriate interval growth of 1 mm per day. Lack of appropriate growth indicates an abnormal sac.

In their opinion paper, *Predicting Pregnancy Failure in Empty Gestational Sacs*, Drs. Nyberg and Filly discuss the importance of establishing *threshold levels* and *discriminatory levels* for the diagnosis of SPL. A threshold level tells us when we "might" be able to discern early pregnancy structures. For instance, we *might* be able to visualize a living embryo at 5.5 weeks. The discriminatory level tells us when we *should* be able to visualize an embryonic structure. Several studies have confirmed that an embryo can be expected to be seen at 6.4 weeks, and that this is the discriminatory level. If an embryo is not detected at 6.4 weeks, the diagnosis of SPL can be made.

Regarding gestational sac values, a gestational sac may be seen as early as 4.3 weeks, the *threshold level*, and must be seen by 5.2 weeks, the *discriminatory level*. Diagnoses of pregnancy failure should always be based on the discriminatory criteria.

Transvaginal sonography is the ideal method to examine the early gestational sac. When the sac measures 8 mm or greater, a definitive yolk sac should be demonstrated. The yolk sac can be expected to grow 0.1 mm per 1 mm of MSD growth up to 15 mm. When the gestational sac measures 16 to 20 mm or greater, an embryo with cardiac activity should be seen. Follow-up examination in 7 to 10 days is recommended if the findings are indeterminate.

Anembryonic Pregnancy (Blighted Ovum)

By definition, **anembryonic pregnancy**, or **blighted ovum**, is a gestational sac in which the embryo fails to develop or stops developing at such an early stage that it is imperceptible by ultrasound (see Table 48-1). The trophoblastic tissue may continue to proliferate despite the failed embryonic growth, the gestational sac will continue to grow, and hCG levels may continue to rise, although not at the expected rate. The typical sonographic appearance of anembryonic pregnancy is a large, empty gestational sac that does not demonstrate a yolk sac, an amnion, or an embryo (Figure 48-4). The MSD increases by 1.13 mm/day in a normal gestation, but the growth rate of an abnormal sac is only 0.70 mm/day. Therefore, abnormal sac growth can be diagnosed when the MSD fails to increase by 0.6 mm/day. In subsequent repeat studies, the sonographer evaluates growth size of the sac, presence of the yolk sac, development of an

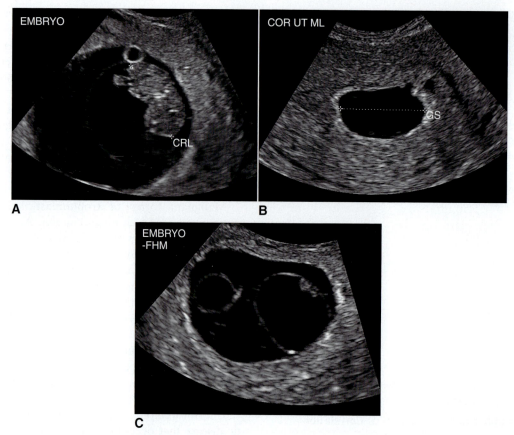

FIGURE 48-4 A, Transvaginal image demonstrating a normal embryo and yolk sac. **B,** Large, empty 6-week gestational sac that does not contain yolk sac, amnion, or embryo. This is consistent with anembryonic pregnancy. **C,** Large, empty gestational sac *(on right)* with an abnormal yolk sac.

embryo, and presence or absence of cardiac activity. Box 48-1 outlines several sonographic intrauterine findings associated with abnormal pregnancies.

Gestational Trophoblastic Disease

Gestational trophoblastic disease is a proliferative disease of the trophoblast that occurs after an abnormal conception. It represents a spectrum of disease from a relatively benign form called hydatidiform (partial, complete, or coexistent) mole to a more malignant form called an invasive mole, or choriocarcinoma. The clinical hallmark of gestational trophoblastic disease is vaginal bleeding in the first or early second trimester. Serum levels of beta-hCG are dramatically elevated and are often greater than 100,000 IU/ml. The patient may also experience symptoms of hyperemesis gravidarum or preeclampsia. Maternal serum alpha-fetoprotein levels will be notably low in pregnancies complicated by a complete hydatidiform mole.

In the United States, gestational trophoblastic disease affects approximately 1 out of every 1000 pregnancies. Associations with women younger than age 20 and older than age 40 with molar pregnancy have been reported. Molar pregnancies are divided into two categories: partial and complete. A partial mole is karyotypically abnormal, usually triploid, and commonly occurs when a normal egg is fertilized by two sperm. Fetal parts may develop concurrently with abnormal trophoblastic tissue. In contrast, genetic studies indicate that a complete hydatidiform mole has a normal diploid karyotype of 46XX, which is usually entirely derived from the father. Complete moles occur when an egg without a nucleus is fertilized by one normal sperm. Trophoblastic tissue proliferates, but no fetal parts ever develop.

Sonographic Findings. The sonographic appearance of molar pregnancy varies with gestational age. The characteristic "snowstorm" appearance of a hydatidiform mole, which includes a moderately echogenic soft tissue mass filling the uterine cavity that is marked with small cystic spaces representing hydropic chorionic villi, may not be apparent initially, but will present with advancing time (Figure 48-5). The appearance of first-trimester molar pregnancy may simulate a missed abortion, incomplete abortion, blighted ovum, or hydropic degeneration of the placenta associated with missed abortion (Figure 48-6).

On transvaginal sonography, the abnormal appearing choriodecidual or trophoblastic reaction consists of a distorted sac shape with a thin, weakly echogenic or irregular choriodecidual reaction and absence of a double decidual sac when the MSD exceeds 10 mm. There is

From Nyberg DA, Laing FC: In Nyberg DA, Hill LM, Bohm-Velez M, et al, editors: *Transvaginal ultrasound,* St Louis, 1992, Mosby.

| **BOX 48-1** | **Sonographic Findings of Gestational Sacs Associated With Abnormal Intrauterine Pregnancies** |

Embryo
- Absence of cardiac motion in embryos 5 mm or larger
- Absence of cardiac motion after 6.5 menstrual weeks

Yolk Sac and Amnion
- Large yolk sac or amnion without a visible embryo
- Calcified yolk sac

Large Gestational Sac
- >18 mm lacking a viable embryo
- >8 mm lacking a visible yolk sac

Shape
- Irregular or misshapen

Position
- Cornual, low, or hour-glassing through cervical os

Trophoblastic Reaction
- Irregular
- Absent double decidual sac finding
- Thin trophoblastic reaction <2 mm
- Intratrophoblastic venous flow

Growth
- Gestational sac growth of <0.6 mm/day
- Absent embryonic growth

Human Chorionic Gonadotropin (hCG) Correlation
- Discrepancy in sac size with hCG levels

---

usually no sign of a viable embryo, and the early developing placenta exhibits multiple abnormal trophoblastic changes. The sonographic examination may reveal a uterus that is larger in size than dates and filled with a heterogeneous complex pattern ("cluster of grapes") along with bilateral adnexal fullness that may represent ovarian enlargement of theca lutein cysts. The trophoblastic reaction may also be seen as a small echogenic mass filling the uterine cavity without the characteristic vesicles. Typically, remarkable increased blood flow is seen with color Doppler, and spectral Doppler shows low-resistive waveforms with high diastolic flow.

The primary treatment of molar pregnancy is uterine curettage followed by serial monitoring of serum hCG levels. Serum hCG level falls toward normal within 10 to 12 weeks after evacuation. The reported incidence of residual disease after curettage is approximately 20%. The use of sonography for direct visualization of the uterine content to ensure complete evacuation during the curettage procedure has been shown to substantially reduce the incidence of residual gestational trophoblastic disease.

A partial mole on sonography has an identifiable placenta, although the placental tissue is grossly enlarged and engorged with cystic spaces, which represent the hydropic villi. An embryo or embryonic tissue may also be identified, but often the embryo is abnormal and is aborted in the first trimester. In later stages of pregnancy (>12 weeks), careful analysis should be performed to look for structural defects, as triploid fetuses usually exist with a partial mole. This includes trisomies 13, 18, and 21.

Bilateral theca lutein cysts have been reported in as many as half of molar pregnancies. Enlarged ovaries may rupture or torse, causing extreme pain for the patient. Theca lutein cysts are well demonstrated on sonography as enlarged ovaries with multiple cystic areas throughout.

Malignant forms of trophoblastic disease include invasive mole and choriocarcinoma. An invasive hydatidiform mole occurs when the hydropic villi of a partial or complete mole invade the uterine myometrium and may further penetrate the uterine wall. This may occur along with the molar pregnancy or may progress after evacuation of the molar tissue has occurred. If this occurs postoperatively, it is referred to as *persistent trophoblastic disease.* Clinically, the patient presents with continued heavy bleeding and highly elevated hCG levels. The sonographic appearance shows an enlarged uterus with multiple focal areas of grapelike clusters throughout.

Choriocarcinoma is a malignant form of trophoblastic disease that occurs in 2% to 3% of molar pregnancies. This tumor is fast-growing and commonly metastasizes to the lungs, liver, and brain. Clinical symptoms include vaginal bleeding, in addition to dyspnea, abdominal pain, and neurologic symptoms, depending on where the metastasis has spread.

ABNORMAL OR ABSENT CARDIAC ACTIVITY

Sonographic differentiation of normal and abnormal appearances of first-trimester pregnancy may be subtle. Distinguishing viable from nonviable gestations is crucial, and demonstration of a living embryo does not necessarily mean a normal outcome. Recent data prospectively looked at 556 pregnancies between 6 and 13 weeks' gestation and identified embryonic heart motion.[4] Overall the pregnancy loss rate after identification of an intrauterine pregnancy with positive cardiac motion was 8.8%. If sonographic abnormalities were detected (subchorionic hematoma being the most frequent), the loss rate was 15.2% compared with 8.8% when sonogram findings were normal. It is of interest that the loss rate after a normal sonogram was similar in symptomatic (10.6%) and asymptomatic patients (9.1%).[4]

Identifying an intrauterine pregnancy with or without cardiac activity is the first conclusive sonographic sign of viability. With transvaginal sonography, a living embryo should be detected by 46 menstrual days. Other sonographic appearances allow the ultrasound clinician to differentiate normal and abnormal findings within the

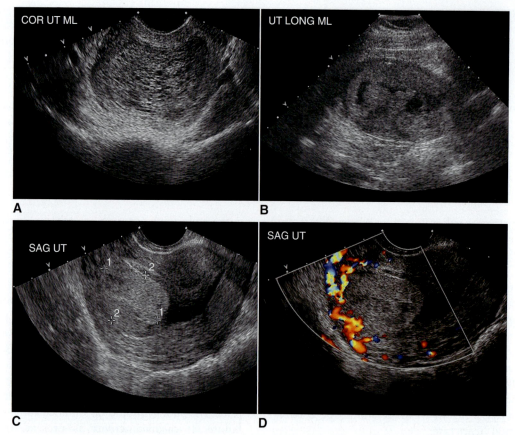

FIGURE 48-5 **A** through **D,** Transvaginal coronal and sagittal image of the pregnant uterus in a patient who presented larger than appropriate for dates and with bleeding. The uterus is filled with tiny grapelike clusters of tissue, which represent a hydatidiform mole.

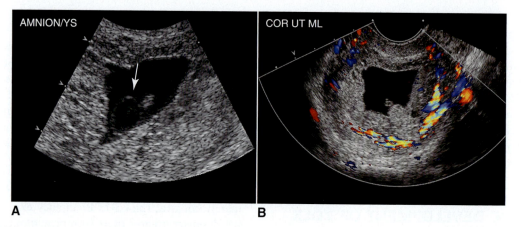

FIGURE 48-6 This patient had a coexistent fetus with a hydatidiform mole *(arrow).* Color Doppler of the molar pregnancy shows high-velocity flow throughout the abnormal tissue.

early gestational period: cardiac rate, gestational sac growth, and yolk sac size and appearance. More than one sonogram may be necessary to establish a normal pregnancy. Sonographic signs are discussed throughout this chapter and are outlined in Table 48-2.

Absent Cardiac Activity

Absence of cardiac activity in the first trimester is the most critical sign for viability of the pregnancy. The heart tube is formed between 3.5 and 5 weeks of conception. If the embryo is visible by sonography but cardiac activity cannot be documented, the prognosis is poor. Caution should be used in interpreting any case that involves a question regarding the accuracy of menstrual dating and in which heart motion is not yet visible by sonography. Usually by the time the embryonic sac measures 9 mm, the presence of cardiac activity is noted. Other studies have noted that with transvaginal sonography, when the crown-rump length (CRL) measures 4 mm, the embryo

TABLE 48-2	First-Trimester Pelvic Mass	
Condition	**Sonographic Findings**	**Differential Considerations**
Corpus luteum cyst	>5 cm in size Internal septations and debris (secondary to hemorrhage) Increased vascularity surrounding corpus luteum	Dermoid Ovarian cancer
Uterine leiomyoma	Increased hormone stimulation growth May compress gestational sac Various sonographic patterns: hypoechoic, echogenic, isoechoic when compared with myometrium Increased size causes uterine endometrial deformity	Uterine contractions Dermoid

should demonstrate cardiac function. Generally, if any doubt exists regarding the measurement, the patient is reexamined after several days for the presence of cardiac activity.

Recall that between 6 and 7 weeks' gestation, the embryo and yolk sac are close in proximity and can be viewed as contiguous structures. After 7 weeks, these structures diverge from one another. Scans should be made with the highest possible transducer frequency to image with the greatest accuracy. The transducer should be very carefully swept through the gestational sac to image the embryo, cardiac motion, and yolk sac. Once cardiac activity is seen, an M-mode should be used to record the actual heart rate.

Embryonic Bradycardia and Tachycardia

Variations in embryonic cardiac rate during the first trimester range between 90 and 170 beats per minute (see Table 48-1). Embryonic cardiac rates of less than 90 beats per minute at any gestational age within the first trimester have been shown to have a poor prognostic finding. In fact, no reported embryo has survived beyond the second trimester with this finding. The fetus with a heart rate greater than 170 beats per minute shows signs of tachycardia, which may lead to heart failure and fetal hydrops (pleural effusion, pericardial effusion, and ascites).

EMBRYONIC DEVELOPMENT OF YOLK SAC AND AMNION

Embryonic Oligohydramnios and Growth Restriction

Growth delay and oligohydramnios within the first trimester have poor outcomes. If the gestational sac measures 5 mm less than the CRL, embryonic oligohydramnios may be suspected, and demise is highly probable.

Embryonic growth restriction can be determined only by relative sonographic dating, either by reliable menstrual history or by growth delay of the embryo or gestational sac in relation to serial sonograms. Chromosome abnormalities, such as triploidy, have been associated with embryonic growth restriction and embryonic oligohydramnios.

Embryonic Yolk Sac Evaluation

The size and appearance of the yolk sac should be evaluated in the first trimester. Expected yolk sac growth is 0.3 mm/day. A normal yolk sac has a maximal diameter of 5.5 mm between 5 and 10 weeks' gestation. An enlarged yolk sac (5.6 mm or greater) has an increased risk for SPL. If the yolk sac is abnormal in appearance, too large for gestational age, misshapen, or highly echogenic, the patient should be watched for early pregnancy failure. If cardiac activity is present, the pregnancy should be followed carefully with ultrasound, as the embryo may continue to grow.

Amnion Evaluation

The amnion is best visualized with transvaginal sonography between the 5th and 7th weeks of gestation as the double bleb sign, the simultaneous side-by-side appearance of the amnion and yolk sac. The amnion should appear as the thinner of the two concentric structures. The embryonic disk lies between the amnion and the yolk sac. Abnormal development is suggested when the amnion becomes very easy to see, or when the thickness and echogenicity approach those of the yolk sac. The mean amniotic sac diameter should be approximately equal to the CRL. Pregnancy exhibiting a mean sac diameter greater than 16 mm without an embryo is consistent with anembryonic pregnancy.

ECTOPIC PREGNANCY

Ectopic pregnancy is one of the most emergent diagnoses made with sonography. An ectopic pregnancy is pregnancy located outside the central/fundal location of the uterus. Approximately 10% of maternal deaths are related to ectopic pregnancy. The occurrence of ectopic pregnancy also has an effect on the future fertility of a patient and increases the risk of a repeat ectopic pregnancy. The incidence of ectopic pregnancy has increased in recent years. Associated risk factors include the rise

in the incidence of pelvic infections, the use of intrauterine contraceptive devices (IUCDs), fallopian tube surgeries, infertility treatments, and a history of ectopic pregnancy.

Clinical findings of pain are nonspecific and may vary. Pelvic pain has been reported in 97% of patients, although pain may be consistent with other pathologic processes, such as appendicitis or pelvic inflammatory disease. The classic clinical findings associated with ectopic pregnancy are vaginal bleeding, an empty uterus, the presence of an adnexal mass, and a positive pregnancy test. These clinical findings are found in nearly 45% of patients.

Pathologically, tubal ectopic pregnancy is diagnosed by the invasion of trophoblastic tissue within the fallopian tube mucosa. This causes the bleeding often associated with ectopic pregnancy, which may cause hematosalpinx, hemoperitoneum, or both.

Ectopic pregnancy occurs within the fallopian tube in approximately 95% of cases. Other sites, such as the ovary, broad ligament, peritoneum, cervix, and cornua, account for the remaining cases (Figure 48-7). When an ectopic pregnancy is found in the interstitial portion of the fallopian tube near the uterine cornu, the risk for massive hemorrhage with rupture that may lead to hysterectomy or even death is increased.

Correlating clinical findings with sonographic findings in ectopic pregnancy is imperative for diagnosis. Specific assays for hCG allow the sonographer/sonologist to discern the sonographic findings. Beta-hCG is quantified from maternal blood by two preparations: the First International Reference Preparation (1st IRP) or the Second International Standard (2IS). It is crucial that the sonographer understand which hCG assay a particular institution or laboratory is using. Quantification of hCG is directly correlated with gestational age throughout the first trimester. Generally, the 1st IRP has hCG quantities double those of the 2IS.

Given the complexities of hCG testing, it is vital that the sonographer have a good understanding of the discriminatory level of hCG and sonographic findings. The discriminatory level of hCG in pregnancy should be thought of as a minimum level of hCG in normal intrauterine or ectopic pregnancy. Using transvaginal techniques, the hCG discriminatory level for detecting an intrauterine pregnancy has been shown to be 800 to 1000 IU/L based on the 2IS, and 1000 to 2000 IU/L based on the 1st IRP.

If discriminatory levels of beta-hCG are met or surpassed and no intrauterine gestational sac is seen, an ectopic pregnancy should be suspected. Caution should be taken if beta-hCG levels are below discriminatory levels. Ectopic gestations do not produce hCG at normal levels (hCG levels double every 2 days) and 90% of ectopic gestations are not viable, and so may not reflect typical correlation between gestational age and hCG levels. Ectopic pregnancy may have a similar appearance to an early intrauterine pregnancy. Thus in nonemergent cases, serial beta-hCG levels are preferred because trending of these levels would demonstrate a continuing pregnancy if hCG levels rise normally, whereas falling hCG levels may indicate missed or incomplete abortion.

Sonographic Findings in Ectopic Pregnancy

The sonographic appearances of ectopic pregnancy have been well documented with both transabdominal and transvaginal techniques (Figure 48-8). The most important finding when scanning for ectopic pregnancy is to determine whether there is a normal intrauterine gestation (reducing the probability of an ectopic pregnancy) or whether the uterine cavity is empty and an adnexal mass is present (Table 48-3). The expectation of visualizing a normal intrauterine gestation is directly correlated with beta-hCG levels. Although the visualization of an intrauterine gestational sac that includes embryonic heart motion firmly makes the diagnosis of intrauterine pregnancy, earlier gestations (5 to 6 weeks) may not demonstrate these findings.

As many as 20% of patients with ectopic pregnancy demonstrate an intrauterine saclike structure known as the **pseudogestational sac.** Although it is challenging, differentiating between normal early gestation and a pseudogestational sac is possible (Figure 48-9) by using the following guidelines: (1) Pseudogestational sacs do not contain a living embryo or yolk sac; (2) pseudogestational sacs are centrally located within the endometrial cavity, unlike the burrowed gestational sac, which is eccentrically placed; and (3) homogeneous level echoes are commonly observed in pseudogestational sacs, unlike in normal gestational sacs. The presence of a yolk sac positively indicates an intrauterine gestation. These

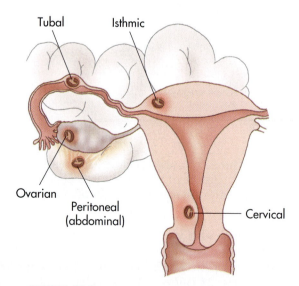

FIGURE 48-7 Potential sites for ectopic pregnancy.

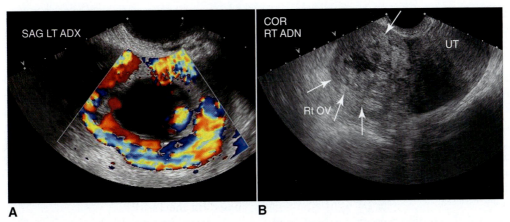

FIGURE 48-8 A, Sagittal sonogram demonstrating high-velocity color flow in the left adnexa that surrounded the ectopic gestational sac. Other images demonstrated an empty uterus with normal endometrial canal. **B,** Coronal sonogram demonstrating uterus *(UT)* and right ovary *(Rt OV)*, with an echogenic concentric ring and embryo seen centrally with fetal heart motion consistent with ectopic pregnancy. *Arrows,* Decidua/trophoblastic villi.

TABLE 48-3	Normal Versus Ectopic Pregnancy
Condition/Sonographic Findings	**Differential Considerations**
Empty uterus	Normal early intrauterine pregnancy (3 to 4 weeks) Recent spontaneous abortion

Normal intrauterine pregnancy (IUP)
  Yolk sac present
  Burrowed gestational sac eccentrically positioned in uterus (usually in the fundus)
  No internal echoes seen within the gestational sac
  Peritrophoblastic flow around sac
  Low-resistive flow pattern	

Ectopic pregnancy with pseudogestational sac
  "Intrauterine" saclike structure
  Yolk sac not present
  Pseudosac seen in central location in uterus
  Homogeneous echoes within pseudosac
  No peritrophoblastic flow
  High-resistive pattern
	Intrauterine debris
	 Incomplete spontaneous abortion
	 Intrauterine blood

Ectopic pregnancy
  Pseudogestational sac
  Extrauterine sac in adnexa with thickened echogenic ring
  Gestational sac or yolk sac
	Incomplete spontaneous abortion
	 Intrauterine blood or fluid in cul-de-sac

Heterotopic pregnancy Simultaneous intrauterine pregnancy and ectopic pregnancy (see findings above for IUP and ectopic pregnancy)	Normal IUP and pelvic mass

Interstitial pregnancy
  Found in segment of fallopian tube
  Rupture with hemorrhage
  Eccentric intrauterine gestational sac with incomplete myometrial mantel surrounding sac
	Ectopic pregnancy
	 Pelvic mass

Nonviable intrauterine pregnancy Pseudogestational sac of ectopic pregnancy	Embryo, no cardiac motion/nonliving intrauterine pregnancy Embryo, cardiac motion/living intrauterine pregnancy

findings are most commonly observed using transvaginal techniques.

Color Doppler imaging and spectral analysis may be helpful in distinguishing a normal sac from a pseudogestational sac with the demonstration of peritrophoblastic flow associated with intrauterine pregnancy. Typically, peritrophoblastic flow demonstrates a low-resistance (high-diastolic) pattern, with fairly high peak velocities (approximately 20 cm/sec). The decidual cast of the endometrium, as seen in the pseudogestational sac,

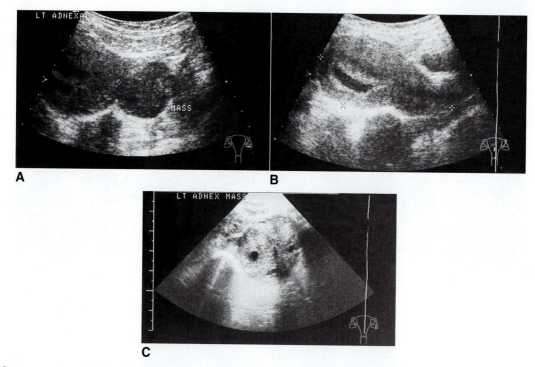

FIGURE 48-9 A young female in her first trimester presented in the emergency room with elevated human chorionic gonadotropin levels, bleeding, and pelvic pain. **A,** Transabdominal scan clearly shows a mass in the left adnexal area separate from the uterus. **B,** Longitudinal scan of the uterus shows the pseudogestational sac in the fundus of the uterus. **C,** Transvaginal scan shows a gestational sac within the left adnexal area.

typically demonstrates a high-resistance pattern (low-diastolic component) with low peak velocities.

Examining the adnexa sonographically is critical in the evaluation of ectopic pregnancy. Identification of a live embryo within the adnexa is most specific for ectopic gestation. Unfortunately, this occurs roughly only 25% of the time. It is important to note that only approximately 10% of live ectopic pregnancies are identified using transabdominal sonography (Figure 48-10).

Identification of an extrauterine sac within the adnexa is one of the most frequent findings of ectopic pregnancy. It has been reported that more than 71% of patients with ectopic pregnancy demonstrate an extrauterine sac or ring, although this study did include living extrauterine ectopic fetuses.[2] The extrauterine gestational sac has sonographic appearances and characteristics similar to those of the intrauterine gestational sac. Extrauterine gestational sacs often demonstrate a thickened echogenic ring, separate from the ovary, which represents trophoblastic tissue or chorionic villi, and there is a possibility that the embryo or yolk sac will be seen (Figure 48-11).

Color flow imaging and Doppler waveforms may also help diagnose extrauterine gestational sacs. One study reported color flow detection in and around 95 of 106 ectopic gestations with a Doppler resistive index of less than 0.40.[3] The positive predictive value of this technique was 96.8%, with sensitivity and specificity of 89.3% and 96.3%, respectively.[3] Other studies must be performed to correlate these criteria.

Adnexal Mass With Ectopic Pregnancy

The risk of ectopic pregnancy can be greater than 90% when an intrauterine gestation is absent and there is a corresponding adnexal mass. Complex adnexal masses, aside from extrauterine gestational sacs, often represent hematoma within the peritoneal cavity, which is usually contained within the fallopian tube (hematosalpinx) or broad ligament. In early gestational ectopic pregnancy, a hematoma may be the only sonographic sign of ectopic pregnancy. It should be distinguished, however, from an ovarian cyst, such as the corpus luteum, which is typically hypoechoic. A hemorrhagic corpus luteum cyst may mimic an extrauterine gestational sac or a distal hematosalpinx.

Often, ovarian processes, such as corpus luteal cysts and endometriomas, can be differentiated based on their location within the ovary, and one can often visualize surrounding ovarian tissue. Although this does not rule out the rare ovarian ectopic gestation, correlation with beta-hCG should help differentiate the two.

It has been reported that approximately 80% of patients with ectopic pregnancy demonstrate at least 25 ml of blood within the peritoneum, caused by blood escaping from the distal tube (fimbria). Approximately 60% of women with an ectopic pregnancy demonstrate intraperitoneal fluid, using transvaginal sonography (Figure 48-12). Studies have correlated an increased risk of ectopic pregnancy with moderate to large quantities

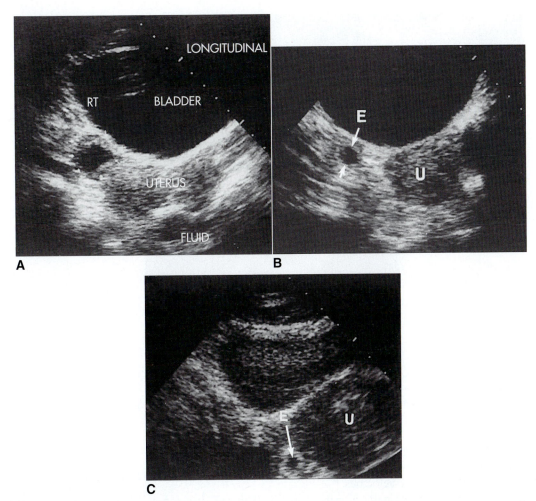

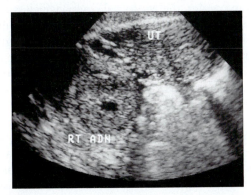

FIGURE 48-10 **A,** Longitudinal scan depicting an empty uterus, fluid in the cul-de-sac, and a "ringlike" cystic mass anterior to the uterus, representing an ectopic gestational sac. *RT,* Right. **B** and **C,** Transverse representations of ectopic gestational sacs *(E).* In **C,** the ectopic sac is in close proximity to the uterine wall. *U,* Uterus.

FIGURE 48-11 Coronal section demonstrating empty uterus *(UT),* and a right adnexal *(RT ADN)* mass with an echogenic ring and a sonolucent center consistent with a gestational sac. This is consistent with ectopic pregnancy with extrauterine sac.

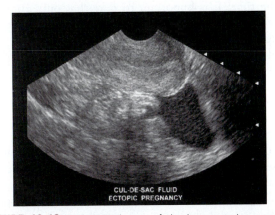

FIGURE 48-12 Transvaginal scan of the lower uterine segment shows the hypoechoic fluid collection in the cul-de-sac secondary to a ruptured ectopic pregnancy. Low-level echoes are suggestive of blood.

of free intraperitoneal fluid and an associated adnexal mass.[11]

The presence of echogenic free fluid has been shown to be highly specific for hemoperitoneum and to be highly correlated with ectopic pregnancy. A 92% risk of ectopic pregnancy with echogenic free fluid has been reported,[5] with 15% of cases demonstrating echogenic free fluid as the only sonographic finding (Figure 48-13). When fluid is present, the sonographer should also look at the abdominal gutters and the right and left upper quadrants to evaluate the extent/volume of fluid present.

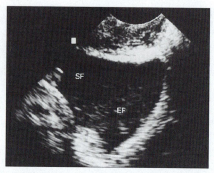

FIGURE 48-13 Transvaginal sonogram demonstrating echogenic free intraperitoneal fluid in an ectopic gestation. *EF,* Echogenic fluid; *SF,* simple fluid.

The combination of an adnexal mass and free pelvic fluid is the most precise sonographic correlation in the diagnosis of ectopic pregnancy.

Although intrauterine and adnexal findings are crucial in diagnosing ectopic pregnancy, it is clear that the described sonographic findings vary in their presentation. One report states that 52.5% of cases with ectopic pregnancy could not accurately demonstrate an adnexal mass or masses.[6] Of that 52.5%, less than half (25.5%) were overshadowed by coexisting findings, such as bowel segments that were echogenic or had isoechoic acoustic properties that did not allow sonographic demarcation of tissue from surrounding ovary or adnexa.[6] Another study demonstrated that in 74% of ectopic pregnancies, a confident diagnosis was made of an intrauterine pregnancy using transvaginal techniques, and that 26.3% of ectopic pregnancies had a normal transvaginal sonogram at initial presentation.[7] A normal transvaginal sonogram as defined in this study had no adnexal masses or pelvic fluid identified and no evidence of intrauterine gestation. These findings reiterate the need for meticulous scanning when looking for evidence of ectopic pregnancy and for an understanding of the limitations of all ultrasound techniques.

Heterotopic Pregnancy

Fortunately, simultaneous intrauterine and extrauterine pregnancies are extremely uncommon, even in patients undergoing an infertility workup. The sonographic observer should be aware that ovulation induction and in vitro fertilization with embryo transfer lead not only to a higher risk of **heterotopic pregnancy** but also to an overall increase in ectopic pregnancies, including bilateral ectopic pregnancies (see Table 48-3).

Interstitial Pregnancy

Interstitial pregnancy, or cornual pregnancy, is potentially the most life-threatening of all ectopic gestations (see Table 48-3). This is because of the location of the ectopic pregnancy, which lies in the segment of the fallopian tube that enters the uterus. This site involves the parauterine and myometrial vasculature, creating life-threatening hemorrhage when rupture occurs. Interstitial pregnancies have been reported to occur in approximately 2% of all ectopic pregnancies. Sonographic identification of an interstitial ectopic pregnancy is difficult, but it has been described as an eccentrically placed gestational sac within the uterus that has an incomplete myometrial mantle surrounding the sac (Figure 48-14). Some institutions measure the myometrial thickness and follow these implantations carefully for evidence of myometrial thinning and uterine rupture.

Cervical Pregnancy

Cervical pregnancy has a reported incidence of 1 in 16,000 pregnancies. Sonographic demonstration of a gestational sac within the cervix suggests a cervical pregnancy, although a spontaneous abortion may have a similar appearance. Several sonographic features can help make the distinction between true cervical pregnancy and spontaneous loss "in situ." An established cervical pregnancy demonstrates a concentric shape with decidual reaction and increased color Doppler flow around the trophoblast. In contrast, SPL appears as a misshapen sac, possibly hour-glassing (the hour-glass sign) through the cervical os, with lack of color flow around the decidual ring. Cervical ectopic pregnancies have an increased risk of complete hysterectomy because of uncontrollable bleeding caused by increased vascularity of the cervix.

Ovarian Pregnancy

An ovarian pregnancy is also very rare, accounting for less than 3% of all ectopic pregnancies. The sonographic diagnosis of ovarian pregnancy may be difficult; reported cases have demonstrated complex adnexal masses that involve or contain the ovary. Thus, distinguishing ovarian pregnancy from a hemorrhagic ovarian cyst or from other ovarian processes may be difficult.

DIAGNOSIS OF EMBRYONIC ABNORMALITIES IN THE FIRST TRIMESTER

Normal embryologic processes that are sonographically visible in the first-trimester embryo have been described in Chapter 47. These normal processes should not be mistaken for anomalies, and the sonographer should be aware of the pathology that can be diagnosed in the first trimester. The development of both high-frequency transvaginal transducers and three-dimensional (3D) technology has significantly increased the sensitivity of ultrasound to detect anomalies in the latter portion of the first trimester. These may include monoamniotic

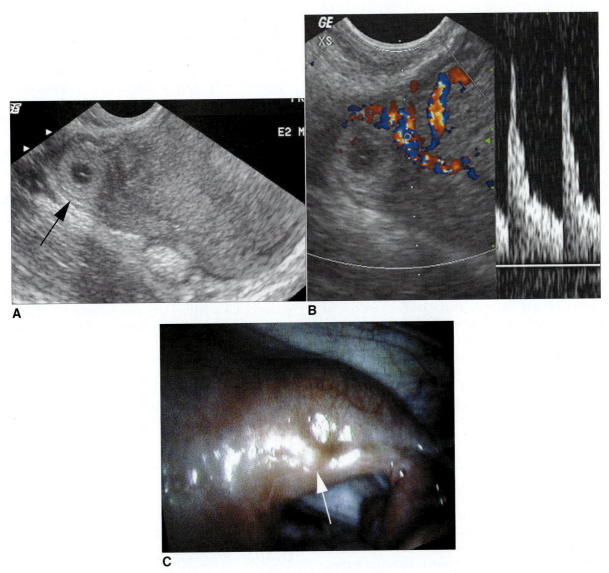

FIGURE 48-14 A 35-year-old G3P1A1 presented without pain but at risk for ectopic pregnancy. **A,** Coronal transvaginal image shows an empty uterus and a tubal ring *(arrow)* immediately adjacent to the uterus. A magnified view of the ring showed a gestational sac with a yolk sac, confirming an ectopic implantation. **B,** Color flow image shows increased vascularity around the sac with high-velocity flow. **C,** At laparoscopy, the ectopic tissue can be seen bulging the isthmus portion of the tube *(arrow)* and was successfully removed via salpingostomy.

twins, conjoined twins, cardiac defects, cystic hygroma, abdominal wall defects, and cranial and spinal defects. Although many abnormalities can be seen at the end of the first trimester, they are more clearly identified as the fetus matures into the second trimester. Other less common abnormalities, such as ectopia cordis, malformations of the skeleton, and complications of multifetal pregnancies, will be discussed in their respective chapters.

Nuchal Translucency

The nuchal translucency is the maximum thickness of the subcutaneous lucency at the back of the neck in an embryo at 11 to 14 weeks' gestation (Figure 48-15). Fluid collection between the skin and the soft tissue over the spine is now an accepted method of assessing genetic risk between 11 and 13 weeks 6 days of fetal life. Original research linked increased nuchal measurement with trisomy 21, although we now know that increased nuchal translucency may be found with trisomies 13 and 18 and in fetuses with cardiac defects and other genetic syndromes. In addition, high-resolution transducers have lowered the threshold of when we are able to sonographically visualize these anomalies. The nuchal translucency measurement is combined with biochemical markers—free beta-hCG and pregnancy-associated plasma protein (PAPP-A)—to assess risk for aneuploidy.

The Fetal Medicine Foundation (FMF) established the following criteria for nuchal measurements, which have become the internationally accepted standard:

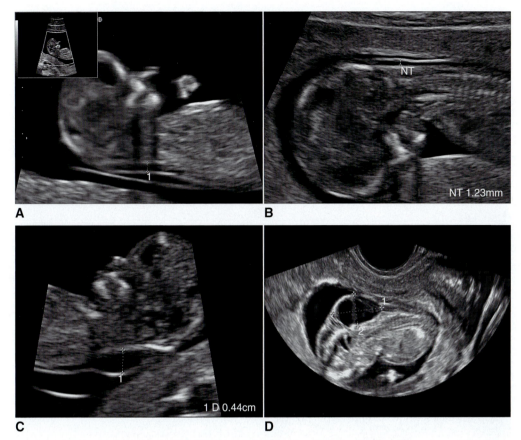

FIGURE 48-15 A, Normal 11-week embryo demonstrating a well-defined neural tube lucency. **B,** Normal 12-week embryo lying face down demonstrates nuchal translucency at the back of the neck. **C** and **D,** Abnormal nuchal thickening is demonstrated in these embryos with a cystic hygroma.

- Fetuses must be between 11 weeks and 13 weeks 6 days.
- The CRL must be between 45 mm and 84 mm.
- The sonographer must obtain an optimal image of the midsagittal plane.
- The embryo must be away from the amniotic membrane with the head in a neutral position, with no hyperextension or flexion.

Further research by the FMF has established that we can evaluate first-trimester fetuses for nuchal thickening, presence or absence of nasal bone, tricuspid regurgitation, abnormal flow in the ductus venosus, and possible abnormalities of the hindbrain.

Cardiac Anomalies

Adoption of the first-trimester scan for aneuploidy and advancements in transducer resolution have given us the opportunity to look for cardiac defects at an earlier gestation than ever before. It is now known that there is a strong relationship between increased nuchal translucency and fetuses with cardiac defects. Researchers are reporting the ability to detect a four-chamber view and great vessels as early as 12 weeks. These fetuses are brought back later in gestation to confirm suspected findings. Markers for cardiac defects include increased nuchal translucency, tricuspid regurgitation, and reversal (or absence) of flow in the ductus venosus. Other cardiac associations that can be detected in the first trimester are ectopia cordis and limb body wall complex.

Cranial Anomalies

Although the embryonic head can be sonographically identified by 7 weeks, the cerebral hemisphere continues to evolve throughout the second trimester. The dominant structure seen within the embryonic cranium in the first trimester is the choroid plexus, which fills the lateral ventricles, which in turn fill the cranial vault (Figure 48-16, *A*). Thus, the diagnosis of hydrocephalus in the first trimester is not possible. However, anomalies of cranial organization, such as holoprosencephaly, have been described in the first trimester. The rhombencephalon-hindbrain is a cystic structure appearing in the embryonic cranium within the posterior aspect at 6 to 8 weeks that should not be confused with an abnormality (Figure 48-16, *B*). A diagnosis of hydranencephaly has been reported during the first trimester; loss of all intracranial anatomy was sonographically demonstrated. (Hydranencephaly is brain necrosis resulting from occlusion of the internal carotid arteries.) In the first trimester,

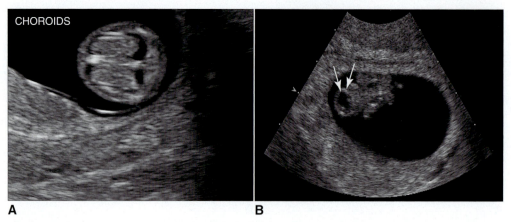

FIGURE 48-16 A, Transvaginal axial scan of the choroid plexus in a first-trimester fetus. **B,** Sonogram of an 8.5-week gestation demonstrating the cystic rhombencephalon within the fetal cranium *(arrows).*

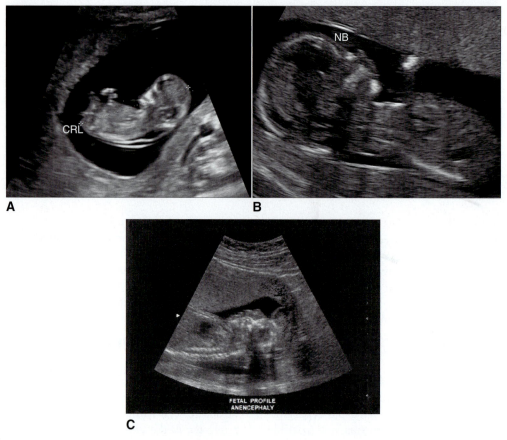

FIGURE 48-17 A, Crown-rump length (CRL) of a normal 11 week 5 day fetus with a well-defined cranial cavity. **B,** The normal cranial cavity is seen in this 13 week 5 day fetus. *NB,* Nasal bone. **C,** Fetal profile of an anencephalic fetus in the early second trimester. The fetus is lying in a vertex position with the spine down. The face is pointing toward the anterior placenta; the skull is absent from the fetal forehead to the top of the cranium.

anencephaly should be diagnosed with caution. Reports have shown normal amounts of brain matter seen in the first-trimester embryo with anencephaly, unlike classic sonographic appearances in the second and third trimesters (Figure 48-17). Ossification of the cranial vault is not complete in the first trimester; the resulting false cranial border definition may give rise to a false-negative diagnosis. Caution is advised if an embryonic

cranial abnormality is suspected (Table 48-4). Because traditional cranial anatomy can be visualized after 12 to 14 weeks' gestation, the sonogram should be repeated at this time to confirm or rule out abnormality.

Acrania. Acrania is the partial or complete absence of the cranium. It is thought to be the predecessor of anencephaly. Ossification of the cranium begins after 9 weeks. Sonography is able to demonstrate abnormal

TABLE 48-4	Cranial Anomalies in the First Trimester
Anomaly	**Sonographic Findings**
Acrania	Abnormal mineralization of bony structures (lack of echogenicity) Abnormally shaped "Mickey Mouse" head
Anencephaly	Absence of cranium superior to orbits with preservation of base of skull and face Brain may project from open cranium
Cephalocele	Midline cranial defect Herniation of brain and meninges
Iniencephaly	Defect in occiput involving the foramen magnum Extreme retroflexion of spine Open spinal defect
Ventriculomegaly	Dilation of ventricular system without enlargement of the cranium Compression of choroid plexus Increased cerebrospinal fluid Dangling choroid in dilated lateral ventricle
Holoprosencephaly	Failure of prosencephalon to differentiate into cerebral hemispheres and lateral ventricles between 4th and 8th weeks Complete to partial failure of cleavage of prosencephalon Facial dysmorphism Remember, brain appears to be single ventricle until falx cerebri develops after 9 weeks
Dandy-Walker malformation	6th to 7th week of gestation Cystic dilation of fourth ventricle Dysgenesis or agenesis of cerebellar vermis and hydrocephaly Elevated tentorium

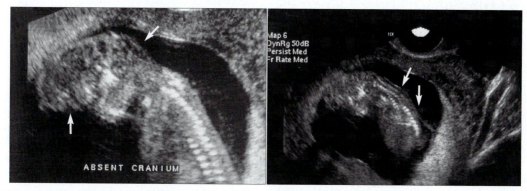

FIGURE 48-18 Acrania. Patient presented with an elevated maternal serum alpha-fetoprotein level. Note the amnion *(arrows)* along the back of the fetus. The amniotic band syndrome was the probable cause of acrania in this fetus.

mineralization of the bony structures: Well-mineralized bone is highly echogenic and is easily imaged with sonography. Acrania has been reported as early as the 12th week of gestation. When this abnormality occurs, the fetus has an abnormally shaped head, referred to as a "Mickey Mouse" head (Figure 48-18).

Anencephaly. Anencephaly is the congenital absence of the brain and cranial vault, with the cerebral hemispheres missing or reduced to small masses. This abnormality may be seen near the end of the first trimester, when there is an absence of the cranium superior to the orbits with preservation of the base of the skull and facial features. The brain may be seen as it projects from the open cranial vault.

Cephalocele. A cephalocele is a midline cranial defect in which there is herniation of the brain and meninges.

The cephalocele may also involve the occipital, frontal, parietal, orbital, nasal, or nasopharyngeal region of the head. The prevalence of the lesion is geographic. In the Western hemisphere, the defect is primarily occipital, whereas in the Eastern hemisphere, the frontal defect is more common.

Iniencephaly. Iniencephaly is a rare, lethal anomaly of cranial development whose primary abnormalities include (1) a defect in the occiput involving the foramen magnum, (2) retroflexion of the spine, where the fetus looks upward with its occipital cranium directed toward the lumbar spine, and (3) open spinal defects.

Ventriculomegaly. Ventriculomegaly, or dilation of the ventricular system without enlargement of the cranium, may be seen near the end of the first trimester, generally after 11 weeks. The normal lateral ventricle is quite

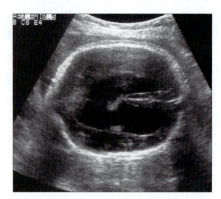

FIGURE 48-19 Ventriculomegaly caused by spina bifida. The near-field lateral ventricle choroid plexus "dangles" into the far-field dilated ventricle.

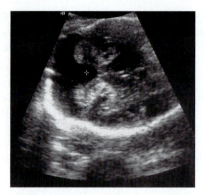

FIGURE 48-20 Dandy-Walker cyst. Note the splayed cerebellar hemispheres. *(Courtesy Ginny Goreczky, Maternal Fetal Center, Florida Hospital, Orlando, FL.)*

prominent in the first trimester and is filled with choroid. Look for compression and thinning of the choroid plexus as increased cerebrospinal fluid accumulates in the ventricular system. The choroid plexus is shown to be "dangling" in the dilated dependent lateral ventricle (Figure 48-19).

Holoprosencephaly. Holoprosencephaly is a malformation sequence that results from failure of the prosencephalon to differentiate into cerebral hemispheres and lateral ventricles between the 4th and 8th gestational weeks. The anomaly ranges from complete to partial failure of cleavage of the prosencephalon with variable degrees of facial dysmorphism. Holoprosencephaly is divided into three types: alobar, semilobar, and lobar. Alobar is the most serious and consists of a single ventricle, a small cerebrum, fused thalami, agenesis of the corpus callosum, and falx cerebri. It is important to remember that before 9 weeks, the normal fetal brain appears to have a "single" ventricle until the falx cerebri develops after 9 weeks.

Dandy-Walker Malformation. This malformation results from cystic dilation of the fourth ventricle with dysgenesis or complete agenesis of the cerebellar vermis, and frequently hydrocephaly. The abnormality occurs around the 6th to 7th week of gestation. In the first trimester, sonographic presentation may include a large posterior fossa cyst continuous with the fourth ventricle, an absent cerebellum, and dilated third and lateral ventricles (Figure 48-20). Dandy-Walker malformation has been reported as early as 11 weeks with transvaginal ultrasound.

Spina Bifida. Spina bifida occurs when the neural tube fails to close after 6 weeks' gestation. Improvements in ultrasound resolution have enhanced our sensitivity to detecting spina bifida, which may be detected at the end of the first trimester. Appearances may include spinal irregularities or bulging within the posterior contour of the fetal spine and extrusion of a mass from the vertebral column. Cranial signs, the lemon sign (scalloping of frontal bones), and the banana sign (curved appearance of the cerebellum) may be appreciated closer to 12 weeks.

New evidence suggests that we may soon be able to evaluate for spina bifida by measuring the fourth ventricle during the 11- to 13.6-week scan.[1] Because the fourth ventricle is usually caudally displaced in spina bifida, the authors sought to measure the hindbrain in the midsagittal view. In normal fetuses, the fourth ventricle appears as an "intracranial lucency" that is measurable. In this study, the four affected fetuses demonstrated a compressed hindbrain, and the intracranial lucency could not be measured. Larger prospective studies are needed to establish the intracranial lucency measurement as a screen for spina bifida.

Abdominal Wall Defects

Although the diagnoses of omphalocele, gastroschisis, and limb–body wall complex have been reported in the first trimester, such diagnoses should be made with care (Figure 48-21). Abdominal wall defects must be distinguished from normal physiologic midgut herniation. As stated previously, normal **bowel herniation** appears sonographically as an echogenic mass at the base of the umbilical cord between 8 and 12 weeks. Because the liver is never normally herniated into the base of the umbilical cord, any evidence of the liver outside the anterior abdominal wall should be considered abnormal. Although the diagnosis of **gastroschisis** in the first trimester may be more difficult, reports have shown the bowel to be separate from the umbilical cord. Gastroschisis is usually visualized as an anterior wall defect, bowel containing, commonly to the right of the umbilical cord. Omphaloceles may contain abdominal organs and bowel and may protrude into the base of the umbilical cord. Bowel-only **omphaloceles** have been reported to have a high association with chromosomal abnormalities and cannot be differentiated from normal physiologic bowel migration until after 12 weeks.

The research of Schmidt et al. suggests that measuring normal gut herniation is possible with transvaginal scanning and ought to be in the range of 6 to 9 mm circumference at 8 weeks, decreasing to 5 to 6 mm circumference

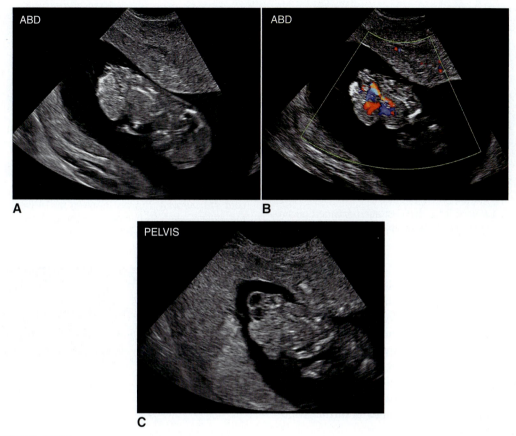

FIGURE 48-21 **A** through **C,** An 11-week fetus with bowel herniation as part of the limb–body wall complex.

at 9 weeks. Any gut herniation larger than 6 mm should be considered suspicious and should be followed for resolution after 11 weeks 5 days.[8]

Obstructive Uropathy

The fetal urinary bladder becomes sonographically apparent at 10 to 12 weeks' gestation. Obstructive uropathy, especially when it occurs at the level of the urethra, results in a very large urinary bladder and is well imaged with sonography. The bladder may be large enough to extend out of the pelvis into the fetal abdomen, presenting as a cystic mass, or it may protrude outside the body (bladder exstrophy). Other anomalies reported in the first trimester include bladder outlet obstruction, megacystis, and cloacal anomalies.

Cystic Hygroma

Cystic hygroma is one of the most common abnormalities seen sonographically in the first trimester (Figure 48-22). Cystic hygromas seen early in fetal life have a high association with chromosomal abnormalities. The most common abnormalities are trisomies 13, 18, and 21. Newer evidence suggests that even if aneuploidy has been ruled out, these fetuses may have other genetic syndromes, deformations, and disruptions.[10] Perinatal

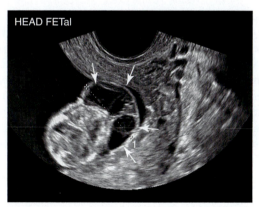

FIGURE 48-22 An 11-week fetus demonstrating sonolucent cystic hygroma with nuchal thickening *(arrows)*.

risk increases significantly when the nuchal translucency reaches 3.5 mm or greater—the 99th percentile.

In fetuses detected with cystic hygroma in the second and third trimesters, **Turner's syndrome** is the most common karyotype abnormality. If the hygroma resolves by 18 weeks and the fetus has a normal targeted ultrasound at 20 to 22 weeks without anomalies, then the perinatal risk is not statistically increased.

Cystic hygromas visualized in the first trimester may vary in size, but all appear on the posterior aspect of the fetal neck and upper thorax (Figure 48-23). Soft tissue

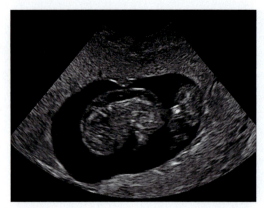

FIGURE 48-23 A 10-week fetus demonstrating enlarged nuchal thickening along the neck and posterior spine representing a cystic hygroma.

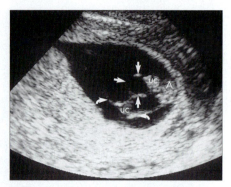

FIGURE 48-24 An 8.5-week gestation demonstrating an umbilical cord cyst *(arrows)*. This cyst resolved by 14 weeks' gestation and the patient went on to normal delivery. *A,* Embryonic abdomen; *UC,* umbilical cord; *curved arrow,* amniotic membrane.

thickening may also be present and should be considered nuchal thickening. Although cystic hygroma and nuchal thickening may be concordant, differentiation may be difficult. Any posterior neck thickness >3 mm, with or without septations, should be followed. Differentiation between cystic hygroma, encephalocele, cervical meningomyelocele, teratoma, or hemangioma should be assessed. If cystic hygroma or nuchal thickening is seen in the first trimester, genetic counseling and further sonographic monitoring are required.

First-Trimester Umbilical Cord Cysts

Sonographic identification of first-trimester umbilical cord cysts has been reported. One study found a 0.4% incidence of umbilical cord cysts between 8 and 12 weeks' gestation.[9] Cyst size varied with a range of 2.0 to 7.5 mm, and embryos whose cysts resolved by the second trimester progressed to normal delivery. Differential considerations of umbilical cord cysts include (1) amniotic inclusion cysts, (2) omphalomesenteric duct cysts, (3) allantoic cysts, (4) vascular anomalies, (5) neoplasms, and (6) Wharton's jelly abnormalities. Umbilical cord cysts that persist through the second trimester or are associated with other abnormalities warrant further investigation and genetic evaluation (Figure 48-24).

FIRST-TRIMESTER PELVIC MASSES

Ovarian Masses

The **corpus luteum cyst** is the most common ovarian mass seen in the first trimester of pregnancy. Corpus luteum cysts secrete the progesterone necessary to preserve the embryo. The typical corpus luteum cyst measures less than 5 cm in diameter and does not contain septations. Occasionally, corpus luteum cysts are large, measuring more than 10 cm, with internal septations and echogenic debris, which are thought to be secondary to internal hemorrhage (Figure 48-25). Because of high

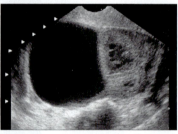

FIGURE 48-25 Transvaginal scan of the adnexal area in a patient in her first trimester shows a large corpus luteum cyst with internal septations and debris.

metabolic activity, color flow imaging may demonstrate a ring of increased vascularity surrounding the corpus luteum, displaying low-resistance (high-diastolic) waveforms on pulsed Doppler imaging. Such findings are similar to decidual flows characterized in ectopic pregnancies, but are intraovarian in location (see Table 48-2).

A hemorrhagic corpus luteum cyst cannot always be differentiated from other pathologic cysts, such as ovarian cancer or dermoid (Figure 48-26). As the pregnancy progresses, corpus luteum cysts regress and typically are not seen beyond 16 to 18 weeks' gestation. If ovarian cystic masses persist beyond 18 weeks' gestation or increase in size, surgical removal may be required because benign and malignant processes cannot be distinguished sonographically. A high incidence of torsion of ovarian masses during the second and third trimesters has been reported. All persistent ovarian masses in pregnancy should be followed closely.

Uterine Masses

Uterine leiomyomas, or fibroids, are common throughout pregnancy. If fibroids coexist with a first-trimester pregnancy, the fibroid should be identified in relation to the placenta and cervix. Fibroids may increase in size throughout the first trimester and early second trimester because of estrogen stimulation. A rapid increase in fibroid size may lead to necrosis of the leiomyoma, a

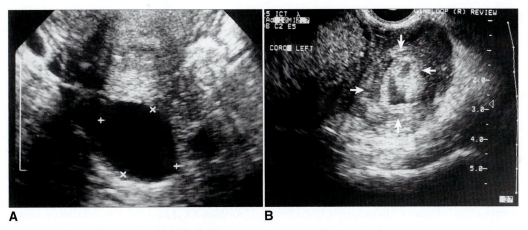

FIGURE 48-26 A, Sonogram demonstrating a typical corpus luteum cyst *(calipers)* within the right ovary in an 8-week gestation. Sonographic characteristics of this cyst are simple, which is typical. **B,** Sonographic example of hemorrhagic corpus luteum cyst *(arrows)*. This may be difficult to differentiate from hematosalpinx, distal tubal ectopic pregnancy, ovarian ectopic pregnancy, or ovarian neoplasms.

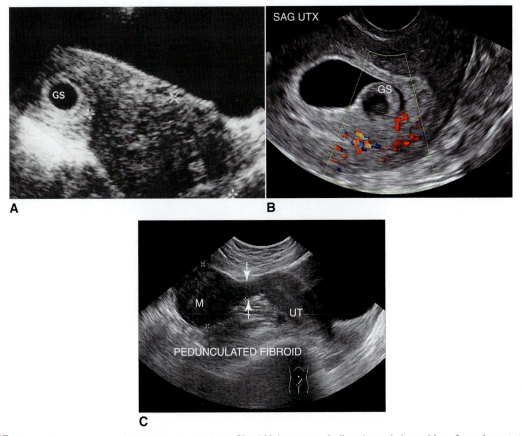

FIGURE 48-27 A, Sagittal sonogram demonstrating an 8-cm fibroid/leiomyoma *(calipers)* coexisting with a 6-week gestational sac *(GS)*. This fibroid continued to grow, compressing this young gestation and causing demise. **B,** Coexisting fibroid with increased color velocity flow is seen posterior to the gestational sac *(GS)*. **C,** A patient with amenorrhea and a pedunculated fibroid may present with a uterus "larger than dates." Sonography demonstrated a normal uterus *(UT)* with a stalk *(arrows)* connecting the pedunculated fibroid superior to the fundus of the uterus. *M,* Mass.

degenerating fibroid that may cause significant pain. Myomectomy is generally avoided during pregnancy owing to the increased vascularity of the uterus and the possibility of marked bleeding. Rapidly growing fibroids may compress the gestational sac, causing spontaneous abortion.

Sonographically, fibroids may be hypoechoic, echogenic, or isoechoic in relation to the myometrium. They typically cause deformity or displacement of the uterus, endometrium, or both. Fibroids are high-acoustic attenuators that give rise to poor acoustic transmission (Figure 48-27). It may be difficult to differentiate fibroid from focal uterine contractions, although preliminary data suggest that color Doppler imaging shows a more hypovascular appearance with uterine contractions than with fibroids. Fibroids may also be differentiated from focal myometrial contractions by observing the focal lesion over time (typically 20 to 30 minutes); the myometrial contraction should disappear, whereas a fibroid persists (see Table 48-2).

REFERENCES

1. Chaoui R, Benoit B, Mitkowska-Wozniak H, et al: Assessment of intracranial translucency (IT) in the detection of spina bifida at the 11-13 week scan, *Ultrasound Obstet Gynecol* 34:249-252, 2009.
2. Fleisher AC, Pennell RG, McKee MS, et al: Ectopic pregnancy: features at transvaginal sonography, *Radiology* 174:375-378, 1990.
3. Kurjak A, Zalud I, Schulman H: Ectopic pregnancy: transvaginal color Doppler of trophoblastic flow in questionable adnexa, *J Ultrasound Med* 10:685-689, 1991.
4. Nyberg DA, Filly RA: Predicting pregnancy failure in empty gestational sacs, *Ultrasound Obstet Gynecol* 21:9-12, 2003.
5. Nyberg DA, Hughes MP, Mack LA, Wang KY: Extrauterine findings of ectopic pregnancy at transvaginal US: importance of echogenic fluid, *Radiology* 178:823-826, 1991.
6. Parvey HR, Maklad W: Pitfalls in the transvaginal sonographic diagnosis of ectopic pregnancy, *J Ultrasound Med* 3:139-144, 1993.
7. Russell SA, Illy RA, Damato N: Sonographic diagnosis of ectopic pregnancy with endovaginal probes: what really has changed? *J Ultrasound Med* 3:145-151, 1993.
8. Schmidt W, Yarkoni S, Crelin ES, et al: Sonographic visualization of physiologic anterior abdominal wall hernia in the first trimester, *Obstet Gynecol* 69:911-915, 1987.
9. Skibo LK, Lyons EA, Levi CS: First trimester umbilical cord cyst, *Radiology* 182:719-722, 1992.
10. Souka AP, von Kaisenberg CS, Hyett JA, et al: Increased nuchal translucency with normal karyotype, *Am J Obstet Gynecol* 192:1005-1021, 2005.
11. Thorsen MK, Lawson TL, Aiman EJ, et al: Diagnosis of ectopic pregnancy: endovaginal vs. transabdominal sonography, *AJR Am J Roentgenol* 155:307-310, 1990.

Sonography of the Second and Third Trimesters

Jean Lea Spitz

OBJECTIVES

On completion of this chapter, you should be able to:
- List the components of a standard obstetric examination in the second and third trimesters and describe the fetal anatomy recommended for review
- Define terminology specific to fetal presentation
- Specify equipment and policies required for facilities performing obstetric sonography
- Describe sonographic techniques used to image specific fetal structures
- Describe normal fetal anatomy visualized in an obstetric sonography examination and variations that may be significant

OUTLINE

The second and third trimesters are the ideal time to obtain sonographic images of detailed fetal anatomy. Fetal anatomy may be accurately assessed after 18 weeks' gestation, although structures may be seen earlier in many pregnancies. Technical factors, such as fetal movement, fluid quantity, fetal position, and maternal wall thickness or obesity, may obscure the anatomy and result in less than optimal images throughout pregnancy.

To perform a complete evaluation of the fetus during the second and third trimesters, the sonographer should follow a specific protocol that includes at a minimum the components recommended for a standard examination. The guidelines for obstetric scanning as outlined by the American Institute of Ultrasound in Medicine (AIUM),

the American College of Radiology (ACR), and the American College of Obstetricians and Gynecologists (ACOG) are described in Chapter 45.

This chapter focuses on the fetal anatomy that the sonographer needs to recognize and analyze within a systematic scanning protocol. A sonographer will screen many normal fetuses when performing standard antepartum obstetric examinations during the second or third trimester of pregnancy. A systematic protocol will ensure a comprehensive review of fetal anatomy in each patient. Thoroughness and experience applied to the recommended components and to additional details, such as facial features, open hands, and fetal situs, will maximize the opportunity to detect fetal anomalies.

> **BOX 49-1** | **Second and Third Trimester Protocol**
>
> - Survey uterus and determine fetal number.
> - Observe fetal cardiac activity.
> - Determine fetal position(s) and placental location(s).
> - Check cervix and lower uterine segment.
> - Survey for uterine or adnexal masses.
> - Assess amniotic fluid.
> - Perform anatomy survey of each fetus.
> - Perform biometric measurements of each fetus.

A SUGGESTED PROTOCOL

The protocol for second- and third-trimester sonography examinations includes a biometric and anatomic survey of the fetus (Box 49-1). The second- and third-trimester sonography examination often includes the following:

1. Observation of fetal viability by visualization of cardiac motion.
2. Demonstration of presentation (fetal lie).
3. Demonstration of the number of fetuses. In multiple gestations, anatomy images are obtained on each fetus, growth parameters of each fetus are obtained and compared, placenta and membrane structures are assessed, and amniotic fluid levels in each sac are documented.
4. Characterization of the quantity of amniotic fluid as normal or abnormal by subjective visualization or by semiquantitative estimates.
5. Characterization of the placenta, including localization and relationship to the internal cervical os. Placenta previa should be excluded by examination of the lower uterine segment.
6. Visualization of the cervix and extension of the examination to include transperineal or transvaginal imaging if the cervix appears shortened, or if the patient complains of regular uterine contractions.
7. Assessment of fetal age through fetal biometry. Fetal growth studies may include a serial growth analysis when serial examinations are performed at intervals that are 2 to 4 weeks apart. Typically, the following fetal measurements are included, and gestational age (GA) correlation from each measure is averaged to assess fetal age by sonography:
   - Biparietal diameter
   - Head circumference
   - Femur length
   - Humerus length
   - Abdominal circumference
8. Evaluation of uterus, adnexa, and cervix to exclude masses that may complicate obstetric management. Maternal ovaries may not be visualized during the second and third trimesters of pregnancy.
9. Anatomic survey of the fetus to exclude major congenital malformations. At a minimum, the anatomy specified in Box 49-1 must be visualized. Specialty or repeat studies may be appropriate if anatomy is not well visualized. Technical difficulty in visualizing anatomy should be recorded and images preserved to document visualization of all required components.

The sonographer should establish a systematic scanning protocol encompassing elements of the protocol outlined previously, all criteria of the guidelines, and any additional views requested in the practice environment. Specialty obstetric sonography examination may be necessary when a fetal anomaly is suspected. An organized approach to scanning ensures completeness and reduces the risk of missing a fetal defect.

EQUIPMENT AND PRACTICES

The second and third trimester standard sonography examination requires current two-dimensional real-time sonography equipment with transabdominal and transvaginal capability. Doppler capabilities facilitate evaluation of amniotic fluid volume, the umbilical cord, and specialty evaluations of the fetal heart and other aspects of fetal and maternal circulation. Three-dimensional equipment can record the volume of a targeted anatomic region and represents an advance in imaging technology. The technical advantage of three-dimensional imaging is that it can acquire, manipulate, and display a number of two-dimensional planes within a volume that may not be accessible with traditional real-time imaging. Three-dimensional equipment is currently only an adjunct to traditional scanning. Until clinical evidence shows a clear medical advantage, three-dimensional sonography is not considered required equipment.

Practice guidelines related to patient education and communication during an examination, competency requirements for sonographers and interpreting physicians, equipment use, scheduling, documentation of results, and image storage specific to obstetric patients will have to be developed at every facility. Practices that receive ultrasound accreditation from the ACR or the AIUM have been shown to improve compliance with published national standards and guidelines.

INITIAL STEPS AND EXAMINATION OVERVIEW

Recognizing normal fetal anatomy is essential to the performance of obstetric sonography. The task of capturing images of standard anatomic planes and organs in a small and mobile fetus poses a considerable challenge for the sonographer. The "eye" and experience required to recognize abnormal structures develop over time.

A key to developing scanning expertise is to become organized and systematic in assessing the fetus, placenta, and amniotic fluid.

The sonographer should initially determine the position of the fetus in relationship to the position of the mother. In determining fetal position and in surveying the uterine contents, the transducer may be systematically moved superior toward the uterine fundus, maintaining a midline path. By angling the probe from side to side, fetal position, cardiac activity, the number of fetuses, the presence of uterine and placental masses, and any obvious fetal anomalies may be recognized and amniotic fluid assessed.

It is important to remember to view cardiac activity at the beginning of each study to ensure that the fetus is alive. If a fetal demise or an obvious anomaly is initially recognized, the sonographer is better prepared to perform the study and involve the physician immediately.

After fetal position is conceptualized, the sonographer determines the left and right sides of the fetus. Being continuously aware of the right and left sides of the fetus is necessary to correctly assess fetal anatomy and situs. Assessment and measurement of the fetus may proceed systematically by moving from fetal head to feet, obtaining anatomy images and measurement at each level. The obstetric sonographer also needs to be prepared to vary this systematic examination and "catch as catch can" when pertinent anatomy presents during fetal movements. The placenta, amniotic fluid, uterus, and adnexa are also examined.

Fetal Presentation

Fetal position may change as a result of fetal movement until actual labor commences. In reality, however, fetal position changes less frequently after 34 weeks. Visualizing nonvertex fetal positions after 34 weeks may be predictive of positional difficulties during labor and delivery. An atypical fetal presentation, such as face, brow, or shoulder presentation, will complicate delivery. Similarly, hyperextension of the fetal head may alter obstetric management.

The fetal lie is described in relation to the maternal long axis. Fetuses generally assume a longitudinal, transverse, or oblique lie within the uterus (Figure 49-1). If the fetus is lying perpendicular to the long axis of the mother, this is described as a **transverse fetal lie.** When the fetus lie is transverse, the sonographer typically reports the position of the fetal head (maternal right or left) and the position of the fetal spine (inferior, superior, anterior, or posterior) (Figure 49-2). When the fetal lie is oblique, it is generally described by stating which quadrant of the uterus contains the fetal head and the direction and position of the fetal spine. If the fetus is lying longitudinal or parallel to the maternal long axis, this is described as a **vertex** (head down) presentation or **breech** (head up) presentation (Figure 49-3).

Vertex. A simple method to determine fetal presentation consists of a midline sagittal scan in the lower uterine segment. Immediately cephalad to the symphysis pubis, the maternal bladder is visualized with the cervix and lower uterine segment posterior. This view allows the sonographer to determine which fetal part is presenting and to check the relationship between the cervix and the placenta. The fetal head is visualized at this level when the fetus is in a vertex or cephalic presentation. Proceeding fundally, if the fetal body is noted to follow the head, a vertex lie is confirmed (Figure 49-4). The fetal body may lie in an oblique axis to the right or left of the maternal midline. If the body is not initially recognized in the midline, the sonographer should direct the transducer from side to side to search for the abdomen. Identification of the vertebral column when entering the cranium further delineates the fetal lie. The position of a fetus in vertex position may be described by stating the relationship of the fetal occiput (back of the head) to the maternal pelvis. If the occiput is adjacent to the left anterior portion of the maternal pelvis, the fetal position is left occiput anterior (LOA). If the occiput is adjacent to the left lateral portion of the maternal pelvis, this is called left occiput transverse (LOT). Similarly, fetuses may be described as left occiput posterior (LOP), occiput posterior (OP), right occiput posterior (ROP), right occiput transverse (ROT), right occiput anterior (ROA), or occiput anterior (OA). Fetuses that are OA (looking straight down) or OP (looking straight up) may present technical difficulties in measuring the fetal head and abdomen and in visualizing fetal cranial anatomy.

Breech. When the lower extremities or buttocks are found to be in the lower uterine segment and the head is visualized in the uterine fundus, a breech presentation is suspected (Figure 49-5). In fetuses near term, determination of the specific type of breech lie provides important clinical information for the obstetrician planning the safest route of delivery. Some fetuses in a breech position, such as those in a frank breech position with the thighs flexed at the hips and the lower legs extended in front of the body and up in front of the head (Figure 49-6), may be safely turned, allowing vaginal delivery. Fetuses in other breech lies, such as complete breech (when both the hips and the lower extremities are found in the lower

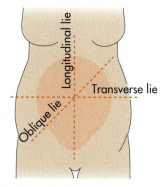

FIGURE 49-1 These vectors demonstrate the three major possible axes that a fetus may occupy. Fetal lie does not necessarily indicate whether the vertex or the breech is closest to the cervix.

FIGURE 49-2 Knowledge of the plane of section across the maternal abdomen (longitudinal or transverse) and the position of the fetal spine and left-side (stomach) and right-side (gallbladder) structures can be used to determine fetal lie and presenting part. **A,** This transverse scan of the gravid uterus demonstrates the fetal spine on the maternal right with the fetus lying with its right side down (stomach anterior, gallbladder posterior). Because these images are viewed looking up from the patient's feet, the fetus must be in longitudinal lie and cephalic presentation. **B,** When the gravid uterus is scanned transversely and the fetal spine is on the maternal left with the right side down, the fetus is in a longitudinal lie and breech presentation. **C,** When a longitudinal plane of section demonstrates the fetal body to be transected transversely, and the fetal spine is nearest the uterine fundus with the fetal left side down, the fetus is in a transverse lie with the fetal head on the maternal left. **D,** When a longitudinal plane of section demonstrates the fetal body to be transected transversely, and the fetal spine is nearest the lower uterine segment with the fetal left side down, the fetus is in a transverse lie with the fetal head on the maternal right. Although real-time scanning of the gravid uterus quickly allows the observer to determine fetal lie and presenting part, this maneuver of identifying specific right- and left-side structures within the fetal body forces one to determine fetal position accurately and to identify normal and pathologic fetal anatomy.

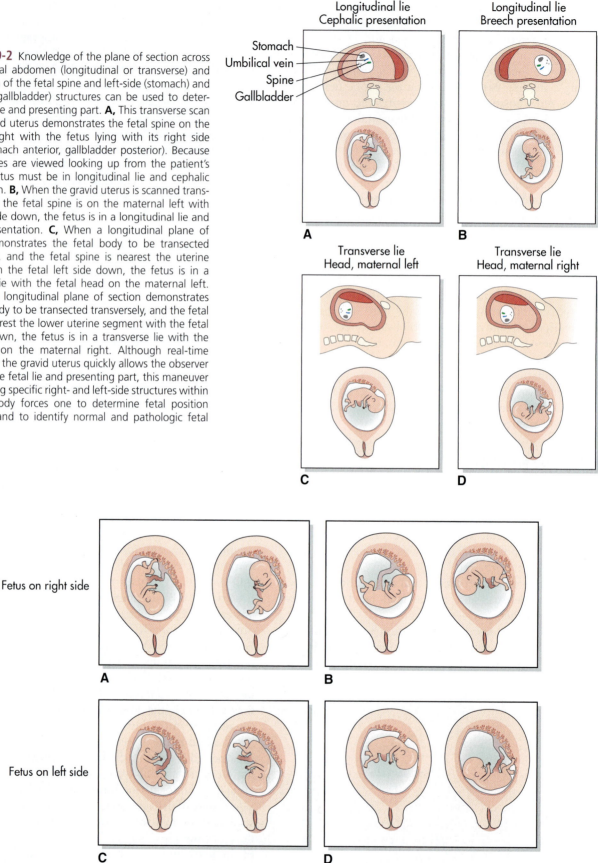

FIGURE 49-3 Fetal positions and the method used to differentiate the left side from the right side. **A,** Fetus lying on the right side; whether the head is up or down, the left side of the fetus is up or closer to the transducer. **B,** Fetus lying on right side in a transverse lie; left side is closer to the transducer. **C,** Fetus lying on the left side; whether the head is up or down, the right side is up or closer to the transducer. **D,** Fetus lying on left side in a transverse lie; the right side is closer to the transducer.

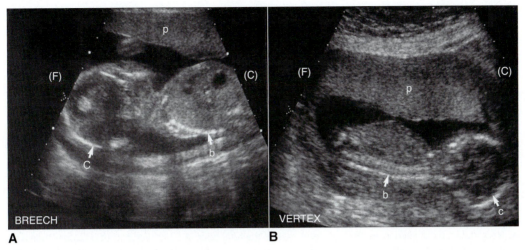

A   **B**

FIGURE 49-4 A, A breech presentation. The body *(b)* is closest in proximity to the direction of the cervix *(C)*, and the cranium *(c)* is directed toward the uterine fundus *(F)*. **B,** A vertex presentation. The cranium *(c)* is closest in proximity to the direction of the cervix *(C)*, and the body *(b)* is directed toward the uterine fundus *(F)*. *p,* Placenta.

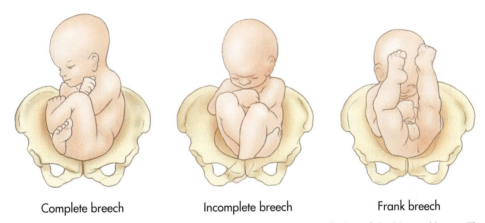

Complete breech   Incomplete breech   Frank breech

FIGURE 49-5 Three possible breech presentations. The complete breech demonstrates flexion of the hips and knees. The incomplete breech demonstrates intermediate deflexion of one hip and knee (single or double footling). The frank breech shows flexion of the hips and extension of both knees.

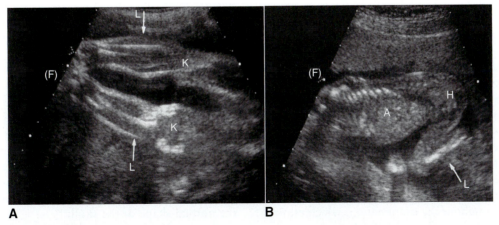

A   **B**

FIGURE 49-6 A, A fetus in a frank breech presentation with both legs extended upward toward the uterine fundus *(F)*. *K,* Knee; *L,* lower leg. **B,** Complete breech presentation with one leg flexed at the hips, with the lower leg *(L)* and foot positioned under the hips *(H)*. The other leg was in a similar position. *A,* Abdomen; *F,* fundus.

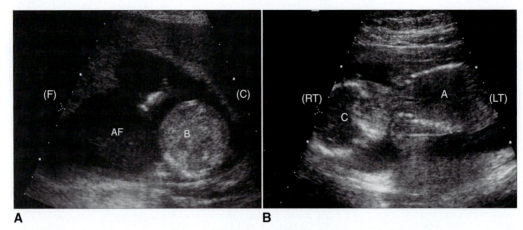

FIGURE 49-7 **A,** A sagittal scan obtained in an 18-week fetus reveals the fetal body in a transverse position rather than a sagittal or coronal orientation (compare with Figure 49-4). *AF,* Amniotic fluid; *B,* body; *C,* toward cervix; *F,* fundus. **B,** In the same fetus, by rotating the transducer 90 degrees, the abdomen may be connected to the head to reveal the transverse lie with the head oriented to the maternal right side *(RT)* and the abdomen *(A)* to the maternal left side *(LT).*

pelvis), need to be delivered by cesarean section. A foot-ling breech is found when the hips are extended and one (single footling) or both feet (double footling) are the presenting parts closest to the cervix. The position of a fetus in breech position may be described by stating the relationship of the fetal sacrum (lower spine) to the maternal pelvis. If the sacrum is adjacent to the left anterior portion of the maternal pelvis, the fetal position is left sacrum anterior (LSA). If the sacrum is adjacent to the left lateral portion of the maternal pelvis, this is called left sacrum transverse (LST). Similarly, fetuses may be described as left sacrum posterior (LSP), sacrum posterior (SP), right sacrum posterior (RSP), right sacrum transverse (RST), right sacrum anterior (RSA), or sacrum anterior (SA). When a fetus is in breech pre-sentation, the shape of the head may appear elongated or *dolichocephalic,* especially in the third trimester.

Transverse. When a transverse cross section of the fetal head or body is noted in the sagittal plane, a transverse lie is suspected (Figure 49-7). By rotating the transducer perpendicular to the maternal axis, the long axis of the fetus may be observed. When a fetus remains in trans-verse lie late in pregnancy, it is important to screen for a mass or placenta previa in the lower uterine segment that is preventing the fetus from moving into a vertex or breech position.

Situs. In addition to determining fetal lie, the right and left sides of the fetus need to be conceptualized to ensure **normal situs** (positioning) of fetal organs. Some sonog-raphers memorize this relationship. For example, if the fetus is in a vertex presentation with the fetal spine toward the maternal right side, the right side of the fetus is down and the left side is up. It is more helpful, however, to practice maintaining a mental picture of the fetal body and position throughout the examination, which allows recognition of the fetal right and left sides.

A sonographer may also differentiate the right from left sides by identifying anatomic landmarks after an initial orientation is verified. For example, if the sonog-rapher initially verifies that the fetal stomach lies on the fetal left side, later in the examination the fetal right and left may be determined in relation to the stomach. The gallbladder on the right side and the **apex** of the heart pointing toward the fetal left side may be verified by their relationship to the stomach. The fetal aorta lies slightly to the left of midline, anterior to the spine, and the infe-rior vena cava is to the right of midline and slightly more anterior to the aorta.

Effective obstetric scanning is founded on the opera-tor's ability to visualize fetal position.

FETAL ANATOMY OF THE SECOND AND THIRD TRIMESTERS

The Cranium

The sonographer must be adept at recognizing the normal appearances and developmental changes of the fetal brain throughout pregnancy. It is imperative to identify neuroanatomy at specific levels where measure-ments are obtained, such as a biparietal diameter or posterior fossa, and to screen for malformations in brain development.

By the 12th week of gestation, the cranial bones ossify. It is important to survey the fetal head to check the contour or outline of the skull bones by sweeping the transducer through the cranium from the highest level (roof) in the brain to the skull base. The cranium appears as a circle at the highest levels and as an oval at the ventricular, peduncular, and basal levels. Extracranial masses (e.g., cephaloceles), central nervous system (CNS) anomalies, skeletal pathology, or fetal death may distort the normal shape of the skull.

Transverse scanning planes are required to evaluate brain anatomy and perform cranial measurements (Figure 49-8). The transducer is aligned in a longitudinal

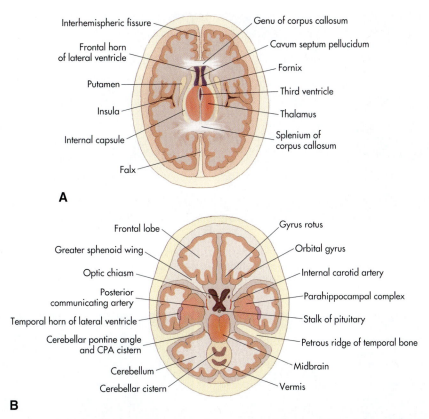

FIGURE 49-8 A, Transverse view of the fetal intracranial anatomy taken at the midsection of the fetal head. **B,** Transverse view inferior to **(A)** taken at the level of the cerebellum and vermis.

or sagittal position over the fetus and then is specifically positioned over the fetal head. Rotation of the transducer perpendicular to the sagittal plane generates transverse sections of the brain. Brain anatomy and measurements are assessed in serial transverse planes. A longitudinal or oblique view of the fetal brain may also be used to locate and assess normal anatomy.

Normal fetal brain parenchyma appears hypoechoic because of the small size reflectors and high water content in the tissue. The sulcus and gyrus are more echogenic. The gyral/sulcal pattern of the brain becomes more complex and more prominent as GA increases. Branches of the anterior cerebral artery run within the midline sulci and may be seen to pulsate within the echogenic structures.

As pregnancy progresses, brain anatomy may be more difficult to visualize owing to increasing calcification of the skull and the position of the fetal head deeper in the pelvis. The calcification of the skull may cause reverberation artifacts in the proximal (near-field) cranial hemisphere that preclude evaluation. Fortunately, most brain anomalies are symmetrical processes, and documentation of the brain may be based on the anatomy seen in the distal hemisphere. In most cases if there is a defect, it is present bilaterally, even though the anatomy may not be adequately discerned. When a brain anomaly is suspected and the fetus is in a vertex presentation, use of a transvaginal probe or transperineal scanning may

allow better visualization of the skull and brain. Magnetic resonance images (MRI) may also be used to evaluate fetal brain anatomy.

Standard obstetric examination guidelines require the sonographer to image and record the cerebellum, the choroid plexus, the cisterna magna, the lateral cerebral ventricles, the midline falx, and the cavum septum pellucidi. It is also suggested that measurement of the nuchal fold may be helpful during a specific age interval to suggest increased risk of aneuploidy. These specific portions of anatomy are described in the following paragraphs in a systematic review of brain structures seen when moving in transverse planes from the roof to the base of the skull.

In a transverse plane, at the most superior level within the skull (Figure 49-9), the contour of the skull should be round or oval and should have a smooth surface. At this level, the interhemispheric fissure, **midline echo (falx),** or falx cerebri is observed as a membrane separating the brain into two equal hemispheres. The midline falx is an important landmark to visualize because its presence implies that separation of the cerebrum has occurred. Lateral and parallel to the midline falx in the superior plane, two linear echoes representing deep venous structures (white-matter tracts) are viewed (see Figure 49-9). It is important to recognize that these white-matter tracts are positioned above the level of the lateral ventricles.

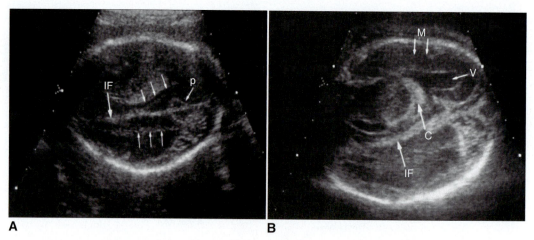

FIGURE 49-9 **A,** Transverse cross section revealing white-matter tracts *(arrows)* coursing parallel to the interhemispheric fissure *(IF)* at 26 weeks' gestation. *P,* peduncles. **B,** The choroid plexus *(c)* is located in the proximal or near hemisphere within the ventricular cavity *(v).* Note the homogeneous appearance of the brain tissue. *M,* Mantle.

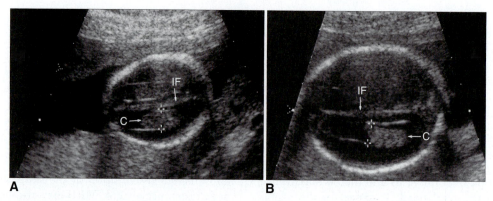

FIGURE 49-10 **A,** Transverse view demonstrating ventricular atrial diameter of 6 mm *(calipers)* at 16 weeks' gestation, representing a normal-size ventricle. *c,* Choroid plexus; *IF,* interhemispheric fissure. **B,** In a 19-week gestation, the atrial diameter of 6 mm corresponds to a normal-size ventricle.

The fetal ventricular system consists of two paired **lateral ventricles,** a midline third ventricle, and a fourth ventricle adjacent to the cerebellum. The ventricular system contains cerebrospinal fluid (CSF), which coats the brain and spinal cord. **Choroid plexus** tissue within the lateral ventricles produces the CSF. Choroid plexus tissue is located within the roof of each ventricle, except at the frontal ventricular horns. This spongelike material is echogenic and is very prominent in early pregnancy. Occasionally, small cysts—which are engorged, spongelike cavities—may be seen in normal pregnancy. It is thought that CSF may become trapped during development within the neuroepithelial folds, resulting in the formation of choroid plexus cysts. This commonly represents a normal fetal development, but these cysts are also known to be associated with trisomy 18. As the cerebral hemispheres grow, the ventricular system and the choroid plexus appear to occupy a much smaller portion of the cranium.

From the lateral ventricles, the fluid travels to the third ventricle through the foramen of Monro. From the third ventricle, the fluid travels through the aqueduct of Sylvius to the fourth ventricle. When the fluid reaches the fourth ventricle, it flows into the cerebral and spinal subarachnoid spaces from the interventricular foramina and the foramen of Luschka. CSF then spreads through the cisterns and surrounds the hemispheres along the subarachnoid spaces. After reaching the arachnoid granulations, it is reabsorbed and enters the venous system (e.g., cranial venous sinuses).

The fetal ventricles are important to assess because **ventriculomegaly** or hydrocephalus (dilated ventricular system) may be a sign of CNS abnormalities. Mild ventriculomegaly may also be associated with congenital anomalies. Aqueductal stenosis at the level of the aqueduct of Sylvius is the most common type of fetal hydrocephaly and will result in excess fluid in the lateral and third ventricles. Dilation of the entire system, including the fourth ventricle, is associated with spinal defects.

The lateral ventricles are viewed at a level just below the white-matter tracts (Figure 49-10). The lumina of the ventricles may be recognized by the bright reflection of their borders and the presence of hyperechoic choroid plexus tissue that fills the cavity of the ventricles early in gestation. The lateral borders of the ventricular chambers are represented as echogenic lines coursing parallel to the midline falx. The lateral ventricle is more easily imaged in the distal hemisphere because of reverberation artifacts in the near field. The ventricular cavity is seen sonographically as a cystic space filled with choroid plexus (Figures 49-11 and 49-12).

The inferior portion of the lateral ventricles connects with the temporal (inferior) and posterior horns. This portion of the ventricle is called the **atrium of the lateral ventricles.** The choroid plexus is tear-shaped. The most inferior portion of the choroid plexus body or glomus marks the site of the atrium. The glomus or body of the choroid plexus will fill the lateral ventricle in a normal pregnancy. If the glomus appears to float or dangle within the cavity, this is a sign of abnormally enlarged or dilated ventricles (ventriculomegaly). Measurements

of the atrium portion of the ventricle are clinically practical because the size of this portion remains the same throughout gestation.

When measuring the ventricle, locate the atrium and measure directly across the posterior portion, measuring perpendicular to the long axis of the ventricle rather than the falx, while placing the calipers at the junction of the ventricular wall and lumen or cavity of the ventricle (see Figure 49-10). The normal atrium measures 6.5 mm. If the atrium measures greater than 10 mm, this warrants serial imaging and further evaluation.

Moving the transducer slightly inferior to the ventricular atrium identifies the area of the thalami and the ambient cisterns. This is the widest transverse diameter of the skull and is therefore the proper level at which to measure the biparietal diameter and head circumference. The midline brain structures (see Figure 49-12) include the **cavum septum pellucidum,** the midline echo, and the

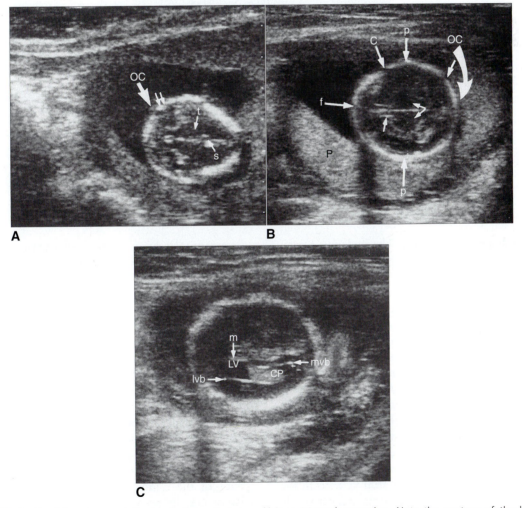

FIGURE 49-11 A, Cranial anatomy at the level of the thalamus *(t)* in a 14-week gestation. Note the contour of the bony calvarium *(double arrows). OC,* occiput; *s,* cavum septum pellucidum. **B,** Cranial anatomy at the same level in an 18-week gestation. *Curved arrow,* Thalamus; *single arrow,* cavum septum pellucidum; *c,* coronal suture; *f,* frontal bone; *OC,* occiput; *P,* placenta; *p,* parietal bones. **C,** Cerebral ventricles at 19 weeks' gestation. The midline echo from the interhemispheric fissure *(m)* is noted. The medial ventricular border *(mvb)* and the lateral ventricular border *(lvb)* are identified. The ventricular cavity *(LV)* and the echogenic choroid plexus *(CP)* are demonstrated.

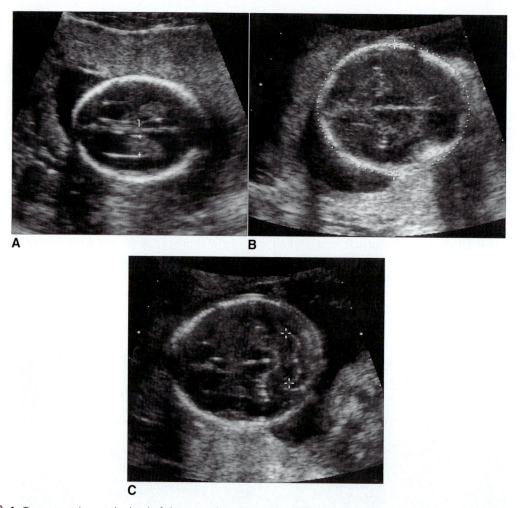

FIGURE 49-12 A, Transverse view at the level of the ventricles. The width of the lateral ventricle is measured from medial to lateral edges *(1)*. **B,** Transverse view slightly inferior to the level of the ventricles, near the thalamus (hypoechoic "heart" structure in the center of the skull). This is the level at which the biparietal diameter and head circumference are measured. **C,** Transverse view inferior to the level of **B;** the cerebellum is demarcated by the calipers.

paired thalami lying on either side. The thalamus resembles a heart with the apex projected toward the fetal occiput.

Between the thalami lies the cavity of the third ventricle (see Figure 49-12). In the same scanning plane, the box-shaped cavum septum pellucidum (CSP) is observed anterior to the thalamus. The CSP is the space between the leaves of the septum pellucidum.

At this transverse level, the frontal horns of the ventricles may be seen as two diverging echo-free structures within the frontal lobes of the brain. The frontal horns are prominent in the presence of ventricular dilation. The **corpus callosum** is an echopenic structure seen in the transverse plane as the band of tissue between the frontal ventricular horns. The corpus callosum can be better appreciated as a linear band in a sagittal view from the top of the fetal head, but this plane is often not accessible in pregnancy.

The ambient cisterns are pulsatile structures vascularized by the posterior cerebral artery bordering the thalamus posteriorly. When scanning laterally in the brain,

the temporal lobe is visible, along with evidence of the insula (i.e., the sylvian cistern complex). The insula appears to pulsate because of blood circulation through the middle cerebral artery, which courses through the insula (see Figure 49-12). The subarachnoid spaces may be seen projecting from the inner skull table.

As the transducer is moved toward the base of the skull, the heart-shaped cerebral peduncles are imaged (Figure 49-13). Although similar to the thalamus in shape, they are smaller. Pulsations from the basilar artery are observed between the lobes of the peduncles at the interpeduncular cistern. The circle of Willis may be seen anterior to the midbrain and appears as a triangular region that is highly pulsatile as a result of the midline-positioned anterior cerebral artery and lateral convergence of the middle cerebral arteries. The suprasellar cistern may be recognized in the center of the circle of Willis.

The *cerebellum* is located in back of the cerebral peduncles within the posterior fossa. The cerebellar hemispheres are joined together by the cerebellar vermis

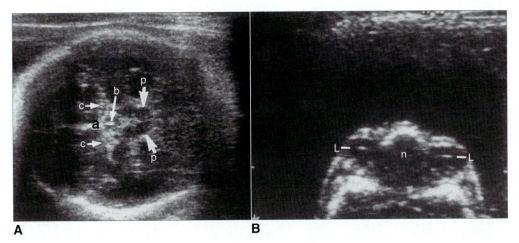

FIGURE 49-13 A, Circle of Willis (*c*) identified anterior to the cerebral peduncles (*p*). Arterial pulsations may be observed from the basilar artery (*b*) and the anterior cerebral artery (*a*) in real-time imaging. The middle cerebral artery pulsations may be seen at the lateral margins of the circle of Willis. **B,** The lenses (*L*) of the eyes are noted when the fetus is looking upward (occipitoposterior position). The nasal cavities are identified (*n*).

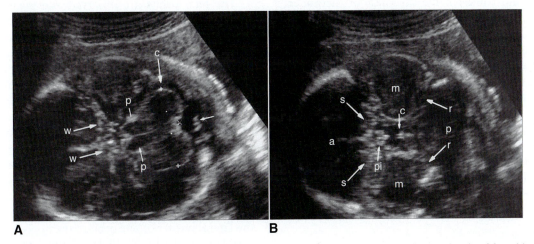

FIGURE 49-14 A, Anatomic depiction at the cerebellar level in a 25-week fetus showing the cerebral peduncles (*p*) positioned anteriorly to the cerebellum (*c*). The circle of Willis (*w*) is outlined. The dural folds that connect the bottom of the falx cerebelli are seen within the cisterna magna (*arrow*). **B,** In the same fetus, at a level slightly below the cerebellar level, the anterior (*a*), middle (*m*), and posterior fossae are shown. Note the sphenoid bones (*s*) and petrous ridges (*r*). *c,* Suprasellar cistern; *pi,* piarachnoid tissue in the basilar cistern.

(Figure 49-14). It is important to recognize the usual configuration of the cerebellum because distortion may represent findings suggestive of an open spina bifida. The *banana sign* is the sonographic term that describes the Arnold-Chiari malformation in which the cerebellum may be small or displaced downward into the foramen magnum. Measurements of transverse cerebellar width allow assessment of fetal age and permit necessary follow-up in fetuses with spinal defects and other anomalies of the cerebellum.

The **cisterna magna** (a posterior fossa cistern filled with CSF) lies directly behind the cerebellum (Figure 49-15). A normal-appearing cisterna magna may exclude almost all open spinal defects. The cisterna magna is almost always effaced (thinned out) or obliterated in fetuses with the Arnold-Chiari malformation changes associated with spina bifida. The cranial changes occur

because tethering of the spinal cord resulting from spina bifida pulls brain tissue downward, obliterating the cisterna magna. In patients at low risk of spinal defect, confirmation of a normal posterior fossa suggests the absence of spina bifida. Because evaluation of the fetal spine remains challenging in excluding small spinal defects, cranial findings associated with this disorder may be very helpful in screening for these lesions.

Enlargement of the cisterna magna may indicate a space-occupying cyst, such as a Dandy-Walker malformation or other abnormalities of the posterior fossa. Enlargement is often a normal variant. The normal cisterna magna measures 3 to 11 mm, with an average size of 5 to 6 mm. Measurements of cisterna magna size are obtained by measuring from the vermis to the inner skull table of the occipital bone. Within the cisterna magna space, linear echoes, which are paired, may be observed

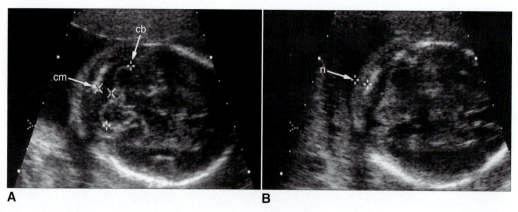

FIGURE 49-15 A, Depiction of a normal cerebellum *(cb)* and cisterna magna *(cm)* in a 24-week fetus. The cerebellum measures 26 mm, and the cisterna magna measures 5 mm in diameter. **B,** In the same fetus, at the same level, the skin behind the neck is measured. A normal nuchal skin fold *(n)* of 5 mm is shown. This measurement is unreliable after 20 weeks' gestation.

posteriorly. These echogenic structures represent dural folds that attach the falx cerebelli (see Figure 49-14).

In the second trimester, the thickness of the **nuchal skin fold** is measured in a plane containing the cavum septi pellucidi, the cerebellum, and the cisterna magna. Values of skin thickness of 5 mm or less up to 20 weeks' GA are normal. Fetuses with thickened nuchal skin are at increased risk for aneuploidy.

At the base of the skull, the anterior, middle, and posterior cranial fossae are observed (see Figure 49-14). The sphenoid bones create a V-shaped appearance as they separate the anterior fossa from the middle fossa, with the petrous bones further dividing the fossa posteriorly. At the junction of the sphenoid wings and the petrous bones lies the sella turcica (site of the pituitary gland).

The Face

The architecture and morphology of the fetal face are easily appreciated after the first trimester of pregnancy. Viewing facial behaviors such as fetal yawning, swallowing, and eye movements not only may be enjoyable but may provide insightful clues to fetal well-being and normal facial anatomy.

The fetal face may be recognized even in the first trimester of pregnancy, and the GA at which the nasal bone first appears may contribute to aneuploidy risk determination. Facial morphology becomes more apparent in the second trimester, but visualization is heavily dependent on fetal positioning, adequate amounts of amniotic fluid, and excellent acoustic windows. Incorporation of three-dimensional ultrasound imaging has enhanced images of facial details and created patient demand for *fetal portraits*.

Fetal Eye Orbits. When scanning inferior to or below the cerebellar plane, the orbits may be visualized. It is important to note that both fetal orbits (and eyes) are present and that the spacing between both orbits appears normal. There are conditions in which eyes may be missing (anophthalmia), fused or

closely spaced (hypotelorism), or abnormally widened (hypertelorism).

The fetal orbits are observed and measured in two planes: (1) a coronal scan posterior to the glabellar-alveolar line (Figure 49-16), and (2) a transverse scan at a level below the biparietal diameter (along the orbito-meatal line) (Figure 49-17). In these views, the individual orbital rings, nasal structures, and maxillary processes can be identified. When the fetus is in an occipitoposterior position (fetal orbits directed up), orbital distances can also be determined. In this view, the orbital rings, lens, and nasal structures may be demonstrated (Figure 49-18). Measurements of the inner orbital distance (IOD) should be made from the medial border of the orbit to the opposite medial border, and the outer orbital (or binocular) distance (OOD) should be measured from the lateral border of one orbit to the opposite lateral wall (see Figures 49-16 to 49-18). **Nomograms** for orbital distance spacing have been published and may confirm impressions of hypertelorism or hypotelorism. Orbital measurements are not used for routine screening because there is a wide range of normal values.

Facial Profile. Views of the fetal forehead and facial profile are achieved by imaging the facial profile (Figure 49-19). In this view, the contour of the frontal bone, the nose, the upper and lower lips, and the chin may be assessed. Profile views of the face are useful in assessing the nasal bone; in excluding forehead malformations such as anterior cephaloceles, abnormal slopes, or **frontal bossing**; and in assessing the chin to exclude an abnormally small chin—**micrognathia**. In a normally proportioned face, each of the segments containing the forehead, the eyes and nose, and the mouth and chin forms approximately one third of the profile.

Nasal Bone. A small nose and midface hypoplasia are recognized components of Down syndrome facies. Studies have shown that the nasal bone is absent during the second trimester in one quarter to one third of Down syndrome fetuses and is present in all normal fetuses. An absent nasal bone is also associated with trisomy 18,

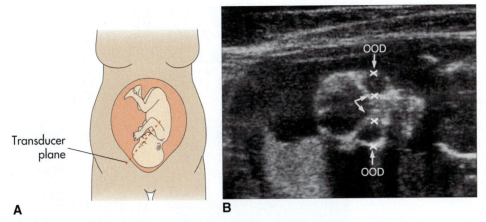

FIGURE 49-16 A, Frontal view. Fetus in a vertex presentation with the fetal cranium in an occipitotransverse position. The transducer is placed along the coronal plane (approximately 2 cm posterior to the glabellar-alveolar line). **B,** This sonogram shows the orbits in the coronal view. The outer orbital diameter *(OOD)* and inner orbital diameter (IOD) *(angled arrows)* are viewed. The IOD is measured from the medial border of the orbit to the opposite medial border *(angled arrows)*. The OOD is measured from the outermost lateral border of the orbit to the opposite lateral border.

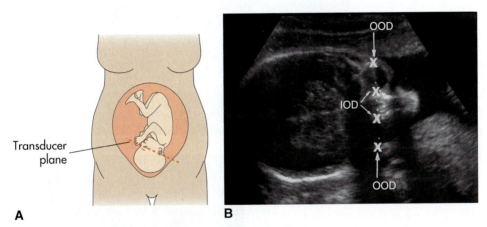

FIGURE 49-17 A, Frontal view demonstrating the fetal cranium in an occipitotransverse position. The transducer is placed along the orbitomeatal line (approximately 2 to 3 cm below the level of the biparietal diameter). **B,** Sonogram demonstrating the orbits in the occipitotransverse position. *IOD,* Inner orbital diameter; *OOD,* outer orbital diameter.

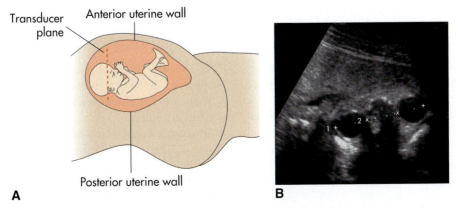

FIGURE 49-18 A, Side view demonstrating the fetus in an occipitoposterior position. The transducer is placed in a plane that transects the occiput, orbits, and nasal processes. **B,** Sonogram of the orbits in an occipitoposterior position.

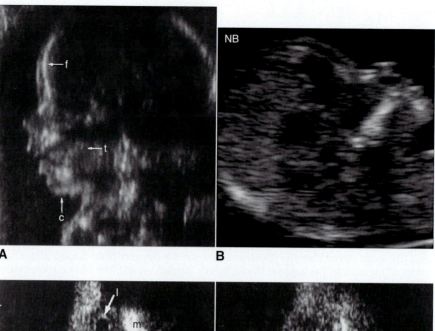

FIGURE 49-19 A, Sagittal view in a 23-week fetus showing the contour of the face in profile. Note the smooth surface of the frontal bone *(f)* and the appearance of the nose and upper and lower lips, tongue *(t),* and chin *(c).* **B,** The fetal nasal bone is seen as a bright linear echo under the linear skin line echo in this profile of the fetus.

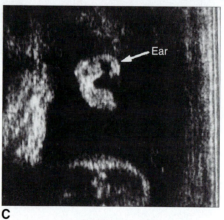

FIGURE 49-20 A, Coronal view showing facial features. *l,* Lens; *ll,* lower lip; *m,* mandible; *n,* nasal bones; *ul,* upper lip; *x,* maxilla; *z,* zygomatic bone. **B,** In the same fetus, the eyelids *(EL)* and mouth *(M)* are shown. **C,** In the same fetus, the ear is shown.

trisomy 13, and monosomy X. The nasal bone appears as a bright echo parallel to the echogenic skin interface in the superior aspect of the nose (see Figure 49-19). It is important that the nasal bone be visualized and documented if present in a midline fetal profile in second-trimester examinations. Nomograms are available for measuring the nasal bone during the second trimester. A shortened nasal bone is a risk factor for aneuploidy.

Frontal bossing is a variation of facial structure where the forehead is more prominent than usual.

It is seen in skeletal dysplasias. Frontal slanting is the opposite of frontal bossing and is characterized by a forehead that slopes backward. Frontal slanting is seen in microcephaly.

Anatomic Landmarks of the Coronal Facial View. By placing the transducer in a coronal scanning plane, sectioning through the face reveals orbital rings, parietal bones, ethmoid bones, nasal septum, zygomatic bone, maxillae, and mandible (Figure 49-20). Scans obtained in an anterior plane over the orbits demonstrate the eyelids and, when directed posterior to this plane, the orbital lens. The eyeglobes, hyaloid artery, and vitreous matter have been sonographically identified.

Fetal Tongue. The oral cavity and tongue are frequently outlined during fetal swallowing (see Figure 49-19). A large tongue that persistently protrudes outside of the mouth is called **macroglossia**. Macroglossia is associated with Beckwith-Wiedemann syndrome and with aneuploidies.

Fetal Lips. The most recent revisions of the obstetric guidelines from AIUM, ACR, and ACOG require visualization of the fetal lip. Coronal/axial views of the face help differentiate the nostrils, nares, nasal septum, maxillae, and mandible (Figure 49-21). This view is helpful in the diagnosis of craniofacial anomalies, such as cleft lip. The soft tissues of the fetal upper lip can be visualized in most fetuses. Visualization improves with advancing gestational age. Visualization of the palate, particularly the hard palate, is more difficult owing to shadowing from the alveolar ridge and interference by the tongue. Sonographers should strive to diagnose cleft lip in utero, as prenatal classes for parents of these children are associated with faster weight gain, quicker surgical intervention, and better outcomes postnatally. It is important to recognize normal facial landmarks that may mimic defects as well.

Fetal Ears. Fetal ears may be defined in the second trimester as lateral protuberances emerging from the parietal bones. Later in pregnancy, the components of the external ear, helix, lobule, and antitragicus (small muscle in the pinna of the ear) may be seen (Figure 49-22). The semicircular canals and the internal auditory meatus have been sonographically recognized. Low-set ears are difficult to diagnose with ultrasound. Some have suggested that if a plane passing through the lower jaw intercepts the ear, they may be low-set. Others have suggested measuring the ears. However, there is a wide range of normal, and visualization of fetal ears has not yet been shown to be sensitive for diagnosis.

Fetal hair is often observed along the periphery of the skull and must not be included in the biparietal diameter measurement (Figure 49-23).

The Vertebral Column

Standard antepartum obstetric examination guidelines require the sonographer to image and record the cervical,

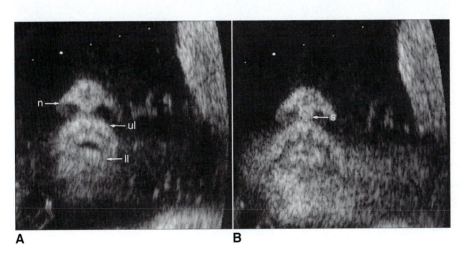

A   B

FIGURE 49-21 A, Axial view through the upper *(ul)* and lower lip *(ll)* in a fetus with an open mouth. Note the nares *(n)* and nasal septum. This view is used to check for a cleft of the upper lip. **B,** In the same fetus, same anatomy viewed with a closed mouth. *s,* Nasal septum.

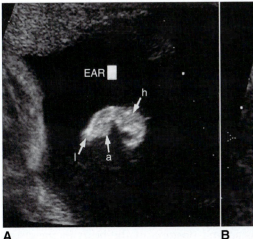
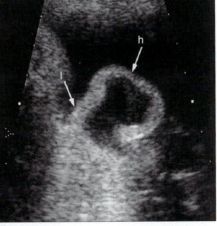

A   B

FIGURE 49-22 A, The external ear observed in a 26-week fetus showing the helix *(h),* lobule *(l),* and antitragicus *(a).* **B,** At 36 weeks' gestation, the lobule *(l)* and helix *(h)* are observed.

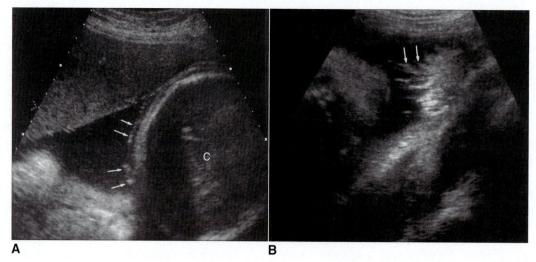

FIGURE 49-23   A, Fetal hair *(arrows)* observed as a series of dots around the periphery of the fetal cranium in a 39-week fetus. *C,* Cranium. **B,** Long hair *(arrows)* observed in a 34-week fetus.

FIGURE 49-24   A, Coronal view of the fetal spine in a 15-week fetus outlining the cervical vertebrae *(cv)* and cranium *(C).* The thoracic vertebrae *(tv)* are visualized distally. The rib *(r)* aids in localizing the thorax. **B,** In the same fetus, a coronal plane outlines the lumbar *(lv)* and sacral vertebrae *(sv). r,* Rib.

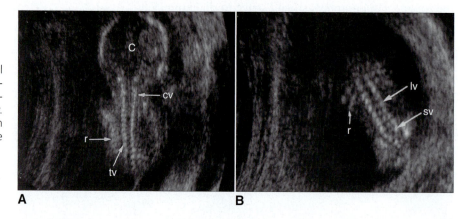

thoracic, lumbar, and sacral spine to better exclude major spinal malformations (e.g., meningomyelocele).

The longitudinal fetal spine is studied in coronal, sagittal, and transverse scanning planes. There are three ossification points in each vertebra. When scanning in the coronal and sagittal planes, only two ossification points are typically seen. In a sagittal section, the spine appears as two curvilinear lines extending from the cervical spine to the sacrum. The normal fetal spine tapers near the sacrum and widens near the base of the skull (Figures 49-24 through 49-26). This double-line appearance of the spine is referred to as the *railway sign* and is generated by echoes from the posterior and anterior laminae and the spinal cord.

In a transverse plane, three ossification points are visible. The three are spaced equidistant, and the spinal column appears as a closed circle, indicating closure of the neural tube. Three echoes form a circle or equilateral triangle that represents the center of the vertebral body and the posterior elements (laminae or pedicles) (Figure 49-27). These elements should be identified in the normal fetus, whereas the pedicles appear splayed in a V-, C-, or U-shaped configuration in a fetus with a spinal defect.

When evaluating the spine, it is imperative for the sonographer to align the transducer in a perpendicular axis to the spinal elements. Incorrect angles may falsely indicate an abnormality. The spinal muscles and the posterior skin border are viewed adjacent to the circular ring of the ossification centers (see Figure 49-27). It is important to note the integrity of the skin surface because this membrane is absent in fetuses with open spina bifida. Inspection of the spine is often impossible when the fetus is lying with the spine against the uterine wall. Optimal viewing of the spine occurs when the fetus is lying on its side in a transverse direction with its back a slight distance from the uterine wall. The sonographer may need to ask the mother to turn slightly in an effort to encourage the fetus to move away from the uterine wall.

The Thorax

Although the fetus is unable to breathe air in utero, the lungs are important landmarks to visualize within the thoracic cavity. The lungs serve as lateral borders for the heart and are therefore helpful in assessing the relationship and position of the heart in the chest.

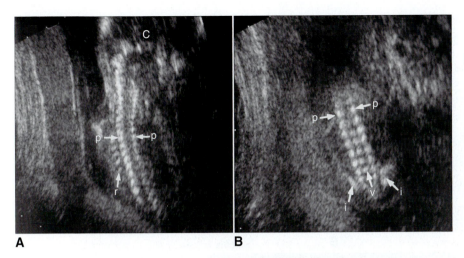

FIGURE 49-25 **A,** Coronal view of the spine in a 19-week fetus, demonstrating the parallel nature of the posterior elements, or laminae *(p)*, of the cervical and thoracic vertebrae. *C*, Cranium; *r*, rib. **B,** In the same fetus, the lumbosacral vertebrae are observed in the coronal plane. The posterior elements *(p)*, or laminae, and the vertebral body *(v)* are noted. In fetuses with spina bifida, widening across the posterior elements may be found (see Chapter 53) *i*, iliac crest.

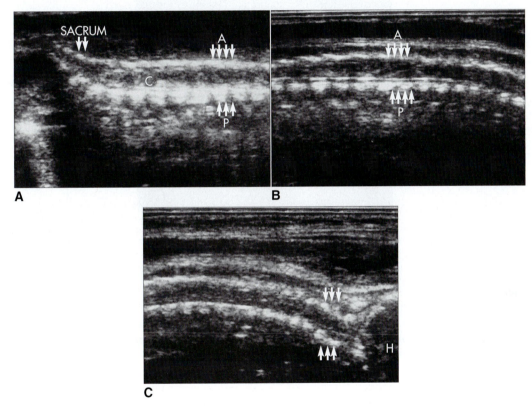

FIGURE 49-26 Longitudinal sections of the lumbosacral **(A)**, thoracic **(B)**, and cervical **(C)** spine in a 37-week fetus displaying the anterior *(A)* and posterior *(P)* elements, or laminae. Note the tapering of the spine at the sacrum **(A)** and the widening at the entrance into the base of the skull (**C,** *H* [head]). Between the posterior elements lie the spinal canal (**A, C**) and cord (may be seen as a linear echo within the spinal canal).

Fetal breathing movements are also observed at this level. Like all fetal organs, the lungs are subject to abnormal development. Lung size, texture, and location should be assessed routinely to exclude a lung mass.

The fluid-filled fetal lungs are observed as solid, homogeneous masses of tissue bordered medially by the heart, inferiorly by the diaphragm, and laterally by the rib cage (Figure 49-28). The heart occupies a midline position within the chest; its displacement warrants further study to exclude a possible mass of the lung or a subdiaphragmatic hernia that may alter the position of the heart.

In sagittal views, lung tissue is present superior to the diaphragm and lateral to the heart (see Figure 49-28). Investigators have attempted to define textural variations of the lung in comparison with the liver. Fetal lung tissue appears more echogenic than the liver as pregnancy progresses.

The ribs, scapulae, and clavicles are bony landmarks of the chest cavity. Because these structures are

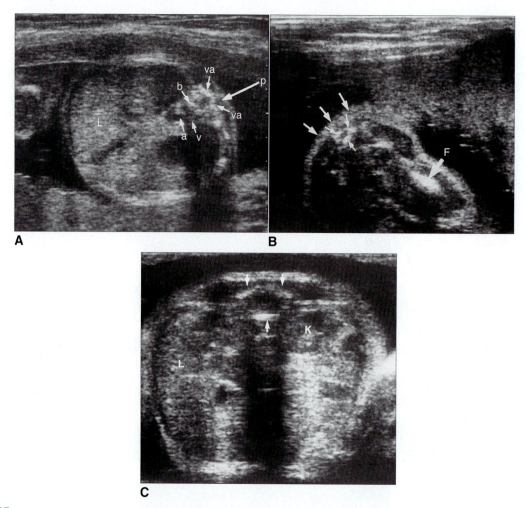

FIGURE 49-27 A, Transverse scans of the vertebral column showing the echogenic ring produced by the vertebral body and posterior elements, or laminae. Thoracic vertebrae with typical landmarks. *L,* liver; *a,* aorta; *b,* body; *p,* posterior vertebral muscles; *v,* vena cava; *va,* vertebral arch or posterior elements. **B,** Sacral vertebra outlined *(small arrows).* Note the intact posterior skin wall in this normal fetus *(large arrows).* **C,** Transverse view through the spine at kidney level *(K)* demonstrating the closed-circle appearance *(arrows)* of the spine created by the intact vertebral arch. *L,* liver.

composed of bone, acoustic shadowing occurs posteriorly. Portions of the rib cage may be identified when sections are obtained through the posterior aspects of the spine and rib cage (Figure 49-29). Oblique sectioning of the ribs reveals the total length of the ribs and floating ribs. On sagittal planes, the echogenic rib interspersed with the intercostal space creates the typical "washboard" appearance of the rib cage (see Figure 49-29). Sound waves strike the rib and are reflected upward, leaving the characteristic void of echoes posterior to the bony element, whereas sound waves pass through the intercostal space.

On a transverse cross section through the chest and upper abdomen, the curvature of the rib may be appreciated below the skin. It is important to differentiate the rib from the skin wall, especially when measuring the abdominal circumference. The entire rib cage is impractical to routinely examine, but study of the ribs is warranted in fetuses at risk for congenital rib anomalies (e.g., rib fractures found in osteogenesis imperfecta).

The clavicles are observed in coronal sections through the upper thorax (Figure 49-30). The clavicular length may aid in determining GA. In this same view, the spinal elements, esophagus, and carotid arteries may be seen. The clavicles may also be demonstrated as echogenic dots superior to the ribs. Measurements of the clavicles may be useful in predicting congenital clavicular anomalies. The clavicles may be shortened with aneuploidy.

The scapula may be recognized on sagittal sections as an echogenic linear echo adjacent to the rib shadows, whereas on transverse sections it is viewed medial to the humeral head (see Figure 49-30). Oblique views demonstrate the entire length of the scapula. The sternum may be seen in axial sections as a bony sequence of echoes beneath the anterior chest wall.

The Heart

Standard antepartum obstetric examination guidelines require the sonographer to image and record a four-

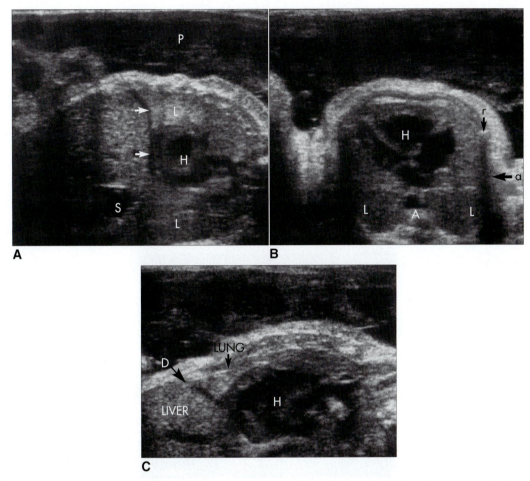

FIGURE 49-28 A, Sagittal scan showing the homogeneous lungs positioned lateral to the heart *(H)* and superior to the diaphragm *(arrows)*. Note the normal placement of the stomach *(S)* inferior to the diaphragm. *L,* lungs; *P,* placenta. **B,** In the same fetus, a transverse section demonstrates the position of the lungs *(L)* in relationship to the heart *(H)*. Note the apex of the heart to the left side of the chest. The base of the heart is in the midline and anterior to the aorta *(A)*. Displacement or shifting of the heart should alert the sonographer to search for a mass of the lungs, heart, or diaphragm. Note the rib *(r)* and resultant acoustic shadow *(a)*. **C,** In the late third trimester of pregnancy, the lung tissue can be observed and compared with the liver texture. *D,* Diaphragm; *H,* heart.

chamber view of the fetal heart. The reader is referred to Chapter 33 for more detailed fetal cardiac anatomy. Many major anomalies of the fetal heart are excluded when cardiac anatomy appears normal in the four-chamber view of the heart. Additional views including outflow tracts may further reduce the risk of cardiovascular anomalies.

The heart lies more transversely in the fetus than in the adult because the lungs are not inflated. The apex of the heart is directed toward the left anterior chest with the right ventricle closest to the chest wall and the left atrium closest to the spine. The four chambers may be seen in a view taken with the beam perpendicular to the septum or in a view with the beam perpendicular to the valves (Figure 49-31). The four-chamber view may be obtained by angling cephalad after obtaining a transverse view of the fetal abdomen that displays the stomach. In a four-chamber view of the heart, it is important to assess the following:

- Cardiac position, situs, and axis. The apex of the heart should point to the fetal left side.
- Presence of the right ventricle and left ventricle (the right ventricle is found when a line is drawn from the spine to the anterior chest wall and is characterized by the presence of moderator bands).
- Equal-sized ventricles. By the end of pregnancy, the right ventricle may be larger than the left ventricle because it is the chamber that pumps blood through the ductus arteriosus to the descending aorta and to the placenta.
- Presence of equal-sized right and left atria, with the foramen ovale opening toward the left atrium as blood is shunted from the right atrium, bypassing the lungs.
- An interventricular septum that appears uninterrupted. The septum appears wider toward the ventricles and thins as it courses cephalad within the heart.

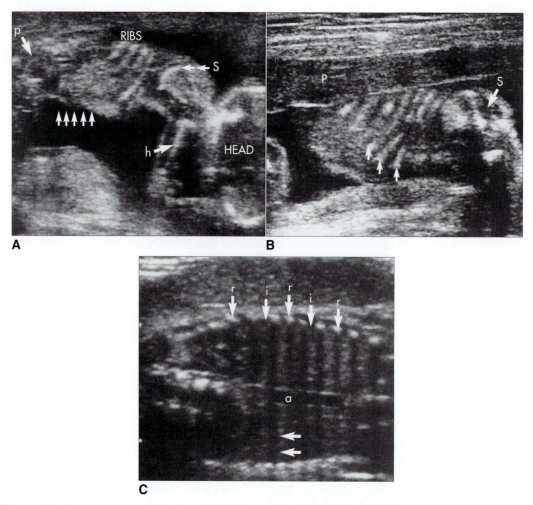

FIGURE 49-29 A, Sagittal view showing the rib cage, scapula *(S)*, anterior abdominal wall *(arrows)*, and humerus *(h)* in a fetus in a back-up position. *p,* pelvis. **B,** Tangential view depicting the length of the ribs *(arrows)*. *P,* placenta; *S,* shoulder. **C,** Sagittal view of the rib cage. Note that sound waves are unable to pass through the bony rib, resulting in a shadow of echoes *(arrows)* posterior to the ribs *(r)*. Sound passes through the intercostal space *(i)*. *a,* Aorta.

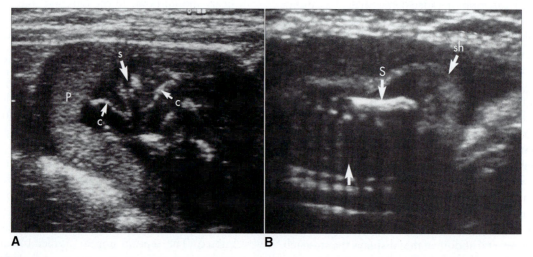

FIGURE 49-30 A, Coronal section of upper thoracic cavity showing the clavicles *(c)* and spine *(s)*. *P,* Placenta. **B,** Sagittal section demonstrating the scapula *(S)* in relationship to the shoulder *(sh)* and ribs *(arrow)*.

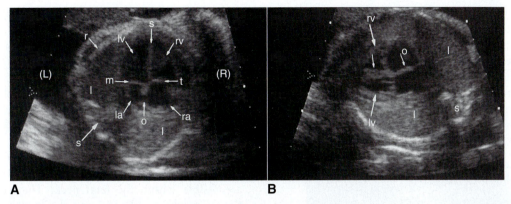

FIGURE 49-31 A, The four-chambered heart view is demonstrated in a 31-week fetus with the spine in the 7 o'clock position. The fetal right side is down and the left side is up. Structures observed are the right *(rv)* and left *(lv)* ventricles; the interventricular septum *(s)*, dividing the two ventricular chambers; and the left *(la)* and right *(ra)* atria. The foramen ovale *(o)*, which allows blood to shunt from the right to left atrium, permits the majority of blood to bypass the lungs. The flap of the foramen ovale is positioned within the left atrium. The atrioventricular valves (mitral and tricuspid) are viewed in systole (closed position). The tricuspid valve allows blood to move from the right atrium to the right ventricle *(rv)*, and the mitral valve *(m)* regulates blood flow from the left atrium to the left ventricle *(lv)*. Note the normal central position of the heart bordered by the lungs *(l)*. The apex of the heart is pointed to the fetal left side *(L)*. When a line is drawn from the spine *(S)* to the anterior chest wall, the right ventricle is found. R, Fetal right side; r, rib. **B,** In a 30-week fetus, the heart is observed in the 5 o'clock position. The fetal left side is down. The lungs *(l)* are viewed bordering the heart laterally. The muscularity of the interventricular septum *(arrow)* is observed along with the foramen ovale *(o)*, separating the atrial chambers. *lv*, Left ventricle; *rv*, right ventricle; *S*, spine.

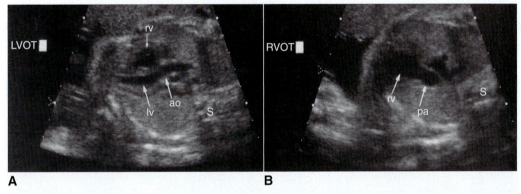

FIGURE 49-32 A, The left ventricular outflow tract *(LVOT)* is observed as the aorta *(ao)* exits the left ventricle *(lv)*. *rv*, Right ventricle. **B,** The right ventricular outflow tract *(RVOT)* is observed as the pulmonary artery *(pa)* exits the right ventricle. The LVOT and RVOT should course perpendicularly to each other. *S*, spine.

- Normal placement of the tricuspid and mitral valves. The tricuspid valve inserts lower, or closer to the apex, than the mitral valve. Both valves should open during diastole and close during systole.
- Normal rhythm and rate (120 to 160 beats per minute).

Guidelines recommend that the standard antepartum obstetric examination include views of the ventricular outflow tracts when this is technically feasible. These views (Figure 49-32) can document that the aortic and pulmonic outflow tracts are similar in size and appropriate in size for GA, that the anterior wall of the aorta is contiguous with the ventricular septum (excludes overriding aorta), and that the great vessels are in normal alignment. These views may provide additional images of the cardiac septum.

An echogenic structure, as bright as bone, that appears within a cardiac chamber and persists despite changes in transducer position is call an **echogenic intracardiac focus (EIF)** (Figure 49-33). This normal variation appears in many normal pregnancies but is associated with increased risk of aneuploidy and cardiac defects. In fetuses at risk for a cardiac anomaly, including those with an EIF, targeted fetal echocardiography may be recommended to further evaluate the outflow tracts, pulmonic valve and veins, and other complex cardiac relationships beyond the scope of a standard obstetric examination. (For further discussion of normal cardiac anatomy, physiology, and targeted echocardiography, see Chapters 33 and 34.)

The Diaphragm and Thoracic Vessels

The diaphragm is the muscle that separates the thorax and abdomen and is commonly viewed in the longitudinal plane. The diaphragm lies inferior to the heart and lungs and superior to the liver, stomach, and spleen

(Figure 49-34). The diaphragm curves gently toward the thorax. If the diaphragm extends outward toward the abdomen, this may be a sign of increased pressure in the thorax as a result of a thoracic mass or effusion. Sonographically, the diaphragm appears as a sonolucent liner structure separating the thorax from the abdomen.

The diaphragm may be more obvious on the right side because of the strong liver interface, but attempts to

observe an intact left diaphragm are encouraged because diaphragmatic defects occur on both sides of the diaphragm. The stomach should be viewed inferior to the diaphragm. Although abdominal contents can move into and out of the thoracic cavity with fetal movement, visualization of the stomach inferior to the diaphragm generally excludes a left-side diaphragmatic hernia. If the fetal heart is displaced to the right, this may be a sign of a left-side diaphragmatic hernia.

Vascular structures may be observed within the thoracic cavity and neck. Vessels emanating from the heart are visible within the fetal neck. The carotid arteries (lateral to the esophagus) and the jugular veins (lateral to the carotid arteries) are frequently noted when the fetal neck is extended (Figure 49-35).

The trachea may be identified as a midline structure in both sagittal and transverse planes. The esophagus and the oropharynx help determine the location of the carotid arteries and are outlined when amniotic fluid is swallowed by the fetus (Figure 49-36).

The aorta, inferior vena cava, and superior vena cava are routinely observed. The aorta is recognized on sagittal planes as it exits the left ventricle and forms the aortic arch (see Figure 49-33). The vessels branching

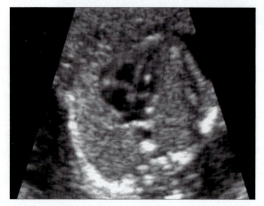

FIGURE 49-33 A four-chamber view of the heart showing an echogenic cardiac focus (EIF) in the left ventricle.

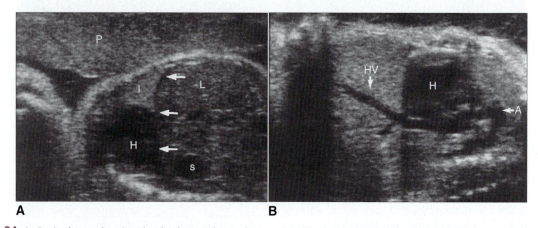

FIGURE 49-34 A, Sagittal scan showing the diaphragm *(arrows)* separating the thoracic and abdominal cavities. *L,* Liver; *l,* lung; *P,* placenta; *s,* stomach. **B,** Sagittal view showing a hepatic vessel *(HV)* coursing through the liver before joining the inferior vena cava as it passes through the diaphragm and empties into the right atrium. Note the aortic arch *(A)* exiting the heart *(H)* superiorly.

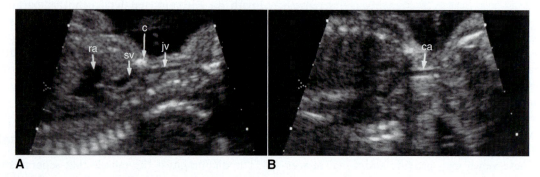

FIGURE 49-35 A, The jugular vein *(jv)* is observed laterally as it empties into the superior vena cava *(sv)* with drainage into the right atrium *(ra)* in a 25-week fetus. This sagittal position is helpful in looking for neck masses such as a goiter (enlarged thyroid gland). *c,* Clavicle. **B,** A carotid artery *(ca)* is observed in a more medial location coursing cephalad into the brain.

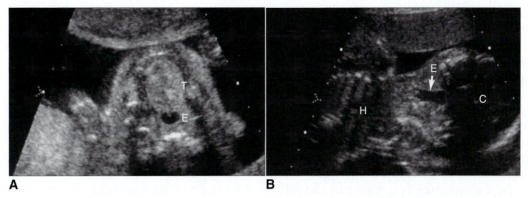

FIGURE 49-36 A, Cross section through the tongue *(T)* and esophagus *(E)* or oropharynx in a 24-week fetus. Recent swallowing of amniotic fluid by the fetus allows visualization of these structures. **B,** Fluid-filled esophagus *(E)* or oropharynx seen in a longitudinal view. The bolus of swallowed amniotic fluid will travel to the stomach. *C,* Cranium; *H,* heart.

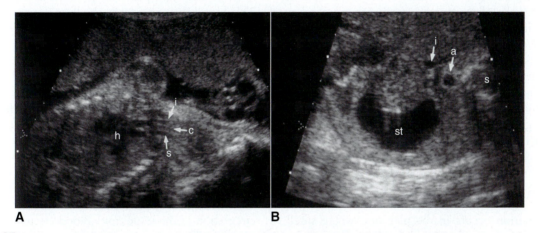

FIGURE 49-37 A, The aortic arch branches are shown in a 35-week fetus with an extended neck. *c,* Left common carotid artery; *h,* heart; *i,* innominate artery; *i,* inferior vena cava; *s,* left subclavian artery; *st,* stomach. **B,** Aorta *(a)* visualized to the left of the spine *(s)* in a transverse cross section.

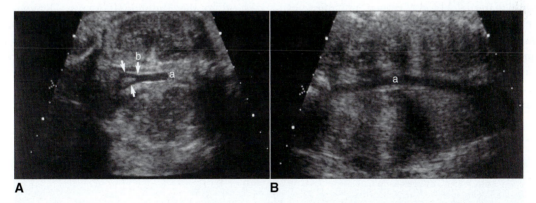

FIGURE 49-38 A, The bifurcation *(b)* of the aorta *(a)* into the common iliac arteries *(arrows)* is viewed in a 32-week fetus. **B,** In the same fetus, a sagittal plane shows the abdominal portion of the aorta *(a)*.

cephalad into the brain may be observed in the cooperative fetus as they arise from the superior wall of the aortic arch. The innominate artery, left common carotid artery, and left subclavian artery may be identified (Figure 49-37).

As the vessels course posteriorly, the thoracic aorta and the descending aorta are observed coursing into the bifurcation of the common iliac arteries (Figure 49-38). The sonographer should recognize the characteristic arterial pulsations from the aorta and its branches. Further divisions of the aorta may be observed as the sonographer views the common iliac vessels, internal iliac vessels, and umbilical arteries that diverge laterally around the bladder (see Figure 49-41). The external iliac arteries are observed as they enter the femoral arteries. The aorta is observed in a transverse plane to the left of the spine.

The inferior vena cava is identified coursing to the right and parallel with the aorta. Transversely, the inferior vena cava is seen anterior and to the right of the spine. It is important to note that the inferior vena cava appears anterior to the aorta within the chest as the vena cava enters anteriorly at the junction of the right atrium.

The hepatic veins may be imaged in sagittal planes or in cephalad-directed transverse planes. The right, left, and middle hepatic vessels are often delineated and followed as they drain into the inferior vena cava (Figure 49-39).

Differentiation of a hepatic and portal vessel may be possible by evaluating the thickness of the vessel wall. In general, the walls of the portal vessels are more echogenic than those of hepatic vessels.

Divisions of the inferior vena cava (i.e., renal veins, hepatic veins, and iliac veins) may be observed. When accessing the presence of renal tissue, color mapping of the renal veins is helpful. The superior vena cava may be outlined entering the right atrium from above the heart. By following the superior vena cava into the neck, the jugular veins may be observed.

Fetal Circulation

Fetal oxygenation occurs in the placenta, where small fetal vessels on the surface of the villi are bathed by maternal blood within the intervillous spaces. Fetal basal metabolic rate and temperature are higher, causing fetal blood levels of essential nutrients to be relatively low compared with maternal blood. Oxygen and nutrients from maternal blood cross by simple diffusion to fetal vessels. Concentrations of waste products, such as urea and creatinine, are higher in fetal blood, and these products diffuse into the maternal circulation.

Fetal circulation differs from postnatal circulation. Fetal circulation bypasses the lungs because the fetal lungs do not oxygenate blood. The ductus arteriosus shunts blood away from the lungs. Fetal circulation shunts oxygenated blood arriving from the placenta away from the abdomen directly to the heart and then to the brain. The hepatobiliary system serves the important function of shunting oxygen-rich blood arriving from the placenta directly to the heart through the ductus venosus (Figure 49-40).

Oxygenated blood from the placenta flows through the umbilical vein, within the umbilical cord, to the fetal cord insertion, where it enters the abdomen (Figure 49-41). From the umbilicus, the umbilical vein courses cephalad along the falciform ligament to the liver, where it connects with the left portal vein (Figure 49-42). The left portal vein courses posteriorly to meet the right anterior and right posterior portal veins (Figure 49-43). This blood then filters into the liver sinusoids, returning to the inferior vena cava by drainage into the hepatic veins.

A special vascular connection, the **ductus venosus**, carries oxygen-rich blood from the umbilical vein directly to the inferior vena cava, which empties directly into the right atrium. This blood bypasses the liver. Inferior vena cava blood flows from the right atrium through the left atrium by way of the foramen ovale. This blood bypasses the lungs. Less oxygenated blood from the superior vena cava and a small portion of blood from the inferior vena cava empty into the right atrium and into the right ventricle. The two ventricles pump blood into the systemic circulation at the same time. Blood ejected from the left ventricle flows to the ascending aorta and to the fetal brain. From the right ventricle, the blood courses from the pulmonary artery into the **ductus arteriosus** and through the descending aorta to provide oxygenated blood to the abdominal organs. Deoxygenated blood exits the fetus through the umbilical arteries, which arise from the fetal iliac arteries. Only 5% to 10% of the blood actually circulates to the lungs. After birth, the foramen ovale, the ductus venosus, and the ductus arteriosus close; fetal circulation converts to this pattern, as seen throughout the rest of life.

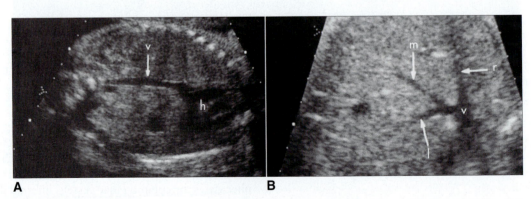

FIGURE 49-39 A, Sagittal view of the inferior vena cava *(v)* entering the right atrium of the heart *(h).* **B,** The left *(l),* middle *(m),* and right *(r)* hepatic veins are shown emptying into the inferior vena cava *(v).*

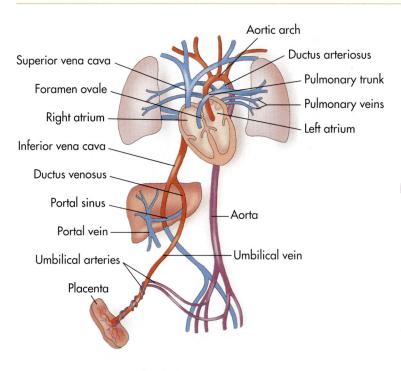

FIGURE 49-40 Fetoplacental circulation.

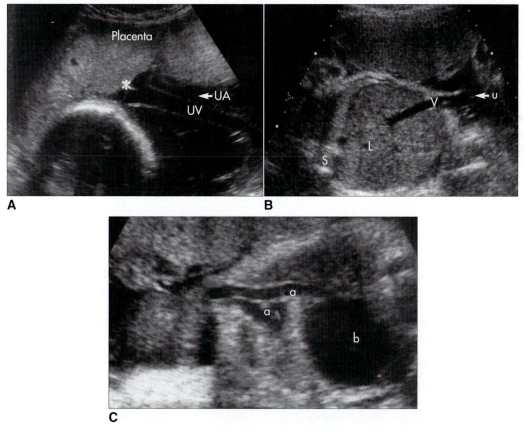

FIGURE 49-41   A, Oxygenated blood leaving the placenta travels through the umbilical vein *(UV)* to the fetal umbilicus. *UA,* umbilical artery; *asterisk,* placental cord insertion. **B,** The umbilical vein *(V)* after entering at the umbilicus *(u)* courses cephalad and into the liver *(L). S,* Spine. **C,** The umbilical arteries *(a)* enter the umbilicus and course laterally around the bladder *(b)* to meet the common iliac arteries.

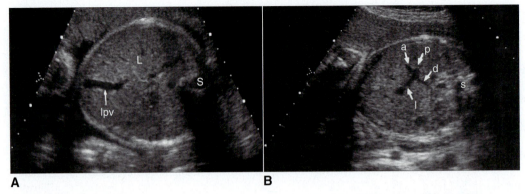

FIGURE 49-42 A, Transverse section of the liver in a 31-week fetus outlining the course of the left portal vein *(lpv)* at its entrance into the liver *(L)* from the fetal umbilical cord insertion. The left portal vein ascends upward and into the liver tissue. *S,* Spine. **B,** The left portal vein *(l)* is shown to bifurcate into the portal sinus, right anterior *(a),* and right posterior *(p)* portal veins. The ductus venosus *(d)* is observed before its drainage into the inferior vena cava.

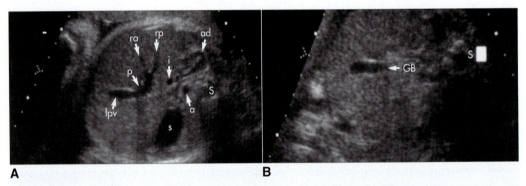

FIGURE 49-43 A, Transverse section of the liver and related structures in a 32-week fetus showing the left portal vein *(lpv)* coursing into the portal sinus *(p).* The blood then moves into the right anterior *(ra)* and right posterior *(rp)* portal veins and ductus venosus. The right adrenal gland *(ad),* fluid-filled stomach *(s),* aorta *(a),* and inferior vena cava *(i)* are shown. **B,** The gallbladder *(GB)* is viewed in the right upper quadrant of the abdomen in a 32-week fetus. The teardrop shape of the gallbladder should be distinguished from the left portal vein. *S,* Spine.

The Hepatobiliary System and Upper Abdomen

The fetal hepatobiliary system includes the liver, portal venous system, hepatic veins and arteries, gallbladder, and bile ducts. Circulation of fetal blood through the ductus venosus in the hepatobiliary system is unique to intrauterine life. The ductus venosus blood flow is a direct link to the fetal heart, and fetal heart failure may be diagnosed by Doppler analysis of flow through the ductus venosus.

The liver is a large organ that fills most of the upper abdomen. The left lobe of the liver is larger than the right lobe because of the large quantity of oxygenated blood flowing through the left lobe. The liver appears pebble-gray and is discerned by its corresponding portal and hepatic vessels. The liver borders may be seen by viewing the diaphragm at the cephalad margin and the small bowel distally in the sagittal plane (Figure 49-44). The fetal liver is the main storage site for glucose and is very sensitive to disturbances in growth; therefore, this is the site at which abdominal measurements reflect liver size.

It is important to check for any collection of fluid around the liver margins because this indicates ascites, that is, fluid retention resulting from anemia, heart failure, or congenital anomalies. Masses of the liver are uncommon but may be detected.

The fetal gallbladder appears as a cone-shaped or teardrop-shaped cystic structure located in the right upper abdomen just below the left portal vein (see Figure 49-43). The gallbladder should not be misinterpreted as the left portal vein. The left portal vein is a midline vessel that appears more tubular and can be traced back to the umbilical insertion.

The fetal pancreas may be seen posterior to the stomach and anterior to the splenic vein when the fetus is lying with the spine down.

The spleen may be observed by scanning transversely and posteriorly to the left of the stomach (Figure 49-45). Recognition of the spleen is helpful when assessing the sensitized pregnancy (anti-D) to check for enlargement resulting from increased blood production (hematopoiesis) or to screen for anomalies of the spleen, such as duplication defects.

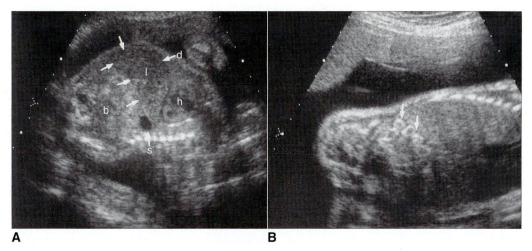

A   **B**

FIGURE 49-44 A, Liver *(l, arrows)* bordered by the diaphragm *(d)* superiorly and the bowel inferiorly in a 29-week fetus. **B,** Small bowel *(arrows)* pictured as small fluid-filled rings. *b,* Bowel; *h,* heart; *s,* stomach.

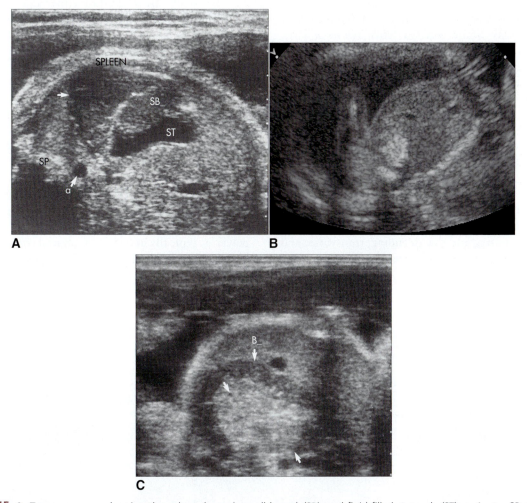

A   **B**

C

FIGURE 49-45 A, Transverse scan showing the spleen *(arrow)*, small bowel *(SB)*, and fluid-filled stomach *(ST)*. *a,* Aorta; *SP,* spine shadow. **B,** Longitudinal view of the fetus demonstrating hyperechoic bowel. **C,** Transverse view of the transverse colon *(B)* and small bowel *(arrows)* in a fetus in a spine-down position.

The Gastrointestinal System

The fetal gastrointestinal tract comprises the esophagus, stomach, and small and large intestines (colon). Guidelines for the standard antepartum obstetric examination require the sonographer to image and document the stomach. The esophagus may be recognized after fetal ingestion of amniotic fluid, which may be traced during swallowing into the oral cavity, through the hypopharynx, and as it travels downward toward the stomach (see Figure 49-36).

The stomach becomes apparent as early as the 11th week of gestation because swallowed amniotic fluid fills the stomach cavity. The full stomach should be seen in all fetuses beyond the 16th week of gestation. Some conditions, such as diminished amounts of amniotic fluid (fetuses with rupture of the membranes) or blockage that prevents the stomach from filling (esophageal atresia), prohibit normal filling of the stomach. On occasion, the stomach has emptied into the small bowel before scanning and is not observed. Repeat studies to confirm the presence of the stomach are warranted. Enlargement of the stomach may occur when a fetus ingests a large quantity of amniotic fluid (non–insulin-dependent diabetic pregnancies), or when a congenital anomaly prohibits normal passage of fluid through the bowel (duodenal atresia).

A normal bowel may be distinguished prenatally by observing characteristic sonographic patterns for each segment. Beyond 20 weeks' gestation, small bowel may be differentiated from large bowel. Small bowel appears to occupy a central position within the lower abdomen, with a cluster appearance of the bowel loops. Peristalsis and even fluid-filled small bowel loops may be observed (see Figures 49-44 and 49-45).

The large intestine and the ascending, transverse, and descending colon and rectum are identified by their peripheral locations in the lower pelvis (see Figure 49-45). The large bowel typically contains meconium particles and may measure up to 20 mm in the preterm fetus and even larger near the time of birth or in the postdate fetus.

The echogenicity of the fetal bowel is typically greater than the echogenicity of the fetal liver. If the fetal bowel is as echogenic as fetal bone, this is known as **hyperechoic bowel** (see Figure 49-45) and is associated with increased risk for aneuploidy and neonatal/childhood pathology.

The Urinary System

Guidelines for the standard obstetric examination require the sonographer to image and document the kidneys and the bladder. The urinary system of the fetus is composed of the kidneys, ureters, and bladder. The adrenal glands are more prominent in the fetus and are seen adjacent to the kidneys.

The kidneys are located on either side of the spine in the posterior abdomen and are apparent as early as the 13th week of pregnancy. The appearance of the developing kidney changes with advancing GA. In the second trimester of pregnancy, the kidneys appear as ovoid retroperitoneal structures that lack distinctive borders. The pelvocaliceal center may be difficult to define in early pregnancy, whereas with continued maturation of the kidneys, the borders become more defined and the renal pelvis becomes more distinct (Figure 49-46). The renal pelvis appears as an echo-free area in the center of the kidney.

The normal renal pelvis appears to contain a small amount of fluid. This most often represents a normal finding during pregnancy. A measurement of the renal pelvis is typically made in a sagittal view of the fetal kidney when fluid is present. The deepest diameter of the

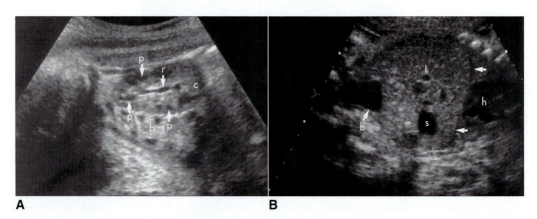

FIGURE 49-46 A, Longitudinal view of the kidney in a 35-week fetus showing the renal cortex *(c)*, pelvis, and pyramids *(p)*. The kidney is marginated by the renal capsule, which is highly visible later in pregnancy because of perirenal fat. *b,* Bowel; *r,* renal pelvis. **B,** Sagittal view of the fluid-filled bladder *(b)* in the pelvis. Note the more cephalic location of the stomach *(s)* in the upper abdomen. *h,* Heart; *L,* liver; *arrows,* diaphragm.

fluid is measured. A renal pelvis that measures greater than 5 mm before 20 weeks' GA, greater than 8 mm between 20 and 30 weeks' GA, and greater than 10 mm beyond 30 weeks' GA is considered abnormal. It is common to see extra fluid within the renal pelvis in fetuses with extra amounts of amniotic fluid and when the mother has a full bladder. Persistent mild bilateral renal pelvis dilation known as **pyelectasis** (Figure 49-47) has been associated with aneuploidy.

By the third trimester of pregnancy, internal renal anatomy becomes clear with observation of the renal pyramids (lining up in sequence in anterior and posterior rows), the cortex or medulla, and renal margins (perirenal and sinus fat at this age allows clear visualization) (see Figures 49-45 and 49-46).

The kidneys appear as elliptic structures when scanning in the longitudinal axis and appear circular in their retroperitoneal locations adjacent to the spine in transverse views. Commonly, in a transverse position, the acoustic spine may shadow the bottom or distal kidney. Rotating to the sagittal plane may image the distal kidney. With the fetus in the spine-up or spine-down position, the kidneys are observed lateral to the spine (see Figure 49-46).

The length, width, thickness, and volume of the kidney have been determined for different GAs. This information is useful when a renal malformation is suspected.

The fetal adrenal glands are most frequently observed in a transverse plane just above the kidneys. The adrenals are seen as early as the 20th week of pregnancy and by 23 weeks assume a rice-grain appearance (Figure 49-48). The center of the adrenal gland appears as a central echogenic line surrounded by tissue that is less echogenic. The central midline interface widens after the 35th week of gestation. The transverse aorta may be used to locate the left adrenal gland because of its close proximity to the anterior surface of the gland. Likewise, the inferior vena cava is helpful in isolating the right adrenal gland. Occasionally, the adrenal glands may be identified in sagittal planes, although rib shadowing may interfere with their recognition.

It is important to realize that adrenal glands may normally appear large in utero and should not be confused with the kidneys. The texture of the adrenal gland is similar to that of the kidney; when a kidney is missing (agenesis), the adrenal may be mistaken for the kidney. Nomograms for normal adrenal size are available.

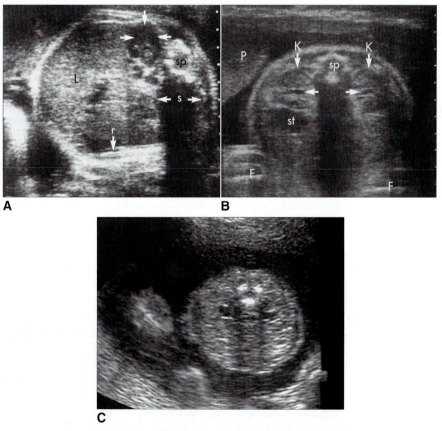

FIGURE 49-47 A, When the fetus is lying on its side, the upper kidney *(arrows)* is observed adjacent to the spine *(sp)*. The kidney on the bottom is shadowed *(s)* by the spine. *L,* liver; *r,* rib. **B,** Kidneys *(K)* observed in a spine-up position *(sp)*. Note the renal pelves *(arrows)*, which are filled with urine—a normal pregnancy finding. The stomach *(st)* is found anterior to the left kidney. Note the spine shadow. *F,* Femora; *P,* placenta. **C,** A transverse image demonstrating bilateral pyelectasis of the kidney.

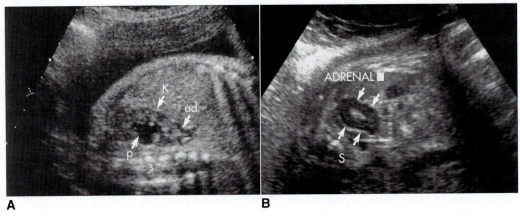

FIGURE 49-48 A, The adrenal gland *(ad)* is observed in a sagittal view in a 32-week fetus. The adrenal is located above the kidney *(K)* in this spine-down *(s)* position. The texture of the adrenal gland is similar to that of the kidney; often, when a kidney is missing (agenesis), the adrenal is mistaken for the kidney. *p,* Renal pelvis. **B,** The rice-grain appearance of the adrenal gland *(arrows)* is depicted in this transverse plane in a 36-week fetus. Note the dense central interface. *S,* Stomach.

Visualization of the renal arteries with color Doppler may be helpful in confirming the presence of kidneys.

At 1 mm, the normal fetal ureter is too small to be recognized. Dilated or obstructed ureters (hydroureter) are readily apparent.

The urinary bladder is visualized in transverse or sagittal sections through the anterior lower pelvis (see Figures 49-41 and 49-46). The bladder is located in midline and appears as a round, fluid-filled cavity. The size of the bladder varies, depending on the amount of urine contained within the bladder cavity. A fetus generally voids at least once an hour, so failure to see the bladder should prompt the investigator to recheck for bladder filling.

The bladder should be visualized in all normal fetuses. The fetal bladder is an important indicator of renal function. When the bladder and amniotic fluid appear normal, one may assume that at least one kidney is functioning. If one fails to identify the urinary bladder in the presence of oligohydramnios (severe lack of amniotic fluid), one should suspect a renal abnormality or premature rupture of the membranes. In some normal situations, the bladder may not be full because of decreased ingestion of fluid. When the bladder empties in utero, it will typically refill within the time frame of an examination.

Fetal bladder size may appear increased in pregnancies complicated by polyhydramnios (large quantities of amniotic fluid).

The Genitalia

Guidelines for the standard antepartum obstetric examination require the sonographer to image and document the stomach, the kidneys, the bladder, the umbilical cord insertion site, and the number of vessels in the umbilical cord. Documentation of gender is not medically necessary in most pregnancies.

Identification of the male and female genitalia is possible provided the fetal legs are abducted and a sufficient quantity of amniotic fluid is present. Providing information regarding gender identification is clinically important when a fetus is at risk for a gender-linked disorder such as aqueductal stenosis or hemophilia and in multiple gestations. In multiple pregnancies, there is a medical indication for determining gender, as it relates to chorionicity.

Information regarding the gender of the fetus may have significant emotional impact; therefore, guidelines should be established within each department regarding its disclosure. Only sonographers with proven gender detection skills should attempt to provide this information and only with consent of the patient.

When attempting to localize the genitalia, the sonographer should follow the long axis of the fetus toward the hips. The bladder is a helpful landmark within the pelvis by which to identify the anteriorly located genital organs. Tangential scanning planes directed between the thighs are useful in defining the genitalia. The gender of the fetus may be appreciated as early as 12 weeks' gestation. When the fetus is in a breech position, gender may be difficult to determine.

The female genitalia may be seen in a transverse plane. The thighs and labia are identified ventral to the bladder, whereas in tangential projections, the entire labial folds and often the labia minora are visible (Figure 49-49). In scans of the perineum obtained parallel to the femora, the shape of the genitalia appears rhomboid (Figure 49-50). Keep in mind that the labia may appear edematous and swollen owing to circulating maternal hormones. This normal finding should not be confused with the scrotum.

The scrotum and penis are fairly easy to recognize in either scanning plane (Figure 49-51). The male genitalia may be differentiated as early as the 12th week of pregnancy. The scrotal sac is seen as a mass of soft tissue

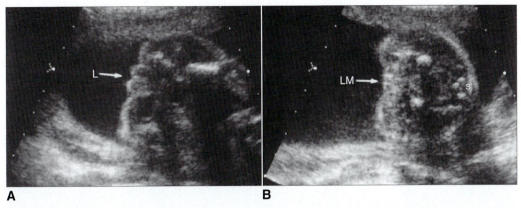

FIGURE 49-49 A, Female genitalia viewed axially in a 23-week fetus showing the typical appearance of the labia majora *(L)*. **B,** In the same fetus, the labia minora *(LM)* are represented as linear structures between the labia majora. *s,* Spine.

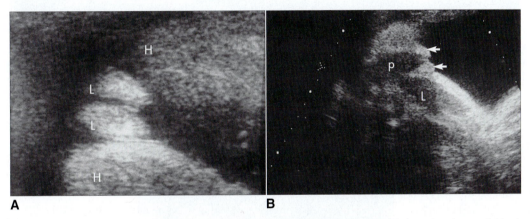

FIGURE 49-50 A, The labia majora *(L)* are imaged in a sagittal plane. *H,* Hips. **B,** The rhomboid-shaped perineum *(p)* is shown in a plane that runs parallel to the femur *(L)*. The labia *(arrows)* are observed in a more frontal plane.

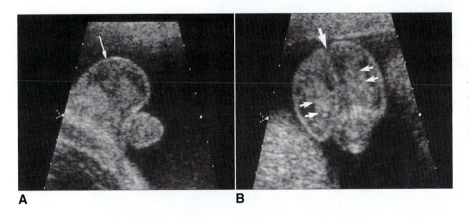

FIGURE 49-51 A, Male genitalia in a 40-week fetus showing the scrotum *(arrow)* and phallus. **B,** Coronal view of the male genitalia outlining descended testicles *(double arrows)* within the scrotum. Note the scrotal septum *(thick arrow)* and phallus.

between the hips, with the scrotal septum and testicles. Fluid around the testicles—hydrocele—is a common benign finding during intrauterine life.

The Upper and Lower Extremities

Guidelines for the standard obstetric examination require the sonographer to verify the presence or absence of legs and arms. The fetal limbs are accessible to both anatomic and biometric surveillance. Bones of the upper and lower skeleton have been described extensively, and many nomograms detailing normal growth patterns for each limb have been generated.

Fetal long-bone measurements help assess fetal age and growth and allow detection of skeletal dysplasias and various congenital limb malformations. Short femora and a short humerus is associated with increased risk for aneuploidy. The sonographer may not only measure fetal limb bones but also survey the anatomic configurations of individual bones whenever possible for evidence of bowing, fracture, or demineralization, as seen in several common forms of skeletal dysplasia.

The upper extremity consists of the humerus, elbow, radius, ulna, wrist, metacarpals, and phalanges.

The humerus is found in a sagittal plane by moving the probe laterally away from the ribs and scapula. The long axis of the humerus should be seen lateral to the scapular echo. The cartilaginous humeral head is noted, as is the cartilage at the elbow (Figure 49-52). The shaft

of the humerus should be seen, along with its characteristic acoustic shadow. The muscles and skin may be noted. Epiphyseal ossification centers may be apparent around the 39th week of pregnancy. In transverse planes, the humerus appears as a solitary bone surrounded by muscle and skin.

By tracing the humerus to the elbow, the radius and ulna are imaged (Figure 49-53; see also Figure 49-52). In transverse sections, two bones are seen as echogenic dots,

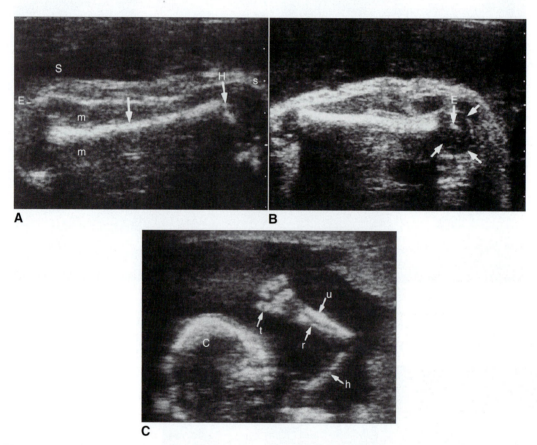

FIGURE 49-52 **A,** Longitudinal scan of the humeral shaft with the humeral head *(H)* near the shoulder *(s).* Note the muscles *(m)* lateral to the bones and the skin interface *(S).* *E,* Elbow. **B,** Similar section of a humerus in a 39-week fetus identifying the proximal humeral epiphysis *(E)* within the humeral cartilage *(arrows).* **C,** Sagittal image of the fetal humerus *(h).* *C,* Cranium; *r,* radius; *t,* thumb; *u,* ulna.

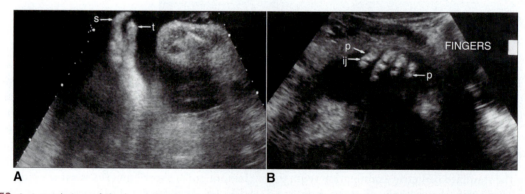

FIGURE 49-53 **A,** Lateral view of the hand showing the thumb *(t)* and second finger *(s)* in a 36-week fetus. **B,** Curvature of the hand in a 30-week fetus showing the phalanges *(p)* of the second through fifth fingers. The thumb is not imaged in this view because it is located slightly lower. Note the interphalangeal joints *(ij)* between the phalanges.

whereas in a sagittal plane, the long axis of each is identified. The laterally positioned ulna projects deeper into the elbow, which is helpful in differentiating this bone from the medially located radius. When the transducer is moved downward, the wrist and hand are observed.

The hands and fingers may be viewed, and it should be noted whether the hands are clenched throughout the examination, or if they open and close normally. When the fingers are viewed in the sagittal plane, individual phalanges, interphalangeal joints, metacarpals, and digits may be observed (Figures 49-54 and 49-55; see also Figures 49-52 and 49-53). Hand movement counts as a positive demonstration of fetal tone that is one component of the biophysical profile. Individual fingers can often be counted even in the first trimester. It is important to observe the hands if an anomaly is suspected, as in chromosome disorders, such as trisomy 18, in which clenching of the hands is common.

Adequate amounts of amniotic fluid are essential in evaluating the hands or feet. With oligohydramnios, the extremities may be difficult to localize. Fetal position may also prevent adequate visualization of the extremities.

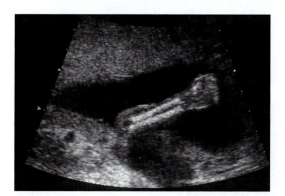

FIGURE 49-54 Long section of the forearm; the radius is shorter than the ulna (seen along the posterior forearm). The closed fist is shown with the thumb closest to the anterior surface.

Nomograms have been generated that relate the lengths of the humerus, radius, and ulna to gestational age assessment. These values are also beneficial in diagnosing abnormal developmental growth of the extremities, as seen in certain skeletal dysplasias.

Similar to the upper extremity, the bones of the lower extremity are visualized and measured both for gestational age dating and for detecting limb anomalies. The femur is the most widely measured long bone and can be found by moving the transducer along the fetal body to the fetal bladder. At this junction, the iliac wings are noted. By moving the transducer inferior to the iliac crests, the femoral echo comes into view. With the transducer centered over the femoral echo, one should rotate the probe until the shaft (diaphysis) of the femur is observed. In this view, the cartilaginous femoral head, muscles, and occasionally the femoral artery are noted (Figure 49-56).

The distal femoral epiphysis is seen within the cartilage at the knee (see Figure 49-56), and this signifies a gestational age beyond 33 to 35 weeks' gestation. At the tibial end, the proximal tibial epiphyseal center is found after the 35th week of pregnancy (Figure 49-57). Medially, the tibia and the laterally positioned fibula (see Figure 49-57) are noted. The tibia is larger than the fibula.

The ankle, calcaneus, and foot are viewed at the most distal point (Figure 49-58). The diagnosis of clubfeet may be suspected when persistent and abnormal flexion of the ankle is seen. Individual metatarsals and toes are frequently seen (see Figure 49-58). Similar to the hands, fetal feet may have malformations, such as extra digits, overlapping, and splaying.

EXTRAFETAL OBSTETRIC EVALUATION

After the fetus has been studied, evaluation of the placenta, amniotic fluid, umbilical cord, and pelvis is recommended.

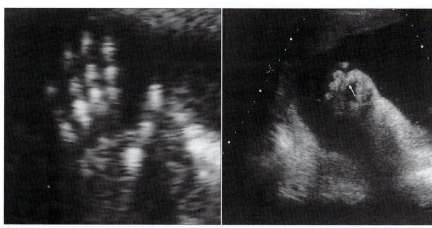

FIGURE 49-55 **A,** An open hand is shown in a 24-week fetus. **B,** A closed hand is viewed in a 38-week fetus with the thumb crossing in front of the palm of the hand *(arrow)*, with the second through fifth digits identified above the thumb.

A   B

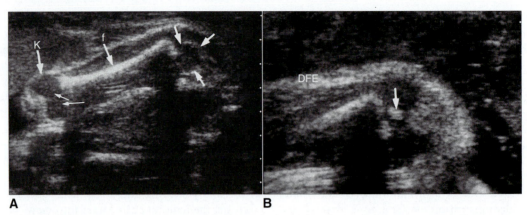

FIGURE 49-56 **A,** Longitudinal section showing the femoral shaft *(f),* with the femoral cartilage *(thick arrows)* and epiphyseal cartilage *(thin arrows)* shown at the knee *(K).* **B,** The distal femoral epiphysis *(arrow)* is clearly shown within the epiphyseal cartilage at the knee in a 42-week fetus. *DFE,* Distal femoral epiphysis.

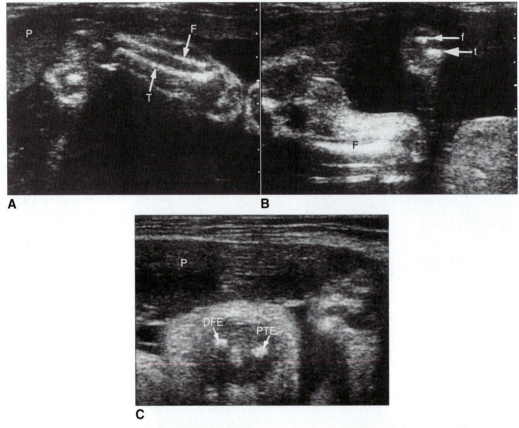

FIGURE 49-57 **A,** Sagittal view of the medially positioned tibia *(T)* and the laterally positioned fibula *(F). P,* Placenta. **B,** In the same fetus, a transverse cross section reveals the two bones. *F,* Fibula; *f,* opposite femur; *P,* placenta; *t,* tibia. **C,** View of the knee in a 42-week fetus showing both the distal femoral epiphysis (DFE) and the proximal tibial epiphysis (PTE).

The Umbilical Cord

Guidelines for the standard antepartum obstetric examination require the sonographer to image and document the umbilical cord insertion site and the number of vessels in the umbilical cord. The normal human umbilical cord contains an umbilical vein and two umbilical arteries (Figure 49-59). The umbilical vein transports oxygenated blood from the placenta, whereas the paired umbilical arteries return deoxygenated blood from the iliac arteries of the fetus to the placenta for purification. The umbilical cord is identified at the cord insertion into the placenta and at the junction of the cord into the fetal umbilicus. The arteries spiral with the larger umbilical vein, which is surrounded by Wharton's jelly (material that supports the cord) (Figure 49-60). Absent cord twists may be associated with a poor pregnancy outcome. The cord is easily imaged in both sagittal and transverse

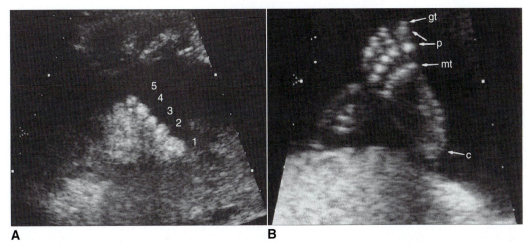

FIGURE 49-58 **A,** Five toes (*1* to *5*) viewed on end in a 38-week fetus. Note the continuity and shape of each toe. Extra toes, webbing, or clefts are considered abnormal. **B,** Plantar foot view in a 20-week fetus showing five toes and ossified metatarsals *(mt)* and phalanges *(p). c,* Calcaneus; *gt,* great toe.

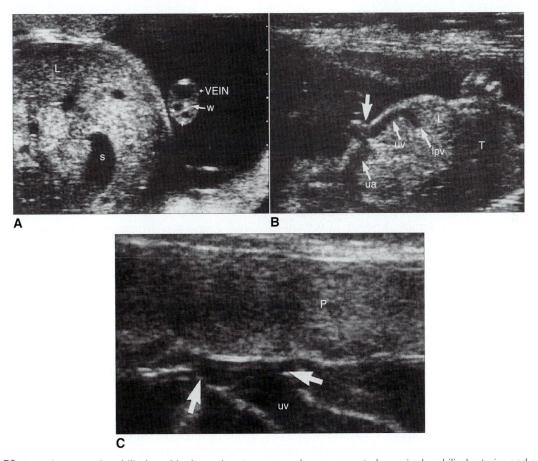

FIGURE 49-59 **A,** A three-vessel umbilical cord is shown in a transverse plane represented as paired umbilical arteries and a single larger umbilical vein. The vessels are supported by the gelatinous Wharton's jelly *(w).* A cross section of the liver *(L)* and stomach *(s)* is in view. **B,** Fetal insertion of the umbilical cord into the umbilicus in a sagittal plane *(large arrow).* The umbilical vein *(uv)* courses superiorly to enter the liver *(L)* and becomes the left portal vein *(lpv),* whereas the umbilical arteries *(ua)* course posteriorly to join the hypogastric arteries. *T,* Thoracic cavity. **C,** Placental insertion of the umbilical cord showing the umbilical vein *(uv)* at this junction *(arrows). P,* Anterior placenta.

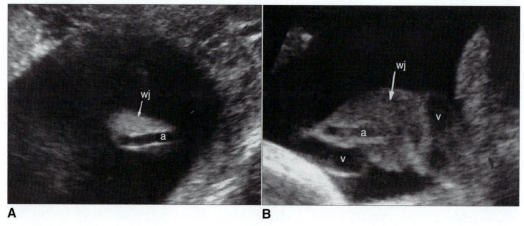

FIGURE 49-60 **A,** Wharton's jelly *(wj)* observed in a 30-week fetus. One of the umbilical arteries *(a)* is in view. **B,** Wharton's jelly is present adjacent to one of the umbilical arteries *(a)*, and the single umbilical vein *(v)* is observed in a 35-week fetus. Wharton's jelly is an important structure to recognize in performing cordocentesis procedures when the needle is directed into the cord vessels.

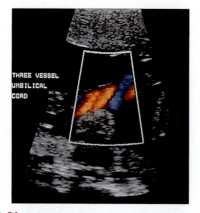

FIGURE 49-61 Color Doppler image showing the cord insertion into the fetal abdomen.

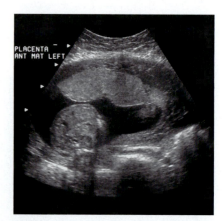

FIGURE 49-62 The homogeneous placenta is shown along the anterior wall of the uterus. The fetal abdomen is seen in cross section.

sections. The umbilical vein diameter increases throughout gestation, reaching a maximum diameter of 0.9 cm by 30 weeks' gestation.

When cord is seen on both sides of the fetal neck, color Doppler may be used to visualize nuchal cord or encirclement of cord around the fetal neck. Multiple loops of nuchal cord have been identified with color Doppler.

Identification of the placental insertion of the cord is important in choosing a site for amniocentesis and in selecting the appropriate site for other invasive procedures. Rarely, the umbilical insertion is atypically located (velamentous insertion).

Insertion of the cord into the fetal umbilicus should be routinely scrutinized in all fetuses because anterior abdominal wall defects are present at this level. Use of color Doppler imaging at this location may demonstrate two umbilical arteries traveling on either side of the fetal bladder toward the iliacs. This image confirms two arteries and aids in three-vessel identification (Figure 49-61).

The uterus and ovaries should be scrutinized for large masses, such as fibroids or ovarian masses that may

alter pregnancy management. This evaluation may be accomplished by surveying the lateral borders of the uterus from the cervix to the fundus along both lateral margins while following both sagittal and transverse axes.

The Placenta

The major role of the placenta is to permit the exchange of oxygenated maternal blood (rich in oxygen and nutrients) with deoxygenated fetal blood. Maternal vessels coursing posterior to the placenta circulate blood into the placenta, whereas blood from the fetus reaches this point through the umbilical cord.

The substance of the placenta assumes a relatively homogeneous pebble-gray appearance during the first part of pregnancy and is easily recognized with its characteristically smooth borders (Figure 49-62). The position of the placenta is readily apparent on most obstetric ultrasound studies. The placenta may be located within the fundus of the uterus along the anterior, lateral, or posterior uterine walls (Figure 49-63), or it may be

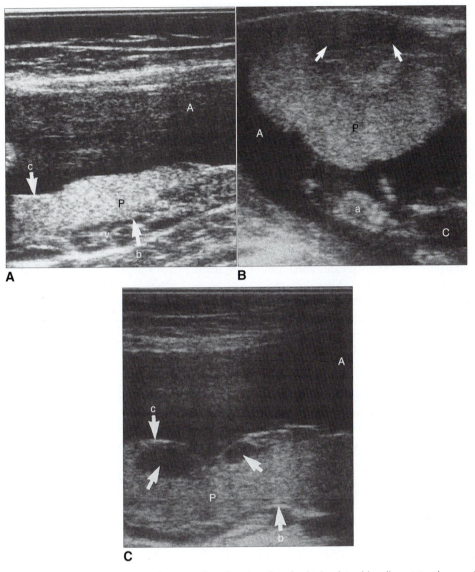

FIGURE 49-63 A, Posterior placenta *(P)* at 21 weeks' gestation showing the chorionic plate *(c)*, adjacent to the amniotic cavity *(A)*, and the basal plate *(b)*, closest to the maternal (endometrial) vessels *(v)*. **B,** Anterior placenta *(P)* at 14 weeks' gestation with evidence of a Braxton-Hicks contraction *(arrows)*. *A,* Amniotic fluid; *C,* fetal cranium; *a,* fetal abdomen. **C,** Posterior placenta *(P)* at 26 weeks' gestation showing several subchorionic cystic spaces *(arrows)* that represent blood vessels or fibrin deposits. *A,* Amniotic fluid; *b,* basal plate; *c,* chorionic plate.

implanted over or near the cervix. The sonographer should attempt to carefully define the entire length of the placenta and should document both upper and lower margins of this organ.

The placenta may originate close to the fundus and extend along the anterior wall (anterior placenta) or along the posterior uterine wall (posterior placenta). When the placenta appears to lie on both anterior and posterior uterine walls, check for a laterally positioned placenta. By moving the transducer laterally, one should be able to define the lateral placenta.

The Amniotic Fluid

Amniotic fluid serves several important functions during intrauterine life. It allows the fetus to move freely within the amniotic cavity while maintaining intrauterine pressure and protecting the developing fetus from injury. The umbilical cord and membranes, lungs, skin, and kidneys all contribute to the production of amniotic fluid. Fetal urination into the amniotic sac accounts for most of the total volume of amniotic fluid by the second half of pregnancy, and the quantity of fluid is directly related to kidney function. A fetus lacking kidneys or with malformed kidneys produces little or no amniotic fluid. The amount of amniotic fluid is regulated not only by the production of amniotic fluid but also by removal of fluid by swallowing, by fluid exchange within the lungs, and by the membranes and cord. Normal lung development is critically dependent on the exchange of amniotic fluid within the lungs. Inadequate lung development may occur when severe oligohydramnios is present, placing the fetus at high risk for developing small or hypoplastic lungs.

The volume of amniotic fluid increases until the 34th week of gestation and then slowly diminishes. The investigator must be aware of relative differences in amniotic fluid volume throughout pregnancy. During the second and early third trimesters of pregnancy, amniotic fluid appears to surround the fetus and should be readily apparent (Figure 49-64). From 20 to 30 weeks' gestation, amniotic fluid may appear somewhat generous, although this typically represents a normal amniotic fluid variant. By the end of pregnancy, amniotic fluid is scanty, and isolated fluid pockets may be the only visible areas of fluid. Subjective observation of amniotic fluid volumes throughout pregnancy helps the sonographer determine the norm and extremes of amniotic fluid.

Several semiquantitative methods of estimating amniotic fluid volume have been developed. Measurement of the deepest vertical pocket of fluid in each of the four quadrants of the uterus and measurement of the single deepest pocket in the sac are two such methods. The deepest vertical pocket is the most commonly used method for biophysical profiles and multiple pregnancy examinations.

Amniotic fluid generally appears echo-free, although occasionally fluid particles (particulate matter) may be seen. Vernix caseosa (fatty material found on fetal skin and in amniotic fluid late in pregnancy) may be seen within the amniotic fluid.

In accordance with the guidelines for obstetric scanning, every obstetric examination should include an evaluation of amniotic fluid volume. When extremes in amniotic fluid volume (polyhydramnios or oligohydram-

nios) are found, targeted studies for the exclusion of fetal anomalies are recommended.

The Membranes

The inner membrane—the amnion—and the outer membrane—the chorion—typically are not seen during the second and third trimesters. The amnion is contiguous with the membrane lining the umbilical cord. At the site of umbilical cord insertion into the placenta, the amnion spreads out over the surface of the chorionic surface of the placenta. At the edge of the placenta, the amnion lies over the smooth chorion lining the uterine wall. When there is a break in the amnion, fluid can infuse between the amnion and chorion. If fluid is seen under a membrane floating on top of the placenta and anchored at the placental cord insertion, this is a subamniotic collection. If fluid is seen under a membrane and fluid collection ends at the edge of the placenta, it is a subchorionic collection.

The Cervix

The uterine cervix in pregnancy can be visualized with abdominal scanning when the maternal bladder is partially full. Image quality is better and the cervical measurements more reproducible when the cervix is visualized and measured using transvaginal or transperineal imaging. When the cervix appears shortened during the abdominal scan, or when the patient is at risk for incompetent cervix or premature delivery, transperineal or transvaginal imaging of the cervix is added to the second-trimester examination. The normal cervix in pregnancy

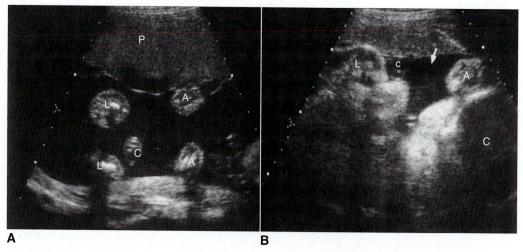

FIGURE 49-64 A, Amniotic fluid in a 20-week pregnancy outlining the legs *(L)* and arms *(A).* This is a typical appearance of the abundance of amniotic fluid during this period of pregnancy. *c,* Umbilical cord; *P,* placenta. **B,** Amniotic fluid *(arrow)* in a 35-week pregnancy demonstrating an amniotic fluid pocket *(arrow)* surrounded by fetal parts and the placenta. The amount of amniotic fluid compared with the fetus and placenta is less at this stage of pregnancy. *A,* Arm; *C,* cranium; *c,* umbilical cord; *L,* leg.

measures 3 cm or longer. If the cervix is shortened, or if the internal os appears to have a V or a U shape, it may be important to monitor and/or intervene.

GENETIC SONOGRAM

A common type of specialized second-trimester obstetric sonography examination is called the **genetic sonogram.** In a genetic sonogram, the patient's individual risk for aneuploidy is adjusted on the basis of sonographic findings. The genetic sonogram includes all elements of the standard obstetric examination with additional attention to anatomic markers for aneuploidy. The markers that are typically evaluated include the nuchal fold, echogenic bowel, humerus length, femur length, EIF, and renal pyelectasis.

Researchers have defined statistical **likelihood ratios** for aneuploidy for each of these *anatomy markers*. For example, a fetus with echogenic bowel may have a risk (or likelihood) for aneuploidy that is increased sixfold. The probability that a fetus with echogenic bowel may have an aneuploidy is six times greater than the probability for a fetus without echogenic bowel. Because these markers are independent and are also independent of age and biochemistry, the probabilities for each element can be multiplied together to determine individual risk.

Patients enter a genetic sonogram with a risk for aneuploidy determined by age or biochemistry. This risk may be increased if a single marker is found by a factor consistent with the likelihood ratio associated with that finding. For example, if a 35-year-old women enters a genetic sonogram with a risk of 1 in 200 and echogenic bowel is found, the risk can be adjusted, that is, increased, to 1 in 33. If two or more anatomic markers are documented, the risk is increased even further.

Somewhat more controversial is lowering risk by a factor of one half or more if no anatomic markers are found. For example, a patient at age 35 with an aneuploidy risk of approximately 1:200 may have that risk lowered by a factor of one half or more with a normal sonogram. This patient would be counseled regarding a risk level of approximately 1 in 400.

The genetic sonogram and risk adjustment based on sonographic findings in the second trimester should be limited to centers with specialty expertise and partnered with genetic counselors and resources. The anatomic markers must be interpreted carefully, and experience can eliminate errors associated with assignment of markers such as hyperechoic bowel or EIF that include subjective assessment of echogenicity.

ACKNOWLEDGMENT

The author would like to acknowledge the work of Kara L. Mayden Argo on a previous edition of this book.

Obstetric Measurements and Gestational Age

Terry J. DuBose and Sandra L. Hagen-Ansert

OBJECTIVES

On completion of this chapter, you should be able to:
- List gestational sac growth and measurements
- Describe how to perform a crown-rump measurement
- Calculate the biparietal diameter, head circumference, abdominal circumference, and extremity measurements

- Assess fetal parameter measurements and fetal growth
- Describe when other measurements should be used to provide additional clinical information
- Evaluate the fetal growth series for IUGR and growth disturbances

OUTLINE

Reliably assessing gestational age and the growth of the fetus has long posed a challenge to all who care for pregnant women. Although not without value, clinical parameters lack the necessary consistency for optimal perinatal care. With recent advances in diagnostic sonography, however, fetal age and growth can be assessed with high accuracy.

The difference between menstrual age and fetal age is important to establish in clinical obstetrics. *Fetal age* begins at the time of conception and is also known as *conceptional age*. Conceptional age is restricted to pregnancies in which the actual date of conception is known, as found in patients with in vitro fertilization or artificial insemination. If conceptual age is already known, the menstrual age may be found by adding 14 days to the conceptual age.

Obstetricians date pregnancies in menstrual weeks, which are calculated from the first day of the **last** normal **menstrual period (LMP).** This method is called *menstrual age* or *gestational age.* The student of sonography must understand that gestational ages are estimated from measurements of fetal parameters and are not the actual age of the parameters. The estimated ages are no more accurate than the measurements taken, and all parameters in a fetus will not result in the same fetal age because fetuses have different proportions: some are long; some are short; some are fat; some are thin.

It is clinically important to know the menstrual age of a patient because this information is used for the following reasons:

- In early pregnancy to schedule invasive procedures (chorionic villus sampling and genetic amniocentesis)
- To interpret maternal serum alpha-fetoprotein screening
- To plan date of delivery
- To evaluate fetal growth

Before the use of sonographic determination of fetal growth, menstrual age was calculated by three factors: (1) the menstrual history, (2) physical examination of the fundal height of the uterus, and (3) postnatal physical examination of the neonate. This process was not always reliable if the patient could not recall the date of her last period or if other factors—such as oligomenorrhea, implantation bleeding, use of oral contraceptives, or irregular menstrual cycle—were present.

GESTATIONAL AGE ASSESSMENT: FIRST TRIMESTER

Gestational Sac Diameter

Transvaginal sonography enables visualization and evaluation of intrauterine pregnancies earlier than was previously thought possible. The earliest sonographic finding of an intrauterine pregnancy is thickening of the decidua. Sonographically, this appears as an echogenic, thick filling of the fundal region of the endometrial cavity occurring at approximately 3 to 4 weeks of gestation (Box 50-1, Figure 50-1).

At approximately 4 weeks of menstrual age, a small hypoechoic area appears in the fundus or midportion of the uterus, known as the *double decidual sac sign.* As the sac embeds further into the uterus, it is surrounded by an echogenic rim and is seen within the choriodecidual tissue. This is known as the **chorionic** or **gestational sac.**

At 5 weeks, the average of the three perpendicular internal diameters of the gestational sac—calculated as the mean of the anteroposterior diameter, the transverse diameter, and the longitudinal diameter—can provide an adequate estimation of menstrual age. A gestational sac should be seen within the uterine cavity when the beta human chorionic gonadotropin (beta hCG) is above 500 mIU/ml (second international standard). This becomes especially important when evaluating a pregnancy for ectopic implantation.

The sac grows rapidly in the first 10 weeks, with an average increase of 1 mm per day. According to one report, a gestational sac growing less than 0.7 mm per day is associated with impending early pregnancy loss.[16] Even the most experienced sonographer may incorporate a measuring error; therefore, the beta-hCG test in conjunction with a sonographic evaluation is suggested in a sequential time frame.

When the gestational sac exceeds 8 mm in mean internal diameter, a yolk sac should be seen (Figure 50-2). The yolk sac is identified as a small, spherical structure with an anechoic center within the gestational sac. It provides early transfer of nutrients from the trophoblast to the embryo. It also aids in the early formation of the primitive gut and vitelline arteries and veins and in the production of the primordial germ cells. Yolk sac size has not been correlated with gestational age determination. Normal yolk sac size should be less than 6 mm. Yolk sacs greater than 8 mm have been associated with poor pregnancy outcome, as have solid, echogenic yolk sacs. Box 50-2 lists sonographic landmarks for early pregnancy.

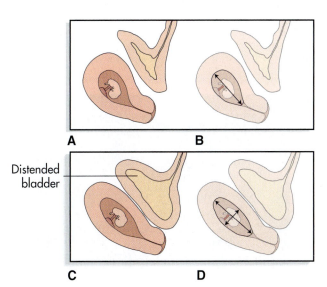

FIGURE 50-1 Gestational sac measurement. **A,** Longitudinal. **B,** The sac length should be measured from inner-to-inner borders. **C,** Longitudinal. **D,** The width of the sac should be measured along the inner-to-inner borders.

BOX 50-1	Gestational Sac Measurements

- A distended urinary bladder affects the gestational sac measurement; it changes its shape from round to ovoid or teardrop.
- If the sac is round, measure one diameter inner to inner.
- If the sac is ovoid, make two measurements inner to inner, one transverse and the other perpendicular to the length.

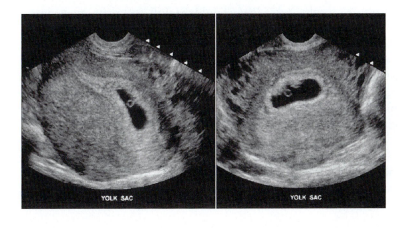

FIGURE 50-2 Sagittal and coronal images of a yolk sac in a 4-week gestation as seen with transvaginal sonography. The small gestational sac is well seen within the endometrial cavity of the uterus.

BOX 50-2	Transvaginal Sonographic Landmarks for Early Pregnancies

- 500 mIU/mL beta-hCG = gestational sac seen
- >8-mm gestational sac = yolk sac seen
- >16-mm gestational sac = embryo seen
- <6-mm yolk sac = normal
- >8-mm yolk sac = abnormal
- >7-mm fetal pole = positive cardiac activity

BOX 50-3	Crown-Rump Length (CRL)

- By transvaginal sonography, the CRL can be measured from 6 to 12 gestational weeks.
- Measurements should be made along the long axis of the embryo from the top of the head (crown) to the bottom of the trunk (rump).
- This is the most accurate fetal age measurement.

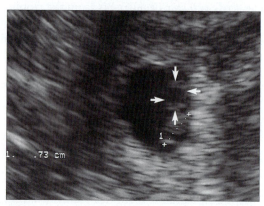

FIGURE 50-3 Transvaginal sonographic measurement of an early crown-rump length (CRL) *(crosses)*. The yolk sac is noted and outlined *(arrows)*. The CRL is consistent with 6.5 weeks.

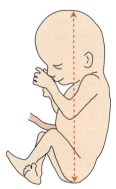

FIGURE 50-5 The crown-rump length should be measured along the long axis of the embryo from the top of the head to the bottom of the trunk.

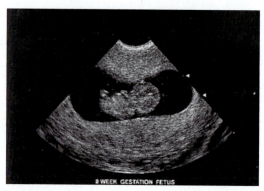

FIGURE 50-4 Transvaginal image of an 8-week gestation showing a developing embryo.

widely used as a determinant of gestational age after more accurate embryonic parameters can be measured (see Chapter 48).

Crown-Rump Length

With transvaginal sonography, embryonic echoes can be identified as early as 38 to 39 days of menstrual age (Box 50-3, Figure 50-5). The **crown-rump length (CRL)** is usually 1 to 2 mm at this stage. The embryo is usually located adjacent to the yolk sac. A CRL is the most accurate sonographic technique for establishing gestational age in the first trimester. The reason for this high accuracy is the excellent correlation between fetal length and age in early pregnancy because pathologic disorders minimally affect the growth of the embryo during this time.

The embryo can be measured easily with real-time dynamic imaging. For transabdominal imaging, the mother's bladder should be full to create an acoustic window. The measurement should be taken from the top of the fetal head to the outer fetal rump, excluding the fetal limbs or yolk sac. The accuracy is ±5 days with a 95% confidence level (Figure 50-6).[19] The average of at least three separate measurements of the CRL should be obtained to determine gestational age.

Cardiac activity should be seen when the CRL exceeds 7 mm, but it may be seen by transvaginal sonography once the CRL reaches 2 mm. It is generally accepted that it is a good idea to follow patients with small CRL and no fetal heartbeat over a few days. In general the CRL should increase at a rate of 8 mm per day. Occasionally

When the mean **gestational sac diameter** exceeds 16 mm, an embryo with definite cardiac activity should be well visualized with transvaginal scanning. This usually occurs by the 6th menstrual week (Figures 50-3 and 50-4) but may be as early as the 5th LMP week with transvaginal sonography. For the transabdominal scanning approach, the maternal urinary bladder must be filled to create an acoustic window. With this technique, the sac shape can vary secondary to bladder compression, maternal bowel gas, or myomas and should not be misinterpreted as abnormal.

Assessing gestational age using a single gestational sac diameter or even up to three averaged diameters yields an accuracy of only ±2 to 3 weeks in 90% of cases.[11] Accordingly, gestational sac diameter has not been

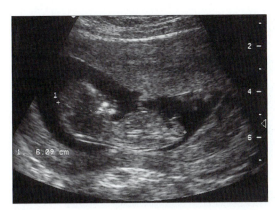

FIGURE 50-6 Transabdominal sonogram demonstrating the proper landmarks for an accurate crown-rump length (CRL) measurement. The calipers should be placed at the top of the fetal head and the bottom of the fetal rump, excluding the legs or yolk sac. The CRL is consistent with a gestation of 12 weeks and 3 days.

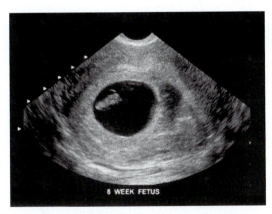

FIGURE 50-7 Transvaginal image of an 8-week gestation that shows a large gestational sac with a small, undeveloped embryo. No cardiac activity was identified.

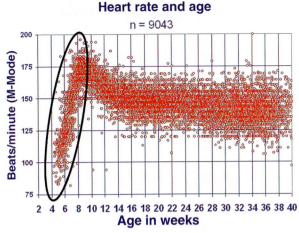

FIGURE 50-8 Scatter plot of 9043 embryofetal heart rates calculated by M-mode throughout gestation. Notice the rapid, linear acceleration in the first month from the early 5th week until the early 9th week. The peak heart rate of 175 beats per minute (mean, ±25) comes at 9.2 LMP weeks.

BOX 50-4	Embryonic Heart Rate (EHR)

- By transvaginal sonography, the EHR can be measured by M-mode to estimate age from the early 5th to early 9th gestational weeks when the CRL is less than 25 mm.
- The most accurate EHR measurements can be obtained by enlarging the 2D image and using a fast sweep speed for the M-mode tracing. Measure from repeating distinct points on the M-mode.
- The EHR age will be accurate to within ±6 days. An EHR age that trails the CRL age by more than 6 days may be associated with impending first-trimester failure and warrants follow-up.
- The normal EHR accelerates linearly at 3.3 beats per minute per day, which is approximately 10 beats every 3 days, or 100 beats in the first month of beating.

an embryo is seen with no visible cardiac activity and a small CRL for menstrual age. It is advisable to wait a week and rescan to see if the patient spontaneously aborts the products of conception or if she needs medical intervention, such as a dilation and curettage procedure. Infrequently an appropriate fetal CRL and positive cardiac activity are seen after the week's wait (Figure 50-7). Why this happens is not known, but experienced sonographers have observed it.

Absence of an embryo by 7 to 8 weeks of gestation is consistent with an embryonic demise or an anembryonic pregnancy. If a nomogram is not readily available to identify gestational age, a convenient formula is gestational age in weeks = CRL in cm + 6. After the 12th week, a CRL is no longer considered accurate because of flexion and extension of the active fetus; therefore, other biometric parameters should be used.

Embryonic Heart Rate

The **embryonic heart rate** (EHR) accelerates linearly during the first month of beating between the 5th and 9th gestational weeks (Figure 50-8). This linear acceleration correlates well with the embryonic age before the CRL reaches 2.5 cm or before approximately 9.2 LMP weeks. The mean rate of acceleration is 3.3 beats per minute per day, 10 beats per minute every 3 days, or approximately 100 beats per minute between the start of beating until the early 9th week (Box 50-4). The embryonic age in days can be estimated with the following formula:

$$\text{LMP age in days} = \text{EHR} \times 0.3 + 6 \text{ days}$$

The result of this estimation will be within ±6 days in 95% of normal pregnancies.[6] If the age estimated by the CRL leads the age by EHR by more than 1 week, it may be prognostic for first-trimester failure and warrants follow-up. Because the heart rate is accelerating so rapidly during the embryonic period, accurate M-mode measurements are desirable. The greatest accuracy can be achieved by magnifying the embryo as much as possible and using a fast M-mode tracing to stretch out the

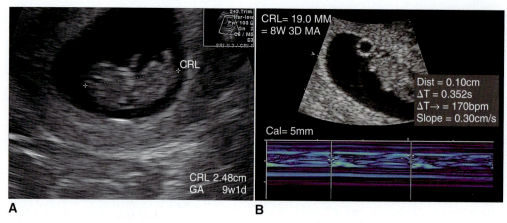

FIGURE 50-9 A, Transvaginal image measuring the CRL at 24.8 mm or 9.1 weeks. **B**, EHR of an embryo measured by M-mode to be 170 beats per minute, which calculates to 8.1 weeks. The CRL of 19.1 mm calculates to 8.4 weeks. The three-tenths week difference in the ages is equal to 50 hours, or about 2 days' difference, and is normal. (EHR age in days = 170 × 0.3 + 6 = 57.0 days = 8.14 weeks. (**A,** *Courtesy of Jyl Rogers, BS, RDMS.* **B,** *Courtesy of Lindley Diacon, MD, RDMS.*)

heartbeats for more precise cursor placement. The cursors should be carefully placed on identifiable, repeating locations of the M-mode tracing (Figure 50-9).

GESTATIONAL AGE ASSESSMENT: SECOND AND THIRD TRIMESTERS

Fetal Measurements

In the second trimester, the gestational age parameters extend to the biparietal diameter, head circumference, abdominal circumference, femur length, and other parameters that may be used. It is critical for the sonographer to know precisely which landmarks are necessary to determine these measurements. Proper gain settings, instrumentation, and fetal lie all influence the accuracy of measurements used to estimate the gestational age.

Biparietal Diameter. In the second trimester, the **biparietal diameter (BPD)** was the first and is the most widely accepted means of measuring the fetal head and estimating fetal age. As the pregnancy enters the third trimester, an accurate measurement of fetal age becomes more difficult to obtain because the fetus begins to drop into the pelvic outlet cavity. The reproducibility of the BPD is ±1 mm (±2 standard deviations). When dating a pregnancy between 17 and 26 weeks of gestation, the predictive value is ±11 days in 95% of the population.[19] After 26 weeks, the correlation of BPD with gestational age decreases because of the increased biologic variability. The predictive value decreases to ±3 weeks in the third trimester. The growth of the fetal skull slows from 3 mm per week in the second trimester to 1.8 mm per week in the third trimester.

When measuring the BPD, it is important to determine the landmarks accurately (Box 50-5, Figures 50-10 and 50-11). The fetal head should be imaged in a transverse axial section, ideally with the fetus in a direct occiput transverse position. The BPD should be

BOX 50-5	Biparietal Diameter

- Obtain biparietal leading edge–to–leading edge diameter (BPD) of the fetal head at the transverse level of the midbrain: falx, cavum septi pellucidi, and thalamic nuclei.
- Make sure the head is symmetric and oval.
- Measure from the outer to the inner margins of the skull.
- In the third trimester, the BPD is not as accurate in predicting fetal age; may approach ±3 to 3.5 weeks.

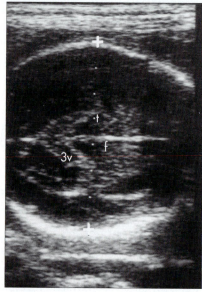

FIGURE 50-10 The biparietal diameter of the fetal head is made at the transverse level of the midbrain at the level of the falx *(f)*, cavum septi pellucidi, and thalamic nuclei *(t)*. *3v,* Third ventricle.

measured perpendicular to the fetal skull at the level of the thalamus and the cavum septi pellucidi. Intracranial landmarks should include the falx cerebri anteriorly and posteriorly, the cavum septi pellucidi anteriorly in the midline, and the choroid plexus in the atrium of each

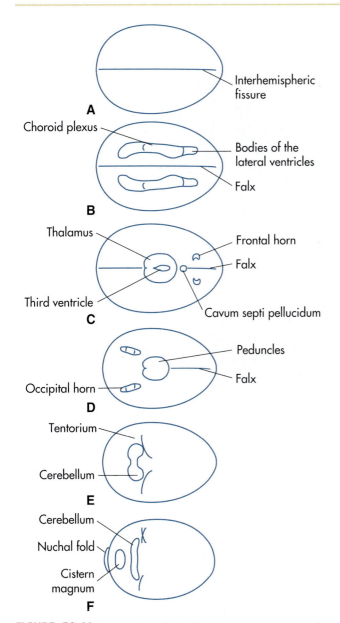

FIGURE 50-11 Progression of the fetal head anatomy in the transaxial plane from the level of the **A,** interhemispheric fissure; **B,** choroid plexus, falx, and bodies of the lateral ventricles; **C,** falx, thalamus, third ventricle, cavum septi pellucidum, frontal horns; **D,** falx, peduncles, occipital horns; **E,** tentorium, cerebellum; and **F,** cerebellum, cistern magnum, nuchal fold.

lateral ventricle (Figure 50-12). With real-time sonography, one can identify the middle cerebral artery pulsating in the insula.

The head shape should be ovoid, not round (**brachycephaly**), because this can lead to overestimation of gestational age, just as a flattened or compressed head (**dolichocephaly**) can lead to underestimation of gestational age estimated from the BPD measurement. The calipers should be placed from the leading edge of the parietal bone to the leading edge of the opposite parietal bone (known as "outer edge to inner edge"). The parietal bones should measure less than 3 mm each. On the outer edge of the fetal head, the soft tissue should not be

included; measuring should begin from the skull bone, excluding the scalp. Gain settings should not be set too high because this can produce a false thickening and incorrect measurement. A reference curve should be applicable to the local population. BPD should not be used to date a pregnancy in cases of severe ventriculomegaly, which may alter the head size and produce macrocephaly, or when microcephaly or skull-altering head lesions are present. In these cases, other biometric parameters should be used.

If the fetus is too large for an accurate CRL but too early for a BPD with the proper landmarks identified, an approximation of the BPD can be obtained by incorporating the following landmarks: a smooth, symmetric head; visible choroid plexuses; and a well-defined midline echo that is an equal distance from both parietal bones (Figure 50-13).

One technique to adjust for the biologic variability of fetal head growth uses the fetus as its own control. Two separate BPD measurements are obtained, the first between 20 and 26 weeks and the second between 31 and 33 weeks. The growth interval was compared with average growth. This technique has been termed **growth-adjusted sonar age (GASA).**[18] The fetus is then categorized into a small, average, or large growth percentile. The developers of this method claim the use of GASA reduces the range in gestational age from ±11 days to ±3 days in 90% of fetuses and to ±5 days in approximately 97% of fetuses.[19] Although GASA compensates for the biologic variability in the individual fetus, it does not take into consideration other factors, such as dolichocephaly, brachycephaly, and **oxycephaly** caused by molding, variations in head shape, or the standard error of measurement.

Head Circumference. Prenatal compression of the fetal skull is common. It occurs more often in fetal malpresentation, such as breech, or in conditions of intrauterine crowding, such as multiple pregnancies. The fetal skull can also be compressed in vertex presentations without any obvious reason or as a result of an associated uterine abnormality, such as leiomyoma. The transverse head circumference (HC) is less affected than BPD by head compression, so the HC is a valuable tool in assessing gestational age (Box 50-6, Figure 50-14).

The HC measurement is taken in the transverse plane at the level of the BPD and can be calculated from the same frozen image. Most modern sonographic equipment has built-in electronic calipers that open to

BOX 50-6	Transverse Head Circumference (HC)

- Use the transverse plane at the level of the BPD to calculate head circumference (HC).
- Place area calipers along the outer margin of the skull to obtain circumference.
- Accurate to ±2 to 3 weeks.

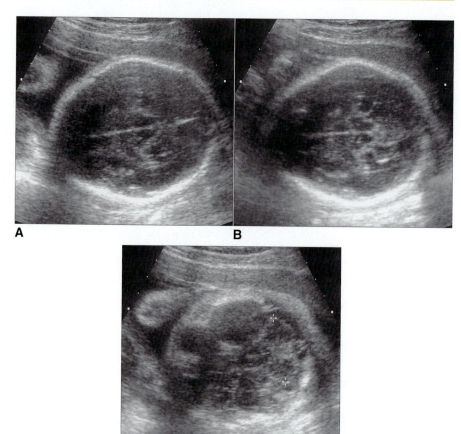

FIGURE 50-12 Transverse section through the fetal head taken at the level of the thalamus and the cavum septum pellucidi. **A,** The biparietal diameter (BPD) is measured from the outer border of the proximal skull to the inner border of the distal skull, or leading edge to leading edge. **B,** The head should be oval in shape because too round or too flat of a head leads to overestimation or underestimation of fetal age. **C,** Inferior angulation from the BPD shows the posterior fossa with the cerebellum *(crossbars)*.

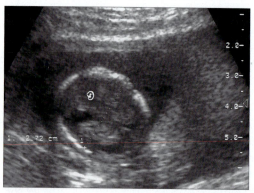

FIGURE 50-13 This 14-week fetus is too big for a crown-rump length measurement yet too small to distinguish the proper biparietal landmarks in the fetal head. At this gestational age, it is acceptable to measure the fetal head at the level of the choroid plexus, which is echogenic and fills most of the head at this time. The same measurement criteria of outer border to inner border should be used.

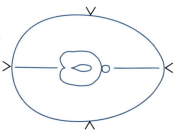

FIGURE 50-14 Head circumference should be taken at the level of the biparietal diameter; the calipers should be placed along the outer margin of the skull to obtain the measurement.

the outline of the fetal head. If this feature is not available, the measurement can be obtained with a light pen, map reader, or electronic planimeter or by manually measuring with the electronic calipers. To measure the widest transverse diameter of the skull manually, the BPD level should be measured with the calipers on the outer border of each side (D1). The length of the occipital frontal diameter (OFD) should then be measured (D2). This is done by measuring from the outer border of the occiput to the outer border of the frontal bone (Figure 50-15). To obtain an accurate HC measurement, 60% to 70% of the skull outline should be displayed on the screen. HC can then be calculated by the following formula:

$$AC = \frac{D1 + D2 \times \pi}{2}$$

Therefore,

$$AC = (D1 + D2) \times 1.57$$

Vertical Cranial Diameter, Coronal View, and 3D BPD Correction. The coronal view of the fetal head is useful for viewing anatomy and assessing the degree of head molding and biologic changes in shape. Modern three-dimensional sonographic equipment can produce perpendicular orthogonal planes, which makes it relatively easy to perform this assessment of overall head shape; however, the coronal view is also easily acquired with standard two-dimensional machines. The proper coronal view should be perpendicular to the standard transverse head circumference (HC) view passing through the thala-

mus. Box 50-7 and Figure 50-16 demonstrate orthogonal planes of the fetal head.

The primary observation is that the coronal section of the fetal skull will be a perfect circle in normally shaped heads. In the presence of dolichocephaly, the vertical cranial diameter (VCD) may be exaggerated, resulting in some degree of oxycephaly, whereas brachycephaly will often be associated with **platycephaly** because the VCD is compressed or shortened. The VCD is the height of an isosceles triangle, the base of which is an imaginary line tangential to the caudal edges of the circles around the bilateral hippocampal gyri, and the VCD will lie along the midline from the middle of the triangle base to the cranial vertex (see Figure 50-16). The coronal view of the normal fetal skull will be a perfect circle, and the coronal triangle will be an equilateral, isosceles triangle. New three-dimensional (3D) orthogonal perpendicular planes will make these assessments easier (Figure 50-17).

In cases where the coronal skull is not a perfect circle, a 3D BPD correction can be obtained by averaging the OFD, BPD, and VCD. In the presence of molding, this 3D BPD correction will be the equivalent to the BPD for a normally shaped head at the same gestational age.

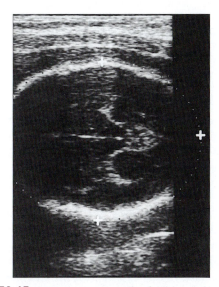

FIGURE 50-15 Transverse section of a fetal head demonstrating the ellipse method of measuring fetal head circumference (HC). The biparietal diameter and HC measurements can be taken from the same frozen image because the same anatomic landmarks are used. The calipers should be placed outside the entire perimeter of the fetal skull *(dotted line)*. This measurement is less affected by head shape than the BPD.

BOX 50-7	Coronal Head Circumference (CHC)

- Use the plane perpendicular to the transverse head circumference (THC). This plane should include the thalamus and brain stem.
- Place area calipers at the midedge of the skull to delineate the coronal triangle; the base of the triangle is tangential to the circles around the hippocampal gyri.
- The height of the triangle is the vertical cranial diameter (VCD). The average of the BPD, OFD, and VCD is the 3D-BPD correction for fetal skull molding.
- The 3D-BPD is accurate to ±1 to 2 weeks.

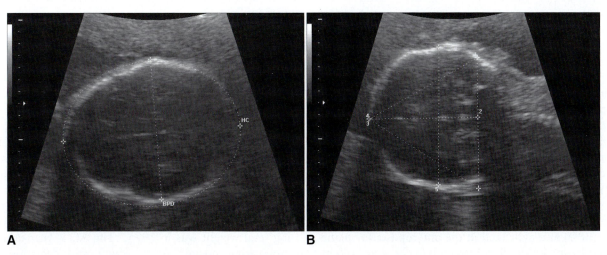

FIGURE 50-16 A, Transverse head circumference (HC) measured outer perimeter, and BPD measured leading edge to leading edge. BPD = 58.7 mm = 24.0 weeks; HC = 216.7 mm = 23.7 weeks; AA = 22.8. **B,** In the same fetus, a coronal head circumference (CHC) showing the coronal triangle and vertical cranial diameter (VCD) as the height of the triangle. The 3D-BPD correction = (58.7 + 76.8 + 47.5)/3 = 61.0 mm = 24.3 weeks. This is a normally shaped fetal skull.

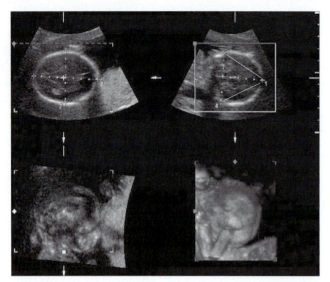

FIGURE 50-17 Three-dimensional orthogonal planes showing the transverse and coronal head circumferences. The sagittal plane *(lower left)* and 3D surface rendering are less useful in this case.

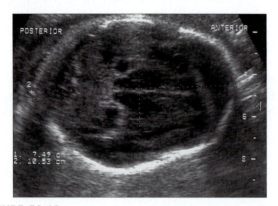

FIGURE 50-18 A biparietal diameter (BPD) with dolichocephaly. The head is elongated in the anteroposterior diameter and falsely shortened in the transverse diameter. The BPD is mean for 29 weeks and the head circumference is mean for 30.3 weeks, but the actual gestational age is 32 weeks.

The student of sonography must realize that as the profession enters the era of true 3D imaging modalities, all parameter measurements may not be the same from all researchers and on all machines. Already the fetal cranium alone has had proposed 3D measurements using outer, mid, and inner bone cursor placement. When using the sonographic instrument's measurement and age calculation packages, the operator is responsible for understanding the proper measurement end points used in that machine's software.

Cephalic Index. Two frequently noted alterations in head shape are dolichocephaly and brachycephaly. In dolichocephaly, the head is shortened in the transverse plane (BPD) and elongated in the anteroposterior plane (OFD) (Figure 50-18). In brachycephaly the head is elongated in the transverse diameter (BPD) and shortened in the anteroposterior diameter (OFD) (Figure 50-19). One can underestimate gestational age from a dolichocephalic

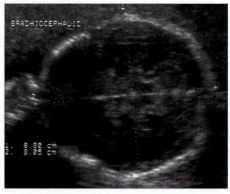

FIGURE 50-19 This biparietal diameter (BPD) is consistent with brachycephaly. The fetal head is falsely wider in the transverse diameter, yet shortened in the anteroposterior plane. The BPD overestimates the gestational age, but the head circumference (HC) remains relatively unaffected. The BPD is mean for 26.7 weeks, and the HC is mean for 24.9 weeks, but the actual gestational age is 23.5 weeks.

head or overestimate with brachycephaly. Because of these variations in fetal head shape, a cephalic index (CI) has been devised to determine the normality of the fetal head shape:

$$CI = BPD/OFD \times 100$$

A normal cephalic index is 80% ±1 standard deviation. The range of normal CI is 75% to 85% (±1 SD ~ 68% of the population). A CI of greater than 85% suggests brachycephaly and one of less than 75% suggests dolichocephaly. In one case report, the CI changed from a high normal of 83% to a significantly abnormal index of 63% during a 2½-week period.[8] This change would normally take approximately 7 weeks. Fetal death resulted. The authors of the report concluded that an abnormal CI may be an early indication of impending fetal death.

The BPD and transverse head circumference do not account for changes in the vertical cranial diameter (VCD). The VCD is a relatively dynamic parameter because pressure on the vertex of the cranium as the fetus stretches and pushes the head against the uterine wall or maternal pubic bone will compress the VCD and exaggerate the BPD and HC in compensation, often resulting in a CI indicating brachycephaly. Conversely, if the BPD is compressed in dolichocephaly, the VCD will increase to compensate.[9,12] Unfortunately, this fact has been ignored for the most part, but as true 3D sonography becomes available, these measurements will come into use.[5]

Abdominal Circumference. The first description of the use of the fetal **abdominal circumference (AC)** in predicting fetal weight was in 1975.[2] The AC is very useful in monitoring normal fetal growth and detecting fetal growth disturbances, such as **intrauterine growth restriction (IUGR)** and macrosomia. It is more useful as a growth parameter than in predicting gestational age.

The fetal abdomen should be measured in a transverse plane at the level of the liver where the umbilical vein branches into the left portal sinus (Box 50-8, Figures 50-20 and 50-21). In this plane, the left portal vein and the right portal vein form a *J* shape. The stomach bubble may be seen at this level on the left side of the fetal abdomen. The abdomen should be more circular than oval because an oval shape indicates an oblique cut resulting in a false estimation of size. Fetal kidneys usually should not be seen when the proper plane is imaged. The AC may change shape with fetal breathing activity, transducer compression, or intrauterine crowding (as in multiple pregnancies or oligohydramnios) or secondary to fetal position, as in a breech presentation. When discrepancies do occur in AC measurements, multiple measurements should be taken and averaged to ensure accuracy. This is also true for other fetal measurements.

The AC can be measured with the same instruments used to measure the HC. The calipers should be placed along the external perimeter of the fetal abdomen to include subcutaneous soft tissue. The following formula can be used to calculate the AC:

$$AC = \frac{D1 + D2 \times \pi}{2}$$

Therefore,

$$AC = (D1 + D2) \times 1.57$$

In this equation, D1 is the diameter from the skin line behind the fetal spine to the outer skin line of the anterior abdominal wall, and D2 is the transverse diameter perpendicular to D1. Unlike in the fetal head, there is no consistent relationship between the anteroposterior and transverse diameters. Sonographers must be sure to measure the AC at the skin line and not to the more obvious rib, spine, and peritoneal echoes.

Of the four basic gestational age measurements, AC has the largest reported variability and is more affected by growth disturbances than the other basic parameters. Later in gestation, the AC correlates more closely with fetal weight than with age.

> **BOX 50-8** | **Abdominal Circumference (AC)**
>
> - The AC should be taken from a round transverse image, perpendicular to the fetal spine, with the umbilical portion of the left portal vein midline within the liver.
> - The outer margin of the abdominal wall should be measured.
> - The abdominal wall measurement is the least accurate for fetal age.

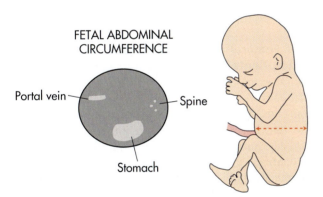

FETAL ABDOMINAL CIRCUMFERENCE

FIGURE 50-20 The abdominal circumference should be taken from a round transverse image at the level of the umbilical vein as it joins the left portal vein within the liver.

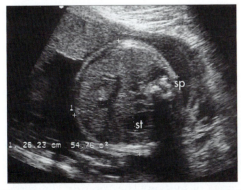

FIGURE 50-21 Transverse section of a fetal abdominal circumference (AC) at 30.3 weeks. The measurement should be taken at the level where the umbilical vein branches into the left portal sinus and forms a J shape. The fetal stomach *(st)* would be seen on the left at this level. One set of calipers should measure the distance from the fetal spine *(sp)* to the anterior abdominal wall. The other set should be placed perpendicular, measuring the widest transverse diameter. When tracing or using an ellipse to measure the AC, the calipers should be placed along the external perimeter of the fetus to include the skin.

Bone Lengths

Femur. The most widely measured and easily obtainable of all fetal long bones is the femur. It usually lies at 30 to 70 degrees to the long axis of the fetal body. **Femur length (FL)** is about as accurate as BPD in determining gestational age. Femur length is an especially useful parameter that can be used to date a pregnancy when a fetal head cannot be measured because of position or when there is a fetal head anomaly (Box 50-9).

The technique for measuring with real-time sonography is fairly simple. First, the lie of the fetus should be determined and the fetal body followed in a transverse section until the fetal bladder and iliac crests are identified. The iliac crests are echogenic and oblique to the fetal bladder. The transducer is moved slightly and rotated to visualize the full length of the femur. The ends of the femur should be distinct and blunt, not pointed, and an acoustic shadow should be cast because of the absorption of the sound waves into the bone (Figure 50-22).

Sonographers measure the femoral diaphysis, which is the calcified portion from end to end. The femoral head is not taken into account even when it is visible.

BOX 50-9	Femur Measurement

- The hyperechoic linear structure represents the ossified portion of the femoral diaphysis and corresponds to femoral length measurement from the greater trochanter to the femoral condyles. These are imaged as rounded hypoechoic masses at each end of the diaphysis called the epiphyseal cartilages; they should not be included in the femoral length measurement. Do not include the distal femoral point (DFP).
- The normal femur has a straight lateral border and a curved medial border.
- Femur length may be used with the same accuracy as BPD to predict gestational age.
- Femur length may indicate skeletal dysplasias or intrauterine growth restriction.

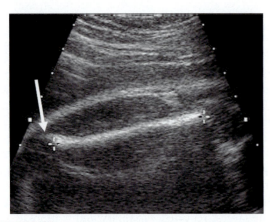

FIGURE 50-22 Longitudinal section through a fetal femur at 31.0 weeks. The longest section of bone should be obtained. The calipers should be placed from the major trochanter to the external condyle, excluding the DFP *(arrow)*. Note the shadow cast posterior to the bone, appropriately demonstrating the absorption of the sound waves into the fetal bone.

After 32 weeks, the distal femoral epiphysis is seen, but it is not included in the femur length measurement. Often an echo from the near side of the cartilaginous distal femoral condyles will be seen, called the "distal femoral point" (DFP), and should not be included in the measure of the diaphysis.

Overestimating the length of the femur by high gain settings or by including the femoral head or distal epiphysis in the measurement is possible. Underestimation can result from using incorrect plane orientation and not obtaining the full length of the bone.

In any routine obstetric evaluation, the femur is usually the only long bone measured, but if there is a 2-week or greater difference between femur length and all the other biometric parameters, all fetal long bones should be measured and a targeted examination of the fetal anatomy should be performed. Three studies found an association between shortened femur and humerus lengths and trisomy.[1,10,17] Dwarfism is also a possibility. Constitutional hereditary growth factors should also be considered. Other bone lengths are sometimes valuable in assessing gestational age.

BOX 50-10	Tibia and Fibula Measurements

- The tibia is longer than the fibula.
- The fibula is lateral to the tibia and thinner.
- Measure the length point to point.

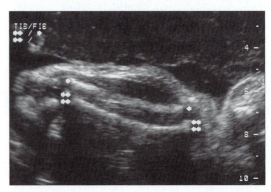

FIGURE 50-23 The tibia and fibula are demonstrated here at 21 weeks. The tibia can be distinguished from the fibula because the tibia is larger *(multiple arrows)* than the small tapering fibula *(single arrow)*.

Distal Femoral and Proximal Tibial Epiphyseal Ossification Centers. One report has correlated the distal femoral epiphyseal ossification (DFE) and the proximal tibial epiphyseal ossification (PTE) with advanced gestational age.[3] The DFE and PTE appear as a high-amplitude echo that is separate but adjacent to the femur or the tibia. The authors of the report found that the DFE can be identified in gestations greater than 33 weeks, and that the PTE is identified in gestations greater than 35 weeks. It is not necessary to measure these ossifications; they are either present or absent. These assessments can be helpful when other growth parameters are compromised because of congenital anomalies or when differentiating an incorrectly dated fetus from a fetus that is **small for gestational age (SGA),** or one with intrauterine growth restriction (IUGR).

Tibia and Fibula. The tibia and fibula can be measured by first identifying the femur, then following it down until the two parallel bones can be identified. The tibia can be identified because the tibial plateau is larger than the fine, tapering fibula. The tibia is located medial to the fibula (Box 50-10, Figure 50-23).

Humerus. Humeral length is sometimes more difficult to measure than femur length. The humerus is usually found very close to the fetal abdomen, but it can exhibit a wide range of motion. The "up side" humerus, or the humerus closest to the transducer, falls in the near-field zone, where detail is not always focused and the acoustic shadow is less clear. The opposite, or "down side," humerus may be obscured because of the overlying fetal spine or fetal ribs (Box 50-11, Figure 50-24). The cartilaginous humeral head surface is also acoustically shiny and may produce specular reflections that should not be included in the measurement of the humeral diaphysis.

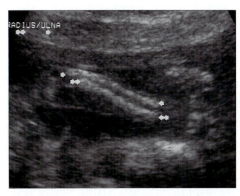

FIGURE 50-25 Longitudinal section through the radius *(two arrows)* and ulna *(one arrow)* at 20.3 weeks of gestation. The calipers should be placed at the most distal portion of each individual bone. The ulna can be distinguished from the radius because the ulna is larger and penetrates much deeper into the elbow.

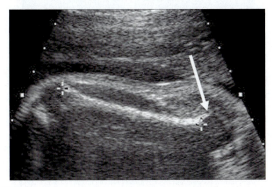

FIGURE 50-24 Longitudinal section through a fetal humerus at 32.4 weeks. The calipers should be placed at the most distal ends of the bone, excluding the PHP *(arrow)*. The anterior, or "up side," humerus is measured here; the humeral head can be observed with the specular echoes of the PHP and exhibiting acoustic enhancement beyond the head.

These specular reflections from the cartilaginous head of the humerus are called the proximal humeral point (PHP) as a corollary to the DFP of the femur. Both the DFP and the PHP, when observed, will always be on the side of the acoustically shiny cartilage proximal to the transducer.

Radius and Ulna. The radius and ulna can be recognized by following the humerus down until two parallel bones are visualized and then rotating the transducer slightly until the full length of the bones is identified. The forearms are commonly found near the fetal face. The ulna can be distinguished from the radius because it penetrates much deeper into the elbow (Box 50-12, Figure 50-25). The ulna is larger and anatomically medial.

Using Multiple Parameters

No single parameter is perfect in predicting gestational age, and estimates of fetal age may improve significantly when two or more parameters are used. However, use of multiple parameters in estimating fetal age is appropriate when the fetus is growing normally or in growth assessment time-series studies. Congenital anomalies of the head, abdomen, skeleton, and functional disturbances must be taken into consideration before using multiple parameters. In a normal population, the various ages estimated from the parameters of the fetal cranium exhibit about half the variation (±5% of age), as do the ages from the fetal torso and extremity parameters (±10% of age).

A birth weight table was developed based on measurements from a group of neonates who had accurate gestational dating using prenatal first-trimester sonography to improve the accuracy of neonatal birth weight percentiles.[4] Prenatally, weight tables are used in conjunction with sonographically estimated fetal weight to help guide obstetric management decisions, especially those concerning the timing of delivery. Fetal weight estimation is a useful parameter in following IUGR fetuses.

A study compared 3D sonographic birth weight predictions with 2D methods and found a significant correlation existed between thigh volume and birth weight at term gestation.[13] Thigh volumes that included the soft tissue mass may represent important markers for fetal growth. The 3D sonography may be an important predictor of growth-restricted fetuses, and the volume measurements may be able to be applied to each fetus to monitor growth.

One author used the technique of averaging the BPD, HC, AC, and FL to determine gestational age.[10] The value of using multiple parameters is that as fetuses individuate, some are longer or shorter, fatter or thinner, and an **average age (AA)** of multiple fetal parameters will result in the best estimation of age. In addition, any of the measurements may be technically incorrect, and it is very unlikely that all of the measurements are overestimated or underestimated.

Age Range Analysis

An extension of the AA of multiple fetal parameters is the **age range analysis (ARA)**. The concept of average ages is based on the fact that not all fetal parameters grow at the same rate; therefore, a fetus with an average age of 30 weeks may have an estimated femoral age of 31 weeks, whereas the AC could measure to be 29 weeks. This fetus would be relatively long and thin but may be normal. By studying large populations using multiple fetal parameter ages, two different groups found that for the same fetus at a given time in gestation, the range of ages of all parameters should be about ±8% to ±10% (±2 SD) of the average age of all the parameters.[7] This means that the range of ages for a fetus with an average age of 20 weeks for all parameters should fall between 18 and 22 weeks, using the ±10%, which is easiest to calculate. Moreover, at 30 weeks all parameter ages should fall between 27 and 33 weeks in normal fetuses (95% of the population). The ARA is a simple way of assessing proportionalities of fetal parameters and is a graphic way of presenting growth-series studies and individual variations, which is also attempted by the GASA method.

Table 50-1 can be used to calculate the ARA for a fetus and to record time-series growth studies to assess for growth disturbances and parameter proportions. The location of a parameter in the normal distribution in standard deviations may be estimated using the Z score formula in this table.

In cases of IUGR growth disturbances, the fetal AA by sonography will lag behind the LMP age. As the case is followed in serial studies, the differences between the sonographic AA and LMP ages will increase as the IUGR becomes more pronounced later in gestation. In cases of normal but small for gestational age (SGA) fetuses, the sonographic AA may lag to some degree behind the LMP age, but the differences of the ages should not increase with time in gestation.

Other Parameters

Numerous other nomograms have been used to correlate almost every aspect of fetal anatomy with gestational age. Among the most interesting of these parameters are the orbits, the cerebellum, the fetal epiphyseal ossification centers, and cranial volume. In general, it can be stated that parameters that normally grow to larger sizes at term will have a more rapid growth trajectory and will generally produce the most accurate fetal age estimates.

Orbits. Another parameter useful in predicting gestational age is the fetal orbit measurements. The orbital diameter (OD), **binocular distance (BD)**, and interocular distance (IOD) can be measured. Gestational age can best be predicted from the BD. This measure is more strongly related to the BPD and gestational age than are the other orbital parameters. The fetal orbits should be measured in a plane slightly more caudal than the BPD. The orbits are accessible in every head position except the occipitoanterior position (i.e., face looking down). All measurements should be taken from outer border to

BOX 50-13	Orbital Measurements

- Orbital diameter increases from 13 mm at 12 weeks to 59 mm or greater at term.
- Measure outer-to-outer diameter (BD).
- Measure inner-to-inner diameter (IOD).

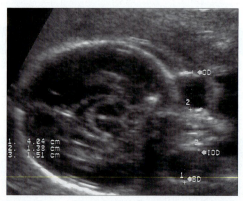

FIGURE 50-26 Transverse section through the fetal head at the level of the orbits at 25.3 weeks. *OD* is the measure of a single fetal orbit. The binocular diameter *(BD)* is a measure of both the orbits at the same time, and the inner orbital diameter *(IOD)* is a measure of the distance between the two orbits. These measurements are especially useful when ruling out hypotelorism or hypertelorism.

outer border (Box 50-13, Figure 50-26). The OD measures a single fetal orbit. The BD includes both fetal orbits at the same time, whereas the IOD measures the length between the two orbits. One view states that (1) both eyes should have the same diameter, (2) the largest diameter of the eyes should be used, and (3) the image should be symmetric. Care should be taken not to underestimate the measurement when there is oblique shadowing from the ethmoid bone. This parameter is especially useful when other fetal growth parameters are affected, such as in ventriculomegaly or skeletal dysplasia. With careful sonographic examinations, the fetus with **hypotelorism, hypertelorism, anophthalmos,** or **microphthalmos** can be diagnosed.

Cerebellum. One study found the fetal cerebellum to be a more accurate reflection of gestational age than the BPD in cases of oligohydramnios, dolichocephaly, breech presentation, or twins or in the presence of a uterine anomaly.[14] The authors of the study claim this is true because the posterior fossa is not affected by any of these conditions. The cerebellum can be measured from the level at which the BPD is obtained by angling back into the posterior fossa to include the full width of the cerebellum. The cerebellum should have a dumbbell or heart shape, depending on the angle of the plane of view.

The widest transverse diameter of the cerebellum should be measured (Box 50-14, Figure 50-27). Authors have described the **banana** and **lemon signs** that associate an abnormally shaped cerebellum with detection of fetal **spina bifida.**[15] In the presence of spina bifida, the fetal cerebellum is displaced downward into the foramen

TABLE 50-1 Fetal Age and Age Range Analysis*—BASIC BABY©

LMP Week	E/FHR b/m	GSD mm	CRL mm	BPD mm	3D-BPD mm	OFD mm	VCD mm	CV ml or cc	THC* mm	Hadlock HC** mm	CHC mm	CERB mm	BIOD mm	FSL mm	Fem mm	Hum mm	ADA mm	AC mm	LMP WEEK	ARA Time-line
Data>																				<Data
41				100	96	123	66	482	349	356	260			74	79	70	120	376	41	
40				97	96	119	70	451	339	350	264		60	73	77	67	118	371	40	
39				95	93	116	66	421	331	344	252		58	71	76	67	116	365	39	
38				93	91	116	66	397	328	340	249	51	60	69	73	65	114	359	38	
37				91	90	113	65	376	320	330	244	50	59	67	73	63	110	342	37	
36				89	88	111	64	351	314	324	240	47	59	65	71	62	103	325	36	
35				87	86	109	63	329	307	316	234	43	57	63	68	60	99	310	35	
34				85	84	106	62	307	299	309	230	41	55	61	66	58	95	299	34	
33				83	82	104	60	289	294	303	224	40	52	59	64	56	92	289	33	
32				80	80	101	58	260	285	294	217	39	51	56	62	55	89	281	32	
31				78	78	98	57	243	277	285	212	37	50	54	59	53	85	268	31	
30				75	75	95	55	220	268	277	205	36	48	52	57	51	81	253	30	
29				73	73	93	55	204	260	269	200	34	46	49	55	50	77	243	29	
28				71	71	89	52	181	251	260	192	32	46	47	53	48	74	231	28	
27				68	68	86	51	166	242	251	187	30	44	45	50	46	71	'221	27	
26				65	66	83	49	146	233	241	178	28	43	43	48	44	68	212	26	
25				62	63	79	47	127	221	231	171	27	41	41	46	43	65	205	25	
24				59	60	76	45	110	211	221	163	25	40	39	43	40	61	191	24	
23				56	56	71	42	93	199	210	154	24	38	37	40	38	58	181	23	
22				53	53	67	40	78	188	199	146	22	36	34	37	36	54	170	22	
21				49	50	62	38	65	175	188	137	21	34	32	35	34	51	160	21	
20				46	47	59	35	54	165	175	129	19	32	30	32	31	47	149	20	
19			130	44	44	55	33	44	155	163	121	19	30	28	29	29	44	138	19	
18			121	40	40	50	31	35	142	149	112	18	28	25	26	26	40	126	18	
17			113	37	37	46	29	28	131	135	104	17	25	22	23	23	36	113	17	
16			104	34	34	42	25	20	118	121	93	15	23	20	20	20	33	103	16	
15			92	30	30	37	23	14	105	105	83	14	21	17	16	16	29	91	15	
14	150		83	27	26	33	20	10	93	90	73	12	17	15	13	13	25	78	14	
13	152		71	23	23	28	17	6	81		63	10	15	13	10	10	21	68	13	
12	159		58	20	20	24	14	3.8	69		54		13	11	7	7	18	57	12	
11	163		46	16	17	20	13	2.4	56		47		13		6	5	15	48	11	
							Embryonic Period													
10	167	53	37	13	13	17	9	1.2	42		45			9	4	4	13	40	10	
9	185	44	25	11	11	13	8	0.7	31		30						10	30	9	
8	165	34	17	7	7	9	5	0.2	19		19						7	22	8	
7	142	26	10	5															7	
6	114	18	5																6	
5	98	11	2																5	
4			4																4	

Growth Series Dating	Exams:	Date		LMP age		Ave. Age		Age Range	
	1st								
	2nd								
	3rd								
	4th								

*THC and CHC are measured at the mid-cranial bones. Data from DuBose T: *Fetal sonography*, Philadelphia, 1996, Saunders. This table is a manual version of BASIC BABY © fetal size/analysis software.

**Hadlock HC is an outer cranial bones perimeter measurement. Hadlock HC data from Hadlock, Deter, Harrist, Park: Fetal head circumference: relation to menstrual age, *AJR* 138:649, 1982.

TABLE 50-1	Fetal Age and Age Range Analysis—BASIC BABY©—cont'd		
Table legend			
Parameter	Symbols	Parameter Name	Measurements in mm
GSD	G	Gestational sac diameter	Mean of two diameters
CRL	R	Crown-rump length	Top of head to rump; do not include legs
E/FHR	E	Embryofetal heart rate	M-mode beats per minute
BPD	B	Biparietal diameter	Leading edge to leading edge (outer to inner)
BPD 3D	3	3D BPD correction	Average (OFD + BPD + VCD)/3 = BPD
OFD	O	Occipitofrontal diameter	Middle of frontal to middle of occipital bones
VCD	V	Vertical cranial diameter	Height of coronal triangle in fetal head
THC	T	Transverse head circumference	THC = (OFD + BPD) × 1.57
CV	V	Cranial volume in ml or cc	CV = OFD x BPD × VCD × 0.0005555
CHC	C	Coronal head circumference	CHC = (VCD + BPD) × 1.57
CERB	c	Cerebellar transverse diameter	Transverse cerebellar diameter
BD	b	Binocular diameter	Outer-to-outer edges of the binocular globes
FSL	S	Fractional spine length	Seven thoracolumbar vertebral bodies and spaces
Fem	F	Femur length	Length of femoral diaphysis
Hum	H	Humerus length	Length of humeral diaphysis
AC	a	Abdominal circumference	AC = d1 + d2 × 1.57
ADA	D	Abdominal diameter average	Average transverse and AP diameters (d1 + d1)/2
Ave. Age	AA	Average age in LMP weeks	Average of multiple parameter's ages
LMP	M	Last menstrual period age	May be estimated from first sonographic study
Range	[ ]	Range of ages	Range normally is less than 20% of Ave. Age

Instructions

To perform age range analysis (ARA) for each examination:

Measure parameters and mark the parameter's sizes in the table to determine each parameter's age, and average all parameter ages; interpolate for more accuracy. Use a straight edge to place symbols in the timeline. Normal fetuses will form a cluster about the LMP age estimated from first sonographic examination. Use a single table to track growth series for each fetus. IUGR will trail LMP age. Range should be < ±10% (20%) of AA.

ARA: To determine the relative location of any parameter in the time-line distribution, use the following formula:

$$(\text{Parameter age} - \text{AA})/(\text{AA} \times 0.05) = \text{Location in standard deviations (SDs)}$$

BOX 50-14	Cerebellar Dimensions

- *Posterior fossa.* In the transaxial image of the head, obtain the BPD (cavum septi pellucidi and thalamus) and then angle the transducer inferior toward the base of the skull to image the posterior fossa.
- Obtain the length of the cerebellum at the level of the cerebellum, vermis, and fourth ventricle.
- Angle the transducer slightly more inferior from the cerebellum to record the cistern magnum and nuchal fold area.
- The depth of the cisterna magna is from the posterior aspect of the cerebellum to the occipital bone measured 5 mm ± 3 mm; measurements >10 mm are abnormal.
- The nuchal fold should measure <3 mm.

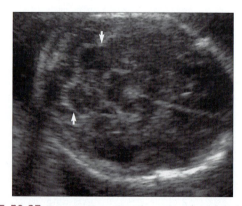

FIGURE 50-27 Transverse section through a fetal head demonstrating the fetal cerebellum. This image is obtained at the same anatomic level as the biparietal diameter, angling back into the posterior fossa of the fetal head. Note the classic dumbbell shape of the normal cerebellum. The widest diameter of the cerebellum should be measured *(arrows)*.

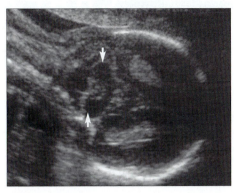

FIGURE 50-28 Coronal section of a fetal cerebellum, which can be used when the traditional views cannot be obtained.

magnum, altering its shape to appear oblong or banana shaped. The frontal bones of the fetal skull also give in to this reduced pressure, collapsing and giving the fetal head a lemon shape. This association is known as the Arnold-Chiari malformation type II.

The fetal cerebellum should not be used as a gestational dating parameter in the presence of a cerebellar or spinal abnormality. A more recent report states that the coronal or other views are just as accurate as long as the transverse width of the cerebellum is measured, especially in fetal heads when the traditional views are unobtainable (Figure 50-28).[20]

REFERENCES

1. Benacerraf B, Neuberg D, Frigoletto FD: Humeral shortening in second trimester fetuses with Down syndrome, *Obstet Gynecol* 77:223, 1991.
2. Campbell S, Wilkin D: Ultrasonic measurement of the fetal abdominal circumference in the estimation of fetal weight, *Br J Obstet Gynecol* 82:689, 1975.
3. Chinn D, et al: Ultrasonic identification of fetal lower extremity epiphyseal ossification centers, *Radiology* 147:815, 1983.
4. Doubilet PM, et al: Improved birth weight table for neonates developed from gestations dated by early ultrasonography, *J Ultrasound Med* 16:241, 1997.
5. Dubose TJ: Reliability and validity of three-dimensional fetal brain volumes, *J Ultrasound Med* 21:709-711, 2002.
6. Dubose TJ, Cunyus JA, Johnson L: Embryonic heart rate and age, *J Diagn Med Sonogr* 6:151-157, 1990.
7. Dubose TJ, Poole E, Butschek C: Range of multiple fetal parameters, *J Ultrasound Med* 7:S205-S206, 1988.
8. Ford K, McGahan J: Cephalic index: its possible use as a predictor of impending fetal demise, *Radiology* 143:517, 1982.
9. Goldberg BB, Kurtz AB: *Atlas of ultrasound measurements*, St. Louis, 1990, Mosby.
10. Hadlock FP, Deter RL, Harris RB: Sonographic detection of abnormal fetal growth patterns, *Clin Obstet Gynecol* 27:342, 1984.
11. Hohler CW: Ultrasonic estimation of gestational age, *Clin Obstet Gynecol* 27:2, 1984.
12. Kurtz AB, Goldberg BB: Fetal head measurements. In Kurtz AB, Goldberg BB, editors: *Obstetrical measurements in ultrasound: a reference manual*, St. Louis, 1988, Mosby.
13. Lee W, et al: Birthweight prediction by three-dimensional ultrasonographic volumes of the fetal thigh and abdomen, *J Ultrasound Med* 16:799, 1997.
14. Mcleary R, Kuhns L, Barr M: Ultrasonography of the fetal cerebellum, *Radiology* 151:441, 1984.
15. Nicolaides KH, et al: Ultrasound screening for spina bifida: cranial and cerebellar signs, *Lancet* 1:72, 1986.
16. Nyberg DA, Laing FC, Filly RA: Threatened abortion: sonographic distinction of normal and abnormal sacs, *Radiology* 158:397, 1986.
17. Rodis JF, et al: Comparison of humerus length with femur length in fetuses with Down syndrome, *Am J Obstet Gynecol* 165:1051, 1992.
18. Sabbagha RE, Hughey M, Depp R: Growth-adjusted sonographic age (GASA): a simplified method, *Obstet Gynecol* 51:383, 1978.
19. Sabbagha RE, Tamura RK, Dal Campo S: Fetal dating by ultrasound, *Sem Roentgenol* 17:3, 1982.
20. Sarno AP, Rose GS, Harrington RA: Coronal transcerebellar diameter: an alternate view, *Ultrasound Obstet Gynecol* 2:158, 1992.

Fetal Growth Assessment by Sonography

Terry J. DuBose and Sandra L. Hagen-Ansert

OBJECTIVES

On completion of this chapter, you should be able to:
- Describe how intrauterine growth restriction may be detected by sonography
- Differentiate between symmetric and asymmetric intrauterine growth restriction
- List which growth parameters should be used to assess intrauterine growth restriction
- Describe how to assess amniotic fluid volume

- Describe how to perform a biophysical profile on a fetus
- Discuss quantitative and qualitative Doppler measurements as applied to obstetrics
- Analyze the significance of macrosomia in a fetus
- Discuss the multiple fetal parameters and calculated ages used to assess the fetal somatic proportions and growth.

OUTLINE

Fetal growth assessment is very important to the perinatologist and obstetric physician. Before the availability of sonographic determination of fetal growth, physicians had to rely on their physical assessment of the neonate to determine what occurred during fetal development. The physician's assessment would determine if the fetus was born **preterm** (before 38 menstrual weeks), at term (between 38 and 42 menstrual weeks), or **postterm** (later than 42 menstrual weeks). Contemporary fetal growth assessment by early sonographic dating and subsequent growth series examinations are most accurate. Further classification dictated whether the fetal birth weight was **small for gestational age (SGA)**, appropriate for gestational age, or **large for gestational age (LGA)**. This determination allowed the clinicians to recognize the increase in perinatal morbidity and mortality for the preterm or postterm and SGA or LGA fetus.

INTRAUTERINE GROWTH RESTRICTION

Intrauterine growth restriction (IUGR) is best described as a decreased rate of fetal growth. IUGR complicates 3% to 7% of all pregnancies. It is most commonly defined as a fetal weight at or below 10% for a given gestational age. It often becomes difficult to differentiate the fetus that is constitutionally small (small for gestational age [SGA]) from one that is growth restricted. IUGR babies are at a greater risk of antepartum death,

| BOX 51-1 | Maternal Factors for Intrauterine Growth Restriction (IUGR) |

- Previous history of fetus with IUGR
- Significant maternal hypertension
- History of tobacco use
- Presence of uterine anomaly
- Significant placental hemorrhage
- Placental insufficiency

| BOX 51-2 | Clinical Observations and Actions for Intrauterine Growth Restriction (IUGR) |

Clinical signs. Decreased fundal height and fetal motion.
Key sonographic markers. Grade 3 placenta before 36 weeks or decreased placental thickness.
Sonographer action. Alert the physician, determine the cause (maternal history, habits, environmental exposure, viruses, diseases, drug exposure), and carefully evaluate placenta and fetal anatomy with sonography.
Assessment of umbilical artery Doppler for increased resistance to flow. S/D > 3.0 after 30 LMP weeks is considered abnormal.

perinatal asphyxia, neonatal morbidity, and later developmental problems. Mortality is increased sixfold to tenfold, depending on the severity of the condition.

The most significant maternal factors for IUGR are the history of a previous fetus with IUGR, significant maternal hypertension or smoking, the presence of a uterine anomaly (bicornuate uterus or large leiomyoma), and significant placental hemorrhage (Box 51-1). Constitutional factors such as the gender of the infant, race of the mother, parity, body mass index, and environmental factors can affect the distribution of normal birth weight in any population.

Before abnormal growth can be diagnosed, the gestational age of the pregnancy must be accurately determined. In the prenatal period, an accurate last menstrual period or a first-trimester sonographic age can be used, and both are important for comparison to subsequent sonographic studies for growth assessment. If first-trimester sonography was not performed, then in the second or third trimester the standard biparietal diameter (BPD), head circumference (HC), abdominal circumference (AC), femur length (FL), and other fetal parameters should be used in conjunction with other tests of fetal well-being (e.g., biophysical profile [BPP] and fetal Doppler velocimetry).

In the postnatal period, several other body dimensions can be used. These include head circumference, crown-heel length, weight-height ratios, ponderal index (PI), and skinfold thickness. Other considerations include maternal size and race and the gender of the neonate. The standards for fetal growth have been incorporated with sonographic computer software, and different programs exist that can be applied to a variety of geographic locations.

The reader should not confuse IUGR with small for gestational age (SGA). SGA describes the fetus with a weight below the 10th percentile without reference to the cause. Fetal growth restriction describes a subset of the SGA fetuses with a weight below the 10th percentile as a result of pathologic processes resulting from a variety of maternal, fetal, or placental disorders. The classification of IUGR is based on the morphologic characteristics of the fetuses studied. There are two basic clarifications: symmetric and asymmetric IUGR. The SGA fetus may simply be normal, but constitutionally small, but a fetus with IUGR is ill and not following a normal growth trajectory. IUGR is often progressive,

with the fetal size lagging farther and farther behind the expected growth rate.

Symmetric IUGR is usually the result of a first-trimester insult, such as a chromosomal abnormality or infection. This results in a fetus that is proportionately small throughout the pregnancy. Approximately 20% to 30% of all IUGR cases are symmetric. The timing of the pathologic insult is recognized as more important than the actual nature of the underlying pathologic process.

Asymmetric IUGR begins late in the second or third trimester and usually results from placental insufficiency. This fetus usually shows head sparing at the expense of abdominal and soft tissue growth. The fetal length (FL) exhibits varying degrees of compromise. An early diagnosis of IUGR and close fetal monitoring (BPP, Doppler, and fetal growth evaluation) are of significant help in managing a pregnancy suspected of IUGR. Clinical observations and appropriate actions for IUGR are listed in Box 51-2.

Symmetric Intrauterine Growth Restriction

Symmetric growth restriction is characterized by a fetus that is small in all physical parameters (e.g., BPD, HC, AC, and FL), which is usually the result of a severe insult in the first trimester. The causes may include low genetic growth potential, intrauterine infection, severe maternal malnutrition, fetal alcohol syndrome, chromosomal anomaly, or severe congenital anomaly. One study demonstrated early IUGR in 9 of 11 fetuses with trisomy 13, 2 of 5 fetuses with 45 XO, and only 2 of 18 fetuses with trisomy 17.[10] Another report described two cases of triploidy in association with early symmetric IUGR.[15] Because of the increased association of chromosomal abnormalities, prenatal testing to rule out aneuploidy should be considered (Figure 51-1).

Asymmetric Intrauterine Growth Restriction

Asymmetric growth restriction is the more common form of IUGR and is usually caused by placental insufficiency. This may be the result of maternal disease, such

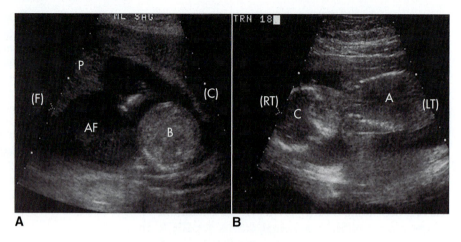

FIGURE 51-1 A, Second-trimester fetus with trisomy 18 shows symmetric intrauterine growth restriction. Both the head and abdomen measured well below expected growth curves. Echogenic bowel *(B)* is seen. **B,** Image shows the small cranium *(C)* and abdomen *(A)*. *F,* fundus; *C,* toward the cervix; *AF,* amniotic fluid; *(LT),* left; *P,* placenta; *(RT),* right.

as diabetes (classes D to F), chronic hypertension, cardiac or renal disease, abruptio placentae, multiple pregnancy, smoking, poor weight gain, drug usage, or uterine anomaly. It should be noted that IUGR fetuses have been born to mothers who have no high-risk factors; therefore, all pregnancies undergoing sonographic examinations should be evaluated for IUGR.

Asymmetric IUGR is characterized by an appropriate BPD and HC and a disproportionately small AC. This reinforces the brain-sparing effect, which states that the last organ to be deprived of essential nutrients is the brain. The BPD and HC may be slightly smaller, but this usually does not happen until the late third trimester.

A proposed third type of IUGR suggests that fetuses with long FL (90th percentile or above) and small AC (at or below the 5th percentile) may be nutritionally deprived even though their estimated fetal weight (ETW) falls at least in the lowest 10%.[5] The theory is that in asymmetric IUGR the fetal length is well preserved, whereas the soft tissue mass is deprived. The FL to AC ratio or PI would be abnormally low. The proponents of this theory claim this occurs in less than 1% of IUGR cases but stress the importance of detection because these cases of IUGR have an estimated fetal weight (EFW) within the limits of normal.[5]

DIAGNOSTIC CRITERIA

The IUGR multiple parameters are shown in Box 51-3.

Biparietal Diameter

The BPD is not a reliable predictor of IUGR for many reasons. The first is the head-sparing theory, which is associated with asymmetric IUGR. Fetal blood is shunted away from other vital organs to nourish the fetal brain, giving the fetus an appropriate BPD (plus or minus 1 standard deviation) for the true gestational age.

The second problem is the potential alteration in fetal head shape secondary to oligohydramnios. Oligohydramnios is a decreased amount of amniotic fluid often

---

> **BOX 51-3** **Multiple Parameters for Intrauterine Growth Restriction (IUGR)**
>
> *BPD.* Imaged in the transverse plane using the cavum septi pellucidi, thalamic nuclei, falx cerebri, and choroid plexus as landmarks. The BPD can be misleading in cases associated with unusual head shapes. Used alone, it is a poor indicator of IUGR.
>
> *HC to AC ratio.* High false-positive rate for use in screening general population. The HC to AC ratio is useful in determining the type of IUGR.
>
> *FL to AC ratio.* Not dependent on knowing gestational age. The FL to AC ratio has a poor positive predictive value.
>
> *FL.* May decrease in size with symmetric IUGR.
>
> *AC.* Measure at level of portal-umbilical venous complex. When growth is compromised, AC is affected secondary to reduced adipose tissue and depletion of glycogen storage in liver. AC is the single most sensitive indicator of IUGR.

associated with IUGR. Dolichocephaly, or a falsely shortened BPD, can lead to underestimation of the fetal weight, and brachycephaly, or a falsely widened BPD, can lead to overestimation of the EFW. The HC measurement is a more consistent parameter, but a combination of all growth parameters (BPD, HC, AC, and FL) should be used when diagnosing a fetal growth discrepancy.

Abdominal Circumference

Because of the variability of fetal proportion and size, the AC is a poor predictor of gestational age but is valuable for assessing fetal size. In IUGR, the fetal liver is one of the most severely affected body organs, which therefore alters the circumference of the fetal abdomen.

Head Circumference to Abdominal Circumference Ratio

The HC to AC ratio was first developed to detect IUGR in cases of uteroplacental insufficiency. The HC to AC ratio is especially useful in differentiating symmetric and asymmetric IUGR. For each gestational age, a ratio is assigned with standard deviations. In an appropriate-for-gestational-age (AGA) pregnancy, the ratio should decrease as the gestational age increases.

In the presence of IUGR and with the loss of subcutaneous tissue and fat, the ratio increases. This is counterintuitive because as the fetal AC decreases, the HC : AC ratio increases, and *vice versa*. The HC to AC ratio is at least 2 standard deviations above the mean in approximately 70% of fetuses affected with asymmetric IUGR. The HC to AC ratio is not very useful, however, in predicting symmetric IUGR, because the fetal head and fetal abdomen are equally small. This can be further complicated in cases of fetal infections (TORCH infections), which can produce organomegaly with enlargement of the liver or spleen and the resulting increase in the abdominal circumference in the presence of fetal IUGR.

Estimated Fetal Weight

The most reliable **estimated fetal weight (EFW)** formulas incorporate several fetal parameters, such as BPD, HC, AC, and FL. This is important because an overall reduction in the size and mass of these parameters naturally gives a below-normal EFW. An EFW below the 10th percentile is considered by most to be IUGR.

There are numerous formulas for estimating fetal weights. One method uses the BPD and AC to derive the fetal weight, with an accuracy of plus or minus 20%. This formula does not take into consideration HC and FL, which contribute to fetal mass. It also ignores the fact that BPD can be altered slightly because of normal variations in head shape, such as brachycephaly or dolichocephaly. These variations can occur in association with oligohydramnios, which may be found with IUGR.

Another method uses three basic measurements: HC, AC, and FL. The use of the HC instead of the BPD has improved the predictive value to plus or minus 15%.

A third method defines three zones of EFW. Each zone has a different prevalence of IUGR. In zone 1, the EFW is above the lower 20% confidence limit and IUGR is ruled out. In zone 3, the EFW is below the lower 0.5% confidence limit and yields an 82% prevalence of IUGR. Patients in this zone should be delivered as soon as lung maturity can be proven. If the EFW is between zone 1 and zone 3, it falls into zone 2, which has a 24% prevalence of IUGR. Patients in this zone should have serial sonograms and fetal heart rate monitoring.

Numerous other growth curves are available, but the one chosen must be appropriate for the population of patients (e.g., sea level versus above sea level). It is also important to remember that symmetric IUGR cannot be diagnosed in a single examination. The interval growth can be plotted on a graph or chart to show the growth sequence (see Table 50-1). Ethnicity, previous obstetric history, paternal size, fetal gender, and the results of tests

of fetal well-being must be considered before IUGR, rather than a healthy SGA, can be diagnosed.

A computer-generated antenatal chart is available that can be customized for individual pregnancies, taking the mother's characteristics and birth weights from previous pregnancies into consideration. Through review of 4179 pregnancies with sonographically confirmed dates, one study showed that in addition to gestation and gender, maternal weight at first antenatal visit, height, ethnic group, and parity were significant determinants of birth weight in the study population.[8] Correction factors were calculated and entered into a computer program to adjust the normal birth weight percentile limits. With adjusted percentiles, the researchers found that 28% of babies that conventionally fit the criteria for SGA (less than the 10%), and 22% of those who were LGA (greater than the 90%) were in fact within normal limits for the pregnancy. Conversely, 24% and 26% of babies identified as small or large, respectively, with adjusted percentiles were missed by conventional unadjusted percentile assessment.[8]

AMNIOTIC FLUID EVALUATION

The association between IUGR and decreased amniotic fluid (oligohydramnios) is well recognized (Box 51-4). Oligohydramnios has also been associated with fetal renal anomalies, poor renal perfusion, rupture of the intrauterine membranes, and postdate pregnancy. One method, developed for evaluating and quantifying amniotic fluid volume at different intervals during a pregnancy, divides the uterine cavity into four equal quadrants by two imaginary lines running perpendicular to each other. The largest vertical pocket of amniotic fluid, excluding fetal limbs or umbilical cord loops, is measured. The sum of the four quadrants is called the **amniotic fluid index (AFI)**. Normal values have been calculated for each gestational age (plus or minus 2 standard deviations). Normal is 8 to 22 cm; decreased is less than 5 cm; and increased is greater than 22 cm (Figure 51-2).

Not every laboratory has adapted the AFI technique, and it is still quite acceptable to use the "eyeball technique," which is simply a subjective evaluation by an experienced sonographer of the overall amount of amniotic fluid. Various other criteria have been described for defining oligohydramnios, such as occurring when the largest vertical pocket is less than 3 cm, less than 1 cm, or less than 0.5 cm. Whichever technique is chosen,

---

BOX 51-4	Key Points for Intrauterine Growth Restriction (IUGR)

- Oligohydramnios occurs if the fetal urine output is reduced.
- Polyhydramnios develops if the fetus cannot swallow.
- Amniotic fluid pocket less than 1 to 2 cm may represent IUGR.
- Not all oligohydramnios is associated with IUGR.

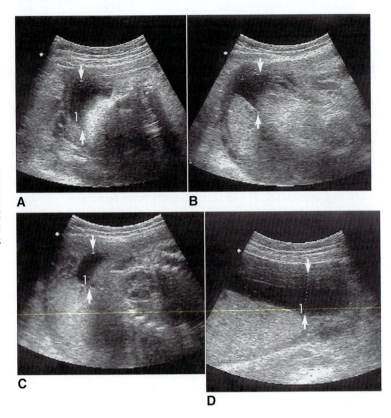

FIGURE 51-2 The four-quadrant technique of amniotic fluid assessment. This technique produces an amniotic fluid index (AFI). The uterus is divided into four equal parts, and the largest vertical pocket of amniotic fluid in each quadrant is measured, excluding fetal limbs or umbilical cord. The sum of the four quadrants is the AFI, which, in this case, equals 14.2 cm at 31 weeks. This is within normal limits.

coworkers in the same sonographic laboratory should use it consistently. The AFI is very helpful in a busy laboratory where multiple sonographers evaluate patients and may have varying opinions on the appearance of normal, decreased, or increased amniotic fluid.

In the presence of oligohydramnios, care should be taken when evaluating fetal growth parameters because they can be compressed. Because the fetus lacks the surrounding fluid protecting it, the circumferences can actually be changed by transducer pressure on the maternal abdomen. This in turn may alter the EFW.

TESTS OF FETAL WELL-BEING

Early diagnosis and estimation of fetal well-being are the main problems in managing IUGR. Fetal breathing motion and urine production were the first functional tests to be assessed. The fetal urine production rate was first described in 1973. The fetal bladder was measured in three dimensions, and the volume was calculated. This was repeated hourly, and the increase was calculated. Because of the time and cumbersome technique involved, this method has not been adopted for widespread use.

Biophysical Profile

The **biophysical profile (BPP)** was originally described by Manning and associates in 1980.[13] Since that time, numerous modifications and variations have been contributed by others. The BPP was adapted to form a linear

relationship with the assessment of multiple fetal biophysical variables, such as the Apgar score in the newborn infant or vital signs in the adult. Five biophysical parameters were assessed individually and in combination. Each test had a high false-positive rate that was greatly reduced when all five variables were combined.

The five parameters are as follows:

1. Cardiac nonstress test (NST)
2. Observation of fetal breathing movements (FBM)
3. Gross fetal body movements (FM)
4. Fetal tone (FT)
5. Amniotic fluid volume (AFV)

The BPP has a specified time limit (30 minutes) to observe these parameters (Box 51-5). Each variable is arbitrarily assigned a score of 2 when normal and 0 when abnormal. A BPP score of 8 to 10 is considered normal. A score of 4 to 6 has no immediate significance. A score of 0 to 2 indicates either immediate delivery or extending the test to 120 minutes.

Fetal Breathing Movements. A true breathing movement is described as simultaneous inward movement of the chest wall with outward movement of the anterior abdominal wall during inspiration (Figure 51-3). An alternative area to watch for breathing is the fetal kidney movement in the longitudinal plane. Two points are given if the practitioner notes one episode of breathing lasting 30 seconds within a 30-minute period. If this is absent, no points are given. The fetal central nervous system initiates and regulates the frequency of fetal breathing movements; these patterns vary with sleep-wake cycles.

Fetal Body and Trunk Gross Movements. At least three definite extremity or trunk movements must be observed within the 30-minute period to score 2 points (Figure 51-4). Fewer than three movements scores zero

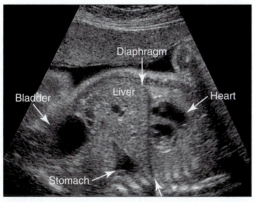

FIGURE 51-3 Fetal breathing may be seen as the chest wall moves inward and the anterior abdominal wall moves outward; breathing may also be seen by watching the movement of the kidney in the longitudinal plane. This coronal-oblique view shows the relationship of the urinary bladder, stomach, diaphragm, and heart.

points. The intact nervous system controls gross fetal body movements; these patterns vary with sleep-wake cycles.

Fetal Tone. Fetal tone is characterized by the presence of at least one episode of extension and immediate return to flexion of an extremity or the spine (Figure 51-5). One active extension and flexion of an open and closed hand would be a good example of positive fetal tone (Figure 51-6). Such a movement would score two points. Abnormal fetal tone is noted by a partial extension or flexion of an extremity without a quick return and would score zero points.

Amniotic Fluid Volume. Amniotic fluid volume is related to the fetal-placental unit and is not influenced by the fetal central nervous system. Premature aging of the placenta (grade III) may contribute to oligohydramnios of IUGR syndrome. Evaluation of the four-quadrant amniotic fluid volume is considered normal if the pockets (quadrants) of fluid measure at least 2 cm or more in two planes and a score of two points is given. The transducer must be perpendicular to the center of the pocket of fluid in the center of the screen, and the uterine wall, cord, or fetal parts cannot be included as part of the fluid measurement.

Decreased amniotic fluid may represent IUGR or intrauterine stress, and serial growth parameters may need to be assessed. Fluid that is decreased near term indicates that the baby may need to be delivered earlier than planned. Decreased fluid means the blood is redistributed to the head and the heart; a decrease in renal perfusion and the resulting reductions in urine output cause the AFI to decrease.

Nonstress Test

The **nonstress test (NST)** is done using Doppler to record fetal heart rate and its reactivity to the stress of uterine contraction. The time expended for this portion of the examination is usually 40 minutes. Fetal motion is detected as a rapid rise on the recording of uterine activity or the patient noting fetal movements. The following conditions indicate a reactive, or normal, NST and score of two points:

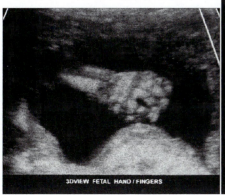

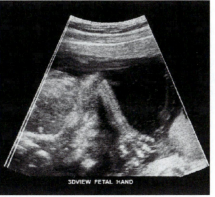

FIGURE 51-4 At least three definite extremity or trunk movements must be seen within the 30-minute period in a normal fetus. **A,** Open fetal hand and wrist. **B,** Elbow, forearm, and wrist.

A

B

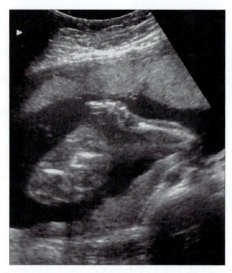

FIGURE 51-5 Fetal tone is characterized by the presence of at least one episode of extension and immediate return to flexion of an extremity or the spine. This view of the upper extremity is shown in flexion.

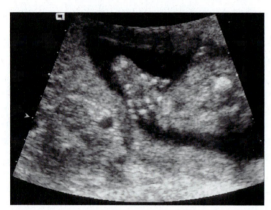

FIGURE 51-6 One active extension and flexion of an open and closed hand is a good example of positive fetal tone. This image shows the hand wide open, with all fingers and thumb extended.

- Two fetal heart rate accelerations of 15 beats per minute or more
- Accelerations lasting at least 15 seconds
- Gross fetal movements noted over 20 minutes without late decelerations

These fetal heart accelerations with fetal movements are a positive sign of fetal well-being; late reductions in rate or decelerations indicate a poor prognosis. Zero points are awarded if two fetal heart rate accelerations with gross fetal movements are not seen during a 40-minute period. Forty minutes is arbitrarily used to accommodate the fetal sleep-wake cycles.

The test is considered normal when all the variables monitored by sonography are normal (FBM, FM, FT, AFV) without the performance of the NST.

The goal of the BPP is to find a way to predict and manage the fetus with hypoxia. One study analyzed the BPP variables based on the gradual hypoxia concept.

This concept states that dynamic biophysical activities (FT, FM, FBM, and fetal heart rate reactivity) are controlled by neural activity arising in distinct anatomic sites in the brain. These become functional at different stages of development, with the later-developing centers requiring higher oxygen levels. The fetal tone center develops at 7.5 to 8.5 weeks. The fetal movement center develops at 9 weeks, and regular diaphragmatic motion develops by 20 to 21 weeks. Heart rate reactivity is the last to occur; it appears by the late second to early third trimester. The hypothesis of gradual hypoxia further supposes that centers that develop later are more sensitive to acute hypoxia. It is therefore expected that the loss of cardiac reactivity and suppression of fetal breathing movements will occur with relatively mild hypoxia. Cessation of FM and eventually loss of FT will occur with progressively more profound hypoxemia.

Doppler Ultrasound

Obstetric Doppler velocimetry (Doppler flow studies) is often used when a fetus has IUGR. The waveforms may show that blood flow in the umbilical vessels of the fetus with IUGR is decreased, which would indicate that the fetus may not be receiving enough blood, nutrients, and oxygen from the placenta.

Two basic types of Doppler are used in sonography. The simplest technique is continuous wave (CW) Doppler. The second is pulsed wave (PW) Doppler. With CW Doppler, a single transducer has two separate piezoelectric crystals, one that continuously transmits signals and one that simultaneously receives signals. Because the crystals are either emitting or receiving sound, CW Doppler measures no specific range or depth resolution (i.e., it records all velocities along the designated line of interrogation). No intrauterine imaging is available with CW, but it may be used in conjunction with a real-time sonographic system to locate or confirm a vessel sampling site. CW is limited to the study of superficial vessels because it cannot discriminate between signals arising from different structures along the beam path.

In **pulsed wave (PW) Doppler**, short bursts of ultrasonic energy are emitted at regular intervals. The same piezoelectric crystal both sends and receives the signals, which allows for range or depth discrimination. The depth of the target is calculated from the elapsed time between transmission of the pulse and reception of its echoes, assuming a constant speed of sound in tissue. In PW Doppler, a sonographer can electronically steer the insonating Doppler beam with the trackball or joystick on the keyboard, along with transducer position and angle manipulations. This permits sampling of vessels at specific anatomic locations.

In one study, CW and PW Doppler were compared using the patient as the control.[14] The systolic to diastolic (S/D or A/B) ratios were obtained from the umbilical artery and the maternal uterine arteries with both CW and PW Doppler systems. The results were comparable. Laboratories can use either a CW or PW Doppler system effectively.

Up to the present, Doppler, or real-time, ultrasonic energy has not been associated with any ill effect to the mother or the fetus when used at the manufacturer's recommended safety level. U.S. Food and Drug Administration guidelines state that the spatial peak-temporal average intensity (SPTA, a unit used to measure ultrasonic intensity) must be less than 94 milliwatts per square centimeter (mW/cm²) in situ. Most commercial equipment uses variable acoustic outputs between 1 and 46 mW/cm². The power output of a given unit should be known before the unit is used on a fetus. Newer sonographic equipment now allows the user to display this information on the screen as the examination is being performed. The mechanical index (MI) and thermal index (TI) are used to indicate the relative acoustic output intensities. The TI is an estimation of the acoustical power that may result in an increase of tissue temperature 1° C. The MI is an indication of the likelihood of causing cavitation, or micro gas bubbles, in the tissues.[24]

Quantitative and Qualitative Measurements. Two main types of measurements can be taken from a Doppler waveform: quantitative and qualitative. Quantitative Doppler flow measurements include blood flow and velocity, whereas qualitative measurements look at the characteristics of the waveform that indirectly approximate flow and resistance to flow. Qualitative measurements include **systolic to diastolic (S/D) ratio, resistance index (RI),** and **pulsatility index (PI)** (Box 51-6). The S/D ratio measures peak systole to end-diastolic blood flow. The RI is calculated as systole minus diastole divided by systole. The pulsatility takes the difference between peak-systole and end-diastole and divides this by the mean of the maximum frequency over the whole cardiac cycle.

Doppler sonography has shown that in fetuses with asymmetric IUGR, vascular resistance increases in the aorta and umbilical artery and decreases in the fetal middle cerebral artery. This reinforces the head-sparing theory, which describes the assurance of blood flow to the fetal brain at the expense of the extremities and the rest of the body.

Increased vascular resistance is reflected by an increased S/D ratio or pulsatility index. Some authors consider an S/D ratio of more than 3.0 in the umbilical artery after 30 weeks to be abnormal, and it is demonstrated by increased resistance in the fetal circulation.[19] The maternal uterine artery S/D ratio should be below 2.6 (Figures 51-7 and 51-8). A ratio above 2.6 suggests increased vascular resistance and indicates a decreased maternal blood supply to the uterus.

In the umbilical circulation, extreme cases of elevated resistance causing absent or reverse end-diastolic flow velocity waveforms are associated with high rates of morbidity and mortality. One report demonstrated that an SGA fetus with an increased umbilical artery S/D ratio is at much higher risk for poor perinatal outcome than a small fetus with a normal S/D ratio (Figures 51-9 and 51-10).[22]

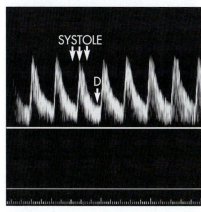

FIGURE 51-7 Typical umbilical artery Doppler waveform representing a normal systolic to diastolic ratio. The ratio measures peak-systolic to end-diastolic flow. The calipers should be placed at the top of the systolic peak and at the bottom of the diastolic trough. Note the normal amount of diastolic flow. *D,* Diastole.

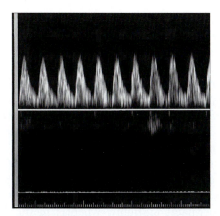

FIGURE 51-8 Umbilical artery Doppler waveform demonstrating increased vascular resistance (less diastolic flow) in the fetal umbilical circulation. The systolic to diastolic (S/D) ratio is 3.8. Some authors consider an S/D ratio of more than 3.0 after 30 weeks of gestation to be abnormal.

BOX 51-6	Doppler Measurements

Resistive Index (RI) = maximum systolic velocity – diastolic velocity/systolic velocity

Systolic/Diastolic Ratio (S/D) = maximum systolic velocity/diastolic velocity

Pulsatility Index (PI) = maximum systolic velocity – diastolic velocity/mean velocity

Acceleration time (ACC) = time from beginning of systole to peak systole

Deceleration time (DCC) = time from peak systole to end diastole

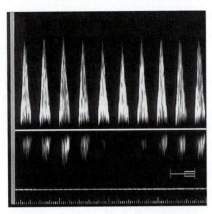

FIGURE 51-9 Umbilical artery waveform with absent end-diastolic velocity (AEDV). The S/D ratio cannot be measured in these cases because of the missing diastolic flow. The patient should be followed closely because AEDV has been associated with adverse perinatal outcome.

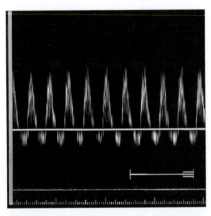

FIGURE 51-10 This umbilical Doppler waveform is the most severe Doppler finding and has been associated with adverse fetal outcomes. This finding is called *complete reversal of end-diastolic velocity.* Note how the diastolic flow dips below the baseline. These results should be reported immediately to the patient's physician.

In one series a growth-restricted fetus with an abnormal S/D ratio was found to be at risk for early delivery, reduced birth weight, decreased amniotic fluid at birth, admission to the neonatal intensive care unit, neonatal complications associated with IUGR, and a prolonged hospital stay.[2] Other authors have reported similar results.[17,22]

Abnormal umbilical artery S/D velocity waveforms have been shown to improve with the patient on bed rest in the left lateral position. The patients were closely monitored with serial Doppler, BPP, and fetal growth evaluation. Of 128 pregnant women, 66 (51.5%) reverted to normal flow in 4.5 weeks, ±1.5 weeks. Another group (48.5%) exhibited persistent abnormal flow.[20] None of the improved group exhibited fetal distress or perinatal mortality, whereas in the abnormal flow group 24% experienced fetal distress and 13% experienced perinatal mortality. The report of the study proposes that a subset of patients with abnormal Doppler velocimetry improves with bed rest and has a better

perinatal outcome, whereas patients with persistent abnormal flow are at risk for poor perinatal outcome.

Combining multiple fetal parameters for an average age of all parameters produces a more accurate fetal age than any single parameter used alone.[9] In addition, it has been found that the range of the parameter ages used for the average age should not vary, in a normal population, more than +/– 8% to 10% of the age. This means that at 20 LMP weeks, all parameters should calculate to an estimated age of +/– 10% of 20 weeks or between 18 and 22 weeks (using the easier 10% calculation). At 30 LMP weeks, all parameters should be between 27 and 33 weeks estimated age. Parameters that fall outside this +/– 10% of age should be rechecked for accuracy of measurements, or malproportions may be considered. The age range analysis (ARA) can be facilitated by recording serial growth studies as shown in Table 50-1 and comparing the parameter ages and average to the LMP age. IUGR is often a progressive process in which the fetal growth rate and sonographic age will lag farther behind the LMP age as the gestation progresses. However, a normal but constitutionally small SGA fetus may lag behind the LMP age at a relatively constant rate.

Of note is that the sonographic age is an estimate from the sonographic parameter measurements and is not the actual parameter age. It is possible for a normally growing fetus to have a 19-week femoral length and a 20-week abdominal circumference, yet both parameters are the same actual LMP age. This means that the parameter's sonographic age estimate is a "surrogate" for the parameter's measurement in the same way that the Doppler calculated estimated velocity is a "surrogate" for the actual measured Doppler frequency shift.

In conclusion, the best method of solving the puzzle of whether a fetus has IUGR or is constitutionally small is to combine an evaluation of all parameters. A normal umbilical artery, maternal uterine artery, and fetal middle cerebral artery help in evaluating the fetus that is well and normal but just small, rather than small secondary to IUGR. The practitioner also must consider the family history of birth weights and ethnicity. For example, it is almost invalid to use the standard EFW growth curves when plotting the fetal growth of a constitutionally small ethnic group, such as some Southeast Asians. A fetus could be labeled as SGA, although its size might be totally appropriate for its heritage. Use of all the fetal surveillance tests (i.e., EFW, AFI, placental grading, BPP, NST) may allow better evaluation of the in utero environment.

MACROSOMIA

Macrosomia is traditionally defined as a birth weight of 4000 g or greater, or above the 90th percentile for estimated gestational age. With respect to delivery, however, any fetus that is too large for the pelvis through which it must pass is macrosomic. Macrosomia has shown to be 1.2 to 2 times more frequent than normal in women who are multiparous, are 35 years or older, have a pre-pregnancy weight of more than 70 kg (154 lb), have a PI in the upper 10%, have pregnancy weight gain of 20 kg (44 lb) or greater, have a postdate pregnancy, or have a history of delivering an LGA fetus.

Macrosomia is also a common result of poorly controlled maternal diabetes mellitus. The frequency of macrosomia in the offspring of mothers with diabetes ranges from 25% to 45%. It is widely accepted that increased levels of glucose and other substrates result in fetal hyperinsulinemia, which promotes accelerated somatic growth. Macrosomic infants of insulin-dependent diabetic mothers are usually heavy and show a characteristic pattern of organomegaly. In addition to adipose tissue, the liver, heart, and adrenals are disproportionately increased in size, which can be reflected by an increased AC. Not all infants of diabetic mothers are larger than average; diabetic mothers with severe vascular disease may in fact be growth restricted.

Malformation syndromes in which fetal increase in size, with or without organomegaly, is a feature include Beckwith-Wiedemann syndrome, Marshall-Smith syndrome, Sotos' syndrome, and Weaver's syndrome.

The macrosomic fetus has an increased incidence of morbidity and mortality as a result of head and shoulder injuries and cord compression. One study found an increasing incidence of shoulder dystocia as birth weight increased.[1] The incidence was 10% in fetuses less than 4500 g and increased to 22.6% in fetuses more than 4500 g. Another study also found an increase, but the overall percentiles were less.[18] This study reported that shoulder dystocia occurred in 4.7% of study fetuses greater than 4000 g and 9.4% of fetuses greater than 4500 g.

Clavicular fractures, facial and brachial palsies, meconium aspiration, perinatal asphyxia, neonatal hypoglycemia, and other metabolic complications are significantly increased in macrosomic pregnancies.

Timing and mode of delivery of the potential macrosomic fetus are of great concern to the obstetrician. One study demonstrated that the incidence of macrosomia increased from 1.7% at 36 weeks to 21% at 42 weeks.[3] A retrospective study evaluated 406 women by sonography late in the third trimester to see if the diagnosis of LGA altered the management of labor and delivery.[12] The sonographic prediction of LGA fetuses had a sensitivity, specificity, and positive predictive value of 50%, 90%, and 52%, respectively. Although there were no significant differences in the rate of induction, use of oxytocin, or use of forceps, women with a sonographic diagnosis of an LGA fetus more frequently received epidural anesthesia and had more cesarean deliveries than women without that diagnosis. The sonographic prediction of EFW in this series was incorrect in half of the cases, with the EFW both underestimating and overestimating the actual birth weight.

Clinical considerations of macrosomia should include the genetic constitution (e.g., familial traits) and environmental factors (e.g., maternal diabetes or prolonged pregnancy).

Two terms relating to macrosomic fetuses are *mechanical macrosomia* and *metabolic macrosomia*. Three types of mechanical macrosomia have been identified: (1) fetuses that are generally large, (2) fetuses that are generally large but with especially large shoulders, and (3) fetuses that have a normal trunk but a large head. The first type can result from genetic factors, prolonged pregnancy, or multiparity. The second type is found in the diabetic pregnancy, and the third type can be caused by genetic constitution or pathologic process, such as hydrocephalus. One type of metabolic macrosomia has been identified, which is the group of LGA fetuses based on a standard weight curve appropriate for the population being studied and a normal range extending to 2 standard deviations above the mean.[6]

Biparietal Diameter

Accurate sonographic prediction of macrosomia would be invaluable to the obstetrician in managing and delivering a fetus with macrosomia. The detection of fetal macrosomia by BPD was first described in 1979.[4] The authors found that all fetuses that were appropriate for gestational age (AGA) at delivery had normal antenatal BPD measurements, but that 25 out of 26 fetuses with two or more BPD values above the 97th percentile were large for gestational age (LGA) at delivery.[4] Another study of the normal progression of fetal head growth in diabetic pregnancies found that, in contrast to the fetal liver, the fetal brain is not sensitive to the growth-promoting effects of insulin.[16] Most investigators believe, however, that BPD is not the optimal parameter for prediction of macrosomia.

Abdominal Circumference

As stated before, AC is useful as a parameter to assess fetal size. It is not very predictive of gestational age. It is probably the single most valuable biometric parameter used in assessing fetal growth (Figure 51-11). In one series the authors were able to predict 4 of 4 macrosomic fetuses when a change in the abdominal circumference was greater than or equal to 1.2 cm per week between the 32nd and 39th weeks of pregnancy (<4000 g), 17 out of 21 (81%) of the fetuses with birth weights between 4000 and 4499 g, and 5 out of 6 (83%) of the fetuses with birth weights exceeding 4500 g.[11] When the abdominal growth was less than 1.2 cm per week (between 32 and 39 weeks), normal fetal growth was correctly identified in 89.1% of cases.

One study found that in fetuses with birth weights less than 4000 g, both the BPD and AC were within the standard deviation for the gestational age.[16] In fetuses

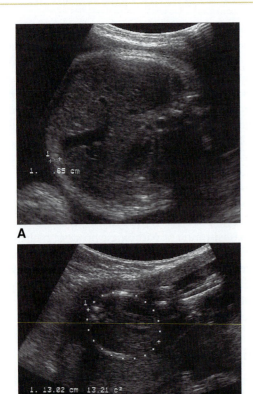

FIGURE 51-11 A, Transverse section through a macrosomic fetal abdomen. Note the fat rind *(calipers)* encircling the entire abdomen compared with a severely intrauterine growth-restricted fetus **(B),** whose growth is 8 weeks behind. The fetal skin is almost transparent and difficult to differentiate from other surrounding organs.

greater than 4000 g, normal BPD values were found, but the AC values were greater than 2 standard deviations above the norm after 28 to 32 weeks.[16]

Estimated Fetal Weight

Sonographic estimation of fetal weight to determine macrosomia is of some value. According to one study, EFWs above the 90th percentile are considered macrosomic.[21] A significant number of false-positive and false-negative results can be expected unless the actual weight is either less than 3600 g or greater than 4500 g. The reason for this may be that currently available formulas to estimate fetal weight assume a uniform density of tissue. Because fat tissue is less dense than lean body mass, it can be hypothesized that sonographic overestimation of fetal weight, particularly in diabetic mothers, is the consequence of an elevated proportion of body fat. This results in a lower body density.

In one report, the pulsatility index (PI) and skinfold thickness were both significantly greater in infants whose sonograms overpredicted the fetal weight compared with those whose sonograms underpredicted the fetal weight.[2] The PI and skinfold thickness are indexes to directly measure fat. The study reported that estimating fetal fat would provide a correction to formulas predicting fetal weight and improve the accuracy of the estimation.

Femur Length to Abdominal Circumference

Another approach to detecting macrosomia is the femur length to abdominal circumference (FL-AC) ratio. This is a time-independent proportionality index. A study of 156 fetuses within 1 week of delivery was done using a cutoff of less than 20.5% (the 10th percentile).[9] Prenatal FL-AC values less than the 10th percentile and newborns with birth weights above the 90th percentile were classified as macrosomic, both prenatal and postnatal. The authors were only able to predict 63% of fetuses that were macrosomic, which suggests that this ratio has a limited clinical application. Current studies fail to show a significant increase in the length of the femur in the macrosomic infant.

Chest Circumference

Chest circumference has been described as a useful parameter in detecting the LGA fetus, with reported detection rates of 80% and 47% in relation to the 90th and 95th percentiles, respectively, for macrosomic fetuses.[23] The sonographic technique of the study is not used frequently. It appears that fetal chest measurements are taken just below the area where cardiac pulsations were identified at the level of the upper fetal abdomen.

Macrosomia Index

A macrosomic index can be calculated by subtracting the BPD from the chest diameter. Chest circumference is measured at the level of the upper fetal abdomen. In a study involving subtraction of the BPD from the chest diameter, 87% of infants weighing more than 4000 g had a macrosomic index of 1.4 cm or greater.[7] Fetal weight of less than 4000 g was predicted accurately in 92% of infants who had a macrosomic index of 1.3 or less. Although this test appears to be quite sensitive, only 61% of those with a positive result were found to be macrosomic at birth.

Other Methods for Detecting Macrosomia

In addition to the numerous biometric parameters useful for detecting macrosomia discussed, there are other sonographic observations that can help rule out the possibility of fetal macrosomia. Mothers with diabetes may accumulate more amniotic fluid (polyhydramnios) than nondiabetic patients. The presence of polyhydramnios in the nondiabetic patient could alert the physician to the presence of undiagnosed maternal glucose intolerance.

The possibility of a fetal anomaly should not be excluded; polyhydramnios has been associated with open neural tube defects and other conditions that may limit fetal swallowing of amniotic fluid.

The placentas of the macrosomic fetus can become significantly large and thick because they are not immune to the growth-enhancing effects of fetal insulin. A placental thickness greater than 5 cm is considered thick when the measurement is taken at right angles to its long axis.

REFERENCES

1. Acker DB, Sachs BP, Freidman EA: Risk factors for shoulder dystocia, *Obstet Gynecol* 66:762, 1985.
2. Bernstein I, Catalano P: Influence of fetal fat on the ultrasound estimation of fetal weight in diabetic mothers, *Obstet Gynecol* 79:561, 1992.
3. Boyd ME, Usher RH, Mclean FH: Fetal macrosomia: prediction, risks, proposed management, *Obstet Gynecol* 61:715, 1983.
4. Crane JP, Kropa MM: Prediction of intrauterine growth retardation via ultrasonically measured head/abdominal circumference ratios, *Obstet Gynecol* 54:597, 1979.
5. Dal Compo S, Sabbagha RE: Intrauterine growth retardation. In Berman M, editor: *Obstetrics and gynecology,* New York, 1991, JB Lippincott.
6. Deter RL, Hadlock FP: Use of ultrasound in the detection of macrosomia: a review, *J Clin Ultrasound* 13:519, 1985.
7. Elliott JP, et al: Ultrasound prediction of fetal macrosomia in diabetic patients, *Obstet Gynecol* 60:159, 1982.
8. Gardosi J, et al: Customized antenatal growth charts, *Lancet* 339:283, 1992.
9. Hadlock FP, et al: Estimation of fetal weight with the use of head, body, and femur measurements: a prospective study, *Am J Obstet Gynecol* 15:333, 1985.
10. Joupilla P, et al: Ultrasonic abnormalities associated with the pathology of fetal karyotype results during the early second trimester of pregnancy, *J Ultrasound Med* 7:218, 1988.
11. Landon M, et al: Sonographic evaluation of fetal abdominal growth: predictor of the large-for-gestational age infant in pregnancies complicated by diabetes mellitus, *Am J Obstet Gynecol* 160:115, 1989.
12. Levine AB, et al: Sonographic diagnosis of the large for gestational age fetus at term: does it make a difference? *Obstet Gynecol* 79:55, 1992.
13. Manning FA, Platt LP, Sypus L: Antepartum fetal evaluation: development of a biophysical profile, *Am J Obstet Gynecol* 136:787, 1980.
14. Mehalek K, et al: Comparison of continuous wave and pulsed wave S/D ratios of umbilical and uterine arteries, *Am J Obstet Gynecol* 72:603, 1988.
15. Nicolaides KH, Rodeck CH, Goslen CM: Rapid karyotyping in non-lethal fetal malformations, *Lancet* 1:283, 1986.
16. Ogata ES, et al: Serial ultrasonography to assess evolving fetal macrosomia, *JAMA* 243:2405, 1980.
17. Phelan JP, et al: Amniotic fluid volume assessment with the four quadrant technique at 36-42 weeks gestation, *J Reprod Fertil* 32:540, 1987.
18. Sandmire MF, O'Halloin TJ: Shoulder dystocia: its incidence and associated risk factors, *Int J Gynecol Obstet* 26:65, 1988.
19. Schulman H, et al: Umbilical velocity wave ratio in human pregnancy, *Am J Obstet Gynecol* 148:985, 1984.
20. Sengupta S, et al: Perinatal outcome following improvement of abnormal umbilical artery velocimetry, *Obstet Gynecol* 78:1062, 1992.
21. Shephard MJ, et al: An evaluation of two equations for predicting fetal weight by ultrasound, *AM J Obstet Gynecol* 142:47, 1982.
22. Trudinger BJ, et al: Flow velocity waveforms in the material uteroplacental and fetal umbilical placental circulations, *Am J Obstet Gynecol* 152:155, 1985.
23. Wladimeroff JW, Bloemsma CA, Wallenberg HCS: Ultrasonic diagnosis of the large-for-dates infant, *Obstet Gynecol* 52:285, 1978.
24. Zagzebski JA: *Essentials of ultrasound physics,* pp. 168-171, St. Louis, 1996, Mosby.

Sonography and High-Risk Pregnancy

Carol Mitchell and Barbara Trampe

A high-risk obstetric patient is one who is at an increased risk for an adverse pregnancy outcome. At its extreme, *adverse* would mean maternal or fetal injury or death. When identifying the high-risk pregnant patient, both the mother and the fetus must be considered. Therefore, this chapter discusses both maternal and fetal high-risk factors.

SCREENING TESTS

Screening tests, as opposed to diagnostic tests, are offered to low-risk populations to identify patients whose risk is high enough for them to be offered diagnostic testing.

Screening for fetal anomalies can be performed in either the first or second trimester. In the first trimester, testing is performed by looking for the pattern of biochemical markers associated with plasma protein A (PAPP-A) and free BhCG. These lab values are used in conjunction with an ultrasound (performed between 11 and 14 weeks) to measure the nuchal translucency. Based on the patient's PAPP-A and free BhCG lab value, age, and nuchal translucency measurement, a more accurate risk calculation can be made for having a child with a chromosomal abnormality. To offer this screening, ultrasound labs must become accredited for first trimester screening. This requires the sonographers and physicians performing the test to attend a specialized training course and perform 40 to 50 first-trimester nuchal translucency measurement exams, which are sent to a core lab for evaluation and monitoring. The advantage to parents with first-trimester screening is that they can evaluate their risk for having a child with a chromosomal problem much earlier in pregnancy and then choose to undergo invasive testing with chorionic villus sampling (CVS) or amniocentesis to obtain tissue for chromosomal analysis.

Second-trimester screening can be performed with the maternal serum quad screen lab value and a targeted ultrasound exam. The **maternal serum quad screen** looks at four serum markers: alpha-fetoprotein (AFP), human chorionic gonadotropin (hCG), unconjugated estriol (uE3), and inhibin-A. The targeted ultrasound is a detailed evaluation of all fetal anatomy that can be seen at the time of exam. Many labs prefer to perform the targeted exam between 18 and 20 weeks gestation. This time period is chosen because it often yields the best view of fetal anatomy based on size. The targeted ultrasound exam includes but is not limited to the evaluation of the anatomy shown in Table 52-1.

Based on the results of the screening maternal serum quad screen and the targeted ultrasound, the patients risk for having a child with a chromosomal anomaly or neural tube defect can be reassessed. Parents are counseled with this information and then can choose to have a diagnostic amniocentesis to obtain fluid for chromosomal analysis, if desired.

MATERNAL FACTORS IN HIGH-RISK PREGNANCY

Advanced Maternal Age

By definition, advanced maternal age (AMA) describes a patient who will be 35 or older at the time of delivery. Advanced maternal age can be an indicator for high-risk pregnancy. For example, the incidence of Down syndrome increases with age. The risk of a 35-year-old woman conceiving a fetus with Down syndrome is 1 in 385, but the risk rises to 1 in 32 at age 45.[1] Maternal age alone, however, fails to detect approximately 80% of fetuses with Down syndrome[1] because these babies are being born to younger women without known risk factors for chromosomal abnormalities. In the United States, it is now standard practice to offer AMA women genetic counseling and invasive prenatal testing for karyotypic analysis. The American College of Obstetrics and Gynecology (ACOG) guidelines recommend that maternal serum screening for neural tube defects and Down syndrome be offered to all women.

Immune and Nonimmune Hydrops

Hydrops fetalis is a condition in which excessive fluid accumulates within the fetal body cavities. This fluid accumulation may result in anasarca, ascites, pericardial effusion, pleural effusion, placental edema, and polyhydramnios. There are two classifications of fetal hydrops: immune hydrops and nonimmune hydrops. By ultrasound evaluation, both types are characterized by extensive accumulation of fluids in fetal tissues or body cavities. Nonimmune hydrops is unrelated to the presence of maternal serum IgG antibody against one of the fetal blood cell antigens.

Immune Hydrops. Blood group isoimmunization is diagnosed on routine antenatal laboratory evaluation, which tests for the presence of a variety antibodies. Any significant antibodies are evaluated for strength of

TABLE 52-1	Targeted Ultrasound in High-Risk Pregnancy
Anatomy	**What to Document**
Central Nervous System (CNS)	**Brain**
	Choroid plexus
	Lateral ventricle (measured at the level of the atrium)
	Thalamus
	Third ventricle
	Cerebellum (measure)
	Cisterna magna (measure)
	Nuchal thickness
	Biparietal diameter (BPD)
	Head circumference (HC)
	Spine
	Longitudinal (cervical, thoracic, lumbar, sacral)
	Transverse (cervical, thoracic, lumbar, sacral)
Face	Orbits
	Upper lip
	Palate
	Nose
	Profile
Heart	**Heart**
	Four-chamber view
	Left ventricular outflow
	Right ventricular outflow
	Three-vessel view
	Aortic arch
	Ductus arteriosus
Gastrointestinal (GI) System	Stomach
	Diaphragm
	Measure abdominal circumference (AC)
Genitourinary (GU) System	Kidneys
	Bladder
Abdominal Wall	Cord insertion
Three-Vessel Cord	Umbilical cord as it enters the abdomen and each artery courses around the bladder
Four Extremities	Humerus (measure)
	Femur (measure)
	Both hands
	Both feet
Placenta	Location
	Absence of previa
Amniotic Fluid Volume	Single largest pocket until 24 weeks
	Amniotic fluid index after 24 weeks
Cervix	Screening evaluation abdominally after 16 weeks
	Transvaginal evaluation of length should be greater than 3 cm

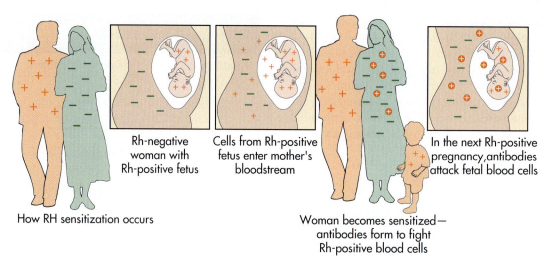

Rh-negative woman with Rh-positive fetus

Cells from Rh-positive fetus enter mother's bloodstream

In the next Rh-positive pregnancy, antibodies attack fetal blood cells

How RH sensitization occurs

Woman becomes sensitized—antibodies form to fight Rh-positive blood cells

FIGURE 52-1 Diagram illustrating the concept of Rh sensitization.

antibody response, which is reported in a titer format (i.e., 1:4, 1:16). If an antibody titer is detected, the pregnancy should be monitored.

Immune hydrops is initiated by the presence of maternal serum immunoglobulin G (IgG) antibody against one of the fetal red blood cell antigens in a process known as sensitization. An antigen is any substance that elicits an immunologic response such as production of an antibody to that substance. In pregnancy this can occur anytime a mother is exposed to red blood cell antigens different from her own. For example, if a father and fetus are Rh+ and a mother is Rh−, and there is a maternal–fetal hemorrhage (mixing of blood), maternal antibodies can be produced against the Rh antigen. In subsequent pregnancies, these antibodies can pass through the placenta and destroy fetal blood cells, resulting in fetal anemia (Figure 52-1). Today, this condition is rare and can be prevented, if RhoGAM is given any time there is potential mixing of the maternal and fetal circulation.

When a sensitized gravid uterus is not treated with RhoGAM, the mother develops an antibody called maternal IgG. This antibody is able to cross the maternal fetal barrier and enter fetal circulation. It attaches to the fetal red blood cells (RBC) and destroys them in a process called hemolysis. Hemolysis can result in fetal anemia, leading to congestive heart failure and **anascara** (Figure 52-2). The severity of fetal anemia can be determined by sonographic surveillance, amniocentesis, and cordocentesis.

Sonographic Surveillance. Sonographic surveillance for an isoimmunized pregnancy should include (but not be limited to) assessment for signs of hydrops. Sonographic findings of hydrops are scalp edema (Figure 52-3), pleural effusion (Figure 52-4), pericardial effusion, ascites (Figure 52-5), polyhydramnios (Figure 52-6), and thickened placenta. Hydrops can be due to fetal anemia. Another ultrasound tool available to predict fetal anemia is Doppler evaluation of the middle cerebral artery (MCA) (Figure 52-7). Because there are fewer red

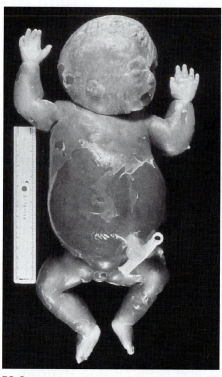

FIGURE 52-2 Hydropic, Rh-sensitized fetal demise. Note the edema of the extremities and protuberant abdomen.

blood cells with anemia, the viscosity of the blood is decreased. A decrease in viscosity results in a decrease in resistance to flow, which can be detected by an increase in velocity in the MCA.

Amniocentesis. Amniocentesis can be used in two ways to monitor the pregnancy. The first is to obtain a sample of amniotic fluid in which direct Rh testing of the fetus can be done. The second way is to monitor the isoimmunized pregnancy with delta optical density 450 (ΔOD450) analysis of amniotic fluid. Bilirubin is a by-product of the hemolysis associated with fetal anemia, and it stains the amniotic fluid. Bilirubin absorbs light

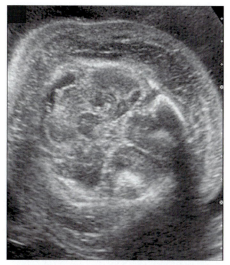

FIGURE 52-3 Scalp edema.

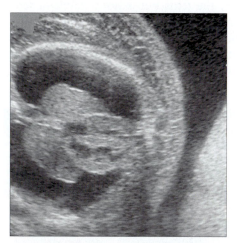

FIGURE 52-4 Pleural effusion.

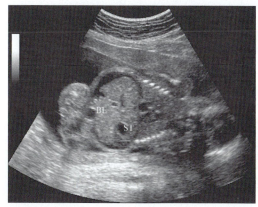

FIGURE 52-5 Coronal view of the fetal abdomen with ascites. *BL,* bladder; *ST,* stomach.

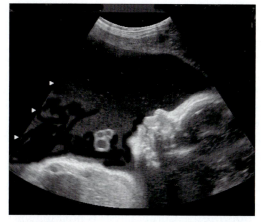

FIGURE 52-6 Fetal profile and polyhydramnios.

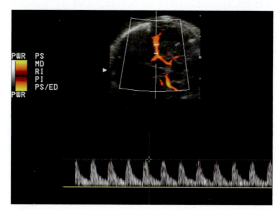

FIGURE 52-7 Doppler of the middle cerebral artery.

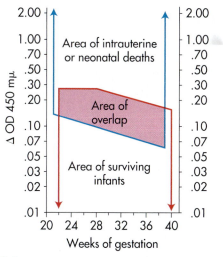

FIGURE 52-8 The Liley curve illustrates perinatal outcome based on *delta* OD450 values.

at the 450-nm wavelength. A spectrophotometric analysis of the fluid to check light absorption of this level indirectly measures the amount of bilirubin present in the fluid and therefore gives a measure of the degree of hemolysis. The gestational age at which the first amnio-

centesis is performed depends on past obstetric history and clinical presentation. Once the amniocentesis is performed and the amniotic fluid is sent for spectrophotometric analysis, the ΔOD450 is categorized into three zones on the Liley curve (Figure 52-8):

1. *Low zone.* Rh-negative and mildly affected fetuses are found in the low zone. They should be followed expectantly and delivered at term.
2. *Midzone.* A downward trend within the midzone indicates the fetus is probably affected but will survive, and delivery should occur at 38 weeks of gestation. A horizontal or rising trend indicates that the fetus is in danger of intrauterine or neonatal death and that preterm delivery or intrauterine transfusion and preterm delivery are indicated.
3. *High zone (fetal death zone).* The fetus in the high zone requires immediate treatment or death will result.

Cordocentesis. Cordocentesis is procedure in which a needle is placed into the fetal umbilical vein to obtain a blood sample. The lab evaluates this sample for fetal blood type, hematocrit, and hemoglobin. If indicated, a fetal transfusion may be performed. There are two methods of transfusing a fetus. The first, intraperitoneal transfusion, uses ultrasound guidance to place a needle in the peritoneal cavity of the fetus. Blood is transfused into the peritoneal space where it is slowly absorbed by the fetus. The second method is direct intravascular transfusion via the umbilical vein (cordocentesis). Using ultrasound guidance, a fine needle is directed through the maternal abdomen toward the umbilical vein where it enters the placenta (Figure 52-9). Red blood cells are transfused directly into the umbilical vein. This method is preferred because a specimen of fetal blood can be obtained before transfusion to confirm that the fetus is truly isoimmunized. A specimen can be obtained after transfusion to document that the fetal hematocrit is adequate.

Alloimmune Thrombocytopenia. In a rare circumstance, a mother may develop an immune response to fetal platelets, much as one might develop an immune response to red blood cells. When this occurs, she develops antibodies to the fetal platelets. The result can be a fetus with a dangerously low platelet count (thrombocytopenia). Infants born with this condition are at increased risk for intracerebral hemorrhage in utero and spontaneous bleeding. Cordocentesis is performed in these cases to document fetal platelet counts before vaginal delivery is attempted. Ultrasound can also be useful to look for evidence of in utero fetal intracerebral hemorrhage.

Nonimmune Hydrops. Nonimmune hydrops (NIH) describes a group of conditions in which hydrops is present in the fetus but is not a result of fetomaternal blood group incompatibility. Numerous fetal, maternal, and placental disorders are known to cause or be associated with NIH (Box 52-1). The incidence of NIH is approximately 1 in 2500 to 1 in 3500 pregnancies, but

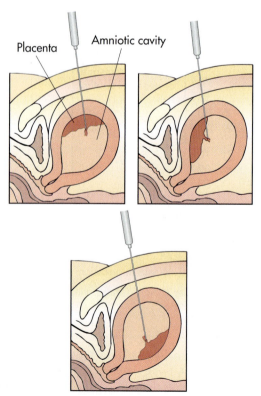

FIGURE 52-9 Possible needle paths in cordocentesis depending on placental position.

BOX 52-1	Disorders Associated with Nonimmune Hydrops

Cardiovascular Problems	**Respiratory Problems**
Tachyarrhythmia	Diaphragmatic hernia
Complex dysrhythmia	Cystic adenomatoid malformation of the lung
Congenital heart block	Tumors of the lung
Anatomic defects	
Cardiomyopathy	**Gastrointestinal Problems**
Myocarditis	Jejunal atresia
Intracardiac tumors	Midgut volvulus
Chromosomal Problems	Meconium peritonitis
Trisomy 21	
Turner's syndrome	**Liver Problems**
Other trisomies	Hepatic vascular malformations
XX/XY mosaicism	Biliary atresia
Triploidy	
Twin Pregnancy	**Infectious Problems**
Twin-to-twin transfusion	Cytomegalovirus
Hematologic Problems	Syphilis
α-Thalassemia	Herpes simplex
Arteriovenous shunts	Rubella
In utero closed-space hemorrhage	Toxoplasmosis
	Congenital hepatitis
	Parvovirus B19
Glucose-6-phosphate deficiency	
Urinary Problems	**Placenta/Umbilical Cord Problems**
Obstructive uropathies	Chorioangioma
Congenital nephrosis	Fetomaternal transfusion
Prune belly syndrome	Placental and umbilical vein thrombosis
Ureterocele	Umbilical cord anomalies

NIH accounts for about 3% of fetal mortality.[7] The exact mechanism for why occurs is unclear, although the same processes described for the hydrops associated with Rh sensitization may apply to NIH.

A variety of maternal, fetal, and placental problems are known to cause or have been found in association with NIH (see Box 52-1). Cardiovascular lesions are the most frequent causes of NIH. Congestive heart failure may result from functional cardiac problems, such as dysrhythmias, tachycardias, and myocarditis, as well as from structural anomalies, such as hypoplastic left heart and other types of congenital heart disease. Obstructive vascular problems occurring outside of the heart, such as umbilical vein thrombosis, and pulmonary diseases, such as diaphragmatic hernia and CCAM–congenital cystic adenomatoid malformation, can cause NIH. Large vascular tumors functioning as arteriovenous shunts can also result in NIH.

Severe anemia of the fetus is another well-recognized etiology for NIH. Although anemia is not caused by isoimmunization, the result is the same. Severe anemia may occur in a donor twin of a twin-to-twin transfusion syndrome, thalassemia, or significant fetomaternal hem-orrhage. To make the diagnosis of NIH, isoimmunization is ruled out with an antibody screen.

Sonographic Findings The fetus may appear similar to a sensitized baby. In addition to ascites (Figures 52-10 and 52-11), scalp edema and pleural and pericardial effusions may be present. Other abnormal findings may also be present that would indicate the cause of the hydrops. If the hydrops is a result of a cardiac tachyar-rhythmia, a heart rate in the range of 200 to 240 is common. If a diaphragmatic hernia is present, bowel will be visible in the chest cavity.

Many times an etiology for NIH cannot be deter-mined. If an etiology is found, treatment is dependent on the cause. As an example, if hydrops results from a tachycardia, medicine can be given to the mother in an attempt to slow the fetal heart rate. Ultrasound can be useful in monitoring the progress of the fetus. Resolution of ascites and gross edema has been documented after the fetal heart was converted to a normal rhythm. If the fetus is anemic because of twin-to-twin transfusion, intrauterine transfusion will not solve the anemia problem because most of the fetal blood is being shunted to the recipient twin (Figure 52-12). Ultrasound can help

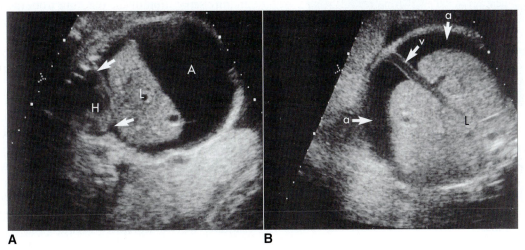

FIGURE 52-10 Transverse sections of fetal abdomen showing ascites in a fetus with nonimmune hydrops. **A,** Sagittal plane. *A,* Ascites; *H,* heart, *L,* liver. **B,** Transverse plane. *a,* ascites; *L,* liver, *v,* umbilical vein.

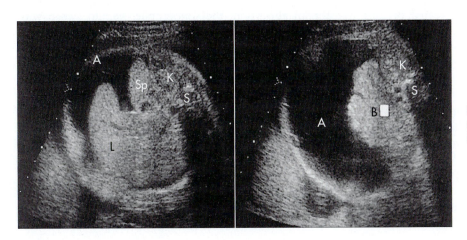

FIGURE 52-11 Cross section of fetal abdomen showing ascites. *A,* ascites; *B,* bowel; *K,* kidney; *L,* liver; *S,* spine.

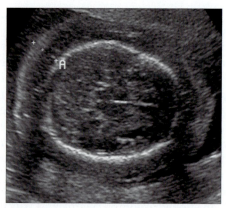

FIGURE 52-12 Twin-twin transfusion syndrome showing hydropic twin with scalp edema.

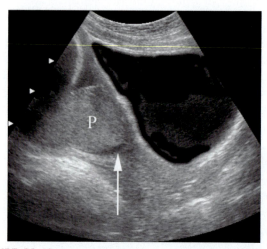

FIGURE 52-13 Placenta previa. *P,* placenta, covering cervical os *(arrow).*

the clinician assess how sick the fetus is by indicating the severity of the hydrops and by biophysical profile. The clinician can then make an informed choice about when to deliver the fetus.

A thorough examination of the fetus, along with fetal echocardiography, must be carried out because abnormalities of almost every organ system have been described with NIH. In addition to the ultrasound examination, genetic amniocentesis for karyotype is indicated, because chromosomal abnormalities have been described as etiologies for NIH.

Vaginal Bleeding

Vaginal bleeding in the second and third trimesters can be associated with placental anomalies like placenta previa and placenta abruption. Placenta previa is the main cause of third-trimester bleeding. In this condition, the placenta covers the internal cervical os and prohibits the delivery of the fetus (Figure 52-13). If the cervical os dilates with labor, there is a significant risk of the placenta detaching from the uterus, resulting in maternal

hemorrhage as well as loss of oxygen and blood supply to the fetus. Transvaginal sonography is the best way to evaluate the relationship of the cervical os to the placental edge. Early in pregnancy the placenta is often lying low, but as the uterus grows, the placenta will appear to migrate away from the cervical os. If this distance is less than 2 cm, the condition may be classified as a marginal or partial placental previa. Even though the placenta may not entirely cover the internal os, the risk for blood loss from the low-lying placental vessels remains. It is important to identify a placenta previa so that a cesarean section may be planned if the previa persists until delivery.

Vasa previa is rare condition in which the umbilical cord is the presenting part. This condition is important to recognize, as it is life threatening to the fetus. This condition is associated with a velamentous cord insertion or succenturiate lobe. Ultrasound is used to assess for vasa previa by utilizing color Doppler to evaluate any structures in front of the cervical os to see if they are vascular. Transvaginal sonography may also assist in identifying this entity.

Placental abruption is another entity that may cause vaginal bleeding during pregnancy. Abruption is the premature separation of the placenta from the uterine wall. When evaluating for placenta abruption, the sonographer should be looking at the area between the placenta and uterine wall. Normally this area is hypoechoic and only 1 to 2 cm thick. If this area is thicker than 1-2 cm, it may be due to an abruption or uterine contraction. Uterine contractions should resolve within 20 to 30 minutes and typically have central blood flow. Abruptions can be difficult to diagnose because clotted blood has the same sonographic appearance as the placental tissue. If bleeding from the abruption has been recent, the sonographer may notice a thin echolucent area between the placenta and the uterus. However, there may be no sonographic signs of an abruption at all. Another way to search for an abruption is to use color flow Doppler. Blood clots from an abruption will not exhibit any color flow. The retroplacental area is hypoechoic because of a large number of blood vessels (mainly veins) located here. Therefore, when evaluating for an abruption, the sonographer should sweep with color Doppler retroplacentally looking for a flow void. If a flow void is present, one should be suspicious of abruption.

MATERNAL DISEASES OF PREGNANCY

Diabetes

Insulin-dependent diabetic mellitus (IDDM) mothers are at an increased risk for pregnancy related complications that include early and late-trimester pregnancy loss and congenital anomalies (Box 52-2). Diabetic pregnancies may be complicated by frequent hospitalizations for

BOX 52-2	Congenital Anomalies in Infants of Diabetic Mothers

Skeletal and Central Nervous System
- Caudal regression syndrome
- Neural tube defects excluding anencephaly
- Anencephaly with or without herniation of neural elements
- Microcephaly

Cardiac
- Transposition of the great vessels with or without ventricular septal defect
- Ventricular septal defect
- Atrial septal defect
- Coarctation of the aorta with or without ventricular septal defect
- Cardiomegaly

Renal
- Hydronephrosis
- Renal agenesis
- Ureteral duplication

Gastrointestinal
- Duodenal atresia
- Anorectal atresia
- Small left colon syndrome

Other
- Single umbilical artery

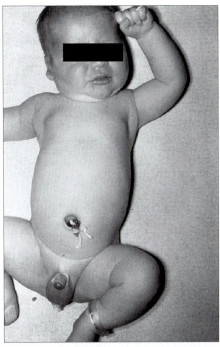

FIGURE 52-14 Macrosomia. A 5280-g (11-lb) infant of a diabetic mother.

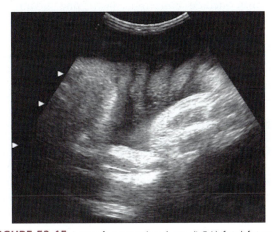

FIGURE 52-15 Large for gestational age (LGA) fetal fat rolls.

glucose control, serious infections such as pyelonephritis, and problems at the time of delivery. These mothers need to be monitored frequently for adequate nutritional and fluid intake, especially if they are experiencing hyperemesis in the first trimester.

Glucose is the primary fuel for fetal growth. If glucose levels are very high and uncontrolled (which happens in diabetes resulting from not being able to produce enough insulin), the fetus may also become macrosomic. Macrosomia is defined as a fetus whose weight is greater than the 90 percentile for gestational age. A macrosomic infant (Figure 52-14) may become too large to fit through the mother's pelvis, necessitating a cesarean section. If delivery is accomplished vaginally, however, the physician may have difficulty delivering the shoulders of the baby after the head has delivered, a condition termed *shoulder dystocia*. Brachial plexus nerve injuries may result from the traction placed on the head and neck in attempts to get the remainder of the baby out.

Once delivered, an infant of a diabetic mother may experience problems with glucose control in the nursery necessitating intravenous glucose administration.

Sonographic Findings. Because correct dating is so important, pregnancy dates should be confirmed with ultrasound. There is an increased risk of early fetal demise, so the presence of a fetal heart beat should be confirmed prior to initiating maternal diabetic protocols. There also is an increased risk of third-trimester loss as well as other pregnancy complications that may neces-

sitate the induction of labor before term when the fetal lung maturity is demonstrated. A diabetic baby delivered preterm may have respiratory distress syndrome and require placement in the high-risk nursery.

Polyhydramnios can be seen with elevated blood sugars and macrosomic fetuses. Polyhydramions can predispose to premature labor, **premature rupture of membranes (PROM)** and maternal discomfort. The fetus of a diabetic mother may measure large for gestational age, making late pregnancy dating inaccurate. Increased adipose tissue may be seen on the fetus in utero (Figures 52-15 and 52-16). Monthly ultrasounds can give the clinician important information regarding fetal growth. If the estimated fetal weight is greater than 4500 g at

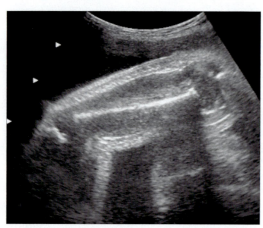

FIGURE 52-16 Large for gestational age (LGA) fetus with adipose tissue in the fetal upper arm.

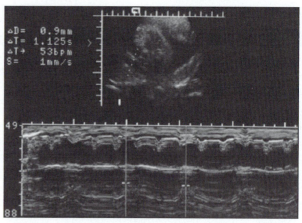

FIGURE 52-17 M-mode demonstrating a ventricular heart rate of 53 bpm in a fetus with complete heart block.

term, the clinician will be alert to the problems of dystocia with a vaginal delivery and may prefer cesarean delivery.

Ultrasound plays a very important role in scanning for fetal anomalies. **Caudal regression syndrome** (lack of development of the caudal spine and cord) is seen almost exclusively in diabetic individuals. Other associated anomalies include congenital heart and neural tube defects. In diabetics who have vasculopathy, fetuses may be at risk for intrauterine growth restriction (IUGR). Sonographic findings with this condition may include small-for-gestation growth patterns and an elevated S/D ratio.

Hypertension

Hypertension is a medical complication of pregnancy that occurs frequently in high-risk populations. Hypertension places both mother and fetus at risk. Hypertensive pregnancies may be associated with small placentas because of the effect of the hypertension on the blood vessels. If the placenta develops poorly, the blood supply to the fetus may be restricted, possibly leading to growth restriction. Growth-restricted fetuses are at increased risk of fetal distress and death in utero.

There are various forms of hypertensive disease during pregnancy. In the past, the term *toxemia* was used to describe hypertensive disorders, because it was believed that a "toxin" in the mother's bloodstream caused the hypertension. Currently, **pregnancy-induced hypertension (PIH)** is thought to be caused by prostaglandin abnormalities.

The terminology currently used in clinical practice to describe hypertensive states during pregnancy includes (1) pregnancy-induced hypertension (preeclampsia, severe preeclampsia, and eclampsia) and (2) chronic hypertension, which was present before the woman became pregnant. Preeclampsia is a pregnancy condition in which high blood pressure develops with proteinuria

(protein in the urine) or edema (swelling). If the hypertension is neglected, the patient may develop seizures that can be life-threatening to both mother and fetus. Severe preeclampsia may develop in some cases and refers to the severity of hypertension and proteinuria. Severe preeclampsia generally indicates that the patient must be delivered immediately. **Eclampsia** represents the occurrence of seizures or coma in a preeclamptic patient. Chronic hypertension is diagnosed in patients in whom high blood pressure is found before 20 weeks of gestation. Chronic hypertension can result from primary essential hypertension or from secondary hypertension (renal, endocrine, or neurologic causes).

Sonographic Findings. The ultrasound team may be called on to perform serial scans for fetal growth and to monitor for the adequacy of amniotic fluid. If fetal growth is falling off the normal growth curve or oligohydramnios occurs, the obstetrician may intervene and deliver the fetus, fearing that intrauterine fetal demise is imminent. Doppler ultrasound can also give the physician information regarding the fetal and maternal circulatory status, which may help determine the pregnancies at risk for developing intrauterine growth restriction.

Systemic Lupus Erythematosus

Systemic lupus erythematosus (SLE) is a chronic autoimmune disorder that can affect almost all organ systems in the body. It is most common in women of childbearing age and may cause multiple peripartum complications. The incidence of spontaneous abortion and fetal death is 22% to 49% in patients with SLE.[2,6] The placenta is affected by the immune complex deposits and inflammatory responses in the placental vessels and may account for the increased number of spontaneous abortions, stillbirths, and intrauterine growth restricted fetuses. The fetus must be monitored to rule out congenital heart block (Figure 52-17) and pericardial effusion.

Other Maternal Disease

Hyperemesis. Ultrasound can be useful in the workup of excessive vomiting in the pregnant woman. **Hyperemesis gravidarum** exists when a pregnant woman vomits so much that she develops dehydration and electrolyte imbalance. When this occurs, hospitalization with intravenous fluid administration is usually necessary. The physician must ensure that the vomiting results strictly from pregnancy and not other disease, such as gallstones, peptic ulcers, or trophoblastic disease. Trophoblastic disease can easily be ruled out by demonstrating a viable intrauterine pregnancy. Gallstones can be ruled out by careful sonographic examination of the gallbladder.

Urinary Tract Disease. Ultrasound can also be useful in the workup of urinary tract disease. Approximately 4% to 6% of pregnant women have asymptomatic bacteriuria. If left untreated, the bacteriuria can develop into pyelonephritis in some women. Although pyelonephritis usually presents with flank pain, fever, and white blood cells in the urine, hydronephrosis is another condition that presents with flank pain. Pregnancy is normally associated with mild hydronephrosis. The hydronephrosis may result from a combination of effects. First, progesterone has a dilatory effect on the smooth muscle of the ureter. Second, the enlarging uterus also compresses the ureters at the pelvic brim, causing a hydronephrosis or obstruction. If a woman presents with more than one episode of pyelonephritis or has continued flank pain, ultrasound examination may provide information as to the etiology.

Adnexal Cysts. Physiologic ovarian cysts may be associated with early pregnancy. These cysts may be large, ranging from 8 to 10 cm, and may be associated with pelvic pain. The cyst should diminish as the pregnancy progresses. If the cyst does not resolve, surgical exploration may be necessary to rule out other ovarian pathology like endometriomas, dermoid cysts (Figure 52-18), and even cancers. Periodic ultrasound examinations are necessary for follow-up of a cyst.

Obesity. Maternal obesity has been associated with an increased incidence of neural tube defects and may be attributed to a deficiency in diet. Obese women start their pregnancy with existing chronic hypertension more often than do women who start their pregnancy at a normal weight. Moreover, obese women are at an increased risk for pregnancy-induced hypertension. Likewise, obese women are at an increased risk for severe eclampsia. Multiple births and urinary tract infections have also been reported to be higher in obese women.[9]

Uterine Fibroids. Finally, pregnant women may periodically present with problems related to uterine fibroids. Fibroids are actually benign tumors of uterine smooth muscle that may be stimulated to excessive growth by the hormones of pregnancy, specifically estrogen. If the growth is very rapid, the fibroid may outgrow its blood supply and undergo necrosis, which may cause pain and premature labor. Ultrasound examination of the uterus in a pregnant woman may detect uterine fibroids (Figure 52-19). It is important to document the size and location of these fibroids, as they may obstruct a clear pathway for fetal delivery. If the placenta implants over a fibroid, it may lead to poor placental profusion in that area, which can be a cause of intrauterine growth restriction.

ULTRASOUND IN LABOR AND DELIVERY

Preterm Labor

Preterm, or premature, labor is the onset of labor before 37 weeks of gestation (Box 52-3). It is an obstetric complication occurring in 15% to 20% of all pregnancies.[5] Premature infants are at greater the risk for having problems, such as respiratory distress syndrome, intracranial hemorrhage, bowel immaturity, and feeding problems.

Potential etiologies of preterm labor include premature rupture of membranes, intrauterine infection, bleeding, fetal anomalies, polyhydramnios, multiple pregnancy, growth restriction, maternal illness (diabetes or hypertension), incompetent cervix, and uterine abnormalities.

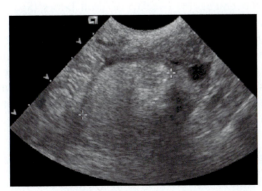

FIGURE 52-18 Dermoid cyst.

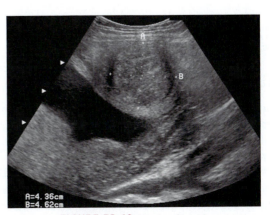

FIGURE 52-19 Uterine fibroid.

BOX 52-3	**Warning Signs of Preterm Labor**

- Menstrual-like cramps (constant or intermittent)
- Low, dull backache
- Pressure (feels like baby is pushing down)
- Abdominal cramping (with or without diarrhea)
- Increase of change in vaginal discharge (contains mucus or is watery, light, or bloody)
- Fluid leaking from the vagina
- Feeling poorly
- Uterine contractions

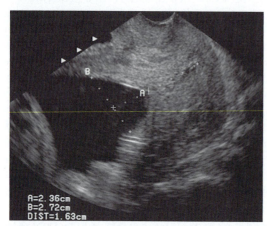

FIGURE 52-20 Incompetent cervix in a patient with triplets.

Epidemiologic factors such as socioeconomic class; maternal age, weight, and height; late prenatal care; smoking; coitus; a history of cervical injury or surgery; and a poor previous obstetric history are presumed etiologies as well. Another patient population at increased risk for preterm labor is patients with multiple gestations. In about half of all cases, no cause or association can be identified for the preterm labor.

Sonographic Findings. Ultrasound assessment of the preterm labor patient should include, but not be limited to, amniotic fluid assessment, cervical assessment (Figure 52-20), fetal number, placental assessment, and targeted ultrasound (see Table 52-1). The sonographer should be aware of the potential causes of preterm labor and tailor the exam accordingly.

FETAL FACTORS IN HIGH-RISK PREGNANCY

Fetal Death

Intrauterine fetal death accounts for roughly half of all perinatal mortality. Although the cause of death cannot be determined in approximately half of the cases, known causes are infection (usually associated with premature rupture of membranes), congenital or chromosomal abnormalities, preeclampsia, placental abruption, diabetes, growth restriction, and blood group isoimmunization.

Fetal death may occur in any trimester of pregnancy. The overall miscarriage rate is reported as 15% to 20%, which means 15% to 20% of recognized pregnancies result in miscarriage. About 80% of miscarriages occur within the first trimester. In the first trimester, embryonic causes of spontaneous abortion are the predominant etiology. Genetic abnormalities within the embryo are the most common cause of spontaneous abortion and account for 50% to 65% of all miscarriages. The most common single chromosomal anomaly is 45,X karyotype, with an incidence of 14.6%. Trisomies are the single largest group of chromosomal anomalies and account for approximately half of all anomalies associated with miscarriage. Approximately 20% of genetic abnormalities are triploidies.

Clinically, first-trimester pregnancy loss may be diagnosed when the patient presents to her physician with vaginal bleeding, cramping, or passage of tissue. Ultrasound examination may reveal a blighted ovum or a fetus with no heart motion. As the pregnancy progresses into the second trimester, pregnancy landmarks become important for determining whether the pregnancy is proceeding normally. Fetal heart tones should be heard with Doppler at approximately 10 to 12 weeks of gestation. At 20 weeks of gestation, the uterine fundal height should have risen to the umbilicus and the uterus should measure approximately 20 cm above the symphysis pubis. The mother should also perceive fetal movements on a daily basis beginning between 16 and 20 weeks of gestation. Failure to achieve any one of these landmarks may prompt the clinician to obtain an ultrasound examination.

As the pregnancy progresses, the clinician will follow the pregnant woman at regular intervals, listening to fetal heart tones and measuring the uterine fundal height at each visit. The mother will be questioned about fetal movements. The absence of a fetal heart rate usually prompts the clinician to obtain an ultrasound examination. Cessation of fetal movements should prompt an immediate search for fetal heart tones. If none are present, ultrasound examination will confirm or rule out intrauterine fetal demise.

Sonographic Findings. Sonographic findings associated with fetal death are (1) absent heartbeat, (2) absent fetal movement, (3) overlap of skull bones (**Spalding's sign**), (4) an exaggerated curvature of the fetal spine (Figure 52-21), and (5) gas in the fetal abdomen. A brief ultrasound examination of the fetus for structural anomalies should be performed and biometry obtained to determine estimated weight for delivery. Care should be taken and consideration given to the family to not add to their emotional stress during this difficult time.

Large for Gestational Age

When a fetus is measuring large for gestational age, the sonographer is asked to evaluate for fetal macrosomia.

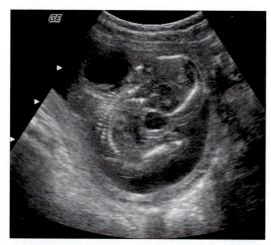

FIGURE 52-21 Extreme curvature of the fetal spine in a fetal demise.

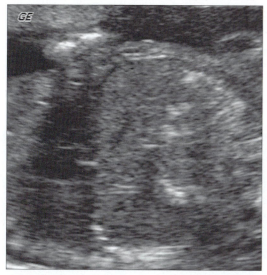

FIGURE 52-22 Liver calcifications in a pregnancy affected by cytomegalovirus (CMV).

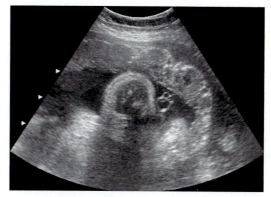

FIGURE 52-23 Placental calcifications.

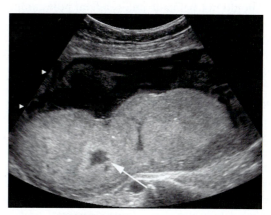

FIGURE 52-24 Placental infarct.

Macrosomia is accelerated growth in utero and is defined as an estimated birth weight greater than 4000 grams. Macrosomia can be symmetric or asymmetric. Symmetric macrosomia is usually due to prolonged pregnancy or to genetics. Asymmetric macrosomia is often seen in diabetic mothers; the fetus will have an abdominal girth larger relative to head size and length. The significance of macrosomia is that there is increased morbidity associated with it due to birth trauma (birth asphyxia). These findings are usually associated with a fetus whose estimated fetal weight is greater than 4000–4500 g (8 lbs 13 oz to 9 lbs 15 oz).

Small for Gestational Age

Small for gestational age can be due chromosomal anomalies, intrauterine infection (Figure 52-22), genetics, or placental insufficiency (Figure 52-23 and 52-24). If chromosomal anomalies are the etiology for the fetus measur-

ing small, growth is often affected symmetrically, meaning that all the fetal measurements will be smaller than expected for gestational age. When placental insufficiency is the cause, fetuses often develop an asymmetrical intrauterine growth restriction pattern. This pattern results in a normal head measurement with a small abdominal circumference and smaller-than-expected limb growth. The clinical significance of recognizing a growth-restricted fetus is that these pregnancies are at an increased risk for perinatal morbidity and mortality compared to normal weight fetuses, and neurologic and intellectual impairment when delivered at term. If the IUGR fetus is recognized early, bed rest can be instituted in an attempt to increase maternal uterine profusion and potentially increase fetal blood supply. Fetal growth and behaviors can be monitored for signs of worsening profusion, and early delivery can be induced if necessary for fetal well-being. Infants delivered at 34 to 35 weeks of gestation have a better chance of catching up to their peers by 2 years of age than growth-restricted fetuses delivered at term.

MULTIPLE GESTATION PREGNANCY

Ultrasound is an extremely valuable tool in the assessment of multiple gestation pregnancies. It may be used to monitor the growth of the fetuses and for guidance of diagnostic and therapeutic procedures. The mother with a multiple gestation is at increased risk for obstetric complications, such as **preeclampsia**, third-trimester bleeding, and prolapsed cord. The fetuses are at increased risk of premature delivery and congenital anomalies. As a result, a twin has a five times greater chance of perinatal death than a singleton fetus.[8] Physicians follow multiple gestations closely with ultrasound.

Before the routine use of obstetric ultrasound, as many as 60% of twin pregnancies went undiagnosed before delivery.[10] Now most multiple gestations are diagnosed before the onset of labor. During the first trimester, multiple gestations can be identified by visualizing more than one gestational sac within the uterus. A firm diagnosis should not be made unless a fetal pole can be seen within each sac, regardless of the number of sacs that are seen.

In the second and third trimesters, several clinical findings may prompt an ultrasound examination. The patient's uterus may be larger on examination than expected for dates. **Maternal serum alpha-fetoprotein (MSAFP)** screening is performed routinely to detect neural tube defects. By virtue of having two fetuses rather than one, twin pregnancies are associated with elevations of MSAFP. Therefore, a patient with elevated MSAFP may present for a scan to rule out neural tube defects and be found to be carrying twins. The physician may detect two fetal heart beats or palpate two heads, prompting an ultrasound examination. Finally, the twins may be unsuspected and found serendipitously.

Once a multiple gestation has been identified, a targeted ultrasound examination should be performed to look specifically for fetal anomalies. In each multiple gestation evaluated by ultrasound, the sonographer needs to evaluate placentation type (Box 52-4). This refers to the number of chorions (chorionicity) and amnions (amnionicity). In a twin pregnancy, this depends on the number of zygotes and, in monozygotic twinning, the timing of zygotic division (Figures 52-25, 52-26, and 52-27).

Dizygotic Twins

There are two types of twins: dizygotic (fraternal) and monozygotic (identical). **Dizygotic** twins arise from two separately fertilized ova. Each ovum implants separately in the uterus and develops its own placenta, chorion, and amniotic sac (diamniotic, dichorionic). The placentas may implant in different parts of the uterus and be distinctly separate or may implant adjacent to each other and fuse. Although the placentas are fused, their blood circulations remain distinct and separate from each other.

Monozygotic Twins

Monozygotic twins (identical) arise from a single fertilized egg, which divides, resulting in two genetically

BOX 52-4	Types of Placentation

- All *dizygotic* pregnancies are dichorionic/diamniotic
- Of *monozygotic* pregnancies, 25% are dichorionic (two placentas); the majority (75%) are monochorionic (one placenta)
- In *dichorionic* pregnancies, whether monozygotic or dizygotic, two layers of amnion and two layers of chorion separate the fetuses

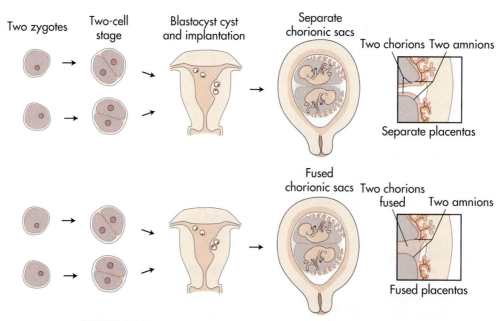

FIGURE 52-25 The dichorionicity and diamnionicity of dizygotic twins.

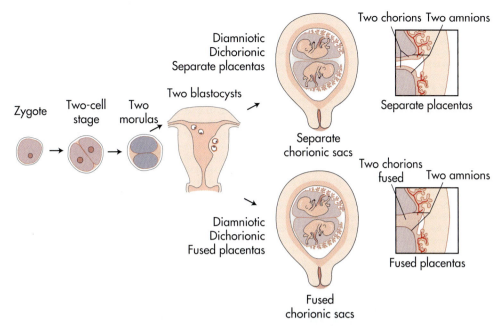

FIGURE 52-26 Possible dichorionicity and diamnionicity of monozygotic twins.

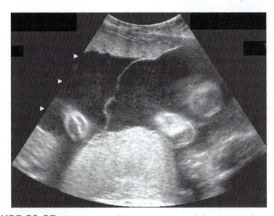

FIGURE 52-27 This image demonstrates a dichorionic, diamniotic twin gestation.

identical fetuses. Depending on whether the fertilized egg divides early or late, there may be one or two placentas, chorions, and amniotic sacs. If the division occurs early, 0 to 4 days postconception, there will be two amnions and two chorions (dichorionic, diamniotic). If the division occurs at 4 to 8 days, there will be one chorion and two amniotic sacs (monochorionic, diamniotic) (Figures 52-28 and 52-29). If the division occurs after 8 days, two fetuses will be present but only one chorion and one amnion (monochorionic, monoamniotic) (Figures 52-30, 52-31, and 52-32). If the division occurs after 13 days, the division may be incomplete and **conjoined twins** may result. The twins may be joined at a variety of sites, including head, thorax, abdomen, and pelvis (Figure 52-33, 52-34, and 52-35). Monozygotic twins present a very high-risk situation. Besides an association with an increased incidence of fetal anomalies, if there is only

one amniotic sac, the twins may entangle their umbilical cords, cutting off their blood supply. In these monochorionic diamniotic pregnancies, only the two layers of amnion separate the twins. Because the circulations of the monozygotic twins communicate through a single placenta, they are at increased risk for a syndrome known as twin-to-twin transfusion, which is discussed later.

One obstacle to imaging twins is the phenomenon of the vanishing and appearing twin. One twin may die in utero and the other one continue to grow. One study showed that 70% of pregnancies that began with twins ended with a singleton.[3] Many of these losses occur very early and are never detected. Others are detected early when the patient presents with vaginal bleeding in the second trimester and two sacs are visualized, one with a healthy fetus and one with a demise (Figure 52-36). If the demise occurs very early, complete resorption of both embryo and gestational sac or early placenta may occur. This phenomenon is sometimes referred to as the "vanishing" twin, because once reabsorbed, the products of conception of this twin will no longer be seen on ultrasound. If the fetus dies after reaching a size too large for resorption, the fetus is markedly flattened from loss of fluid and most of the soft tissue. This is termed **fetus papyraceous** (Figure 52-37).

Just as a twin may appear to vanish, one may also "appear." The appearing twin is seen when ultrasound exams are performed very early in gestation (5 to 6 weeks) and undercounting of the gestation sacs occurs. Undercounting can occur because of a discrepancy in gestational sac size, the locations of sacs, if the patient is scanned before yolk sacs are seen, in cases of monochorionic, monoamniotic gestation without crown-rump

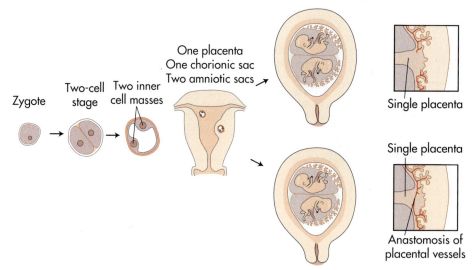

FIGURE 52-28 A monochorionic, diamniotic, monozygotic twin gestation.

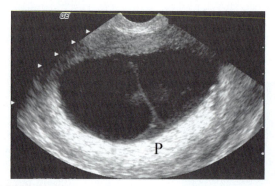

FIGURE 52-29 A monochorionic, diamniotic twin gestation.

FIGURE 52-30 A monochorionic, monoamniotic, monozygotic twin gestation.

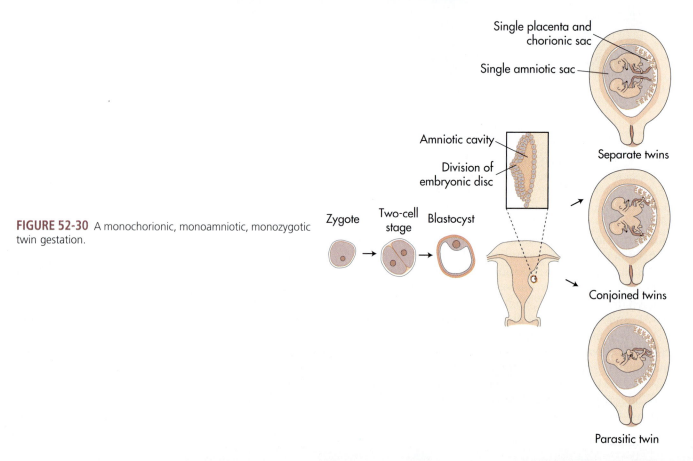

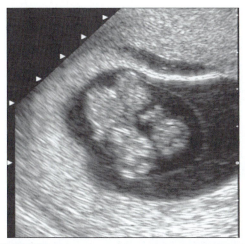

FIGURE 52-31 A monochorionic, monoamniotic twin gestation.

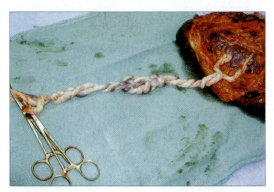

FIGURE 52-32 Gross illustration of monochorionic, monoamniotic placenta with two tangled amniotic cords.

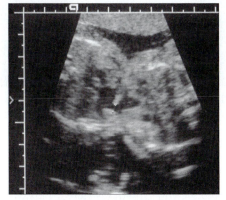

FIGURE 52-33 A set of conjoined twins connected at the thorax. Note they share a single four-chamber heart.

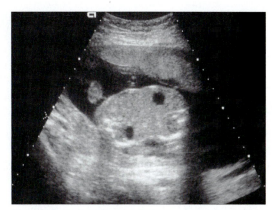

FIGURE 52-34 A set of conjoined twins connected at the abdomen. Note the stomach bubbles visualized on each twin.

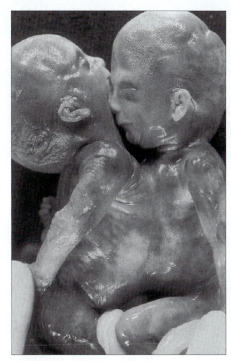

FIGURE 52-35 Thoracoabdominal conjoined twins.

lengths, and failure of the operator to identify a second gestational sac.

Anomalies Specific to Twin Pregnancies

As stated previously, multiple gestations have a high rate of anomalies, and a careful search must be performed to rule out birth defects. It is also important for sonographers to understand which abnormalities are unique to multiple gestations they should be screening for. Several abnormalities are specific to multiple gestations. They are poly–oligo sequence, acardiac anomaly, and conjoined twins.

Poly-Oli Sequence ("Stuck Twin"). Poly-oli sequence, also known as "stuck twin" syndrome, is characterized by a diamniotic pregnancy with polyhydramnios in one sac and severe oligohydramnios and a smaller twin in the other sac (Figure 52-38). This syndrome usually manifests between 16 to 26 weeks' gestation. Most involve monochorionic gestations. Stuck-twin syndrome may result from a fetal anomaly in one sac resulting in polyhydramnios, compressing the blood flow in the normal twin's placenta and resulting in oligohydramnios; placental insufficiency in one placenta; and twin-twin transfusion syndrome. When oligohydramnios exists in one sac and polyhydramnios in the other, the

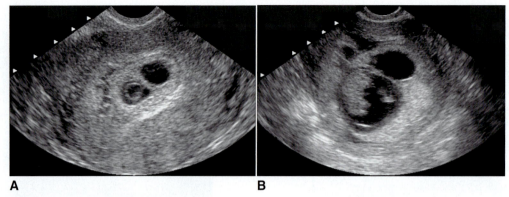

FIGURE 52-36 A, An early twin gestation. **B,** Same patient further into pregnancy demonstrates vanishing twin phenomenon.

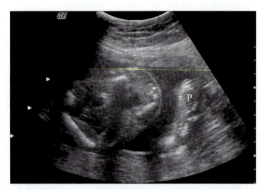

FIGURE 52-37 The demise of one twin resulting in a fetus papyraceous, *P*.

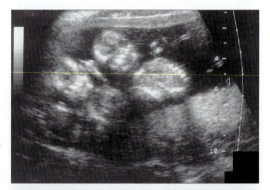

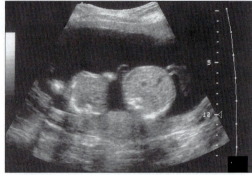

FIGURE 52-39 Multiple gestation affected by twin-to-twin transfusion syndrome (TTS). Note the size discrepancy between the two fetuses.

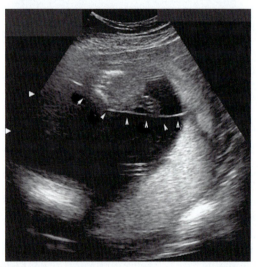

FIGURE 52-38 A "stuck twin." Arrowheads point to the amnion surrounding the stuck twin.

small twin may appear stuck in position within the uterus, hence the term "stuck twin." In the event that twin-to-twin transfusion exists, the growth of the twins will be discordant, with the donor twin falling off the growth curve (Figure 52-39).

Twin-to-twin transfusion syndrome (TTS) exists when there is an arteriovenous shunt within the placenta. The arterial blood of one twin is pumped into the venous

system of the other twin. As a result, the donor twin becomes anemic and growth restricted. This twin has less blood flow through its kidneys, urinates less, and develops **oligohydramnios**. The recipient twin, however, gets too much blood flow. The twin may be normal or large in size. This fetus has excess blood flow through its kidneys and urinates too much, leading to **polyhydramnios**. This twin may even go into heart failure and become hydropic.

If twin-to-twin transfusion exists, both twins are at risk of dying—the smaller one because its nutritional and oxygen-rich blood supply is severely restricted, and the larger one because of heart failure. Depending on the gestational age, the obstetric specialist may be forced to deliver the fetuses early if it appears one or both of the twins are at risk of dying in utero. Fetal surveillance is increased when growth discordance, oligohydramnios, or polyhydramnios is discovered. Treatments for stuck twin syndrome include serial amniocentesis, selective feticide, umbilical cord ligation of one twin, and laser occlusion of anastomosing placental vessels.

Acardiac Anomaly. By definition, a cardiac anomaly is a rare anomaly, occurring in monochorionic twins, in which one twin develops without a heart and often without the upper half of the body (Figure 52-40). It has been suggested that this occurs because of an artery-to-artery connection in the placenta that leads to perfusion of the abnormal twin via the co-twin. The reversed direction of blood flow in the abnormal twin alters the hemodynamic properties needed for normal cardiac formation. On ultrasound, one will see a monochorionic twin gestation with one normal fetus and one fetus with an absent heart. The abnormal twin also has other anomalies such as absent head, absent organs in the thorax and abdomen, and absent or abnormal limbs.

Conjoined Twins. This condition occurs when there is an incomplete division of the embryo after 13 days from conception. Five types of conjoined twins have been described: thoracopagus (joined at the thorax), omphalopagus (joined at the anterior wall), craniopagus (joined at the cranium, syncephalus, conjoined twins with one head) pygopagus (joined at the ischial region), and ischiopagus (attached at the buttocks). On ultrasound, one will see a monochorionic, monoamniotic gestation with two fetuses connected.

Scanning Multiple Gestations

Multiple gestations have many potential risks, so the sonographer must do a complete job of scanning the fetuses. In addition to the anatomy listed in Table 52-1, the ultrasound report should include the following information:

1. Number of sacs
2. Number and location of placentas
3. Gender of the fetuses
4. Biometric data
5. Presence of anomalies

The fetal gestational sacs should be assigned a label (typically an alphabetical letter) to consistently identify them in following exams. The sac and fetus directly over the internal os is labeled A. Sacs above that should be additionally identified by their placental location or additional identifying information such as left or right side of the uterus. This is will be important in future exams to consistently evaluate the growth of each fetus against its own previous growth, not that of another sibling.

During the first trimester, the sonographer must be careful to analyze the uterine contents for the presence of multiple gestations. Multiple gestations may be initially undercounted in early pregnancies of less than 6 weeks performed with transvaginal ultrasound. After 6 weeks' gestational age, determining pregnancy number is easily accomplished by counting embryos in the uterus. Before 6 weeks the embryo is not consistently visualized and the sonographer must count the gestational sacs and small yolk sacs. An article reported that the frequency of undercounting multiple gestations on a 5.0- to 5.9-week sonogram was highest for monochorionic twins (86%), followed by higher-order gestations (16%), and last by dichorionic twins (11%).[4] The authors of the report reasoned that some of the gestational sacs may differ in size or the yolk sac may be too small to adequately image so early. This may account for the "vanishing twin" or "appearing twin" phenomenon.

When scanning multiple gestations, the sonographer should always try to determine whether there are one or two amniotic sacs by locating the membrane that separates the sacs. If two sacs are seen, the pregnancy is known to be diamniotic, but sonography will not be able to indicate whether the twins are identical. As noted before, both monozygotic and dizygotic twins may have two amniotic sacs.

Documentation of a membrane separating the fetuses confirms the presence of a diamniotic pregnancy. The membrane, composed of amnion with or without chorion, exhibits a characteristic appearance that permits distinction from other membranes of pregnancy. In a twin pregnancy with two separate placentas, the membrane extends between the fetuses obliquely across the uterus from the edge of the placenta to the contralateral edge of the other placenta. If only one placental site exists, the membrane extends between the fetuses away from the central portion of the placental site. The fetus may touch the membrane but does not cross it, and the membrane does not adhere to entrap the fetus. The membrane has no free edge within the amniotic fluid. These features distinguish the normal membrane separating

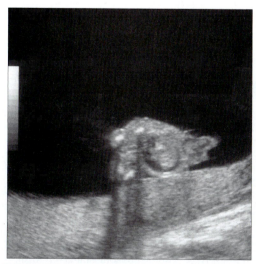

FIGURE 52-40 An acardiac, acephalic twin gestation.

twins from other membranes or membrane-like structures within the amniotic fluid (i.e., uterine synechiae, partial uterine septations, or amniotic bands).

Failure to image the membrane separating the twin fetuses does not reliably predict the presence of a monoamniotic pregnancy. If only one placenta is seen and a membrane cannot be visualized, other features may assist in the prediction of amnionicity, chorionicity, and zygosity. A male and female fetus is dizygotic, diamniotic, and dichorionic. A twin pregnancy with intertwined umbilical cords, conjoined twins, or more than three vessels in the umbilical cord is found in a monozygotic pregnancy that is monoamniotic and monochorionic.

The location of the placenta should be determined. An attempt also should be made to determine the number of placentas. Occasionally, clearly separate placentas may be identified. If two placentas are implanted immediately adjacent to each other and fuse, it may be difficult to determine whether there are one or two placentas. The body of the placenta should be scanned to determine whether a line of separation can be seen.

The twins should each then be scanned for corroboration of dates and size, measuring parameters that include biparietal diameter (BPD), head circumference (HC), abdominal circumference (AC), and femur length (FL).

Dolichocephaly can be common in twin pregnancies as a result of crowding. In dolichocephaly the BPD is shortened and the occipitofrontal diameter (OFD) is lengthened because of compression. Therefore, the BPD underestimates gestational age with dolichocephaly. The sonographer should always determine the cephalic index (CI) (CI = BPD/OFD × 100). CI of less than 75% suggests dolichocephaly. The normal CI is 75% to 85%.

Because the growth of twins is similar to that of singletons early in pregnancy, singleton growth charts are generally used. It is important to keep in mind that a fetus from a multiple gestation is usually smaller than a singleton fetus. It is known that twins are smaller in size at birth than singleton fetuses of comparable gestational age. Of concern is the ability to detect growth restriction in one or both fetuses. When attempting to determine whether only one twin is growth restricted, differences between the measurements of the two twins must be examined. A difference in estimated fetal weight of more than 20%, a difference in BPD of 6 mm, a difference in AC of 20 mm, and a difference in femur length of 5 mm have been reported as predictors of discordance of growth between twins.[10]

The gender of the fetuses is important to determine. If there is growth discordance between the twins but one is a male and one is a female, then twin-to-twin transfusion cannot exist. If both twins are of the same sex, however, and growth discordance exists, twin-to-twin transfusion syndrome may be a possibility.

Umbilical cord Doppler may be useful for fetal surveillance. During the fetal cardiac cycle, there is umbilical blood flow during both the pumping (systole) and

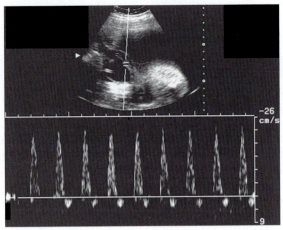

FIGURE 52-41 Reversal of diastolic flow in a twin gestation with TTS.

filling (diastole) phases of the heartbeat. No flow (absent end-diastolic flow) and reverse flow during diastole (reverse end-diastolic flow) (Figure 52-41) are signs of fetal jeopardy and may prompt the obstetrician to do further fetal well-being testing or even to deliver the fetuses.

One report suggests that most cases of twin transfusion syndrome are identified in the second semester.[11] Abnormal Doppler studies in twin pregnancies should prompt a search for other findings seen in this syndrome, such as polyhydramnios, stuck twin, or hydrops. When Doppler flow patterns are abnormal, careful follow-up should be used to determine if shunting exists.

The multifetal pregnancy reduction method has been used on pregnancies of more than four fetuses to improve the survival chances of the remaining fetuses. The procedure is performed toward the end of the first trimester by ultrasound-guided injection of potassium chloride into the thoraxes of the fetuses to be aborted.

ACKNOWLEDGMENTS

The author acknowledges the contribution of Sandra Hagen-Ansert, Kara L. Mayden-Argo and Laura J. Zuidema to this chapter in the previous editions of this book.

REFERENCES

1. Beckman CRB, Ling FW, Laube DW, Smith RP, et al: *Obstetrics and gynecology*, ed 4, Philadelphia, 2002, Lippincott Williams & Wilkins, pp. 39-62.
2. Classen SR, Paulson PR, Zacharias SR: Systemic lupus erythematosus: perinatal and neonatal implications, *J Obstet Gynecol Neonat Nurs* 27:493, 1998.
3. Doubilet PM, Benson CB: "Appearing twin": undercounting of multiple gestations on early first trimester sonograms, *J Ultrasound Med* 17:199, 1998.
4. Doubilet PM: *Sonography of multiple gestations. Syllabus update in Ob/Gyn ultrasound, vol II, June 1-3*, Laurel, MD, 1997, American Institute of Ultrasound in Medicine, pp. 19-24.

5. Gravett M: Causes of preterm delivery, *Sem Perinatol* 8:246, 1984.
6. Harvey CJ, Verklan T: Systemic lupus erythematous: obstetric and neonatal complications, *NAACOG Clin Issues Perinat Women Health Nurs* 1:177, 1990.
7. Holzgreve W, Curry CJ, Golbus HS, et al: Investigation of nonimmune hydrops fetalis, *Am J Obstet Gynecol* 150:805, 1984.
8. Mari G, Adrignolo A, Abuhamad AZ, et al: Diagnosis of fetal anemia with Doppler ultrasound in the pregnancy complicated by maternal blood group immunization, *Ultrasound Obstet Gynecol* 5:400, 1995.
9. Morin KH: Perinatal outcomes of obese women: a review of the literature, *J Obstet Gynecol Neonat Nurs* 27:431, 1998.
10. Newton ER, Cetrulo SL: Management of twin gestation. In Cetrulo CL, Sbaria AJ, editors: *The problem-oriented medical record for high risk obstetrics*, New York, 1984, Plenum.
11. Pretorius DH, Manchest D, Barkin S, et al: Doppler ultrasound of twin transfusion syndrome, *J Ultrasound Med* 7:117, 1988.

Prenatal Diagnosis of Congenital Anomalies

Charlotte G. Henningsen

ALPHA-FETOPROTEIN AND CHROMOSOMAL DISORDERS

A major congenital anomaly is found in 3 of every 100 births, and an additional 10% to 15% of births are complicated by minor birth defects. Because prenatal ultrasound has become the investigative tool for the obstetrician to access the developing fetus, it is likely that the fetus with an anomaly will be subjected to ultrasound at some time during pregnancy. The role of the sonographer is to screen for the unsuspected anomaly and to study the fetus at risk for an anomaly. The benefits of the examination are greatest when the sonographer is adept at detecting congenital anomalies and understands the cause, progression, and prognosis of the common congenital anomalies.

When a fetal anomaly is found antenatally, a multidisciplinary team approach to managing the fetus, mother, and family is preferable because the fetus may need special monitoring (e.g., serial ultrasound), delivery, postnatal care, and surgery. This multidisciplinary team includes the perinatologist (maternal-fetal medicine

specialist), neonatologist (specialist for critically ill infants), sonologist, perinatal sonographer, pediatric surgeon, other pediatric specialists, geneticist, obstetrician, perinatal and pediatric social workers, and other support personnel. Consultation with specialists is recommended when diagnosis is uncertain. Once an anomaly is found, these specialists can work as a team to optimize clinical management, to prepare the patient and family for possible surgery, to provide the patient and family with emotional support, and to plan for delivery. Most fetuses with major birth defects are delivered in perinatal regional centers where the specialized physicians, nurses, equipment, treatment, and postnatal surgery are available.

GENETIC TESTING

Chorionic Villus Sampling

Chorionic villus sampling (CVS) is an ultrasound-directed biopsy of the placenta or chorionic villi (chorion frondosum). The chorion frondosum is the active trophoblastic tissue that becomes the placenta. Because the chorionic villi are fetal in origin, chromosomal abnormalities may be detected when cells from the villi are grown and analyzed. Other conditions, such as biochemical or metabolic disorders, thalassemia, and sickle cell disease (hemoglobinopathies), may also be diagnosed using chorionic villi.

CVS is an alternative test used to obtain a fetal karyotype by the culturing of fetal cells similar to amniocentesis. The advantage of CVS includes the following: (1) it is performed early in pregnancy (10 to 14 weeks), (2) results are available within 1 week, and (3) earlier results allow more options for parents.

CVS is performed transcervically or transabdominally (Figure 53-1). Ultrasound performed before the actual procedure aids in a number ways: (1) It determines the relationship between the lie of the uterus and cervix and path of the catheter. Bladder fullness influences this relationship. Filling or emptying of the bladder may be necessary to facilitate the catheter route. (2) It assesses the fetus in terms of life, normal morphology, and age. (3) It identifies uterine masses or potential problems that may interfere with passage of the catheter.

Transvaginal CVS is performed in the dorsolithotomy position (pelvic examination position). The sonographer aids the obstetrician in determining the correct route to pass the catheter through the cervix to the placenta. A guiding stylet is initially introduced to check uterine and placental position. A flexible catheter is then introduced and directed into the placental tissue (Figure 53-2). The placental cells are aspirated through the catheter. The villi are collected and transported to the cytogenetics technician for analysis. Additional retrievals often are necessary. The sonographer should monitor the fetal heart rate and check for procedural bleeding.

The transabdominal CVS approach entails using a syringe and needle inserted into the placenta to withdraw the villi. The procedure is performed in a manner similar to amniocentesis (see the discussion of amniocentesis).

The risk of fetal loss because of CVS is approximately 0.05% to 1.0%. There has been some association with limb reduction defects when CVS is performed before 8 weeks of gestation. $Rh_o(D)$ immune globulin (RhoGAM) should be administered to Rh-negative unsensitized women to prevent sensitization problems in subsequent pregnancies.

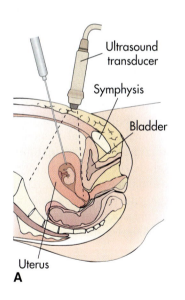
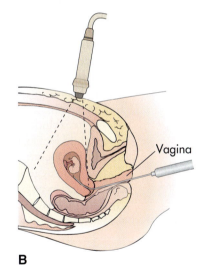

FIGURE 53-1 **A,** Transabdominal chorionic villus sampling. **B,** Transcervical chorionic villus sampling.

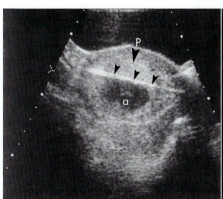
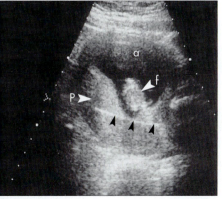

FIGURE 53-2 **A,** Transcervical chorionic villus sampling at 10 weeks of gestation demonstrating the placement of the sampling catheter *(arrowheads)* within an anterior placenta *(P)* or chorion frondosum. *a,* Amniotic cavity. **B,** Transcervical chorionic villus sampling at 11 weeks of gestation showing the placement of the sampling catheter *(arrowheads)* within a posterior placenta *(P)*. Note the fetal abdomen *(f)* within the amniotic cavity *(a)*.

Amniocentesis

Amniocentesis was first used as a technique to relieve polyhydramnios, to predict Rh isoimmunization, and to document fetal lung maturity. In the mid-1960s, amniocentesis was used to study fetal cells from amniotic fluid that allowed the analysis of fetal chromosomes (Figure 53-3). Normal and abnormal chromosomal patterns (Figures 53-4 and 53-5) could be identified.

Amniocentesis is a test offered to expectant patients who are at risk for a chromosomal abnormality or biochemical disorder that may be prenatally detectable. The results are available between 1 and 3 weeks; however, if rapid results are desired, fluorescence in situ hybridization (FISH) provides a limited analysis within 24 hours for the most common chromosomal anomalies. The FISH assay most commonly evaluates for numeric abnormalities of chromosomes 21, 13, 18, X, and Y.

Advanced maternal age is a common reason for performing amniocentesis. All pregnant women are at risk for having a child with a chromosomal defect, but the risk is greater in a woman of advanced maternal age. The risk of having a fetus with Down syndrome is 1 in 365 in a woman who is 35 years of age, whereas the risk for a woman who is 21 years of age is only about 1 in 2000. The risk of having a fetus with any chromosomal anomaly is 1 in 180 in the woman who is 35 years of age versus 1 in 500 for the woman who is 21 years of age.

Other indications for genetic amniocentesis include a history of a balance rearrangement in a parent or previous child with a chromosomal abnormality, a history of an unexplained abnormal alpha-fetoprotein (AFP) level or an abnormal triple screen, and a fetus with a congenital anomaly.

Amniocentesis for genetic reasons is ideally performed between 15 and 20 weeks of gestation. Amniocentesis may be done as early as 12 weeks, but it may lead to the development of fetal scoliosis or clubfoot secondary to the reduced amount of amniotic fluid. The rate of miscarriage in early amniocentesis is not clearly defined. Some studies have shown that the loss rate is similar to midtrimester amniocentesis, whereas others have shown a higher loss rate. The fetal loss rate of midtrimester amniocentesis is reported as 1/200 in the United States.[2] Amniocentesis performed beyond 20 weeks of gestation is possible but may be associated with poor cell growth.

The amniocentesis procedure should include a fetal survey to exclude congenital anomalies. A fetal examination should be performed, and targeted areas of anatomy should be documented to exclude the physical features that would suggest a chromosomal anomaly (e.g., hand clenching, **hypoplasia** of the fifth middle phalanx, choroid plexus cysts, ventriculomegaly, thickened nuchal fold, cardiac anomalies, omphalocele, spina bifida, or foot anomalies).

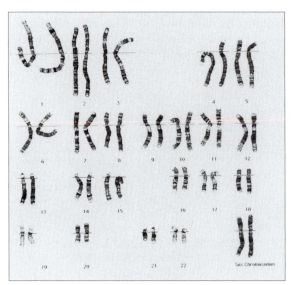

FIGURE 53-3 Normal karyotype demonstrating 46 chromosomes in a female fetus (46, XX).

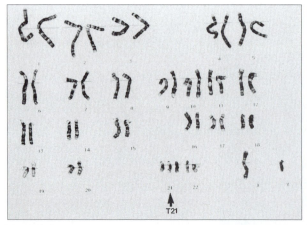

FIGURE 53-4 Karyotype of trisomy 21 (Down syndrome) in a male fetus (47, XY, 21). Note the extra chromosome at the 21st position (*arrow*). Note the sex chromosomes indicating a male fetus.

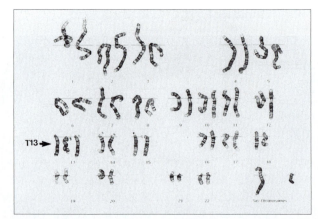

FIGURE 53-5 Karyotype of trisomy 13 (47, XY 13) (*arrow*) male fetus.

The sonographer will also assist the physician in the amniocentesis procedure. The optimal collection site for amniotic fluid should be away from the fetus, away from the central portion of the placenta, away from the umbilical cord, and near the maternal midline to avoid the maternal uterine vessels.

Technique of Genetic Amniocentesis

Ultrasound-monitored amniocentesis is a technique that allows the continuous monitoring of the needle during the amniocentesis procedure. Using this technique, the maternal skin is prepared with a povidone-iodine solution.

The transducer is placed in a sterile cover or sterile glove to allow monitoring on the sterile field during the procedure. Sterile coupling gel may be applied to the maternal skin to ensure good transmission of the sound beam. The amniocentesis site is rescanned to confirm the amniotic pocket, and then the site and pathway for the introduction of the needle are determined. The distance to the amniotic fluid may be measured with electronic calipers, which may be useful in obese patients in whom

a longer needle may be necessary. In many instances, a new site is chosen as a result of fetal movement or a myometrial contraction in the proposed site, and the transducer is moved to a new sterile area. On successful identification of the amniocentesis site, a finger is placed between the transducer and the skin to produce an acoustic shadow. The needle is then inserted under continuous ultrasound observation (Figure 53-6). Inserting the needle in a plane perpendicular to the transducer will allow for a bright reflection of the needle tip, so that it can be easily observed (Figure 53-7) at the edge of the uterine wall and then as it punctures the uterine cavity. When incorrectly directed, the needle may be repositioned.

Amniotic fluid is aspirated through a syringe connected to the needle hub. Approximately 20 ml of amniotic fluid will be collected for chromosomal analysis and AFP evaluation. In advanced pregnancies, additional amniotic fluid may be required. When amniocentesis is performed because of a known fetal anomaly, acetylcholinesterase and viral studies (**TORCH** titers) may be ordered. Following aspiration of amniotic fluid, the needle is removed from the uterus under sonographic guidance.

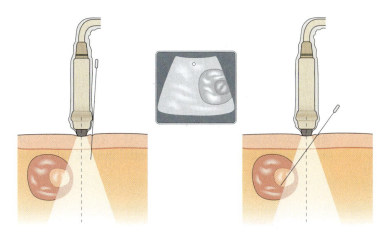

FIGURE 53-6 If the needle is inserted parallel to the transducer, only the tip will be represented. If the needle is inserted at an angle with the transducer, the beam will intersect the needle, but it will not demonstrate its tip, which could be in a harmful position. Notice that in both cases the image on the screen is the same. Angling the needle is a dangerous procedure that should be avoided.

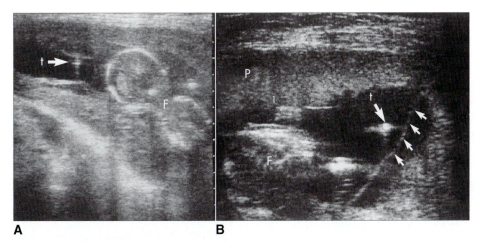

FIGURE 53-7 A, Genetic amniocentesis at 15.6 weeks of gestation using direct visualization method. The needle tip *(t)* is identified within the amniotic cavity. *F,* Fetus. **B,** Genetic amniocentesis at 16 weeks of gestation in a twin pregnancy. The needle tip *(t)* is identified within the sac above the amniotic membrane *(arrows)*. *F,* Fetus; *P,* placenta. *1,* Umbilical cord insertion into placenta.

After the amniocentesis has been completed, fetal cardiac activity should be identified and documented. If the placenta has been traversed, the site should be monitored for bleeding. The use of videotaping can allow for continuous recording and documentation of the fetal examination, the amniocentesis, and postamniocentesis ultrasound evaluation.

The continuous monitoring with ultrasound during amniocentesis is invaluable in cases of oligohydramnios, anterior placental position, and premature rupture of membranes. Ultrasound imaging can help achieve a successful amniocentesis when only small pockets of fluid are available.

Genetic Amniocentesis and Multiple Gestations

Amniocentesis in multiple gestations warrants special consideration. Preliminary sonographic examination for each fetus should be performed to include a survey of fetal anatomy and growth profiles. Determination of whether the pregnancy is monozygotic or dizygotic should be made. It should be determined if there are multiple sacs, and the amount of amniotic fluid within each sac should be assessed.

The amniocentesis technique for multiple gestations is similar to the singleton method, except that each fetal sac is entered. To be certain that amniotic fluid is obtained from each sac, indigo carmine dye can be injected into the first sac. The presence of clear amniotic fluid indicates that the second sac has been penetrated when the second pass is made. If dye-stained fluid is visible, it indicates that the first sac has been penetrated a second time. Documentation of each amniocentesis and meticulous labeling of fluid samples are recommended. It is desirable to avoid the placenta in patients who are Rh-negative. In all Rh-negative patients, RhoGAM is administered within 72 hours of the procedure.

Cordocentesis

Cordocentesis is another method in which chromosomes are analyzed. Fetal blood is obtained through needle aspiration of the umbilical cord. Karyotype results can be processed within 2 to 3 days; however, the availability of FISH has decreased the need for cordocentesis for chromosomal analysis. Cordocentesis is more commonly used for guidance for transfusions to treat fetal isoimmunization

MATERNAL SERUM MARKERS

Alpha-Fetoprotein

Alpha-fetoprotein (AFP) is the major protein in fetal serum and is produced by the yolk sac in early gestation and later by the fetal liver. AFP is found in the fetal spine, gastrointestinal tract, liver, and kidneys. This protein is transported into the amniotic fluid by fetal urination and reaches maternal circulation or blood through the fetal membranes (Figure 53-8). AFP may be measured in the maternal serum (MSAFP) or from amniotic fluid (AFAFP).

AFP levels are considered abnormal when elevated or low. Neural tube defects, such as anencephaly and open spina bifida, are common reasons for high AFP levels. In both instances, AFP leaks from the defect to enter the amniotic fluid and then diffuses into the maternal bloodstream (see Figure 53-8). AFP elevations will not be found when there is closed spina bifida (occulta) because there is no opening to allow leakage.

Monitoring of AFP is a screening test for neural tube defects and other conditions (Box 53-1). Evaluation is usually based on 2.0 to 2.5 multiples of the median (MOM), but false positives do occur. MSAFP screening detects approximately 88% of anencephalics and 79% of open spina bifida cases when 2.5 multiples of the median (MOM) are used.[10]

MSAFP levels increase with advancing gestational age and peak from 15 to 18 weeks of gestation (the ideal sampling time). AFAFP, in contrast, decreases with fetal age. A common reason for elevations is incorrect dates. Because AFP levels vary with gestational age, if the fetus is older or younger than expected, AFP levels will be reported as increased or decreased.

Other reasons for elevations are acrania and encephalocele (which may occur in association with Meckel-Gruber syndrome), with AFP leakage from the exposed membranes and tissue. The concentration of AFP correlates with the size of the defect. AFP levels tend to be significantly higher in fetuses with anencephaly than

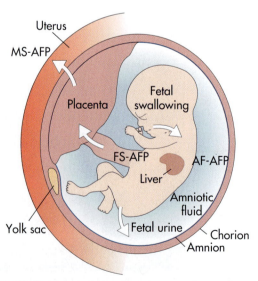

FIGURE 53-8 Schematic drawing showing the production and distribution of alpha-fetoprotein (AFP) into its three components: fetal tissues, amniotic fluid, and maternal serum. *AF-AFP,* Amniotic fluid AFP; *FS-AFP,* fetal serum AFT; *MS-AFP,* maternal serum AFP.

BOX 53-1 Reasons for Elevation of Alpha-Fetoprotein and Acetylcholinesterase

Neural Tube Defects
Anencephaly
Exencephaly (acrania)
Encephalocele (including Meckel-Gruber syndrome)
Spina bifida
Sacrococcygeal teratoma

Abdominal Wall Defects
Omphalocele
Gastroschisis
Limb-body wall complex
Amniotic band syndrome
Bladder or cloacal exstrophy
Ectopia cordis

Multiple Gestation
Twin with a co-twin death
Acardiac twin
Fetus papyraceous

Gastrointestinal Obstruction
Annular pancreas
Duodenal atresia
Esophageal atresia

Renal Anomalies
Congenital nephrosis
Hydronephrosis
Polycystic kidney disease (including Meckel-Gruber syndrome)
Urinary tract obstruction
Prune belly syndrome
Urethral atresia

Placental and Cord Abnormalities
Chorioangioma
Placental or cord hematoma

Umbilical cord hemangioma
Hydatidiform mole

Fetal Heart Failure
Hydrops or ascites
Lymphangiectasia
Rh isoimmunization

Neck Masses
Cystic hygroma
Noonan's syndrome (with hygroma)

Liver Disease
Hepatitis
Maternal herpes virus (fetal liver necrosis and skin lesions)
Hepatocellular carcinoma
Hamartoma of liver

Miscellaneous Causes
Incorrect dates
Fetal demise
Oligohydramnios
Unexplained
Hereditary overproduction of alpha-fetoprotein
Blood in amniotic fluid
Chromosome abnormalities (trisomies 18 and 13, Turner's syndrome, triploidy)
Cystadenomatoid malformation
Epignathus
Intracranial tumor
Pilonidal cyst
Skin defects
Hydrocephalus
Congenital heart defects
Viral infections (cytomegalovirus [CMV], parvovirus)

Modified from Milunsky A, editor: *Genetic disorders and the fetus: diagnosis, prevention and treatment,* ed 3, Baltimore, 1992, Johns Hopkins University Press; Nyberg DA, Mahony BS, Pretorius DH, editors: *Diagnostic ultrasound of fetal anomalies, text and atlas,* St. Louis, 1990, Mosby.

with spina bifida because more tissue is exposed. It is important to remember that approximately 20% of spina bifida lesions are covered by skin, so AFP elevations will not be detected in serum or amniotic fluid. Sacrococcygeal teratomas are also known to be associated with high AFP levels.

Two common abdominal wall defects, omphalocele and gastroschisis, produce elevations of AFP. With an **omphalocele,** AFP leaks through the membrane encasing the herniated bowel or liver. In gastroschisis, AFP diffuses directly into the serum and amniotic fluid from the herniated bowel, which lacks a covering membrane; thus, AFP levels are higher in a fetus with gastroschisis than in a fetus with an omphalocele.

Other abdominal wall defects cause leakage in the same manner. Bladder or cloacal exstrophy, ectopia cordis (herniation of the heart out of the chest), limb-body wall complex, and amniotic band syndrome are examples of other anomalies that may present with an elevated AFP level.

It is expected that the AFP level in a twin pregnancy will be twice that of a singleton pregnancy because two fetuses make twice the AFP. In multiple gestations in which there is death of a co-twin (fetus papyraceous) or when one twin is an acardiac twin, AFP may be higher than normal.

Obstructions of the gastrointestinal tract may cause reduced clearance of AFP. This may explain elevations with anomalies, such as an annular pancreas, esophageal atresia, and duodenal atresia.

A fetus with a kidney lesion may produce increased AFP. In congenital nephrosis, the kidneys excrete extremely high levels of AFP. Polycystic kidneys and urinary tract obstruction may also lead to higher levels of AFP because there is abnormal clearance or filtration of AFP because of kidney maldevelopment and urinary tract leakage.

Placental lesions, such as chorioangiomas, hemangiomas, and hematomas, are known to be responsible for AFP elevations. Placental problems in general may explain the prevalence of growth restriction, fetal death, and abruption in patients with unexplained AFP elevations.

In heart failure, faulty diffusion of AFP may lead to an abnormal AFP increase when hydrops, ascites, or lymphangiectasia are present. Severely sensitized fetuses with Rh isoimmunization may have heart failure because of severe anemia. In the fetus with a **cystic hygroma,** obstructed lymph sacs lead to AFP diffusion through the hygroma into the bloodstream and amniotic fluid.

Liver disease in the mother or fetus may cause high AFP levels. Hepatitis, maternal herpes virus and resultant fetal liver necrosis, skin lesions, hepatocellular carcinoma, and fetal liver tumors (hamartomas) are rare causes of elevated AFP.

Other causes include chromosomal abnormalities associated with fetal anomalies or placental problems that permit the abnormal passage of AFP. Fetuses with trisomy 13 or trisomy 18 may also have renal anomalies, neural tube defects, ventral wall defects, or skin lesions that cause elevations in the AFP level. Fetuses with Turner's syndrome often present with cystic hygromas. In triploidy, abnormal placental molar degeneration leads to increased AFP diffusion.

Cystic adenomatoid malformations cause rises in AFP because of excessive leakage from the lungs. Pilonidal cysts of the back and various skin disorders and tumors, such as epignathus and intracranial lesions, are also associated with high AFP levels. Rarely the fetus manufactures excessive amounts of AFP as a hereditary condition.

Fetal death is a frequent cause of a high MSAFP level. Pregnancies complicated by oligohydramnios may have higher concentrations of AFP because there is less amniotic fluid to diffuse the protein.

Contamination of an amniotic fluid specimen by blood may also falsely increase the level of AFP.

In utero viral infections (cytomegalovirus and parvovirus) are reported to permit excessive AFP leakage because the maternal-fetal surface may be irritated and disrupted by inflammation.

Unexplained elevations in MSAFP suggest that the pregnancy is at increased risk for complications and poor outcomes, including low birth weight and stillbirth. Preeclampsia, hypertension, and abruptio placentae are other third-trimester complications associated with these elevations.

Mothers with elevated MSAFP values and normal AFAFP values are potentially at risk for other fetal anomalies unrelated to neural tube defects. Hydrocephalus, without a spinal defect (increased cerebrospinal fluid allows increased diffusion), and congenital heart disease (probable altered perfusion of blood flow through placenta) are reported in conjunction with unexplained, non-neural tube defect problems.

Low AFP levels have been found with chromosomal abnormalities, such as trisomy 21, trisomy 18, and trisomy 13 (Box 53-2). Other causes include incorrect patient dates (fetus younger than expected), fetal death, hydatidiform moles, spontaneous abortion, and a nonpregnant state. In some cases, the cause may remain unknown.

Amniocentesis may be offered when MSAFP levels are elevated and ultrasound reveals no obvious explanation. Amniotic fluid tests usually include karyotyping for chromosomal abnormalities, AFAFP levels, and acetylcholinesterase. AFAFP is more specific for detecting levels of AFP. Acetylcholinesterase is specific for detecting an open neural tube. Beyond 20 weeks of gestation, acetylcholinesterase is the preferred test because AFP analysis is no longer sensitive.

When AFP is elevated (greater than 3 MOM) and the cranium (ventricles and cisterna magna) and spine appear normal, the risk of the fetus actually having a small spinal defect is approximately halved. The overall risk of miscarriage from an amniocentesis is 1 in 200, so it is important to weigh the risk of complication with the possible yield of identifying an abnormality.

Prenatal scanning and amniocentesis are used to evaluate the fetus with a low AFP value to exclude any physical features that may suggest a chromosomal abnormality. Such findings might include choroid plexus cysts, hand anomalies, or cardiac defects.

BOX 53-2	Common Sonographic Features of Chromosomal Anomalies			
Trisomy 21	**Trisomy 18**	**Trisomy 13**	**Triploidy**	**Turner's Syndrome**
Nuchal thickness	Heart defects	Holoprosencephaly	Hydatidiform placental	Cystic hygroma
Heart defects	Choroid plexus cysts	Heart defects	degeneration	Heart defects
Duodenal atresia	Clenched hands	Cleft lip and palate	Heart defects	Hydrops
Shortened femurs	Micrognathia	Omphalocele	Renal anomalies	Renal anomalies
Mild pyelectasis	Talipes	Polydactyly	Omphalocele	
Mild ventriculomegaly	Renal anomalies	Talipes	Cranial defects	
Echogenic bowel	Cleft lip and palate	Echogenic chordae tendineae	Facial defects	
	Omphalocele	Renal anomalies		
	CDH	Meningomyelocele		
	Cerebellar hypoplasia	Micrognathia		

Quadruple Screen

Another biochemical screening test used in the early second trimester is known as the quadruple screen. Formally known as the triple test or triple screen, this biochemical screening test combines three serum markers: AFP, human chorionic gonadotropin (hCG), and unconjugated estriol. This blood test improved the detection rate for trisomy 21 over MSAFP testing alone. Biochemical screening in trisomy 21 fetuses reveals high hCG levels and decreased AFP and estriol levels. Additionally, biochemical screening may suggest trisomy 18 when hCG, AFP, and estriol levels are all decreased. The quadruple screen added another maternal serum marker, dimeric inhibin A, improving the sensitivity in detecting Down fetuses. The risk for a neural tube defect or chromosomal problem is calculated for each mother. A patient may elect to undergo ultrasound with or without amniocentesis based on the risk for chromosomal or neural tube defects.

FIRST TRIMESTER SCREENING

Pregnancy-Associated Plasma Protein A

A first-trimester serum marker used to detect anomalies is pregnancy-associated plasma protein A (PAPP-A). PAPP-A is a glycoprotein derived from the trophoblastic tissue that is then diffused into the maternal circulation. PAPP-A levels increase in maternal serum throughout pregnancy. PAPP-A levels have been found to be decreased in pregnancies affected by aneuploidy.

Free Beta Human Chorionic Gonadotropin

Free beta-hCG is also a glycoprotein derived from the placenta that can be assessed in maternal serum in the first trimester to evaluate for increased risk of Down syndrome. Free beta-hCG and PAPP-A are being evaluated in combination with nuchal translucency measurements in the first trimester as a sensitivity screening tool for Down syndrome. When PAPP-A and hCG assessments are combined with information regarding maternal age and nuchal translucency, the detection rates for Down syndrome have been reported to be equal to or greater than the quadruple screen, and the information can be provided to women at a much earlier gestational age.

First-trimester assessment techniques that utilize sonographic evaluation for the detection of aneuploidy are discussed further in Chapter 47.

MEDICAL GENETICS

A normal karyotype consists of 46 chromosomes, 22 pairs of autosomes, and a pair of sex chromosomes (see Figure 53-3). Aneuploidy is an abnormality of the number of chromosomes. One of the most common aneuploid conditions is Down syndrome, in which an individual has an extra chromosome number 21 (see Figure 53-4). The cause of trisomy is usually nondisjunction, the failure of normal chromosomal division at the time of meiosis. The cause of nondisjunction is unknown, although there is strong association with maternal age.

A chromosomal disorder is caused by too much or too little chromosome material. A dominant disorder is a condition caused by a single defective gene (autosomal dominant). It is usually inherited from one parent (who is also affected), but it may arise as a new mutation (spontaneous gene change). An inherited dominant disorder carries a 50% chance that each time pregnancy occurs, the fetus will have the condition. An example of an autosomal-dominant condition is osteogenesis imperfecta (types 1 and 4).

A recessive disorder (autosomal recessive) is caused by a pair of defective genes, one inherited from each parent. With each pregnancy, the parents have a 25% chance of having a fetus with the disorder. An example of an autosomal recessive condition is infantile polycystic kidney disease.

Boys inherit X-linked disorders from their mothers. Affected males do not transmit the disorder to their sons, but all of their daughters will be carriers for the disorder. The sons of female carriers each have a 50% chance of being affected, and the daughters each have a 50% chance of being a carrier. Whereas an X-linked gene is located on the female sex chromosome (the X), an autosomal gene is located on one of the numbered chromosomes. An example of an X-linked condition occurring in male fetuses is aqueductal stenosis. Aqueductal stenosis, however, may also occur in females.

A multifactorial condition is an abnormal event that arises because of the interaction of one or more genes and environmental factors. Anencephaly is an example of a multifactorial disorder.

Mosaicism is the occurrence of a gene mutation or chromosomal abnormality in a portion of an individual's cells. It is difficult to predict the types of problems that will occur when mosaicism is found.

CHROMOSOMAL ABNORMALITIES

Chromosomal abnormalities are found in 1 of every 180 live births.[5] There is a high prevalence of chromosomal abnormalities in patients referred for second-trimester amniocentesis because of advanced maternal age, abnormal AFP, abnormal quadruple screen (hCG, AFP, estriol, and inhibin A), or ultrasound detection of multiple fetal anomalies. It is important to become familiar with and to search for the physical features (see Box 53-2) that would suggest trisomies 13, 18, and 21, triploidy, and Turner's syndrome.

Nuchal Translucency

An abnormal fluid collection behind the fetal neck has been strongly associated with aneuploidy. This nuchal translucency (NT) has been reported as a late first-trimester finding identified between 10 and 14 weeks of gestation.[6] The NT increases with gestational age, so the NT measurement should be compared with the gestational age or crown-rump length to determine risk for aneuploidy and combined with maternal age and first trimester serum screening. A thickened NT is associated with chromosomal abnormalities, such as trisomies 13, 18, 21; triploidy; and Turner's syndrome (Figure 53-9). This first-trimester finding is not a precursor to the development of a cystic hygroma or second-trimester edema. Even in fetuses with normal chromosomes, an increased nuchal translucency has been associated with an increased incidence of structural defects, such as cardiac, diaphragmatic, renal, and abdominal wall anomalies. In addition to the increased risk of chromosomal abnormality and other anomalies, an increased nuchal translucency has also been associated with spontaneous miscarriage and perinatal death. The criteria used in measuring the nuchal translucency are defined in Chapter 47.

Trisomy 21

Trisomy 21, also known as Down syndrome, occurs in 1.21 in 1000 live births.[9] It is one of the most common chromosomal disorders and is characterized by an extra chromosome number 21. There is an association with advanced maternal age; however, this anomaly may affect infants born to women of all ages. Trisomy 21 is associated with an abnormal nuchal translucency, an abnormal first trimester screen and an abnormal quadruple screen.

Infants with trisomy 21 may present with a variety of physical features (Figure 53-10) including brachyceph-

aly; epicanthal folds (a fold of skin that covers the inner corner of the eye); a flattened nasal bridge; round, small ears; broad neck with extra skin (nuchal fold); and a protruding tongue. Other anomalies that have been associated with Down syndrome include heart defects (septal defects, endocardial cushion defect, tetralogy of Fallot), duodenal atresia, esophageal atresia, anorectal atresia, and omphalocele (Figure 53-11). Cystic hygroma, nonimmune hydrops, hydrothorax, and echogenic intracardiac foci may also be observed. Skeletal anomalies may be present, including shortened extremities, space between the first and second toes, hypoplasia of the middle fifth phalanx (Figure 53-12), and clinodactyly of the fifth finger (inward curving). A single palmar (hand) crease is found in approximately 30% of affected infants.[4]

The prognosis for survival depends on associated anomalies, with heart anomalies a major cause of mortality in infancy. Mental retardation is always present, with IQ ranges between 25 and 50 in childhood. In

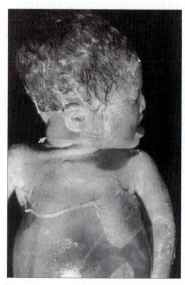

FIGURE 53-10 Postmortem photograph of a neonate with trisomy 21 (Down syndrome). Duodenal atresia was found. Note the nuchal thickening *(arrow)*.

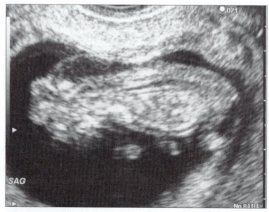

FIGURE 53-9 This fetus with trisomy 13 presented with a thickened and septated nuchal translucency and anencephaly in the late first trimester of pregnancy.

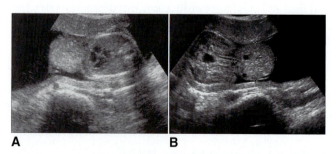

A B

FIGURE 53-11 A, A 22-week fetus with tetralogy of Fallot (ventricular septal defect [VSD], overriding aorta, pulmonary stenosis, right ventricular hypertrophy). Only the VSD is appreciated in this four-chamber view. **B,** Omphalocele in same fetus. These findings together are highly suggestive of a chromosomal anomaly.

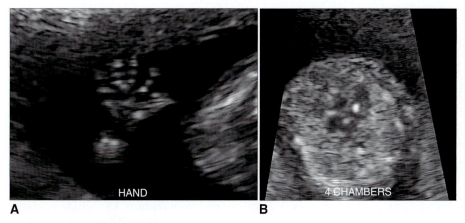

FIGURE 53-12 A, Absent fifth middle phalanx in a fetus with trisomy 21. **B,** In the same fetus, an echogenic intracardiac focus is observed. Other anomalies were an AV canal defect and thickened nuchal fold.

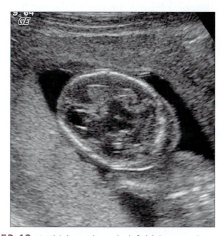

FIGURE 53-13 A thickened nuchal fold is seen in a fetus with trisomy 21.

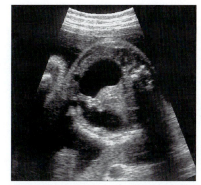

FIGURE 53-14 The double bubble sign is identified in this case of duodenal atresia. This is a significant finding associated with trisomy 21.

addition to heart failure, alimentary defects can also be life threatening. Respiratory problems, eye problems, and premature aging are common.

Sonographic Findings. Ultrasound diagnosis of trisomy 21 is limited because of the subtleness and infrequency of some of the phenotypic expressions. Anomalies that may be identified with Down syndrome include the following:

- Nuchal fold of 6 mm or greater (Figure 53-13)
- Extremity anomalies (hypoplasia of the middle phalanx or clinodactyly of the fifth finger; space between first and second toes)
- Shortened femur or short humerus (< the 5th percentile)
- Duodenal atresia (Figure 53-14)
- Heart defects (Figure 53-15) (present in approximately 30% to 40%)
- **Intrauterine growth restriction (IUGR)**
- Mild pyelectasis (≥ 4 mm in anteroposterior diameter)
- Echogenic bowel (Figure 53-16)
- Mild ventriculomegaly (Figure 53-17)

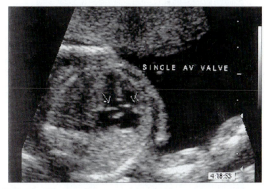

FIGURE 53-15 This endocardial cushion defect (atrioventricular canal) presented with an atrial septal defect, ventricular septal defect, and common valve.

- Echogenic intracardiac focus (tip of mitral valve apparatus)
- Absence of the nasal bone between 11 and 14 weeks

Trisomy 18

Trisomy 18, also known as Edwards' syndrome, is the second most common chromosomal trisomy, occurring in 3 of 10,000 live births.[11] This karyotype demonstrates

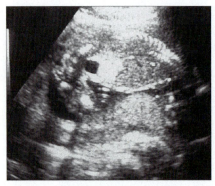

FIGURE 53-16 Echogenic bowel, bowel with the same echogenicity as fetal bone, is a subtle finding associated with trisomy 21.

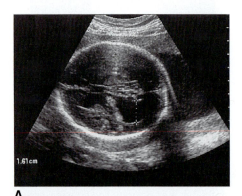

A

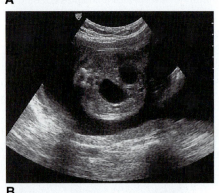

B

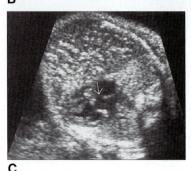

C

FIGURE 53-17 A female with fetus presented at 26 weeks of gestation with an uncertain last menstrual period. Ultrasound revealed ventriculomegaly **(A)** and duodenal atresia **(B). C,** Subsequent ultrasound examination also identified an atrial septal defect. There was fetal demise in utero at 35 weeks of gestation.

an extra chromosome 18. Trisomy 18 is associated with an abnormal quadruple screen.

Physical features that have been identified in fetuses with trisomy 18 (Figure 53-18) include cardiac anomalies, which are present in the majority of fetuses with this chromosomal anomaly. Cranial anomalies that have been identified are dolichocephaly, microcephaly, hydrocephalus, agenesis of the corpus callosum, cerebellar hypoplasia, encephalocele, a strawberry-shaped head, and choroid plexus cysts (Figure 53-19). Facial abnormalities include low-set ears, **micrognathia,** and cleft lip (Figure 53-20) and palate. Abnormal extremities identified with trisomy 18 include persistently clenched hands (Figure 53-21), talipes, rocker-bottom feet, and radial aplasia. Other anomalies associated with Edwards' syndrome include omphalocele, congenital diaphragmatic hernia (Figure 53-22), neural tube defects, cystic hygroma, and renal anomalies.

The fetus with trisomy 18 will often spontaneously abort. Infants are profoundly retarded. It is considered a lethal anomaly, with 90% of infants dying within the first year of life.[1]

▶ **Sonographic Findings.** Sonographic features of trisomy 18 are evident in 90% of affected fetuses, and, in addition to the features listed previously, may also

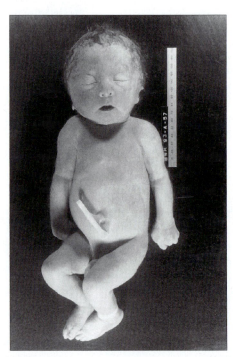

FIGURE 53-18 Neonate with trisomy 18. Note the clenched hands and rocker-bottom feet. Prenatal ultrasound revealed a supratentorial cyst confirmed after autopsy.

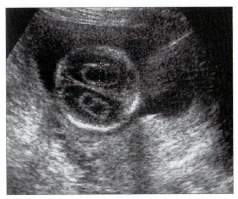

FIGURE 53-19 Bilateral choroid plexus cysts were identified in a pregnancy referred for triple screen suggestive of trisomy 18. Amniocentesis confirmed Edwards' syndrome.

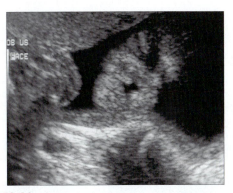

FIGURE 53-20 Cleft lip and palate are associated with aneuploidy. A median cleft, as in this example, and bilateral clefts carry a greater risk than a unilateral cleft.

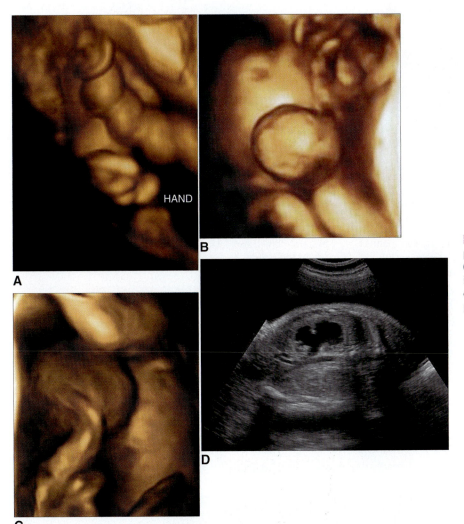

FIGURE 53-21 This fetus with trisomy 18 presented with persistently clenched hands **(A)** and an omphalocele **(B)**. Note the cord insertion into the abdominal wall defect is consistent with omphalocele **(C)**. Hydronephrosis was also present **(D)**.

include polyhydramnios, IUGR, single umbilical artery, and nonimmune hydrops.

Trisomy 13

Trisomy 13, also known as Patau's syndrome, occurs in 1 in 5000 to 20,000 births.[12] It is the result of an extra chromosome 13. This extremely severe anomaly consists of multiple anomalies, many of which involve the brain.

The physical features (Figure 53-23) characteristic of trisomy 13 include holoprosencephaly (Figure 53-24), a common finding in fetuses with trisomy 13. Other cranial anomalies include agenesis of the corpus callosum and microcephaly. Facial anomalies may be associated with

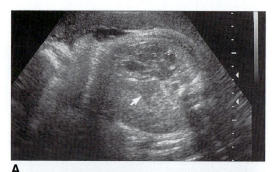

A

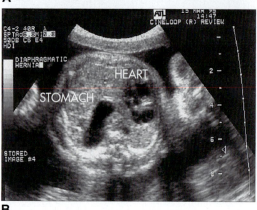

B

FIGURE 53-22 Congenital diaphragmatic hernia (CDH) is associated with aneuploidy. **A,** This is an unusual presentation of CDH in that the stomach was not identified in the thorax, even though it was a left-side defect. Note the malposition of the heart. There is the bowel adjacent to the heart. Karyotype revealed normal chromosomes. The baby died shortly after birth because of respiratory complications. **B,** A common ultrasound presentation of CDH with the stomach evident within the thorax. Note the displacement of the heart.

the presence of holoprosencephaly and include **hypotelorism**, proboscis, cyclopia (Figure 53-25), and nose with a single nostril. Cleft lip and palate, microphthalmia, and micrognathia may also be present. Heart defects are present in 90% of fetuses and may include ventricular septal defect, atrial septal defect, and hypoplastic left heart. Other anomalies associated with trisomy 13 include omphalocele, renal anomalies (Figure 53-26), and meningomyelocele. Associated limb anomalies (Figure 53-27) include **polydactyly**, talipes,

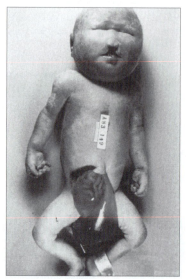

FIGURE 53-23 Neonate with trisomy 13. Note the hypotelorism, bilateral cleft lip and palate, bowel-filled omphalocele, and polydactyly of the hands.

FIGURE 53-24 Multiple anomalies were identified in this pregnancy consistent with alobar holoprosencephaly. Amniocentesis confirmed trisomy 13. Ultrasound findings included a single ventricle characteristic of holoprosencephy and splaying of the cerebellar hemispheres consistent with a Dandy-Walker malformation was also noted **(A).** Polydactyly was identified on right **(B)** and left hands **(C),** and an omphalocele was also identified **(D).**

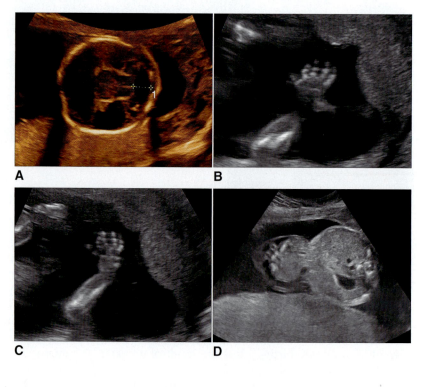

A   **B**

C   **D**

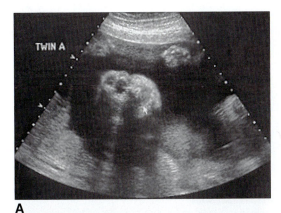

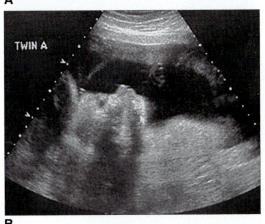

FIGURE 53-25 The facial anomalies associated with trisomy 13 include cyclopia **(A)**. The nose was also absent **(B)**.

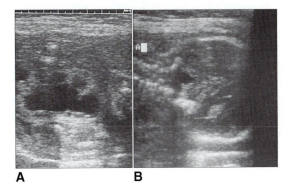

FIGURE 53-26 A fetus with trisomy 13 presents with hydronephrosis **(A)** and Dandy-Walker malformation **(B)**.

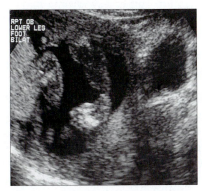

FIGURE 53-27 Limb anomalies associated with aneuploidy include talipes (clubfoot).

rocker-bottom feet, and overlapping fingers. Cystic hygroma and echogenic chordae tendineae (Figure 53-28) may also be identified.

The prognosis for trisomy 13 is extremely poor, with 80% of infants dying within the first month. It is considered a lethal anomaly. Survivors are profoundly retarded, with multiple deficits and problems.

Sonographic Findings. Sonographic features are evident in 90% of fetuses with trisomy 13. In addition to the features listed previously, trisomy 13 may also be associated with IUGR, single umbilical artery, and polyhydramnios. Trisomy 18 and Meckel-Gruber syndrome (encephalocele, cystic kidneys, polydactyly) may have a similar sonographic appearance.

Triploidy

Triploidy is the result of a complete extra set of chromosomes. It often occurs as the result of an ova being fertilized by two sperm. It is estimated to occur in approximately 1% of conceptions, although most fetuses will spontaneously abort in the first trimester.[3] Only 1 in 5000 will continue to 16 to 20 weeks of gestation.[8]

Physical features of triploidy include heart defects, renal anomalies, omphalocele, and meningomyelocele. Cranial defects associated with triploidy include holoprosencephaly, agenesis of the corpus callosum, hydrocephalus, and Dandy-Walker malformation. Facial anomalies may be present and include low-set ears, **hypertelorism**, cleft lip and palate, and micrognathia. Cryptorchidism, ambiguous genitalia, syndactyly, and talipes may also be observed.

Triploidy is considered a lethal condition, with those surviving the gestational period dying shortly after birth. A mosaic form of triploidy may be compatible with survival, although these infants are affected with mental retardation.

Sonographic Findings. Sonographic features of triploidy include the previously described findings in

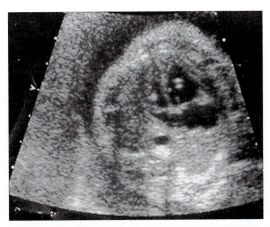

FIGURE 53-28 Isolated echogenic foci may be insignificant. When in the right ventricle or bilateral as seen in this image, aneuploidy should be considered. Chromosomal analysis revealed trisomy 13.

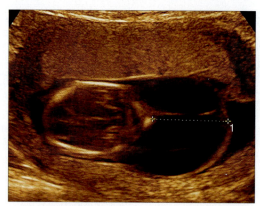

FIGURE 53-29 A cystic hygroma was identified in a fetus with Turner's syndrome.

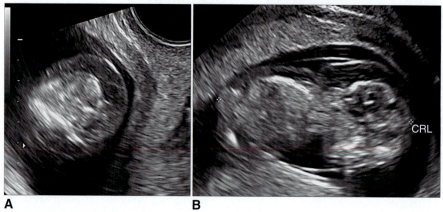

A   B

FIGURE 53-30 Turner's syndrome. **A,** A septated cystic hygroma is noted in the nuchal region in a 12-week fetus. **B,** Significant edema was also evident around the fetal abdomen. This fetus died shortly thereafter.

addition to severe IUGR and placental changes (hydatidiform degeneration). Oligohydramnios is often present and may hamper adequate visualization of the fetus.

Turner's Syndrome

Turner's syndrome (45 X) is a genetic abnormality marked by the absence of the X or Y chromosome. It is not associated with advanced maternal age. It occurs in 1 of every 2500 live births.[7] Patients may present with an elevated MSAFP when a cystic hygroma is present.

Cystic hygroma (Figure 53-29) is one of the most pathognomonic findings for this disorder. Other physical features include cardiac anomalies, of which coarctation of the aorta is the most common. General lymphedema and hydrops may also be present. Renal anomalies, such as horseshoe kidney, renal agenesis, hydronephrosis, and hypoplastic kidney, may coexist. Short femurs are also associated with Turner's syndrome.

Most fetuses with Turner's syndrome will spontaneously abort. The prognosis is especially grave when the fetus presents with a large cystic hygroma and edema or hydrops (Figure 53-30). If the hygroma is isolated, it may regress in utero. The prognosis after birth depends on the severity of associated anomalies. Female infants who survive will have immature sexual development, amenorrhea, short stature, a webbed neck, cubitus valgus (abnormal elbow angle), and a shield chest with widely spaced nipples. They may also have poor hearing, and hormone replacement is necessary for sexual development. Turner's syndrome children usually have normal intelligence.

Sonographic Findings. The previously listed ultrasound findings for Turner's syndrome may also include oligohydramnios, especially when severe renal anomalies are present.

ACKNOWLEDGMENTS

I would like to acknowledge the sonographers Maria Roman, Lucy Burgos, Jamie Prieto, and Lori Sisk at the Maternal Fetal Center, Orlando, Florida, for continually sharing their interesting cases with me, so that I am able to share a piece of their knowledge. I would also like to thank the perinatologist Dr. Fuentes for allowing me to continue to expand my skills and knowledge under his mentoring.

REFERENCES

1. Benacerraf BR: *Ultrasound of fetal syndromes*, ed 2, Philadelphia, 2008, Churchill Livingstone.
2. Callen PW: *Ultrasonography in obstetrics and gynecology*, ed 5, Philadelphia, 2008, Saunders.
3. Jauniaux E, Brown R, Rodeck C, et al: Prenatal diagnosis of triploidy during the second trimester of pregnancy, *Obstet Gynecol* 88:983, 1996.
4. Jeanty P: Prenatal detection of simian crease, *J Ultrasound Med* 9:131, 1990.
5. Nyberg DA, Mahony BS, Pretorius DH, editors: *Diagnostic ultrasound of fetal anomalies: text and atlas*, St. Louis, 1990, Mosby.
6. Pandya PP, Kondylios A, Hilbert L, et al: Chromosomal defects and outcome in 1015 fetuses with increased nuchal translucency, *Ultrasound Obstet Gynecol* 5:15, 1995.
7. Papp C, Beke A, Mezei G, et al: Prenatal diagnosis of Turner syndrome, report on 69 cases, *J Ultrasound Med* 25:711-717, 2006.
8. Rijhsinghani A, Yankowitz J, Strauss RA, et al: Risk of preeclampsia in second trimester triploid pregnancies, *Obstet Gynecol* 90:884, 1997.
9. Szigeti Z, Sdaba A, Pete B, et al: Correlation of prenatal sonographic diagnosis and norphologic findings of fetal autopsy in fetuses with trisomy 21, *J Ultrasound Med* 26:61-68, 2007.
10. United Kingdom collaborative study on alpha-fetoprotein in relation to neural tube defects: maternal serum alpha-fetoprotein measurement in antenatal screen for anencephaly and spina bifida in early pregnancy, *Lancet* 1:1323, 1977.
11. Watson WJ, Miller RC, Wax JR, et al: Sonographic findings of trisomy 18 in the second trimester of pregnancy, *J Ultrasound Med* 27:1033-1038, 2008.
12. Watson WJ, Miller RC, Wax JR, et al: Sonographic findings of trisomy 13 in the first and second trimesters of pregnancy, *J Ultrasound Med* 26:1209-1214, 2007.

3D and 4D Evaluation of Fetal Anomalies

Dennis Wisher

OBJECTIVES

On completion of this chapter, you should be able to:
- Describe the difference between manual and automatic 3D acquisition
- List the applications of gynecologic and obstetric 3D acquisition
- Describe the difference between the multi-slice view and the oblique view
- Define the concept of multivolume rendering
- Describe the mirror view used in multivolume rendering

OUTLINE

Three-Dimensional (3D) Technology
Acquisition
Multiplanar Display

Three-Dimensional Rendering
Multi-slice View
Oblique View

Multivolume Rendering
Conclusion

Although three-dimensional ultrasound has been commercially available since the 1990s, many sonographers and physicians still perceive 3D as being new. All too often, the perceived value of 3D ultrasound is limited to creating pretty pictures of the fetal face. To broaden diagnostic awareness, it is necessary to understand the basic clinical and technical concepts of 3D ultrasound. The focus of this chapter is three-fold: (1) to introduce the sonographer to the technical concepts of 3D ultrasound, (2) to acquaint the sonographer with the 3D tools that are currently available, and (3) to provide clinical examples that illustrate the integration of 3D ultrasound into conventional sonographic examinations. Although three-dimensional ultrasound has demonstrated diagnostic value in a variety of medical specialties, this chapter focuses on the obstetric and gynecologic applications of three-dimensional ultrasound.

The 3D concepts and interactive tools discussed in this chapter are built on the fundamental concepts of 2D technology and therefore require a confident understanding of 2D gray-scale ultrasound as a prerequisite. Conventional 2D ultrasound requires sonographers to master a variety of intricate probe movements in order to perform sonographic examinations. The sonographer then *mentally* assimilates the 2D real-time images into a three-dimensional representation. Unfortunately, the ability to mentally assimilate accurate anatomic spatial relationships becomes more challenging as anatomy and pathology become more complicated.

THREE-DIMENSIONAL (3D) TECHNOLOGY

The basic conceptual protocol of three-dimensional ultrasound requires a method of collecting, storing, and displaying patient anatomy as 3D volume data. Storing patient anatomy as 3D volume data allows the sonographer to perform detailed retrospective reviews of complex anatomy and pathology after the patient has left the ultrasound lab.

Three-dimensional technology has steadily improved since the mid-1990s, and during that time it has demonstrated significant clinical potential as an effective adjunct to conventional 2D scanning. The degree to which 3D is integrated depends on the examination being performed.

The advantages of 3D are many and include the following:

- Decreased patient scan times
- Documentation of image planes not attainable using conventional 2D ultrasound
- Retrospective review of stored patient anatomy
- Rotation of anatomic scan planes
- More accurate volume measurements
- More standardized documentation
- Decreased repetitive probe motions

Acquisition

Acquisition is the method of collecting patient anatomy as a series of slices, which are then processed and stored for display as 3D volume data. There are two main methods of acquisition: manual acquisition (also called "free-hand" acquisition) and automatic acquisition.

Manual Acquisition. **Manual acquisition** is the original 3D method of collecting anatomy. It required the sonographer to manually slide the probe along the patient's skin to collect anatomy as a series of slices. Manual acquisition assumes a specific number of slices will be collected during a specific time and distance. Unfortunately, manually sliding the probe at a consistent speed over a given distance often proved to be difficult for even the most experienced of 2D sonographers, and this method was often perceived as being tedious and time consuming. Manual acquisition often resulted in "nonuniform" data sets containing questionable spatial relationships between anatomic structures.

Automatic Acquisition. Today, the majority of manufacturers have replaced manual acquisition probe technology with specialized 3D probes capable of performing a more efficient method of acquisition called automatic acquisition. Unlike manual techniques, **automatic acquisition** allows the sonographer to collect patient anatomy as a series of slices without having to manually move the probe during the acquisition process. Because there is no manual movement, the acquisition process is consistent, providing uniform data sets with exact spatial relationships between the collected anatomic structures. The precision of the automatic acquisition process also allows accurate measurements to be performed on each of the displayed multiplanar images.

Automatic acquisition is made possible by a small motor connected to the element array housed within the 3D ultrasound probe. The motor, governed by computer precision, sweeps the element array in a single fanlike motion within the probe, thus collecting patient anatomy (within the field of view) as a series of 2D slices. The acquired slices are then instantaneously processed and displayed as 3D volume anatomy.

The amount of anatomy collected during the acquisition process is determined by the sonographer who selects the depth of the 2D image and the size of the acquisition angle. Proper selection of the acquisition angle dictates the size of the sweep motion of the internal element array. The speed of the automatic sweep mechanism is also sonographer dependent. Slower acquisition speeds provide higher resolution, whereas faster acquisition sweeps result in decreased image quality. (Most ultrasound systems in use today perform "slow" acquisitions in 2 to 3 seconds.)

The precision and consistency of automatic acquisition eliminates the need for manual probe movement during the acquisition process and elevates the potential for efficient integration of 3D into conventional 2D examinations. The 3D transvaginal probe is an excellent example of the successful integration of 3D technology into conventional 2D ultrasound examinations. The entire uterus can be acquired in as little as 2 to 3 seconds using automatic acquisition probes, decreasing patient scan times and improving patient acceptance of transvaginal examinations.

Multiplanar Display

After acquisition, patient anatomy may be reviewed using the **multiplanar display**, which demonstrates anatomy as three simultaneous orthogonal scan planes: longitudinal, transverse, and the coronal plane. The coronal plane is often referred to as the "C-plane" and frequently displays views of anatomy that are unattainable using conventional 2D ultrasound.

It is important to understand that planar images display an orthogonal relationship. That is to say, images display 90 degrees to each other. This (orthogonal) relationship acts as the cornerstone in the diagnostic foundation of the multiplanar display providing exact spatial relationships between planar anatomy. The sonographer may also rotate the planar images to provide more comprehensive review of complex anatomy or pathology. A significant advantage of multiplanar imaging is the ability to perform retrospective reviews of stored patient anatomy.

Gynecologic Application of Multiplanar Imaging. The nongravid uterus is an excellent clinical example of the diagnostic potential of multiplanar technology. The American Institute of Ultrasound in Medicine (AIUM) has suggested documentation of specific anatomic structures when performing conventional 2D sonographic gynecologic examinations. Two-dimensional pelvic anatomy can also be documented as three simultaneous scan planes, depicting conventional longitudinal and transverse images, as well as the unique coronal (C-plane) image (Figure 54-1). Careful observation of the C-plane reveals the diagnostic value of this unique image. The "normal" inverted triangular shape of the endometrium is clearly seen demonstrating both cornual angles along with the lower uterine segment. The surrounding myometrium also displays with clarity, allowing confident documentation regarding the number, size and location of fibroid tumors.

The endometrial fundus and serosal uterine fundus clearly display, providing confident documentation and differentiation of Müllerian duct anomalies such as septate and bicornuate uteri. Müllerian duct patients often present with a history of reproductive complications, including infertility and recurrent miscarriage. Differentiation of septate from bicornuate is an essential part of patient management and preoperative planning, if surgical correction is chosen. Surgical correction of septi uteri is usually performed using hysteroscopic technique to remove the internal septum, returning the endometrial cavity to a more "normal" triangular shape. Bicornuate uteri, on the other hand, require more complicated surgical intervention (metroplasty), as compared to septate uteri (Figure 54-2).

The precision of the multiplanar display also proves advantageous when evaluating the location of an intrauterine device (IUD). Unlike conventional 2D ultra-

sound, which is limited to viewing the IUD in longitudinal and transverse planes, C-plane images allow sonographers to visualize both the actual "T-shape" of the IUD and its specific location within the endometrial cavity. Optimal IUD placement displays as midline with the "T-arms" in close proximity to the endometrial fundus. Improper IUD positioning is easily detected using the C-plane. Planar images also allow sonographers to more specifically interrogate the location of the "T-arms" of the IUD to determine if any portions of the "arms" extend beyond the walls of the endometrium.

Not all IUD images display as echogenic (bright white). The sonographic appearance depends on the specific model of IUD visualized. The ParaGard Copper T380A IUD displays as an echogenic "T-shape" structure, but the Mirena (hormonal) IUD displays as an

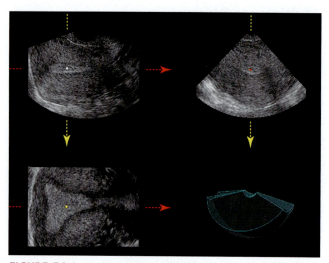

FIGURE 54-1 Normal uterus displays as three simultaneous scan planes using the multiplanar display, including the longitudinal, transverse, and unique coronal planes.

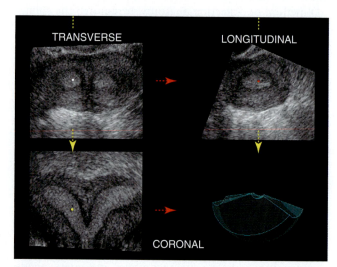

FIGURE 54-2 The multiplanar display provides additional diagnostic value when documenting Müllerian duct anomalies by providing clear visualization of both the endometrial shape and the serosal uterine fundus. Here septate uteri are shown.

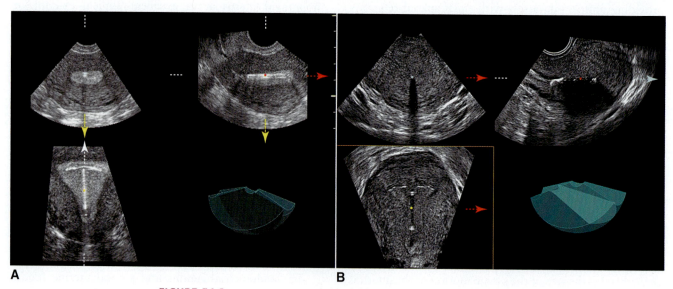

A   B

FIGURE 54-3 Multiplant images of the ParaGard **(A)** and Mirena **(B)** IUDs.

anechoic (black) shaft with thin echogenic "T-arms" (Figure 54-3). The significant difference in sonographic appearance is due to the materials used to construct the IUD. Although both are made of plastic, the shaft of the ParaGard is wound with copper wire that creates an echogenic sonographic appearance. The shaft of the Mirena does not contain copper wire; instead it contains a reservoir tube coated with barium flake, which gives it an anechoic shadowing appearance.

In addition to detailed documentation of uterine anatomy, three-dimensional ultrasound also provides confident documentation of ovary and adnexal pathology, including wall irregularities, septations, and solid components constituting adnexal masses in views often not attainable using conventional 2D scanning.

Sonohysterography. The combination of automatic acquisition probe technology and multiplanar imaging make 3D technology an excellent adjunct when performing conventional 2D sonohysterography examinations. Patient preparation, catheter placement, and infusion of saline remain the same as when performing the 2D sonohysterogram procedure; the difference is incorporating the 3D transvaginal probe to acquire the contents of endometrial cavity (saline and polyp). The 3D transvaginal probe obviates the need for excessive probe movements. The resultant C-plane provides exceptional images depicting the shape, size, and contents of the endometrial cavity, thus providing more confident documentation of polyps and tumors (Figure 54-4). In addition to more comprehensive documentation, the ability to acquire the entire uterus in seconds (automatic acquisition) significantly decreases the time needed to perform the procedure, resulting in better patient acceptance.

Obstetric Applications of Multiplanar Imaging. As previously stated, the diagnostic value of multiplanar imaging is as an adjunct to (not a replacement of) conventional 2D ultrasound imaging. Keeping this in mind, multiplanar imaging provides detailed evaluation of the fetus including face, brain, abdomen, heart, and skeletal anatomy.

Fetal Face. The fetal face is a good example of the potential value of 3D integration. Routinely visualized as part of conventional 2D examinations, the eyes, nose, lips, and chin are evaluated when documenting the fetal face. Although 2D ultrasound has successfully documented facial anomalies for many years, it is limited to viewing the face as a single flat image. Three-dimensional imaging, on the other hand, can provide more detailed documentation of spatial relationships by utilizing the precision of multiplanar imaging (as well as 3D surface rendering). For example, viewing three simultaneous scan planes allows a much better determination of the true midsagittal plane essential for documenting anomalies such as micrognathia. The literature has cited that what appears to be the "true" midsagittal plane is all too often incorrect. Confident determination of the "true" midsagittal plane is essential when performing measurements as not to underestimate anatomic dimensions (Figure 54-5).

Though conventional 2D ultrasound has proven effective for the diagnosis of cleft lip and palate, experienced sonographers are aware of the limitations often associated with 2D, like the difficulty of displaying the secondary palate. Conventional documentation using 2D ultrasound usually depicts coronal images of the fetal nose and lips, as well as axial images of the primary palate (with maxillary alveolar ridge and tooth buds). If

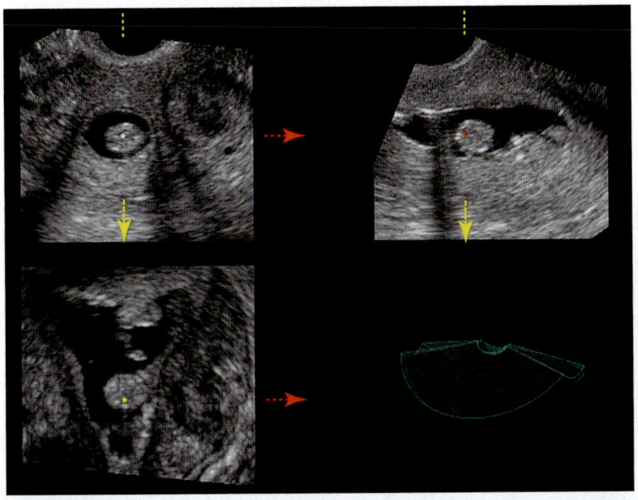

FIGURE 54-4 Three-dimensional ultrasound is an excellent adjunct complimenting conventional 2D sonohysterography examinations, providing detailed documentation regarding the shape and contents of the endometrium when viewed in the unique C-plane. Multiple echogenic polyps display within the endometrial cavity; a large hypoechoic fibroid is also seen in the adjacent myometrium.

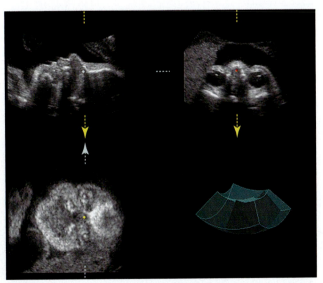

FIGURE 54-5 Displaying the fetal face as three orthogonal scan planes provides more confident determination of the "true" midsagittal plane.

the alveolar ridge appears to be intact (displaying an echogenic horseshoe shape), the secondary palate is then often assumed to be intact as well. Unfortunately, this assumption is not always accurate. Published literature has shown that it is possible to have a defect in the soft palate (velum) but still maintain a normal appearance to the primary palate. The limited visualization of the secondary palate is often attributed to two factors. The first is shadowing from the primary palate (maxillary alveolar ridge), which obscures visualization of the secondary palate. The second is the natural downward curvature of the soft palate that does not allow for optimal perpendicular reflection of the ultrasound beam, which results in suboptimal 2D visualization.

Although multiplanar technology is an excellent adjunct to conventional 2D sonography, it is important to recognize the significance of probe positioning during the acquisition process when attempting to acquire images of the fetal secondary palate. All too often, positioning of the probe (ultrasound beam) perpendicular to the lips results in posterior shadowing from the maxilla obstructing visualization of the secondary palate. However, positioning the probe so the ultrasound beam strikes the palate from a more inferior angle of insonation (30 to 45 degrees instead of 90 degrees) will often improve the clarity of the resultant planar palate images. Keeping this in mind, multiplanar imaging provides the ability to systematically progress through stored 3D anatomy assisting with more comprehensive documentation of facial defects such as cleft lip and palate (Figure 54-6).

Central Nervous System. One single acquisition performed at the level of the BPD in the axial plane or at the level of the cerebellum (axial plane) captures the anatomy of the entire fetal brain. Although the acquisition was performed in the axial plane, anatomy can be reviewed in any desired image plane, including longitu-

dinal, transverse (axial), and coronal. This ability allows sonographers to evaluate many landmark intracranial structures often difficult to attain using conventional 2D ultrasound.

Documentation of the corpus callosum is a good example of the value of planar imaging for the sonographic evaluation of the fetal brain. When attempting to determine agenesis (complete absence) of the corpus callosum or dysgenesis (partial absence), many sonographers will make an effort to document the midsagittal view of the fetal brain by utilizing the frontal suture as an acoustic window. Accomplishment of this task depends on fetal positioning often making the transfrontal (sagittal midline) image difficult to attain using conventional 2D scanning techniques. However, incorporating 3D technology, the fetal brain is collected from one axial acquisition. Utilization of planar rotations allows the sonographer to display specific anatomic structures located within the 3D data set. Therefore, anatomy located in the midsagittal plane displays, even though the acquisition was performed in the axial plane (Figure 54-7).

The corpus callosum viewed using the transfrontal view (sagittal midline) displays as a curved hypoechoic structure with well-defined borders following along the curvature of the cavum septi pellucid (CSP). However, the same corpus callosum—when acquired from an axial (transverse) plane and then reconstructed to display the midsagittal view—depicts the corpus callosum as an *echogenic* curved linear structure representing the interface of the corpus callosum and cavum septi pellucidi. Often, the corpus callosum cannot be specifically distinguished from the border of the cavum septi pellucidi in this reconstructed scan plane, instead displaying as an echogenic curved linear "complex" representing both the corpus callosum and CSP. Nevertheless, this planar view provides important diagnostic information regarding the

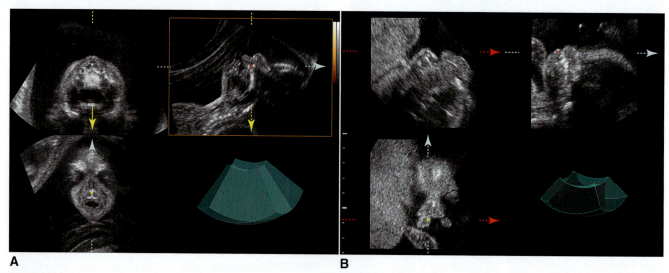

A   B

FIGURE 54-6 A, This image depicts the normal lip and palate as three orthogonal scan planes using the multiplanar display. **B,** Demonstration of the lip and palate defect as planar images.

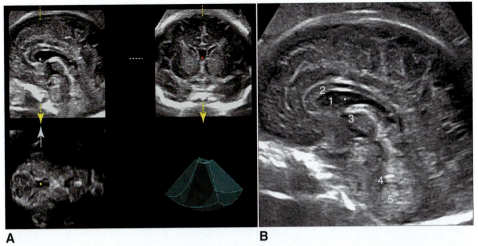

FIGURE 54-7 A, The multiplanar image represents a 34-week fetus and was attained using one single acquisition in the midsagittal plane. **B,** The midsagittal image displays the *(1)* cavum septi pellucidi with cavum vergae, *(2)* corpus callosum, *(3)* third ventricle, *(4)* fourth ventricle, and *(5)* cerebellar vermis.

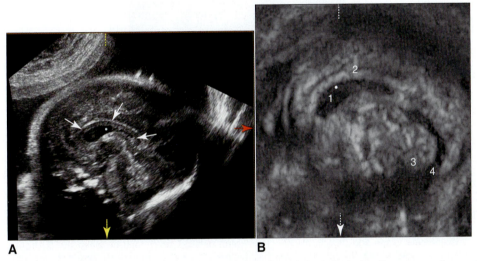

FIGURE 54-8 A, This image was created using the midsagittal plane (transfrontal view) displaying the corpus callosum *(arrows)* as a curved hypoechoic structure with well-defined borders following along the superior of the CSP. **B,** The corpus callosum image was initially acquired from an axial (transverse) plane and then reconstructed to display the midsagittal plane. An echogenic curved linear structure representing the interface of the corpus callosum and the CSP displays. This image displays the *(1)* cavum septi pellucidi, *(2)* corpus callosum, *(3)* cerebellar vermis, and *(4)* posterior fossa. Both the transfrontal view and the reconstructed midsagittal view can be used as effective tools when documenting agenesis of the corpus callosum.

presence of midsagittal anatomy essential when attempting to document intracranial anomalies, including agenesis of the corpus callosum (Figure 54-8).

Although 3D acquisitions collect a vast amount of intracranial anatomy, the sonographer may not be familiar with every minute anatomic structure in the fetal brain. Keeping this in mind, as a general statement, documentation of the fetal brain using three distinct axial image planes (transventricular, transthalamic, and transcerebellar) proves effective for the majority of intracranial anomalies. These image planes are readily assessable using the multiplanar display when acquired in the axial plane utilizing a transabdominal acquisition of the obstetric patient (Figure 54-9).

The precision of multiplanar imaging also provides confident assessment for a variety of central nervous system (CNS) anomalies, including Dandy Walker malformations, anencephaly, and cephalocele. Planar imaging also acts as an effective adjunct when documenting neural tube defects (such as spina bifida), as the fetal spine can be rotated into standardized planes allowing for confident determination regarding the specific level of the vertebral defect (Figure 54-10).

Skeleton and Limbs. The same systematic precision used when documenting fetal neural tube defects can also be incorporated into examinations of fetal skeletal and limb anomalies like scoliosis, hemivertebra, and club feet. Planar imaging also provides more comprehensive

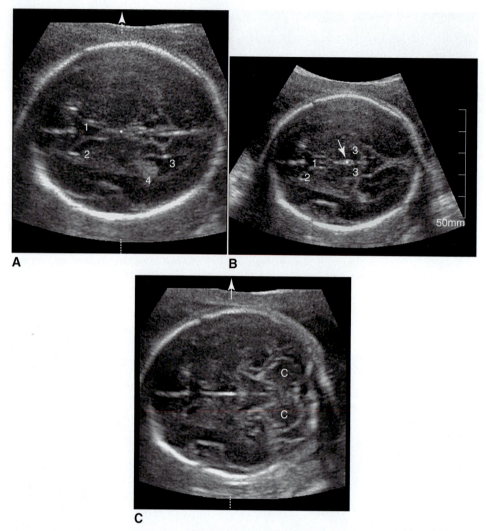

FIGURE 54-9 A, This planar image displays the transventricular plane demonstrating the *(1)* cavum septi pellucidi, *(2)* anterior horns of lateral ventricle, and *(3)* atria of lateral ventricles with *(4)* the choroid plexus. **B,** This image displays the transthalamic plane, which is located just inferior to the transventricular plane and depicts the *(1)* cavum septi pellucidi positioned between the *(2)* frontal horns of the lateral ventricles *(arrow),* the third ventricle, and *(3)* thalami. The transthalamic plane is used when performing BPD or head circumference measurements. **C,** This planar image depicts the transcerebellar plane, displaying the posterior fossa and cerebellar hemispheres *(c).* The cerebellar vermis may also display in this plane. The transcerebellar plane is located inferior to the transthalamic plane.

evaluations when counting the number of digits and documenting the structure of the hand, wrist, and forearm.

THREE-DIMENSIONAL RENDERING

Renderings display a three-dimensional representation of the anatomy of interest. To better comprehend the concept of three-dimensional (3D) rendering, it is necessary once again to return to the concept of the 2D gray-scale image. Two-dimensional images are composed of small picture elements called pixels, and each pixel has an assigned gray-scale value depending on the strength of the received 2D echo. The 3D data set is conceptually similar, composed of three-dimensional pixels called **voxels**. Voxels also have assigned gray-scale

values depending on the strength (amplitude) of the returning 2D echoes.

Three-dimensional renderings are often described as though a light were projected from back to front along a specific line of voxels within the data set (also called "ray casting"). That is, specific gray-scale voxel values are identified and displayed ("projected") onto the 2D monitor (Figure 54-11).

Images rendered in 3D are usually classified into two groups: *surface* or *transparent renderings.* Surface renderings display the surface detail of anatomy as seen in the example of the fetal face, whereas transparent renderings look beyond the surface of the anatomy to reveal structures located within. Transparent renderings are usually composed of one of the following rendering modes: *maximum, minimum,* or *x-ray.* Maximum mode

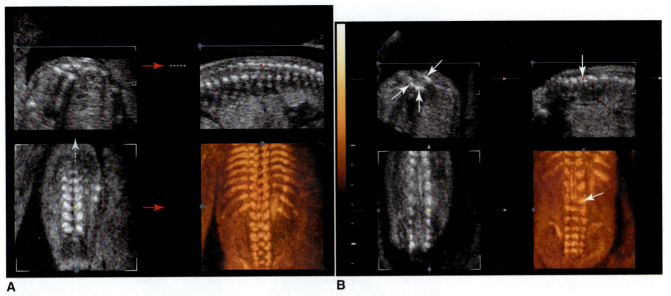

A   **B**

FIGURE 54-10 A, The multiplanar image displays the normal fetal spine with clarity documented as three orthogonal scan planes; the 3D-rendered spine displays as well. **B,** The image provides detailed documentation of a spinal defect using the multiplanar display and 3D rendering.

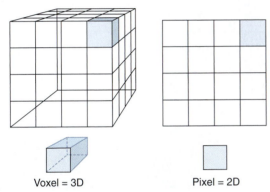

Voxel = 3D   Pixel = 2D

FIGURE 54-11 A 2D gray-scale image is composed of small picture elements called *pixels*. The 3D data set is composed of three-dimensional pixels called *voxels*. Voxels have assigned gray-scale values depending on the amplitude of the received 2D echo.

displays bright echoes hidden within the data set, advantageous when documenting the fetal spine. Minimum mode displays the black (anechoic) echoes hidden within the data set, advantageous when documenting vessels, fluid, or cystic structures. X-ray mode displays the mean value of the dark and bright echoes located within the data set, usually creating a soft haze appearance on displayed 3D-rendered anatomy.

Although patient anatomy may have initially been stored as a multiplanar display, the sonographer can still change the display format without performing a second acquisition. Keeping this in mind, the same 3D anatomy previously viewed using the multiplanar display may also exhibit as a 3D-rendered image, if desired, during the retrospective review.

All too often, the perception of 3D rendering is limited to that of the fetal face, even though 3D rendering has potential to be an effective diagnostic adjunct to both 2D as well as multiplanar examinations. When performed correctly, 3D rendering provides detailed documentation of fetal limb anomalies, facial and palate defects, abdominal wall, and neural tube defects. As discussed, the acquisition process collects the anatomy of interest, but the aesthetic appearance of that anatomy is directly dependent on the rendering modes selected by the sonographer (Figure 54-12). The 3D-rendered images are often used as effective consultative tools when explaining the severity of an anomaly to a patient or medical professional.

Multi-slice View

Multi-slice view displays 3D anatomy as a series of sequential parallel images similar in display format to that of computed tomography (CT) and magnetic resonance imaging (MRI). The sonographer determines the number of images to be displayed, as well as the interval between the displayed images. The sonographer may also rotate multi-slice view images to display optimal diagnostic perspectives.

Although conventional 2D ultrasound is perceived as being an excellent noninvasive diagnostic tool, it is often criticized as lacking reproducibility. Multi-slice view empowers the sonographer with the ability to increase consistency and precision by displaying anatomy as a series of sequential slices. This concept proves to be especially helpful when documenting complex pathology or when documenting serial examinations for changes in size and shape of focal masses.

Documentation as a series of sequential images is especially helpful when evaluating obstetric and gynecologic anatomy, as the multi-slice view improves

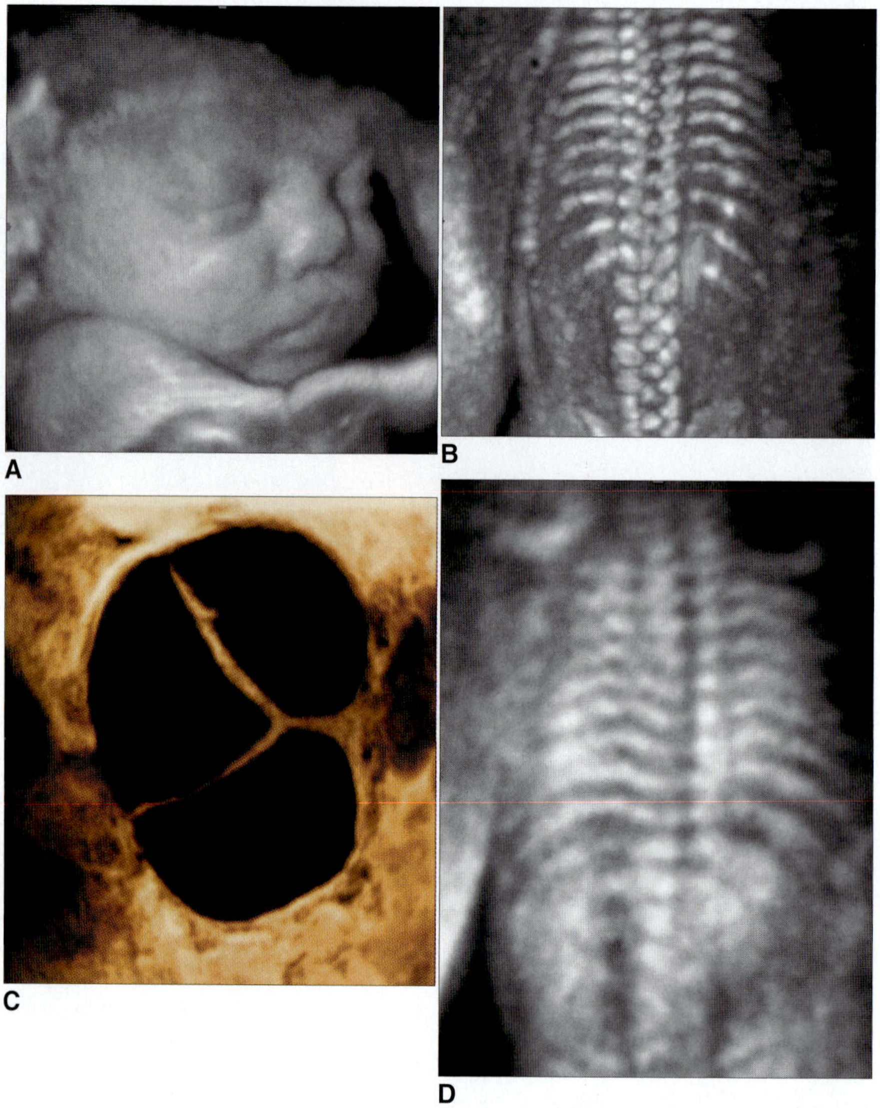

FIGURE 54-12 A, The 3D-rendered image displays the detail of the fetal face using surface mode. **B,** The rendered image displays the fetal spine and ribs using maximum mode. **C,** The image displays a cyst containing multiple septations using minimum mode. **D,** The image displays the fetal spine with a softer appearance using x-ray mode.

comprehension of spatial relationships. For example, one single (2-second) acquisition performed at the level of the transverse fetal abdominal circumference routinely yields comprehensive documentation of the fetus depicting the AIUM-suggested anatomy in sequential order from inferior to superior, including bladder, gender, femur, stomach, cord insertion, kidneys, and four-chamber heart (Figure 54-13). Equally as impressive, axial (transverse) acquisitions performed at the BPD level display fetal brain anatomy as parallel sequential images including posterior fossa, both cerebellar hemispheres, cerebellar vermis, thalami, cavum septi pellucidi, lateral ventricles, choroid plexus, and interhemispheric fissure (Figures 54-14).

Multi-slice view also provides detailed documentation of cleft lip and palate defects displaying craniofacial anomalies as a series of sequential parallel images in axial (transverse), sagittal, and coronal views.

The combination of automatic acquisition transvaginal probes and multi-slice view imaging provides

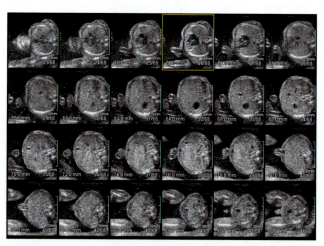

FIGURE 54-13 One single acquisition yields comprehensive multi-slice view documentation of the fetus, as seen in this example depicting the AIUM-suggested anatomy (genitals, bladder, stomach, cord insertion, kidneys, and four-chamber heart). If desired, the sagittal and coronal images can also be displayed from this same single acquisition.

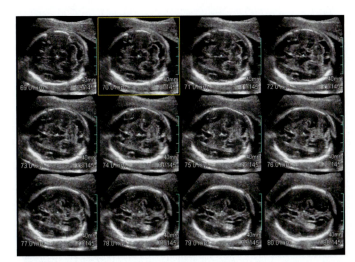

FIGURE 54-14 Multi-slice view displays acquired anatomy as a series of parallel sequential images as seen in this example of the fetal brain. All scan planes (axial, sagittal, and coronal) as well as any oblique scan planes may be displayed from one single acquisition.

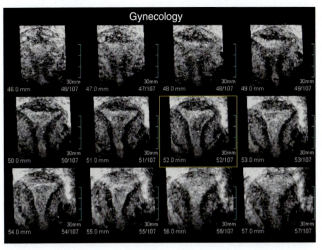

FIGURE 54-15 This multi-slice view image displays uterine anatomy as a series of parallel sequential images in the unique C-plane. The shape of the endometrium, as well the adjacent myometrium and serosal fundus, display with clarity.

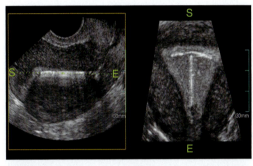

FIGURE 54-16 Oblique view displays the corresponding cross-sectional image from within the acquired 3D data set. In this example the unique coronal image of the uterus with IUD displays with clarity.

effective integration of 3D technology and conventional (2D) pelvic ultrasound examinations. As previously stated, all displayed sequential images result from a single acquisition (usually 2 to 3 seconds), thus benefiting the sonographer by reducing the need for excessive repetitive stress probe movements during the sonographic examination, as well as improving patient acceptance of the transvaginal procedure through decreased scan times.

Multi-slice view also displays the unique C-plane, providing detailed images of the endometrial cavity, both cornual angles as well as a lower uterine segment display (within the C-plane). In addition to endometrial detail, the sequential display of images provides more comprehensive documentation of the myometrium as well. The multi-slice view also proves to be an effective adjunct for confident documentation of Müllerian duct anomalies, as both the serosal and transmetrial fundus display with clarity (Figure 54-15).

Oblique View

From its inception, 2D ultrasound has dictated documentation of anatomy or pathology in two orthogonal scan planes (usually longitudinal and transverse). This basic sonographic rule helps to increase diagnostic confidence when documenting suspected anomalies. **Oblique view** incorporates this basic concept when interacting with 3D anatomy. Using a dual screen display format, the sonographer positions the oblique-view line (from any position) through the anatomy of interest; the corresponding cross-sectional image displays on the adjacent screen. The sonographer is also able to trace along the curvature of the anatomy of interest to display the corresponding cross-sectional view from within the 3D data set (Figure 54-16).

Multivolume Rendering

To date, the newest advancement to 3D technology is called multivolume rendering. Continued advancements in computer processing capabilities combined with advanced digital signal processing permits multiple rendered images to display simultaneously in the same amount of time previously required to create just one single render. Three interactive tools incorporating this technology—volume slice, mirror view, and oblique view extended (OVIX)—will be discussed.

Volume Slice. Volume slice displays seven sequential 3D-*rendered* volume images simultaneously. This should not be confused with multi-slice view, which displays sequential *planar* images. Each 3D-rendered image displays a different anatomic depth from within the data set, which is advantageous when documenting fetal face anomalies, spinal defects, and uterine anomalies. Figure 54-17 demonstrates the spinal defect from the skin line through the vertebral anatomy using a series of sequential volume rendered images, each using an offset depth interval of 1 mm. Sequential 3D-rendered images help to

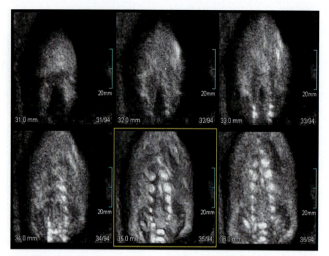

FIGURE 54-17 Volume slice displays anatomy as a series of sequential 3D volume rendered images, starting at the skin line and extending through the vertebral anatomy. Each rendered image displays at a different depth interval, providing improved spatial comprehension and documentation of the spinal defect *(arrows)*.

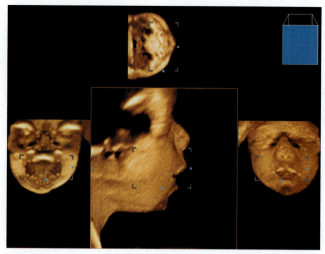

FIGURE 54-19 Mirror view simultaneously displays the anatomy of interest from four different volume viewing perspectives in real time: the front view of the fetal face, the coronal "reverse face" with hard palate, the profile, as well as the axial palate simultaneously display in real time.

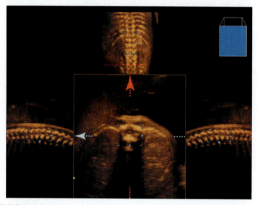

FIGURE 54-18 Mirror view simultaneously displays the 3D-rendered spine from four different viewing perspectives in real time. The sonographer is able to rotate the displayed 3D-rendered images to display the desired diagnostic perspectives.

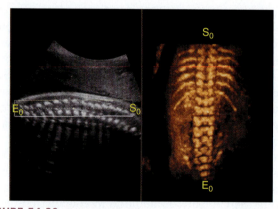

FIGURE 54-20 OVIX provides the corresponding 3D volume slice from within the acquired data set. Using the acquired planar image as a reference, the sonographer places the OVIX line through the sagittal spine; the corresponding 3D-rendered image of the fetal coronal spine displays with clarity.

improve spatial comprehension of three-dimensional anatomy and pathology.

Mirror View. Improvements in computer processing speed and digital signal processing have made possible a new 3D tool called **mirror view,** which displays simultaneous rendered volume images from four different perspectives in real time (Figures 54-18). Using the fetal face as an example, the nose and lips, the coronal hard palate (seen in the so-called reverse face view), as well as the profile and axial secondary palate simultaneously display (Figure 54-19). Mirror view has the potential to be an effective adjunct to conventional 2D ultrasound when documenting anomalies of the fetal face and palate.

Oblique View Extended (OVIX). As previously noted, evaluation of anatomy and pathology using conventional 2D ultrasound requires documentation in two different image planes (traditionally, longitudinal and transverse). This foundational concept has been incorporated into

3D ultrasound as well. After acquiring patient anatomy, the sonographer positions a so-called OVIX line through the anatomy of interest to display the correlating volume slice from within the acquired 3D volume data set. The sonographer determines the thickness of the correlating anatomic volume slice. **Oblique view extended (OVIX)** is similar in concept to oblique view, with the distinction being that oblique view displays the corresponding cross-section *planar* image, whereas OVIX displays the corresponding *volume* slice.

OVIX provides detailed three-dimensional images of the anatomy of interest, especially helpful when documenting 3D-rendered images of the fetal spine (Figure 54-20).

Fetal Heart. Perceived as a screening tool, the four-chamber heart image is documented as an essential part of (2D) fetal sonographic examinations. Although the four-chamber view provides essential information regarding the number and size of atria and ventricles, it does not provide direct visualization of the left ventricular outflow tract (LVOT) or right ventricular outflow tract (RVOT). Three-dimensional ultrasound has the potential to elevate the four-chamber view to a more effective screening tool by using basic automatic acquisition techniques or implementing spatial temporal imaging correlation (STIC) acquisitions.

Automatic acquisitions performed in the axial plane at the level of the four-chamber view routinely capture the entire fetal heart in 2 to 3 seconds. The dynamic motion of the fetal heart makes it is necessary for the sonographer to adjust the speed of acquisition (faster acquisition) in order to avoid or minimize the possibility of motion artifacts. The sonographer also adjusts the acquisition angle to acquire anatomy from fetal stomach up through the heart and trachea.

Once acquired, the fetal heart can be displayed using a variety of 3D interactive tools including, multiplanar imaging, 3D rendering, oblique view, multi-slice view, volume slice, mirror view, and volume slice imaging. Multiplanar imaging is most commonly used. It displays cardiac anatomy as three orthogonal image planes from a single transverse acquisition taken at the level of the four-chamber view (Figure 54-21). The sonographer then displays landmark cardiac anatomy including LVOT and RVOT using a variety of planar rotation techniques.

Multi-slice view also proves to be an effective complement to the four-chamber view by displaying the fetal heart as a series of parallel image slices. This display format yields comprehensive documentation of cardiac anatomy. Careful observation of the multi-slice view image in Figure 54-22 demonstrates the four-chamber view, the five-chamber view, the three-vessel view, and the three-vessel trachea view (3VT).

Comprehension of the axial plane anatomy depicted within the three-vessel view and the three-vessel trachea view prove advantageous when utilizing 3D ultrasound as an adjunctive screening tool for the assessment of the fetal heart. Changes in configuration or size of the three circular structures representing the main pulmonary artery, ascending aorta, and superior vena cava increase awareness as to the presence of possible cardiac anomalies.

Figure 54-23 demonstrates the so-called three-vessel view, depicting three anechoic circular structures. The first and largest circle represents the (1) main pulmonary artery, the middle circle represents the (2) ascending aorta, and the last and smallest circle represents the (3) superior vena cava. A connection between the (1) main

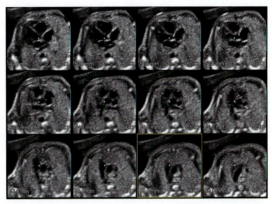

FIGURE 54-22 The multi-slice view image displays the four-chamber view image in the upper left corner, followed by the five-chamber view in the upper right corner. The bifurcation of the pulmonary arteries displays as the last image on observer's right in the middle row. The three-vessel view with ductus arteriosus displays in the lower left corner, and the three-vessel trachea view with aortic arch displays as the third image toward the right on the bottom row. The transverse aortic arch displays as the lower right corner image.

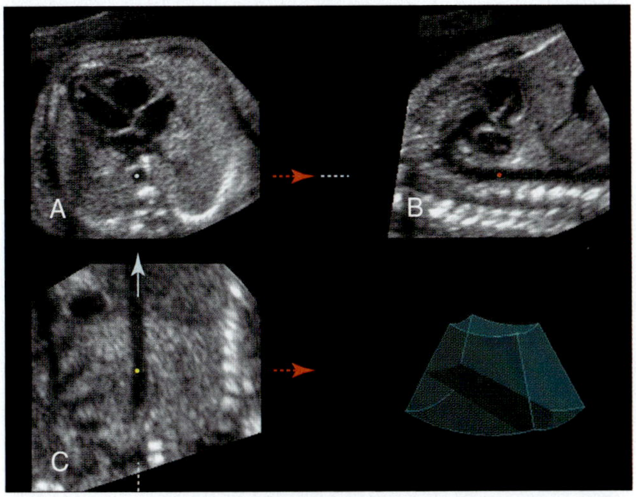

FIGURE 54-21 Fetal heart displayed as three orthogonal image planes using the multiplanar display. **A,** Planar image of the four-chamber view. **B,** The sagittal aortic arch. **C,** The coronal aorta, as well as fetal stomach.

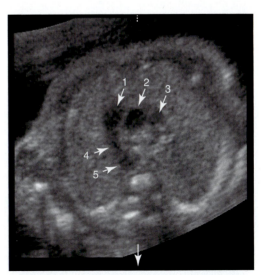

FIGURE 54-23 The three-vessel view displays the *(1)* main pulmonary artery, *(2)* ascending aorta, *(3)* superior vena cava, *(4)* ductus arteriosus, and *(5)* descending aorta.

pulmonary artery and the (5) descending aorta representing the (4) ductus arteriosus is also seen within the three-vessel view image.

The sonographer may also display the bifurcation of the main pulmonary artery by locating the axial plane positioned just caudal to the ductus arteriosus image; the (1) main pulmonary artery, (2) ascending aorta, (3) superior vena cava, (4) left pulmonary artery, (5) right pulmonary artery, and (6) descending aorta display with clarity (Figure 54-24). This author strongly recommends documentation of the pulmonary bifurcation, as it provides confident differentiation of the pulmonary artery from the aorta, especially if structures are abnormally positioned.

The three-vessel trachea view (3VT) displays the same structures present in the three-vessel view, as well as the aortic arch, which is seen as a connection between the middle circle (ascending aorta) and the circle just anterior to the fetal spine (descending aorta). The trachea displays as a slitlike structure adjacent to the aorta. Changes in size or spatial relationships of the three circular structures representing the main pulmonary artery, ascending aorta, and superior vena cava suggests the possibility of a cardiac anomaly (Figure 54-25).

In addition to multi-slice view imaging, the multiplanar display also allows the sonographer to transition among the four-chamber view, to the five-chamber view, to the three-vessel view, and finally to the three-vessel trachea view by moving from inferior to superior through the axial planes of the heart. Additional viewing perspectives of fetal cardiac anatomy (including LVOT and RVOT) can also be identified and documented using the multi-slice view or the multiplanar display by implementing a variety of scrolling and rotational techniques.

Spatial Temporal Imaging Correlation (STIC). Basic automatic acquisition techniques usually require 2 to 3 seconds to collect patient anatomy. **Spatial temporal imaging correlation (STIC)** acquisitions, on the other hand, require a much longer acquisition time, usually 12 to 15 seconds. The longer acquisition collects a greater amount of cardiac anatomic data. Then, using a sophisticated repositioning process, the acquired heart images are realigned to represent specific portions of the cardiac cycle. These are then displayed as a continuous 3D cine loop representing one cardiac cycle in motion (Figure 54-26). STIC heart anatomy can be reviewed using the

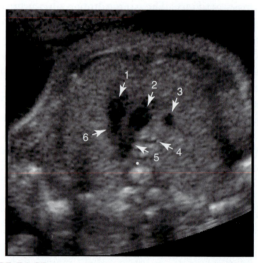

FIGURE 54-25 Three-vessel trachea view displaying the (1) main pulmonary artery, (2) ascending aorta, (3) superior vena cava, (4) trachea, (5) aortic arch, and (6) ductus arteriosus.

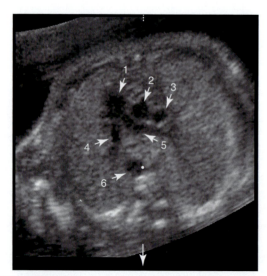

FIGURE 54-24 Good differentiation of pulmonary artery from aorta is achieved when documenting the pulmonary bifurcation, which is helpful when great vessels are abnormally positioned.

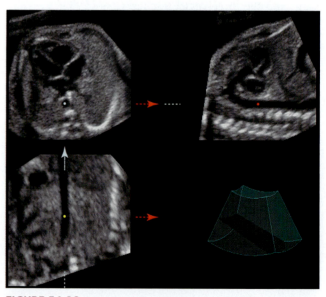

FIGURE 54-26 STIC technology displays one fetal heart cycle as a continuous 3D cine loop. The moving STIC cine loop provides more comprehensive documentation of fetal heart wall contractility and valve motion.

multiplanar display, 3D rendering, multi-slice view, oblique view, OVIX, and volume slice imaging.

STIC technology has its advantages and disadvantages. One definite advantage is that the moving STIC cine loop provides more a comprehensive understanding of fetal heart wall contractility and valve motion. The beating (STIC) heart can also be rotated to display desired landmark cardiac anatomy including LVOT, RVOT, aortic, and ductal arch views. In addition, STIC acquisitions can be performed using color Doppler, displaying both gray-scale anatomy and color Doppler as four-dimensional cine STIC images in motion.

One potential disadvantage associated with STIC technology is the length of time needed to perform the acquisition. As previously stated, non-STIC acquisitions usually require 2 to 3 seconds, whereas STIC acquisitions require 10 to 15 seconds. The considerably longer (STIC) acquisition time invites the opportunity for motion artifact within the data set if the fetus were to change position during the acquisition process.

As with any new technology, a moderate learning curve is required to facilitate effective integration of STIC into conventional (2D) fetal cardiac examinations. Appreciation of multiplanar imaging and 3D rendering techniques are mandatory prerequisites (in addition to comprehensive knowledge of fetal cardiac anatomy)

before implementing STIC as an effective diagnostic tool. Regardless of technique (STIC or basic automatic acquisition), three-dimensional ultrasound has demonstrated diagnostic potential as an effective adjunct to conventional 2D fetal heart ultrasound examinations. Both techniques elevate the diagnostic potential of four-chamber view as an effective screening tool.

CONCLUSION

The medical community has embraced 2D ultrasound for many years, yet it has also often criticized 2D ultrasound for lacking reproducibility and consistency. The "artistic individuality" associated with 2D ultrasound has provided diagnostic documentation but has lacked reproducibility when compared to other imaging modalities such as computed tomography (CT) and magnetic resonance imaging (MRI). Three-dimensional ultrasound is not meant to replace 2D ultrasound, but it can be an effective adjunct. Three-dimensional technology has the potential to combine the "individuality" of conventional 2D ultrasound with the consistency and reproducibility of CT and MR through the incorporation of 3D tools such as multi-slice view and volume slice. The first step toward effective 3D integration is comprehension of basic 3D interactive tools.

The Placenta

Pamela M. Foy

OBJECTIVES

On completion of this chapter, you should be able to:
- Describe embryogenesis of the placenta
- List the functions of the placenta
- List and describe imaging techniques and sonographic findings for the placenta
- Identify the placental position and describe its importance
- Describe the sonographic findings and clinical significance of placental pathologies
- Recognize placental abruption on ultrasound

OUTLINE

The placenta is a temporary organ of pregnancy. Its development has long been of interest to anatomists, researchers, and obstetricians. Most sonographers have not had as great an interest in the placenta because the fetus is more engaging. But valuable information regarding placental configuration, location, pathology, and maturation can be assessed. The placenta is effectively evaluated by antenatal ultrasound.

The major role of the placenta is to permit the exchange of oxygenated maternal blood (rich in oxygen and nutrients) with deoxygenated fetal blood. Maternal vessels coursing posterior to the placenta circulate blood into the placenta, and blood from the fetus reaches this point through the umbilical arteries, which are within the umbilical cord.

It is recognized that the anatomic components of the placenta are discernible from as early as the 7th to 8th week of gestation. By the end of the first trimester, sonography can be used to determine the location, position, and identify specific components of the placenta. Combined studies using transvaginal ultrasonography, hysteroscopy, chorionic villus sampling, and hysterectomy specimens from the first trimester of pregnancy have recently indicated the absence of continuous blood flow in the intervillous space before 12 weeks of gestation.

EMBRYOGENESIS

The transformation of endometrial cells into glycogen and lipoid cells characterizes the decidual reaction that occurs in response to ovarian hormones (estrogen and progesterone). After fertilization, the development of the placenta is seen in the changes in the decidua (Box 55-1).

The chorion, amnion, yolk sac, and allantois constitute the embryonic or fetal membranes. These membranes develop from the zygote. Implantation of the blastocyst occurs 6 to 7 days after fertilization. Enlargement of trophoblasts helps to anchor the blastocyst to the endometrial lining, or *decidua*. The placenta has two components: the maternal portion, the **deciduas basalis**, formed by the endometrial surface (Figure 55-1); and the fetal portion, which develops from the **chorion frondosum**.

The fetal chorion is the fusion of the trophoblast and extraembryonic mesenchyme. There are two types of trophoblastic cells. The syncytiotrophoblast is the outer layer of multinuclear cells, and the cytotrophoblast is the inner layer of mononuclear cells (Box 55-2).

The major functioning unit of the placenta is the chorionic villus (Figure 55-2). Within the chorionic villus are the intervillous spaces. The maternal blood enters these intervillous spaces. As the embryo and membranes grow, the **decidua capsularis** is stretched. The **chorionic villi** on the associated part of the chorionic sac gradually atrophy and disappear (smooth chorion or chorion laeve). The chorionic villi related to the decidua basalis increase rapidly in size and complexity (villous chorion or chorion frondosum).

The maternal surface of the placenta, which lies contiguous with the **deciduas basalis**, is termed the **basal plate**. The fetal surface, which is contiguous with the surrounding chorion, is termed the **chorionic plate**. The cotyledons are cobblestone in appearance and composed of several mainstem villi and their branches. They are covered with a thin layer of the **deciduas basalis**.

Before birth, the fetal membranes and placenta perform the following functions and activities: protection, nutrition, respiration, and excretion (Box 55-3). At birth or *parturition*, they separate from the fetus and are expelled from the uterus as the afterbirth.

Fetal-Placental-Uterine Circulation

An understanding of maternal-fetal circulation is necessary. Oxygenated maternal blood is brought to the placenta through 80 to 100 end branches of the uterine arteries, the spiral arteries. Maternal blood enters the intervillous space near the central part of each placental lobule where it flows around and over the surface of the villi. Maternal blood returns through a network of

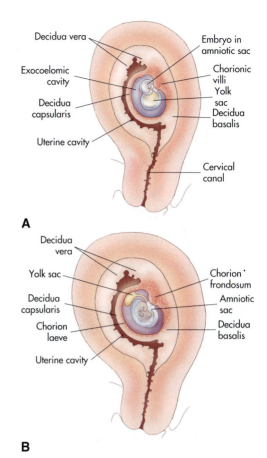

A

B

FIGURE 55-1 A, The placenta has two components: the fetal portion, developed from the chorion frondosum (chorionic plate); and a maternal portion, the decidua basalis, formed by the endometrial surface. **B,** The chorionic villi gradually atrophy and disappear (chorion laeve). The chorionic villi in the decidua basalis increase rapidly in size and complexity.

basilar, subchorial, interlobular, and marginal veins. A very thin layer normally separates the fetal blood from the maternal blood. This layer is composed of the capillary wall, the trophoblastic basement membrane, and a thin rim of cytoplasm of the syncytiotrophoblast. The fetal placenta is anchored to the maternal placenta by the cytotrophoblastic shell and anchoring villi. It provides a large area where materials may be exchanged across the placental membrane and interposed between fetal and maternal circulation.

Oxygen-rich blood passes through the umbilical vein into the fetal abdomen. Some of the blood is distributed

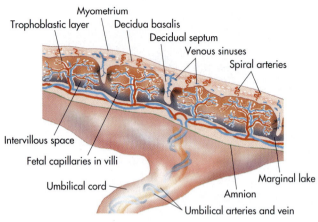

Myometrium
Trophoblastic layer
Decidua basalis
Decidual septum
Venous sinuses
Spiral arteries
Intervillous space
Fetal capillaries in villi
Umbilical cord
Marginal lake
Amnion
Umbilical arteries and vein

FIGURE 55-2 The major functioning unit of the placenta is the chorionic villus. The spiral arteries, venous sinuses, and uterine arteries line the periphery of the placenta.

BOX 55-3 | Functions of the Placenta

Respiration
Transfer of oxygen from maternal blood across the placental membrane into fetal blood is by diffusion. Carbon dioxide passes in the opposite direction. The placenta acts as "fetal lungs."

Nutrition
Water, inorganic salts, carbohydrates, fats, proteins, and vitamins pass from maternal blood through the placental membrane into fetal blood.

Excretion
Waste products cross membrane from fetal blood and enter maternal blood. Excreted by mother's kidneys.

Protection
Some microorganisms cross the placental border.

Storage
Carbohydrates, proteins, calcium, and iron are stored in placenta and released into fetal circulation.

Hormonal Production
Produced by syncytiotrophoblast of placenta: human chorionic gonadotropin, estrogens, progesterone.

---

into the liver, whereas the rest passes through the ductus venosus into the IVC and continues to the heart through the right atrium across the foramen ovale and into the left atrium. Blood then passes into the left ventricle, ascending aorta, and this blood supplies the brain and upper part of body through the brachiocephalic circulation. Unoxygenated blood from the SVC passes into the right atrium, through the right ventricle and across the main pulmonary artery. A minor portion of blood from the RV supplies the lungs whereas the majority of the blood passes through a fetal shunt, the ductus arteriosus, into the aorta arch. This shunt protects the lungs against circulatory overload. The fetal blood continues inferiorly through the descending aorta, the internal iliac arteries, to the umbilical arteries and into the umbilical cord to

return to the placenta for respiratory and nutrient exchange. By term, approximately 40% of the fetal cardiac output is directed through the umbilical circulation.

The placenta is dedicated to the survival of the fetus. Even when exposed to a poor maternal environment (e.g., when the mother is malnourished, diseased, smokes or abuses drugs), the placenta can often compensate by becoming more efficient. Unfortunately, there are limits to the placenta's ability to cope with external stresses. Eventually, if multiple or severe enough, these stresses can lead to placental damage, fetal damage, and even intrauterine death and pregnancy loss.

Maternal placental circulation may be reduced by a variety of conditions that decrease uterine blood flow, such as severe hypertension, renal disease, or placental infarction. Placental defects can cause intrauterine fetal growth restriction (IUGR). The net effect is that there is a reduction of flow between the fetal and maternal blood.

Placental Membrane. The placental membranes are often called a barrier because there are a few compounds, endogenous and exogenous, that are unable to cross the placental membranes in detectable amounts.

Cordal Attachments

The attachment of the cord is usually near the center of the placenta. Abnormal cordal attachments to the placenta are battledore and velamentous placenta. A **battledore placenta** refers to the insertion of the umbilical cord at the margin of the placenta, within 10 mm of the edge (Figure 55-3). A **velamentous placenta** refers to an umbilical cord that inserts on the membranes (Figure 55-4). This is best demonstrated with color Doppler. These submembranous vessels are fragile and in a small number of cases (less than 2%) may be associated with significant fetal hemorrhage, especially if the membrane carrying the vessels is positioned across the internal os (**vasa previa**).

Yolk Sac

The secondary yolk sac forms after the regression of the primary yolk sac on the ventral surface of the embryonic disk at 28 menstrual days. The yolk sac has a role in the transfer of nutrients to the embryo during the 2nd and 3rd weeks of gestation while the uteroplacental circulation is developing. It is connected to the midgut by a narrow yolk stalk. Before 5 menstrual weeks, the amniotic sac and secondary yolk sac have been pressed together with the embryonic disk between them. This structure is suspended within the chorionic cavity. The yolk sac becomes displaced from the embryo and lies between the amnion and the chorion (see Figure 55-1). By 9 weeks, the yolk sac has diminished to less than 5 mm in diameter.

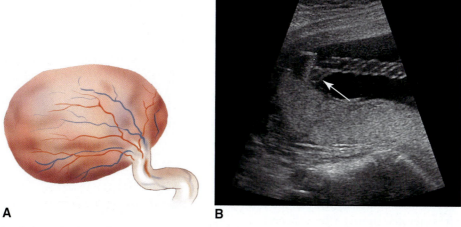

FIGURE 55-3 A, A battledore placenta refers to the insertion of the umbilical cord at the margin of the placenta. **B,** This sagittal transabdominal image reveals a marginal cord insertion 7.6 mm from the edge of the placenta (*arrow*).

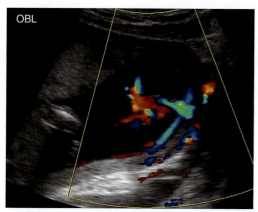

FIGURE 55-4 Oblique view of uterus with color Doppler demonstrates a placental cord inserting into the membranes (a velamentous insertion).

Implantation of the Placenta

Normally the placenta will implant on the anterior, fundal, posterior, or lateral wall of the uterus. Occasionally, placental implantation will occur within the lower uterine segment, resulting in a condition called **placenta previa.**

Membranes

The fetal membranes consist of the chorion, amnion, allantois, and yolk sac. The chorion originates from the trophoblastic cells and remains in contact with the trophoblasts throughout pregnancy. The amnion develops at the 28th menstrual day and is attached to the margins of the embryonic disk. As the embryo grows and folds ventrally, the junction of the amnion is reduced to a small area on the ventral surface of the embryo to form the umbilicus.

Expansion of the amniotic cavity occurs with the production of amniotic fluid. Usually, by 16 weeks'

gestation the amnion fuses with the chorion and can no longer be seen with ultrasound as two separate membranes. If the amnion/chorion separation extends beyond 16 weeks' gestation, it may be associated with polyhydramnios, aneuploidy, or prior amniocentesis. Hemorrhage may also have this appearance.

The secondary yolk sac forms after regression of the primary yolk sac at 28 menstrual days on the ventral surface of the embryonic disk. Before 5 menstrual weeks, the amniotic sac and secondary yolk sac have been pressed together with the embryonic disk between. This structure is suspended within another membrane (the chorion) by the connecting stalk. The yolk sac becomes displaced from the embryo and lies between the amnion and the chorion (see Figure 55- 1).

THE AMNIOTIC SAC AND AMNIOTIC FLUID

The amnion forms a sac that contains amniotic fluid. The sac encloses the embryo and forms the epithelial covering of the umbilical cord. Most of the amniotic fluid comes from the maternal blood by diffusion across the amnion from the decidua parietalis and intervillous spaces of the placenta.

In the first trimester the fetus begins to excrete urine to fill the amniotic cavity. The fetus swallows the amniotic fluid, and this cycle continues throughout pregnancy. The amniotic fluid has many functions including permitting the fetus room to move, assisting in maintaining a constant fetal body temperature, serving as a protective buffer for the fetus, and allowing the lungs to develop properly.

THE PLACENTA AS ENDOCRINE GLAND

The chronic villi are the functional endocrine units of the placenta. A central core with abundant capillaries is surrounded by an inner layer, cytotrophoblast, and an outer layer, syncytiotrophoblast. The inner layer produces neuropeptides, and the outer layer produces the protein hormones human chorionic gonadotropin (hCG) and human placental lactogen (hPL), along with the sex steroids estrogen and progesterone.

After the 7th week of gestation, most progesterone is produced by the syncytiotrophoblast from maternally derived cholesterol precursors. Progesterone production is exclusively a maternal-placental interaction, with no contribution from the fetus. The production of placental estrogen involves an intricate pathway requiring maternal, placental, and fetal contributions.

The function of hCG is to maintain the corpus luteum in early pregnancy. It is elevated shortly after conception and peaks at 8 to 10 weeks. The hPL is responsible for the promotion of lipolysis and an anti-insulin action that serves to direct nutrients to the fetus.

THE UMBILICAL CORD

The umbilical cord forms during the first 5 weeks of gestation. The cord is surrounded by a mucoid connective tissue called **Wharton's jelly**. The intestines grow at a faster rate than the abdomen and herniate into the proximal umbilical cord at approximately 7 weeks' gestation and remain there until approximately 10 weeks' gestation. The insertion of the cord into the ventral abdominal wall is an important sonographic anatomic landmark because scrutiny of this area can reveal abdominal wall defects such as omphalocele, gastroschisis, or limb-body wall complex.

The normal umbilical cord has one large vein and two smaller arteries. A single umbilical artery (SUA) is found in approximately 1% of all singleton births and 7% of twin gestations. Congenital malformations (genitourinary, cardiovascular, facial, and musculoskeletal) are seen in 25% to 50% of infants with a single umbilical artery. There is a reported association with abnormal fetal growth, specifically intrauterine growth restriction, or a small-for-gestation-age fetus. For this reason, it may be warranted to obtain a growth ultrasound in the third trimester to evaluate fetal size. Single umbilical artery is seen more commonly in the fetuses of insulin dependent diabetic women.

Sonographic Evaluation of the Umbilical Cord

The vessels of the cord may be followed with real-time ultrasound from the placenta to the fetal abdomen and the sonographer should document the cord insertion into the placenta (Figure 55-5). The intra-abdominal portion of the umbilical vein courses superiorly. The **ductus venosus** shunts a significant amount of the oxygenated blood from the umbilical vein directly into the inferior

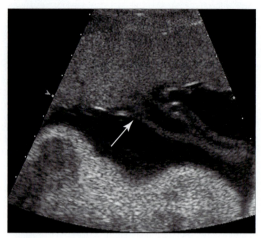

FIGURE 55-5 Umbilical cord is seen at placental insertion site *(arrow)*.

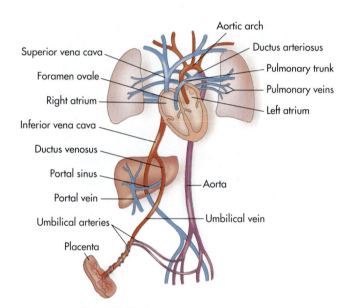

FIGURE 55-6 Fetal circulation diagram.

vena cava. A portion of the umbilical venous blood also supplies the liver (Figure 55-6).

Sonographically, the ductus venous appears as a thin intrahepatic channel with echogenic walls branching from the umbilical vein (Figure 55-7). It lies in the groove between the left lobe and the caudate lobe of the liver. The ductus venosus is patent during fetal life until shortly after birth, when closure occurs. After closure, the remnant of the ductus venosus is known as the **ligamentum venosum**.

The two umbilical arteries carry deoxygenated blood from the fetus to the placenta. They ascend into the umbilical cord and are a branch of the internal iliac arteries. Their normal position is adjacent to the fetal bladder. There are two acceptable ways to document both umbilical arteries. The first approach, which is

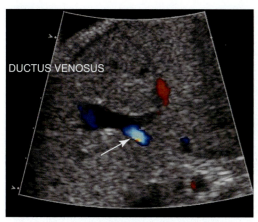

FIGURE 55-7 Axial view of fetal abdomen identifies the ductus venosus (*arrow*) as it branches off the umbilical vein.

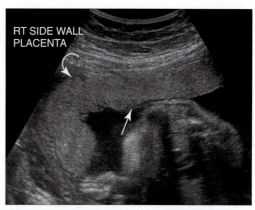

FIGURE 55-8 An anterior right side wall placenta demonstrates the smooth homogeneous texture of the organ. The chorionic plate (*arrow*) can be seen on the fetal surface of the placenta. The basal surface (*curved arrow*) of the placenta is seen along the myometrial surface of the uterus.

easier to obtain second trimester, is to image the fetal pelvis in an axial scanning plane at the level of the fetal bladder. The umbilical arteries will be seen as they course along the lateral aspect of the fetal bladder. Color and power Doppler can be used to visualize the umbilical arteries. A second approach for the sonographer is to evaluate a free loop of cord in a short axis plane to visualize the umbilical vein and two smaller arteries. After birth, the umbilical arteries become the superior vesical arteries.

SONOGRAPHIC EVALUATION OF THE NORMAL PLACENTA

The two surfaces of the placenta merit special attention because they are important in assessing normal placental anatomy and evaluating for placental abruption. The fetal surface of the placenta (portion of the placenta adjacent to the amniotic cavity) is the echogenic chorionic plate that courses along the placental tissue and is found at the junction with the amniotic fluid. This linear echogenicity is further enhanced by the strong interface of the amnion covering the chorionic plate (Figure 55-8).

The second surface is the basal plate or maternal portion of the placenta, which lies at the junction of the myometrium and the substance of the placenta (see Figure 55-8). Maternal blood vessels from the endometrium (endometrial veins) run behind the basal plate and may be confused with placental abruption. This represents normal vascularity, however. The endometrial veins are more apparent sonographically when the placenta is positioned fundally or posteriorly within the uterine cavity.

The placenta can be identified with sonography as early as 8 menstrual weeks. The substance of the placenta assumes a relatively homogenous midlevel gray appearance between 8 and 20 weeks of gestation and is easily recognized with its characteristically smooth borders. After 20 weeks' gestation, the intraplacental

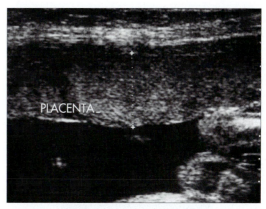

FIGURE 55-9 The AP thickness of the placenta measures over 7 cm in this Rh-sensitized pregnancy. Calipers should be placed perpendicular to the placental borders.

sonolucencies (e.g., venous lakes or intervillous thrombi) and placental calcification may begin to appear. The thickness of the placenta varies with gestational age, but is usually 2 to 3 cm in fetuses greater than 23 weeks' gestation. The thickness of a normal placenta will rarely exceed 4 cm. When evaluating placental thickness, the sonographer must acquire a perpendicular measurement of the placental substance in relation to the myometrial wall. Enlarged placentas may be associated with Rh sensitization, diabetes of pregnancy, or congenital anomalies (Figure 55-9).

Several sonolucent areas within the placenta may confuse the sonographer unfamiliar with the wide range of placental variants. Cystic structures representing large fetal vessels are commonly observed coursing behind the chorionic plate and between the amnion and chorion layers (Figure 55-10). Observation with real-time or color Doppler of blood flow (Figure 55-11) helps to differentiate these vessels. Deposits of fibrin may also be found in the intervillous space posterior to the chorionic

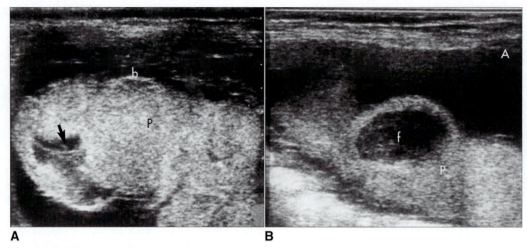

FIGURE 55-10 A, Subchorionic cystic area of the placenta at 29 weeks of gestation. Blood flow was obvious under real-time imaging *(arrow). b,* Basal plate; *p,* placenta. **B,** Subchorionic cystic area at 24 weeks of gestation, with internal echoes, representative of blood flow *(f).* Color Doppler imaging may aid in detecting areas of blood flow. *A,* Amniotic fluid; *p,* placenta.

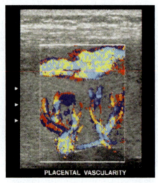

FIGURE 55-11 Color Doppler shows the normal vascularity of the marginal lakes, capillaries, and basal area of the placenta.

plate, and blood flow will not be seen in fibrinous areas. A heterogenous placenta may be more commonly observed in women with elevated maternal serum alpha-fetoprotein or a history of first trimester bleeding.

Placental sonolucencies may also be seen within the placental substance. These have been referred to as placental lakes and are most often a normal finding. These areas may change dramatically in shape and size during the course of the ultrasound examination, especially if there is a change in maternal position. Frequently, blood flow will not be detected with color Doppler, but with real-time sonography, slow swirling flow can be appreciated.

The placenta is separated from the myometrium by a subplacental venous complex. These veins (basilar and marginal) can become very prominent, especially for lateral and posterior placentas, and should not be confused for a retroplacental or marginal hemorrhage. The myometrium is a thin, hypoechoic layer posterior to the basilar veins. The basalar veins pand the myometrium measure as much as 9 to 10 mm in average thickness.

The placenta increases in size and volume with gestational age, but the maximum thickness does not exceed 4 cm.

Placental Position

A survey of the placenta transabdominally should always be performed scanning longitudinally from side to side and transversely from inferior to superior so that the placental position and size can be evaluated. The insertion of the cord into the placental substance should be visualized and described as midplacental, marginal, or velamentous. The inferior edge of the placenta should be documented to evaluate its relationship to the internal cervical os.

The position of the placenta is readily apparent on most obstetric ultrasound examinations. The placental location varies but may be seen along the fundus, anterior, posterior, or lateral uterine wall (Figure 55-12). Specific names are given to the placenta according to its point of origin, such as fundus of the uterus along the anterior wall *(fundal anterior placenta)* or along the posterior uterine wall *(fundal posterior placenta).* Occasionally the placenta may be dangerously low, implanted over or near the cervix, (placenta previa) (Figure 55-13). The location of a placenta can appear to change dramatically with the development of focal myometrial contractions called Braxton-Hicks. **Braxton-Hicks contractions** (normal contractions of pregnancy) should not be confused with placental pathology. The appearance of these contractions may distort the uterine contour, but they will resolve with time (Figure 55-14). This area should be rescanned after 15 to 20 minutes to see if the uterine contour has returned to normal. Sonographically a uterine myoma will appear as a hypoechoic uterine wall mass. If the placenta is implanted upon a myoma, it will

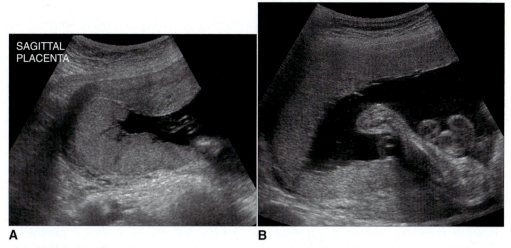

FIGURE 55-12 **A,** Sagittal view of the uterus reveals a posterior fundal placenta **B,** Transverse view of the uterus demonstrates a right side wall placenta that extends along the anterior wall of the uterus.

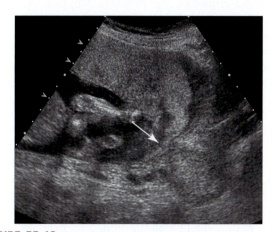

FIGURE 55-13 Transabdominal image of Placenta previa. *Arrow* points to the placenta implanted over the internal cervical os.

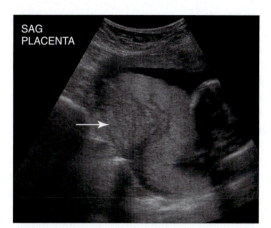

FIGURE 55-14 Braxton Hicks. Uterine contraction (*arrow*) is seen distorting the placenta.

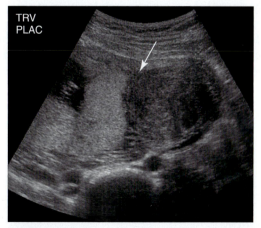

FIGURE 55-15 Myoma. Transverse view of the uterus reveals a hypoechoic uterine myoma (*arrow*). The left sidewall placenta is implanted on the myoma.

have poor perfusion, which will increase the risk for placental abruption (Figure 55-15).

For the sonographer to visualize the internal os of the cervix, a sagittal image of the **lower uterine segment (LUS)** and cervix should be obtained. In this way, the relationship of the placenta to the internal os can be visualized (Figure 55-16). If the maternal bladder is full, a normally implanted placenta may appear to be covering the internal cervical os because the cervix is falsely elongated, giving the false impression of a placenta previa. Emptying the maternal bladder reduces the pressure on the lower uterine segment and allows the cervix to assume a more normal position. Another method to better demonstrate the internal cervical os when scanning transabdominally is to tilt the patient in a slight Trendelenburg position (head lower than body). This relieves the pressure of the uterus on the lower uterine segment.

Transvaginal sonography is the best imaging tool to identify the lower uterine segment, especially when evaluating the inferior edge of the placenta. The sonographer should acquire a midline sagittal image of the cervix and lower uterine segment to show the internal cervical os free of placenta. A measurement can be obtained to show the distance from the cervix. If transvaginal sonography is not available or possible, the cervix can be evaluated with the transperineal or translabial technique.

Describing the location of the placenta has clinical importance. A placenta previa noted on ultrasound alerts the obstetrician that a pelvic examination should not be performed. A finger inadvertently pushed through an unknown previa can result in vaginal bleeding. If a placenta is noted to be a low-lying early in pregnancy, the placenta location can be followed with consecutive scans to see whether this location persists.

When the placenta appears to lie on both the anterior and posterior uterine walls, the sonographer needs to scan laterally for a connection that would make this a sidewall placenta. If the anterior and posterior placenta does not appear to communicate, a **succenturiate placenta** should be considered. A succenturiate, or accessory lobe placenta, is when there are additional placental lobes joined to the main placenta by blood vessels. The sonographer can differentiate the main lobe from the accessory lobe by locating the placental cord insertion site, which will identify the main placenta. There is a slight risk that these connecting blood vessels may rupture or that an extra lobe may be inadvertently left in the uterus after delivery; therefore, the clinician should be notified of this finding.

The concept that the placenta changes its position within the uterine cavity has been termed **placental migration**, implying that the placenta actually moves and relocates. There are different theories as to why the placenta appears to migrate. One theory suggests that the placenta actually does not move but that the position appears changed because of the physiologic growth and development of the lower uterine segment. Another theory postulates that the low blood supply in the lower uterine segment causes the placenta in that area to atrophy and disappear while the areas of rich blood supply toward the fundus and midportion of the uterus causes the placenta to hypertrophy.

Although the majority of placentas that appear to be previas in the early second trimester will not be a previa by the third trimester, there are exceptions. If the placenta is a complete previa in the early second trimester,

it is unlikely to change its position drastically. In all likelihood, during the third trimester, such a placenta will remain a complete previa. A placenta previa should not be diagnosed before 20 weeks' gestation.

DOPPLER EVALUATION OF THE PLACENTA

Color, power, and pulsed Doppler can be used to assess placental function. The uterine artery sonographically reveals a high-resistance flow pattern in the first trimester, which should become a low-resistance flow pattern in the second trimester. The normal trophoblastic invasion of the spiral arteries produces this low-resistance Doppler pattern. In the first trimester, the flow velocity waveform shows a notched appearance in early diastole. This notch usually disappears by 24 weeks' gestation. In the second trimester, the obtained Doppler signals of the uterine arteries are variable depending on the location of the placenta. The lowest resistance in the uterine arteries is seen on the placental side. (Figure 55-17) Abnormal trophoblastic invasion of the spiral arteries of the maternal uteroplacental circulation is associated with a range of pregnancy complications, including placental insufficiency, IUGR, preeclampsia, and placental abruption.

To acquire a uterine artery waveform transabdominally, the sonographer should scan in a sagittal scanning plane, superior to the symphis pubis. The transducer is moved laterally and manipulated to find the main branch of the uterine artery where it crosses the external iliac artery. With color Doppler the image is magnified, and to obtain a pulsed Doppler waveform, the image is optimized with the correct gate size and placement, gain, and

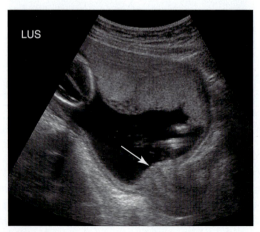

FIGURE 55-16 Ultrasound clearly shows the internal cervical os *(arrow)*. The placenta is implanted away from the os.

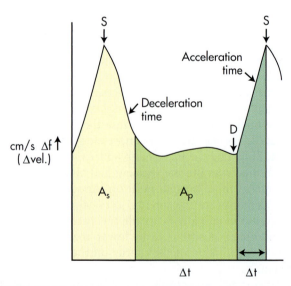

FIGURE 55-17 Waveform analysis. After 24 weeks, the uterine artery Doppler typically shows a high-flow, low-resistance pattern, particularly for the uterine artery on the same side as the placenta.

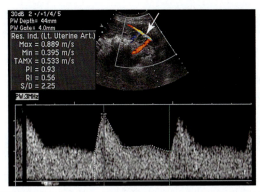

FIGURE 55-18 Pulsed Doppler gate is seen (*arrow*) within the uterine artery after it crosses the external iliac artery. Corresponding normal uterine artery waveform is demonstrated.

scale (Figure 55-18). Both right and left uterine arteries are evaluated, and it is necessary to record if they are the placental or nonplacental waveform. The waveform should be measured and evaluated for the presence or absence of a diastolic notch. The resistance index, pulsatility index, and S/D ratio can be obtained.

The umbilical artery can also be evaluated sonographically, and the normal waveform should always have antegrade diastolic flow. The sonographer should acquire an umbilical artery waveform in a midsegment of cord, making certain that the fetus is in an inactive state. Color Doppler should be utilized to visualize the umbilical cord vessels. The image should be magnified and then optimized with the correct gate size and placement, gain, and scale to obtain the pulsed Doppler waveform. The waveform should be measured and evaluated. The resistance index, pulsatility index, and S/D ratio can be obtained.

EVALUATION OF THE PLACENTA AFTER DELIVERY

The normal-term placenta has several characteristics at delivery. It measures about 15 to 20 cm in diameter, is discoid in shape, weighs about 600 g, and measures less than 4 cm in thickness. The clinician ascertains that the placenta has been delivered intact to avoid complications of postpartum hemorrhage or infection. Membranes of the amnion and chorion are inspected for color and consistency, with attention to meconium staining or signs of infection. The length of the umbilical cord is noted (and measured in the pathology laboratory). Short umbilical cords may result in traction during labor and delivery, leading to tearing of the cord, abruption, or inversion of the uterus. Long umbilical cords are more likely to prolapse, become twisted around the fetus, or tie in true knots.

Fibrin Deposition

Fibrin is a protein derived from fibrinogen. It is found throughout the placenta, but it is most pronounced in the floor of the placenta (in the septa) and increases continuously throughout pregnancy. Fibrin deposits on the villi may increase their mechanical stability; the deposits may be the result of eddies in the turbulent flow—more flow equals increased fibrin deposits. Fibrin may also be attributed to the regulation of intervillous circulation.

Sonographic Findings. On ultrasound examination, this fibrin deposition (subchorionic) appears as hypoechoic areas beneath the chorionic plate of the placenta. Differential diagnosis of fibrin deposition includes a venous lake or a subchorionic hematoma. A venous lake will have slow flow that can be appreciated with real-time sonography. It may be difficult to distinguish fibrin deposits from a hematoma on ultrasound.

ABNORMALITIES OF THE PLACENTA

The major pathologic processes seen in the placenta that can adversely affect pregnancy outcome include intrauterine bacterial infections, decreased blood flow to the placenta from the mother, and immunologic attack of the placenta by the mother's immune system. Intrauterine infections (most commonly the result of migration of vaginal bacteria through the cervix into the uterine cavity) can lead to severe fetal hypoxia as a result of villous edema (fluid buildup within the placenta itself). Both chronic and acute decreases in blood flow to the placenta can cause severe fetal damage and even death.

In addition to supplying the fetus with nutrition, the placenta is a barrier between the mother and fetus, protecting the fetus from immune rejection by the mother, a pathologic process that can lead to intrauterine growth restriction or even demise. In addition to these major pathologic categories, many other insults—such as placental separation, cord accidents, trauma, viral and parasitic infections—can adversely affect pregnancy outcome by affecting the function of the placenta (Table 55-1).

Placentomegaly

Placentomegaly is an enlarged placenta weighing more than 600 g. On ultrasound examination, the placenta appears abnormally thick and measures greater than 4 cm. Measurement should extend from the subplacental veins to the amniotic fluid junction. Seen with maternal and fetal disorders, maternal diabetes and Rh incompatibility are primary causes for placentomegaly (Box 55-4).

Placenta Previa

Placenta previa is the implantation of the placenta over the internal cervical os. The placenta normally implants in the body or fundus of the uterus; however, in 1 of 200 pregnancies, the placenta implants over or near to the

TABLE 55-1 | Lesions of the Placenta

Lesion Significance	Incidence Etiology	Clinical Findings
Intervillous thrombosis	36%: Bleeding from fetal vessels	Fetal-maternal hemorrhage
Massive perivillous fibrin deposition	22%: Pooling and stasis of blood in intervillous space	None
Infarct	25%: Thrombosis of maternal vessel or retroplacental bleed and associated condition	Depends on extent
Subchorionic fibrin	20%: Pooling and stasis of blood in subchorionic space	None
Hydatidiform change	< 1%: Complete mole < 1%: Partial mole	Predisposes to choriocarcinoma Associated with symptoms of preeclampsia
Chorioangioma	1%: Vascular malformation	Usually none, depends on size

BOX 55-4 | Placenta Size

Placentomegaly
Maternal diabetes
Maternal anemia
α-Thalassemia
Rh sensitivity
Fetomaternal hemorrhage
Chronic intrauterine infections
Twin-twin transfusion syndrome
Congenital neoplasms
Fetal malformations

Small Placenta
Intrauterine growth restriction
Intrauterine infection
Aneuploidy

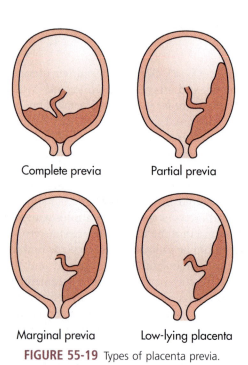

Complete previa   Partial previa

Marginal previa   Low-lying placenta

FIGURE 55-19 Types of placenta previa.

internal os of the cervix. The risk increases for women with a history of cesarean delivery.

The placenta may be considered (1) a complete or total previa, (2) a partial previa, (3) a marginal previa, or (4) low lying (Figure 55-19). With complete placenta previa, the cervical internal os is completely covered by placental tissue; this occurrence has been found in 20% of patients with previa. This previa may be symmetric or asymmetric. A partial previa only partially covers the internal os. A marginal previa does not cover the os, but its edge comes to the margin of the os, hence the term *marginal placenta previa*. Although a low-lying placenta is implanted in the lower uterine segment, its edge does not reach the internal os. A low-lying placenta does not usually have symptoms associated with it.

A pregnancy complicated by placenta previa is considered high risk because of the danger of life-threatening hemorrhage. During the third trimester of pregnancy, two very important changes occur. First, the lower uterine segment is developing–that is, thinning and elongating in preparation for labor. As the lower uterine segment develops, the placental attachment to the lower uterine wall may be disrupted, resulting in bleeding. Second, the cervix softens and some dilation can occur before the onset of labor. Cervical dilation may also disrupt the attachment of a placenta located over or near the cervical os.

Before 20 weeks' gestation, "complete previa" may be noted in about 5% of second-trimester pregnancies, with 90% resolving by term with the growth of the lower uterine segment. A good rule of thumb is that if the placenta is covering the cervix but also extends to the uterine fundus second trimester, it will usually not be covering the cervix by the third trimester. Asymptomatic partial previas are seen in as many as 45% of early second-trimester pregnancies, with over 95% resolving before delivery.

Multiple factors are associated with placenta previa: advanced maternal age, smoking, cocaine abuse, prior placental previa, multiparity, and prior cesarean section or uterine surgery. Complications of placenta previa include preterm delivery, maternal hemorrhage, increased risk of placental invasion, increased risk of postpartum hemorrhage, and IUGR.

Clinically, the patient may present with painless, bright red vaginal bleeding in the third trimester. About 25% of patients will present with bleeding during the first 30 weeks. Twenty percent of cases are associated with uterine focal myometrial contractions. Abnormal lie (either transverse or breech) is also associated with placenta previa.

When a patient presents with third-trimester bleeding, diagnosis is imperative because the treatment will differ based on the clinical diagnosis. If the diagnosis is placenta previa, the fetus is preterm, and the mother is not bleeding heavily, clinical management may be conservative: bed rest, maternal transfusion, if necessary, and close observation until the point where delivery is necessary. Cesarean section delivery is needed in the majority of cases. With marginal placental previas, a minority of patients may deliver vaginally. The pressure of the fetus as it passes through the cervix and birth canal may compress the part of the placenta that has been disrupted (Box 55-5).

◢ **Sonographic Findings.** The sonographer needs to examine the location of the placenta in relation to the lower uterine segment and cervix. The maternal urinary bladder may be used as a landmark to identify the location of the internal cervical os. The sonographer should be cautious about misinterpreting a low-lying placenta covering the internal os secondary to an overdistended bladder. The patient should be asked to empty her bladder, and the lower uterine segment should be rescanned transabdominally to see the inferior edge of the placenta in relation to the os.

If the fetus is in a cephalic presentation in the last trimester of pregnancy, the sonographer should examine the fetal head in relationship to the posterior wall of the uterus and the mother's sacrum. A distance of less than 1.5 cm indicates there will not be enough room for the placenta to be between the fetal head and posterior uterine wall (Figure 55-20).

If there is any question of a placenta previa transabdominally, the patient should be evaluated with transvaginal sonography. The transducer should be prepared as for a transvaginal examination, with a protective covering. The transvaginal transducer is ideal for this approach, with the probe inserted only into the vaginal fornix. If the edge of the placenta covers the internal cervical os more than 15 mm, it will probably not resolve (Figure 55-21). Color Doppler can be utilized to evaluate for vasa previa. Pulsed Doppler can be used to differentiate fetal vessels from maternal vessels. The transperineal/translabial approach is also useful for evaluating the lower uterine segment when the definition of the placenta needs to be clarified and transvaginal sonography is unavailable. The transducer is placed along the maternal labia to demonstrate the maternal bladder, the internal os (directed in a vertical orientation), the lower uterine segment, the fetal head, and the placenta (if previa). Longitudinal and transverse scans are obtained to delineate the relation of the placenta to the cervical os.

Vasa Previa

Vasa previa is a potentially life-threatening fetal complication that occurs when large fetal vessels run in the fetal membranes across the cervical os. These vessels are at

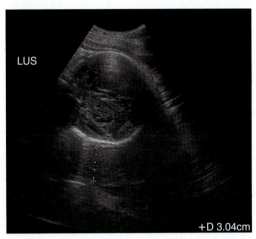

FIGURE 55-20 A lower uterine segment (LUS) in the longitudinal plane shows the placental tissue (30 mm) lying between the maternal sacrum and the fetal head. This woman had a complete placenta previa.

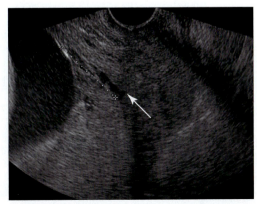

FIGURE 55-21 Complete previa. Transvaginal image of cervix reveals a posterior placenta covering ICO (*arrow*) and extending 29.5 mm anteriorly. This complete previa persisted until delivery.

BOX 55-5	Predisposing Factors for Abnormal Placental Adherence

- Placenta previa
- Chronic endometritis
- Prior cesarean section
- Submucosal leiomyomas
- Uterine scars
- Intrauterine synechiae

risk of rupture and life-threatening hemorrhage. Its occurrence is found in 1 of 2500 deliveries. The two most common causes of vasa previa are (1) velamentous insertion of the umbilical cord into placental membranes, which cross over the cervix (2) when a succenturiate lobe is present and the connecting vessels traverse the cervix. When delivery is imminent, the unsupported fetal vessels are prone to tear as the cervix dilates, which can result in exsanguination of the fetus. A rapid cesarean delivery may prevent fetal demise.

Sonographic Findings. Vasa previa is diagnosed with sonography when the implanted fetal umbilical vessels are seen to cover the cervix. Color Doppler and transvaginal sonography allows visualization of these vascular structures as they cover the cervical os (Figure 55-22).

Placental Invasion

Placental invasion is defined as an abnormal penetration of placental tissue beyond the endometrial lining of the uterus. There are three variants of placenta invasion. With **placenta accreta,** the chorionic villi attach *to* the myometrium without muscular invasion. Placenta accreta occurs in approximately 1 in 2500 deliveries. **Placenta increta** is further extension of the chorionic villi *into* (in-) the myometrium. **Placenta percreta** is penetration of the chorionic villi *through* (per-) the uterus.

The risk of placenta accreta increases in patients with placenta previa and uterine scar from previous cesarean section. The risk of increta is 10% to 25% in women with one previous cesarean section when the placenta is implanted over the scar and exceeds 50% in women with placenta previa and multiple cesarean deliveries (Table 55-2).

Placenta increta results from underdeveloped decidualization of the endometrium. The association of

placenta previa reflects the thin, poorly formed deciduas of the lower uterine segment that offers little resistance to deeper invasion by the trophoblast. The previous cesarean scar permits the trophoblastic invasion. High maternal mortality and morbidity are associated with placenta increta/percreta, so accurate prenatal diagnosis is critical.

Sonographic Findings. Almost all cases of placental invasion have a placenta previa in the anterior location in a woman with a previous history of cesarean deliveries. There is usually a loss of the subplacental hypoechoic zone, which is representative of the myometrium. Multiple, hypoechoic placental vascular lacunae will be seen with real-time imaging.

Sonographers need to pay careful attention to the placenta and myometrium in any patient with a placental previa and prior history of cesarean section. The sonographer should evaluate the placenta previa to look for the loss of the subplacental hypoechoic zone. A transvaginal ultrasound should be performed, but *do not* have the patient empty her bladder. The probe should be angled toward the maternal urinary bladder to evaluate the uterine-bladder interface (Figure 55-23). Color

TABLE 55-2	Placental Invasion	
Type of Bleeding	**Invasion of Chorionic Villi Has Occurred**	**Blood Loss**
Placenta accreta	Superficially *to* myometrium	Mild
Placenta increta	Deep *into* myometrium	Moderate
Placenta percreta	*Through* the myometrium	Severe

Data from http://telpath2.med.utah.edu/WebPath/PLACHTML/PLACO70.html.

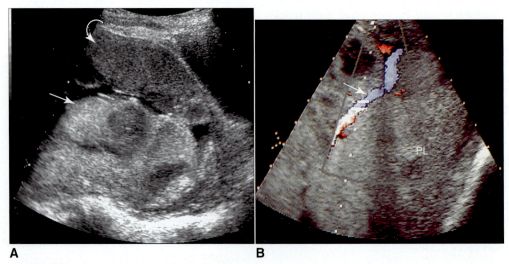

A   B

FIGURE 55-22 A, Vasa previa. Transabdominal image of succenturiate lobe anterior (*arrow*) and main placenta posterior (*curved arrow*). **B,** Transvaginal image reveals fetal vessel (*arrow*) crossing cervical os.

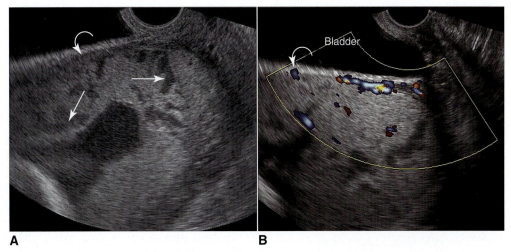

FIGURE 55-23 A, Transvaginal image of placenta and bladder. *Arrows* are showing hypoechoic vascular lacunae. *Curved arrow* is pointing at loss of the subplacental hypoechoic zone. **B,** Color Doppler demonstrates vessels in the thinned subplacental zone (*curved arrow*).

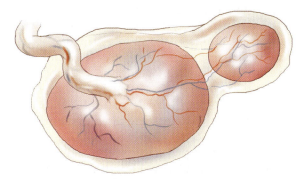

FIGURE 55-24 A succenturiate placenta is the presence of one or more accessory lobes connected to the body of the placenta by blood vessels.

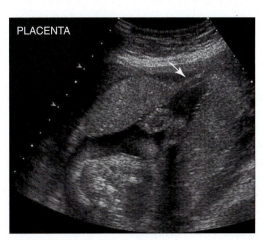

FIGURE 55-25 Transverse image of the uterus reveals a left side wall placenta. Vessels (*arrow*) can be seen connecting the accessory lobe, which is anterior.

Doppler will define vessels that have extended into the wall of the urinary bladder. The perineal scanning approach may also help the sonographer further define the lower uterine segment and the vascularity of the placenta in relationship to the maternal bladder.

Succenturiate Placenta

The succenturiate placenta is the presence of one or more accessory lobes connected to the body of the placenta-by-placenta vessels (Figure 55-24). The incidence occurs in 3% to 6% of pregnancies.

Normally, the placenta is oval with a shape that varies somewhat depending on its site of implantation and areas of atrophy. When the placenta develops a secondary lobe or several other smaller lobes, they are called succenturiate lobes. These lobes have a tendency to develop infarcts and necrosis (50% of deliveries). They may create a "placenta previa" or be retained after delivery.

The retention of the succenturiate lobe at delivery may result in postpartum hemorrhage and infection.

Rarely, rupture of the connecting vessels may occur during delivery, causing fetal hemorrhage and demise.

◢ **Sonographic Findings.** The sonographer should look for a discrete lobe that has "placenta texture" but is separate from the main body of the placenta. (Figure 55-25) Color Doppler can be used to help identify communicating vessels. The succenturiate placenta varies in appearance; it may be as large as or smaller than the main lobe of the placenta. Placental cord insertion is usually on the main placenta.

Circumvallate/Circummarginate Placenta

A **circumvallate/circummarginate placenta** is the attachment of the placental membranes to the fetal surface of the placenta rather than to the underlying villous placental margin (Figure 55-26). This abnormality occurs in 1% to 2% of pregnancies. It results in placental villi

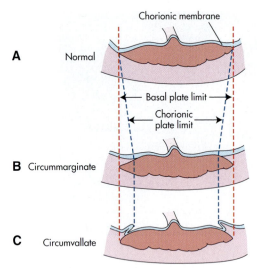

FIGURE 55-26 Comparison of extrachorial placentas with a normal placenta **(A)**. The transition of membranous to villous chorion is at the placental edge. **B,** Circummarginate placenta. The transition of membranous to villous chorion occurs central to the edge of the placenta, but the chorionic surface remains smooth. **C,** Circumvallate placenta. The chorionic membrane is folding.

around the border of the placenta that are not covered by the chorionic plate. A circumvallate placenta is diagnosed when the placental margin is folded, thickened, or elevated with underlying fibrin and hemorrhage. It is associated with premature rupture of the membranes, preterm labor, intrauterine growth restriction, and placental abruption.

Placental Hemorrhage

Hemorrhage may occur within or around the placenta and is more commonly seen than a placental abruption. Placental hemorrhage refers to bleeding from the placenta from any cause. The locations of placental hemorrhage include retroplacental, subchorionic, subamniotic, and intraplacental sites. A hemorrhage seen in the first trimester does not carry the same risk as hemorrhage in the third trimester. First trimester hemorrhages are more likely to resolve spontaneously if bleeding subsides.

Sonographic Findings. The sonographic appearance of placental hemorrhage varies greatly with the location, size, and age of onset of the hemorrhage. Upon examination of the placenta, the sonographer will notice an abnormality in the texture and size of the placenta. If a hemorrhage is present, the echogenicity depends on the age of the hemorrhage; the acute bleed is similar to the echogenicity of the placenta, whereas the subacute and chronic bleed becomes more hypoechoic. The bleed may be retroplacental or subchorionic. Careful analysis should be made from the normal villus attachment of the placenta to the uterine wall to detect an abnormal collection of blood secondary to hemorrhage. For all types

of abruption, the sonographer needs to evaluate fetal heart rate, as a poor outcome will be seen when fetal bradycardia is present.

PLACENTAL ABRUPTION

Placental abruption refers to the separation of a normally implanted placenta prior to term delivery. Placental abruption is a premature placental detachment and occurs in 1 in 120 pregnancies. Bleeding in the decidua basalis occurs with separation (Figure 55-27). The mortality rate ranges from 20% to 60% and accounts for 15% to 25% of perinatal deaths. Clinically the patient may present with any of the following signs: vaginal bleeding, abdominal or back pain, preterm labor, fetal distress or demise, and uterine irritability. The detection of acute abruptions with ultrasound is not sensitive, as the hemorrhage may have the same echogenicity as the placenta. **Abruptio placenta** may be further classified as retroplacental or marginal. With abruption, bleeding into the deciduas basalis is apparent. An expanding hematoma can lead to loss of surface area for respiratory and nutrient exchange, placing the fetus at risk for hypoxia and even sudden fetal death.

Maternal hypertension is seen in approximately 50% of severe abruptions associated with fetal demise. Hypertension is chronic in half of these cases; in the other half, it is pregnancy induced. Other risk factors for abruption include a prior abruption, short umbilical cord, uterine anomaly, myomas, abdominal trauma, placenta previa, tobacco use, and cocaine abuse. The recurrence of placental abruption ranges from 5% to 16% in subsequent pregnancies.

Retroplacental Abruption

Retroplacental abruption results from the rupture of spiral arteries and is a "high-pressure" bleed. It is associated with hypertension and vascular disease. The hematoma is between the placenta and the uterus and is quite worrisome. If the blood remains retroplacental, the patient may have no vaginal bleeding. Acute sonographic findings show thickening of the placenta. Older

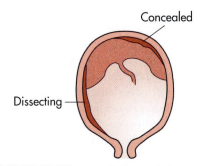

FIGURE 55-27 Types of placental abruption.

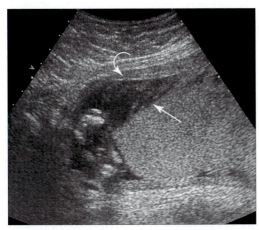

FIGURE 55-28 Hypoechoic hematoma is seen separating the placenta (*arrow*) from the uterine wall (*curved arrow*).

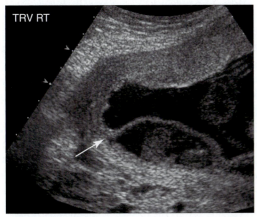

FIGURE 55-29 Subchorionic bleed can be seen arising from the edge of the placenta (*arrow*).

hematomas tend to be hypoechoic when compared to the placenta, and the visual sonographic clue is separation of the placenta substance from the uterine wall (Figure 55-28).

Marginal Abruption

Marginal abruptions are the most common type of abruption and are also known as subchorionic bleeds. This type of hemorrhage results from tears of the marginal veins and represents a "low-pressure" bleed. This hemorrhage arises from the edge of the placenta, dissects beneath the placental membranes, and is associated with little placental detachment. A subchorionic hemorrhage accumulates at the site of the separation from the placenta. Women may continue to bleed after the initial hemorrhage when blood tracks behind the membranes and through the cervix. This will be old blood and frequently brownish in color. The sonographer needs to carefully scan along the edge of the placenta to identify a marginal abruption. (Figure 55-29).

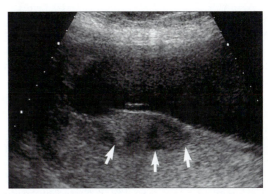

FIGURE 55-30 Thrombus within the intervillous spaces occurs in one third of the pregnancies. The inhomogeneity of the placenta is seen with sonolucent areas within the texture of the placenta (*arrow*).

Intervillous Thrombosis

The presence of thrombus within the intervillous spaces occurs in one third of pregnancies. It results from intraplacental hemorrhage caused by breaks in the villous capillaries. Usually there is little risk to the fetus, although the condition is associated with Rh sensitivity and elevated alpha-fetoprotein levels from a fetal-maternal hemorrhage.

Sonographic Findings. On ultrasound examination, sonolucencies are seen within the homogeneous texture of the placenta. These sonolucencies increase with advanced gestational age and indicate maturity of the placenta (Figure 55-30).

Placenta Infarcts

Placental infarction is a focal discrete lesion caused by ischemic necrosis. Infarcts are common, found in 25% of pregnancies, and are usually small with no clinical significance. Large infarcts may reflect underlying maternal vascular disease. Infarcts within the placenta evolve through acute, subacute, and chronic stages. The majority of infarcts are hypoechoic in the acute stage and ultrasound may be unable to distinguish from intraplacental hemorrhages. Calcification may occur over time. Maternal floor infarction is a complication of the third trimester; large amounts of fibrin are deposited in and around the maternal plate with extension into the intervillous space and entrapment of chorionic villi.

PLACENTAL TUMORS

Gestational Trophoblastic Disease

Gestational trophoblastic disease, also known as a **molar pregnancy**, encompasses disease processes that originate in the placenta. They may be benign or malignant and include complete or partial mole, choriocarcinoma, and invasive mole. Complete moles generally have a diploid karyotype and have no fetal tissue. Clinical symptoms include nausea and vomiting (from elevated hCG levels), vaginal bleeding, and uterine size larger than dates. In this group, 12% to 15% will develop malignant gestational trophoblastic disease (choriocarcinoma). This disease is covered more thoroughly in Chapter 48.

Partial or incomplete moles usually have a triploid karyotype and fetal tissue is often present. Clinically these women may present with vaginal bleeding. Malignancy is diagnosed in 2% to 3% of partial hydatidiform moles. Twinning with a complete mole and fetus is rare, but the fetus will have a normal placenta

Sonographic Findings. The sonogram of a complete mole reveals excessive uterine size, no embryo, and an inhomogeneous intrauterine mass with cystic structures completing filling the uterine cavity (Figure 55-31). Bilateral ovarian theca lutein cysts are seen secondary to ovarian hyperstimulation related to the elevated hCG hormone levels. Because most pregnant women have a first-trimester ultrasound, this diagnosis is usually made in the first trimester.

A partial mole carries little malignant potential. It is associated with an abnormal fetus or fetal tissue. On ultrasound examination, a reduced amount of amniotic fluid is noted. The placenta is thick with multiple intraplacental cystic spaces (Figure 55-32).

Chorioangioma

A chorioangioma is a benign vascular tumor of the placenta. Second to trophoblastic disease, chorioangioma is the most common tumor of the placenta, occurring in 1% of pregnancies. The tumor is usually small and consists of a benign proliferation of fetal vessels; the majority are capillary hemangiomas that arise beneath the chorionic plate. Large tumors can act as arteriovenous malformations shunting blood from the fetus, thus causing complications. Fetal complications include polyhydramnios, hydrops, anemia, cardiomegaly, IUGR, and demise. The maternal serum alpha-fetoprotein may be elevated in the amniotic fluid or maternal serum, especially from vascular tumors. Preterm labor is another complication of large chorioangiomas and is thought to be related to polyhydramnios.

Sonographic Findings. Ultrasound examination shows a circumscribed solid (hyperechoic or hypoechoic) or complex mass that protrudes from the fetal surface of the placenta (Figure 55-33). It may be located near the umbilical cord insertion site. The majority of these benign tumors are small and incidentally noted at delivery. Those larger than 5 cm are usually detected prenatally and are more likely to have complications. Color Doppler can help make the diagnosis, although the amount of flow in the tumor varies. When a placental mass is seen, the sonographer should evaluate the fetus for polyhydramnios, hydrops, IUGR, and signs of anemia. Excessive amniotic fluid occurs as a result of transudation through the wall of abnormal tumor vessels. Differential diagnosis for solid placental masses includes gestational trophoblastic disease, teratoma, or maternal tumor metastatic to the placenta.

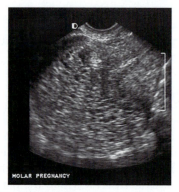

FIGURE 55-31 A hydatidiform mole is seen on ultrasound as multiple tiny vesicles throughout the uterine cavity.

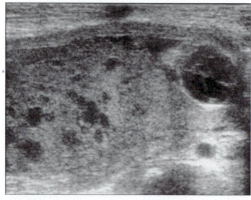

FIGURE 55-32 Partial mole. Thickened placenta with cystic changes is seen.

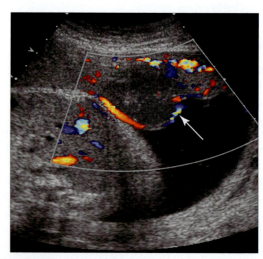

FIGURE 55-33 The hypoechoic mass compared to the normal placenta parenchyma is a chorioangioma (*arrow*). Vascularity is demonstrated with color Doppler.

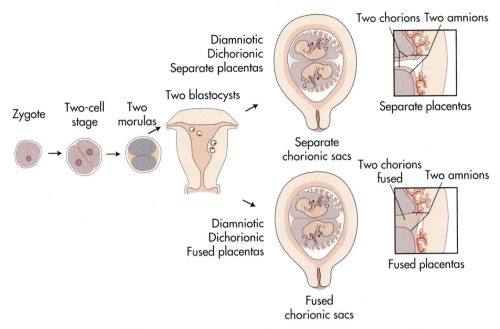

FIGURE 55-34 Possible dichorionicity and diamnionicity of monozygotic twins.

The Placenta in Multiple Gestation

Monozygotic twins are associated with all three types of membranes: dichorionic/diamniotic (di/di), monochorionic/diamniotic (mono/di), or monochorionic/monoamniotic (mono/mono), depending on when the twinning event occurred. If the membranes are di/di, the pregnancy is probably dizygotic (97% chance), with only a 3% chance that it is a monozygotic pregnancy. The diamniotic/dichorionic two placentas can also occur in monozygotic pregnancies when the division occurs during the first 4 days of gestation. If the membranes are mono/di or mono/mono, they are from a monozygotic pregnancy (Box 55-6).

Sonographic Findings. The sonographer should be able to carefully scan the uterus to determine the site and number of placentas to help differentiate the type of multiple gestations. Refer to Chapter 52 for further discussion of multiple gestations (Figure 55-34).

BOX 55-6	Multiple Gestation Pregnancies and Placentas

Dizygotic (Fraternal Twins)
Derived from two zygotes
Diamniotic/dichorionic/two placentas
Occurs during first 4 days of gestation

Monozygotic (Identical Twins)
Derived from one zygote
Diamniotic/dichorionic/two placentas
Monochorionic/diamniotic/one placenta
Occurs during 1st week of gestation
Monochorionic/monoamniotic/one placenta
Occurs during 2nd week of gestation

Risks Involved
Monochorionic
Placental vascular anastomosis

Monoamniotic
Entanglement of umbilical cord

The Umbilical Cord

Sandra L. Hagen-Ansert

OBJECTIVES

On completion of this chapter, you should be able to:
- Describe the development and normal anatomy of the umbilical cord
- Predict obstetric problems that may be associated with abnormal umbilical cord dimensions
- Discuss the umbilical cord disorders presented in this chapter, including causes and clinical significance
- Differentiate how the sonographer may distinguish tumors and cysts from a true knot in the umbilical cord

OUTLINE

DEVELOPMENT AND ANATOMY OF THE UMBILICAL CORD

The umbilical cord is the essential link for oxygen and important nutrients among the fetus, the placenta, and the mother. The amnion covers the cord and blends with the fetal skin at the umbilicus. The umbilical cord comprises two arteries and one vein surrounded by gelatinous stroma. Vascular connections within the cord serve a reverse function in the fetus; the vein carries oxygenated blood to the fetus, whereas the arteries bring venous blood back to the placenta.

The umbilical cord can be visualized with sonography from the 8th gestational week until term. The amniotic membrane covers the fetal surface of the placenta and the multiple vessels that branch from the umbilical vein and arteries. The cord should normally insert into the center of the placenta.

Embryologic Development

The umbilical cord forms during the first 5 weeks of gestation (7 menstrual weeks) as a fusion of the omphalomesenteric (**yolk stalk**) and **allantoic ducts.** An outpouching from the urinary bladder forms the urachus, which projects into the connecting stalk to form the allantois. The allantoic vessels become the definitive umbilical vessels. The umbilical cord acquires its epithelial lining as a result of enlargement of the amniotic cavity and envelopment of the cord by amniotic membrane. The intestines grow at a faster rate than the abdomen; they herniate into the proximal umbilical cord at approximately 7 weeks and remain there until approximately 10 weeks. The insertion of the umbilical cord into the ventral abdominal wall is an important sonographic anatomic landmark because scrutiny of this area will reveal abdominal wall defects, such as omphalocele, gastroschisis, or limb–body wall complex.

Normal Anatomy

The umbilical cord is covered by the amniotic membrane. The cord includes two umbilical arteries and one umbilical vein (Figure 56-1) and is surrounded by a homogeneous substance called Wharton's jelly. **Wharton's jelly** is a myxomatous connective tissue that varies in size and may be imaged with high-frequency ultrasound transducers. The diameter of the cord usually measures 1 to 2 cm (variations in cord diameter are usually attributed to Wharton's jelly). The normal length of the cord is 40 to 60 cm; it is difficult to assess the length reliably with ultrasound.

The umbilical arteries arise from the fetal internal iliac arteries, course alongside the fetal bladder, and exit the umbilicus to form part of the umbilical cord. The paired umbilical arteries course along the entire length of the cord in a helicoidal fashion surrounding the umbilical vein. The umbilical arteries branch along the chorionic plate of the placenta.

The umbilical vein is formed by the confluence of the chorionic veins of the placenta, with its primary purpose to transport oxygenated blood back to the fetus. The umbilical vein enters the umbilicus and joins the left portal vein as it courses through the liver. The intra-abdominal portions of the umbilical vessels degenerate after birth; the umbilical arteries become the lateral ligaments of the bladder, and the umbilical vein becomes the round ligament of the liver.

Sonographic Evaluation of the Umbilical Cord

The umbilical cord has one large vein and two smaller arteries (Figure 56-2). The umbilical vein transports oxygenated blood from the placenta, and the paired umbilical arteries return deoxygenated blood from the fetus to the placenta for purification. The umbilical cord is identified at the cord insertion into the placenta and at the junction of the cord into the fetal umbilicus. The arteries spiral with the larger umbilical vein (Figure 56-3), which is surrounded by Wharton's jelly (Figure 56-4). Absent cord twists may be associated with decreased fetal movement and a poor pregnancy outcome.

The umbilical vein diameter increases throughout gestation, reaching a maximum diameter of 0.9 cm by 30 weeks' gestation. The umbilical cord has been found to be significantly larger in fetuses of mothers with gestational diabetes than in the normal population; the increase in width is attributed mainly to an increase in Wharton's jelly content.

In the second and third trimesters, the two arteries and the vein can be clearly seen. The number of umbilical arteries can be clearly seen and should be documented. The three vessels of the cord may be followed with real-time ultrasound as they enter the abdomen and travel toward the liver and iliac arteries (Figure 56-5). From the left portal vein, umbilical blood may flow through the **ductus venosus** to the systemic veins (inferior vena cava or hepatics), bypassing the liver, or through the right portal sinus to the right portal vein. The ductus venosus forms the conduit between the portal system and the systemic veins.

Sonographically, the ductus venosus appears as a thin intrahepatic channel with echogenic walls. It lies in the groove between the left lobe and the caudate lobe. The ductus venosus is patent during fetal life until shortly after birth, when transformation of the ductus into the ligamentum venosum occurs (beginning in the 2nd week after birth).

The umbilical arteries may be followed caudally from the cord insertion, in their normal path adjacent to the

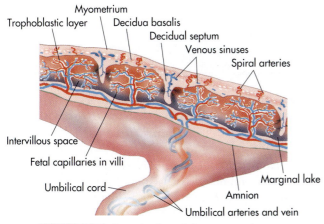

FIGURE 56-1 Organization of the mature placenta.

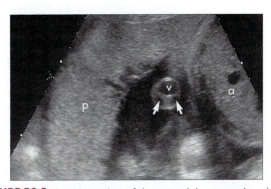

FIGURE 56-2 Transverse view of the normal three-vessel cord. The umbilical vein *(v)* is the largest vessel, with two smaller arteries *(arrows)* spiraling around the vein. *a,* Abdomen; *p,* placenta.

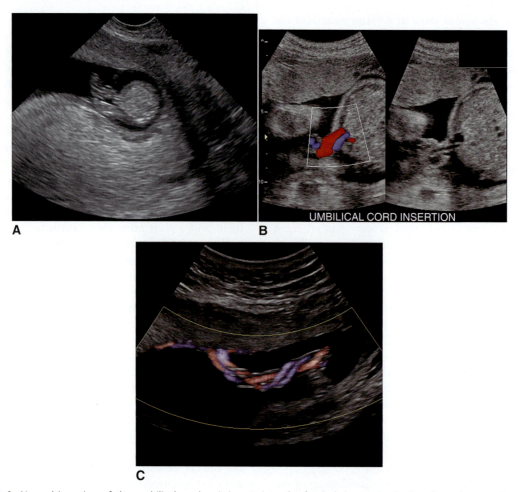

FIGURE 56-3 **A,** Normal insertion of the umbilical cord as it inserts into the fetal abdomen in the late first trimester. **B,** Insertion of the umbilical cord in the late second trimester. Color Doppler is helpful to identify the cord insertion. **C,** The umbilical cord may be seen as it exits the placental surface.

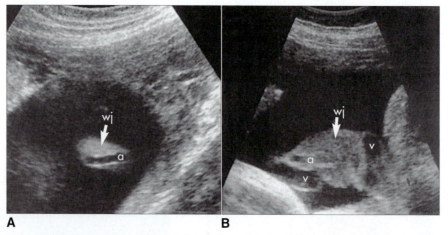

FIGURE 56-4 **A,** Wharton's jelly *(wj)* observed in a 30-week fetus. One of the umbilical arteries *(a)* is in view. **B,** Wharton's jelly *(wj)* is present adjacent to one of the umbilical arteries *(a)*, and the single umbilical vein *(v)* is observed in a 35-week fetus. Wharton's jelly is an important structure to recognize when performing cordocentesis procedures in which the needle is directed into the cord vessels.

fetal bladder, to the iliac arteries. On sonography, the sonographer may look at the cord in a transverse plane to see one large umbilical vein and two smaller umbilical arteries. Another sonographic approach to viewing the arteries is to look lateral to the fetal bladder in a transverse or coronal plane. The umbilical arteries run along the lateral margin of the fetal bladder and are well imaged with color flow Doppler (Figure 56-6). In the postpartum stage, the umbilical arteries become the **superior vesical arteries.**

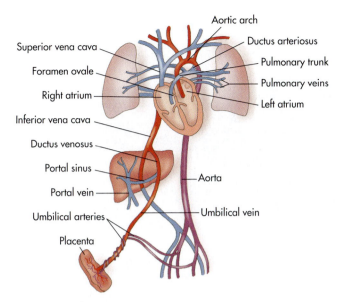

FIGURE 56-5 The umbilical vein leaves the placenta to deliver nutrients to the fetus. From the left portal vein, the umbilical blood flows through the ductus venosus to the inferior vena cava or hepatics, or through the right portal sinus to the right portal vein. The iliac arteries drain into the umbilical arteries.

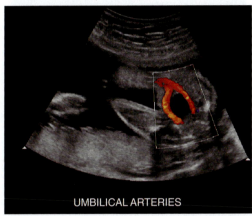

UMBILICAL ARTERIES

FIGURE 56-6 The umbilical arteries *(red)* are shown along the lateral margins of the fetal bladder.

ABNORMAL UMBILICAL CORD DIMENSIONS

Although the umbilical cord varies normally in length and width, researchers have found specific problems associated with a cord that varies from standard dimensions. In the first trimester, the length is approximately the same as the crown-rump length. The normal cord measures 40 to 60 cm in length and is difficult to assess reliably with sonography (Figure 56-7).

A short umbilical cord measures less than 35 cm in length. This condition is associated with or is predisposed to the following:

- Oligohydramnios
- Restricted space (as in multiple gestations)

- Intrinsic fetal anomaly
- Tethering of the fetus by an amniotic band
- Inadequate fetal descent
- Cord compression
- Fetal distress

Coiling of the umbilical cord is normal and is related to fetal activity. The normal cord may coil as many as 40 times, usually to the left and near the fetal insertion site. The helical twisting of the cord can be easily determined by gross pathologic inspection. With the cord held vertically, vessels along the anterior surface that spiral downward from high left to low right, angled like the left side of the letter V, indicate a left helix (Figure 56-8, A). The incidence of a "left" twist of the cord in pregnancy is found at a rate of 7:1. The significance of this is that a fetus with a "right" twist in the cord has a higher incidence of fetal anomalies than one with a "left" twist (Figure 56-8, B).

The absence of cord twisting is an indirect sign of decreased fetal movement (Figure 56-9). This event occurs in a small (4.3%) number of deliveries; however, it may lead to increased mortality and morbidity. Other obstetric problems seen with a short umbilical cord include preterm delivery, decreased heart rate during delivery, meconium staining secondary to fetal distress, and fetal anomalies. If the cord is completely atretic, the fetus is attached directly to the placenta at the umbilicus, and an omphalocele is always present.

It has been theorized that the length of the umbilical cord is determined in part by the amount of amniotic fluid present in the first and second trimesters, and in part by fetal mobility. Therefore the presence of oligohydramnios, amniotic bands, or limitation of fetal movement for any reason may impede umbilical cord growth.

A long umbilical cord measures longer than 80 cm and may be associated with or predisposed to the following:

- Polyhydramnios
- Nuchal cord (occurs in 25% of deliveries)
- True cord knots (occur in 0.5% of deliveries); may be difficult to distinguish from "false" cord knot or redundancy of cord; true knots cause vascular compromise and fetal demise
- Umbilical cord compression, cord presentation, and prolapse of the cord leading to fetal distress
- Umbilical cord stricture or torsion resulting from excessive fetal motion

The diameter of the umbilical cord measures from 2.6 to 6.0 cm. Variations in cord diameter are usually attributed to diffuse accumulation of Wharton's jelly. This condition has been associated with maternal diabetes, edema secondary to fetal hydrops, Rh incompatibility, and fetal demise.

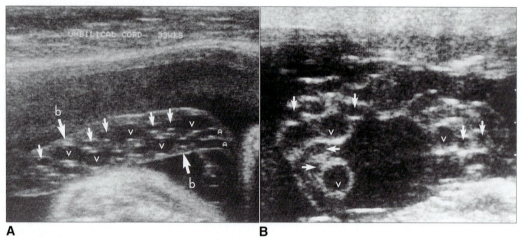

A   B

FIGURE 56-7 A, The umbilical cord is shown in a sagittal plane in a 33-week fetus, outlining the cord borders (*b*), the umbilical vein (*v*), and the arteries *(arrows)*. The spirals of the cord vessels and Wharton's jelly are outlined. Abnormal cord twists may indicate a higher risk for stillbirth. **B,** Cross sections of the umbilical cord.

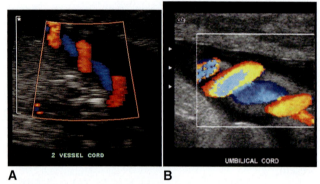

A   B

FIGURE 56-8 A, As the cord is held vertically, vessels along the anterior surface spiral downward from high left to low right, angled like the left side of the letter *V,* to indicate a left helix. **B,** This two-vessel cord has a right twist; the fetus has multiple congenital anomalies.

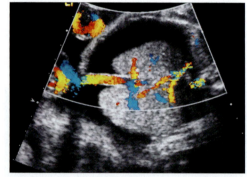

FIGURE 56-9 This hydropic fetus showed decreased movement over 24 hours. The cord is shown without its usual twisting and coiling, indicating decreased fetal movement.

UMBILICAL CORD MASSES

Umbilical cord masses are not very common in the fetus. Many of the "masses" seen on ultrasound may be attributed to focal accumulation of Wharton's jelly and may be isolated or associated with an omphalocele or cyst. Cystic masses in the cord are usually omphalomesenteric or allantoic in origin. These are generally small (less than 2 cm), tend to occur near the fetal end of the cord, and resolve by the second trimester. Cysts that persist beyond the first trimester usually are associated with other fetal anomalies and aneuploidy.

Other masses associated with the umbilical cord include

- Omphalocele (cord runs through the middle of this mass as it protrudes from the umbilicus)
- Gastroschisis (mass is usually found to the right of this cord)
- Umbilical herniation
- Teratoma of the umbilical cord

- Aneurysm of the cord
- Varix of the cord (may be intra-abdominal)
- Hematoma of the cord (usually iatrogenic—cordocentesis or amniocentesis)
- True knot of the cord
- Angioma of the cord (well-circumscribed echogenic mass that may cause increased cardiac failure and hydrops; alpha-fetoprotein level is increased; associated with a cyst caused by transudation of fluid from a hemangioma)
- Thrombosis of cord secondary to compression or kinking, focal cord mass, true cord knots, velamentous cord insertion, or cord entanglement in monoamniotic twins (commonly seen with fetal demise)

Omphalocele

Omphalocele occurs 1 in 5000 births and results from failure of the intestines to return to the abdomen. The hernia may consist of a single loop of bowel, or it may contain most of the intestines (Figure 56-10). The

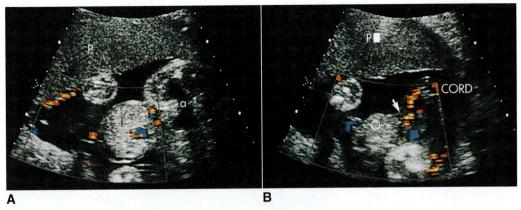

FIGURE 56-10 A, Image of a liver-filled omphalocele in a 26-week fetus showing hepatic vessel flow within the herniated liver *(l). a,* Abdomen; *P,* placenta. **B,** In the same fetus, color enhancement aids in the confirmation of the cord vessels entering the base of the omphalocele *(O, arrow); P,* placenta. No other anomalies were found, and the karyotype was normal.

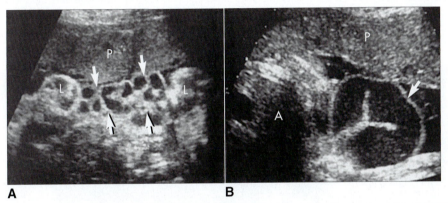

FIGURE 56-11 A, Gastroschisis showing herniated bowel *(arrows)* in the amniotic cavity. Cesarean section was performed at 36 weeks' gestation because of a nonreactive nonstress test with variable decelerations and absent breathing. A small for gestational age infant with a left-side gastroschisis was delivered. *L,* Limbs; *P,* placenta. **B,** Isolated bowel segment *(arrow)* observed in another fetus with gastroschisis at 29 weeks' gestation. Bowel dilatation (29 mm) and obstruction (meconium ileus) are shown. Note the haustral markings within the obstructed bowel. *A,* Abdomen; *P,* placenta.

covering for the hernia sac consists of epithelium from the umbilical cord.

Gastroschisis

Gastroschisis is usually a right paraumbilical defect involving all layers of the abdominal wall and usually measuring 2 to 4 cm. The small bowel always eviscerates through the defect (Figure 56-11). The loops of bowel are never covered by a membrane; thus they are directly exposed to amniotic fluid and elevated alpha-fetoprotein levels. Other organs that may eviscerate are large bowel, stomach, a portion of the gastrointestinal system, and, rarely, liver.

Umbilical Herniation

Umbilical herniation occurs when the intestines return normally to the abdominal cavity and then herniate prenatally or postnatally through an inadequately closed umbilicus (Figure 56-12).

Omphalomesenteric Cyst

Omphalomesenteric cyst is a cystic lesion of the umbilical cord caused by persistence and dilatation of a segment of the omphalomesenteric duct lined by epithelium of gastrointestinal origin. During the third week of early development, the omphalomesenteric duct joins the embryonic gut and the yolk sac. This is closed by the 16th week of gestation; however, in some cases, small vestigial remnants of the duct may be found in normal umbilical cords (Figure 56-13). The omphalomesenteric cyst is found closer to the fetal cord insertion and may vary in size (up to 6 cm). This condition affects females more frequently than males, at a rate of 5:3. In addition, an associated condition of Meckel's diverticulum may be noted.

Hemangioma of the Cord

A hemangioma of the cord arises from the transepithelial cells of the vessels of the umbilical cord. Pathologically,

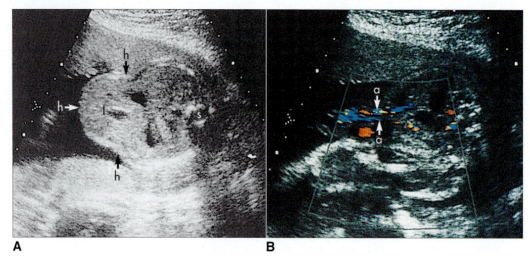

FIGURE 56-12 A, Umbilical hernia *(h, arrows)* observed in a fetus with Carpenter's syndrome (acrocephalopolysyndactyly). *l,* Liver; *s,* spine. **B,** In the same fetus, at the cord insertion level using color imaging, the umbilical arteries are observed entering the abdomen *(a)* in a normal location. This excludes the diagnosis of omphalocele.

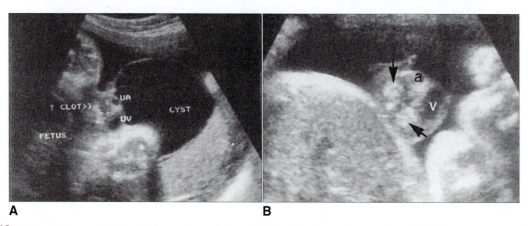

FIGURE 56-13 A, Omphalomesenteric cyst observed in a 34-week fetus. Clot formation was found within one artery. A single umbilical artery *(UA)* was viewed in proximal sections of the cord close to the cyst, and three vessels were noted distally. *UV,* Umbilical vein. **B,** In the same fetus, clot is observed *(arrows)*. At birth, a 10-cm, serous-filled cyst consistent with omphalomesenteric cyst was confirmed. The cyst weighed 1 lb.

this angiomatous nodule is surrounded by edema and myxomatous degeneration of Wharton's jelly. The sites of origin are the main vessels of the umbilical cord, and the nodule may involve more than one vessel. This condition is rare; however, when found near the placental end of the cord, the size varies from small to large (up to 15 cm). The fetus may develop nonimmune hydrops.

Hematoma of the Cord

Trauma to the umbilical vessels occasionally may cause extravasation of blood into Wharton's jelly. This usually occurs near the fetal insertion of the cord. The umbilical vein is most frequently involved. If the blood clot is new, the mass is hyperechoic on ultrasound; if the clot is old, the mass is hypoechoic and septated. Complications have been reported at rates as high as 47% to 52% with fetal mortality.

Thrombosis of the Umbilical Vessels

Thrombosis of the umbilical vessels is defined as occlusion of one or more vessels of the umbilical cord; primarily it occurs in the umbilical vein. The incidence is higher in infants of diabetic mothers than in infants of nondiabetic mothers. Thrombosis may be primary or may occur secondary to torsion, knotting, looping, compression, or hematoma. The sonographer should look for aneurysmal dilatation of the cord and the presence of fetal hydrops. Other maternal factors are phlebitis and arteritis. The prognosis is poor in the fetus with umbilical vein thrombosis.

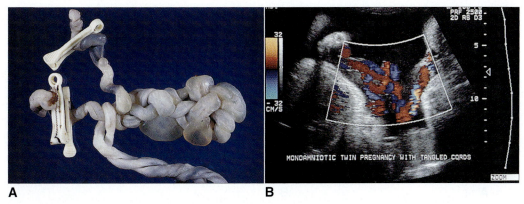

FIGURE 56-14 **A,** Pathologic specimen of an umbilical cord with multiple knots. **B,** Ultrasound image of a monoamniotic twin pregnancy showing multiple knots and tangles within the cord. Doppler flow shows decreased velocity in the blood flow.

UMBILICAL CORD KNOTS

True Knots of the Cord

True knots of the umbilical cord have been associated with long cords, polyhydramnios, intrauterine growth restriction, and monoamniotic twins. The knots may be single or multiple, with increased incidence of congenital anomalies (Figure 56-14). The mortality rate is 8% to 11%. In these cases, a flattening or dissipation of Wharton's jelly is seen, with venous congestion distal to the knot and vascular thrombi within the cord.

The knot may be formed when a loop of cord is slipped over the infant's head or shoulders during delivery. Usually, the umbilical vessels are protected by Wharton's jelly and are not constricted enough to cause fetal anoxia in this condition.

Color Doppler is useful for recording absence of blood flow within the umbilical cord. When Doppler is used to image a false knot, flow is not completely constricted but may appear to show constriction secondary to fetal activity and tension on the cord as the fetus moves.

False Knots of the Cord

False knots of the umbilical cord are seen when the blood vessels are longer than the cord. Often they are folded on themselves and produce nodulations on the surface of the cord (Figure 56-15).

Nuchal Cord

Nuchal cord is the most common cord entanglement in the fetus. Multiple coils may be seen around the fetal neck (Figure 56-16). A single loop of cord has been reported in more than 20% of deliveries; two loops have been documented in 2.5%. Trouble begins as the fetus descends into the birth canal during delivery and the coils tighten sufficiently enough to reduce the flow of blood through the cord. Fetal heart deceleration, meconium-stained amniotic fluid, and babies requiring

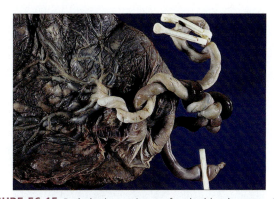

FIGURE 56-15 Pathologic specimen of a double placenta with a false knot.

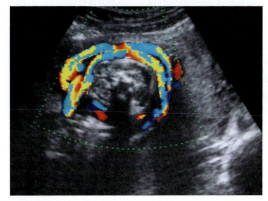

FIGURE 56-16 Nuchal cord is well demonstrated by color Doppler as it wraps multiple times around the fetal neck.

resuscitation are seen more frequently when a cord entanglement occurs.

UMBILICAL CORD INSERTION ABNORMALITIES

Marginal Insertion of the Cord (Battledore Placenta)

The differential proliferation of placenta villi may result in eccentric insertion of the umbilical cord into the

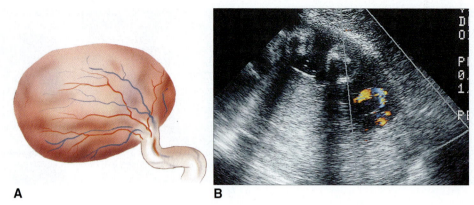

A   **B**

FIGURE 56-17 **A,** Battledore placenta with insertion of cord at the margin of the placenta. **B,** Color Doppler shows the marginal insertion of the cord into the edge of the placenta instead of into the middle of the placenta.

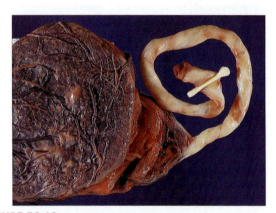

FIGURE 56-18 Pathologic specimen of the membranous insertion of the cord into the membranes of the placenta.

placenta. The cord implants into the edge of the placenta (**battledore placenta**) instead of into the middle of the placenta (Figure 56-17). This is significant when the cord is inserted near the internal os because labor may cause the cord to prolapse or be compressed during contractions. The marginal insertion occurs in 2% to 10% of singleton births, 20% of twins, and 18% of pregnancies with a single umbilical artery.

Membranous or Velamentous Insertion of the Cord

Membranous or velamentous insertion of the cord occurs when the cord inserts into the membranes before it enters the placenta, rather than inserting directly into the placenta (Figure 56-18). This condition occurs in 1% of singleton births, 12% of twins, and 9% of pregnancies with a single umbilical artery. Risk of thrombosis, cord rupture during delivery, or vasa previa is increased.

Velamentous insertion may occur when most of the placental tissue grows laterally, leaving the initially centrally located cord in an area that becomes atretic. Another theory shows a defect in the implantation of the cord that occurs at the site of the trophoblast in front of the decidua capsularis, instead of at the area of trophoblast that forms the placental mass. Implantation occurs in the chorion leave, where the umbilical vessels lie on the membranous surface.

Velamentous umbilical cord insertion is associated with higher risk of low birth weight, small for gestational age, preterm delivery, low Apgar scores, and abnormal intrapartum fetal heart rate pattern.

Associated anomalies occur in less than 10% of pregnancies with velamentous insertion of the cord. These anomalies include esophageal atresia, obstructive uropathies, congenital hip dislocation, spina bifida, ventricular septal defect, and cleft palate. An increased risk has been reported for intrauterine growth restriction and premature birth.

VASA PREVIA AND PROLAPSE OF THE CORD

Prolapse of the umbilical cord occurs when the cord lies below the presenting part. This condition may exist whenever the presenting part does not fit closely and fails to fill the pelvic inlet; further risk is incurred if the membranes rupture early. Compression of the cord reduces or cuts off the blood supply to the fetus and may result in fetal demise. Abnormal fetal presentation occurs in nearly half of prolapse cord cases. A slightly higher risk is incurred when the fetus is in a transverse or breech presentation.

Vasa previa is defined as the presence of umbilical cord vessels crossing the internal os of the cervix. Mortality may be high, ranging from 60% to 70% for vaginal delivery, and results from rupture of the vessels and fetal exsanguination. Color Doppler is the best method of detection in the ultrasound examination. Vasa previa may be due to many factors, including velamentous insertion of the cord, succenturiate lobe of the placenta, or low-lying placenta with marginal insertion of the cord near the internal os.

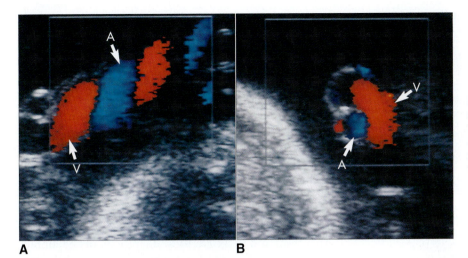

A   B

FIGURE 56-19 Color flow imaging of a single umbilical artery in sagittal **(A)** and transverse **(B)** images. The single umbilical artery *(A, blue)* and umbilical vein *(V, red)* are shown. The fetus had posterior urethral valve syndrome.

Cord Presentation and Prolapse

Cord presentation with prolapse of the umbilical cord through the cervix into the vagina occurs in 0.5% of deliveries. An occult prolapse occurs when the cord lies alongside the presenting part. The perinatal mortality rate of 25% to 60% is due to cord compression during vaginal delivery. Conditions predisposing to cord presentation and prolapse are as follows:

- Abnormal fetal presentation
- Nonengagement of the fetus because of prematurity
- Long umbilical cord
- Abnormal bony pelvic inlet
- Leiomyomas
- Polyhydramnios
- Vasa previa
- Velamentous insertion of the cord
- Marginal insertion of the cord in a low-lying placenta
- Incompetent cervix with premature rupture of the membranes

Prematurity

Two factors contribute to failure of the fetus to fill the pelvic inlet cavity: small presenting part and increased frequency of abnormal presentation in premature labor. Fetal mortality is high in the premature population secondary to birth trauma and anoxia.

Multiple Pregnancy

Multiple pregnancy factors include failure of adequate adaptation of the presenting part to the pelvis, higher incidence of abnormal presentation, polyhydramnios, and premature rupture of the membranes of the second twin when it is unengaged.

Obstetric Procedures

One third of cord prolapse problems are produced during obstetric procedures:

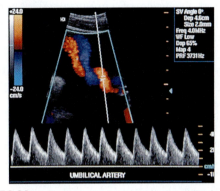

FIGURE 56-20 Color Doppler shows normal umbilical artery flow in a fetus with a two-vessel cord.

- Artificial rupture of membranes
- Disengaging the head
- Flexion of an extended head
- Version and extraction

SINGLE UMBILICAL ARTERY

A **single umbilical artery** occurs in 0.08% to 1.9% of singleton births and 3.5% of twin pregnancies; it is more frequent in miscarriages and autopsy series (Figures 56-19 and 56-20). Reports have found single umbilical artery in 18% of pregnancies with marginal insertion of the cord and in 9% with membranous insertion of the cord. The probable cause is atrophy of one of the umbilical arteries in the early development stage. The left umbilical artery is absent a slightly higher percentage of time than the right.

Single umbilical artery has been associated with the following[1]:

- Congenital anomalies in 20% to 50% of cases
- Increased incidence of intrauterine growth restriction (small placenta) (Figure 56-21)
- Increased perinatal mortality

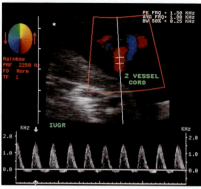

FIGURE 56-21 Doppler waveform of the fetus with intrauterine growth restriction (IUGR) shows no diastolic flow and prominent systolic flow in the Doppler waveform.

- Increased incidence of chromosomal abnormalities (trisomies 18, 13, and 21; Turner's syndrome; and triploidy)

Infants with single umbilical arteries have associated anomalies that affect other organ systems, such as the following:

- Musculoskeletal (23%)
- Genitourinary (20%)
- Cardiovascular (19%)
- Gastrointestinal (10%)
- Central nervous system (8%)

Multiple studies have investigated normal measurements of the vessels within the umbilical cord. A three-vessel cord showing artery-to-artery difference of more than 50% was defined as hypoplastic umbilical artery. A study of 100 pregnancies found that at between 20 and 36 weeks' gestation, all pregnancies with a single umbilical artery had a transverse umbilical artery diameter greater than 4 mm, and all pregnancies with two umbilical arteries had a transverse umbilical arterial diameter less than 4 mm. In another study, the diameter of the umbilical artery was greater than 50% of that of the umbilical vein in the fetus with a single umbilical artery.[2]

Sonographic detection of a single umbilical artery (SUA) should prompt the investigation of further fetal anomalies. The incidence of associated anomalies has been reported to range from 25% to 50%. Major anomalies have included cardiac defects, skeletal abnormalities, abdominal wall defects, diaphragmatic hernia, holoprosencephaly, and hydrocephalus. The diagnosis of an SUA in the second and third trimesters has increased with routine visualization of the number of vessels within the cord. A characteristic sonographic finding of the two-vessel cord is disconcordance of the two vessels on cross section. Once the transducer is rotated to record the long axis view, the two-vessel cord appears straight and non-coiled, although occasionally the single artery may loop around the vein. Visualization with color of the umbili-

cal artery alongside the bladder may provide further confirmation that only one artery is present.

Another variation that may be seen is discordant size between the two arterial vessels, with one being more hypoplastic than the other. Discordant blood flow would be seen in the umbilical artery Doppler. The resistive index is almost always higher in the smaller artery, and end-diastolic flow may be absent.

Variations in the number of umbilical arteries have been reported. The presence of more than three vessels in the cord has been documented in conjoined twins.

VARIX OF THE UMBILICAL VEIN

Aneurysm and varix are focal dilatations of the umbilical vessels affecting the umbilical artery and vein, respectively. Focal dilatation of the umbilical vein is nearly always intra-abdominal, but extrahepatic in location. A varix appears on sonography as a dilated intra-abdominal, extrahepatic portion of the umbilical vein. Color Doppler shows continuity with the umbilical vein. Usually, the prognosis is for a normal outcome in a fetus with a varix of the umbilical vein.

PERSISTENT INTRAHEPATIC RIGHT PORTAL VEIN

Persistence of right portal vein rather than normal left-sided portal vein is called persistent intrahepatic right portal vein. The development of the venous drainage is somewhat complex. At 5 to 6 weeks' gestational age, paired umbilical veins carry blood from the placenta to the primitive heart. The veins join an anastomotic venous network formed by the omphalomesenteric veins in the developing liver to establish the umbilical-portal venous connection. By 6 weeks, the right umbilical vein regresses, and the left umbilical vein enlarges to accommodate the increasing flow. The umbilical vein now enters the left portal vein directly. The right umbilical vein usually regresses at 6 weeks' gestation and is not seen by sonography.

Persistence of the right umbilical vein is rare and may be related to an involution of the left umbilical vein. If it persists, the right umbilical vein enters the right lobe of the liver to join the right portal vein. At least 50% of patients with this condition have other fetal anomalies as well. On sonography, the umbilical vein curves toward the left-sided stomach rather than toward the liver.

REFERENCES

1. Dudiak CM, Salomon CG, Posniak HV, Olson MC, Flisak ME: Sonography of the umbilical cord, *Radiographics* 15:1035-1050, 1995.
2. Sepulveda W, Peek MJ, Hassan J, Hollingsworth J: Umbilical vein to artery ratio in fetuses with single umbilical artery, *Ultrasound Obstet Gynecol* 8:23-26, 1996.

Amniotic Fluid, Fetal Membranes, and Fetal Hydrops

Mitzi Robert

OBJECTIVES

On completion of this chapter, you should be able to:
- Describe the derivation, production, and functions of amniotic fluid
- Discuss the methods for assessing amniotic fluid volume
- Determine abnormal volumes of amniotic fluid
- Discuss the etiology, prognosis, and clinical and sonographic findings of abnormal conditions of fetal membranes
- Define immune hydrops fetalis and nonimmune hydrops fetalis
- Identify the causes of hydrops and describe its sonographic features

OUTLINE

Amniotic fluid plays a vital role in fetal growth and serves several important functions during intrauterine life. Amniotic fluid allows the fetus to move freely within the amniotic cavity while maintaining intrauterine temperature and protecting the developing fetus from injury. Abnormalities of the fluid may interfere with normal fetal development and cause structural abnormalities, or may be an indirect sign of an underlying anomaly such as neural tube defect or gastrointestinal disorder. This section will focus on the production and sonographic patterns of amniotic fluid, assessment and disorders of amniotic fluid volume, and use of amniotic fluid volumes in the diagnosis of fetal disorders.

DERIVATION

The **amniotic cavity** forms early in fetal life and is filled with **amniotic fluid.** The fluid completely surrounds and protects the embryo and later, the fetus. Amniotic fluid is produced by the umbilical cord, the membranes, lungs, skin, and kidneys. The amount of amniotic fluid present at any one time reflects a balance between amniotic fluid production and amniotic fluid removal. The mechanisms of amniotic fluid production and consumption, and the composition and volume of amniotic fluid, depend on gestational age.

Early in gestation, the major source of amniotic fluid is the amniotic membrane, a thin membrane lined by a single layer of epithelial cells. During this stage of development, water crosses the membrane freely, and the production of amniotic fluid is accomplished by active transport of electrolytes and other solutes by the amnion, with passive diffusion of water following in response to osmotic pressure changes.

As the fetus and placenta mature, amniotic fluid production and consumption change. Changes include movement of fluid across the chorion frondosum and fetal skin, fetal urine output and fetal swallowing, and gastrointestinal absorption. The chorion frondosum, the portion of the chorion that develops into the fetal portion of the placenta, is a site where water is exchanged freely between fetal blood and amniotic fluid across the amnion. Fetal skin is also permeable to water and some solutes to permit direct exchange between the fetus and amniotic fluid until keratinization occurs between 24 and 26 weeks. Fetal production of urine and the ability to swallow begin between 8 and 11 weeks' gestation. The amount of urine produced is most significant at approximately 18 to 20 weeks' gestation. Fetal urination into the amniotic sac accounts for nearly the total volume of amniotic fluid by the second half of pregnancy, so the quantity of fluid is directly related to kidney function. Therefore, a fetus with malformed kidneys or renal agenesis is surrounded by little or no amniotic fluid. The fetus swallows amniotic fluid, which is absorbed by the digestive tract.

CHARACTERISTICS OF AMNIOTIC FLUID

Amniotic fluid performs the following six functions:

1. Acts as a cushion to protect the fetus
2. Allows embryonic and fetal movements
3. Prevents adherence of the amnion to the embryo
4. Allows symmetrical growth
5. Maintains a constant temperature
6. Acts as a reservoir to fetal metabolites before their excretion by the maternal system

Quantity of Fluid

The amount of amniotic fluid is regulated not only by the production of fluid but also by removal of the fluid by swallowing, by fluid exchange within the lungs, and by the membranes and cord (Figure 57-1). Normal lung

development depends critically on the exchange of amniotic fluid within the lungs. Inadequate lung development may occur when the amount of amniotic fluid is severely low, placing the fetus at high risk for developing small or hypoplastic lungs.

The volume of amniotic fluid increases progressively until about 33 weeks' gestation, with an average increment per week of 25 ml from the 11th to the 15th week, and 50 ml from the 15th to the 28th week of gestation. In the last trimester, the mean amniotic fluid volume does not change significantly (Box 57-1). The sonographer must be aware of the relative differences in amniotic fluid volume throughout pregnancy. During the second and early third trimesters of pregnancy, amniotic fluid appears to surround the fetus and should be readily visible. From 20 to 30 weeks' gestation, amniotic fluid may appear rather generous, although this typically represents a normal amniotic fluid variant. By the end of pregnancy, the amniotic fluid is scanty, and isolated fluid pockets may be the only visible areas of fluid. Toward the end of the pregnancy, at between 38 and 43 weeks' gestation, a general decline is seen in the amniotic fluid.

Sonographic Findings. Amniotic fluid generally appears echo-free, although occasionally echogenic fluid particles may be seen (Figure 57-2). The fluid particles may represent a normal variant, particulate matter, **vernix caseosa**, intra-amniotic blood, or intrauterine meconium passage. It should be noted that the term *amniotic sludge* has been used to describe a dense collection of echogenic particles within the fluid at the level of the cervix. The presence of sludge may be related to intrauterine infection and is associated with risk of preterm premature rupture of membranes, chorioamnionitis, and preterm delivery. In cases of intrauterine meconium passage, the amniotic fluid may take on a "snowstorm" appearance.

ASSESSMENT OF AMNIOTIC FLUID

In accordance with the guidelines for obstetric scanning, every obstetric examination should include a thorough evaluation of amniotic fluid volume. Abnormal amounts of amniotic fluid are described as hydramnios (polyhydramnios) and oligohydramnios. Hydramnios refers to an increase in amniotic fluid for gestational age, whereas

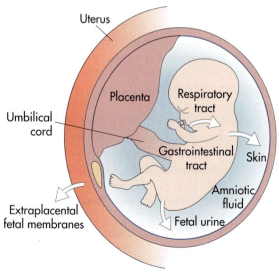

FIGURE 57-1 Schematic drawing of amniotic fluid formation.

Uterus

Placenta

Umbilical cord

Respiratory tract

Gastrointestinal tract

Skin

Amniotic fluid

Extraplacental fetal membranes

Fetal urine

BOX 57-1	Amniotic Fluid Volume Regulation

- Amniotic fluid volume increases rapidly during first trimester.
- Fetus swallows fluid, which is reabsorbed by gastrointestinal tract and recirculates through the kidneys.
- By 20 weeks' gestation, amniotic fluid volume increases by 10 ml/day.
- Amount of fluid produced by fetal urination slightly exceeds amount removed by fetal swallowing; >40% of fluid increase originates from other sources.

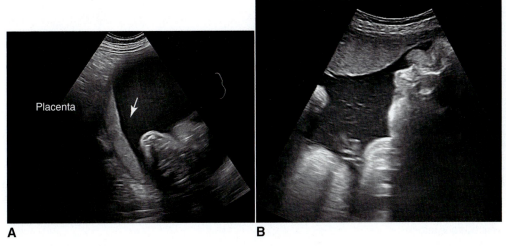

FIGURE 57-2 A, Amniotic fluid revealing echo-free fluid appearance and a flattened placenta due to polyhydramnios. **B,** At 37 weeks' gestation, the amniotic fluid is mixed with particulate matter or vernix.

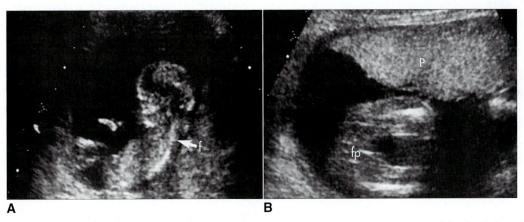

FIGURE 57-3 A, Amniotic fluid around a 13-week fetus in a sitting position. Note the hand in front of the fetal chest. Amniotic fluid appears in black. *f,* Fetus. **B,** Amniotic fluid around an 18-week fetus. The fetus appears to be surrounded by amniotic fluid *(black areas).* *P,* Placenta; *fp,* fetal pelvis.

oligohydramnios refers to a decreased amount of amniotic fluid. When extremes in amniotic fluid volume (hydramnios or oligohydramnios) are seen, targeted studies for the exclusion of fetal anomalies are recommended. In some instances, the abnormal fluid levels may be associated with maternal factors, unknown etiologies, or correlation with fetal weight (small for age fetus has decreased amniotic fluid, whereas large for age fetus has increased volume of fluid).

Several methods are used to calculate an amniotic fluid measurement. Each obstetric center may use one or a combination of these methods. Each department should have clear guidelines for sonographers to use when assessing amniotic fluid. These guidelines will aid in proper amniotic fluid assessments when multiple sonographers are monitoring the same patient.

Subjective Assessment

Subjective assessment is performed as the sonographer initially scans "through" the entire uterus to perform the visual "eye-ball" assessment of the fluid present, the lie of the fetus, and the position of the placenta (Figure 57-3). When amniotic fluid is assessed subjectively, decreased amniotic fluid is identified by an overall sense of crowding of the fetus and obvious lack of amniotic fluid and/or inability to identify any significant pockets of fluid in any sector of the uterus (Figure 57-4). Excessive fluid is defined subjectively when there is an obvious excess of fluid, the fetus appears in the most dependent portion of the uterus, or the fetus appears to move excessively for gestational age (Figure 57-5). This subjective assessment is more successful in the hands of experienced sonographers than in the hands of a beginner. Generally, this method will lead the sonographer to use a more quantitative method to document the amount of amniotic fluid present.

Amniotic Fluid Index

The **amniotic fluid index (AFI)** method is used most frequently for evaluating and quantifying amniotic fluid

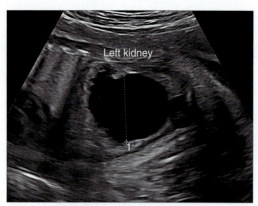

FIGURE 57-4 Obvious lack of fluid surrounding this 26-week fetus presenting with a bladder outlet obstruction. The left kidney is visualized with severe hydronephrosis.

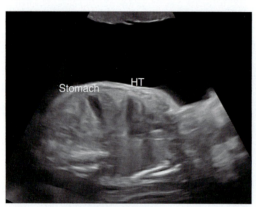

FIGURE 57-5 Fetus presents with severe polyhydramnios at 30 weeks' gestation. *HT,* heart.

volume at different intervals during a pregnancy. The AFI method is a valid and reproducible technique. With this method, the uterine cavity is divided into four equal quadrants by two imaginary lines perpendicular to each other (Figure 57-6). The largest vertical pocket of amniotic fluid, excluding fetal limbs or umbilical cord loops, is measured.

The sonographer should hold the transducer in the sagittal plane and perpendicular to the table (not the curved skin surface) when assessing these pockets of fluid. Each quadrant should be evaluated to reflect the most accurate display of fluid. The transducer should be moved until the cord loops and/or fetal limbs are not within the pocket of fluid (Figure 57-7). Care must be taken not to include the thickness of the maternal uterine wall in the measurement or to apply too much pressure to the skin, causing the pocket of fluid to appear smaller. Slight adjustment of the gain will aid in visualization of the uterine wall or of the umbilical cord within the fluid. Color Doppler technology can be used to document a pocket of fluid free of the umbilical cord or any fetal parts.

Normal values have been calculated for each gestational age (plus or minus 2 standard deviations). The

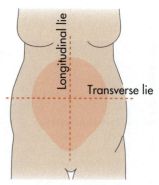

FIGURE 57-6 The amniotic cavity is divided into quadrants by two imaginary lines perpendicular to each other. The largest pocket of fluid is measured in each quadrant.

values are relatively stable after 20 weeks until the end of the third trimester. The AFI peaks late in the third trimester of pregnancy, with a rapid decline near term.

- Normal amniotic fluid correlates with AFI of 10 to 20 cm.
- Borderline values of 5 to 10 cm indicate low fluid, and values of 20 to 24 cm indicate increased fluid.
- Oligohydramnios correlates with an AFI of less than 5 cm, with the largest vertical pocket measuring 2 cm or less.
- Polyhydramnios correlates with an AFI of greater than 24 cm, with the largest vertical pocket measuring 8 cm or more.

Single-Pocket Assessment

The **maximum vertical pocket** assessment of amniotic fluid is done by identifying the largest pocket of amniotic fluid (Figure 57-8), which should measure greater than 1 cm. The pocket of fluid should be clear of fetal components and of the umbilical cord. As with the AFI, the gain should be adjusted for clear visualization of the uterine wall, and minimum pressure should be applied to the abdomen. The depth of the pocket is measured at right angles to the uterine contour and is placed into one of three categories:

1. Less than 2 cm, indicating oligohydramnios
2. 2 to 8 cm, indicating normal amniotic fluid
3. Greater than 8 cm, indicating polyhydramnios

As a general rule, the AFI may be approximated by multiplying the largest pocket of amniotic fluid times three.

Two-Diameter Pocket Assessment

The two-diameter pocket determination uses the largest pocket of amniotic fluid. Horizontal and vertical dimensions of the maximum vertical pocket are multiplied together to obtain a single volume. A two-diameter

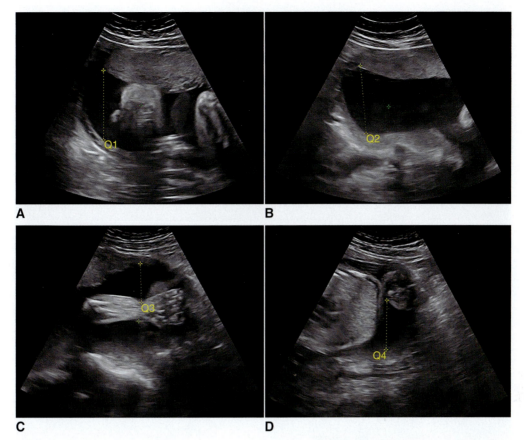

FIGURE 57-7 A through **D,** The deepest vertical pocket is measured in each quadrant free of any fetal components.

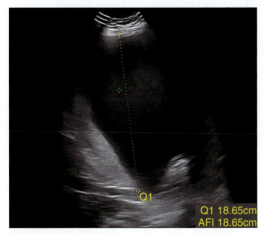

FIGURE 57-8 A single largest vertical pocket is noted, measuring 18.65 cm.

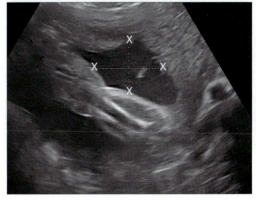

FIGURE 57-9 Demonstrates the two-diameter measurement technique.

pocket of 15 to 50 cm is considered normal (Figure 57-9).

Amniotic Fluid Assessment in Twin Pregnancies

In twin pregnancies, it is important to assess each sac independently when performing amniotic fluid determinations (Figure 57-10). Twin pregnancies have a slightly lower median AFI value than singleton pregnancies. The two-diameter pocket measurement appears to be a better predictor of oligohydramnios than the AFI or the largest vertical pocket. However, in cases of polyhydramnios, the largest vertical pocket has been reported to be more accurate (Figure 57-11). Although the AFI gives an overall assessment of the pregnancy, it does not accurately show differences between sacs. The only method used for accurately determining the amount of amniotic fluid is the dye-determined method, which can be used in singleton or multiple gestations. The dye technique

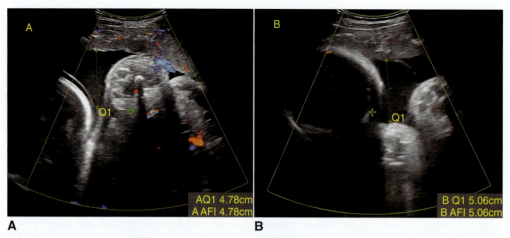

FIGURE 57-10 A, Measurement of the largest vertical pocket of fluid for Twin A. Color Doppler is used to ensure that the cord is not present within the pocket (+ indicates body of fetus A). **B,** Measurement of the largest vertical pocket of fluid for Twin B. Note the visualization of the dividing membrane (+ indicates head of fetus B).

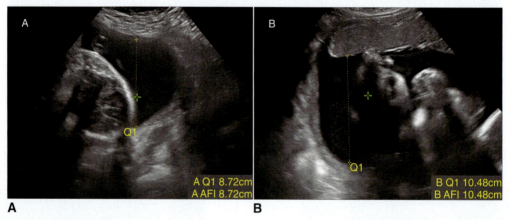

FIGURE 57-11 A and **B,** Single vertical pocket measurements are utilized in this twin pregnancy at 30 weeks' gestation with polyhydramnios.

requires injection of dye into the sac(s) via amniocentesis. After 20 minutes, another amniocentesis is performed, in which 1 ml of fluid greater than the injected dye is removed and frozen. Finally, the fluid/dye mixture is evaluated to identify the amount of concentrate that determines the amniotic fluid volume.

ABNORMAL AMNIOTIC FLUID VOLUMES

Polyhydramnios

Polyhydramnios (also known as *hydramnios*) is defined as an amniotic fluid volume of greater than 2000 ml. The finding of polyhydramnios is associated with increased perinatal mortality and morbidity and maternal complications. By clinical definition, polyhydramnios is an excessive amount of fluid that causes the uterine size to be larger than expected for gestational dates. Often the patient will present for a sonographic examination with the clinical finding of uterus larger than dates (rule out multiple gestation, molar pregnancy, or fetal size greater than dates).

Etiology. The amniotic fluid compartment is in dynamic equilibrium with the fetal and maternal compartments. In polyhydramnios, the equilibrium shifts so that a net transfer of water into the amniotic space occurs. As discussed earlier, many factors are involved in the regulation of amniotic fluid volume (e.g., swallowing, urination, uterine-placental blood flow, fetal respiratory movements, fetal membrane physiology).

Clinical Findings. Increased amniotic fluid volume produces uterine stretching and enlargement that may lead to preterm labor and various other maternal symptoms. In addition, acute onset of hydramnios may be painful, compress other organs or vascular structures, cause hydronephrosis of the kidneys, or produce shortness of breath from compression of the organs on the diaphragm.

Often polyhydramnios may be diagnosed sonographically before it is clinically suspected. Chronic hydramnios characteristically develops between the 28th week of gestation and term. Polyhydramnios may develop acutely over a few days or chronically over weeks. Acute polyhydramnios occurs in the second trimester and accounts for only 2% of cases. Usually, the cause of acute polyhydramnios is twin–twin transfusion syndrome; however, other congenital anomalies may be responsible.

Polyhydramnios is often associated with central nervous system disorders and/or gastrointestinal problems. Central nervous system disorders cause depressed swallowing. With gastrointestinal abnormalities, a blockage (atresia) of the esophagus, stomach, duodenum, or small bowel often results in ineffective swallowing. Fetal hydrops, skeletal anomalies, and some renal disorders (usually unilateral) may also be associated with hydramnios. Other forms of polyhydramnios that cannot be explained by congenital anomalies are considered idiopathic (Box 57-2). Maternal conditions such as diabetes mellitus, obesity, Rhesus incompatibility, anemia, congestive cardiac failure, and syphilis have been associated with polyhydramnios.

Prognosis. Once polyhydramnios has been diagnosed, the prognosis for pregnancy is guarded. Perinatal mortality and morbidity are increased, as are maternal morbidity and mortality. The mother has an increased risk of developing pregnancy-induced hypertension, preterm labor, or postpartum hemorrhage. Other conditions associated with increased amniotic fluid volume include maternal diabetes mellitus, fetal macrosomia, and Rh

---

BOX 57-2 | Congenital Anomalies Associated With Polyhydramnios

Gastrointestinal System
Esophageal atresia and/or tracheoesophageal fistula
Duodenal atresia
Jejunoileal atresia
Gastroschisis
Omphalocele
Diaphragmatic hernia
Meckel's diverticulum
Congenital megacolon
Meconium peritonitis
Annular pancreas
Pancreatic cyst

Head and Neck
Cystic hygroma
Goiter
Cleft palate
Epignathus

Respiratory System
Cystic adenomatoid malformation
Congenital hydrothorax
Extralobar sequestration
Primary pulmonary hypoplasia
Congenital pulmonary lymphangiectasia
Pulmonary cyst
Asphyxiating thoracic dystrophy

Cardiovascular System
Arrhythmias
Coarctation of the aorta
Myxomas and hemangiomas
Ectopia cordis
Cardiac tumor
Heart anomaly with hydrops

Central Nervous System
Anencephaly
Hydrocephaly
Microcephaly
Iniencephaly
Hydranencephaly
Holoprosencephaly
Encephalocele
Spina bifida
Dandy-Walker malformation

Genitourinary System
Ureteropelvic junction obstruction
Posterior urethral valves
Urethral stenosis
Multicystic kidney disease
Large ovarian cyst
Mesoblastic nephroma
Bartter syndrome
Megacystis microcolon hypoperistalsis syndrome

Skeletal System
Thanatophoric dwarf
Camptomelic dwarf
Osteogenesis imperfecta
Heterozygous achondroplasia
Arthrogryposis multiplex
Klippel-Feil syndrome
Nager acrofacial dysostosis
Achondrogenesis

Congenital Infections
Cytomegalovirus
Toxoplasmosis
Listeriosis
Congenital hepatitis

Miscellaneous
Sacrococcygeal teratoma
Cranial teratoma
Cervical teratoma
Congenital sarcoma
Placental chorioangioma
Cavernous hemangioma
Metastatic neuroblastoma
Myotonic dystrophy
Fetal acetaminophen toxicity
Retroperitoneal fibrosis
Multisystem anomalies
Pena-Shokeir syndrome
Cutaneous vascular hemarthrosis
Twin reversed arterial perfusion sequence/acardiac anomaly

From Nyberg DA, Mahony BS, Pretorius DH: *Diagnostic ultrasound of fetal anomalies: text and atlas,* St Louis, 1990, Mosby.

isoimmunization. Diabetes mellitus is associated with an increased frequency of hydramnios and represents the most common maternal cause of elevated amniotic fluid volume, especially when poorly controlled.

Sonographic Findings. Serial sonographic examinations are indicated to monitor the progression of amniotic fluid. Because amniotic fluid production is a dynamic process, changing maternal, fetal, or placenta conditions may dramatically affect the volume index.

Visual criteria for polyhydramnios include an obvious discrepancy between the size of the fetus, the size of the uterus, and the amount of amniotic fluid. During the second trimester, the amniotic fluid completely surrounds the fetus; however, as the pregnancy progresses, the fetal parts consume the majority of the uterine space; therefore the amount of amniotic fluid appears to be less than in the first and second trimesters. Serial scans may be necessary when the amniotic fluid appears to be more generous than normal at a particular gestational age. Sonographic signs of polyhydramnios are as follows:

- Appearance of a freely floating fetus within the swollen amniotic cavity (the fetus commonly will be seen lying on his or her back, while freely moving in the amniotic fluid)
- Accentuated fetal anatomy as increased amniotic fluid improves image resolution
- AFI equal to or greater than 20 cm

Polyhydramnios may be further defined as mild when the single largest pocket is greater than 8 cm; moderate, when greater than 12 cm; and severe, when greater than 16 cm. The AFI may also be further qualified as mild polyhydramnios, greater than 20 cm; moderate, greater than 24 cm; and severe, greater than 25 cm (Figure 57-12).

Oligohydramnios

Oligohydramnios is an overall reduction in the amount of amniotic fluid, resulting in fetal crowding and decreased fetal movement. The incidence of oligohydramnios is estimated to be between 0.5% and 5.5% of all pregnancies, depending on the population tested and the criteria used for diagnosis.

Etiology. The development of oligohydramnios may be attributed to one of five causes: congenital anomalies (Box 57-3), intrauterine growth restriction, postterm pregnancies, ruptured membranes, and iatrogenesis. Second-trimester oligohydramnios is associated with a poor prognosis, especially if the maternal serum alpha-fetoprotein level is concurrently elevated. Maternal conditions associated with oligohydramnios include hypertension, preeclampsia, chronic cardiac or renal disease, connective tissue disorders, and treatment with indomethacin.

Clinical Findings. The association of intrauterine growth restriction (IUGR) with decreased amniotic fluid (oligohydramnios) is well recognized. Fetal hypoxemia may produce growth restriction and oligohydramnios. A fourfold increased risk of growth delay is seen when oligohydramnios is present. Doppler evaluation of the growth-restricted fetus shows abnormal umbilical flow in patients with oligohydramnios.

Placental insufficiency may cause IUGR associated with oligohydramnios. Placental insufficiency causes redistribution of fetal blood flow away from the kidneys and toward the brain to counterattack the hypoxia. This results in decreased urine output, which decreases fluid volume.

The postterm pregnancy is defined as a gestational age of 42 or more weeks. Oligohydramnios is a common complication of postdate pregnancies (remember the decrease in amniotic fluid production near the end of pregnancy) and is associated with diminished placental function. It is also associated with arterial redistribution of fetal blood flow with a brain-sparing effect.

Iatrogenic causes of oligohydramnios include medications, insensible fluid loss, maternal intravascular fluid depletion, and prior procedures such as chorionic villous sampling. Medications associated with oligohydramnios include nonsteroidal anti-inflammatory drugs, angiotensin-converting enzyme inhibitors, calcium

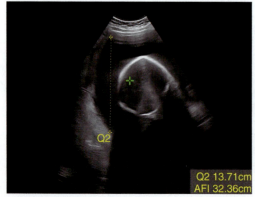

Q2 13.71cm
AFI 32.36cm

FIGURE 57-12 Fetus presenting at 29 weeks' gestation with duodenal atresia. The single vertical pocket measurement of 13.71 cm suggests polyhydramnios. An amniotic fluid index (AFI) measurement of 32.36 cm supports the findings (+ indicates fetal head).

BOX 57-3	Causes of Oligohydramnios

Nonanomalous Conditions
Intrauterine growth restriction
Premature rupture of membranes
Postdate pregnancy (42 weeks)
Chorionic villous sampling

Fetal Anomalous Conditions
Infantile polycystic kidney disease
Renal agenesis
Posterior urethral valve syndrome
Dysplastic kidneys
Chromosomal abnormalities

channel blockers, and nitrous oxide. The nonsteroidal drugs are prostaglandin synthetase inhibitors that inhibit renal vascular flow and decrease glomerular filtration. The angiotensin-converting enzyme inhibitors reduce fetal blood pressure and decrease renal perfusion.

Prognosis. The development of oligohydramnios may cause potential complications, such as fetal demise, pulmonary hypoplasia, and various skeletal and facial deformities resulting from compression of the fetus on the uterine wall. Fetal deformations, such as clubbing of the hands or feet, pulmonary hypoplasia, hip displacement, and phenotypical features of Potter's sequence have been reported. The fetus that presents with oligohydramnios in the second trimester has a higher prevalence of structural malformations than the fetus that presents in the third trimester.

Persistent oligohydramnios in the second trimester carries a poor prognosis, regardless of the cause. Severe oligohydramnios with a single-pocket measurement of less than 1 cm lasting 14 days after spontaneous premature rupture of the membranes at less than 25 weeks' gestation is associated with an extremely high mortality rate.

Maternal hydration has been shown to improve amniotic fluid for patients with oligohydramnios and in women with normal amniotic fluid volumes. If fetal anomalies or premature ruptured membranes are present, maternal hydration will have little effect. One study was conducted to see if maternal hydration would increase the AFI in women with low AFI values. The control group was instructed to drink a normal amount of fluid; the hydration group was instructed to drink 2 L of water, in addition to the usual amount of fluid, 2 to 4 hours before the posttreatment AFI was determined. The mean posttreatment AFI was significantly greater in the hydration group. Findings suggested that maternal oral hydration increased the amniotic fluid volume in women with decreased fluid levels.

⬛ **Sonographic Findings.** Criteria for oligohydramnios are based on subjective experience and estimations of the AFI. Oligohydramnios may be defined as a single pocket of fluid with a depth of less than 2 cm or an AFI of less than 5 cm. A gray zone for decreased fluid ranges from 5 to 9 cm when a four-quadrant approach is used. Poor scanning resolution is common in pregnancies complicated by oligohydramnios, and limited anatomy surveys are expected (Figure 57-13). The sonographer should consider examining the fetus with transvaginal sonography to better define fetal anatomy in efforts to detect the anomaly causing the oligohydramnios.

If intrauterine membranes are not ruptured and oligohydramnios is present before 28 weeks' gestation, the fetal renal system should be carefully evaluated by the sonographer to rule out renal agenesis, infantile polycystic disease, or posterior urethral valve syndrome. If oligohydramnios is severe in a fetus with posterior urethral valves, the prognosis is not good. The renal area may be

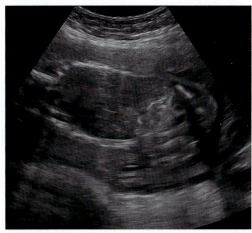

FIGURE 57-13 Fetal anatomy is difficult to evaluate owing to oligohydramnios.

difficult to identify in the presence of severe oligohydramnios, and the use of color Doppler to demarcate the renal arteries may be helpful for the sonographer in determining whether or not the kidneys are present.

In the presence of oligohydramnios, care should be taken when evaluating fetal growth parameters, because the fetal head and abdomen can be compressed when the fluid level is low. The fetus lacks surrounding fluid to protect it; therefore, circumferences can actually be inaccurately measured because of increased transducer pressure on the maternal abdomen. This pressure, in turn, may alter the estimated fetal weight through erroneous measurements. Evaluation of blood flow in the umbilical cord, the placenta, and the cerebrovascular system with color and Doppler techniques is critical in determining the presence or absence of intrauterine growth retardation.

FETAL MEMBRANES

The primary fetal membranes are the amnion and chorion. The chorion is derived from the outer layer of the developing blastocyst, specifically, the chorion levae and the chorion frondosum. The amnion is derived from the inner cell mass of the blastocyst and is attached to the embryonic disk at the insertion of the umbilical cord. The chorionic membrane is always in contact with the developing decidua and is separated from the amnion by fluid early in embryonic development (Figure 57-14). The amniotic membrane is very thin (.02 and .5 mm) and echogenic. It is seen most often as a small line, although under certain circumstances, it may appear as a circular membrane surrounding the embryo (Figure 57-15). The amnion can be visualized within the chorionic cavity with transvaginal sonography between 4 and 5 weeks' gestation. The amnion will grow approximately 1 mm per day and will fuse with the chorion between 12 and 16 weeks' gestation (Figure 57-16). Fusion results in development of the amniotic cavity (bag of water)

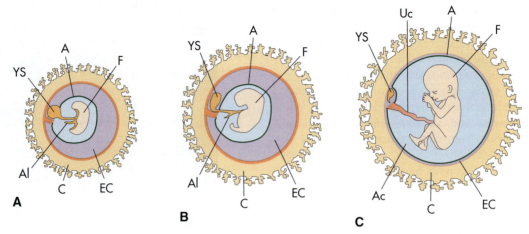

FIGURE 57-14 A, Four weeks' gestation. The amnion is formed from cells found on the interior of the developing cell mass that is to become the fetus and placenta. *F,* Fetus; *YS,* yolk sac; *C,* chorion; *Al,* allantois; *A,* amnion; *EC,* extraembryonic coelom. **B,** Six weeks' gestation. **C,** Eight weeks' gestation. *Ac,* Amniotic cavity; *Uc,* umbilical cord

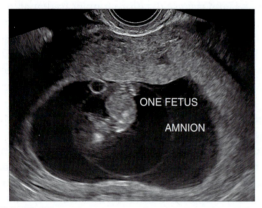

FIGURE 57-15 Transverse scan demonstrating the amnion dividing the amniotic cavity and the chorionic cavity at 10 weeks' gestation.

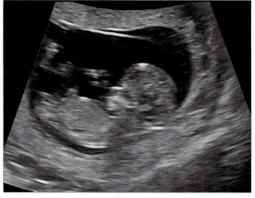

FIGURE 57-16 In this image of a 12-week fetus, the amnion can be seen as an echogenic line unattached from the chorion anteriorly.

surrounded by the chorioamniotic membrane. Abnormalities involving the fetal membranes can occur at multiple points in the pregnancy. It is important for sonographers to evaluate the membranes, differentiate membranes from abnormalities, and identify abnormalities associated with disruption in the membranes.

Ruptured Fetal Membranes

The tissue of the chorioamniotic membrane (fused chorion and amnion) is composed of several types of cells. The integrity and makeup of the cells aid in determination of the strength of the membrane. Under normal conditions, the chorioamniotic membranes rupture as the result of normal cell death activation of enzymes and mechanical forces. Normally, the membranes will rupture after the onset of labor. **Premature rupture of membranes (PROM)**, **preterm premature rupture of membranes (PPROM)**, and **spontaneous premature rupture of membranes (SPROM)** describe conditions in which the mem-

branes rupture ("water breaks") abnormally, resulting in loss of amniotic fluid and/or oligohydramnios.

Etiology. Rupture of membranes too soon, prior to labor, or at both times has numerous causes. It may result from normal cell death, activation of enzymes, or mechanical forces present, just as in normal cases. However, multiple underlying pathologic processes have been associated with abnormal ruptured membranes. Research has indicated that several other factors may play a role in increasing the risk of abnormal ruptured membranes. These risks include smoking, history of sexually transmitted disease, African American descent, vaginal bleeding, previous preterm delivery, lower socioeconomic status, presence of intrauterine infection, and pregnancy-related invasive procedures.

Clinical Findings. Patients suspected of having rupture of the membranes (ROM) present clinically with sudden gushing or leaking of fluid. Upon physical examination, a nitrazine paper and fern test is used as a screening tool to assess for the presence of amniotic fluid in vaginal secretions. The patient is also checked for cervical dilatation, as well as leaking of fluid with coughing or fundal pressure. It has been documented that an amniocentesis may be performed to inject an indigo carmine dye into the amniotic sac. If the membranes are truly ruptured, the patient will leak blue dye from the vagina. To estimate the amount of amniotic fluid present and to evaluate fetal well-being, a sonogram is performed.

Prognosis. The prognosis of a fetus affected by abnormal ruptured membranes is dependent on fetal gestational age, fetal status, and the ability to control uterine contractions. In general, abnormal rupture of the membranes is associated with preterm delivery (common), fetal and neonatal death, neonatal respiratory distress, prolapsed umbilical cord, chorioamnionitis, and placental abruption. It has been found that approximately one third of all preterm births are associated with PROM.

Pregnancy management for patients presenting with ROM includes hospitalization, fetal monitoring (nonstress test and biophysical profile [BPP]), bed rest, administration of antibiotics (for **chorioamnionitis**), and **corticosteroid therapy**. Although variations in treatment occur among patients presenting with ROM, pregnancy management may include the following:

- Delivery is indicated with active labor, consistent abnormal fetal heart tracings, evidence of amniotic infection, placental abruption, or prolapsed cord.
- If rupture of the membranes occurs at 24 to 33 weeks' gestation, the follow-up procedure includes administration of corticosteroids and antibiotics and delivery at approximately 34 weeks' gestation.
- An amniocentesis is performed to verify fetal lung maturity in cases in which the fetus needs to be delivered before 34 weeks' gestation.
- If the fetus is between 34 and 36 weeks' gestation, antibiotics are usually given, followed by delivery.
- It is common for term patients who experience ROM to move into active labor within 24 hours.

Sonographic Findings. The role of sonography in patients presenting with ROM includes documenting the integrity of the placenta, fetal size, amniotic fluid volume, fetal well-being, and fetal Doppler studies. The information gathered is important in determining pregnancy management. Not all patients with ROM will present for sonography; however, it is common for patients to be evaluated every day to assess fetal well-being and fluid volumes.

The integrity of the placenta, fetal growth, and the BPP should be evaluated. Placental abruption is associated with ROM. Sonographers should pay close attention to the retroplacental complex and the anterior/posterior diameter of the placenta. The sonographic appearance of abruptions will vary, but a few key findings may be helpful in identifying abruption. These findings include areas of increased diameter, areas of questionable echo-genicity, an interrupted retroplacental complex, and an abnormal continuum of the attachment of the placenta to the uterine wall. Placental location is important when documenting the integrity of the placenta. Abnormal location of the placenta such as circumvallate placenta is associated with placental abruption and oligohydramnios. Documentation of the placenta should be followed by fetal growth measurements. Sonography is not reliable in determining fetal growth from day to day; it is usually most reliable when measurements are taken at 2-week intervals. Initial weight and age estimations provided by sonography will help physicians plan pregnancy management and will help them be prepared to provide to the mother and other health care providers vital information for delivery preparation. The longer the pregnancy can be maintained, the more sonography can aid in providing fetal growth information. Along with evaluating the placenta and fetal growth, assessing fetal well-being plays a significant role in the management of pregnancy. Fetal well-being should be evaluated sonographically by performing a BPP. These tests are usually done daily to monitor the fetus for amniotic fluid volumes, fetal breathing movements, fetal tone, and fetal gross body movements. Abnormal results or sudden changes may indicate fetal distress, thus changing the course of pregnancy management.

Patients diagnosed with ROM may present with oligohydramnios. Oligohydramnios may be defined as a single pocket of fluid with a depth of less than 2 cm, or an AFI of less than 5 cm (Figure 57-17). It has been noted that patients presenting with less than 2 cm of fluid have been diagnosed with intrauterine infections. Although the significance of infection is increased in patients with severe oligohydramnios, other findings should be considered. Other findings associated with intrauterine infection or chorioamnionitis include changes in fetal heart rate (tachycardia) and fetal behavioral states (specifically, lack of fetal breathing). One should also note that maternal clinical symptoms may be present. These symptoms include fever, tachycardia, tender uterus, possible abnormal white blood cell count, and abnormal vaginal discharge.

Color and spectral Doppler are used to indicate alterations in blood flow that can help determine the degree of fetal distress. Umbilical artery, umbilical vein, middle cerebral artery, and ductus venosus blood flow aid in determining fetal distress. In cases of ROM, fetuses are at risk for umbilical cord compression or prolapse. These conditions may be indicated first by variable decelerations on fetal heart monitor tracings, as well as lack of fetal movement reported by the mother. The use of color and spectral Doppler can provide information regarding blood perfusion in the fetus. If compression or prolapsed cord is evident, an amnioinfusion (saline is injected directly into amniotic sac) may be helpful in decompressing the cord. However, if the fetus is in continued distress, delivery is indicated.

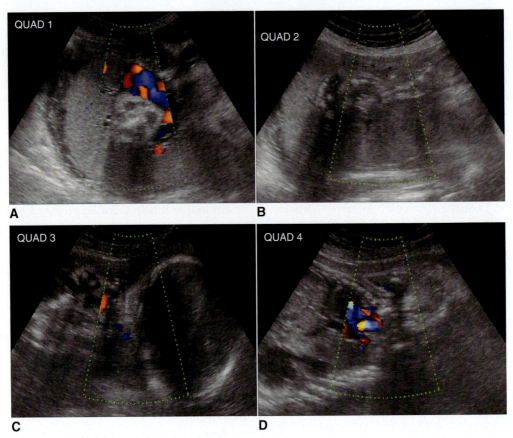

FIGURE 57-17 A through **D,** Patient presents at 30 weeks' gestation with rupture of membranes (ROM). Amniotic fluid index (AFI) reveals severe oligohydramnios. Color Doppler was used to ensure that the anechoic fetal cord was not misrepresented as fluid.

Amniotic Band Syndrome

Amniotic band syndrome (ABS) is associated with an abnormality in the fetal membranes. It is a common, nonrecurrent cause of various fetal malformations involving the limbs, craniofacial region, and trunk. Numerous synonyms have been documented to describe the disruption of fetal tissue due to the presence of amniotic bands. Some of these terms include *ADAM complex* (amniotic deformities, adhesion, mutilation), *amniotic band sequence, aberrant tissue bands,* and *congenital constricting bands.*

Etiology. The most widely accepted theory for the formation of amniotic bands is that rupture of the amnion during early pregnancy leads to subsequent entanglement of various embryonic or fetal parts by fibrous mesodermic bands, which emanate from the chorionic side of the amnion. Entrapment of fetal parts by the bands may cause lymphedema, amputation, or slash defects in nonembryologic distributions. The amnion, which is contiguous with the fetal skin at the umbilicus, is thought to protect the fetus from contact with the chorion. When disruption of the amnion occurs, the fetus may adhere to and fuse with the chorion, with subsequent maldevelopment of subjacent fetal tissue. This theory suggests that when gastroschisis results in exteriorization of the liver, the amniotic band syndrome

should be strongly considered. Rupture of the amnion may be associated with exposure to teratogens, genetic factors, multifactorial conditions, chorionic villous sampling, and amniocentesis. However, the exact etiology is unknown.

Clinical Findings. Various congenital malformation syndromes are thought to be caused by compression of the fetus by "amniotic bands"; this results in developmental abnormalities or fetal death. Amniotic band syndrome may represent a milder form of limb–body wall complex and may be predicted by amniotic bands (fibrous tissue strands) that entangle or amputate fetal parts. Facial clefts, asymmetrical encephaloceles, constriction or amputation defects of the extremities, and clubfoot deformities are common findings. The site where the amniotic band cuts across the fetus is usually evident after birth.

Prognosis. The prognosis of a fetus diagnosed with amniotic band syndrome is dependent on the extent of the malformations. Minor soft tissue malformations or lethal malformations may be present. Patients should be counseled on all malformations identified and should be given appropriate options. In some cases, intrauterine fetal surgery to remove the bands is an option. These cases are typically limited to fetuses in which the benefit of the surgery outweighs the risks. It is common for bands to be found around upper and lower extremities.

If Doppler evaluation indicates that the band is constricting blood flow to a portion of an extremity, endoscopic intrauterine surgical removal (intrauterine lysis) of the band may be performed to avoid limb dysfunction or amputation.

Sonographic Findings. Sonography can be very useful in determining the extent of malformation of a fetus affected by amniotic band syndrome; however, it should be noted that research indicates that minor deformities may be identified only after birth. Sonographers first should be suspicious of the abnormality if echogenic bands are present within the amniotic cavity (Figure 57-18). Following the band closely with real-time scanning will allow the sonographer to observe where the band is attached to the uterine wall and what, if any, constriction is placed on the fetus (Figure 57-19). Moreover, careful observation with real-time scanning lets the sonographer observe whether the fetus is free from the band, or if movement is restricted. All extremities and all soft tissues should be closely evaluated to identify whether interference of fetal development or amputation has occurred. Entanglement of the bands around soft tissue is usually seen as an indentation of the soft tissue surrounded by edema (Figure 57-20). Use of three-dimensional sonography and advanced techniques has helped to improve the visualization of bony and soft tissue malformations (Figure 57-21). Other malformations include anencephaly, exencephaly, gastroschisis, limb or digit amputation, facial clefts, encephaloceles, and any slash defect.

Amniotic Sheets

Amniotic sheets, shelves, or folds are identified as echogenic nonfloating bands that cross through the amniotic cavity. They are thicker than bands associated with amniotic band syndrome, do not cause fetal malformations, and most likely signify uterine synechiae.

Etiology. Visible amniotic sheets are believed to be caused by uterine scars (**synechiae**) from previous instrumentation used in the uterus (usually curettage), cesarean section, or episodes of endometritis. When pregnancy begins to progress in the uterine cavity, expanding membranes encounter the scar and wrap around it. The flat

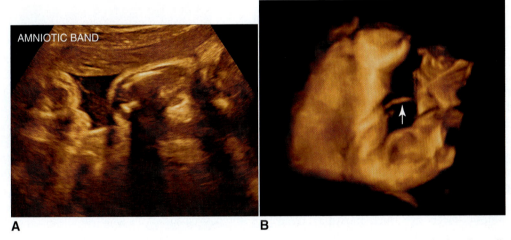

FIGURE 57-18 A, An echogenic band is noted floating in the amniotic fluid. The echogenic band was attached to the wall of the gestational sac. **B,** Three-dimensional imaging with reformatting demonstrates the band (*arrow*).

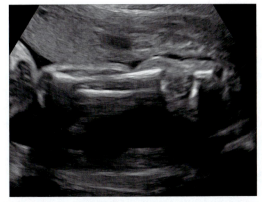

FIGURE 57-19 In the same patient seen in Figure 57-18, the band was followed through the sac and appeared to be attached to the right forearm.

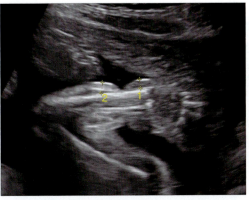

FIGURE 57-20 Soft tissue edema is seen in the forearm, where the band is constricting the soft tissue.

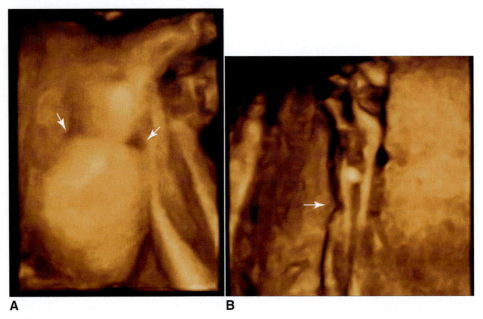

A   **B**

FIGURE 57-21 A, Constriction of the soft tissue is easily seen upon four-dimensional evaluation (*arrows*). **B,** Additional rendering of the three-dimensional image demonstrates the depth of the constricted soft tissue as it relates to the ulna and radius of the forearm (*arrow*).

portion of the sheet consists of apposed layers of chorion and amnion. The free edge of the sheet is defined by the course of the synechia itself, which may produce a bulbous appearance. Amniotic sheets arise because of redundant amnion-chorion, which, in turn, may be related to bleeding and subchorionic hemorrhage.

Clinical Findings. Patients with a history of endometrial dilatation and curettage (D&C), intrauterine infection, endometritis, removal of fibroids or endometrial polyps, or prior cesarean section are at risk for the development of uterine scars (synechiae). Synechiae have been associated with infertility and miscarriage. Patients who present with uterine synechiae and infertility are often diagnosed with **Asherman's syndrome.**

Prognosis. Amniotic sheets are thick muscular tissue bands that are not associated with fetal malformations. Surgical removal of the scars may be indicated for those patients with recurrent pregnancy loss or infertility.

▶ **Sonographic Findings.** Sonographic findings in patients with amniotic sheets may show a fine echo-dense line in the uterine cavity separated from the uterine wall by an echolucent space. The membrane may completely surround the fetus, or the membrane may be freely mobile in the amniotic cavity. The membranes can appear anywhere in the uterine or cervical cavity. They may be seen extending from one side of the uterus to the other, oblique across the uterus, or as multiple echogenic lines (Figure 57-22). Color and spectral Doppler can be used to aid in visualization and documentation of maternal blood flow within the synechiae. Amniotic sheets are present in 0.6% of patients undergoing screening obstetric ultrasound examinations. Care should be taken to separate the diagnosis of amniotic sheets from amniotic bands or circumvallate placenta. In circumvallate pla-

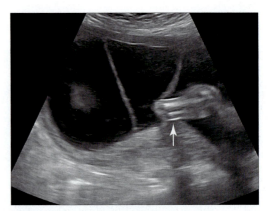

FIGURE 57-22 Twenty-two week fetus. Two echogenic uterine synechiae are seen within the anechoic amniotic sac. Note the fetal arm pushing against the synechiae (*arrow*).

centa, the chorion and the attached amnion form a raised ridge of tissue at the junction of the chorion and the basal plate. Beyond this ridge, normal vessels on the fetal surface are absent; after delivery, these redundant membranes are described as being adherent to the fetal surface, rather than projecting from it.

Both the circumvallate placenta and amniotic sheets appear as a thick membrane projecting into the amniotic fluid. Circumvallate placental membranes originate from the edge of the fetal surface of the placenta, whereas amniotic sheets attach to the uterine wall itself.

HYDROPS FETALIS

In cases of **hydrops fetalis,** a disparity is seen between the amount of serous fluid being produced and the amount being absorbed. This disparity leads to the accumulation of fluid or edema within a fetus in at least two areas. Edema can manifest as pleural effusions, ascites, cardiac effusion, skin edema, or anasarca. Other fetal findings seen with hydrops include an enlarged umbilical cord, polyhydramnios, placental edema, and an enlarged liver and spleen. The fetus and the mother can be affected by the presence of fetal hydrops. In many cases, fetal hydrops is highly associated with mortality. Diagnosis and determination of cause are essential in providing proper pregnancy management. Hydrops is categorized as immune-related and non–immune-related. Sonographically, hydrops is identified by the presence of abnormal collections of fluid.

- **Ascites** can be seen as anechoic fluid surrounding abdominal and pelvic organs and the umbilical cord insertion (common site of early ascites) (Figure 57-23). Careful attention should be paid to avoid mistaking normal hypoechoic abdominal musculature for ascites (pseudoascites).
- **Pleural effusion** can be seen as anechoic fluid filling the thoracic cavity or outlining the fetal lungs (Figure 57-24).
- Skin edema can occur as increased skin thickening around the skull, neck, extremities, or abdomen. In

some reports, a measurement of greater than 5 to 6 mm for soft tissue thickness is utilized for diagnosis. When skin edema is massive, encasing most of the body, the term *anasarca* is typically used to describe the condition (Figure 57-25).
- **Pericardial effusion** is seen as excess anechoic fluid in the pericardial cavity. Normally, a small amount of fluid is noted in this cavity, particularly in the apex. However, if the fluid collection measures greater than 2 mm, pericardial effusion is considered (Figure 57-26).
- Placental edema can be identified as a thickened placenta measuring greater than 4 to 4.5 cm in true anterior/posterior diameter.

Maternal clinical presentations in most cases include those associated with polyhydramnios. Symptoms include preterm labor, PPROM, and supine hypotension syndrome. In a few cases, maternal clinical symptoms may mimic the clinical features of the hydropic fetus. This is known as mirror syndrome, Ballantyne syndrome,

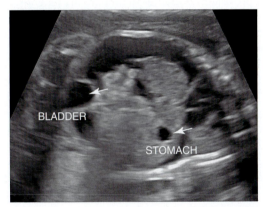

FIGURE 57-23 Ascites is noted in this fetus throughout the abdominopelvic cavity.

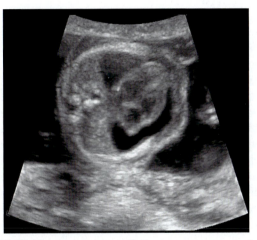

FIGURE 57-24 Bilateral pleural effusions are seen surrounding the heart and lungs.

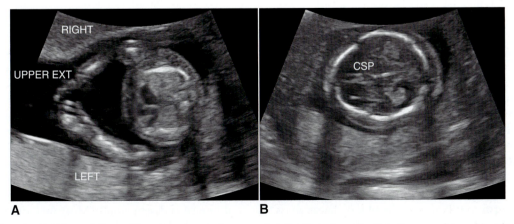

FIGURE 57-25 A, In this 16-week fetus, skin edema is noted surrounding the thoracic cavity. **B,** In the same fetus, skin edema is also noted surrounding the skull.

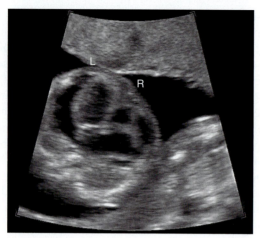

FIGURE 57-26 Pericardial effusions are identified around the abnormal fetal heart.

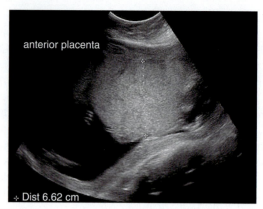

FIGURE 57-27 A thickened placenta is identified in a fetus with hydrops. The anterior-posterior diameter of the placenta measured 6.62 cm.

or pseudotoxemia. The mother will exhibit features of edema, rapid weight gain, hypertension, and mild proteinuria.

Immune Hydrops

Immune hydrops fetalis (IHF) is associated with alloimmune hemolytic disease (erythroblastosis fetalis) or rhesus (Rh) isoimmunization. Maternal blood sampling and a history of a previously affected fetus is extremely important for pregnancy management.

Etiology. Because immune hydrops is associated with Rh isoimmunization (sensitization or development of antibodies), blood serum tests are taken from the mother for evaluation of antibodies and blood typing. Maternal blood tests involve evaluating the blood for the presence of Rh-D antigen (positive blood grouping) or the absence of Rh-D antigen (negative blood grouping). The risk of isoimmunization is not apparent when the mother's blood test results indicate the Rh-D positive blood group. However, patients presenting with Rh-D negative blood grouping are at risk for developing antibodies that can attack a fetus that is Rh-D positive. The production of antibodies contributes to fetal anemia progressing into immune hydrops. This typically occurs with the second and subsequent pregnancies because of the lack of sufficient quantities of the Rh-antigen to stimulate the maternal immune system.

The risk of development of hydrops in the second and subsequent pregnancies is increased owing to the formation of immunoglobulin G (IgG) antibody during the first pregnancy. The IgG antibody was produced by the maternal lymphocytes formed during the first pregnancy to recognize Rh-D antigen. If maternal serum blood tests indicate a positive IgG antibody, further evaluation of blood titers is required. Blood titers aid in determining the levels of specific antibodies in the blood. These titers are evaluated multiple times throughout the pregnancy to determine whether IgG has crossed into the fetus and

is destroying fetal blood cells. If at any point the titer results are greater than 1:16, an amniocentesis is performed to evaluate for fetal anemia and to assess the severity of fetal hemolysis.

It should be noted that multiple types of blood compatibilities and alloimmunizations are present, other than those listed previously. It is important for sonographers to understand the possible sonographic features and appropriate follow-up in all patients diagnosed with a form of Rh incompatibility.

Prognosis. In general, the diagnosis of Rh incompatibility, fetal anemia, or hemolytic disorders is associated with high prenatal and perinatal morbidity. Few treatments and preventive measures can be used to reduce poor fetal outcomes. For instance if maternal blood serum indicates an Rh-D negative blood group, the mother should be given an anti-D immunoglobulin such as Rhogam to protect the Rh-positive fetus from Rh-negative maternal antibodies. The medication is usually given at around 28 weeks' gestation and has proved successful in decreasing perinatal mortality and morbidity. In cases in which severe fetal anemia is diagnosed, intrauterine blood transfusions are given to help correct the anemia. Research has shown that fetuses treated with blood transfusions before the onset of hydrops have an increased survival rate compared with those in whom hydrops has developed.

Sonographic Findings. Sonography reveals evidence of ascites, pleural effusion, and/or skin edema. Other findings include a thickened placenta and hydramnios (Figure 57-27). Fetal ascites may be the first fluid collection seen within the fetus (Figure 57-28). In addition to gray-scale imaging, spectral Doppler analysis of the middle cerebral artery (MCA) should be used to monitor the fetus for anemia. Doppler evaluation of the MCA includes recording peak velocity measurements of the artery. The artery should be sampled at the proximal end and at a zero-degree angle. Most facilities obtain velocities from the MCA in closest proximity to the transducer. It should be noted that research has provided support

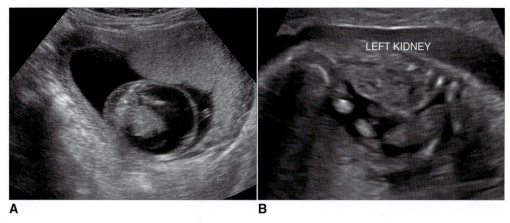

FIGURE 57-28 A, Massive ascites is seen surrounding the liver. **B,** In this image of the left kidney, ascites is noted around the kidney and intestines.

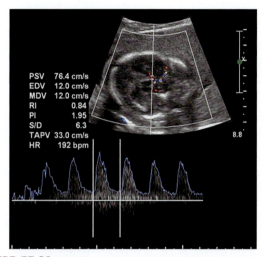

FIGURE 57-29 Middle cerebral artery (MCA) color and spectral Doppler analysis in this anemic fetus indicates an abnormal peak velocity of 76.4 cm/sec and a heart rate of 192 bpm.

for sampling both MCAs. If the peak velocity is 50 cm/sec after 30 weeks' gestation, fetal anemia is likely indicated (Figure 57-29). Other forms of measurement are available that calculate the multiples of the mean for the MCA. The MCA should be evaluated every 1 to 2 weeks in fetuses at risk for developing anemia. In addition to recording the velocities of the MCA, peak systolic measurement of the aorta has been found to be useful in diagnosing anemia. Peak velocity measurements of the aorta greater than 1 cm/sec are considered a clinical finding for anemia. Fetal anemia may be present with or without hydrops. Conclusive evidence of anemia is further evaluated by means of amniocentesis (evaluation of amniotic fluid) or cordocentesis (evaluation of fetal blood via the umbilical cord).

Nonimmune Hydrops

Nonimmune hydrops fetalis (NIHF) describes the presence of abnormal accumulations of fluid in the fetal body

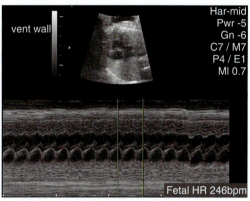

FIGURE 57-30 Tachycardia was identified in this patient with a heart rate of 246 bpm.

and/or skin. It is associated with numerous conditions and causes.

Etiology. Nonimmune hydrops may be a sporadic condition or may be associated with numerous other causes. Cardiac insufficiency, one of the most common causes, can result from cardiac anomalies (cardiac tumors) or arrhythmias (tachycardia) (Figure 57-30). Fetal anomalies associated with decreased venous return to the heart, structural lymphatic obstruction, and hypoproteinuria constitute other causes.

Prognosis. Prognosis for a fetus presenting with NIHF is poor. It has been noted that the overall mortality rate is 50% to 98%. This varying percentage rate is directly related to the etiology of the hydrops. In some cases of anemia or tachycardia, the cause can be treated, thereby reducing or resolving the hydrops. Laser therapy has been used to treat hydrops in cases of twin–twin transfusion syndrome involving NIHF. Fetuses born with NIHF typically are very distressed and require immediate medical attention.

Sonographic Findings. Sonographically, all abnormal fluid collections should be documented and measured. The fetus should be thoroughly evaluated for anomalies that may be associated with NIHF. Anomalies that may

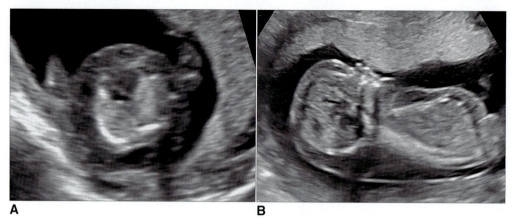

FIGURE 57-31 A and **B,** Massive skin edema was visualized in this fetus with trisomy 21.

be present include fetal tumors (heart or liver), cardiac anomalies, cystic adenomatoid malformations of the lung, and chorioangiomas of the placenta. Sonographic findings associated with characteristics of trisomy 21, 45X (Figure 57-31) and fetal infections (TORCH) should be documented because of their relationship with NIHF.

ACKNOWLEDGMENTS

To Roy Bors-Koefoed, MD, Janet Thweatt, BHS, RT(R), RDMS, Patricia Williams, RDMS, Christina Taff, BHS, RDMS, and Terri Vest, RN, RDMS, for their contributions of sonographic images for this chapter.

The Fetal Face and Neck

Diana M. Strickland and Sandra L. Hagen-Ansert

Congenital anomalies of the face affect 1 in 600 births. Cleft lip, hypotelorism, hypertelorism, and micrognathia are examples of facial problems that may be found by ultrasound during pregnancy. Many anomalies of the face and neck can be caused by maternal drug use (Table 58-1). As in other investigations, the detection of subtle facial malformations depends on the sonographer's skill and ability to recognize facial pathology, the position of the fetus, and the amount of amniotic fluid near the face.

EMBRYOLOGY OF THE FETAL FACE AND NECK

In its 4th week, the embryo has characteristic external features of the head and neck area in the form of a series of branchial arches, pouches, grooves, and membranes. These structures are referred to as the *branchial apparatus* and bear a resemblance to gills.

There are six branchial arches, but only the first four are visible externally (Figure 58-1, *A*). The arches are separated by branchial grooves, and each is composed of a core of mesenchymal cells. The mesenchyme forms the cartilage, bone, muscle, and blood vessels.

The first branchial arch is also known as the mandibular arch; it forms the jaw, zygomatic bone, ear, and temporal bone (Figure 58-1, *B*). The second branchial arch contributes to the hyoid bone.

The branchial arches consist of mesenchymal tissue derived from intraembryonic mesoderm covered by ectoderm and containing transderm. Neural crest cells migrate into the branchial arches and proliferate, resulting in swelling that demarcates each arch. The neural crest cells develop the skeletal parts of the face, and the mesoderm of each arch develops the musculature of the face and neck.

The maxillary prominences arise from the first branchial arch and grow cranially just under the eyes and the mandibular prominence, which grows inferiorly. The primitive mouth is an indentation on the surface of the ectoderm (referred to as the stomodeum) (Figure 58-2). By the 5th week of development, five prominences are identified: the frontal nasal prominence, forming the upper boundary of the stomodeum; the paired maxillary prominences of the first branchial arch, forming the lateral boundaries of the stomodeum; and the paired mandibular prominences, forming the caudal boundary.

The nasal pits are formed as the surface ectoderm thickens into the nasal placodes on each side of the frontal nasal prominence; as these placodes invaginate, the nasal pits are formed (Figure 58-3). Until 24 to 26 days' gestation, the stomodeum is separated from the pharynx by a membrane that ruptures by about the 26th day to place the primitive gut in communication with the amniotic cavity.

TABLE 58-1	Potential Fetal Malformations Associated With Maternal Drug Use and Infectious Disease
Drug	**Fetal Malformation(s)**
Albuterol	Tachycardia
Alcohol (ethanol)	Microcephaly, micrognathia, cleft palate, short nose, hypoplastic philtrum, cardiac defects (VSD, ASD, double-outlet right ventricle, pulmonary atresia, dextrocardia, tetralogy of Fallot), IUGR, diaphragmatic hernia, pectus excavatum, radioulnar synostosis, scoliosis, bifid xiphoid, NTDs
Amantadine	Cardiac defects (single ventricle with pulmonary atresia)
Aminopterin	NTDs, hydrocephalus, incomplete skull ossification, brachycephaly, micrognathia, clubfoot, syndactyly, hypoplasia of thumb and fibula, IUGR
Angiotensin-converting enzyme (ACE) inhibitors	Hypocalvaria, oliogohydramnios, neonatal renal failure, hypotension, pulmonary hypoplasia, joint contractures, IUGR, stillbirth
Antithyroid drugs	Goiter
Aspirin (Bayer, St. Joseph)	Slight increased risk for gastroschisis; premature closure of the ductus arteriosus; intracranial hemorrhage in premature or LBW infants
Bromides	Polydactyly, clubfoot, congenital hip dislocation
Busulfan	Pyloric stenosis, cleft palate, microphthalmia, IUGR
Caffeine	Musculoskeletal defects, hydronephrosis
Captopril	Leg reduction
Carbamazepine	NTDs, cardiac defects (atrial septal defect), nose hypoplasia, hypertelorism, cleft lip, congenital hip dislocation
Carbon monoxide	Cerebral atrophy, hydrocephalus, fetal demise
Chlordiazepoxide	Microcephaly, cardiac defects, duodenal atresia
Chloroquine	Hemihypertrophy
Chlorpheniramine	Hydrocephalus, polydactyly, congenital hip dislocation
Chlorpropamide	Microcephaly, dysmorphic hands and fingers
Clomiphene	NTDs, microcephaly, syndactyly, clubfoot, polydactyly, esophageal atresia
Cocaine	Spontaneous abortion, placental abruption, prematurity, IUGR, possible cardiac defects, skull defects, genitourinary anomalies
Codeine	Hydrocephalus, head defects, cleft palate, musculoskeletal defects, dislocated hip, pyloric stenosis, respiratory malformations
Cortisone	Hydrocephalus, cardiac defects (VSD, coarctation of aorta), clubfoot, cleft lip
Coumadin	NTDs, cardiac defects, scoliosis, skeletal deformities, nasal hypoplasia, stippled epiphyses, chondrodysplasia punctata, short phalanges, toe defects, incomplete rotation of gut, IUGR, bleeding
Cyclophosphamide	Cardiac defects, cleft palate, flattened nasal bridge, four toes on each foot, syndactyly, hypoplastic midphalanx, craniosynostosis, microcephaly, hypotelorism, blepharophimosis, microphthalmos, shallow orbits with proptosis, malformed ears, flat nasal bridge with bulbous nasal tip
Cytarabine	NTDs, cardiac defects, lobster claw hand, missing digits of feet, syndactyly
Cytomegalovirus	Microcephaly, ventricular dilatation, cerebral calcification, ascites, hepatosplenomegaly, chorioretinitis, IUGR
Diazepam	NTDs, cardiac defects, absence of arm, syndactyly, absence of thumbs, cleft lip and palate
Diethylstilbestrol	Structural abnormalities of the cervix, vagina, uterine cavity; epididymal cysts, hypoplastic testes, cryptorchidism
Diuretics	Respiratory malformations
Estrogens	Cardiac defects, limb reduction
Fluorouracil	Radial aplasia, absent thumbs, aplasia of esophagus and duodenum, hypoplasia of lungs
Fluconazole	Brachycephaly, micrognathia, trigonocephaly, low ears, abnormal calvarial development, cleft palate, femoral bowing, thin ribs, humeral-radial fusion, arthrogryposis, heart defects
Heparin	Bleeding
Imipramine	NTDs, cleft palate, renal cysts, diaphragmatic hernia
Indomethacin	Fetal demise, hemorrhage
Lithium	NTDs, cardiac defects (VSD, Ebstein's anomaly, mitral atresia, dextrocardia)
Lymphocytic choriomeningitis virus	Hydrocephalus, intracranial calcifications, chorioretinitis
Methotrexate	Oxycephaly, absence of frontal bones, large fontanels, micorgnathia, long, webbed fingers, low-set ears, IUGR, dextrocardia
Methyl mercury	Microcephaly, asymmetrical head
Metronidazole	Midline facial defects
Oral contraceptives	NTDs, cardiac defects, vertebral defects, limb reduction, IUGR, tracheoesophageal malformation
Parovirus B19	Hydrocephalus, myocarditis, hydrops, stillbirth
Penicillamine (Cuprimine, Depen)	Cutis laxa
Phenobarbital (Luminal)	Hypoplastic fingernails, epicanthal folds, broad, depressed nasal bridge, short nose with long philtrum, increased risk for heart disease, oral clefts, urinary tract defects, hemorrhage

Drug	Fetal Malformation(s)
TABLE 58-1	**Potential Fetal Malformations Associated With Maternal Drug Maternal Drug Use and Infectious Disease—cont'd**
Phenylpropanolamine (Acutrim, Dexatrim, Phenyldrine)	Slightly increased risk for gastroschisis; theoretic risk for bradycardia
Phenytoin (Dilantin, Phenytek)	Coarctation of aorta, cardiac septal defects, microcephaly, wide anterior fontanelle, ocular hypertelorism, broad, depressed nasal bridge, short nose with bowed upper lip, short neck, cleft lip and palate, hypoplastic fingernails, growth deficiency
Primidone	Cardiac defects (VSD), webbed neck, small mandible
Pseudoephedrine (Sudafed)	Slightly increased risk for gastroschisis
Quinine	Hydrocephalus, cardiac defects, facial defects, vertebral anomalies, dysmelias
Rubella	Microcephaly, cataract, glaucoma, corneal opacity, chorioretinitis, microphthalmos, strabismus, patent ductus arteriosus, pulmonic stenosis, septal defects, growth deficiency, occasionally—hypospadias and cryptorchidism
Sulfasalazine (Azulfidine)	Slightly increased risk for heart defects, oral clefts, and urinary tract defects
Tetracycline	Limb hypoplasia, clubfoot
Thalidomide	Cardiac defects, spine defects, limb reduction (amelia), phocomelia, hypoplasia, duodenal stenosis or atresia, pyloric stenosis
Thioguanine	Missing digits
Tobacco	IUGR
Toluene	IUGR, neonatal hyperchloremia acidosis, possible mental dysfunction, cardiac defects, dysmorphic facies
Trifluoperazine	Cardiac defects, phocomelia
Trimethadione	Microcephaly, low-set ears, broad nasal bridge, cardiac defects (ASD, VSD), IUGR, cleft lip and palate, esophageal atresia, malformed hands, clubfoot
Valproic acid	NTDs, microcephaly, wide fontanelle, cardiac defects, IUGR, cleft palate, hypoplastic nose, low-set ears, small mandible, depressed nasal bridge, polydactyly
Varicella	Microcephaly, chorioretinitis, limb hypoplasia (with or without digits), clubfoot, cutaneous scars, growth deficiency
Warfarin (Coumadin)	Nasal hypoplasia, depressed nasal bridge, stippling of uncalcified epiphyses, mild hypoplasia of nails, shortened fingers

From Nyberg DA, Mahoney BS, Pretorius DH: *Diagnostic ultrasound of fetal anomalies: text and atlas,* St Louis, 1990, Mosby and from Nyberg DA, McGahan JP, Pretorius DH, Pilu G (eds), *Diagnostic imaging of fetal anomalies,* ed 2, Philadelphia, 2003, Lippincott, Williams, and Wilkins.
IUGR, intrauterine growth restriction; *ASD,* atrial septal defect; *LBW,* low birth weight; *NTDs,* neural tube defects; *VSD,* ventricular septal defect.

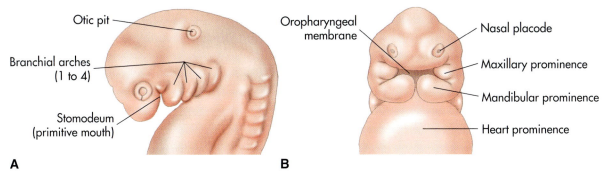

FIGURE 58-1 A, Lateral view of the embryo at 28 days shows four of the six branchial arches, otic pit, and stomodeum. **B,** Frontal view of the embryo at 24 days demonstrates the nasal placode, maxillary prominence, and mandibular prominence.

The maxillary prominences grow medially between the 5th and 8th weeks. This growth compresses the medial nasal prominences together toward the midline. The two medial nasal prominences and the two maxillary prominences lateral to them fuse together to form the upper lip (Figure 58-4). The medial nasal prominences form the medial aspect of the lip, which is the origin of the labial component of the lip, the upper incisor teeth, and the anterior aspect of the primary palate. The lateral nasal prominences form the alae of the nose. The maxillary prominences and lateral nasal prominences are separated by the nasolacrimal groove. The ectoderm in the floor of this groove forms the nasolacrimal duct and lacrimal sac.

The nose is formed in three parts. The bridge of the nose originates from the frontal prominence, the two medial nasal prominences form the crest and tip of the nose, and the lateral nasal prominences form the sides, or alae. The mandibular prominences merge at the end of the 4th to 5th week and form the lower lip, chin, and mandible.

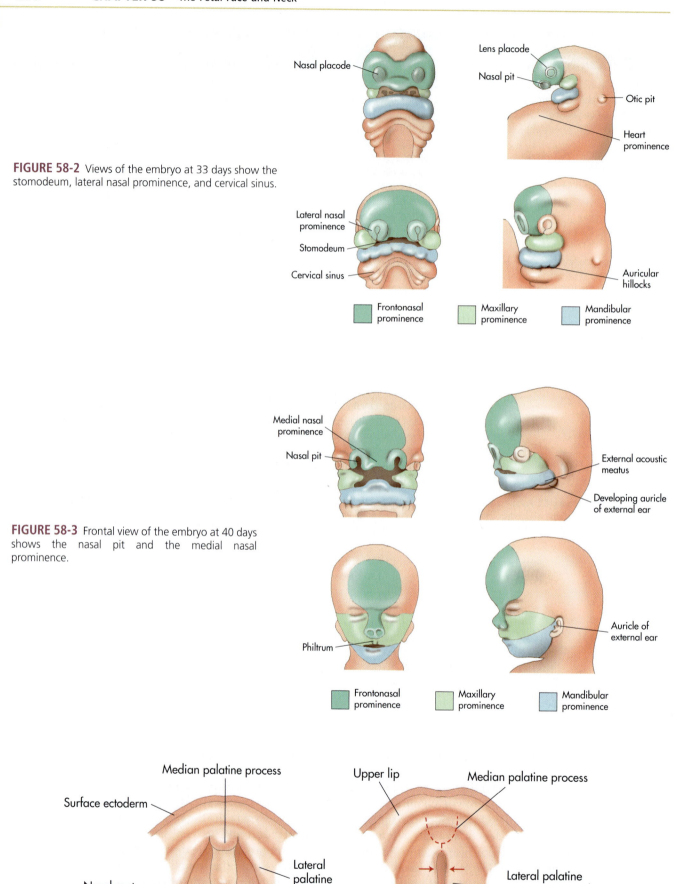

FIGURE 58-2 Views of the embryo at 33 days show the stomodeum, lateral nasal prominence, and cervical sinus.

FIGURE 58-3 Frontal view of the embryo at 40 days shows the nasal pit and the medial nasal prominence.

FIGURE 58-4 First-trimester development of the roof of the mouth showing formation of the upper lip and palate.

SONOGRAPHIC EVALUATION OF THE FETAL FACE

Fetal facial evaluation is not routinely included in a basic fetal scan; however, when there is a family history of craniofacial malformation, or when another congenital anomaly is found, the face should be screened for a coexisting facial malformation. Many fetuses with a facial defect also have chromosomal abnormalities. Extensive facial screening may be hindered by bone shadowing, poor fetal position, oligohydramnios, or maternal obesity. Certain facial anomalies often indicate a specific syndrome or condition (e.g., orbital fusion and a **proboscis** suggest alobar holoprosencephaly). The use of three- and four-dimensional ultrasound reconstruction has been shown in recent years to be a useful adjunct to conventional two-dimensional assessment of the fetal face (Box 58-1 and Figures 58-5 to 58-8).

Facial anomalies are heterogeneous and occur as isolated defects or as part of a syndrome. A family history of a facial anomaly (e.g., cleft lip) may prompt a targeted study, although recurrence risks are relatively low (less than 5%). Hemangiomas and teratomas may occur anywhere on the body, and the fetal head and neck are no exception. Any mass should be investigated with color Doppler to delineate any vascular characteristics (Figure 58-9).

ABNORMALITIES OF THE FACE AND NECK

Abnormalities of the Facial Profile

Forehead. The fetal forehead may be appreciated by evaluation of the profile. This is achieved by a series of midsagittal scans through the face. The fetal forehead

---

BOX 58-1	Sonographic Points to Remember

- Features of the fetal face can be identified at the end of the first trimester.
- The fetal profile is well imaged with transvaginal sonography beginning late first trimester to early second trimester (make sure adequate amniotic fluid surrounds the face) (Figure 58-5).
- The modified coronal view is best for imaging the cleft lip and palate (Figure 58-6).
- The maxilla and orbits are well imaged in a true coronal plane.
- The lens of the eye is seen as a small echogenic circle within the orbit (Figure 58-7).
- The longitudinal view demonstrates the nasal bones, soft tissue, and mandible (useful to rule out micrognathia, anterior encephalocele, or nasal bridge defects; examine upper lip) (Figure 58-8).
- Transverse view shows orbital abnormalities and intraorbital distances (useful to evaluate the maxilla, mandible, and tongue).

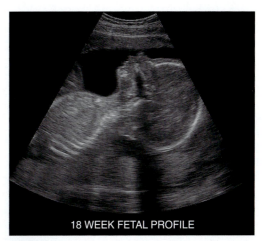

18 WEEK FETAL PROFILE

FIGURE 58-5 The fetal profile is well seen with amniotic fluid surrounding the face. This is a useful plane to image the forehead, nose, lips, and chin.

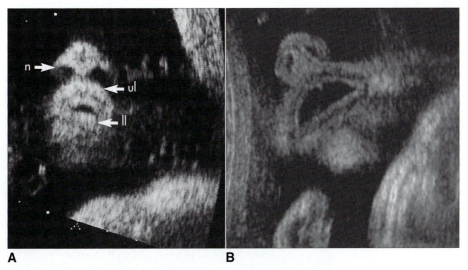

A   B

FIGURE 58-6 A, Axial view through the upper (*ul*) and lower lip (*ll*) in a fetus with an open mouth. Note the nares (*n*) and nasal septum. This view is used to check for a cleft of the upper lip. **B,** In another fetus, the nasal septum is well seen and the vermilion tissue of the lips can be differentiated.

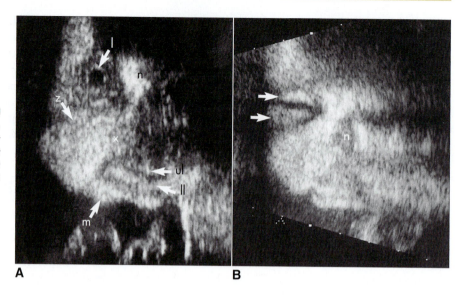

FIGURE 58-7 A, Coronal view showing facial features. Lens *(l),* zygomatic bone *(z),* maxilla *(x),* upper lip *(ul),* lower lip *(ll),* mandible *(m),* nasal bones *(n).* **B,** In the same fetus, in a more anterior coronal view, the upper and lower eyelids *(arrows)* and the nose *(n)* are shown.

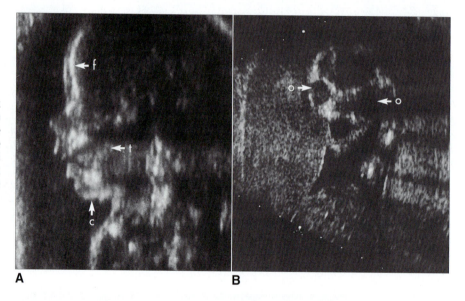

FIGURE 58-8 A, Sagittal view in a 23-week fetus showing the contour of the face in profile. Note the smooth surface of the frontal bone *(f)* and the appearance of the nose, upper and lower lips, tongue *(t),* and chin *(c).* **B,** Coronal facial view in an 18-week fetus revealing a wide-open mouth. Note the nasal bones between the orbits *(o).*

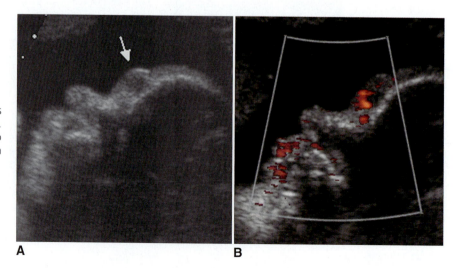

FIGURE 58-9 A, A soft tissue mass is seen overlying the fetal forehead *(arrow).* **B,** Color Doppler demonstrates the mass to have vascular flow within, suggesting a hemangioma.

(frontal bone) appears as a curvilinear surface with differentiation of the nose, lips, and chin seen inferiorly. This view allows diagnosis of anterior **cephaloceles**, which may arise from the frontal bone or midface. Anterior cephaloceles may cause widely spaced orbits (hypertelorism) (Boxes 58-2 and 58-3).

Off-axis, or nonmidline, encephaloceles have also been reported with amniotic band syndrome. This occurs when the amnion disrupts early in the embryonic period, leaving strands of tissue within the uterus that may lead to malformation of the fetus.

Skull. Craniosynostosis (premature closure of any or all six of the cranial sutures) causes the fetal cranium to become abnormally shaped. *Clover-leaf skull* (Kleeblattschädel) appears as an unusually misshapen skull with a clover-leaf appearance in the anterior view. Clover-leaf skull has been associated with numerous skeletal dysplasias (most notably, thanatophoric dysplasia) and ventriculomegaly (Figure 58-10). **Trigonocephaly** (premature closure of the metopic suture) may cause the forehead to have an elongated (tall) appearance in the sagittal plane and appear triangular shaped in the axial plane (Figure 58-11). Three-dimensional imaging has been shown to be useful in evaluating fetal cranial sutures. *Frontal bossing* may be observed in a fetus with a lemon-shaped skull (from spina bifida) or with skeletal dysplasias. Any irregularities in the contour of the forehead should prompt the investigator to search for other malformations.

Midface Hypoplasia. Midface hypoplasia, or maxillary hypoplasia with depressed or absent nasal bridge, is an underdevelopment of the middle structures of the face. The flat facies that this defect produces are more easily noted with coexisting frontal bossing. Midface hypoplasia may be seen in fetuses with chromosome anomalies, such as trisomy 21; craniosynostosis syndromes, such as Apert's syndrome; and limb and skeletal abnormalities, such as achondroplasia, chondrodysplasia punctata, asphyxiating thoracic dysplasia, and others (Figure 58-12). The fetal nasal bone may be small or absent with certain chromosome anomalies, particularly trisomy 21. Recent studies have evaluated the presence or absence of the fetal nasal bone as a predictor of chromosome anomalies (Figure 58-13).

Frontonasal Dysplasia. Frontonasal dysplasia is a median cleft face syndrome consisting of a range of midline facial defects involving the eyes, forehead, and nose. Abnormalities include ocular hypertelorism, a variable bifid nose, a broad nasal bridge, a midline defect of the frontal bone, and extension of the frontal hairline to

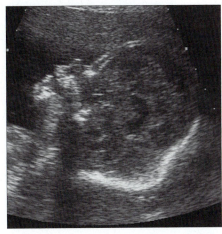

FIGURE 58-10 Sagittal view of a fetus with thanatophoric dysplasia with a clover-leaf skull or Kleeblattschädel.

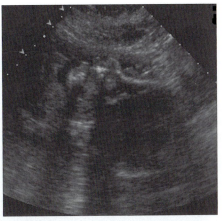

FIGURE 58-11 Sagittal view of a fetus with premature closure of the metopic suture, which elongated and flattened the fetal forehead.

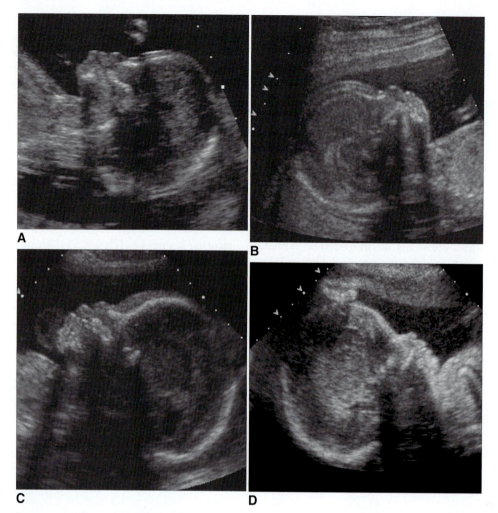

FIGURE 58-12 Midline sagittal views. **A,** A fetus affected by familial midface hypoplasia. **B,** A fetus with trisomy 21 (Down syndrome); note flattened facies. **C,** A fetus with a skeletal dysplasia demonstrates mild frontal bossing and midface hypoplasia. **D,** A fetus with neonatal progeroid syndrome; note smallness of facial profile compared with the head. Cranial biometry was consistent with gestational age.

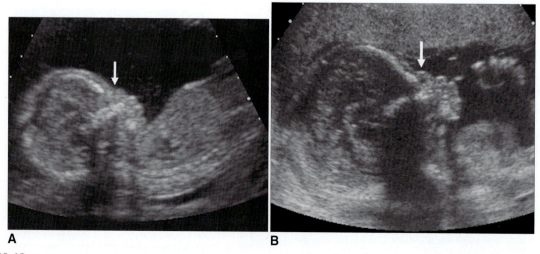

FIGURE 58-13 **A,** Trisomy 21 fetus with absent nasal bone *(arrow).* **B,** Another fetus with trisomy 21 with absent nasal bone *(arrow).*

form a widow's peak. The cause of frontonasal dysplasia is unknown, and its occurrence is sporadic.

By ultrasound, the primary finding will likely be hypertelorism. If one cranial abnormality is found, the sonographer should carefully look for additional dysmorphic features (Figure 58-14).

Nuchal Area. The association of first-trimester fetal **nuchal lucency** with aneuploidy is well established and is dependent on the size and extent of the nuchal abnormality. The latest studies of nuchal translucency (NT) thickness have attempted to delineate the exact role of this measurement as a screening tool for chromosome anomalies. In a review of recent studies,[2] it was shown that when fetal NT is performed in conjunction with maternal biochemical screening (maternal serum free-[beta]-human chorionic gonadotropin and pregnancy-associated plasma protein-A, or PAPP-A), the detection

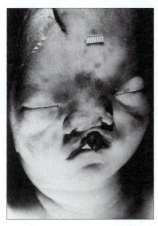

FIGURE 58-14 Postmortem photograph of neonate with median cleft facial syndrome (frontonasal dysplasia). Note the hypertelorism and mass of the upper lip. Other abnormalities observed prenatally include severe ventriculomegaly with a shift of the interhemispheric fissure.

rate of chromosome anomalies is 87%, as opposed to 76.8% with the fetal NT measurement alone. The optimal gestational age for the measurement of fetal NT is 11 weeks of gestation to 13 weeks, 6 days of gestation. Fetal crown-rump length should be within the range of 45 to 84 mm. It is important to adjust the depth and image magnification, so that the head and upper torso account for 75% of the image field. In a midline sagittal plane, care should be taken to ensure delineation of the amnion and nuchal borders by waiting for the fetus to move, or by gently bouncing the transducer on the maternal abdomen. Calipers should be placed on the borders of the NT and not in the nuchal fluid area. A measurement greater than 3 mm is abnormal, and the thicker the fetal NT is above 3 mm, the greater is the chance that the fetus will be affected by a chromosome anomaly or another defect, such as congenital heart disease (Figure 58-15).

Nose and Upper Lip. Masses of the nose and upper lip may distort the facial profile and indicate a cleft lip. Tumors such as an **epignathus** or a teratoma may disrupt the facial contour in the sagittal plane. These anomalies will be discussed in greater detail in later sections.

Tongue. Tongue protrusion may suggest **macroglossia** (enlarged tongue), a condition found in **Beckwith-Wiedemann syndrome** (congenital overgrowth of tissues) (Figure 58-16). Organomegaly is also a feature of this syndrome. Some glycogen storage diseases may also exhibit macroglossia and organomegaly (Figure 58-17).

Mandible. Congenital **micrognathia** should be suspected when a small chin is observed. Most cases of micrognathia are detected from the subjective appearance of a small chin when imaging the fetal profile (Figure 58-18). Several authors have proposed more objective methods of evaluation of the fetal mandible such as providing quantitative data to assess the size of the mandible either by an index or according to

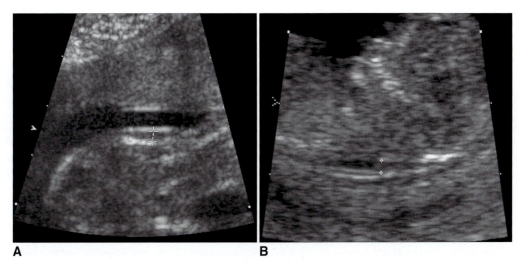

A   **B**

FIGURE 58-15 **A,** A 13-week, 6-day fetus. Caliper placement demonstrates the measurement of a normal fetal nuchal translucency. **B,** An 11-week, 4-day fetus. Fetal nuchal translucency measurement from an anteroposterior sagittal plane.

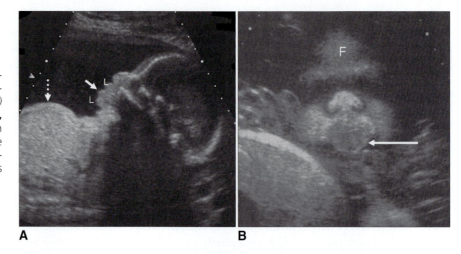

FIGURE 58-16 **A,** A fetus with Beckwith-Wiedemann syndrome. Note tongue protruding from mouth *(arrow)* between lips *(L)* and enlarged fetal liver *(dotted arrow).* **B,** Another fetus with Beckwith-Wiedemann syndrome. Coronal view of the fetal face demonstrates a protruding tongue suggesting macroglossia *(arrow).* The fetal liver was also enlarged in this fetus. *F,* forehead.

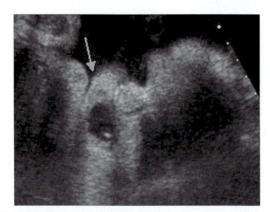

FIGURE 58-17 Coronal view of fetal face showing a hypoechoic mass in the fetal mouth. A sublingual cyst was noted to move into and out of the fetal mouth in the sagittal plane *(arrow).*

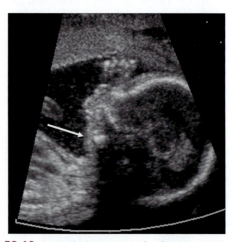

FIGURE 58-18 Sagittal plane view of a fetus with micrognathia *(arrow).*

gestational age. Mandibular width is measured in an axial plane laterally from rami to rami. Mandibular length, or AP diameter, is assessed by measuring from the mentum of the mandible to the bisection of the lateral width line (Figure 58-19). Paladini and others have proposed the use of an established jaw index using the anteroposterior diameter of the mandible and the biparietal diameter (AP Diam/BPD × 100) for diagnosing micrognathia.[3] An index of 21 or less yielded a 100% positive predictive value. Lee and others believed that three-dimensional (3D) imaging added complementary information to 2D imaging of the chin, and that a true midline plane could be better achieved using 3D reconstructed images.[1] Micrognathia is associated with many conditions that can be subdivided into three groups of anomalies: chromosome anomalies, such as trisomy 18 and triploidy; skeletal dysplasias; and primary mandibular disorders, such as **Pierre Robin syndrome** and **Treacher Collins syndrome.** An abnormally small chin may be so severe that polyhydramnios occurs because of the inability of the fetus to swallow; airway obstruction may be a complication at delivery.

Ear. The fetal ears may be imaged in a parasagittal plane or in a coronal plane (Figure 58-20). Ear malformations

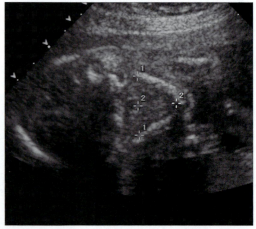

FIGURE 58-19 Axial view of a normal fetal mandible demonstrating mandibular width *(1)* and mandibular anterior-posterior (AP) diameter *(2).*

are rarely predicted prenatally. Low-set ears may be appreciated in a longitudinal or coronal view when placement of the ear appears lower than usual in many craniofacial malformations and syndromes. Ear malformation may be observed in Goldenhar's syndrome with anophthalmia (absent eye) and **hemifacial microsomia** (abnormal smallness of one side of the face). Small ears (Roberts' syndrome) and inadequate development of the ear (Nager acrofacial dysostosis syndrome and Treacher Collins syndrome) may be observed prenatally. **Otocephaly** is a rare anomaly whereby absence of the mandible causes the ears to form close together anteriorly and toward the neck.

Abnormalities of the Orbits

Orbital architecture has become increasingly important in the evaluation of craniofacial anomalies. The anatomy of the orbits, the use of orbital measurements in gestational age assessment, and the role of ultrasound in detecting ocular abnormalities have been investigated (Figure 58-21).

The sonographer must document the presence of both eyes and assess the overall size of the eyes to exclude **microphthalmia** (small eyes) and **anophthalmia** (absent eyes). Masses of the orbit (periorbital) and of the eye (intraocular) may be excluded with careful scanning of

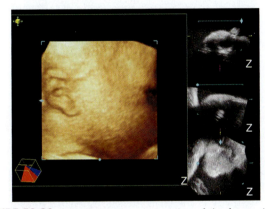

FIGURE 58-20 A multiplanar reconstruction of the fetus with the ear lobe well seen.

the eyes. Periorbital masses, such as lacrimal duct cysts (**dacryocystoceles**), dermoids, and hemangiomas, have been reported (Figure 58-22). In a laterally approached axial plane, the hyaloid artery may be observed within the fetal eye. The hyaloid artery, which regresses in the third trimester, is a branch of the primitive dorsal ophthalmic artery. It extends from the optic nerve through the vitreous cavity to the lens to aid in its development (Figure 58-23).

Transvaginal sonography has aided in early detection of ocular anomalies and other intracranial abnormalities. The fetal eyes are evaluated on transvaginal sonography in a transverse section of the fetal skull at the orbital plane. In addition, an oblique tangential section from the nasal bridge is used to detect the hypoechogenic circles lateral to the nose, in the anterior part of the orbits, representing the fetal lens. Using this method, ocular abnormalities, including **strabismus,** microphthalmia, divergence of lens, **exophthalmia,** and cataracts, have been demonstrated.

Orbital distance measurements are helpful in the diagnosis of fetal conditions in which hypotelorism or hypertelorism is a feature (Figure 58-24). Both of these conditions are associated with other anomalies, and often the orbital problem aids in the diagnosis of which type of cranial anomaly or genetic syndrome is present. An anatomic and biometric evaluation of the fetal orbits should be attempted in fetuses at risk for abnormal orbital distance.

Hypotelorism. **Hypotelorism** is a condition characterized by decreased distance between the orbits (Figures 58-25 and 58-26). It is associated with several syndromes and other anomalies, including **holoprosencephaly, microcephaly,** craniosynostoses, and **phenylketonuria (PKU).**

Obvious hypotelorism will be seen in ethmocephaly and cebocephaly or may be so severe that a single orbit is demonstrated with a fused or single eye, as is seen in

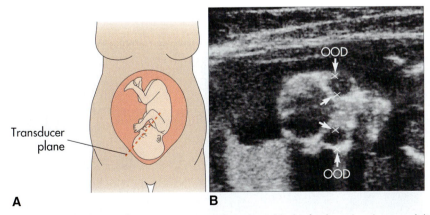

FIGURE 58-21 **A,** Frontal view demonstrating a fetus in a vertex presentation with the fetal cranium in an occipitotransverse position. The transducer is placed along the coronal plane (approximately 2 cm posterior to the glabella-alveolar line). **B,** Sonogram demonstrating the orbits in the coronal view. The outer orbital diameter *(OOD)* and inner orbital diameter (IOD) *(angled arrows)* are viewed. The IOD is measured from the medial border of the orbit to the opposite medial border *(angled arrows)*. The OOD is measured from the outermost lateral border of the orbit to the opposite lateral border.

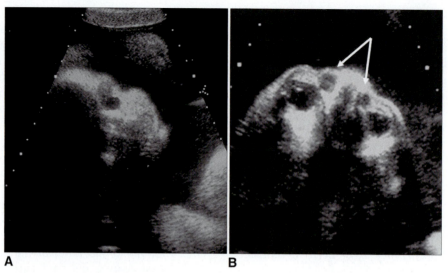

FIGURE 58-22 A, A coronal view of the fetal face reveals a small hypoechoic mass just inferomedial to the eye. **B,** In the transverse plane, bilateral lacrimal duct cysts are exhibited *(arrows)*.

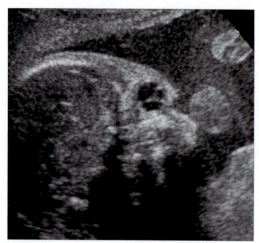

FIGURE 58-23 An axial view of the fetal head demonstrates the hyaloid artery seen as a linear structure within the vitreous cavity of the eye.

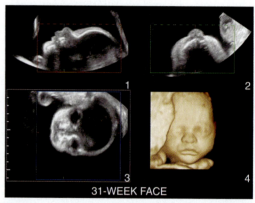

31-WEEK FACE

FIGURE 58-24 Multiplanar reconstruction through the fetal orbits may allow the correct placement of calipers to measure the outer-to-outer distance of the orbits, sometimes referred to as the binocular measurement, and the inner-to-inner orbital measurement.

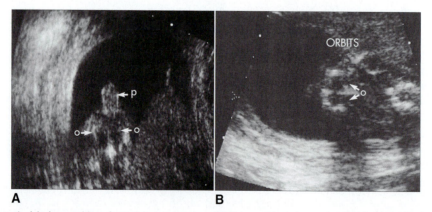

FIGURE 58-25 A, Proboscis *(p)* observed in a frontal facial view in a midline position above the closely spaced orbits *(o)* in a 20-week fetus with ethmocephaly. **B,** In the same fetus, the orbits *(o)* are observed. A single eye with fused orbits was found. Trisomy 13 was noted after delivery.

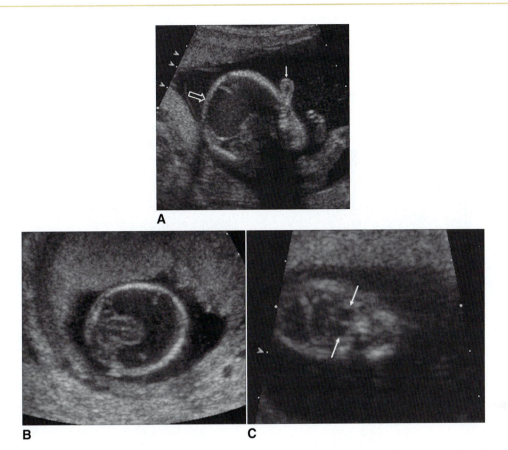

FIGURE 58-26 **A,** A midline sagittal view of the face in a fetus with holoprosencephaly shows a proboscis *(arrow);* a dorsal sac (sometimes seen with holoprosencephaly) can be seen in the posterior fetal cranium *(open arrow).* **B,** An axial view of the same fetus displays the monoventricle seen with holoprosencephaly. **C,** Coronal view of the same fetus reveals hypotelorism *(arrows).*

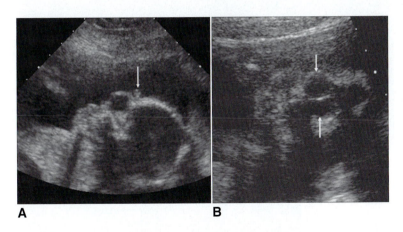

FIGURE 58-27 **A,** A midline sagittal plane view through the face of a fetus with holoprosencephaly demonstrates cyclopia with a small proboscis *(arrow)* above the central eye. **B,** The coronal view of the same fetus shows two asymmetrically sized eyes within one orbit *(arrows).*

cyclopia (Figures 58-27 and 58-28). Measurements of orbital width may identify fetuses with hypotelorism.

Hypertelorism. Hypertelorism is characterized by abnormally wide-spaced orbits. Hypertelorism is found in several abnormal fetal conditions, genetic syndromes, and chromosomal anomalies. Fetuses exposed to phenytoin (Dilantin) during pregnancy may manifest signs of hypertelorism as part of the fetal phenytoin syndrome (microcephaly; growth abnormalities; cleft lip and/or palate; cardiac, genitourinary, central nervous system, and skeletal anomalies). In Pfeiffer syndrome and Apert's syndrome, hypertelorism and brachycephaly have been

described as a result of abnormal closure of the cranial sutures (craniosynostosis). In both syndromes, ventriculomegaly may be present. Other conditions that manifest with hypertelorism and premature suture closure include Crouzon syndrome, cephalosyndactyly, acrocephalopolysyndactyly, and **oculodentodigital dysplasia.**

Fetal hypertelorism may be diagnosed by orbital distances that fall above normal ranges for gestational age.

Recognition of hypertelorism may provide evidence for a particular genetic syndrome or concurrent anomalies. Frontal cephaloceles may widen the space between the eyes (Figure 58-29). The reader is referred to comprehensive sources for a detailed list of conditions associated with hypertelorism.

Frontonasal dysplasia (median cleft facial syndrome) was diagnosed in a fetus with ventriculomegaly based on sonographic findings of hypertelorism and cleft lip (see Figure 58-14).

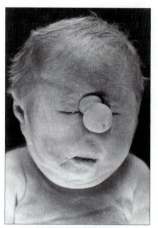

FIGURE 58-28 Postmortem photograph of a neonate with ethmocephaly. Note the proboscis and hypotelorism. The mouth appeared normal. A common ventricle and absent optic and ophthalmic nerves were noted. The chromosomes were consistent with trisomy 13.

Abnormalities of the Nose, Maxilla, Lips, and Palate

The nose, maxilla, lips, and palate may be viewed by placing the transducer in a lateral coronal plane or sagittal profile plane, and in modified tangential maxillary view or modified coronal view (inferior-superior projection) (Figure 58-30, A). In the lateral coronal view, the integrity of the nasal structures in relationship to the orbital rings and maxillae is studied. In a profile plane, the contour of the nose, upper and lower lips, and chin is observed. This is an important view in assessing the presence or absence of the nose, lips, and chin. Irregularities in nasal contour may indicate a particular syndrome. Tangential cuts, with the transducer angled inferiorly to superiorly through the maxilla, demonstrate the nasal septum and nostril openings, or nares (Figures 58-30 and 58-31). In holoprosencephaly, nasal anomalies range from absence of the nose (**arhinia**) to the presence of a proboscis to a single-nostril nose (cebocephaly) (Figure 58-32).

Evaluation of the nasal triad should assess (1) nostril symmetry, (2) nasal septum integrity, and (3) continuity of the upper lip, to exclude cleft lip and palate. The sonographer should not mistake the normal nostrils or frenulum for a cleft. The maxilla marks the posterior

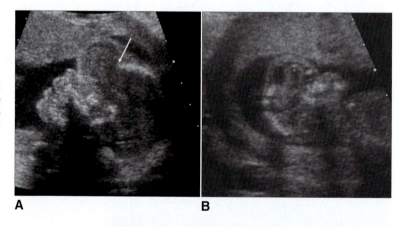

FIGURE 58-29 A, Midline sagittal view of a fetus with an anterior (frontal) encephalocele and delineation of the bony defect *(arrow).* **B,** Midline sagittal image of a large frontal encephalocele that also involved facial structures.

A   B

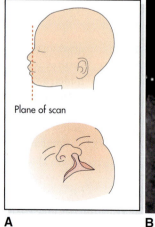
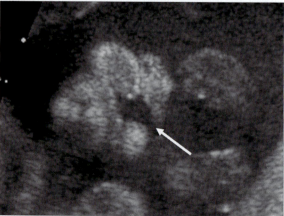

FIGURE 58-30 A, Facial cleft. This drawing illustrates a plane of section that visualizes clefts of the upper lip. **B,** A modified coronal plane demonstrates a unilateral cleft lip *(arrow).* The cleft extended into the fetal nose, and an associated cleft palate was present.

Plane of scan

A   B

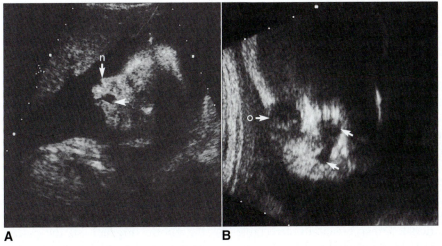

FIGURE 58-31 A, Unilateral cleft lip in the fetus shown in Figure 58-10, with clefting defect extending through the palate into the nasal cavity *(arrow)* in a sagittal plane in a 25-week fetus. Note the globular appearance of the tissue under the nose *(n)* (premaxillary protuberance). **B,** In the same fetus, a coronal plane illustrates the extent of clefting *(arrows)*. Note the defect extending from the upper lip to the nasal cavity. *O,* orbit.

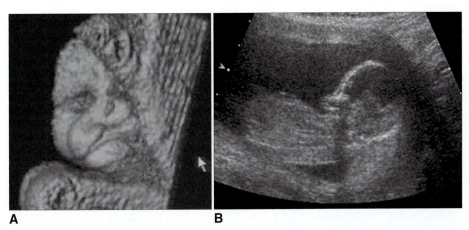

FIGURE 58-32 A, An early three-dimensional image of a median facial cleft seen with holoprosencephaly. **B,** Fourteen-week fetus midline sagittal view demonstrates midface anomalies, which include hypotelorism and arhinia as well as median facial cleft, which assisted in the early detection of holoprosencephaly.

border of the nose and is a landmark used in assessing the fetus at risk for premaxillary protuberance, as seen in Roberts' syndrome.

Lip and Palate. Cleft lip with or without cleft palate represents the most common congenital anomaly of the face. The frequency of cleft lip with or without a cleft palate shows ethnic variation. This disorder occurs in 1 per 600 births in Caucasians, in 1 per 3000 births in African Americans, in 1 per 350 births in Asians, and in 1 per 150 to 1 per 250 births in Native Americans. Cleft lip occurs because of failure to fuse the primary and secondary palate, resulting in a cleft defect coursing anteriorly through the upper lip and alveolus. Cleft palate occurs when the lateral palatine processes fail to fuse at the midline. Cleft lip and palate occur together when both fusions are absent.

A facial cleft may involve only the upper lip or may extend to involve the alveolus, posterior hard palate, and soft palate. Clefts may be unilateral or bilat-eral and may occur in isolation or in association with other anatomic and karyotypic abnormalities. Isolated posterior cleft palate is recognized as a distinct entity, separate from isolated cleft lip alone or cleft lip and palate.

Clefts of the face may occur along various facial planes. Defects range from clefting of the lip alone to involvement of the hard and soft palate, which may extend into the nose and in rare cases to the inferior border of the orbit. In rare instances, lateral clefts (may be called macrostomia if bilateral) may be observed when clefting courses laterally from the corner of the mouth and in severe cases may extend to the ear. Additionally, oblique and asymmetrical clefts may occur with amniotic band syndrome.

Isolated cleft lip may occur as a unilateral or bilateral defect and, when unilateral, commonly originates on the left side of the face. When a bilateral lesion is present, cleft palate is found in up to 85% of neonates. When unilateral, cleft palate may be seen in 70% of infants. Isolated cleft palate is a separate disorder from cleft lip associated with cleft palate. More than 200 facial cleft syndromes are known, and counseling regarding recurrence is challenging (Figure 58-33). It has been reported that when a cleft palate is present, fetal breathing may be observed with color Doppler in both the nasopharynx and the oropharynx. In the presence of a normal palate, color flow should be observed only in the fetal nasopharynx when the mouth is closed (Figure 58-34).

A majority of cleft lip and/or palate occurrences are thought to have multiple causes. Causes that may be detected prenatally include a familial predisposition or chromosomal abnormalities (trisomies 13, 18, 21; triploidy; and translocations). Other prenatally detectable clefting conditions include acrocephalopolysyndactyly, amniotic band syndrome, anencephaly, congenital cardiac disease, diastrophic dysplasia, holoprosencephaly, Kniest dysplasia, spondyloepiphyseal dysplasia congenita, and Meckel-Gruber, Roberts', and multiple pterygium syndromes. A premaxillary protrusion or a premaxillary mass suggests the presence of a bilateral cleft lip and palate, even when only a unilateral defect is suspected sonographically. This premaxillary mass of tissue corresponds to abnormal anterior herniation of the hard palate and teeth caused by defects in the alveolar ridge (Figure 58-35).

Sonographically, visualization of the hard and soft palates remains a diagnostic challenge because of considerable bony shadowing. The sonographer needs to use a systematic approach when examining the fetal face for clefts in the coronal and axial planes. The addition of 3D and 4D reconstruction may complement the 2D assessment of facial anomalies, in particular, facial clefts. It has been shown to be valuable in enhancing understanding of the extent of abnormalities and in helping the plastic surgeon and the patient to understand the fetal defect suspected. A caution about 3D imaging: When viewing 3D images, patients may be able to recognize abnormalities before the doctor has had the opportunity to clarify the diagnosis and counsel them (Figure 58-36, Box 58-4).

Abnormalities of the Oral Cavity

Few congenital malformations of the oral cavity exist. The normal fetus may exhibit various behavioral patterns, such as swallowing, protrusion and retrusion of the tongue, and hiccoughing. Abnormal positioning of the tongue may be indicative of a mass of the oral cavity, an obstructive process, or macroglossia (large tongue in Beckwith-Wiedemann syndrome).

The antenatal sonographic diagnosis of epignathus has been reported. An epignathus is a teratoma located in the oropharynx. These masses may be highly complex and contain solid, cystic, or calcified components. In fetuses with epignathus, swallowing may be impaired, resulting in hydramnios. In these cases, a small stomach may be present (Figure 58-37).

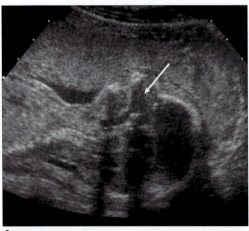
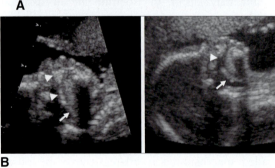

FIGURE 58-33 A, Sagittal image of a fetus with a bilateral cleft lip and palate. Fluid is seen in the common oropharynx-nasopharynx area, suggesting a cleft palate *(arrow)*. **B,** Midline sagittal plane of a normal palate in a 29-week fetus *(left)* and a 21-week fetus *(right)*. The hard palate can be seen adjacent to the fetal tongue *(arrowheads)*, and the fetal soft palate can be visualized between the oropharynx and nasopharynx *(arrows)*. Observation of the fetus while swallowing and moving the mouth may aid in delineation of these structures.

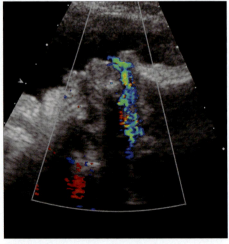

FIGURE 58-34 Color Doppler image of fetal breathing in a fetus with a normal palate, demonstrating color seen only in the nasopharynx.

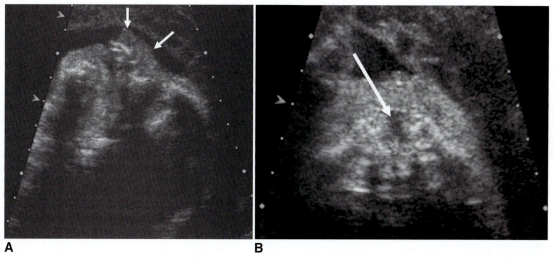

A   **B**

FIGURE 58-35 A, Sagittal image of a fetus with a cleft lip and palate. The fetal profile is distorted by a premaxillary mass *(lower arrow)*. Fetal nose *(upper arrow)*. **B,** Axial view of the maxilla in the same fetus delineates the bony defect of the maxilla *(arrow)*.

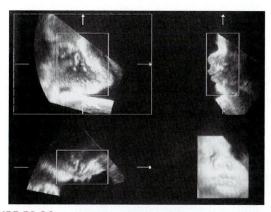

FIGURE 58-36 Three-dimensional reconstruction of the fetal face in a 34-week fetus. The *x, y,* and *z* axes are aligned to reproduce the three-dimensional image on the lower right.

BOX 58-4	Sonographic Findings of Cleft Lip and Palate

- Median cleft lip: caused by incomplete merging of the two medial nasal prominences at the midline
- Oblique facial cleft: failure of maxillary prominence to merge with the lateral nasal swelling, with exposure of the nasolacrimal duct
- Complete bilateral cleft lip and palate: large gap in upper lip on modified coronal view; nose is flattened and widened; a premaxillary mass may be present
- Unilateral complete cleft lip and palate: incomplete fusion of maxillary prominence to the medial prominence on one side; modified coronal view
- Incomplete cleft: nose is intact; modified coronal view of lip

Abnormalities of the Neck

Congenital anomalies of the neck are rare but when present may represent life-threatening disorders. Neck masses are usually large and obvious because their presence causes distortion of the neck contour and adjacent structures. The most common neck mass is cystic hygroma colli (lymphatic obstruction). Rarer lesions include cervical meningomyelocele, hemangiomas, teratomas, goiter, sarcoma, and metastatic adenopathy. **Branchial cleft cysts** (Figure 58-38) are prenatally detectable.

Clinically, a fetal neck mass is cause for concern. When a large tumor exists, delivery of the infant is complicated because the tumor may cause delivery dystocia (inability to deliver the trunk once the head has been delivered) and obstruction of the airway, which may require an EXIT procedure at delivery. The EXIT procedure, or *ex utero intrapartum treatment* procedure, is a specialized surgical procedure used to deliver babies who have airway compression.

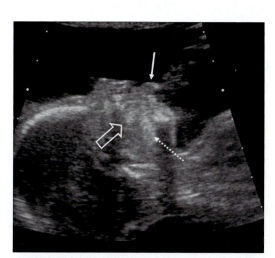

FIGURE 58-37 Sagittal view of a fetus with a small epignathus: external portion of the mass *(solid arrow)*, mass erupting from the maxilla *(open arrow)*, and tongue compressed against the lower jaw *(dotted arrow)*.

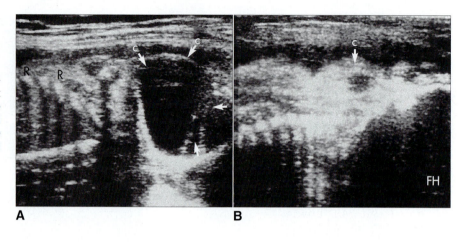

FIGURE 58-38 A, Branchial cleft cyst represented as a large unilateral septated cystic neck mass *(c, arrows)*. *R,* Rib. **B,** In the same fetus, the branchial cleft cyst *(c)* at term had almost completely resolved. The neonate had no complications after birth. *FH,* Fetal head.

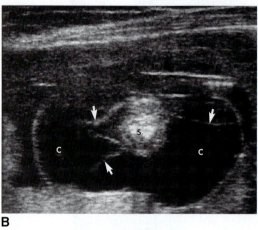

FIGURE 58-39 A, Lymphatic system in a normal fetus *(left)* with a patent connection between the jugular lymph sac and the internal jugular vein, and a cystic hygroma and hydrops from a failed lymphaticovenous connection *(right)*. **B,** Transverse neck view showing large posterolateral cystic masses *(c)* representing cystic hygromas in a fetus with Turner's syndrome. Note the multiple septations within the hygromas *(arrows)*. *s,* Cervical spine.

A goiter observed prenatally suggests that the mother may have thyroid disease. When cystic hygroma is found, there is a high risk for Turner's syndrome (45 X). Other chromosomal defects are also associated with cystic hygroma. Cystic hygroma or lymphangiectasia may result from heart failure (e.g., because of a cardiac malformation or abnormal cardiac function).

Cystic Hygroma. Fetal **cystic hygroma** results from a malformation of the lymphatic system that leads to single or multiloculated lymph-filled cavities around the neck. Normally, the lymphatic vessels empty into two sacs lateral to the jugular veins (jugular lymph sacs) that communicate with the jugular veins and form the right lymphatic duct and thoracic duct. Failure of the lymphatic system to properly connect with the venous system results in distention of the jugular lymph sacs and accumulation of lymph in fetal tissue. This abnormal collection of lymph causes distention of the lymph cavities, which may lead to fetal hydrops and even fetal death (Figure 58-39). About 70% of cystic hygromas involve the neck (usually arising from the posterior aspect of the neck bilaterally, but more rarely arising from the anterior or lateral surface), and up to 20% involve the axillae (atypical cystic hygroma). Cystic hygromas may present as isolated small cystic cavities with or without septations. Fifty percent of cystic hygromas are associated with chromosomal anomalies; therefore, identification should be accompanied by a thorough anatomic survey (Figure 58-40, *A, B*).

Cystic hygromas may be small and may regress because alternate routes of lymph drainage eventually develop. With this type of hygroma, webbing of the neck and swelling of the extremities may be appreciated after birth (Figure 58-40, *C*). These features are frequently seen in neonates with Turner's syndrome (45 X). Females are of short stature and are sterile because they develop only ovarian streaks. Cardiac and renal diseases are common. If the posterior neck skin appears thick without significant fluid-filled areas, this may represent a thickened nuchal fold, as seen with other chromosomal

anomalies such as trisomy 21. This area should be measured in a suboccipital-bregmatic view (a tangential axial image that includes the anterior fontanelle, or bregma, and the cerebellum) at between 15 and 21 weeks. A measurement that is 6 mm is considered abnormal, and the fetus should undergo further prenatal genetic screening testing.

Large fetal cystic hygromas have a typical sonographic appearance. They appear as bilateral large cystic masses at the posterolateral borders of the neck that in severe cases may surround the neck and head and upper trunk. Typically, a dense midline septum divides the hygroma, with septations noted within the dilated lymph sacs. Because of an accumulation of lymph in the fetal tissue, fetal hydrops may result. Cystic hygroma with fetal hydrops carries 100% mortality. Pericardial or pleural effusions, edema of thoracic and abdominal skin, ascites, and limb edema are common. Heart failure commonly

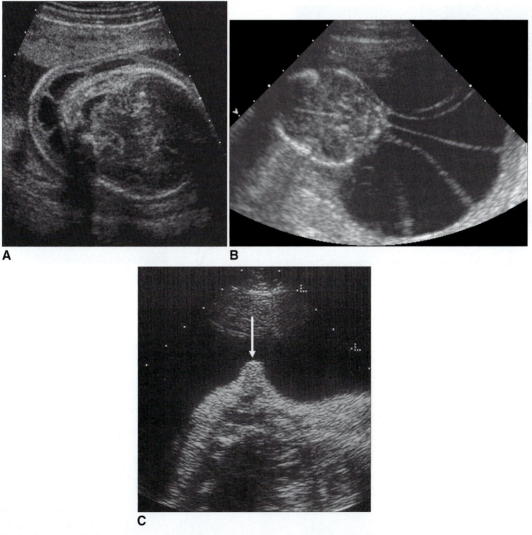

FIGURE 58-40 A, A transverse view of the neck demonstrates a small cystic hygroma. **B,** The large septated compartments seen in a fetus with a large cystic hygroma. **C,** Transverse view of the fetal neck demonstrates the remaining "webbing" from resolution of a cystic hygroma *(arrow).*

results in intrauterine death (Figures 58-41, 58-42, and 58-43). The differential considerations for cystic hygroma include meningomyelocele, encephalocele, nuchal edema, branchial cleft cyst, cystic teratoma, hemangioma, and thyroglossal duct cyst (Figure 58-44).

Fetal Goiter. Whenever maternal thyroid disease is present, the fetal thyroid should be evaluated. A **fetal goiter (thyromegaly)** usually appears as a symmetrical (bilobed), solid, homogeneous mass arising from the anterior fetal neck in the region of the fetal thyroid gland (Figure 58-45). The esophagus may be obstructed in the instance of a large goiter and hyperextended fetal neck, resulting in hydramnios and a small or absent stomach. When a goiter is suspected, the fetus may be hypothyroid or hyperthyroid. Circulating maternal antibodies (i.e., thyroid-stimulating immunoglobulin [TSI] and/or thyrotrophic binding inhibiting immunoglobulin [TBII]) determine whether fetal thyroid function is inhibited (hypothyroid) or stimulated (hyperthyroid). However, if both antibodies coexist, fetal thyroid function cannot be assessed accurately. Fetal thyroid function may then be determined by performing percutaneous umbilical blood sampling (PUBS) of the umbilical vein. If the fetus is found to be hypothyroid, then intrauterine fetal therapy may involve the weekly instillation of thyroxine via

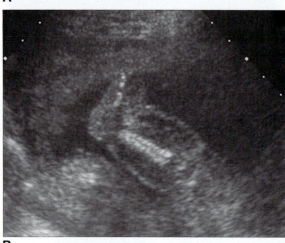

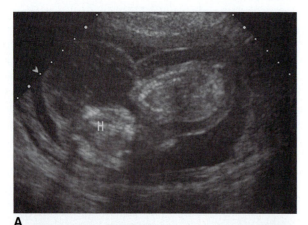

FIGURE 58-41 A, Fifteen-week fetus with a large cystic hygroma *(H)* that extends to include most of the fetal trunk. **B,** Limb edema in a fetus with cystic hygroma and generalized anasarca.

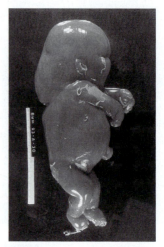

FIGURE 58-43 In the neonate shown in Figure 54-24, a side view shows the posterior lateral positioning of the cystic hygromas.

FIGURE 58-42 A, In the fetus shown in Figure 58-25, at 26 weeks' gestation, fetal movements were decreased, prompting ultrasound evaluation, which revealed a fetal demise. Note the helmet-like appearance of the scalp edema *(arrows)*. *FH,* Fetal head. **B,** In the same fetus, sagittal views revealed the posterolateral cystic hygroma *(arrows)* caused by lymphangiectasia from heart failure. *FH,* Fetal head; *s,* spine. Tetralogy of Fallot was revealed on autopsy.

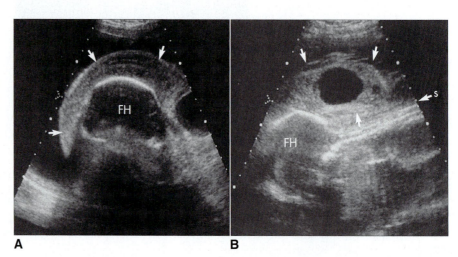

amniocentesis, or may result in an increase in maternal medication (propylthiouracil [PTU]) for the hyperthyroid fetus because these drugs cross the placenta very readily. With intrauterine therapy, most fetal goiters regress and the physical examination is normal at birth. Follow-up studies of fetuses with goiter should include assessment of fetal thyroid size, signs of fetal tachycardia (if fetus is hyperthyroid), and amniotic fluid volume.

Teratoma. Neck **teratomas** are usually unilateral and located anteriorly. They may have complex sonographic (cystic, solid, echogenic) patterns similar to teratomas of other organs (Figure 58-46). Color Doppler may help differentiate this mass from atypical hygromas or other more cystic masses.

The neck is often difficult to assess when amniotic fluid is decreased, when the fetus is in an unfavorable position, or when the neck is in close proximity to the placenta. Nonetheless, evaluation of the neck should be routinely attempted. Box 58-5 lists the questions the sonographer should answer about fetal neck masses.

BOX 58-5 Questions for the Sonographer Evaluating a Fetal Neck Mass

- What is the position of the mass (anterior, posterior, lateral, or midline)?
- Is it a unilateral or bilateral lesion?
- Is a nuchal ligament present?
- What are the Doppler properties? (Hemangiomas have arterial and venous characteristics.)
- Is there polyhydramnios?
- Is heart failure or hydrops present?
- Are there coexisting anomalies?
- Is there hyperextension, which may suggest neck mass or iniencephaly (fusion of occiput to spine)?

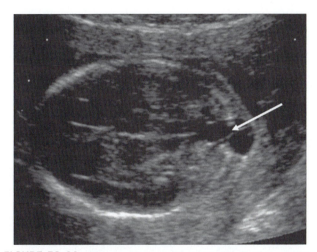

FIGURE 58-44 A fetus with a small encephalocele that could be mistaken for a small cystic hygroma. Identification of a bony defect suggests an encephalocele *(arrow).*

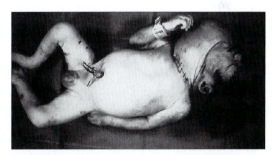

FIGURE 58-46 A large teratoma was found to arise from the posterior neck on this neonate. Multiple ultrasound studies demonstrated the mass to be complex in texture.

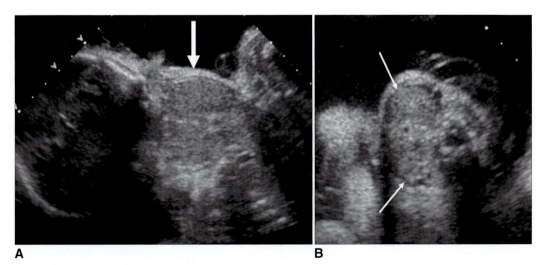

A   B

FIGURE 58-45 **A,** Axial image of the fetal neck, which reveals the bilobed enlarged fetal thyroid gland *(arrow).* **B,** A coronal view of the same fetus with the enlarged thyroid gland *(arrows).*

REFERENCES

1. Lee W, McNie B, Chaiworapongsa T, et al: Three-dimensional ultrasonographic presentation of micrognathia, *J Ultrasound Med* 21:775-781, 2002.

2. Nicholaides KH: Nuchal translucency and other first-trimester sonographic markers of chromosomal abnormalities, *Am J Obstet Gynecol* 191:45-67, 2004.

3. Palladini D, Morra T, Teodoro A, et al: Objective diagnosis of micrognathia in the fetus: the jaw index, *Ultrasound Obstet Gynecol* 93:382-386, 1999.

The Fetal Neural Axis

Charlotte G. Henningsen

OBJECTIVES

On completion of this chapter, you should be able to:
- Describe the embryology of the neural tube fetal brain development
- Discuss the anomalies that can occur in the fetal head and spine
- Recognize the sonographic appearance of fetal head and spine anomalies

EMBRYOLOGY

The central nervous system (CNS) arises from the ectodermal neural plate at around 18 gestational days. The cephalic neural plate develops into the forebrain, and the caudal end forms the spinal cord. The midbrain and hindbrain then form, and the neural plate begins to fold. The cranial and caudal neuropores represent unfused regions of the neural tube that will close between 24 and 26 gestational days. The forebrain will continue to develop into the prosencephalon, the midbrain will become the mesencephalon, and the hindbrain will form the rhombencephalon.

At the end of the 3rd week, the cephalic end of the neural tube will bend into the shape of a C (cephalic flexure), with the area of the mesencephalon having a very prominent bend. The brain then folds back on itself, and by the beginning of the 5th week another prominent bend, the cervical flexure, appears between the hindbrain and the spinal cord. The brain that originally was composed of three parts has now further divided into five parts. The prosencephalon divides into the telencephalon, which becomes the cerebral hemispheres, and the diencephalon, which eventually develops into the epithalamus, thalamus, hypothalamus, and infundibulum. The rhombencephalon also subdivides

into the metencephalon, which ultimately becomes the cerebellum and pons, and the myelencephalon, which transforms into the medulla. The fundamental organization of the brain is represented in these five divisions that persist into adult life.

The primitive spinal cord divides into two regions. The alar plate region matures into the sensory region of the cord, and the basal plate region develops into the motor region of the cord. These regions further subdivide into specialized functions. Initially, the spinal cord and the vertebral column extend the length of the body. After the first trimester, the posterior portion of the body grows beyond the vertebral column and spinal cord, and growth of the spinal cord lags behind that of the vertebral column. At birth, the spinal cord terminates at the level of the third lumbar vertebra, although by adulthood, the cord will end at the level of the second lumbar vertebra.

Neural function begins at 6 weeks' gestation and commences with primitive reflex movements at the level of the face and neck. By 12 weeks' gestation, sensitivity has spread across the surface of the body except at the back and top of the head. The fetus begins to have defined periods of activity and inactivity at the end of the 4th month. Between the 4th and 5th months, the fetus can grip objects and is capable of weak respiratory movements. At 6 months' gestation, the fetus displays the sucking reflex, and by about 28 weeks, significant changes in brain wave patterns have occurred.

Many of the congenital malformations of the CNS result from incomplete closure of the neural tube. A wide range of defects may affect the spine and/or brain. The remainder of this chapter presents anomalies of the CNS (Table 59-1).

Correctly identifying anomalies of the fetal head and spine can be a complex task. Some of the distinguishing characteristics that help define specific anomalies are listed in Table 59-2.

ANENCEPHALY

Anencephaly, also known as aprosencephaly or atelencephaly, is the most common neural tube defect, with an overall incidence of approximately 1 in 1000 pregnancies in the United States. The incidence varies with geographic location, with a much higher prevalence in the

TABLE 59-1	Anomalies Most Frequently Associated With Ventriculomegaly
Anomaly	**Distinguishing Characteristics**
Spina bifida	Deformed cranium "lemon sign"; usually disappears in third trimester Obliteration of cisterna magna Open spinal defect
Cephalocele	Open cranial defect; usually occipital skull base Obliteration of the cisterna magna Occasional lemon sign
Holoprosencephaly	Absent/incomplete midline Single ventricular cavity Facial anomalies
Dandy-Walker complex	Midline posterior fossa cyst Defect in cerebellar vermis
Agenesis of corpus callosum	Absent cavum septi pellucidi Elevated third ventricle Interhemispheric cyst/lipoma
Arachnoid/ glioependymal cyst	Intracranial cyst with regular contours displacing/compressing cortex
Porencephaly	Intracranial cyst with jagged outline often communicating with lateral ventricles
Schizencephaly	Clefts in cortical mantle
Intracranial hemorrhage	Echogenic/complex mass in lateral ventricles/brain parenchyma
Microcephaly	Small head
Vascular malformations	Fluid-filled lesion with blood flow at Doppler examination
Craniostenosis	Abnormal skull shape
Lissencephaly	Absent/reduced cerebral convolutions
Infection	Intracranial/periventricular echogenicities

From Nyberg D: *Diagnostic imaging of fetal anomalies,* Philadelphia, 2003, Lippincott, Williams & Wilkins.

United Kingdom. The incidence also varies with gender and race, with a female prevalence of 4 to 1 over males, and a prevalence of white over black of 6 to 1. A significant recurrence risk of 2% to 3% for subsequent pregnancies has been documented for a woman with a history of a prior pregnancy with an open neural tube defect.

Anencephaly, which means absence of the brain, is caused by failure of closure of the neural tube at the cranial end. The result consists of absence of the cranial vault, complete or partial absence of the forebrain, which may partially develop and then degenerate, and presence of the brain stem, midbrain, skull base, and facial structures. The remnant brain is covered by a thick membrane called *angiomatous stroma* or *cerebrovasculosa.*

Anencephaly is a lethal disorder, with up to 50% of cases resulting in fetal demise. The remainder die at birth or shortly thereafter. Because of the severity of this disorder, early diagnosis is preferred. Prenatal diagnosis is often made with ultrasound following referral for increased maternal serum alpha-fetoprotein levels, which are extremely high with this defect because of the absent skull and exposed tissue.

Causes of neural tube defects, including anencephaly, are numerous. Anencephaly may result from a syndrome, such as Meckel-Gruber (i.e., cystic kidneys, occipital encephalocele and/or polydactyly [postaxial], microcephaly, microphthalmia, cleft palate, and genitourinary anomalies), or a chromosomal abnormality, such as trisomy 13 and trisomy 18. Risk is increased in patients with diabetes mellitus, including those whose disorders are well controlled. Environmental and dietary factors, including hyperthermia, folate and vitamin deficiencies, and teratogenic levels of zinc, may also increase the prevalence of neural tube defects. Other teratogens associated with neural tube defects include valproic acid, methotrexate, and aminopterin. Another cause of neural tube defects is amniotic band syndrome, which may manifest with clefting defects.

Sonographic Findings. Anencephaly may be detected with ultrasound as early as 10 to 14 weeks' gestation, although the only sonographic feature may be acrania. The crown-rump length may be normal because degeneration of the fetal brain is progressive, leading to a reduction in the crown-rump length with advancing gestation. Second-trimester identification of anencephaly is more obvious, with absent cerebral hemispheres evident, along with absence of the skull.

Sonographic features of anencephaly include the following:

- Absence of the brain and cranial vault (Figure 59-1)
- Rudimentary brain tissue characterized as the cerebrovasculosa (Figure 59-2)
- Bulging fetal orbits, giving the fetus a froglike appearance (Figure 59-3)

Other sonographic findings associated with anencephaly include polyhydramnios, which is commonly seen

TABLE 59-2	Differential Considerations for Central Nervous System Anomalies		
Anomaly	Sonographic Findings	Differential Considerations	Distinguishing Characteristics
Anencephaly	Absence of brain and cranial vault Froglike appearance Cerebrovasculosa	Microcephaly Acrania Cephalocele	No calvarium above vault orbits
Cephalocele	Extracranial mass Bony defect in calvarium	Cystic hygroma	Defect in skull
Dandy-Walker malformation	Posterior fossa cyst Splaying of cerebellar hemispheres	Arachnoid cyst Cerebellar hypoplasia	Cerebellar hemispheres will be splayed
Vein of Galen aneurysm	Midline cystic structure Turbulent Doppler flow	Arachnoid cyst Porencephalic cyst	Doppler flow in the cystic space
Porencephalic cyst	Cyst within brain parenchyma No mass effect Communication with ventricle	Arachnoid cyst	No mass effect Cyst communicating with ventricle
Hydranencephaly	Absence of brain tissue Fluid-filled brain Absent or partially absent falx	Hydrocephaly Holoprosencephaly	Lack of intact falx No rim of brain tissue

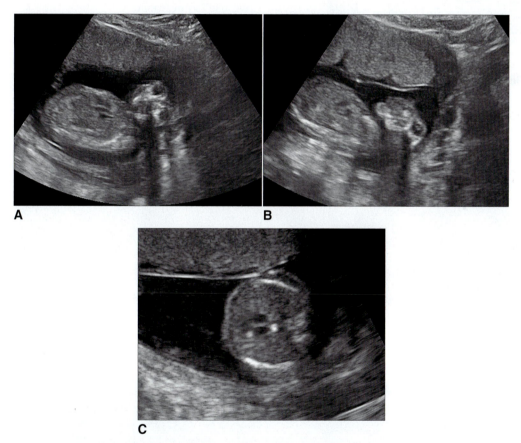

FIGURE 59-1 A, An anencephalic fetus; absence of the brain and calvarium is identified. Note the froglike appearance. **B,** A profile of the anomaly. **C,** Echogenic foci were noted in the heart; amniocentesis revealed trisomy 13.

but may not be present until after 26 weeks' gestation, although oligohydramnios may occasionally be identified. Coexisting spina bifida and/or craniorachischisis may be identified in fetuses with anencephaly. Additional anomalies include cleft lip and palate, hydronephrosis, diaphragmatic hernia, cardiac defects, omphalocele, gastrointestinal defects, and talipes.

When severe, microcephaly may be confused with anencephaly, although the presence of the cranium should aid in a definitive diagnosis. Other defects that may mimic anencephaly include acrania (brain is abnormal but present), cephalocele (brain herniation), and amniotic band syndrome (usually asymmetrical cranial defects).

ACRANIA

Acrania, also known as exencephaly, is a lethal **anomaly** that manifests as absence of the cranial bones with the presence of complete, although abnormal, development of the cerebral hemispheres. This anomaly occurs at the beginning of the 4th gestational week, when the

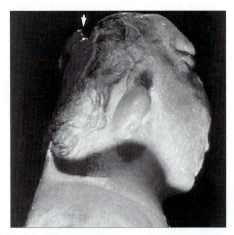

FIGURE 59-2 Postmortem photograph of anencephaly. The *arrow* points to the rudimentary brain (cerebrovasculosa).

mesenchymal tissue fails to migrate and does not allow bone formation over the cerebral tissue. The prevalence of acrania is rare, with only a few cases reported in the literature. In addition, acrania usually progresses to anencephaly as the brain slowly degenerates as a result of exposure to amniotic fluid.

Acrania may be confused with anencephaly, although the presence of significant brain tissue and the lack of a froglike appearance should establish the diagnosis. Other disorders that may mimic acrania include hypophosphatasia and osteogenesis imperfecta, both of which result in hypomineralization of the cranium. Identification of additional findings, such as long bone fractures, should help to distinguish these disorders from acrania. In addition to the lack of other skeletal anomalies, lack of a calvarium allows differentiation of the cerebral hemispheres within the amniotic fluid, giving the fetal head a bilobed appearance. This bilobed brain is best identified in the first trimester and has been described as a "Mickey Mouse" appearance.

Sonographic Findings. Sonographic features of acrania include the following:

- The presence of brain tissue without the presence of a calvarium (Figure 59-4)

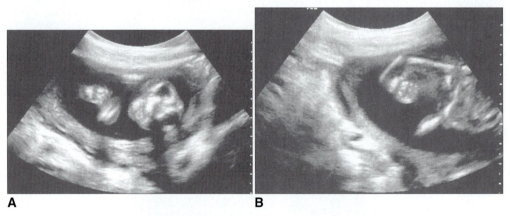

A   **B**

FIGURE 59-3 **A,** Anencephaly was identified in a fetus with **(B)** a radial ray defect and tetralogy of Fallot. A chromosomal anomaly was suspected.

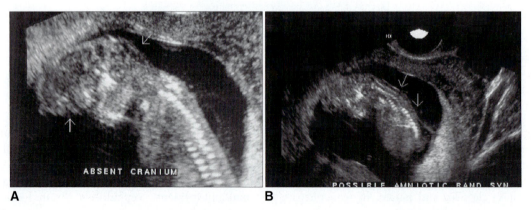

A   **B**

FIGURE 59-4 Acrania. Patient presented with an elevated maternal serum alpha-fetoprotein. Note the amnion *(arrows)* along the back of the fetus. Amniotic band syndrome was the probable cause.

- Disorganization of brain tissue
- Prominent sulcal markings (Figures 59-5 to 59-7)

Acrania may be associated with other anomalies, including spinal defects, cleft lip and palate, talipes, cardiac defects, and omphalocele. Acrania has also been associated with amniotic band syndrome (see Figure 59-4, B).

CEPHALOCELE

A cephalocele is a neural tube defect in which the meninges alone or the meninges and brain herniate through a defect in the calvarium. *Encephalocele* is the term used to describe herniation of the meninges and brain through the defect; *cranial meningocele* describes the herniation of only meninges (Figure 59-8). Cephaloceles occur at a rate of 1 to 3 in 10,000 live births.

Cephaloceles involve the occipital bone (Figure 59-9) and are located at the midline in 75% of cases, although

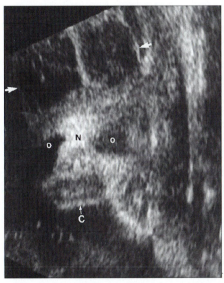

FIGURE 59-5 Coronal facial view showing absence of the parietal bones *(arrows)*, with highly visible brain tissue *(arrows)* representing acrania or exencephaly. *c,* Chin; *N,* nose; *o,* orbits.

they may also involve the parietal, frontal, and temporal regions or other bones of the calvarium.

The prognosis for the infant with a cephalocele varies based on the size, location, and involvement of other brain structures. The presence of brain in the defect dictates a poor prognosis. Microcephaly and other associated anomalies worsen the outcome. An infant with an isolated cranial meningocele has a 60% chance of normal mentation.

Sonographic Findings. The sonographic appearance of a cephalocele largely depends on the location, size, and involvement of brain structures. Cephaloceles containing meninges only; brain tissue only; meninges and brain tissue; and meninges, brain tissue, and lateral ventricles are referred to as meningocele, encephalocele, encephalomeningocele, and encephalomeningocystocele, respectively. According to the size of the lesion, cephaloceles are classified as occipital cephaloceles, which occur when the defect lies between the lambdoid suture and the foramen magnum; parietal cephaloceles, which occur between the bregma and the lambda; and anterior cephaloceles, which lie between the anterior aspects of the ethmoid bone. Anterior cephaloceles are further classified into frontal and basal varieties. The frontal cephaloceles are always external lesions that occur near the root of the nose. Basal cephaloceles are internal lesions that occur within the nose, the pharynx, or the orbit.

Sonographic features of cephaloceles include the following:

- An extracranial mass (Figure 59-10), which may be fluid-filled (cranial meningocele) or contain solid components (encephalocele)
- A bony defect in the skull
- Ventriculomegaly, which is more commonly identified with an encephalocele

Another sonographic finding associated with cephaloceles is polyhydramnios. Coexisting anomalies include microcephaly, agenesis of the corpus callosum, facial

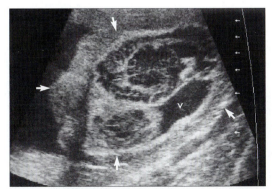

FIGURE 59-6 In the fetus shown in Figure 59-5, a transverse view shows the disorganized and freely floating brain tissue *(arrows)*. The brain anatomy is enhanced because of the absence of skull bones. Note the herniated ventricle *(v)* and sulcal markings.

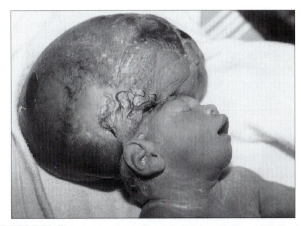

FIGURE 59-7 Same neonate shown in Figures 59-5 and 59-6, with acrania shortly after birth. The infant died within a few hours.

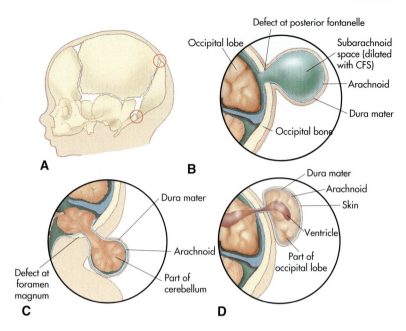

FIGURE 59-8 Schematic drawings illustrating cranium bifidum (bony defect in the cranium) and various types of herniation of the brain and/or meninges. **A,** Sketch of the head of a newborn infant with a large protrusion from the occipital region of the skull. The upper circle indicates a cranial defect at the posterior fontanelle, and the lower circle indicates a cranial defect near the foramen magnum. **B,** Meningocele consisting of a protrusion of the cranial meninges that is filled with cerebrospinal fluid. **C,** Meningoencephalocele consisting of a protrusion of part of the cerebellum that is covered by meninges and skin. **D,** Meningohydroencephalocele consisting of a protrusion of the part of the occipital lobe that contains part of the posterior horn of a lateral ventricle.

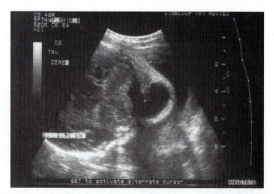

FIGURE 59-9 Neonate with a posterior occipital encephalocele.

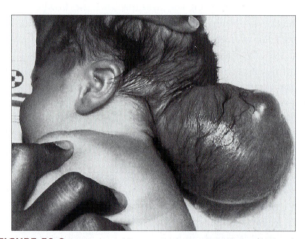

FIGURE 59-10 Cranial meningocele. The sac protruding from the cranium is fluid-filled.

clefts, spina bifida, cardiac anomalies, and genital anomalies. Chromosomal anomalies and syndromes have been identified with cephaloceles, including trisomy 13 and Meckel-Gruber syndrome, which is an autosomal-recessive disorder characterized by encephalocele,

polydactyly, and polycystic kidneys (Figure 59-11). Other syndromes linked with cephalocele include Chemke, cryptophthalmos, Knobloch, dyssegmental dysplasia, von Voss, Roberts', and Walker-Warburg. Cephaloceles located off midline are usually the result of amniotic band syndrome and may be further distinguished by associated limb anomalies and abdominal wall defects.

Cephaloceles may be confused with **cystic hygromas,** although they lack a cranial defect. Anencephaly may be difficult to distinguish from encephaloceles of significant size, and the presence of the cranial vault with encephalocele should establish the diagnosis. Frontal encephaloceles may be difficult to distinguish from a facial teratoma.

SPINA BIFIDA

Spina bifida encompasses a wide range of vertebral defects that result from failure of neural tube closure. The meninges and neural elements may protrude through this defect. The defect may occur anywhere along the vertebral column but most commonly occurs along the lumbar and sacral regions. The incidence of this defect has declined as a result of campaigning by the U.S. Public Health Service, which encourages women to increase their intake of folic acid before becoming pregnant, and the subsequent mandate by the Food and Drug Administration to add folic acid to cereal grain products. Decreases in the prevalence of anencephaly and encephalocele have been noted.

The term *spina bifida* means that there is a cleft or opening in the spine (Figure 59-12). When covered with skin or hair, it is referred to as *spina bifida occulta,* an anomaly that is associated with a normal spinal cord and nerves and normal neurologic development. Spina bifida occulta is extremely difficult to detect in the fetus.

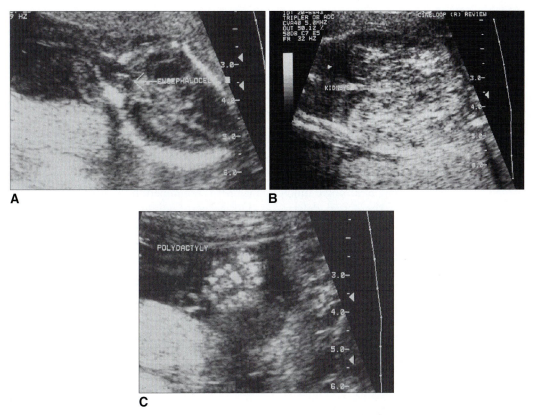

FIGURE 59-11 Encephalocele as part of Meckel-Gruber syndrome. **A,** Brain tissue herniating from the occipital region. **B,** Large echogenic kidneys consistent with autosomal-recessive polycystic kidney disease (ARPKD). **C,** Polydactyly was noted on the hands.

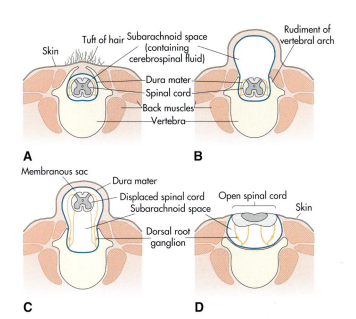

FIGURE 59-12 Diagrammatic sketches illustrating various types of spina bifida and commonly associated malformations of the nervous system. **A,** Spina bifida occulta. About 10% of people have this vertebral defect in L5 and/or S1. It usually causes no back problems. **B,** Spina bifida with meningocele. **C,** Spina bifida with meningomyelocele. **D,** Spina bifida with myeloschisis. The types illustrated in **B** through **D** are often referred to collectively as *spina bifida cystica* because of the cystic sac that is associated with them.

Because the defect is covered by skin, the maternal serum alpha-fetoprotein level will be normal.

When the defect involves only protrusion of the meninges, it is termed a *meningocele.* More commonly, the meninges and neural elements protrude through the defect. This is called a *meningomyelocele.* If the defect is very large and severe, it is termed *rachischisis.* These defects are commonly associated with increased maternal serum alpha-fetoprotein.

Spina bifida is also associated with varying degrees of neurologic impairment, which may include minor anesthesia, paraparesis, or death. Fetuses with myelomeningoceles often present with cranial defects associated with the Arnold-Chiari (type II) malformation, which is identified in 90% of patients. The Arnold-Chiari II malformation presents invariably with hydrocephalus caused by the cerebellar vermis, which becomes displaced into the cervical canal. This changes the shape of the cerebellum, giving it a "banana" appearance, and leads to obliteration of the cisterna magna. In addition, caudal displacement of the cranial structures causes scalloping of the frontal bones of the skull, making the fetal head resemble a lemon.

Management of a fetus with spina bifida usually includes serial ultrasound examinations to monitor progression and extent of ventriculomegaly and to follow fetal growth. Fetuses may be delivered early for ventricular shunting, usually by cesarean section to preserve as much motor function as possible. Surgical repair of these defects in utero is being performed in a randomized clinical trial to determine whether surgery decreases the incidence of hindbrain herniation, thus decreasing the incidence of hydrocephalus and subsequent shunting. Risks incurred with this procedure include premature delivery, maternal morbidity, and fetal mortality.

The prognosis for an infant with spina bifida varies greatly according to the type, size, and location of the defect. Rachischisis is invariably lethal, and higher lesions (Figure 59-13) tend to have a worse prognosis. When intervention is desired, surgical closure of the defect is performed to preserve existing neurologic function. In addition to management of the actual defect, attention to any hydrocephalus, urinary tract anomalies or dysfunction, and orthopedic issues may be part of the long-term care required for this child.

Sonographic Findings. Sonographic examination of the fetal spine should include a methodical survey of the spine in the sagittal and transverse planes (Figure 59-14). The normal fetal spine should demonstrate the posterior ossification centers completing a spinal circle. The survey of the fetal spine may be impeded when the spine is down, when the fetus is in the breech position, when oligohydramnios is present, and when maternal obesity precludes adequate visualization.

Sonographic features of spina bifida include the following:

- Splaying of the posterior ossification centers with a V or U configuration (Figure 59-15)
- Protrusion of a saclike structure that may be anechoic (meningocele) or contain neural elements (myelomeningocele) (Figure 59-16)
- A cleft in the skin (Figure 59-17)

After a spinal defect has been identified, the level and extent of the defect, the presence or absence of neural elements contained in the protruding sac, and associated intracranial findings should be documented.

Associated sonographic cranial findings include the following:

- Flattening of the frontal bones, giving the head a "lemon" shape (Figure 59-18)
- Obliteration of the cisterna magna
- Inferior displacement of the cerebellar vermis, giving the cerebellum a rounded, "banana" shape (see Figure 59-18)
- Ventriculomegaly (Figures 59-19 and 59-20)

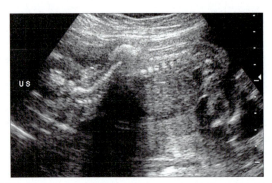

FIGURE 59-13 A large spinal defect at the thoracic level is seen in the fetus. The prognosis was expected to be extremely poor.

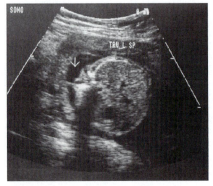

FIGURE 59-15 Meningomyelocele with spinal splaying appearing as a V.

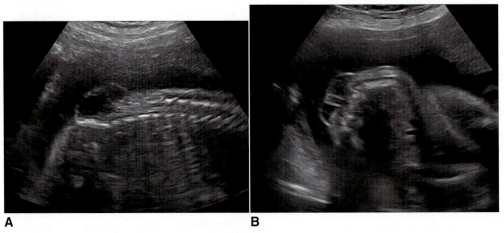

A   B

FIGURE 59-14 Sagittal **(A)** and transverse **(B)** views of the fetal spine *(arrows)* demonstrate this defect in the lumbar region consistent with a myelomeningocele.

The "lemon sign" is not specific for spina bifida, and similar head shapes have been described with other CNS malformations, such as encephalocele, and with non-CNS malformations, such as thanatophoric dysplasia. This appearance may also be indistinguishable from the "strawberry sign" described in association with trisomy 18.

Other sonographic findings associated with spina bifida include talipes, cephaloceles, cleft lip and palate, hypotelorism, heart defects, and genitourinary anomalies (Figures 59-21 and 59-22). Spina bifida has also been associated with multiple syndromes and chromosomal anomalies, including trisomy 18. Fetuses exposed to teratogens, such as valproic acid (Figure 59-23), carbamazepine, methotrexate, and aminopterin, are also at greater risk for developing spina bifida. Maternal diabetes, maternal obesity, hyperthermia, and folic acid deficiency have been associated with spina bifida as well. A family history of spina bifida or anencephaly is a significant risk factor for the occurrence of spina bifida.

DANDY-WALKER MALFORMATION

Dandy-Walker malformation (DWM) is a defect that may have varying degrees of severity. It manifests with agenesis or hypoplasia of the cerebellar vermis with resulting dilatation on the fourth ventricle and enlargement of the posterior fossa. The occurrence rate is 1 in 25,000 to 35,000, and the condition accounts for 4% of

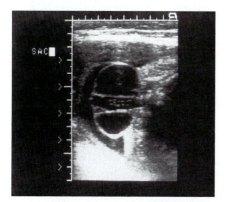

FIGURE 59-16 Meningomyelocele identified in a fetus with mild ventriculomegaly. Note the neural elements protruding into the sac.

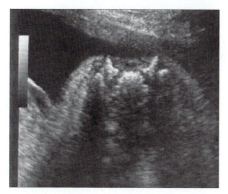

FIGURE 59-17 Spina bifida with a U-shaped configuration and an open cleft in the skin.

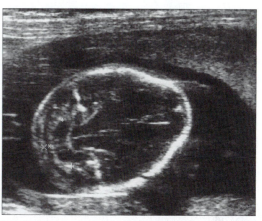

FIGURE 59-18 Abnormally shaped cerebellum "banana sign" (calipers [+]) in a 21-week fetus with a lumbosacral meningomyelocele. Note the lemon-shaped frontal bones consistent with frontal bossing.

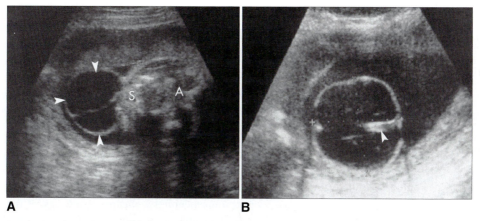

A   B

FIGURE 59-19 A, Lumbosacral meningomyelocele (arrows) shown in a 21-week fetus, detected on a basic fetal scan. A, Abdomen; S, spine. B, Lumbosacral meningomyelocele measuring 6 cm (calipers) observed in a 33-week fetus during a basic fetal scan. Note the spinal elements (arrow) within the meningomyelocele sac. Additional anomalies include clubbing of the feet and inward rotation of the legs. Ventriculomegaly was present, but effacement of the cisterna magna was not apparent.

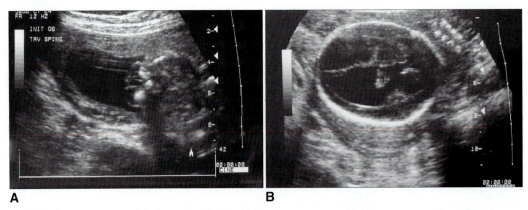

FIGURE 59-20 A, A fetus of 24.6 weeks' gestation with a meningomyelocele. Neural elements were identified in the sac. **B,** A significant amount of ventricular dilatation was identified within the fetal head.

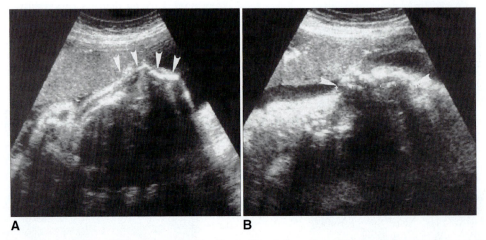

FIGURE 59-21 A, Thoracic meningomyelocele demonstrated with significant disruption of the bony elements *(arrows)*. **B,** In the same fetus, another view demonstrating the spinal defect. Coexisting anomalies included significant ventriculomegaly of 27 mm, unilateral renal agenesis, and a single umbilical artery.

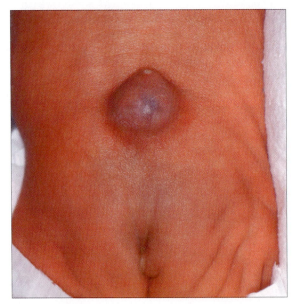

FIGURE 59-22 A neonate with a lumbar myelomeningocele.

hydrocephalus in infants. Dandy-Walker complex encompasses the three main types of posterior fossa malformations. DWM is described here and also includes an elevated tentorium; Dandy-Walker variant (DWV) manifests with cystic dilatation of the fourth ventricle and hypoplasia of the cerebellar vermis without an enlarged posterior fossa; megacisterna magna (MCM) is defined as an enlarged cisterna magna.

Development of the cerebellar vermis begins during the 9th week; however, communications between the fourth ventricle and the cisterna magna are not complete until the 18th week of gestation. Because of this, diagnosis of agenesis and hypoplasia of the cerebellar vermis should not be made prior to the 18th week of gestation.

DWM is associated with other intracranial anomalies about 50% of the time. These include agenesis of the corpus callosum, aqueductal stenosis, microcephaly, **macrocephaly,** encephalocele, gyral malformations, heterotopias, and lipomas. Chromosomal anomalies that may be associated with DWM include trisomies 13, 18, and 21 and triploidy. DWM has been associated with several syndromes, including Meckel-Gruber syndrome,

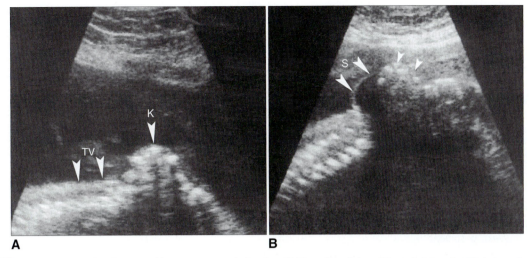

FIGURE 59-23 A, Meningomyelocele caused by a teratogen (valproic acid [Depakene]) in a 26-week fetus. Sagittal view showing thoraco-lumbar meningomyelocele with marked kyphosis *(K)* of the spinal elements. *TV,* Thoracic vertebrae. **B,** In the same fetus, a meningomyelocele sac *(S)* is observed and marked disruption and malalignment of the vertebrae are outlined *(small arrowheads)*. This mother was given valproic acid for a seizure disorder during the first trimester of pregnancy. Valproic acid is a known teratogen that may produce neural tube defects. Elevated levels of maternal serum alpha-fetoprotein prompted the fetal study. Coexisting anomalies included ventriculomegaly, small cranium, and a unilateral clubfoot.

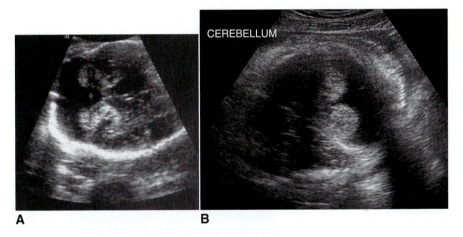

FIGURE 59-24 A, Dandy-Walker cyst. Note the splayed cerebellar hemispheres. **B,** This Dandy-Walker malformation was not associated with ventriculomegaly; amniocentesis revealed normal chromosomes.

Walker-Warburg syndrome, and Aicardi's syndrome, and has been linked with congenital infection and maternal diabetes.

The prognosis for DWM depends on the presence or absence of associated anomalies and on the degree of hypoplasia of the cerebellar vermis, as this correlates with the severity of mental retardation. Mortality depends highly on other anomalies. Many infants with isolated DWM have a subnormal IQ, although some may have normal function.

Sonographic Findings. Sonographic survey may reveal extracranial anomalies that are also associated with DWM, including cardiac anomalies, polydactyly, facial clefts, and urinary tract anomalies.

Sonographic features of DWM include the following:

- A posterior fossa cyst that can vary considerably in size (Figure 59-24)

- Splaying of the cerebellar hemispheres as a result of complete or partial agenesis of the cerebellar vermis
- An enlarged cisterna magna caused by the cerebellar vermis anomaly and posterior fossa cyst
- Ventriculomegaly (Figure 59-25)

Differential considerations should include the arachnoid cyst, but identification of the splayed cerebellar hemispheres may help to confirm DWM. Cerebellar hypoplasia should also be considered when the cisterna magna is enlarged; however, confirming the small cerebellum may make this diagnosis.

HOLOPROSENCEPHALY

Holoprosencephaly encompasses a range of abnormalities resulting from abnormal cleavage of the prosencephalon (forebrain). The incidence is 1 in 10,000 to 20,000 live births, although the incidence in embryos has

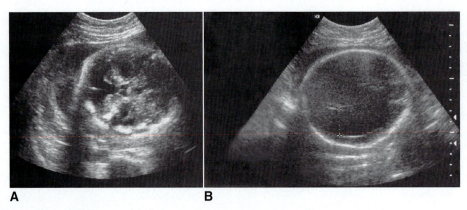

A   **B**

FIGURE 59-25 This patient had a history of elevated maternal serum alpha-fetoprotein. Follow-up in a maternal fetal center for a history of hydrocephalus revealed a Dandy-Walker malformation **(A)** and ventriculomegaly **(B).** The fetus was 30 weeks and 4 days, with a head size typical of 36 weeks' gestation.

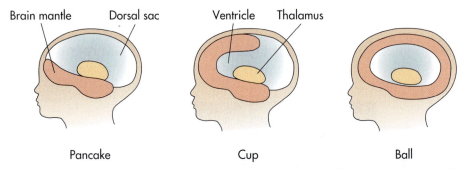

Pancake   Cup   Ball

FIGURE 59-26 Diagram of three morphologic types of alobar holoprosencephaly (and semilobar holoprosencephaly) in sagittal view. In the pancake type, the residual brain mantle is flattened at the base of the brain. The dorsal sac is correspondingly large. The cup type has more brain mantle present, but it does not cover the monoventricle. In the ball type, the brain mantle completely covers the monoventricle, and a dorsal sac may or may not be present.

been much higher (1 in 250). Holoprosencephaly has been associated with chromosomal anomalies in up to 50% of cases; however, it may also be a sporadic event or may be associated with syndromes, genetic factors, and teratogens. The recurrence risk has been reported as high as 13% to 14% when identified as a sporadic event.[1]

Three forms of holoprosencephaly are known. The most severe form is classified as alobar, the intermediate form as semilobar, and the mildest form as lobar. Identification of the specific form depends on the degree of failed hemispheric division.

Alobar holoprosencephaly is characterized by a singular monoventricle brain tissue that is small and may have a cup, ball, or pancake configuration (Figure 59-26); fusion of the thalamus; and absence of the interhemispheric fissure, cavum septum pellucidum, corpus callosum, optic tracts, and olfactory bulbs. Semilobar holoprosencephaly (Figure 59-27) presents with a singular ventricular cavity with partial formation of the occipital horns, partial or complete fusion of the thalamus, a rudimentary falx and interhemispheric fissure, and absent corpus callosum, cavum septum pellucidum, and olfactory bulbs. In lobar holoprosencephaly, almost complete division of the ventricles is seen with a corpus callosum that may be normal, hypoplastic, or absent,

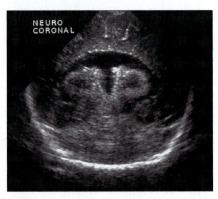

FIGURE 59-27 A neonatal ultrasound in a newborn revealed semilobar holoprosencephaly. There was no history of a prenatal ultrasound because of the normal course of the pregnancy. The infant lived for only a few weeks.

although the cavum septum pellucidum will still be absent.

The cause of holoprosencephaly varies. It is frequently sporadic but has been associated with chromosomal anomalies, most specifically, trisomy 13; however, trisomy 18 and triploidy have been identified, along with anomalies of chromosomes 7, 3, and 11. Rare familial patterns have been transmitted in autosomal dominant and autosomal recessive forms. Multiple syndromes have also been associated with holoprosencephaly, including Meckel-Gruber syndrome, Aicardi's syndrome, Fryns syndrome, and hydrolethalus syndrome. Teratogens reported to produce holoprosencephaly include alcohol, phenytoin, retinoic acid, maternal diabetes, and congenital infection. Holoprosencephaly has also been associated with radiation exposure, and in rare instances, with the use of oral contraceptives and aspirin during the first trimester.

The prognosis for holoprosencephaly is considered uniformly poor. In its most severe forms, fetuses die at birth or shortly thereafter. In the least severe form, survival is possible, although usually with severe mental retardation.

◗ Sonographic Findings. Sonographic features of holoprosencephaly include the following:

- A common C-shaped ventricle that may or may not be enlarged (Figure 59-28)
- Brain tissue with a horseshoe shape as it surrounds the monoventricle
- Fusion of the thalamus with absence of the third ventricle
- Absence of the interhemispheric fissure
- A dorsal sac with expansion of the monoventricle posteriorly
- Absence of the corpus callosum
- Absence of the cavum septum pellucidum

Holoprosencephaly is often associated with facial abnormalities, especially with the most severe forms (Figure 59-29). The facial anomalies identified include cyclopia, hypotelorism (Figure 59-30, *A*), an absent nose, a flattened nose with a single nostril, and proboscis (Figures 59-30, *B* and 59-31). **Cebocephaly** consists of the combination of hypotelorism with a normally placed nose with a single nostril. Ethmocephaly consists of severe hypotelorism with a proboscis superior to the eyes. In addition, facial clefts may be present, with median or bilateral clefting most commonly observed.

Other sonographic findings associated with holoprosencephaly include hydrocephaly, microcephaly, polyhydramnios, and intrauterine growth restriction (IUGR). In addition, renal cysts or dysplasia, omphalocele, cardiac defects, spina bifida, talipes, and gastrointestinal anomalies have been identified in the presence of holoprosencephaly. Chromosomal anomalies must also be considered if holoprosencephaly is present, especially trisomy 13.

AGENESIS OF THE CORPUS CALLOSUM

The corpus callosum is a fibrous tract that connects the cerebral hemispheres and aids in learning and memory. Dysgenesis of the corpus callosum describes a range of complete to partial absence of the callosal fibers that cross the midline, forming a connection between the two hemispheres. The incidence is reported to be 1 to 3 in 1000 births.

The corpus callosum begins to develop at 12 weeks' gestation and development is not complete until 20 weeks. The cause of agenesis of the corpus callosum (ACC) is somewhat unclear but is thought to involve a vascular disruption or inflammatory lesion before 12 weeks. Cases of agenesis of the corpus callosum, also

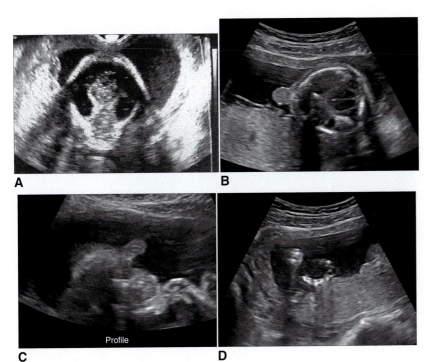

FIGURE 59-28 Holoprosencephaly. **A,** C-shaped monoventricle. **B,** A different fetus with a proboscis. **C,** Note the abnormal-appearing profile. **D,** Polydactyly was also identified on all four extremities, suggesting the possibility of trisomy 13.

known as callosal agenesis, are sporadic. It may be associated with other CNS malformations, including hydrocephalus, gyral anomalies, heterotopias, Dandy-Walker malformation, and holoprosencephaly. It may be transmitted in an autosomal dominant or autosomal recessive manner, and X-linked syndromes have also been identified. Chromosomal anomalies that may accompany agenesis of the corpus callosum include trisomies 21, 13, and 18 and triploidy; multiple syndromes have been associated with ACC, including Aicardi, Apert, Opitz, and Joubert syndromes, to name a few. Maternal diseases such as diabetes, infection, and alcohol abuse are also contributing factors. In addition, extracranial anomalies are associated with ACC.

The prognosis for agenesis of the corpus callosum depends largely on the high incidence of associated anomalies, many of which carry a poor prognosis. As an isolated event, agenesis of the corpus callosum may be asymptomatic or may be associated with mental retardation and/or seizures.

Sonographic Findings. Sonographic features of agenesis of the corpus callosum (Figure 59-32) include the following:

- Absence of the corpus callosum
- Elevation and dilatation of the third ventricle
- Widely separated lateral ventricular frontal horns with medial indentation of the medial walls
- Dilated occipital horns (colpocephaly), giving the lateral ventricles a teardrop shape
- Absence of the cavum septum pellucidum

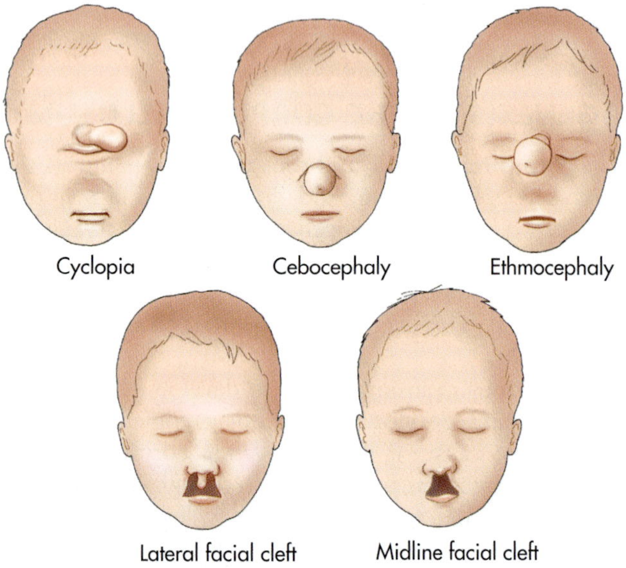

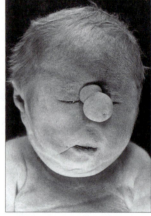

FIGURE 59-31 Postmortem photograph of a neonate with ethmocephaly. Note the proboscis and hypotelorism. The mouth appears normal. A common ventricle and absent optic and ophthalmic nerves were found. The chromosomes were consistent with trisomy 13.

Cyclopia   Cebocephaly   Ethmocephaly

Lateral facial cleft   Midline facial cleft

FIGURE 59-29 Facial features of holoprosencephaly. These drawings illustrate the normal facial features in contrast with the variable facial features of holoprosencephaly. In cyclopia, the proboscis projects from the lower forehead superior to one median orbit, and the nose is absent. Ethmocephaly is very similar to cyclopia but has two narrowly placed orbits with a proboscis and absent nose. In cebocephaly, a rudimentary nose with a single nostril and hypotelorism are present. Hypotelorism may occur with a median cleft lip or a bilateral cleft lip.

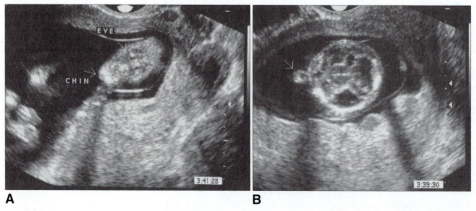

A   B

FIGURE 59-30 A, A fetus with trisomy 13 demonstrates small eyes with hypotelorism. **B,** In the same fetus, a proboscis *(arrow)* is seen above the orbits.

Sonographic findings associated with agenesis of the corpus callosum include other CNS anomalies, such as holoprosencephaly, DWM, cranial lipoma, Arnold-Chiari malformation, septo-optic dysplasia, hydrocephaly, encephalocele, porencephaly, microcephaly, and lissencephaly. Other abnormalities associated with agenesis of the corpus callosum include cardiac malformations, diaphragmatic hernia, lung agenesis or dysplasia, and absent or dysplastic kidneys. Multiple chromosomal anomalies and syndromes have been linked with agenesis of the corpus callosum, including trisomies 13, 18, 11, and 8, and Aicardi's syndrome.

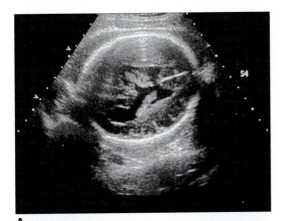

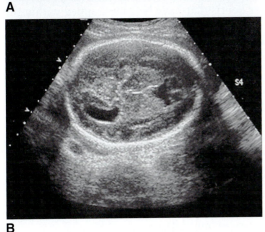

FIGURE 59-32 **A,** Agenesis of the corpus callosum is diagnosed in this fetus with an absent cavum septum pellucidum. **B,** The occipital horn of the lateral ventricle also appears dilated.

AQUEDUCTAL STENOSIS

Aqueductal stenosis results from obstruction, atresia, or stenosis of the aqueduct of Sylvius causing ventriculomegaly. The aqueduct of Sylvius connects the third and fourth ventricles, which explains the enlargement of the lateral ventricles and the third ventricle in the presence of a normal fourth ventricle.

Aqueductal stenosis is usually a sporadic anomaly, but may also result from intrauterine infection, such as cytomegalovirus, rubella, and toxoplasmosis. Cranial masses and ventricular hemorrhage are other contributing factors to acquired obstruction. Primary aqueductal stenosis is usually X-linked and has an autosomal-recessive inheritance.

The prognosis for aqueductal stenosis is considered poor and varies with associated anomalies. Approximately 90% of survivors have an IQ less than 70. Infants with X-linked aqueductal stenosis are profoundly mentally retarded.

Sonographic Findings. Sonographic features of aqueductal stenosis include the following:

- Ventricular enlargement of the lateral ventricles, which may be severe (Figures 59-33 and 59-34)
- Third ventricular dilatation
- Flexion and adduction of the thumb (seen in the X-linked form)

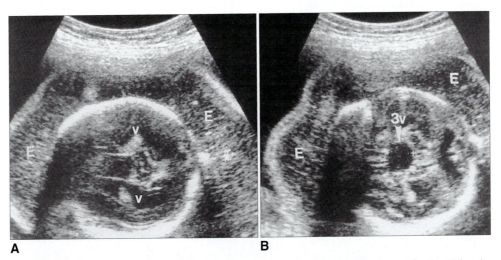

FIGURE 59-33 **A,** Ventricular view in a fetus with acquired aqueductal stenosis caused by parvovirus infection. Dilatation of the ventricular system *(v)* resulted from inflammation, causing obstruction to the flow of cerebrospinal fluid. The fetus was severely hydropic. Note the significant scalp edema *(E)*. **B,** In the same fetus, third ventricle *(3v)* dilatation is demonstrated. Cordocentesis was performed to find a cause for the severe nonimmune hydrops, and parvovirus was detected within the fetal blood. The fetus died shortly after birth. *E,* Scalp edema.

VEIN OF GALEN ANEURYSM

An aneurysm of the vein of Galen, also known as a vein of Galen malformation, is a rare arteriovenous malformation. The vein will be enlarged and will communicate with normal-appearing arteries.

Vein of Galen aneurysm (VAGA) is considered a sporadic event and has a male predominance. It is usually an isolated anomaly, although it has been associated with congenital heart defects, cystic hygromas, and hydrops. VAGA can be associated with neurologic damage, which may result from ischemia, hemorrhage, or a mass effect.

The prognosis for vein of Galen aneurysm is generally poor, especially when associated with hydrops and/or cardiac failure. When symptoms present later in older children and young adults, the prognosis is generally good. Embolization is the primary treatment utilized.

Sonographic Findings. Sonographic features of vein of Galen aneurysm include the following:

- A cystic space that may be irregular in shape and is located midline and posterosuperior to the third ventricle
- Turbulent flow with Doppler evaluation

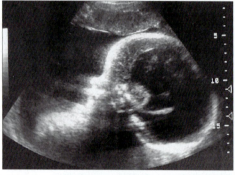

FIGURE 59-34 A sagittal image of a fetus with severe hydrocephaly that was thought to result from aqueductal stenosis.

Other sonographic findings associated with a vein of Galen aneurysm include fetal cardiomegaly and nonimmune hydrops. Ventriculomegaly with resultant macrocephaly may also develop.

The vein of Galen aneurysm may be confused with arachnoid cysts, which are very rare and may occur anywhere within the brain. Doppler evaluation of an arachnoid cyst will reveal no blood flow within the structure. Porencephalic cysts should also be listed in the differential considerations; however, these may be distinguished by the absence of blood flow and by communication of this cyst with the ventricle.

CHOROID PLEXUS CYSTS

Choroid plexus cysts are round or ovoid anechoic structures found within the choroid plexus. These cysts are common, occurring with a frequency of 0.4% to 3.6%. Choroid plexus cysts contain cerebrospinal fluid and cellular debris that have become trapped within the neuroepithelial folds.

Choroid plexus cysts are usually isolated findings without association with other anomalies. Furthermore, they often resolve by 22 to 26 weeks' gestation. Choroid plexus cysts have been identified in association with aneuploidy, most commonly with trisomy 18 and considerably less with trisomy 21.

Sonographic Findings. Sonographic features of choroid plexus cysts include the following:

- Cysts within the choroid plexus ranging in size from 0.3 to 2 cm
- Unilateral or bilateral cysts (Figure 59-35)
- Solitary or multiple
- Unilocular or multilocular
- Enlargement of the ventricle with a large cyst

Careful sonographic survey for anomalies that might suggest aneuploidy should follow identification of a choroid plexus cyst to include nuchal fold measurement, meticulous survey of the heart, and a survey of the feet

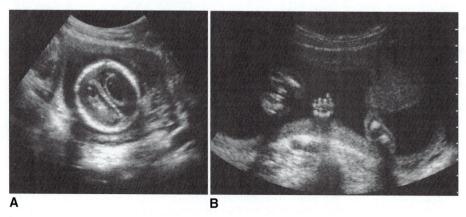

A   B

FIGURE 59-35 A, Bilateral choroid plexus cysts are observed in this fetus with trisomy 18. **B,** The same fetus also had a heart defect and these persistently clenched hands.

and hands to look for abnormal posturing and polydactyly. Amniocentesis for karyotyping may be offered, especially when other factors that may increase the risk for aneuploidy are considered, including maternal age, abnormal triple screen, and other ultrasound findings.

PORENCEPHALIC CYSTS

Porencephalic cysts, also known as porencephaly, are cysts filled with cerebrospinal fluid that communicate with the ventricular system or subarachnoid space. They may result from hemorrhage, infarction, delivery trauma, or inflammatory changes in the nervous system. The affected brain parenchyma undergoes necrosis, brain tissue is resorbed, and a cystic lesion remains.

No associated anomalies are known to occur in fetuses with porencephalic cysts. Postnatal problems may include seizures, developmental delays, motor deficits, visual and sensory problems, and hydrocephalus.

Sonographic Findings. The sonographic features of porencephalic cysts include the following:

- A cyst within the brain parenchyma without mass effect
- Communication of the cyst with the ventricle or subarachnoid space (Figure 59-36)
- Reduction in size of the affected hemisphere, which may cause a midline shift and contralateral ventricular enlargement

Porencephalic cysts may be confused with arachnoid cysts (see Figure 59-40), although the lack of a mass effect seen with porencephaly may aid in differentiating the two.

SCHIZENCEPHALY

Schizencephaly is a rare disorder characterized by clefts in the cerebral cortex. The clefts may be unilateral or bilateral, open-lip or closed-lip defects and are usually noted in the area of the sylvian fissure. Schizencephaly is thought to result from abnormal migration of neurons. These clefts can extend from the ventricle to the outer surface of the brain and are lined with abnormal gray matter.

The cause of schizencephaly remains unclear, although it has been linked with multiple assaults during pregnancy. Schizencephaly has been associated with congenital infection, drugs and other toxic exposures, vascular accidents, and metabolic abnormalities. An association with aneuploidy has also been noted.

The prognosis for patients with schizencephaly varies, ranging from mild to severe outcomes. Open-lip lesions and bilateral clefts carry a worse prognosis. Long-term effects include blindness; motor deficits, which may include spastic quadriparesis; hemiparesis; and hypotonia. Seizures, which may be uncontrollable, mental retardation, and language impairment are also possible. Hydrocephalus may be progressive, requiring shunt placement.

Sonographic Findings. Sonographic features of schizencephaly include the following:

- A fluid-filled cleft in the cerebral cortex extending from the ventricle to the calvarium (Figure 59-37)
- Observation of ventriculomegaly

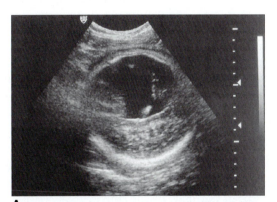

A

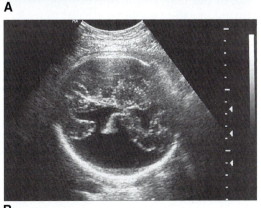

B

FIGURE 59-37 A and B, This patient came for an initial ultrasound at 32 weeks' gestation for late prenatal care. The ultrasound revealed hydrocephaly, and the patient was referred to a maternal-fetal center, where the diagnosis of schizencephaly was made based on the cleft that extends to the calvarium. This diagnosis was confirmed at birth with computed tomography.

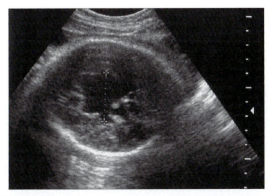

FIGURE 59-36 This patient with a history of hydrocephalus seen on ultrasound examination was referred at 32 weeks' gestation to a fetal diagnostic center. A porencephalic cyst was identified communicating with the lateral ventricle. Ventriculomegaly was also noted. The patient was counseled that this finding carried a poor prognosis.

Schizencephaly is associated with absence of the septum pellucidum and corpus callosum. Septo-optic dysplasia may be present, in addition to other abnormalities of the brain. Hydrocephaly can be seen when ventriculomegaly is present, but microcephaly has also been observed.

HYDRANENCEPHALY

Hydranencephaly is destruction of the cerebral hemispheres by occlusion of the internal carotid arteries. Brain parenchyma is destroyed and is replaced by cerebrospinal fluid. Because the posterior communicating arteries are preserved, the midbrain and cerebellum are present, and the basal ganglia, choroid plexus, and thalamus may be spared. This rare abnormality occurs with a frequency of approximately 1 in 10,000 births.

Hydranencephaly may also be associated with polyhydramnios. No coexisting structural or chromosomal anomalies are associated.

The cause of hydranencephaly usually involves congenital infection or ischemia. Infections associated with hydranencephaly include cytomegalovirus and toxoplasmosis. Brain ischemia may result from maternal hypotension, twin-to-twin embolization, or vascular agenesis, and hydranencephaly has been associated with cocaine abuse. It is believed that hydranencephaly may occur later in pregnancy, and that brain structures may initially be normal. The assault to the brain by infection or an ischemic event subsequently destroys normal brain tissue.

The prognosis for hydranencephaly is grave (Figure 59-38), with death occurring at birth or shortly thereafter; however, some long-term survivors have been reported.

▌ **Sonographic Findings.** Sonographic features of hydranencephaly include the following:

- Absence of normal brain tissue with almost complete replacement by cerebrospinal fluid (Figure 59-39)
- Absent or partially absent falx
- Presence of the midbrain, basal ganglia, and cerebellum
- Possible identification of the choroid plexus
- Possible occurrence of macrocephaly

Hydranencephaly may be confused with severe hydrocephaly, although the presence of an intact falx and surrounding rim of brain parenchyma may help to differentiate hydrocephaly from hydranencephaly. Holoprosencephaly with severe ventriculomegaly may have a similar appearance. However, these three anomalies have extremely poor outcomes.

VENTRICULOMEGALY (HYDROCEPHALUS)

Ventriculomegaly refers to dilatation of the ventricles within the brain. **Hydrocephalus** occurs when ventriculomegaly is coupled with enlargement of the fetal head.

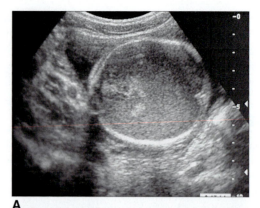

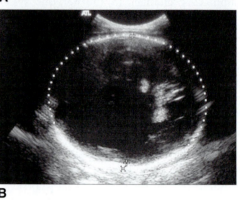

FIGURE 59-38 A, Hydranencephaly was suspected in this young woman with poorly controlled diabetes. The low-level echoes seen in this image of the fetal head swirled on real-time examination. **B,** Follow-up examinations revealed a grossly enlarged head with little identified brain tissue and replacement of low-level echoes by anechoic fluid. The woman presented to labor and delivery near term with absence of movement, and fetal demise was confirmed with ultrasound.

The incidence of hydrocephalus is 0.3 to 1.5 per 1000 live births. Enlargement of the ventricles occurs with obstruction of cerebrospinal fluid flow. This obstruction may be caused by a ventricular defect, such as aqueductal stenosis, and is referred to as *noncommunicating hydrocephalus*. The obstruction may be noted outside of the ventricular system, such as with an arachnoid cyst (Figure 59-40), and is referred to as *communicating hydrocephalus* (Figure 59-41). Rarely, ventriculomegaly results from overproduction of cerebrospinal fluid by a choroid plexus papilloma.

Physiologically, when an obstruction occurs, the ventricles dilate as the flow of cerebrospinal fluid is blocked. This increases the pressure within the ventricular system, which leads to ventricular expansion. Enlarged ventricles may exert pressure on the brain tissue, sometimes producing irreversible brain damage.

Hydrocephalus may be associated with an anomaly, or the cause may remain unknown. Many of the abnormalities linked with ventricular dilatation were discussed earlier in this chapter and include aqueductal stenosis, arachnoid cysts, and vein of Galen aneurysms. Common causes of ventriculomegaly include spina bifida and

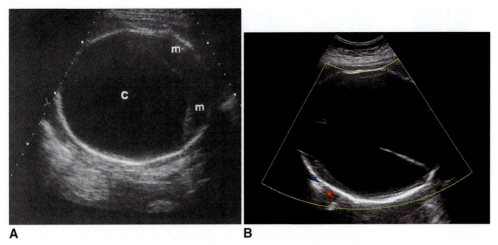

FIGURE 59-39 A, Hydranencephaly *(c)* in a fetus at 33 weeks' gestation showing a massive collection of cerebrospinal fluid. Note the brain tissue in the occipital region *(m)*. **B,** In a different fetus at 37 weeks' gestation, hydranencephaly is identified. The head measurements were greater than the 95th percentile, so the infant was delivered by cesarean section.

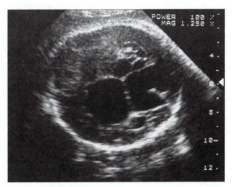

FIGURE 59-40 Multiple arachnoid cysts identified in this fetal head.

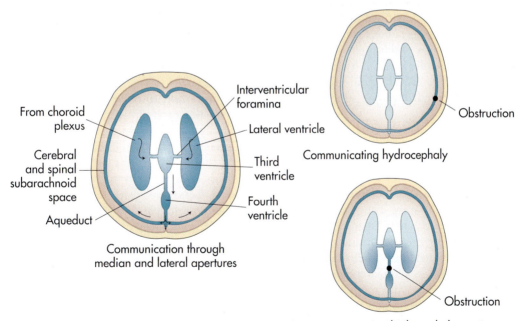

FIGURE 59-41 The course of the cerebrospinal fluid and its obstruction in hydrocephaly. Normally, the cerebrospinal fluid from the choroid plexuses flows through the interventricular foramina to the third ventricle, aqueduct, fourth ventricle, median and lateral apertures, and spinal and cerebral subarachnoid space. It is then taken into the venous system (e.g., the cranial venous sinuses). Obstruction occurs within the ventricular system (e.g., at the aqueduct) in noncommunicating hydrocephaly (i.e., the ventricles and the subarachnoid space do not communicate). Obstruction occurs outside the ventricular system (e.g., in the cranial subarachnoid space) in communicating hydrocephaly (i.e., the ventricles and the subarachnoid space communicate).

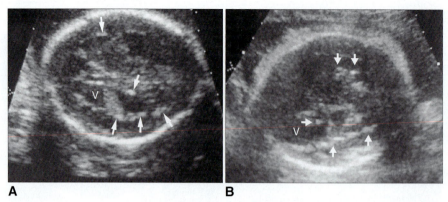

FIGURE 59-42 A, Periventricular calcifications *(arrows)* and ventriculomegaly *(v)* in a 20-week fetus. An infectious cause was suspected. All testing had proved negative. **B,** In the same fetus at 30 weeks' gestation, persistent periventricular calcifications *(arrows)* with ventriculomegaly *(v)* were observed. No other anomalies or complications were present.

encephaloceles. Dandy-Walker malformation, agenesis of the corpus callosum, lissencephaly, schizencephaly, and holoprosencephaly may also present with hydrocephalus. Intracranial neoplasm, such as a teratoma, may cause ventricular dilatation. Ventriculomegaly may also be associated with musculoskeletal anomalies, such as thanatophoric dysplasia and achondroplasia. Ventricular enlargement has also been linked to congenital infection, such as toxoplasmosis or cytomegalovirus (Figure 59-42).

Ventriculomegaly may be a manifestation of a syndrome or chromosomal abnormality. Mild ventriculomegaly has been associated with trisomy 21; ventriculomegaly has also been identified in trisomies 13 and 18. Other syndromes associated with ventriculomegaly include Meckel-Gruber syndrome, Apert's syndrome, Roberts' syndrome, hydrolethalus, Walker-Warburg syndrome, Smith-Lemli-Opitz syndrome, nasal-facial-digital syndrome, and Albers-Schönberg disease.

Fetal ventriculomegaly typically progresses from the occipital horns into the temporal and then the frontal ventricular horns. Ventriculomegaly may be quantitated by measuring the ventricular atrium across the glomus of the choroid plexus. A ventricle is considered dilated when its diameter exceeds 10 mm. The proximal ventricle may be difficult to adequately image because of reverberation artifacts from the calvarium. An effort should be made to determine whether ventricular enlargement is unilateral or bilateral; a unilateral ventriculomegaly, especially when isolated and mild, may have a good prognosis. Transvaginal technique may be used to further clarify the defect when the fetus is in a vertex position.

The mortality for fetuses with hydrocephalus is high. The outcome depends largely on the presence and severity of associated anomalies, and prognosis has improved in those with isolated ventriculomegaly. Survivors may require ventricular shunting to improve survival and intellectual outcome.

Sonographic Findings. Sonographic features of ventriculomegaly include the following:

- Lateral ventricular enlargement exceeding 10 mm (Figure 59-43)
- A "dangling choroid sign" as the gravity-dependent choroid plexus falls into the increased ventricular space (Figure 59-44)
- Possible dilatation of the third and fourth ventricles
- Fetal head enlargement when biparietal and head circumference measurements exceed those for the established gestational age

The fetus should also be surveyed for associated anomalies, which are present in 80% of cases of ventriculomegaly. Obstetric management may include amniocentesis to rule out chromosomal anomalies and laboratory tests to rule out congenital infection. In addition to numerous intracranial abnormalities associated with ventriculomegaly, the fetus should be surveyed for defects involving the face, heart, kidneys, abdominal wall, thorax, and limbs. In the absence of other abnormalities, fetal therapy for shunt placement may be an option. Cesarean delivery may also be necessary because of the large size of the fetal head.

Severe hydrocephaly may be confused with hydranencephaly and holoprosencephaly. Documenting a complete falx and the presence of the choroid plexus in the lateral ventricles, as well as separate third and fourth ventricles, may help to differentiate severe ventriculomegaly from other anomalies.

MICROCEPHALY

Microcephaly is an abnormally small head that falls 2 standard deviations below the mean. It occurs because the brain is reduced in size. Isolated microcephaly occurs

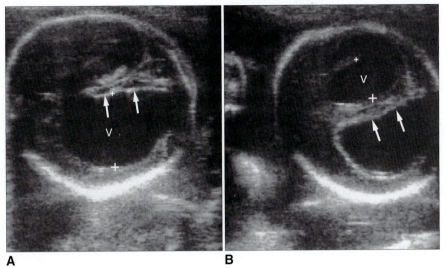

A   **B**

FIGURE 59-43 A, Ventriculomegaly observed in the distal cranial hemisphere in a 25-week twin fetus with severe growth restriction. The ventricle measured 28 mm in diameter. *Arrows,* Interhemispheric fissure. **B,** In the same fetus, the proximal ventricle *(V)* is displayed measuring 17 mm in diameter. Note the asymmetry between ventricles, suggesting a shift of the interhemispheric fissure *(arrows)* and porencephaly. The larger distal ventricle represents the actual porencephalic cyst, whereas the smaller ventricle has dilated in response to the infarction. Premature delivery occurred at 26 weeks' gestation because of chronic twin–twin transfusion syndrome in a monochorionic pregnancy. The twin depicted in these figures died shortly after birth. Autopsy confirmed the occurrence of the porencephalic event as an end result of severe shunting of blood within the placental cotyledons.

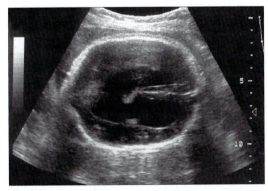

FIGURE 59-44 Ventriculomegaly caused by spina bifida. The anterior choroid plexus "dangles" into the posterior ventricle.

in 1 per 1000 births and is more commonly caused by an associated anomaly.

Microcephaly may result from inheritance of an autosomal dominant or autosomal recessive pattern. Microcephaly may also occur with chromosomal aberrations and various brain anomalies. Teratogens linked with microcephaly include congenital infection (rubella, toxoplasmosis, cytomegalovirus), maternal alcohol abuse, heroin addiction, mercury poisoning, maternal phenylketonuria, radiation, and hypoxia.

The prognosis for fetuses with microcephaly depends to a degree on the cause. About 85% of children with microcephaly are mentally retarded.

Sonographic Findings. Sonographic diagnosis of microcephaly depends on an accurate assessment of fetal

age. Biparietal diameter, occipitofrontal diameter, and head circumference should be used when evaluating for microcephaly. In addition, ratios comparing the head perimeter with abdominal perimeter and the head perimeter with femur length are also useful. Impaired cranial growth should coincide with appropriate growth of the abdominal circumference and femur length. Serial measurements for a fetus at risk for microcephalus should be performed at monthly intervals. Because microcephaly may manifest later in the pregnancy, diagnosis before 24 weeks' gestation may be impossible.

Sonographic features of microcephaly include the following:

- Small biparietal diameter (Figure 59-45)
- Small head circumference
- Abnormal head circumference/abdomen circumference and head circumference/femur length ratios

Other sonographic findings associated with microcephaly may include disorganized brain tissue and ventriculomegaly. A thorough search for evidence of an associated anomaly should ensue, including careful investigation of the fetal heart. Cerebral calcifications may be identified with congenital infection. A fetus with an encephalocele may have microcephaly caused by the amount of brain tissue protruding outside the calvarium. Other cranial anomalies associated with microcephaly include porencephaly, agenesis of the corpus callosum, craniosynostosis, holoprosencephaly, lissencephaly, schizencephaly, macrogyria, microgyria,

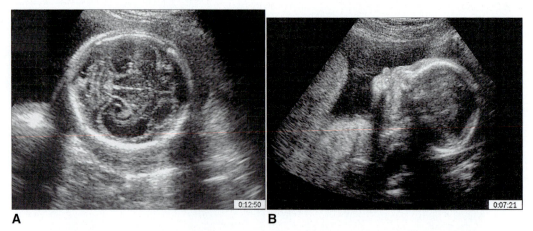

FIGURE 59-45 A, Microcephaly is demonstrated in this fetus with semilobar holoprosencephaly. **B,** In the same fetus, the profile shows the small head; the fetus also had a bilateral cleft lip.

agyria, and Kleeblattschädel defect. Microcephaly has been associated with trisomies 13, 18, 21, and 22 and with triploidy. Numerous syndromes have been linked with microcephaly, including Meckel-Gruber syndrome, Pena-Shokeir syndrome, and Neu-Laxova syndrome.

REFERENCE

1. Bullen PJ, Rankin JM, Robson SC: Investigation of the epidemiology and prenatal diagnosis of holoprosencephaly in the North of England, *Am J Obstet Gynecol* 184:1256-1262, 2001.

The Fetal Thorax

Sandra L. Hagen-Ansert

The detection of thoracic defects is important because many lesions may compromise fetal breathing and require surgery in the immediate neonatal period. Lung and diaphragm disorders are discussed in this section. Heart abnormalities may also cause devastating secondary compression effects (pulmonary hypoplasia) and are discussed in Chapters 33 and 34.

EMBRYOLOGY OF THE THORACIC CAVITY

One of the important determinants of whether the fetus can survive as a neonate in the air-filled, ex utero environment is the adequacy of biochemical and structural development and maturity of the lungs. Adequacy of pulmonary development is probably the single most important determinant of fetal viability, and pulmonary immaturity is the major reason why fetuses younger than 24 weeks' gestation are generally considered nonviable.

In early development, mesenchymal buds from the early trachea form and penetrate the masses destined to become the lungs. The bronchi, bronchioles, alveolar ducts, and alveoli are developed through multiple divisions and budding. Between 16 and 20 weeks, the normal number of bronchi has formed. Between 16 and 24

weeks, a dramatic increase in the number and complexity of air spaces and vascular structures has occurred. After 24 weeks, another important developmental phenomenon occurs: progressive flattening of the epithelial cells lining the air spaces, which allows closer apposition of capillaries to the fluid-filled air space lumen and results in further development of the air-blood barrier necessary for efficient gas exchange after birth.

Breathing movements that occur before birth result in the aspiration of fluid into the lungs. The lungs at birth are about half filled with fluid derived from the amniotic cavity, tracheal glands, and lungs. The fluid present in the lungs at birth clears by three routes: (1) through the mouth and nose, (2) into the pulmonary capillaries, and (3) into the lymphatics and the pulmonary vessels.

NORMAL SONOGRAPHIC CHARACTERISTICS

The fetal thorax is examined by the sonographer in both the transverse and coronal or parasagittal planes. The normal thoracic cavity is symmetrically bell-shaped, with the ribs forming the lateral margins, the clavicles forming the upper margins, and the diaphragm forming the lower margins. The lungs serve as the lateral borders for the

- Transverse, coronal, and/or parasagittal
- Evaluate chest: size, shape, symmetry
- Evaluate heart: position, size, rate, pericardial fluid
- Evaluate pulmonary texture
- Centrally positioned mediastinum

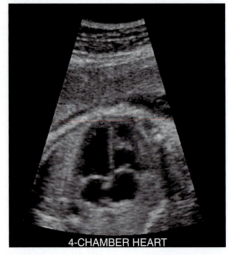

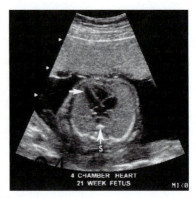

FIGURE 60-2 The ratio of the heart to the thorax is measured in a transverse view of the chest. The heart circumference normally measures at least one third of the thoracic circumference.

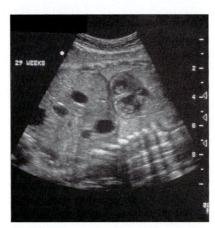

FIGURE 60-1 Longitudinal view of the fetal thorax and abdomen. The lungs are well seen above the diaphragm. Rib shadowing may be seen in the thoracic cavity. The stomach bubble is up, indicating that the left side of the fetus is closer to the maternal uterine wall.

heart and lie superior to the diaphragm. The diaphragm may be observed on sonography as an echogenic smooth hypoechoic muscular margin between the fetal liver or spleen and the lungs (Box 60-1).

Size

The thorax is normally slightly smaller than the abdominal cavity (Figure 60-1). The ratio (thoracic circumference to abdominal circumference) has been reported to remain constant throughout pregnancy (0.94 ± 0.05). Extreme variations in thoracic size should signal the sonographer to look for other anomalies. In the presence of oligohydramnios, resultant pulmonary hypoplasia may be seen with a reduction in overall thoracic size. Chest circumference measurements are made in the transverse plane at the level of the four-chamber view of the heart (Figure 60-2).

A fetus with a significant narrow diameter of the chest may have **asphyxiating thoracic dystrophy.** Several syndromes may be associated with this finding, including thanatophoric dwarfism. The best ultrasonic determination for predicting pulmonary hypoplasia is the chest area (CA) minus the heart area (HA) times 100 divided by the chest area (CA):

$$\frac{CA - HA \times 100}{CA}$$

FIGURE 60-3 Transverse image of the chest shows the apex *(arrow)* of the heart pointing toward the left side of the abdomen. The axis is rotated 45 degrees from midline, which is normal. The spine *(s)* is seen at 6 o'clock, with the aorta just anterior to the spine.

Position

The central portion of the thorax is occupied by the mediastinum, with most of the heart positioned in the midline and left chest. The apex of the heart should be directed toward the spleen; the base of the heart lies horizontal to the diaphragm (Figure 60-3). The location of the heart is important to document in a routine sonographic examination, as detection of abnormal position may indicate the presence of a chest mass, pleural effusion, or cardiac malformation.

Texture

The fetal lungs appear homogeneous on sonography with moderate echogenicity. Early in gestation, the lungs are similar to or slightly less echogenic than the liver (Figure 60-4), and, as gestation progresses, a trend toward increased pulmonary echogenicity relative to the

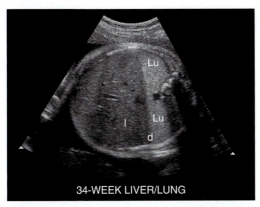

FIGURE 60-4 Longitudinal view of the fetal chest and abdomen shows the homogeneous, moderately echogenic texture of the lungs *(Lu)*, diaphragm *(d)*, and liver *(l)*.

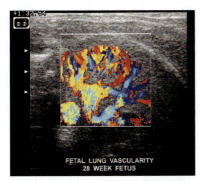

FIGURE 60-5 Color Doppler image of fetal lung vascularity in a 24-week fetus.

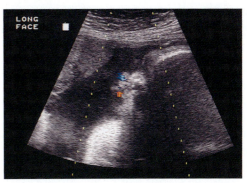

FIGURE 60-6 Color Doppler image of the fetal breathing pattern seen through movement of the nostrils.

liver is observed. Overlying ribs and acoustic enhancement produced by blood in the heart are two important problems that may complicate the exact determination of echogenicity of the lungs. Color Doppler may be used to outline the vascular pattern within the lungs (Figure 60-5). Ultrasound cannot be used to assess lung maturity.

Respiration

Fetal breathing becomes more prominent in the second and third trimesters. The mature fetus spends almost one third of its time breathing. Fetal breathing movements are documented if characteristic seesaw movements of the fetal chest or abdomen are sustained for at least 20 seconds. Fetal breathing movements are considered absent if no such fetal activity is noted during the 20-minute observation period.

Color flow Doppler may be used to detect fetal breathing through the nostrils. The fetal facial profile should be obtained with the nose clearly demonstrated; as color is turned on, flow disturbance movement may be seen to flow from the nostrils (Figure 60-6).

The biophysical profile used by many obstetricians to assess fetal well-being employs the respiration pattern as a factor in its scoring. Fetal respiration may vary in response to maternal activities and substance ingestion; it is stimulated by increased sugar doses and is decreased by smoking.

ABNORMALITIES OF THE THORACIC CAVITY

Abnormalities of the Lungs

To exclude pleural masses, a thorough investigation of lung texture and homogenicity is necessary. Lung masses are separate from the heart and are located above the level of the diaphragm. Lesions of the lungs may be cystic, solid, or complex.

When evaluating the fetus for a lung mass, the sonographer should assess the following: position of the fetal heart, orientation of the cardiac axis, and measurement of the thoracic circumference (which can be evaluated with a thoracic/abdominal ratio growth chart). Cardiac axis may be evaluated in a four-chamber heart view (see Chapter 33) by estimating the angle at which the intraventricular septum crosses the spine at the anterior chest wall (see Figure 60-3). The normal cardiac axis ranges from 22 to 75 degrees (average, 45 degrees). Deviation from the normal axis may suggest the presence of an intrathoracic mass. Measurements of thoracic circumference may aid in estimating the size of the thoracic cavity and may predict an abnormally small chest cavity and secondary pulmonary hypoplasia. Nomograms for thoracic circumference are available (Table 60-1). These data vary from the more recent data of Laudy and Wladimiroff, especially during the end of the last trimester.[2] Methods for measuring the lung include length, area, and volume, with the use of three-dimensional ultrasound. The right lung volume is slightly greater than the left.

When the heart position and axis vary from the normal position, the sonographer should look closely for any abnormality that may be the cause of such displacement (i.e., pleural mass or diaphragmatic hernia). Fetal echocardiography is beneficial for excluding cardiac involvement, and evaluation of an intact diaphragm is

TABLE 60-1	Fetal Thoracic Circumference Measurements*									
Gestational Age (week)	No.	Predictive Percentiles								
		2.5	5	10	25	50	75	90	95	97.5
16	6	5.9	6.4	7.0	8.0	9.1	10.3	11.3	11.9	12.4
17	22	6.8	7.3	7.9	8.9	10.0	11.2	12.2	12.8	13.3
18	31	7.7	8.2	8.8	9.8	11.0	12.1	13.1	13.7	14.2
19	21	8.6	9.1	9.7	10.7	11.9	13.0	14.0	14.6	15.1
20	20	9.5	10.0	10.6	11.7	12.9	13.9	15.0	15.5	16.0
21	30	10.4	11.0	11.6	12.6	13.7	14.8	15.8	16.4	16.9
22	18	11.3	11.9	12.5	13.5	14.6	15.7	16.7	17.3	17.8
23	21	12.2	12.8	13.4	14.4	15.5	16.6	17.6	18.2	18.8
24	27	13.2	13.7	14.3	15.3	16.4	17.5	18.5	19.1	19.7
25	20	14.1	14.6	15.2	16.2	17.3	18.4	19.4	20.0	20.6
26	25	15.0	15.5	16.1	17.1	18.2	19.3	20.3	21.0	21.5
27	24	15.9	16.4	17.0	18.0	19.1	20.2	21.3	21.9	22.4
28	24	16.8	17.3	17.9	18.9	20.0	21.2	22.2	22.8	23.3
29	24	17.7	18.2	18.8	19.8	21.0	22.1	23.1	23.7	24.2
30	27	18.6	19.1	19.7	20.7	21.9	23.0	24.0	24.6	25.1
31	24	19.5	20.0	20.6	21.6	22.8	23.9	24.9	25.5	26.0
32	28	20.4	20.9	21.5	22.6	23.7	24.8	25.8	26.4	26.9
33	27	21.3	21.8	22.5	23.5	24.6	25.7	26.7	27.3	27.8
34	25	22.2	22.8	23.4	24.4	25.5	26.6	27.6	28.2	28.7
35	20	23.1	23.7	24.3	25.3	26.4	27.5	28.5	29.1	29.6
36	23	24.0	24.6	25.2	26.2	27.3	28.4	29.4	30.0	30.6
37	22	24.9	25.5	26.1	27.1	28.2	29.3	30.3	30.9	31.5
38	21	25.9	26.4	27.0	28.0	29.1	30.2	31.2	31.9	32.4
39	7	26.8	27.3	27.9	28.9	30.0	31.1	32.2	32.8	33.3
40	6	27.7	28.2	28.8	29.8	30.9	32.1	33.1	33.7	34.2

From Chitkara U, Rosenberg J, Chervenak FA, et al: Prenatal sonographic assessment of the fetal thorax: normal values, *Am J Obstet Gynecol* 156:1069-1074, 1987.

*Measurements in centimeters.

necessary to exclude diaphragmatic hernia. Abnormalities in cardiac rhythm and fetal hydrops may be present in fetuses with lung masses caused by compression of venous return and cardiac failure. Pleural effusions are commonly found in conjunction with lung masses.

The lungs will not grow or develop properly when a small uterine cavity results from severe oligohydramnios, when the chest cavity is abnormally small, when the balance between tracheal and airway pressure and fluid volume is inadequate, or when the fetus is unable to practice breathing movements.

A mass within the thoracic cavity may have detrimental effects on lung development. The heart and mediastinal structures may be displaced from the normal position, and the lung may be compressed and destroyed. These effects may lead to pulmonary hypoplasia.

Pulmonary Hypoplasia. Pulmonary hypoplasia is caused by a decrease in the numbers of lung cells, airways, and alveoli, with a resulting decrease in organ size and weight. This reduction in lung volume leads to small, inadequately developed lungs. A decreased ratio of lung weight to body weight is a consistent method of diagnosing pulmonary hypoplasia. This condition most commonly occurs after prolonged oligohydramnios or

secondary to a small thoracic cavity caused by a structural or chromosomal abnormality.

Pulmonary hypoplasia may occur when amniotic fluid volume is extremely reduced. Kidney abnormalities (bilateral renal agenesis, bilateral multicystic kidney disease, severe renal obstruction [e.g., posterior urethral valve syndrome], unilateral renal agenesis with contralateral multicystic kidney development or severe obstruction, and infantile polycystic kidney disease) result in lethal pulmonary hypoplasia. Pulmonary hypoplasia may also occur in fetuses with severe intrauterine growth restriction and early rupture of the membranes.

Masses within the thoracic cavity, including pleural effusion, diaphragmatic hernia (and eventration), cystic adenomatoid malformation of the lung, bronchopulmonary sequestration, and other large cysts and tumors of the lung and thorax, may lead to pulmonary hypoplasia. Cardiac defects, some skeletal dysplasias, central nervous system disorders, and chromosomal trisomies (13, 18, and 21) may manifest with pulmonary hypoplasia. A small percentage of infants have pulmonary hypoplasia with no fetal or uterine problem.

Unilateral pulmonary agenesis or hypoplasia is a rare anomaly that is often associated with other fetal malformations. An absent lung should be considered in the differential diagnosis of every fetus with a mediastinal shift and apparent chest mass, especially when it is seen in conjunction with other defects, such as esophageal abnormalities.

The prognosis for infants with pulmonary hypoplasia is grave, with 80% dying after birth. The severity of pulmonary hypoplasia depends on when pulmonary hypoplasia occurred during pregnancy, its severity, and its duration (Box 60-2). Other factors, such as pulmonary fluid dynamics, fetal breathing movements, and hormonal influences, may contribute to pulmonary hypoplasia.

Sonographic Findings. Various methods used to determine the presence of pulmonary hypoplasia include thoracic measurements, various lung measurements, estimation of lung volume, Doppler studies of the pulmonary arteries, and assessment of fetal breathing activity. The sonographer may be able to check for pulmonary hypoplasia by measuring the thoracic circumference at the level of the four-chamber heart view, excluding the skin and subcutaneous tissues. A thoracic circumference below the 5th percentile suggests the possibility of pulmonary hypoplasia. The sonographer should understand that this measurement may not be helpful in conditions in which an intrathoracic mass compresses lung tissue and yet the thoracic circumference remains normal (i.e., diaphragmatic hernia, pleural effusion, and cystic adenomatoid malformations). The sonographer should also look for the finding of small echogenic lungs, as they lie lateral to the cardiac chambers in the fetus with pulmonary hypoplasia.

Cystic Lung Masses. Lung cysts are echo-free masses that replace normal lung parenchyma (Figure 60-7). Lung cysts may vary in size, ranging from small isolated lesions to large cystic masses that may cause notable shifts of intrathoracic structures. Simple cysts may be surgically excised after delivery (Box 60-3).

Bronchogenic Cysts. The most common lung cyst detected prenatally is the **bronchogenic cyst.** Bronchogenic cysts occur as a result of abnormal budding of the foregut and lack any communication with the trachea or bronchial tree. They typically occur within the mediastinum or lung; infrequently they are seen inferior to the diaphragm.

Sonographic Findings. Sonographically, bronchogenic cysts appear as small circumscribed masses with no evidence of a mediastinal shift or heart failure (see Figures 60-7 and 60-8). Amniotic fluid volume is within the normal range.

Pleural Effusion (Hydrothorax). An accumulation of fluid within the pleural cavity that may appear as an isolated lesion or secondary to multiple fetal anomalies is called a **pleural effusion** or **hydrothorax** (see Figure 60-7). The most common reason for a pleural effusion is chylothorax occurring as a right-side unilateral collection of fluid secondary to a malformed thoracic duct. Hydramnios often accompanies chylothorax resulting

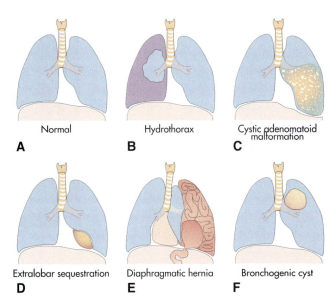

FIGURE 60-7 Schematic drawings of thoracic masses and mass effect. **A,** Normal thorax. The lungs have convex margins anterolaterally. **B,** Hydrothorax. Anechoic pleural fluid displaces the lungs away from the chest wall and compresses the lungs. **C,** Cystic adenomatoid malformation. An intrapulmonary mass of variable echogenicity may shift the mediastinum and create hydrops. **D,** Bronchopulmonary extralobar sequestration. A spherical or triangular echogenic mass is evident in the inferior portion of the thorax or upper abdomen. **E,** Diaphragmatic hernia. A complex mass (usually on the left side) creates mediastinal shift. Peristalsing bowel in the thorax provides convincing evidence of the diagnosis. Displaced stomach or scaphoid abdomen is an ancillary finding. **F,** Bronchogenic cyst. If it causes bronchial compression, a simple cyst near the mediastinum or appearing centrally in the lung may produce a mediastinal shift.

BOX 60-2 Pulmonary Hypoplasia

- Reduction in lung volume resulting in small, inadequately developed lungs
- Occurs from prolonged oligohydramnios or secondary to small thoracic cavity
- Look for chromosome anomalies, renal anomalies, intrauterine growth restriction, premature rupture of membranes, masses within thoracic cavity

---

BOX 60-3 Cystic Lung Masses

Bronchogenic cysts: most common; unilocular or multilocular cysts usually within mediastinum or lung; normal amniotic fluid

Pleural effusions: hydramnios accompanies chylothorax (esophageal compression); may result from immune or nonimmune causes or congestive heart failure; may occur with cardiac mass; lymphangiectasia, cystic adenomatoid malformation (CAM), sequestration, hernia; compression of lung tissue; shift of mediastinal structures

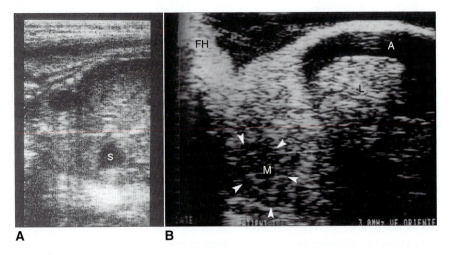

FIGURE 60-8 A, Longitudinal section of the chest revealing a small cystic mass in the lung. Note the relationship of the stomach (s) to the cyst. A benign bronchogenic cyst was found after birth. **B,** Longitudinal scan showing a bulky noncystic mass (M) in the thorax consistent with cystic adenomatoid malformation (type 3). Abdominal ascites (A) is present. L, Liver; FH, fetal head.

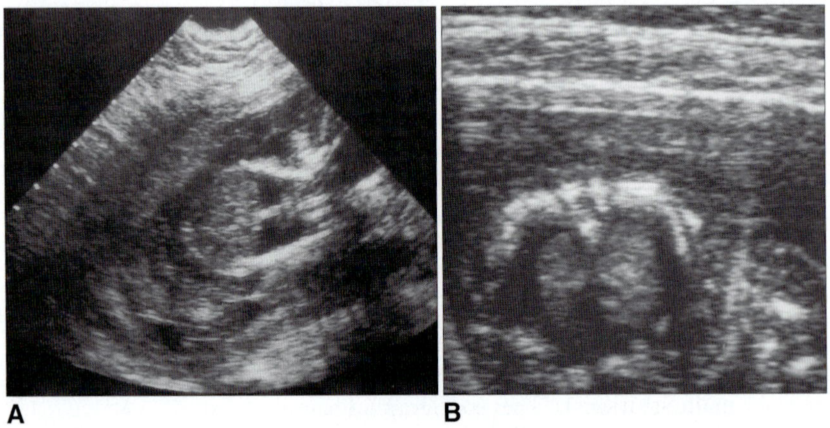

A   **B**

FIGURE 60-9 A, Bilateral pleural effusions in a 23-week fetus. **B,** Transverse view of bilateral pleural effusions.

A   **B**

from esophageal compression. Fetal hydrothorax can be unilateral or bilateral. When it is bilateral, it occurs about equally on the right and left sides.

Pleural effusions may result from immune (e.g., Rh hemolytic disease) or nonimmune causes or from congestive heart failure. Effusions may also occur in fetuses with chromosomal abnormalities (e.g., trisomy 21) and in fetuses with a cardiac mass. Other reasons for pleural effusions include **lymphangiectasia,** cystic adenomatoid malformations, bronchopulmonary sequestration, diaphragmatic hernia, hamartoma, atresia of the pulmonary vein, and other, unknown causes.

▶ **Sonographic Findings.** Sonographically, pleural effusions appear as echo-free peripheral masses on one or both sides of the fetal heart (Figure 60-9). The effusions conform to the thoracic cavity and often compress lung tissue. The lung appears to float in the fluid. Pleural fluid is rarely encountered before the 15th week of gestation, except in association with Down or Turner's syndrome. Compression of lung parenchyma may cause pulmonary hypoplasia, which often represents a life-threatening consequence for the neonate (Figure 60-10).

The presence of a pleural effusion may cause a shift in mediastinal structures, compression of the heart, and inversion of the diaphragm. The shape of the lung appears normal in the presence of a pleural effusion. Once a

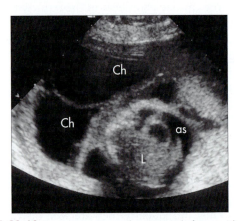

FIGURE 60-10 Transverse scan of a 26-week fetus with a huge cystic hygroma (Ch) and fetal hydrops. Ascites (as) may be seen surrounding the fetal liver (L). The sonographer should also look for the presence of pleural and pericardial effusion.

pleural effusion has been discovered, a careful search for lung, cardiac, and diaphragmatic lesions should be attempted. Likewise, evaluation for signs of hydrops (ascites, scalp edema, and tissue edema) should be performed. Correlation with clinical parameters is warranted to exclude immunologic causes of pleural effusion.

The mortality rate for the infant with a pleural effusion approaches 50%; the prognosis is poorer with associated hydrops. When the pleural effusion is large, lung development is impaired, which may result in pulmonary hypoplasia. Some neonatologists advocate draining a large pleural collection (thoracentesis) by placing a thoracoamniotic shunt within the pleural space. This approach attempts to allow for lung growth when it is performed during the second trimester of pregnancy. Thoracentesis may be performed to determine whether the lung has the ability to reexpand once the fluid is removed, thus excluding pulmonary hypoplasia, lessening the effects of hydramnios, and obtaining a fetal karyotype using lymphocytes from the aspirated lung fluid.

Solid Lung Masses. Solid tumors of the fetal lungs, appearing as echo-dense masses in the lung tissue, have been reported by ultrasound. Pulmonary sequestration and certain types of cystic adenomatoid malformations (CAMs) appear as solid lung masses (see Figure 60-7) (Box 60-4).

Pulmonary Sequestration. Pulmonary sequestration is a supernumerary lobe of the lung, separated from the normal tracheobronchial tree. In **pulmonary sequestration**, extra pulmonary tissue is present within the pleural lung sac (intralobar) or is connected to the inferior border of the lung within its own pleural sac (extralobar). This probably develops from a separate outpouching of the foregut or by separation of a segment of the developing lung from the tracheobronchial tree. This extra lung tissue is nonfunctional and receives its blood supply from the systemic circulation. The arterial supply is usually derived from the thoracic aorta, with venous drainage into the vena cava.

BOX 60-4 | Sonographic Findings in Sequestration

- Echogenic solid mass resembling lung tissue
- Rarely occurs below diaphragm
- Associated with hydrops and polyhydramnios, diaphragmatic hernia, gastrointestinal anomalies
- Normal intra-abdominal anatomy

Sonographic Findings. Sonographically, an echo-dense solid mass resembling lung tissue is observed, usually in the lower lobe of the lung (Figure 60-11). A majority of extralobar defects occur on the left side and rarely below the diaphragm. Intralobar lesions are spherical, and extralobar sequestration appears as a cone-shaped or triangular mass. These lesions may resemble a cystic adenomatoid (type II) malformation. Color Doppler may aid the sonographer in viewing this anomalous circulation. A hypoplastic lung may be observed on the affected side. Hydrops is a frequent finding. Other associated anomalies are diaphragmatic hernia and gastrointestinal and lung anomalies (pulmonary hypoplasia).

The prognosis for intralobar sequestration is highly favorable, whereas extralobar sequestration carries a poor prognosis because of associated anomalies and hydrops.

Laryngeal atresia may be diagnosed when bilateral lung enlargement is observed (Figure 60-12).

Congenital Cystic Adenomatoid Malformation. Congenital cystic adenomatoid malformation (CCAM) is a multicystic mass within the lung consisting of primitive lung tissue and abnormal bronchial and

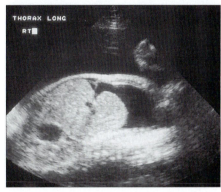

FIGURE 60-11 Longitudinal scan of a 23-week fetus with a right-side pulmonary sequestration. The echogenic mass is well seen in the lower lobe of the thoracic cavity. A large pleural effusion surrounds the mass.

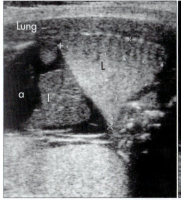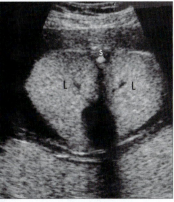

FIGURE 60-12 **A,** Echogenic lung (*L, in calipers*) in a 21-week fetus with severe hydrops. The opposite lung appeared similar in texture. Oligohydramnios and episodes of bradycardia were evident. *a,* Ascites; *l,* liver. **B,** In the same fetus, both echogenic lungs (*L*) are viewed. Laryngeal or tracheal agenesis was suspected. It is believed that excess lung fluid is manufactured by the abnormal lung. *s,* Spine.

bronchiolar-like structures. CCAM, one of the broncho-pulmonary foregut malformations (see Figure 60-7), results from an embryogenetic alteration in the developing lung during the first 8 to 9 gestational weeks. The lesion may involve one or more lobes of the lung or an entire lung, or, in rare cases, may be bilateral. The malformation may communicate with the bronchial tree. The cysts within the mass may be large or small, with a variable texture that may be solid, mixed, or cystic in appearance. Most lesions are unilateral and do not favor either lung.

Three forms of cystic adenomatoid malformation are known. In CCAM type I (macrocystic), one or more large cysts replace normal lung tissue (single or multiple cysts measuring more than 2 cm and up to 10 cm) (Figure 60-13). Type II (macrocystic with a microcystic component) lesions consist of multiple small cysts (less than 1 cm) (Figure 60-14). Type II lesions are associated with fetal and/or chromosomal abnormalities in 25% of cases. These anomalies may include renal agenesis, pulmonary anomalies, and diaphragmatic hernia. Type III (microcystic) malformations are characterized as bulky, large, noncystic lesions appearing as echo-dense masses

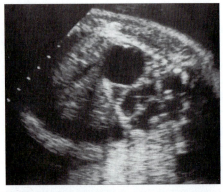

FIGURE 60-13 Type I cystic adenomatoid malformation showing multiple large cystic areas replacing normal lung tissue.

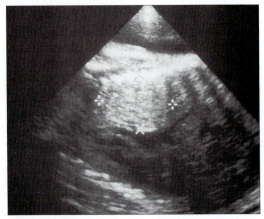

FIGURE 60-14 Type II cystic adenomatoid malformation shows multiple cystic areas measuring less than 1 cm. The mass is echogenic at the base of the thoracic cavity.

of the entire lung lobe (Figure 60-15). When a shift of mediastinal structures occurs, lung compression may occur and hydrops may develop. Hydramnios may be observed secondary to esophageal compression, preventing normal fetal swallowing.

Differentiation among the types of cystic adenomatoid malformations is imperative because prognosis varies depending on the type of lesion. Type I lesions have favorable outcomes, whereas type II and III lesions have poor prognoses.

Sonographic Findings. When a cystic or solid lung mass has been identified, the sonographer should attempt to do the following:

- Determine the number(s) and size(s) of cystic structure(s)
- Check for presence or absence of a mediastinal shift
- Identify and assess the size of the lungs
- Look for fetal hydrops
- Exclude cardiac masses
- Search for other fetal anomalies

Based on these findings, an appropriate prognosis and management plan may be instituted (Box 60-5).

A review of the spontaneous improvement of these thoracic masses in utero indicates the following[1]:

- Sonographically detected fetal chest masses may result in pathologically proven thoracically derived lesions or may resolve, some without sequelae.
- The mass lesions may change in size and echogenicity.
- Sonograms of fetuses with CAM may be normal in the first and second trimesters and only later may show abnormalities on ultrasound.
- The presence of polyhydramnios, hydrops, or notable cardiac deviation predicts poor outcome more accurately than the lesion type.

Congenital Bronchial Atresia. **Congenital bronchial atresia** is a rare pulmonary anomaly that results from the focal obliteration of a segment of the bronchial lumen. It is found most commonly in the left upper lobe and appears on ultrasound as an echogenic pulmonary mass lesion. In normal fetuses, the bronchi are not

BOX 60-5	Sonographic Findings in Cystic Adenomatoid Malformations

- Type I: single or multiple large cysts 2 cm in diameter; good prognosis after resection of affected lung
- Type II: multiple small cysts, <1 cm in diameter, echogenic; high incidence of other congenital anomalies (renal, gastrointestinal)
- Type III: large, bulky, noncystic lesions producing mediastinal shift; poor prognosis
- Usually only one lobe is affected.
- Associated polyhydramnios and anasarca have poor prognosis.

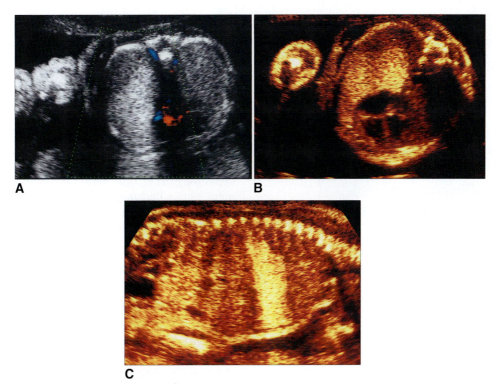

FIGURE 60-15 A fetus is found at 32 weeks to have asymmetry in the lung tissue, which turned out to be type III cystic adenomatoid malformation. This echogenic mass affected the right lung. **A,** Gray-scale transverse scan comparing both textures of the lung. The right lobe is clearly more echogenic. **B,** B-color display of the cystic adenomatoid malformation as it slightly displaces the cardiac axis. **C,** Longitudinal B-color scan of the echo-dense mass just above the diaphragm in the thoracic cavity.

visualized. If a fetal main stem or segmental bronchus can be seen on sonography, this is probably because it is fluid-filled and abnormal.

Other Complex Lung Masses. The internal components of complex lung masses are cystic and solid and appear heterogeneous. At times, compressed adjacent thoracic organs further complicate determination of the type of lesion (pleural effusion surrounding lungs and heart). Congenital dilatation of the bronchial tree may have both cystic and solid characteristics.

Congenital lobar emphysema is lobar overinflation of the lung without destruction of alveolar septa. It usually occurs in the upper left or middle lobe and is located within the normal pleural envelope. This condition may appear identical to microcystic CCAM, presenting as a large solid mass.

Laryngeal and tracheal atresia is an uncommon finding in utero. The sonographic findings show enlarged, bilateral, symmetrically distended echogenic fetal lungs due to fluid distention of tiny air spaces within the lung tissue. The heart may be displaced anteriorly in the midline and may appear engulfed by the prominent lung fields. The trachea and bronchi may be fluid filled. Fetal ascites is usually present without other findings of hydrops. Polyhydramnios may be seen secondary to esophageal compression. Oligohydramnios has also been reported as a result of cardiac compromise or diminished lung fluid efflux into the amniotic space.

Abnormalities of the Diaphragm

The diaphragm is an important muscle separating the thoracic cavity from the abdomen. The diaphragm is specifically studied in fetuses at risk for congenital defects of the diaphragm when there is a shift in the cardiac silhouette, or when atypical structures are found in the fetal chest. In the normal fetus, the diaphragm should appear as a curvilinear hypoechoic structure coursing anteriorly to posteriorly (Figure 60-16). The fetal stomach and liver should be identified caudal to the diaphragm, with the lungs and heart positioned cephalad. Failure to recognize these normal relationships should prompt the sonographer to search for diaphragmatic defects.

Congenital Diaphragmatic Hernia. Congenital diaphragmatic hernia (CDH) is a herniation of the abdominal viscera into the chest that results from a congenital defect in the fetal diaphragm. It is a sporadic defect, occurring in 1 per 2000 to 1 per 5000 births. The muscular diaphragm forms between the 6th and 14th weeks of gestation as a result of a chain of events involving the fusion of four structures: (1) septum transversum (future central tendon), (2) pleuroperitoneal membranes, (3) dorsal mesentery of the esophagus (future crura), and (4) body wall. Normally, the primitive diaphragm is intact by the end of the 8th menstrual week. The most posterior aspect of the diaphragm, derived from the body wall, is

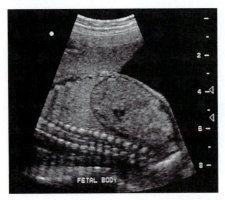

FIGURE 60-16 Longitudinal scan of the diaphragm as it separates the thoracic cavity from the abdominal cavity.

the part of the diaphragm that forms last and is most commonly defective.

During the embryologic phase, when the gut is moving back into the abdominal cavity (around 10 to 12 weeks), sufficient intra-abdominal pressure may be produced, so that if fusion of the primitive diaphragmatic structures is incomplete, abdominal viscera can herniate into the thorax.

The diaphragmatic hernia permits the abdominal organs to enter the fetal chest (see Figures 60-7 and 60-17 to 60-19). The most common type of diaphragmatic defect (accounting for more than 90% of defects) occurs posteriorly and laterally in the diaphragm (herniation through the **foramen of Bochdalek**). This hernia

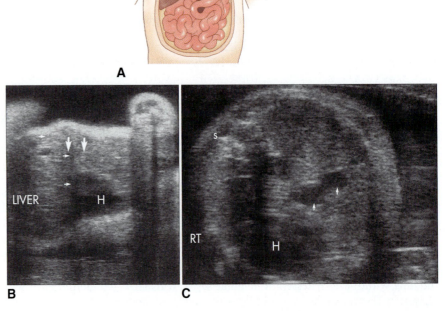

FIGURE 60-17 A, Schematic demonstrating hernia of intestinal loops and part of the stomach into the left pleural cavity. The heart and mediastinum are pushed to the right, whereas the left lung is compressed. **B,** Sagittal view in a fetus with a diaphragmatic hernia. The heart (H) is displaced to the right side of the fetal thorax by herniated bowel (large arrows). Diaphragm (small arrows). **C,** Transverse section in the same patient showing the herniated stomach (arrows) at the level of the heart (H). s, Spine; RT, right.

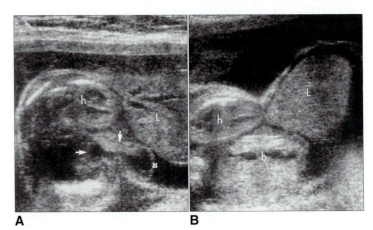

FIGURE 60-18 A, Diaphragmatic hernia in association with omphalocele shown in a 28-week fetus. Displacement of the heart (h) to the right chest is demonstrated. Herniated bowel (arrows) with peristalsis demonstrated by real-time imaging confirmed the diagnosis. L, Lung. **B,** In the same fetus, the liver (L) is shown in close proximity to the heart (h) and bowel (b) because of the absent diaphragm.

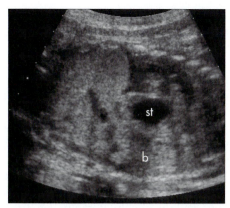

FIGURE 60-19 Longitudinal image of a 25-week fetus with a large left-side hernia. The stomach *(st)* and bowel *(b)* are seen within the thoracic cavity.

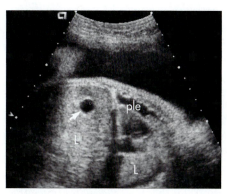

FIGURE 60-20 Longitudinal scan of a right-side diaphragmatic hernia; the liver *(L)* is seen in the thoracic cavity. Pleural effusion *(ple)* is present. The gallbladder *(arrow)* is seen within the liver.

is usually found on the left side of the diaphragm, and in left-side organs (stomach, spleen, and portions of the liver) enter the chest through the opening. The abnormally positioned abdominal organs shift the heart and mediastinal structures to the right side of the chest. Usually the stomach is in the chest near the heart, instead of below the diaphragm. In left-side hernias, the sonographer should look for the stomach, portions of the small and large intestines, and the left lobe of the liver and spleen in the thoracic cavity. Peristalsis of the bowel loops may be seen within the thoracic cavity (Box 60-6).

Diaphragmatic hernias may occur anteriorly and medially in the diaphragm, through the **foramen of Morgagni,** and may communicate with the pericardial sac. In anteromedial defects, the heart may be normally positioned but surrounded by pleural fluid, while the fetal stomach may be located in its normal position in the abdomen (Figure 60-20). Thinning of the diaphragm (eventration) may give rise to sonographic characteristics similar to those of diaphragmatic hernias.

Defects on the right side of the diaphragm allow the right-side abdominal viscera (liver, gallbladder, intestines) to enter the chest. As a consequence of herniated abdominal organs, the lungs are compressed and may become hypoplastic.

The size of the diaphragmatic defects can be variable, ranging from small to large to complete absence of both diaphragms. The smaller defects are difficult to diagnose in utero. Hydrops usually is not present with left-side congenital diaphragmatic hernias unless associated fetal malformations are present. The presence of pulmonary hypoplasia and pulmonary hypertension is the real issue that results from the size of the hernia. The pulmonary arteries become hypertrophied and thickened, resulting in pulmonary hypertension that after birth leads to persistent fetal circulation. Bilateral hernias are very unusual and more difficult to detect with sonography because the degree of cardiomediastinal shift may not be evident. The heart may be slightly displaced anteriorly and superiorly, and the stomach may be found in the left chest.

BOX 60-6	Sonographic Criteria Suggestive of a Diaphragmatic Hernia

- Shift of the heart and mediastinal structures (right shift in left-side defects; left shift in right-side defects)
- Mass within the thoracic cavity (liver, stomach, spleen, and large bowel in left-side defects; liver, gallbladder, intestines in right-side defects)
- Small abdominal circumference resulting from herniated abdominal structures
- Obvious diaphragm defect
- Hydramnios
- More than 50% have structural anomalies or chromosomal abnormalities.
- Structural defects include cardiovascular (tetralogy of Fallot and others), genitourinary (renal agenesis, cystic dysplasia, and ureteropelvic junction obstruction), central nervous system (holoprosencephaly, hydrocephalus, and spinal anomalies), clubbed feet, hemivertebrae and absent ribs, genital (ambiguous genitalia and others), and gastrointestinal (imperforate anus, annular pancreas, and absence of the gallbladder).
- Growth restriction suggests associated anomalies.
- The abdominal circumference below the 5th percentile and the liver in the chest indicate poor prognosis.*

*Data from Teixeira J, Sepulveda W, Hassan J, Cox PM, Singh MP: Abdominal circumference in fetuses with congenital diaphragmatic hernia: correlation with hernia content and pregnancy outcome, *J Ultrasound Med* 16:407-410, 1997.

Sonographic Findings. On sonographic examination, a *left-side congenital diaphragmatic hernia* is usually found when the cardiac silhouette is displaced to the right and an ectopic stomach is in the chest. It is very important to note the cardiomediastinal shift to make the diagnosis of a hernia. The apex of the heart will be abnormally shifted, depending on the size of the CDH defect. The small bowel and colon are commonly intrathoracic but are often collapsed and difficult to identify specifically if peristalsis is not present. The sagittal image of the fetus may allow visualization of the diaphragm, depending on how large the defect is. The fetal lung may be small and compressed.

BOX 60-7	Sonographic Features of Left Congenital Hernia

- Intrathoracic stomach
- Displaced cardiac apex
- Cardiomediastinal shift is critical in making the diagnosis.
- Intrathoracic liver (look for portal venous flow)
- Small right lung
- Small left ventricle of heart
- Evaluate for chromosomal abnormalities.

A portion of the liver herniates into the chest in approximately two thirds of cases, and the presence or absence of intrathoracic liver is important to note because it is associated with a poorer outcome. Color flow may be useful in demarcating the portal vasculature within the liver to ascertain whether the tissue is truly liver or not. Box 60-7 lists the sonographic features of left congenital hernia.

In a *right-side diaphragmatic hernia,* the sonographer will see the liver in the chest, possibly a collapsed bowel, and the heart deviated far to the left. The stomach alignment will be abnormal, but inferior to the diaphragm and moved to the right. Color may help to trace the portal vasculature in the liver as it lies within the chest cavity. The gallbladder may also herniate into the thoracic cavity and appear as a solitary "cystic" mass in the lung. A small amount of ascitic fluid adjacent to the liver may be present with right-side hernias. Pleural fluid is not usually associated with other chest masses, except in sequestration. At birth, respiration may be severely compromised, which may result in death of the newborn.

The amniotic fluid may be normal unless the bowel is obstructed with resulting polyhydramnios. The placenta is normal; the abdominal circumference will be abnormally small. Careful scanning before 18 weeks' gestation is important to identify the normal contour of the diaphragm on sagittal and coronal views. A small defect may not show abnormalities early in the gestational period.

The prognosis is poor for the fetus if the congenital diaphragmatic hernia is detected before birth; if the stomach is found in the chest, especially if it is dilated; if the left heart is underdeveloped; or if congenital heart disease is present. The primary cause of death is pulmonary hypoplasia. If the diagnosis is made before 25 weeks' gestation and polyhydramnios is present, the survival rate is low.

Frequently associated abnormalities include cardiac malformations (20%), central nervous system malformations (30%), renal anomalies, vertebral defects, pulmonary hypoplasia, and facial clefts. In addition, chromosome abnormalities (trisomy 18 and 21) have been associated with diaphragmatic hernia.

It is important to note that when a diaphragmatic hernia is present, the stomach may not be filled when there is concomitant oligohydramnios, or if the fetus is swallowing abnormally. The only clue to a diaphragmatic hernia in this situation may be evidence of a solid mass in the chest. Peristalsis within the herniated intestines confirms the diagnosis. When the sonographer is unable to demonstrate the stomach bubble in the normal anatomic location after repeated observations, a search for a diaphragmatic hernia should be attempted.

Lung and mediastinal masses, in particular, cystic adenomatoid malformations, may be difficult to distinguish from diaphragmatic hernias. The normally positioned peritoneal organs should aid in differentiating between these two conditions.

At birth, most infants with congenital diaphragmatic hernia have pulmonary hypoplasia and secondary respiratory insufficiency. The mortality rate is high (75%) because of the increased frequency of coexisting fetal congenital anomalies. The extracorporeal membrane oxygenation (ECMO) procedure has provided such babies with severe diaphragmatic hernias a chance for survival immediately after delivery. This procedure canalizes the carotid artery (while occluding the opposite carotid artery) in an effort to bypass the pulmonary circulation to provide an opportunity for the lung tissue to mature before circulation demands are in place.

REFERENCES

1. Budorick NE, Pretorius DH, Leopold GR, Stamm ER: Spontaneous improvement of intrathoracic masses diagnosed in utero, *J Ultrasound Med* 11:653-662, 1992.
2. Laudy JA, Wladimiroff JW: The fetal lung. 2. Pulmonary hypoplasia, *Ultrasound Obstet Gynecol* 16:482-494, 2000.

The Fetal Anterior Abdominal Wall

Sandra L. Hagen-Ansert and Denise Spradley

Sonography has proven to be very effective for detecting anterior abdominal wall defects in utero. These defects occur during the first trimester as the midgut elongates and migrates into the umbilical cord. The midgut usually returns into the abdominal cavity by the 11th week of gestation. When this fails to occur, an abdominal wall defect is formed. The two most common defects are omphalocele and gastroschisis. Less common defects are ectopia cordis, limb-body wall complex, and cloacal exstrophy.

EMBRYOLOGY OF THE ABDOMINAL WALL

By the end of the 5th week of development, an embryo is a flat disk consisting of three layers: ectoderm, mesoderm, and endoderm. In the 6th week, a process called *folding* helps the embryo transform itself into a cylindrical shape. This transformation is a critical part of the process of closing the abdominal wall.

As the embryo folds at the cranial end, the base of the yolk sac is partially incorporated as the foregut, which later develops as the pharynx, lower respiratory system, esophagus, stomach, duodenum (proximal to the opening of the bile duct), liver, pancreas, gallbladder, and biliary duct system.

The growth of the neural tube causes the embryo to fold at the caudal end, incorporating part of the yolk sac as the hindgut, which turns into the cloaca. It also causes the connecting stalk (located at the tail) to move to the ventral surface of the embryo, incorporating the allantois into the umbilical cord. The derivatives of the hindgut are the distal part of the transverse colon, the descending colon, the sigmoid colon, the rectum, the superior portion of the anal canal, the epithelium of the urinary bladder, and most of the urethra (Figure 61-1).

The sides of the embryo fold, leading to the formation of the lateral and anterior abdominal wall. The midgut is the primordium of the small intestines (including most of the duodenum), cecum, vermiform appendix, ascending colon, and the right half to two thirds of the transverse colon. The connection of the yolk sac and body stalk will form the umbilical cord at the ventral region of the embryo. Expansion of the amniotic cavity will

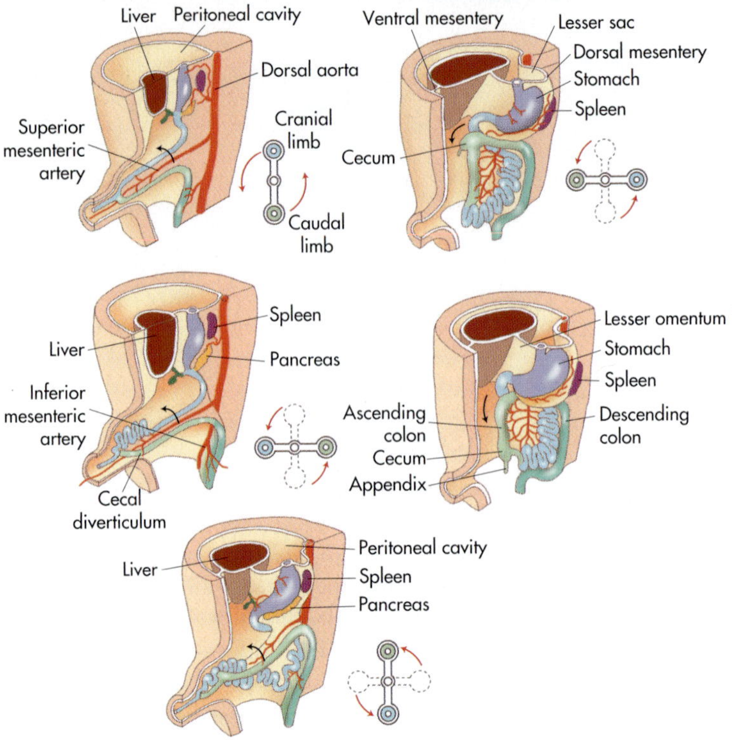

FIGURE 61-1 Development and rotation of the midgut from the 6th to 11th week. The midgut is the primordium of the small intestines, cecum, appendix, ascending colon, and right half to two thirds of the transverse colon. The connection of the yolk sac and body stalk will form the umbilical cord at the ventral region of the embryo.

cover the umbilical cord by the amnion. Fusion of the midline begins during the 7th week of development and is completed by the 8th week.

The umbilical veins drain the placenta, body stalk, and the evolving abdominal wall. During the 7th week, the hepatic bud enlarges, and the right umbilical vein atrophies. The proximal portion of the left umbilical vein between the subhepatic portion and the common cardinal vein also atrophies. Branches of the aorta now replace the nutritive function of the umbilical veins with respect to the developing abdominal wall. The superior mesenteric artery is formed from the right omphalomesenteric artery.

Umbilication hernia of the bowel occurs during the 8th week of development as the midgut extends to the extraembryonic coelom in the proximal portion of the umbilical cord. The midgut grows faster than the abdominal cavity at this stage because of the increased size of the liver and kidneys. Thus, the herniation develops. The intestines return to the abdominal cavity by the 12th week of gestation.

SONOGRAPHIC EVALUATION OF THE FETAL ABDOMINAL WALL

It should be possible to detect abdominal wall defects in utero, as the defects form early in embryologic development. It is very important to image the cord insertion site and the fetal anterior abdominal wall to evaluate for the presence or absence of such defects. If the urinary bladder and pelvis are evaluated closely, the diagnosis of

bladder and cloacal exstrophy may also be made with sonography. The most common types of abdominal wall defects are gastroschisis, omphalocele, and umbilical hernia. Other types of abdominal ventral wall defects include ectopia cordia, bladder and cloacal exstrophy, amniotic band syndrome, and the limb-body wall complex. The following questions should be routinely answered:

1. Is a limiting membrane present?
2. What is the relation of the umbilical cord to the defect?
3. Which organs are eviscerated?
4. Is the bowel normal in appearance?
5. Are other fetal malformations evident?

ABNORMALITIES OF THE ANTERIOR ABDOMINAL WALL

Abdominal wall defects cause distortion of the normal contour of the ventral or anterior surface of the fetal abdomen. Table 61-1 summarizes the typical sonographic features and associated conditions of fetal abdominal wall defects.

The three most common abdominal wall defects are the **omphalocele**, umbilical hernia (a form of omphalocele), and **gastroschisis**. The incidence of omphaloceles is roughly 1 in 4000 live births. Rarer abdominal wall defects include ectopia cordis, pentalogy of Cantrell, limb-body wall complex, amnion rupture sequence, and bladder and cloacal exstrophy. Overall, gastroschisis has

TABLE 61-1	Typical Features of Ventral Wall Defects and Associated Conditions		
Type of Defect	**Description**	**Sonographic Features**	**Other Anomalies**
Gastroschisis	Paraumbilical defect	Typically only bowel is eviscerated; occasionally other organs, but almost never the liver	Associated anomalies are uncommon; high rate of bowel-related complications
Omphalocele	Midline defect, contained by membrane	Variable	High risk of other anomalies and/or aneuploidy
Extracorporeal liver		Typically large	When isolated without other detectable anomalies, risk of aneuploidy is very low; however, high rate of cardiac anomalies
Intracorporeal liver		Typically small	>50% risk of aneuploidy when detected prenatally
Beckwith-Wiedemann syndrome	Syndromic condition	Macroglossia; omphalocele; visceromegaly	Omphalocele is typically intracorporeal liver type
Pentalogy of Cantrell	Omphalocele Anterior diaphragmatic hernia Distal partial sternal defect Pericardial defect Cardiac defect	May appear only as high omphalocele; pleural effusion, even transient, is highly suggestive of diaphragmatic hernia in this situation	None
Absent sternum	Absent sternum	Dynamic heart covered by skin	Rare; usually isolated
Ectopia cordis	Thoracic defect of sternum and skin	Dynamic heart not covered by skin	Rare; high rate of cardiac and other defects; may be associated with high omphalocele
Bladder exstrophy	Eviscerated urinary bladder	Nonvisualization of urinary bladder; soft tissue mass of anterior abdominal wall may be subtle	Increased risk of fetal aneuploidy
Cloacal exstrophy	Eviscerated cloaca with two hemibladders	Nonvisualization of urinary bladder; in one variation, ileal prolapse produces "elephant trunk" appearance	Severe, complex anomaly
Limb-body wall complex	Multiple anomaly condition	Bizarre, complex defect with ventral wall defect, close attachment to placenta, cranial defects, scoliosis	100% lethal, but no risk of aneuploidy

From Nyberg DA, McGahan JP, Pretorius DH, et al, editors: *Diagnostic ultrasound of fetal anomalies: text and atlas,* Philadelphia, 2003, Lippincott, Williams & Wilkins.

an incidence of 12 per 10,000, although only rarely are affected infants born to older mothers. The role of the perinatal team is to distinguish among these lesions because clinical management, associated anomalies, delivery, and postnatal surgical survival vary, depending on the specific type of abdominal wall defect.

Box 61-1 outlines what the sonographer should investigate to distinguish between omphalocele and gastroschisis.

Omphalocele

During the 8th to 12th weeks of development, the fetal bowel normally migrates into the umbilical cord from the abdominal cavity. This normal embryologic herniation of the bowel permits the development of the intraabdominal organs and allows necessary bowel rotation. Because of the lack of space within the abdominal cavity and the large fetal liver and kidneys, the bowel is forced from the abdomen and into the extraembryonic coelom of the umbilical cord. This herniation permits the bowel

BOX 61-1	Differentiation of Omphalocele from Gastroschisis

The sonographer should investigate the following to differentiate an omphalocele from a gastroschisis:
- Look for the presence of a membrane; gastroschisis does not have one.
- Look at the umbilical cord; the cord goes through the omphalocele, whereas gastroschisis is found to the right of the cord.
- Determine which organs are eviscerated.
- Determine if the bowel is normal in texture.
- Look for other anomalies, because omphaloceles often occur with chromosomal abnormalities.

to rotate around the superior mesenteric artery. These herniated loops of bowel normally return and rotate into position within the abdominal cavity by the 12th week of pregnancy. When bowel loops fail to return to the abdomen, a bowel-containing omphalocele occurs (Figure 61-2).

An omphalocele develops when there is a midline defect of the abdominal muscles, fascia, and skin that results in herniation of intraabdominal structures into the base of the umbilical cord (Figure 61-3). This herniation is covered by a membrane that consists of the amnion and peritoneum. The alpha-fetoprotein (AFP) level may be slightly elevated or within normal limits.

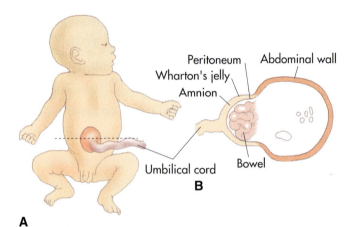

FIGURE 61-2 Typical features of bowel-containing omphalocele (intracorporeal liver) shown on external examination **(A)** and on cross-sectional view **(B).**

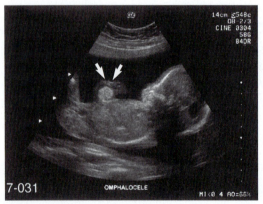

FIGURE 61-3 Longitudinal image of a 14-week fetus showing a small omphalocele with its covering membrane *(arrows)* projecting from the umbilical area.

Omphaloceles are characterized as two types: (1) those that contain the liver within the sac and (2) those that contain a variable amount of bowel without liver.

Fetuses with an omphalocele that contains only a bowel have a higher risk for chromosomal abnormalities and other anomalies (Figures 61-4 and 61-5). Bowel within the omphalocele develops because the intestine fails to return to the abdomen (primitive body stalk remains). A liver omphalocele represents a developmental defect in abdominal wall closure. This type of omphalocele affects the abdominal wall muscles, fascia, and skin. Liver omphaloceles may contain a bowel and demonstrate a relatively large abdominal wall defect in comparison with the abdominal diameter (Figures 61-6 and 61-7).

The prognosis for infants with an omphalocele varies according to the extent of the primary defect and associated structural and chromosomal abnormalities. Perinatal mortality approaches 80% when more than one fetal abnormality exists, and almost all infants die when there is a chromosomal or major heart defect. Without other anomalies, the mortality rate is approximately 10% with an isolated omphalocele.

The mode of delivery for fetuses with an omphalocele varies according to the type of omphalocele and other anomalies. The obstetrician may elect vaginal delivery when a chromosomal abnormality and other major anomalies predict no chance for survival.

Sonographic Findings. The sonographic signs of an omphalocele are as follows:

- Central abdominal wall defect with evisceration of the bowel or a combination of liver and bowel into the base of the umbilical cord. Color flow imaging may aid in viewing the continuity of the umbilical cord into the omphalocele. The stomach may be involved (Figure 61-8). Bowel omphaloceles appear echogenic and must be distinguished from umbilical hernia (covered by skin and fat).
- Membrane consisting of the peritoneum and amnion forms the omphalocele sac encasing the herniated organs.

FIGURE 61-4 Typical features of liver-containing omphalocele shown on external examination **(A)** and on cross-sectional view **(B).**

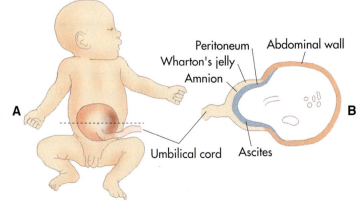

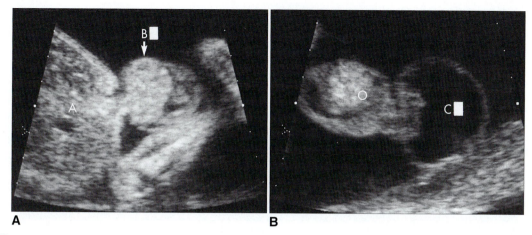

FIGURE 61-5 A, Bowel omphalocele *(B)* in a fetus with trisomy 18. *A,* Abdomen. **B,** In the same fetus, an umbilical cord cyst *(C)* is noted coursing distally into the omphalocele *(O)*. Other anomalies observed include a strawberry-shaped cranium, hypoplastic cerebellum, nuchal fold, and esophageal atresia. Additionally, a large atrial septal defect, hypoplastic left ventricle, single umbilical artery, and hydramnios were found.

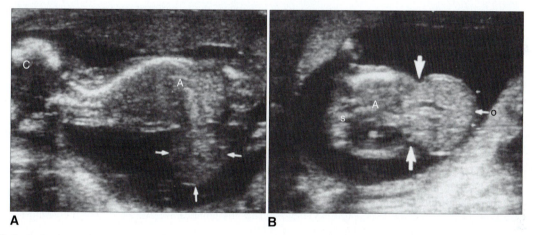

FIGURE 61-6 A, Sagittal scan in an 18-week fetus in a spine-up position with a mass herniating from the anterior abdominal wall representing an omphalocele *(arrows)*. *A,* Abdomen; *C,* cranium. **B,** In the same fetus, in a transverse direction, herniation of the liver into the omphalocele *(o)* is observed. Note the portal vessel within the liver. *A,* Abdomen; *large arrows,* first border of the omphalocele; *s,* spine.

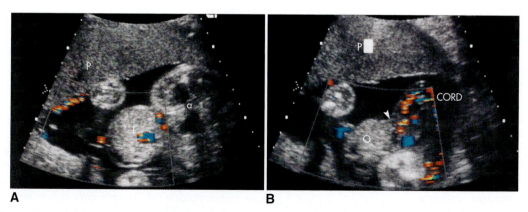

FIGURE 61-7 A, Color flow imaging of a liver-filled omphalocele in a 26-week fetus showing hepatic vessel flow within the herniated liver. *a,* Abdomen; *P,* placenta. **B,** In the same fetus, color enhancement aids in the confirmation of the cord vessels entering the base of the omphalocele *(O, arrow)*; *P,* placenta. No other anomalies were found, and the karyotype was normal.

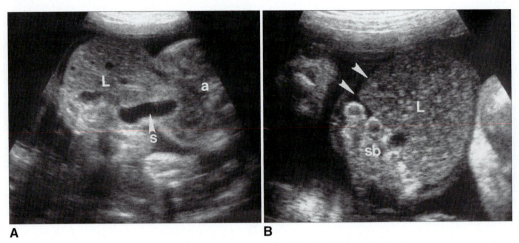

FIGURE 61-8 A, Large, liver-filled (L) omphalocele shown in a 27-week fetus. This omphalocele also contained a portion of the stomach (s) and small bowel. a, Abdomen. The karyotype was normal, and no other sonographic anomalies were detected. **B,** In the same fetus, small bowel (sb) and ascites (arrows) are shown. Surgical repair of the omphalocele was successful after birth. L, Liver.

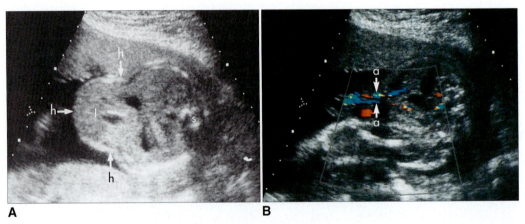

FIGURE 61-9 A, Umbilical hernia (h; arrows) observed in a fetus with Carpenter's syndrome (acrocephalopolysyndactyly). l, Liver; s, spine. **B,** In the same fetus, at the cord insertion level and using color imaging, the umbilical arteries are observed entering the abdomen in a normal location. This excludes the diagnosis of an omphalocele. a, Artery.

- Umbilical hernias may be confused with liver omphaloceles; however, a normal cord insertion suggests hernia (Figure 61-9).
- Ascites may coexist with an omphalocele.
- Hydramnios is found in one third of fetuses.
- Associated anomalies (50% to 70%) include complex cardiac disease (30% to 50%) and gastrointestinal, neural tube, and genitourinary tract anomalies (polycystic kidneys with a small omphalocele may indicate trisomy 13) (Figure 61-10).
- Omphaloceles may occur concurrently with diaphragmatic hernia.
- Chromosomal anomalies occur in 35% to 60% of omphaloceles. Most common are trisomies 13 and 18. Omphaloceles may be found with trisomy 21, Turner's syndrome, and triploidy.
- When scoliosis is found, consider limb-body wall complex (or body-stalk anomaly), a lethal disorder, which also includes severe cranial defects (acrania,

encephalocele), facial clefts, extensive abdominal wall defect of the chest, and abdomen and limb defects. Abnormal fusion of the amnion and chorion extends as a sheet from the cord and adheres to the fetus and placenta (Figures 61-11 and 61-12).
- Amniotic band syndrome may represent a milder form of limb-body wall complex and may be predicted by amniotic bands (fibrous tissue strands) that entangle or amputate fetal parts. Facial clefts, asymmetric encephaloceles, constriction or amputation defects of the extremities, and clubfoot deformities are common findings. Uterine sheets (synechiae) should not be confused with amniotic bands.
- Pentalogy of Cantrell is considered when a large omphalocele, diaphragmatic hernia, ectopia cordis (evisceration of heart), and other heart defects are observed (Figures 61-13 and 61-14).
- Consider bladder or cloacal exstrophy when a low omphalocele is observed. Other anomalies may

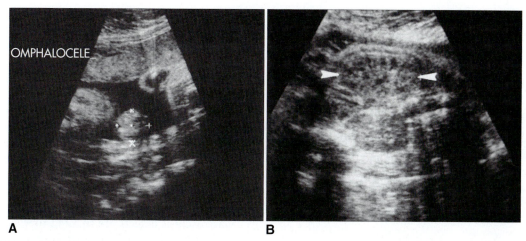

FIGURE 61-10 A, Bowel-filled omphalocele (2 mm) *(calipers)* in a 27-week fetus. **B,** In the same fetus, enlarged polycystic kidneys *(arrows)* were observed bilaterally. Oligohydramnios, an 8-mm nuchal fold, cerebellar hypoplasia, and enlarged cisterna magna with Dandy-Walker malformation and asymmetry of the heart were found. Genetic amniocentesis was declined. Intrauterine growth restriction was apparent by 33 weeks of gestation. Trisomy 13 was suspected. Neonatal karyotype after birth confirmed the diagnosis of trisomy 13 with translocation. The infant died within 1 hour of birth.

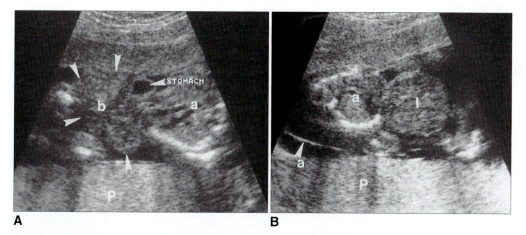

FIGURE 61-11 A, Early amnion rupture sequence or body stalk anomaly in a 17-week fetus, revealing extensive herniation of the abdominal organs. The stomach and bowel *(b)* are eviscerated. *a,* Abdomen; *P,* placenta. **B,** In the same fetus, herniation of the liver *(l)* is noted. Note the amniotic band *(a, arrow)* outlined within the amniotic cavity. Amniocentesis reveals a chromosomally normal infant. *a,* Abdomen.

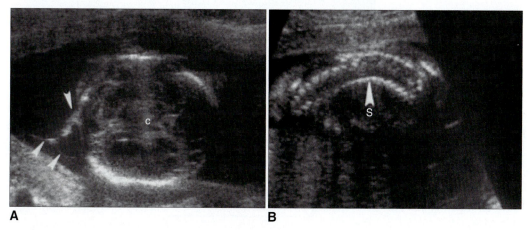

FIGURE 61-12 A, In the fetus depicted in Figure 61-11, amniotic bands *(arrows)* are shown adhering to the cranium *(c).* **B,** In the same fetus, scoliosis *(s)* is demonstrated. The fetus delivered prematurely at 29 weeks of gestation because of premature rupture of the membranes. Autopsy revealed posterior scalp defects with attachment of amniotic bands. Low-set ears and posteriorly rotated ears, bilateral cleft lip and palate, absent toes unilaterally, constriction ring of the thumb and first finger of one hand, and bilateral simian creases were found. The abdominal wall defect included herniation of the stomach, intestine, liver, and two spleens. A wide midline defect that was continuous with the cord was found. Scoliosis was also confirmed.

include anal atresia, spina bifida, and lower-limb defects.

• When organomegaly and macroglossia are observed, Beckwith-Wiedemann syndrome is suspected (occurs in 12% of infants with an omphalocele).

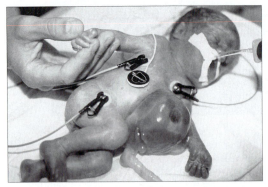

FIGURE 61-13 Neonate depicted in Figure 61-14 with diaphragmatic hernia and an omphalocele.

Gastroschisis

Gastroschisis is a periumbilical defect that nearly always is located to the right of the umbilicus. Gastroschisis is an opening in the layers of the abdominal wall with evisceration (herniation) of the bowel and, infrequently, the stomach and genitourinary organs but rarely the liver (Figure 61-15). It is thought that gastroschisis is a consequence of atrophy of the right umbilical vein or a disruption of the omphalomesenteric artery. Gastroschisis defects are usually not known to be genetically transmitted, although the recurrence risk for gastroschisis has been estimated at 3.5%.

Gastroschisis defects are small (2 to 4 cm in size) and are located next to the normal cord insertion. In the majority of cases, the defect is positioned to the right of the umbilical cord. The insertion of the umbilical cord is normal in fetuses with gastroschisis (Figures 61-16 and 61-17). Small bowel is always found in the herniation.

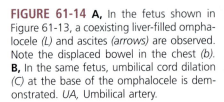

FIGURE 61-14 A, In the fetus shown in Figure 61-13, a coexisting liver-filled omphalocele *(L)* and ascites *(arrows)* are observed. Note the displaced bowel in the chest *(b).* **B,** In the same fetus, umbilical cord dilation *(C)* at the base of the omphalocele is demonstrated. *UA,* Umbilical artery.

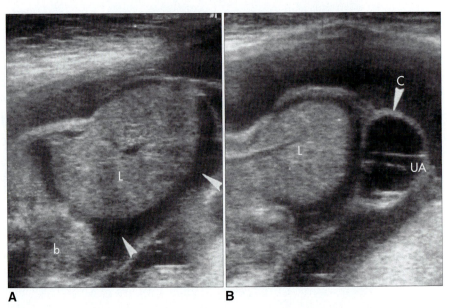

A   B

FIGURE 61-15 Typical features of gastroschisis shown on external examination **(A)** and cross-sectional view **(B).**

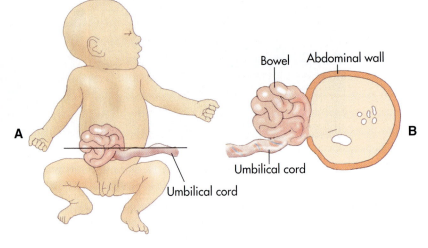

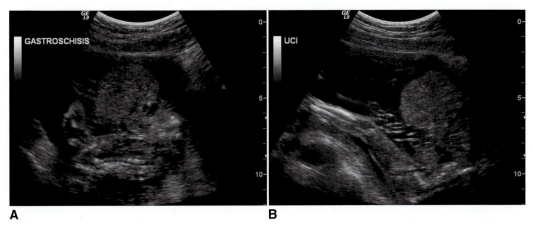

FIGURE 61-16 **A,** Appearance of gastroschisis in a 19-week fetus with elevation of maternal serum alpha-fetoprotein. Note the typical appearance of herniated, free-floating bowel loops. **B,** In the same fetus, a normal cord insertion is shown with a herniated bowel.

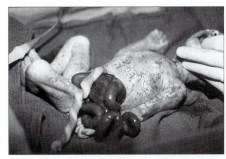

FIGURE 61-17 Neonate with left-side gastroschisis shown in Figure 61-19, *A.* Note the insertion of the cord to the right of the defect.

Other organs that may be involved in the herniation include the large bowel, the stomach, occasionally portions of the genitourinary system, and rarely the liver.

Alpha-fetoprotein levels are significantly higher in gastroschisis compared with an omphalocele because of the exposed bowel. The occurrence of gastroschisis is 1.75 to 2.5 in 10,000 live births. It has been found more frequently in males.

Although coexisting anomalies are rare with gastroschisis, associated gastrointestinal problems may be of considerable medical consequence to the infant. This defect prevents the occurrence of normal bowel rotation, and intestinal atresia or stenosis may ensue because of ischemia (compression of mesenteric vessels or bowel torsion). Ischemia may cause bowel perforation or meconium peritonitis. In several neonatal studies, more than half of the infants with gastroschisis in which ischemia and gangrene of the bowel were present subsequently died.

The obstetrician usually prefers to deliver the infant by cesarean section to prevent bowel damage and contamination from a vaginal delivery. The prognosis for the infant with uncomplicated gastroschisis is excellent. Surgical repair usually occurs within hours of delivery;

with extensive defects, reconstruction is performed in stages using Silastic sheets.

Sonographic Findings. The sonographer may be able to detect gastroschisis after 12 weeks of gestation. The patient usually has a notably elevated maternal serum AFP level. As the sonographer evaluates the area of umbilical cord insertion, multiple loops of the bowel (small bowel and often colon) may be seen outside the abdominal cavity in the area of the cord. The cord is normally inserted into the abdominal wall, and the defect is almost always to the right of the umbilical cord insertion. The edges of the bowel are irregular and free floating without a covering membrane, as is seen with an omphalocele. Ascites is not present in the abdominal cavity.

The sonographic appearance of gastroschisis is as follows:

- Right paraumbilical defect of abdominal wall, rarely a left-side defect (Figure 61-18).
- Free-floating herniated small bowel. Large bowel, stomach, gallbladder, urinary bladder, and pelvic organs may be involved. When organs other than small or large bowel are seen, body stalk anomalies should be suspected.
- A herniated bowel may be mildly dilated with a bowel wall thickening (chemical peritonitis because of irritation by urine within amniotic fluid) (Figure 61-19). Dilatation may be seen in herniated portions of the bowel or within the fetal abdominal cavity.
- Notably dilated bowel may suggest infarction or bowel atresia (Figure 61-20).
- Hydronephrosis, bladder deviation (Figure 61-21), and exstrophy (Figure 61-22) may be observed.
- Consider amniotic band syndrome amputations when clefting of the face or encephalocele is found. Severe body wall defects may be seen in gastroschisis with secondary band formation (Figures 61-23 through 61-25).

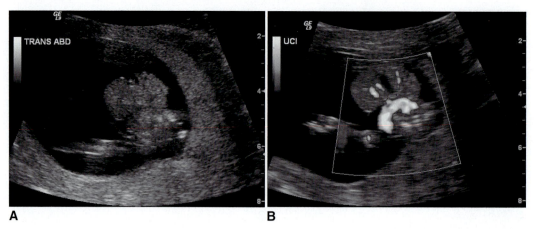

FIGURE 61-18 A, Transverse image of a 22-week fetus with moderate-sized gastroschisis. **B,** The umbilical cord is well seen with color as it enters to the right of the defect.

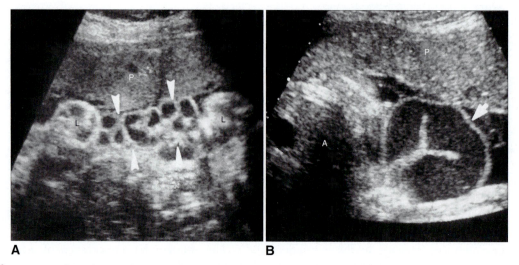

FIGURE 61-19 A, Gastroschisis showing herniated bowel *(arrows)* in the amniotic cavity. Cesarean section was performed at 36 weeks of gestation because of a nonreactive nonstress test with variable decelerations and absent breathing. A small-for-gestational-age infant with left-side gastroschisis was delivered. *L,* Limb; *p,* placenta. **B,** Isolated bowel segment *(arrow)* observed in another fetus with gastroschisis at 29 weeks of gestation. Bowel dilation (29 mm) and obstruction (meconium ileus) are shown. Note the haustral markings within the obstructed bowel. *A,* Abdomen, *p,* placenta.

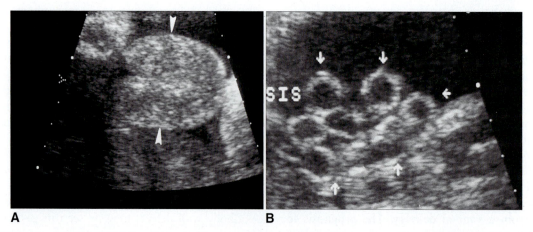

FIGURE 61-20 A, Herniated large intestine *(arrows)* with meconium at 34 weeks of gestation in a fetus with gastroschisis. Note the dilated bowel, which measured 20 mm in diameter. **B,** In the same fetus, portions of the small bowel *(arrows)* are observed with mild dilation.

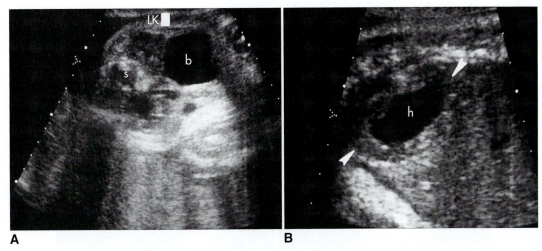

FIGURE 61-21 In a fetus with gastroschisis, concomitant anomalies were detected and included **(A)** deviation of the bladder and **(B)** unilateral hydronephrosis *(h, arrows)*. *LK,* Normal left kidney; *s,* spine; *b,* bladder.

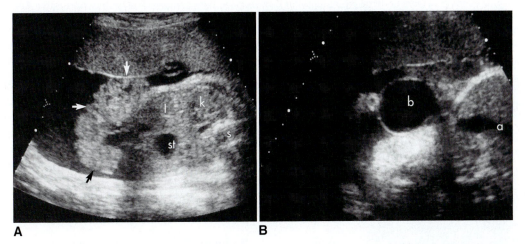

FIGURE 61-22 A, Gastroschisis *(arrows)* evident in a 34-week fetus in a transverse view. Note the intraabdominal position of the stomach *(st),* liver *(l),* and kidney *(k). s,* Spine. **B,** In the same fetus, note that the bladder *(b)* is herniated from the pelvis (exstrophy). The uterus and ovaries were also found to be herniated from the pelvis after delivery. Congenital microcolon was also found. *a,* Abdomen.

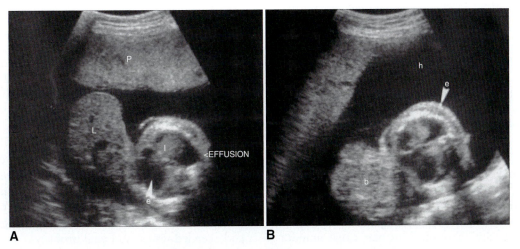

FIGURE 61-23 Gastroschisis with secondary amniotic bands shown in a 28-week fetus. **A,** Eviscerated liver *(L)* and bowel *(b)* are documented. Bilateral pleural effusions *(arrows)* and soft tissue edema *(e)* in **B** are apparent. Note the hydramnios *(h). l,* Lung; *P,* placenta.

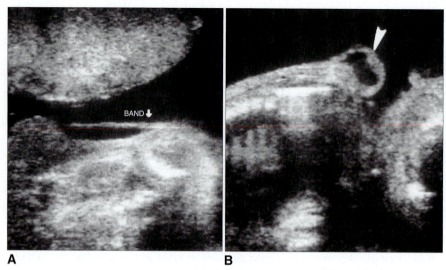

FIGURE 61-24 In the fetus depicted in Figures 61-23 and 61-25, multiple amniotic bands *(BAND)* **(A)** were found adhering to the abdomen with attachment to the shoulder *(arrow)* in **(B)**. Normal chromosomes were found by amniocentesis. Amniotic fluid alpha-fetoprotein was extremely elevated (175 MOM) with positive acetylcholinesterase. The fetus was delivered at 28 weeks of gestation because of worsening hydrops. No resuscitative measures were undertaken. Autopsy findings revealed right paraumbilical gastroschisis with eventration of the liver and intestine. Intestinal malrotation and small-bowel obstruction were found. Moderate fetal hydrops with bilateral pleural effusions and pulmonary hypoplasia were noted. An amniotic band or peritoneal band extended from the liver to the thumb. The defect was consistent with gastroschisis occurring early in embryogenesis because of the intestinal malrotation with secondary amniotic band rupture.

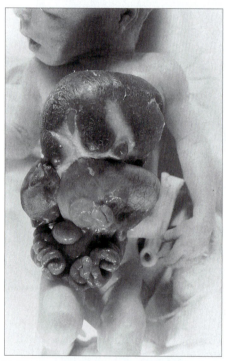

FIGURE 61-25 Neonate depicted in Figures 61-23 and 61-24 with gastroschisis and secondary amniotic band rupture.

Amniotic Band Syndrome

Amniotic band syndrome is the rupture of the amnion, which leads to entrapment or entanglement of the fetal parts by the "sticky" chorion. This may cause amputation or defects in random sites. Early entrapment by the bands may lead to severe craniofacial defects and internal malformations. Late entrapment leads to amputations or limb restrictions. The prevalence of this syndrome is low, occurring in 7.8 in 10,000 births. Anomalies associated with amniotic band syndrome include anomalies of the limbs, cranium, face, thorax, spine, abdominal wall (gastroschisis, omphalocele, bladder exstrophy), and the perineum.

Beckwith-Wiedemann Syndrome

Beckwith-Wiedemann syndrome is a rare group of disorders having in common the coexistence of an omphalocele, macroglossia, and visceromegaly. Most of the cases are sporadic. Beckwith-Wiedemann syndrome is characterized by macrosomia, macroglossia, visceromegaly, embryonic tumors (i.e., Wilms' tumor, hepatoblastoma, neuroblastoma, and rhabdomyosarcoma), an omphalocele, neonatal hypoglycemia, and ear creases. Sonographic findings usually note the presence of an omphalocele, growth acceleration, macroglossia, and visceromegaly. In the third trimester, polyhydramnios may be present.

Bladder and Cloacal Exstrophy

Bladder exstrophy is characterized by a defect in the lower abdominal wall and anterior wall of the urinary bladder. The everted bladder becomes exposed on the lower abdominal wall. The anomaly may be mild or severe (accompanied by an omphalocele, inguinal hernia, undescended testes, and anal problems). **Cloacal exstrophy** is rare and more complex than bladder exstrophy. This condition occurs early in development with involvement of the primitive gut and persistent cloaca. It results in exstrophy of the bladder in which two hemi-bladders are separated by intestinal mucosa.

Sonographic Findings. With bladder exstrophy, the normal urinary bladder is not visible upon sonographic evaluation. Instead, a soft tissue mass, representing the exposed bladder mucosa, may be seen on the surface of the lower abdominal wall. In addition, an anterior abdominal wall defect may be the primary ultrasound finding of cloacal exstrophy.

Pentalogy of Cantrell, Ectopia Cordis, and Cleft Sternum

The **pentalogy of Cantrell** is rare and is the association of a cleft distal sternum, diaphragmatic defect, midline anterior ventral wall defect, defect of the apical pericardium with communication into the peritoneum, and an internal cardiac defect. A high or superumbilical omphalocele is usually the primary finding of pentalogy of Cantrell. If the diaphragmatic defect is large enough to produce a diaphragmatic hernia, displacement of the heart and mediastinum may be observed, but the sternal and pericardial defects are not well seen. The presence of pericardial effusion may be found. Pentalogy of Cantrell may be associated with various cardiac defects, cleft lip (may also have cleft palate), encephalocele, exencephaly, and sirenomelia. In the first trimester, cystic hygroma may be present. This has also been associated with trisomies 13 and 18 and 45 X (Turner's syndrome).

In ectopia cordis, the exposed heart presents outside the chest wall through a cleft sternum. The most dramatic finding is the presence of a heart outside the thoracic cavity; a portion or all of the heart may protrude through the defect in the sternum. Anomalies most frequently associated with ectopia cordis include an omphalocele, cardiovascular malformations, and craniofacial defects.

A cleft sternum may be either partial or absent without ectopia cordis and is typically a superior or total cleft. Dramatic pulsations of the anterior chest wall occur from the heart beating against the chest without the presence of the sternum to protect it. This condition is associated with vascular malformations, including cavernous hemangiomas and an omphalocele.

Sonographic Findings. On sonographic examination, the heart may be seen to lie outside the normal thoracic cavity or bulge through the defective sternum. It is common to see pericardial and pleural effusions. Differential considerations include body stalk anomaly, amniotic band syndrome, and isolated ectopia cordis. The prognosis depends on many factors, including the extent of the defect and the size of the thoracic cavity that allows surgical intervention to place the heart back into the chest.

Limb-Body Wall Complex

The **limb-body wall complex** anomaly is associated with large cranial defects (**exencephaly** or **encephalocele**); facial cleft; body wall complex defects involving the thorax, abdomen, or both; and limb defects. Other anomalies include **scoliosis** and various internal malformations. The limb-body wall complex occurs with the fusion of the amnion and chorion; the amnion does not cover the umbilical cord normally but extends as a sheet from the margin of the cord and is continuous with both the body wall and the placenta. Left-side body wall defects are three times more common than right-side defects.

Sonographic Findings. On ultrasound examination, the defects are large and involve the abdomen and thorax. The eviscerated organs form a complex, bizarre-appearing mass entangled with membranes. The umbilical cord is short and adherent to the placental membranes.

The Fetal Abdomen

Sandra L. Hagen-Ansert

OBJECTIVES

On completion of this chapter, you should be able to:
- Describe the development of the digestive system and list the unique features of the fetal abdomen
- Describe normal development of the stomach and the importance of its sonographic visualization
- Define abnormalities of the fetal gastrointestinal tract and hepatobiliary system and describe their sonographic findings

The fetal abdominal organs—liver, biliary system, spleen, stomach, kidneys, and colon—are well formed by the second trimester. The following differences between the fetal and adult abdomen have been noted:

- The umbilical arteries and veins provide important anatomic landmarks for fetal abdominal anatomy and measurements.
- The ductus venosus is patent and serves as a conduit between the portal veins and systemic veins.
- The proportions of the fetal body differ from those in the adult. The fetal abdomen is larger relative to body length, and the liver occupies a larger volume of the fetal abdomen.
- The fetal pelvic cavity is small; therefore, the urinary bladder, ovaries, and uterus lie in the abdominal cavity.
- The apron of the greater omentum is small, contains little fat, and remains unfused in the fetus. Fetal ascites may therefore separate the omental leaves.

EMBRYOLOGY OF THE DIGESTIVE SYSTEM

The primitive gut forms during the 4th week of gestation as the dorsal part of the yolk sac is incorporated into the embryo during folding. The primitive gut is divided into three sections: foregut, midgut, and hindgut.

The Foregut

The derivatives of the foregut are the pharynx, lower respiratory system, esophagus, stomach, part of the duodenum, liver and biliary apparatus, and pancreas.
Esophagus. The esophagus is short in the beginning, but it rapidly lengthens as the body grows, reaching its final length by the 7th week. The *tracheoesophageal septum* partitions the trachea from the esophagus. **Esophageal atresia,** usually associated with a tracheoesophageal fistula, results from abnormal deviation of the tracheoesophageal septum in a posterior direction.

When this occurs, amniotic fluid cannot pass to the intestines for absorption and hydramnios results.

Esophageal stenosis is the narrowing of the esophagus, usually in the distal third portion. This occurs from incomplete recanalization of the esophagus during the 8th week of development.

Stomach. The stomach appears as a fusiform dilation of the caudal part of the foregut (Figure 62-1). During the 5th and 6th weeks, the dorsal border (greater curvature) grows faster than the ventral border (lesser curvature). The stomach is suspended from the dorsal wall of the abdominal cavity by the dorsal mesentery or dorsal mesogastrium. The dorsal mesogastrium is carried to the left during rotation of the stomach and formation of a cavity known as the omental bursa or lesser sac of the peritoneum. The lesser sac communicates with the main peritoneal cavity or greater peritoneal sac through a small opening, called the epiploic foramen.

Duodenum. The duodenum develops from the caudal part of the foregut and cranial part of the midgut (see Figure 62-1). The two parts grow rapidly and form a C-shaped loop that rotates to the right, where it comes to lie primarily in the retroperitoneum. The junction of the two embryonic parts of the duodenum in the adult is just distal to the entrance of the common bile duct. The duodenum is supplied by branches of the celiac trunk and the superior mesenteric artery.

During the 5th and 6th weeks, the lumen of the duodenum becomes partly or totally occluded (depending on the proliferation of its lining of epithelial cells). Normally the duodenum is recanalized by the end of the 8th week. Partial or complete failure of this process results in either **duodenal stenosis** (narrowing) or **duodenal atresia** (blockage). Usually the third or fourth parts of the duodenal are affected.

Liver and Biliary System. The liver, gallbladder, and biliary ducts arise as a bud from the most caudal part of the foregut in the 4th week (see Figure 62-1). The hepatic diverticulum grows between the layers of the ventral mesentery, where it rapidly enlarges and divides into two parts. The liver grows rapidly and intermingles with the vitelline and umbilical veins, divides into two parts, and fills most of the abdominal cavity. The large cranial part is the primordium of the parenchyma of the liver. The small caudal part gives rise to the gallbladder and cystic duct.

The hemopoietic cells, Kupffer cells, and connective tissue cells are derived from the mesenchyme in the septum transversum. The septum transversum is a mass of mesoderm between the pericardial cavity and the yolk stalk. It forms a major part of the diaphragm and the ventral mesentery.

Hemopoiesis (blood formation) begins during the 6th week and accounts for the large size of the liver between the 7th and 9th weeks of development. By the 12th week, bile formation by the hepatic cells has begun.

Extrahepatic Biliary Atresia. Blockage of the bile ducts results from their failure to recanalize following the solid stage of their development. This malformation may also result from interference with the blood supply of the ducts resulting from infection during the fetal period.

Pancreas. The pancreas develops from the dorsal and ventral pancreatic buds of the endodermal cells that arise from the caudal part of the foregut (see Figure 62-1). When the duodenum grows and rotates to the right, the ventral bud is carried dorsally and fuses with the dorsal bud. The ducts of the two pancreatic buds join. The combined duct becomes the main pancreatic duct that opens with the bile duct into the duodenum. The proximal part of the duct may persist as the accessory pancreatic duct.

Spleen. The spleen is a lymphatic organ that is derived from a mass of mesenchymal cells located between the layers of the dorsal mesogastrium (see Figure 62-1). The spleen is lobulated in the fetal period.

The Midgut

The derivatives of the midgut are the small intestines (including most of the duodenum), the cecum and cloaca exstrophy, the ascending colon, and most of the transverse colon. The superior mesenteric artery supplies all of these structures.

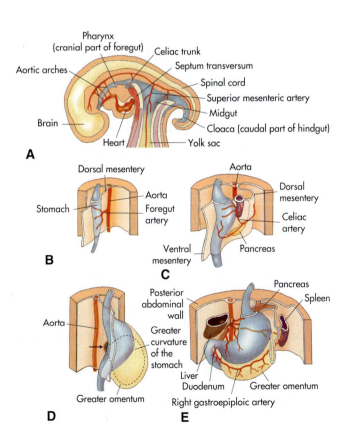

FIGURE 62-1 Development of the digestive system. **A,** Four weeks. **B,** Five weeks. **C,** Six weeks. **D** and **E,** Development of the stomach; seven weeks.

The midgut is suspended from the abdominal wall by an elongated dorsal mesentery. It communicates with the yolk sac via the yolk stalk. While the midgut lengthens and forms a midgut loop, it herniates outside the abdomen into the proximal part of the umbilical cord. Usually by the 10th or 11th week, this midgut herniation returns to the abdomen and undergoes further rotation resulting from the decrease in size of the liver and kidneys and the growth of the abdominal cavity.

After the intestines return to the abdominal cavity, they enlarge, lengthen, and assume their final positions. Their mesenteries are pressed against the posterior abdominal wall. At this time, the ascending colon and descending colon become retroperitoneal. Likewise the duodenum and most of the pancreas also become retroperitoneal structures. At the same time, the small intestines form a new line of attachment that extends from where the duodenum becomes retroperitoneal to the ileocecal junction. The mesentery of the transverse colon fuses with the dorsal mesogastrium to form the posterior wall of the inferior part of the omental bursa. The sigmoid colon retains its mesentery, but it is shorter than in the early fetus.

Malformations of the Midgut

Omphalocele and Gastroschisis. Omphalocele and gastroschisis are defects that occur when the midgut fails to return to the abdominal cavity from the umbilical cord during the 10th week. In an **omphalocele,** coils of intestine protrude from the umbilicus and are covered by a transparent sac of amnion. The umbilical cord pierces the central part of the omphalocele. Conversely, a **gastroschisis** is a condition in which the bowel or organs are free floating from the midline defect. The gastroschisis is usually located to the right of the umbilical cord. (See Chapter 61 for further discussion of omphalocele and gastroschisis.)

Umbilical Hernia. When the intestines return normally to the abdominal cavity and then herniate either prenatally or postnatally through an inadequately closed umbilicus, an umbilical hernia forms. The hernia differs from an omphalocele in that the protruding mass (omentum or loop of bowel) is covered by subcutaneous tissue and skin.

Meckel's Diverticulum. Meckel's diverticulum is the most common malformation of the midgut. A **Meckel's diverticulum** is a remnant of the proximal part of the yolk stalk that fails to degenerate and disappear during the early fetal period. It is usually a small finger-like sac, about 5 cm long, that projects from the border of the ileum.

The Hindgut

The derivatives of the hindgut are the left part of the transverse colon, the descending colon, the sigmoid colon, the rectum, the superior portion of the anal canal, the epithelium of the urinary bladder, and most of the urethra. The inferior mesenteric artery supplies all of these structures.

SONOGRAPHIC EVALUATION OF THE ABDOMINAL CAVITY

The sonographer must carefully evaluate the gastrointestinal system during the routine fetal anatomy sonographic examination. The stomach, liver and vascular structures, cord insertion, small bowel, and colon should be clearly identified.

Gastrointestinal System

Stomach. The stomach should be identified as a fluid-filled structure in the left upper quadrant inferior to the diaphragm. A marked variation in the size of the stomach can be seen, even within the same fetus. Most fetuses older than 14 to 16 weeks should have fluid in their stomach (Figure 62-2). If no fluid is apparent, the stomach should be reevaluated in 20 to 30 minutes to rule out the possibility of a central nervous system problem (swallowing disorders), obstruction, oligohydramnios, or atresia. If fluid is still not noted during the sonographic evaluation, the fetus may be reexamined the following day or week to see if there has been a change in the size of the stomach. Esophageal anomalies are the least common problem for nonvisualization of the stomach.

The fluid within the stomach should be anechoic with linear rugae in the normal fetus. Echogenic debris may sometimes be seen along the dependent wall of the stomach that may represent vernix, protein, or intraamniotic hemorrhage. The presence of an echogenic mass in the fetal stomach in a patient who demonstrates clinical or sonographic evidence of placental abruption should raise the possibility of hematoma formation associated with an intraamniotic hemorrhage.

Although the fetal stomach is usually located on the left of the abdomen, there are conditions in which the stomach will be seen in the right upper quadrant (*situs inversus*). The fetal position must be identified, followed by the identification of the right and left sides of the fetus. If the fetus is in a vertex presentation with the spine up, the aorta and stomach both should be seen to the left of the spine. A total **situs inversus** implies that the stomach and the heart are both on the right side of the body and the liver is on the left. With a **partial situs inversus,** only the heart or the abdominal organs are reversed (dextrocardia or liver on the left; stomach on the right).

Esophagus. The normal esophagus can be visualized in the thorax during the second and third trimesters as two or more parallel echogenic lines ("multilayered" pattern). Sometimes it is possible to see fluid in the esophagus as the fetus swallows the amniotic fluid.

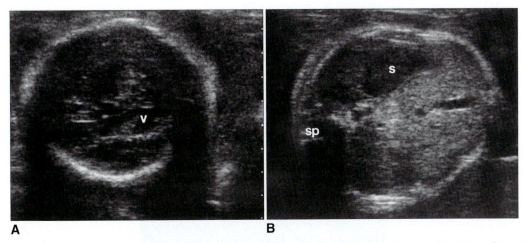

FIGURE 62-2 A 32-week fetus with microcephaly. **A,** Small head and ventricle *(v).* **B,** Transverse image at the level of the stomach *(s)* and spine *(sp).*

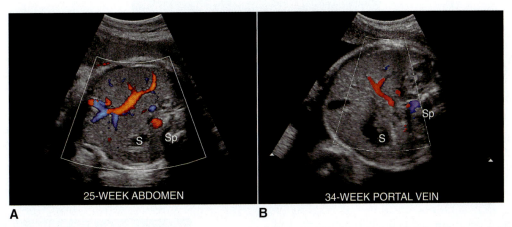

25-WEEK ABDOMEN

34-WEEK PORTAL VEIN

FIGURE 62-3 A and **B,** The abdominal circumference is measured from a transverse image at the level of the portal sinus *(red)* and the umbilical portion of the left portal vein. The stomach *(S)* is seen posterior; the spine *(Sp)* is at 3 o'clock.

Abdominal Circumference. The abdominal circumference is measured at the level of the portal sinus and the umbilical portion of the left portal vein ("hockey stick" appearance on the sonogram) (Figure 62-3). Be careful to avoid oblique scanning of the abdomen that may lead to an incorrect diameter-circumference measurement. The abdomen should be round, not oval. The pressure of the transducer should not compress the abdominal cavity.

Umbilical Cord Insertion. In the fetus, the umbilical vein courses cephalically in the free, inferior margin of the falciform ligament. It joins the umbilical portion of the left portal vein at the caudal margin of the left intersegmental fissure of the liver (Figure 62-4). The insertion of the umbilical cord must be imaged with color because it inserts into both the fetal abdomen and the placenta.

Visualization of the umbilical cord insertion site must be made to rule out the presence of an omphalocele, gastroschisis, hernia, or mass formation. After birth, the umbilical vein collapses and ultimately becomes the ligamentum teres hepatis.

Bowel. Movement of the gastric musculature begins in approximately the 4th to 5th month of gestation. The sonographic appearance of the bowel varies with menstrual age. The fetus is capable of swallowing sufficient amounts of amniotic fluid to permit visualization of the stomach by 11 menstrual weeks. In the second trimester, this movement and fetal swallowing result in the delivery of increased amniotic fluid volume distally into the small bowel and colon where fluid and nutrients are reabsorbed. After the 15th to 16th week, meconium begins to accumulate in the distal part of the small intestine as

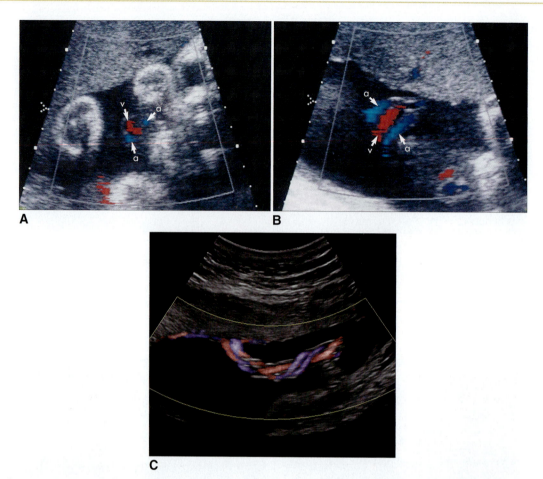

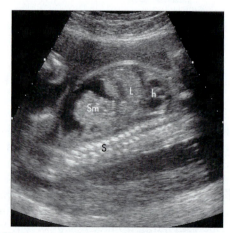

FIGURE 62-4 A, Color representation of the paired umbilical arteries *(a, blue)* and single umbilical vein *(v, red)* in a 30-week fetus viewed in a transverse plane. **B,** Sagittal view of the umbilical arteries *(a, blue)* and umbilical vein *(v, red).* Color flow imaging may highlight vessels that may not be obvious because of fetal position, oligohydramnios, and congenital anomalies. **C,** Color demonstration of the three-vessel cord shows the two umbilical arteries (blue) wrapped around the single umbilical vein.

a combination of desquamated cells, bile pigments, and mucoproteins.

Until the midsecond trimester, the small bowel lumen is quite difficult to demonstrate and appears as an ill-defined area of increased echogenicity in the mid to lower abdomen. The distinction of the large bowel from the small bowel is possible after 20 menstrual weeks. The region of the small bowel can be seen because it is slightly hyperechoic, compared with the liver, and may appear mass like in the central abdomen and pelvis (Figure 62-5). The hyperechoic appearance could be secondary to reflections from the walls of collapsed loops of the small bowel or from mesenteric fat between the loops. This hyperechoic appearance of the small bowel persists throughout the pregnancy. As the pregnancy progresses, the hyperechoic area becomes less prominent, and the small bowel is located more centrally in the abdomen than the colon. After 27 weeks, **peristalsis** of the normal small bowel is increasingly observed. The normal diameter of the small bowel lumen is less than or equal to 5 mm, with a length of 15 mm near term.

The colon is seen near the end of the second trimester as a long tubular hypoechoic structure with well-defined

FIGURE 62-5 Longitudinal scan of a 23-week fetus with abdominal ascites surrounding the small bowel *(Sm). h,* Heart; *L,* liver; *S,* spine.

walls. The **haustral folds** of the colon help to differentiate it from the small bowel. In early gestation, haustral folds appear as thin linear echoes within the lumen of the colon; later, the colon diameter increases and the folds become longer and thicker. Normal measurements of the colon diameter range from 3 to 5 mm at 20 weeks to 23 mm or larger at term. The colon is more peripheral than the small bowel. Hypoechoic echoes from the meconium may be seen within the lumen. The colon does not have peristalsis like the small bowel.

After 14 weeks of gestation, lipid is absorbed from the fetal colon and the remaining contents collect in the colon as meconium. The meconium within the lumen of the colon appears hypoechoic relative to the fetal liver and in comparison with the bowel wall. This is the point where the normal colon can be mistaken for an abnormally dilated small bowel or other pathologic processes, including renal cysts and pelvic masses. This pitfall is more prominent when the meconium has a more sonolucent appearance than usual (reflective of increased water content). The meconium increases slightly in echogenicity as the fetus grows nearer to term delivery.

Hepatobiliary System

Liver. The fetal liver is relatively large compared with the other intraabdominal organs and occupies most of the upper abdomen in the fetus. It accounts for 10% of the total weight of the fetus at 11 weeks and 5% of the total weight at term. The hepatic veins and fissures are formed by the end of the first trimester (Figure 62-6). The left lobe of the liver is larger than the right in utero secondary to the greater supply of oxygenated blood. This of course reverses after birth.

Gallbladder. The normal gallbladder may be seen sonographically after 20 weeks of gestation. Both the gallbladder and portal-umbilical vein appear as oblong fluid-filled structures on the transverse view of the fetal abdomen through the liver (Figure 62-7). The gallbladder is distinguished by its location to the right of the portal-umbilical vein and as an oblong, more oval structure than the "tubular" intrahepatic umbilical vein.

Pancreas. The normal fetal pancreas has been seen in utero, but it is more difficult to routinely recognize because of the lack of fatty tissue within the gland. It lies in the retroperitoneal cavity anterior to the superior mesenteric vessels, aorta, and inferior vena cava (Figure 62-8).

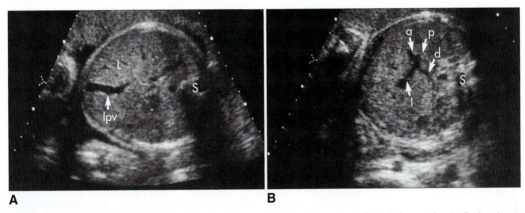

FIGURE 62-6 A, Transverse section of the liver in a 31-week fetus outlining the course of the left portal vein *(lpv)* at its entrance into the liver *(L)* from the fetal umbilical cord insertion. The left portal vein ascends upward and into the liver tissue *(L)*. *S,* Spine. **B,** The left portal vein *(l)* is shown to bifurcate into the portal sinus, right anterior *(a)*, and right posterior *(p)* portal veins. The ductus venosus *(d)* is observed before its drainage into the inferior vena cava. *S,* Spine.

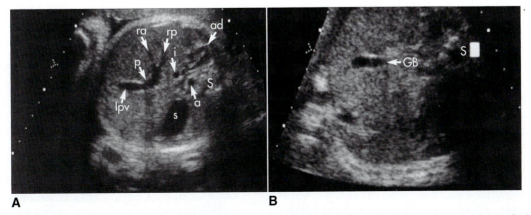

FIGURE 62-7 A, Transverse section of the liver and related structures in a 32-week fetus showing the left portal vein *(lpv)* coursing into the portal sinus *(p)*. The blood then moves into the right anterior *(ra)*, and right posterior *(rp)*, portal veins, and ductus venosus (see Figure 58-6, B). The right adrenal gland *(ad)*, fluid-filled stomach *(s)*, aorta *(a)*, and inferior vena cava *(i)* are shown. *S,* Spine. **B,** The gallbladder *(GB)* is viewed in the right upper quadrant of the abdomen in a 32-week fetus. The teardrop shape of the gallbladder should be distinguished from the left portal vein. *S,* Spine.

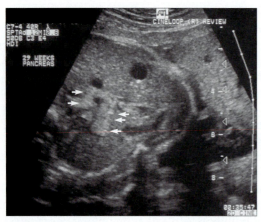

FIGURE 62-8 Transverse image of the fetal abdomen. The fetal spine is shown at 8 o'clock with the pancreas just anterior *(arrows)*.

Spleen. The spleen is homogeneous in texture, similar in echogenicity to the kidney, and slightly less echogenic than the liver. It increases in size during gestation. The spleen is imaged on a transverse plane posterior and to the left of the fetal stomach.

ABNORMALITIES OF THE HEPATOBILIARY SYSTEM

Anomalies of the liver, gallbladder, pancreas, and spleen are rare. Detection of abnormal morphology is beneficial because many lesions may be clinically undetected in the newborn period.

Liver

Although involved in several congenital anomalies (diaphragmatic hernia, omphalocele), the fetal liver is rarely affected by isolated hepatic lesions. Liver parenchymal cysts and hemangiomas of the liver have been reported. The liver enlarges in fetuses with Rh-immune disease in response to increased hematopoiesis (red blood cell production in the liver).

Liver tumors, hamartoma, and hepatoblastoma are uncommon and may be observed prenatally. Other tumors seen with sonography include hepatic teratoma, adenoma, or metastases from neuroblastoma. Although a rare tumor, hemangioendothelioma is the most common, symptomatic, vascular hepatic tumor of infancy and may cause nonimmune hydrops in the fetus.

■ **Sonographic Findings.** Most of these tumors appear as hypoechoic solid masses within the liver, although cystic components have also been reported as mixed with the solid masses. About 5% of benign and malignant liver tumors are calcified.

Liver calcification may be observed as an isolated echogenic focus. This calcification is usually a benign finding; rarely, it may be a hemangioma, multiple foci secondary to infection (transplacental infections, cytomegalovirus, toxoplasmosis), or hepatic necrosis from ischemia. If multiple calcifications are seen within the liver, other organs such as the brain and spleen may also be affected.

Situs Inversus

Situs inversus may present as a total reversal of the thoracic and abdominal organs or as a partial reversal (mirror image of some organs). Partial situs inversus is a more severe disorder and may develop in two different combinations of organ reversals. In partial situs inversus, the thoracic viscera are usually reversed and the abdominal viscera may or may not be reversed. Occasionally, partial situs inversus may involve the abdominal organs only without affecting the heart position in the left chest. Partial situs is divided into asplenia and polysplenia. **Asplenia** (absence of the spleen) is represented by an abnormally positioned stomach and gallbladder (more midline position), a more centrally positioned liver, and an abnormal positioning of the aorta and inferior vena cava on the same side. **Polysplenia** (more than one spleen) is represented by a transposition of the liver, spleen, and stomach and by an absence of the gallbladder. There is interruption of the inferior vena cava and the azygos vein is directly posterior to the heart and in front of the spine. At least two spleens are present along the greater curvature of the stomach (which is on the right side). Heart block is common in polysplenia syndrome. In polysplenia-asplenia, the normal size spleen is not seen on sonography between the stomach and left kidney on the transverse abdominal image

The cause of situs inversus is unclear, but it is thought to occur early in embryogenesis before normal laterality determination (before 3 weeks). Cardiac malformations are particularly common (99%) in asplenia syndrome and are seen with less frequency in polysplenia syndrome (90%). Cardiac defects include endocardial cushion defects, hypoplastic left heart (Figure 62-9), and transposition of the great vessels.

The infant with total situs inversus usually has a normal outcome. About 20% may have Kartagener's syndrome (immotile cilia, bronchiectasis). The mortality rate for partial situs inversus is extremely high, with death occurring in 90% to 95% with asplenia syndrome and 80% with polysplenia syndrome.

■ **Sonographic Findings.** Sonographically, these signs may be observed:

- Total situs inversus (right-side heart axis and aorta; transposition of liver, stomach, and spleen; left-side gallbladder).
- Partial situs inversus (right-side stomach, left-side liver). Dextrocardia with normal stomach position.
- Other anomalies to check for include gastrointestinal, genitourinary, and neural tube defects.

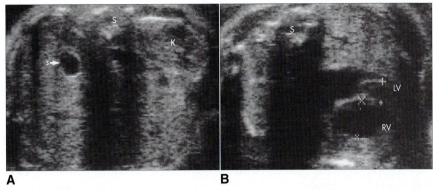

FIGURE 62-9 A, Partial situs inversus observed in a transverse spine-up position. The stomach *(s with arrow)* was found on the right side of the abdomen. *K,* Kidney; *S,* spine. **B,** In the same fetus, a hypoplastic left ventricle *(LV)* is shown. Other findings included bilateral liver, a left-side inferior vena cava, and a right-side descending aorta, right gallbladder, double inlet right ventricle *(RV)*, common atrioventricular valve, atrial septal defect, and one outflow vessel (pulmonary artery). *S,* spine.

Pseudoascites

There are many causes of pseudoascites in the fetus. Gastrointestinal obstruction with bowel perforation may present as meconium peritonitis and ascites. The nongastrointestinal causes include immune and nonimmune hydrops, urinary tract obstruction, congenital infection, and some abdominal tumors.

A sonolucent band near the fetal anterior abdominal wall is commonly identified during routine obstetric examinations in the fetus over 18 weeks of gestation. This band results from normal musculature surrounding the abdominal wall. True ascites is identified within the peritoneal recesses and is interspaced between loops of small bowel (which then causes the bowel loops to appear more echogenic), whereas pseudoascites is always confined to an anterior fetal abdomen and is centrally located. Furthermore, **pseudoascites** never outlines the falciform ligament like true ascites.

Gallbladder

Anomalies of the gallbladder may be detected using prenatal sonographic techniques. **Cholelithiasis** (gallstones) may be identified in the fetus when calcifications are found within the gallbladder. These gallstones resolve spontaneously in utero or in the childhood period (Figure 62-10).

A **choledochal cyst** (dilation of the common bile duct) may be diagnosed when a cystic mass is identified adjacent to the fetal stomach and gallbladder (Box 62-1). Choledochal cysts may be confused with malformations of the stomach or bowel or duodenal atresia. The sonographer should remember that the gallbladder is more anterior than the duodenum and thus a cystic mass attached to the bile duct near the gallbladder would make the mass more likely a choledochal cyst. Choledochal cysts may be associated with intermittent biliary obstruction and severe biliary cirrhosis; therefore, early diagnosis is important. (See Chapter 26 for further information.)

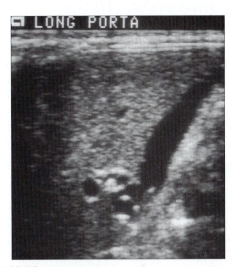

FIGURE 62-10 Longitudinal scan of a neonate with gallstones. Small calcifications with shadowing were seen in the fetal ultrasound in the gallbladder.

BOX 62-1	Sonographic Criteria for Choledochal Cyst

- Close proximity of the cyst to the neck of the gallbladder
- An ovoid right upper quadrant cyst with an entering bile duct
- A cyst and gallbladder that enlarge as gestation progresses
- Absence of peristaltic activity in the cyst

From Schwartz H, et al: Choledochal cyst in a second trimester fetus, J Diagn Med Sonogr 1:10, 1989.

Agenesis of the gallbladder occurs in approximately 20% of patients with biliary atresia. Absence of the gallbladder also can occur in association with polysplenia and rare multiple anomaly syndromes. The ability to visualize the fetal gallbladder routinely increases with gestational age.

Pancreas

Pancreatic cysts are uncommon, but when present, may appear as midline anechoic cystic masses in the fetal abdomen.

Spleen

Evaluation of the fetal spleen for exclusion of splenic anomalies is possible. Asplenia (absence of the spleen) may be amenable to antenatal identification, and in association with congenital heart disease the polysplenia-asplenia syndrome should be considered.

Congenital splenic cysts are rare but have been reported in utero. Enlargement of the spleen (splenomegaly) may be seen on the ultrasound examination. The spleen, like the liver, may enlarge in fetuses with Rh-immune disease. Nomograms are available to detect hepatomegaly and splenomegaly.

ABNORMALITIES OF THE GASTROINTESTINAL TRACT

The majority of gastrointestinal malformations are correctable after birth; consequently, recognition of a gastrointestinal anomaly before delivery may prevent the complications of dehydration, bowel necrosis, and respiratory difficulties that occur when these lesions are unsuspected before delivery. Box 62-2 lists the causes of nonvisualization of the stomach. The fetal bowel can be altered by a number of pathologic processes. A bowel obstruction results in proximal bowel dilation, which is characteristically recognized as one or more tubular structures within the fetal abdomen. Dilated bowel loops are generally sonolucent in texture but may be normal or increased in echogenicity. The most reliable criterion for diagnosing a dilated bowel is the bowel diameter, rather than the sonographic appearance. One should be careful not to mistake a dilated ureter for a dilated loop of the bowel. Most cases of bowel dilation do not become evident on sonography until after 20 weeks of gestation. Polyhydramnios commonly accompanies obstruction of the gastrointestinal tract, and this rarely develops before 20 weeks of gestation as a result of a gastrointestinal cause.

Esophagus, Stomach, and Duodenum

The normal upper esophagus may be seen after amniotic fluid is swallowed. This fluid passes from the esophagus into the fetal stomach. Obstruction of the normal swallowing sequence may occur because of an atretic or obstructive process. Atresias develop when a portion of the bowel grows and infarcts; this can occur anywhere in the gastrointestinal tract. A membrane covering the lumen and intestinal loops enlarges above the obstruction, and bowel loops below the atresia are narrowed (stenotic). This enlargement of the bowel proximal to the obstruction is readily apparent on ultrasound. Blockage results in the backup of amniotic fluid and hydramnios.

Esophageal atresia is a congenital blockage of the esophagus resulting from the faulty separation of the foregut into its respiratory and digestive components (Figure 62-11). The most common form occurs in conjunction with a fistula, communicating between the trachea and esophagus (tracheoesophageal fistula), that allows the passage of amniotic fluid into the stomach. Gastric secretions may contribute to stomach fluid. In some instances, however, a fistula is not present, fluid does not reach the stomach, and the stomach will not be visualized by ultrasound. The combination of polyhydramnios and an absent stomach over repeated studies may be suggestive of esophageal atresia. Esophageal atresia will not be diagnosed in the majority of cases because of a tracheoesophageal fistula.

Esophageal atresia occurs in 1 in 2500 live births. The sonographer may observe the absent stomach and hydramnios (Figure 62-12). However, in more than half of the cases, the stomach is present because a fistula is usually present that leads to fluid filling the stomach. Hydramnios may exist from impaired reabsorption of swallowed fluid and may be associated with esophageal atresia, but it usually does not develop until the third trimester. The upper neck sign has been observed as an additional finding in a patient with esophageal atresia. A fluid-filled, blind-ending esophagus during fetal swallowing has been noted in a 22-week fetus.

Coexisting anomalies are common in 50% to 70% of fetuses with esophageal atresia. The most commonly observed anomaly is anorectal atresia (others include vertebral defects, heart defects, and renal and limb

---

BOX 62-2	Causes of Nonvisualization of the Stomach

- Esophageal atresia or tracheoesophageal fistula
- Diaphragmatic hernia
- Facial cleft
- Central nervous system disorder
- Other swallowing disorders
- Oligohydramnios from other causes

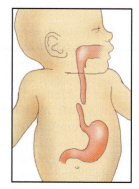

FIGURE 62-11 Esophageal atresia is a congenital blockage of the esophagus. The primary sonographic findings are polyhydramnios and an absence of the stomach bubble.

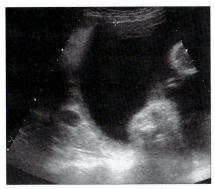

FIGURE 62-12 Longitudinal scan of a patient who had polyhydramnios. This quadrant of fluid measured more than 10 cm, which alone qualifies for an abnormal collection of fluid. The fetus did not show a stomach bubble and was diagnosed with esophageal atresia.

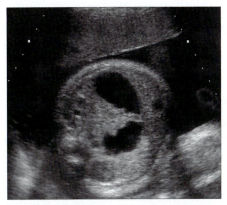

FIGURE 62-14 Transverse image of the fetal abdomen showing two large echo-free structures that communicated on real-time imaging. The fetus had duodenal atresia.

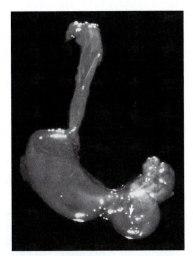

FIGURE 62-13 Gross specimen showing duodenal atresia from a neonate with trisomy 21 (Down syndrome). Note the narrowing at the duodenum *(arrow)*.

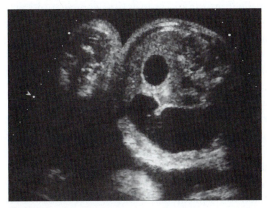

FIGURE 62-15 This 24-week fetus had trisomy 21. The transverse abdomen showed a very dilated stomach with communication into a smaller sac. Thirty percent of trisomy 21 pregnancies will also have duodenal atresia.

BOX 62-3	**Causes of Double Bubble**

- Duodenal atresia
- Duodenal stenosis
- Annular pancreas
- Ladd's bands
- Proximal jejunal atresia
- Malrotation
- Diaphragmatic hernia

anomalies [VACTERL]). Growth restriction is present in 40% of the cases. Chromosomal trisomies (18 and 21) are reported in association. Survival depends on the presence of associated congenital anomalies.

Duodenal atresia is a blockage of the duodenal lumen by a membrane that prohibits the passage of swallowed amniotic fluid (Figure 62-13). Atresia or narrowing of the bowel segment below the obstruction occurs. In duodenal atresia, the amniotic fluid fails to move beyond the obstruction, and consequently, amniotic fluid backs up in the duodenum and stomach.

Sonographic Findings. Two echo-free structures (stomach and duodenum) are found in the upper fetal abdomen and they communicate. This sonographic appearance is termed the double bubble sign (Figure 62-14, Box 62-3). Hydramnios is almost always seen with duodenal atresias later in pregnancy. Most cases of duodenal atresia are found distal to the ampulla and often coexist with annular pancreas.

About 30% of fetuses with duodenal atresia have trisomy 21 (Down syndrome) (Figure 62-15). Cardiovascular anomalies are frequent, and therefore fetal echocardiography is invaluable in excluding cardiac lesions. Anomalies occur in approximately 50% of infants with duodenal atresia. Genitourinary anomalies (horseshoe kidney, ectopic kidneys) may coexist with this condition. Other gastrointestinal abnormalities, such as imperforate anus and atresia of the small bowel, may be present. Esophageal atresia may also be found.

Symmetric growth restriction commonly occurs in fetuses with duodenal atresia. Amniotic fluid alpha-fetoprotein values are commonly elevated in fetuses with duodenal atresia caused by faulty swallowing. Infants with duodenal atresia require immediate surgery after birth to connect the stomach to the jejunum, thus bypassing the obstruction.

Bowel

Intestinal Obstructions. Atresia or stenosis of the jejunum, ileum, or both, and small bowel atresia are slightly more common than duodenal atresia; it occurs in 1 in 3000 to 5000 live births and is thought to be secondary to a vascular accident, sporadic, or secondary to volvulus or gastroschisis. Various fetal malformations may also occur with maternal drug usage (see Table 58-1). The entire length of the bowel is subject to obstruction. Blockage of the jejunum and ileal bowel segments (**jejunoileal atresia** or stenosis) appears as multiple cystic structures (more than two) proximal to the site of atresia within the fetal abdomen. Because these structures are high in the abdomen, hydramnios may be present. The general rule is that the more distal the obstruction, the less severe the hydramnios and the later it will develop. The causes of fetal small-bowel obstruction include malrotation, atresias, volvulus, peritoneal bands, and cystic fibrosis. The dilated bowel loops may be isolated or may be associated with other anomalies, ascites, or meconium peritonitis.

▧ Sonographic Findings. Sonographically, intestinal obstructions appear as cystic bowel loops that are discontinuous with the stomach (Figure 62-16). It is important to remember that bowel loops may be identified in the third trimester of pregnancy. It has been reported that the normal fetal colon progressively increased in diameter after 23 weeks of gestation, although it never exceeded 18 mm in a preterm fetus. Fetal intestinal obstruction should be suspected when clear cystic structures are found in the pelvis. In some instances, echoes within the bowel may be identified in intestinal obstructions but may also represent normal meconium patterns (see Figure 62-16). Vascular restriction may lead to obstruction secondary to a gastroschisis (Figure 62-17).

Meconium Ileus. **Meconium ileus** is a small-bowel disorder marked by the presence of thick meconium in the distal ileum. Meconium ileus is the earliest manifestation of cystic fibrosis, occurring in 10% to 15% of patients, and is the third most common form of neonatal bowel obstruction after atresia and malrotation. Most cases of meconium ileus occur in newborns with cystic fibrosis. Infants with **cystic fibrosis** have multiple medical problems, including pancreatic disease and respiratory problems resulting from long-standing lung disease. Cystic fibrosis is an autosomal-recessive condition.

Meconium begins to accumulate in the fetal bowel in the second trimester, at which time it can be seen sonographically as tiny echogenic reflections within the peristaltic small bowel (Figure 62-18). Because the colon

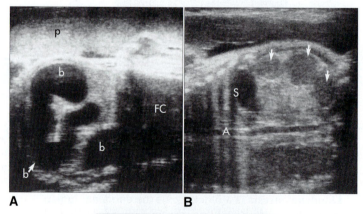

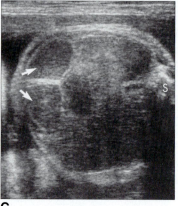

FIGURE 62-16 A, Bowel obstruction secondary to gastroschisis. Note the tubular shape of the cystic bowel loops *(b)*. *FC,* Fetal chest; *p,* placenta. **B,** Bowel obstruction in a fetus with cystic fibrosis at 36 weeks of gestation. Note that the bowel loops in this case are filled with meconium *(arrows)* rather than cystic, as in **A.** *A,* Aorta; *S,* stomach. **C,** In the fetus shown in **B,** echo-filled bowel loops are viewed in a transverse direction *(arrows)*. *S,* Spine.

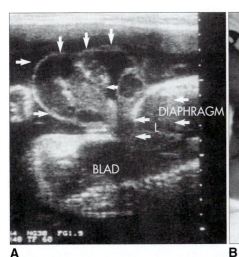

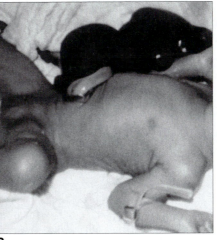

FIGURE 62-17 **A,** Sagittal scan demonstrating anterior abdominal wall defect with protrusion of the entire small bowel in a fetus with a gastroschisis *(arrows)*. Note the obstructed (cystic) components of small bowel. *L,* Liver. **B,** Gastroschisis defect in same patient after birth. Note the normal cord insertion.

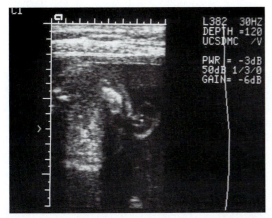

FIGURE 62-18 Meconium accumulates in the fetal bowel in the second trimester and is seen sonographically as echogenic reflections (notice shadowing) within the peristaltic small bowel.

BOX 62-4	Pitfalls in the Diagnosis of Meconium Ileus

- Significant dilatation of the meconium-filled ileum in the meconium ileus can look like the colon in shape, size, and location.
- More proximal small bowel may have the features of active peristalsis and fluid-filled contents.
- Do not be distracted by the difference in diameter between the proximal and distal small bowel when making a diagnosis of small-bowel obstruction or meconium ileus.

does not exhibit peristalsis in utero, the meconium remains suspended at the rectum. The anal sphincter prevents the passage of meconium (meconium plug) into the amniotic fluid unless the fetus is stressed or traumatized.

Sonographic Findings. With meconium ileus, the ileum dilates because of impacted meconium (which appears echogenic) (Figure 62-19). Increased production of mucus by the gastrointestinal organs and electrolyte imbalance explains the overproduction of meconium (characteristic of cystic fibrosis). It is important to realize that the normal small bowel may appear echogenic during the second trimester of pregnancy. Other fetal conditions have been associated with echogenic small bowel (cytomegalovirus and trisomy 21). Meconium peritonitis may occur secondary to perforation of an obstructed bowel. An inflammatory response occurs because of leakage of the bowel contents, which may cause fibrosis of tissue and calcifications. A pseudocyst may develop because of chronic meconium peritonitis (Box 62-4).

Other Small Bowel Obstructions. Rarer small-bowel obstructions, chloridorrhea (life-threatening diarrhea in the newborn) and megacystis-microcolon intestinal hypoperistalsis syndrome (absence of peristalsis), may be observed during pregnancy. In the latter, bladder dilatation and hydronephrosis are characteristic findings in predominantly female fetuses. Amniotic fluid volume is typically normal to increased. Obstruction may also be present when gastroschisis is present (see Figure 62-17). Obstructions of the large intestine diagnosed prenatally include anorectal atresia and Hirschsprung's disease.

Anorectal Atresia. Anorectal atresia presents as a complex disorder of the bowel and genitourinary tract. Imperforate anus (a finding in anorectal atresia) is a disorder that occurs when a membrane covers the anus prohibiting the expulsion of meconium. Anorectal atresia may present as part of the VACTERL association or in caudal regression. The prognosis is poor with anorectal atresia because of associated anomalies. Incontinence of both bowel and bladder is common in the infant.

Sonographic Findings. Anorectal atresia may be diagnosed sonographically by observing dilated colon and calcified meconium. Amniotic fluid is typically normal or may be decreased when there are associated renal problems.

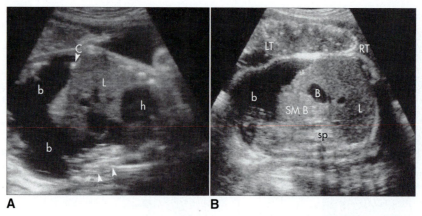

FIGURE 62-19 A, Meconium peritonitis secondary to bowel obstruction is shown with an irregular appearance of the bowel *(b)* in the lower pelvis extending upward toward the chest in a 30-week fetus. Calcifications *(C)* are observed in several locations. Clumping of bowel was observed *(arrows)*. Meconium peritonitis with bowel perforation was suspected. There was a moderate increase in the amniotic fluid volume by 33 weeks of gestation. *h,* Heart; *L,* liver. **B,** In the same fetus, transverse view showing bowel dilation *(b)* in a spine-down position. Note the normal-appearing small bowel *(SM B). L,* Liver; *LT,* left side of abdomen; *RT,* right side of abdomen; *sp,* spine. At birth the neonate was diagnosed with meconium ileus and peritonitis necessitating an ileostomy. At 2 months of age, the infant was discharged on normal formula feedings. Cystic fibrosis was suspected.

Hirschsprung's Disease. Hirschsprung's disease (**megacolon**) is a congenital disorder in which there is abnormal innervation of the large intestine.

▌ **Sonographic Findings.** This condition is difficult to diagnose prenatally but may be suspected when dilated bowel loops are observed.

Meconium Peritonitis. Meconium peritonitis is a condition that may arise when the fetus has a sterile chemical peritonitis secondary to in utero bowel perforation. Hydramnios is present in 65% of the fetuses with meconium peritonitis. A complication may result in the formation of a meconium pseudocyst as the inflammatory reaction seals the perforation.

▌ **Sonographic Findings.** On ultrasound examination, calcifications are seen on the peritoneal surfaces or in the scrotum via the processus vaginalis. The ascitic fluid may also be echogenic. It is unusual to see calcification in the meconium ileus in a fetus with cystic fibrosis.

Hyperechoic Bowel. Hyperechoic bowel is a subjective impression of an unusually echogenic bowel, typically seen during the second trimester. The cause of hyperechoic bowel may be due to decreased water content, alterations of meconium, or both. The decreased water content may be secondary to hypoperistalsis, given that fluid is normally resorbed by the small bowel.

▌ **Sonographic Findings.** The significance of hyperechoic bowel varies with its location in the small bowel or colon, menstrual age, and degree of echogenicity (Box 62-5). The degree of hyperechogenicity may be compared with the iliac wing of the fetus. There are three gradations of the degree of hyperechogenicity of the bowel:

- Grade 1: mildly echogenic and typically diffuse
- Grade 2: moderately echogenic and typically focal

BOX 62-5 | **Causes of Echogenic Areas in the Fetal Abdomen**

Calcified
Peritoneal calcification: Meconium peritonitis, hydrometrocolpos
Intraluminal meconium calcification: Anorectal atresia, small bowel atresia; rarely isolated without bowel obstruction
Parenchymal: Liver, splenic, adrenal, ovarian cyst
Cholelithiasis: gallbladder

Noncalcified
Echogenic meconium
Intraabdominal extrathoracic pulmonary sequestration
Tumors
Adrenal hemorrhage

From Nyberg DA, Neilsen IR: Abdomen and gastrointestinal tract. In Nyberg DA, McGahan JP, Pretorius DH, et al, editors: Diagnostic imaging of fetal anomalies, Philadelphia, 2003, Lippincott Williams & Wilkins.

- Grade 3: very echogenic, similar to that of bone structures

Ascites. True ascites in the fetal abdomen is always abnormal. In the fetus, the ascitic fluid collects between the two leaves of unfused omentum, resulting in a cyst-like appearance in the abdomen (Figure 62-20). The prognosis is poor in nonimmune hydrops. Other conditions that may cause ascites to develop include bowel perforation or urinary ascites secondary to bladder rupture.

▌ **Sonographic Findings.** Ascites usually outlines the falciform ligament and umbilical vein. When ascites is associated with hydrops fetalis, pleural effusions, and pericardial effusion, integumentary edema will often be observed.

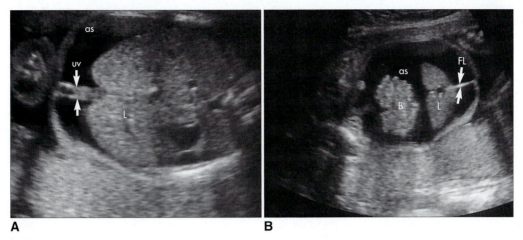

FIGURE 62-20 A, Fetal ascites *(as)* surrounds the umbilical vein *(uv). L,* liver. **B,** Ascites *(as)* completely surrounds the liver *(L)* and falciform ligament *(FL). B,* Bowel.

MISCELLANEOUS CYSTIC MASSES OF THE ABDOMEN

Cystic masses of the lower fetal abdomen may be observed prenatally. It is important for the sonographer to determine the size of the mass, its precise location, and to identify resultant compression of other organ systems (hydronephrosis, hydroureter, fetal hydrops).

When a cystic mass is discovered, attempts should be made to determine the characteristics of the mass. A description of the mass should include the components of the structure, such as (1) an echo-free versus an echo-filled mass, (2) the presence or absence of septations, and (3) coexisting fetal anomalies. The sonographer should systematically investigate all abdominal organ systems to determine the anatomic origin of the mass. The hepatic system (liver, gallbladder, spleen, and pancreatic areas) should be evaluated along with the gastrointestinal system (esophagus, stomach, and intestines) and genitourinary system (kidneys, ureters, and bladder).

Occasionally, cysts arise from the urachus (dilation of remnant allantoic stalk between umbilicus and bladder), fetal ovary, or omentum. Ovarian and omental cysts are generally isolated and well circumscribed. Determination of the fetal gender is beneficial when an ovarian mass is suspected. If abdominal masses are large, they may occupy the entire lower fetal pelvis, making a specific intrauterine diagnosis impossible.

The Fetal Urogenital System

Mitzi Roberts

OBJECTIVES

On completion of this chapter, you should be able to:
- Discuss the development of the urogenital and genital system
- Describe the sonographic appearance of the fetal kidneys and bladder
- Detail the complications of renal agenesis
- Describe the sonographic findings associated with abnormalities of the kidney
- Differentiate types of renal cystic disease
- Distinguish among different types of urinary obstruction
- Identify congenital malformations of the genital system

Prenatal ultrasound is capable of diagnosing many anomalies of the genitourinary system. A complete sonographic examination includes evaluation of both kidneys, documentation of the urinary bladder, and assessment of amniotic fluid. In the presence of oligohydramnios, the sonographer should carefully search the renal areas and

bladder to determine if an obstruction is present that may lead to the diminished production of amniotic fluid. It is also possible for abnormalities of the genitourinary system to be discovered incidentally during the complete obstetric sonogram evaluation. A maternal history of renal disease or drug usage (amitriptyline, amobarbital, caffeine, cocaine, imipramine, sulfonamide) carries an increased risk of urogenital fetal malformations (see Table 58-1).

EMBRYOLOGY OF THE UROGENITAL SYSTEM

Embryologically and functionally, the urogenital system can be divided into two parts: the urinary system and the genital system. Both systems develop from the intermediate mesoderm, and the excretory ducts of both systems initially enter a common cavity called the cloaca. While the embryo bends and folds in the horizontal plane during the 4th week, the intermediate mesoderm forms a longitudinal mass on both sides of the aorta called the *urogenital ridge*. Both the urinary and genital systems develop from the mesoderm in these ridges. The part of the urogenital ridge that gives rise to the urinary system is known as the nephrogenic cord or nephrogenic ridge. The part that gives rise to the genital system is known as the gonadal ridge or *genital ridge*. The urinary system develops first.

The sex of the fetus is determined at the time of fertilization, but there is no morphologic indication of gender until the 9th week of development. Early embryogenesis shows similar development in both sexes. The gonads are derived from the gonadal ridges and are the first parts of the genital system to undergo development. As the genital ridge enlarges and frees itself from the mesonephros by developing a mesentery, the male ridge becomes the mesorchium and the female the mesovarium. At the same time, the coelomic epithelium that covers the primitive gonads proliferates and forms the cords of cells, called primary sex cords, that grow into the mesenchyme of the developing gonads. The primordial germ cells originate in the wall of the yolk sac and migrate into the embryo and enter the primary sex cords to give rise to the ova and sperm.

DEVELOPMENT OF THE GENITOURINARY SYSTEM

Development of the Kidneys

Three sets of excretory organs develop in the embryo: the pronephros, mesonephros, and metanephros. Only the third set remains as the permanent kidneys (Figure 63-1). The first pair of "kidneys," *pronephros*, are rudimentary and nonfunctional. The second pair of "kidneys," *mesonephroi*, function for a short time during the early fetal period and then degenerate after they are replaced by the metanephros or permanent kidneys.

The permanent kidneys (metanephros) begin to develop early in the 5th week while the mesonephroi are still developing (Figure 63-2). Urine formation begins toward the end of the first trimester, around the 11th to 12th week, and continues actively throughout fetal life.

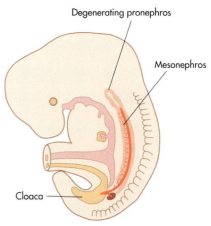

FIGURE 63-1 Five-week embryo showing three sets of kidneys that developed in the embryo. The pronephros is rudimentary and nonfunctional. The mesonephros functions for 2 weeks and then degenerates. The metanephros develops into the permanent kidney.

Urine is excreted into the amniotic cavity and forms a major part of the amniotic fluid. The kidneys do not need to function in utero because the placenta eliminates waste from the fetal blood. The kidneys must be able to assume their waste excretion role after birth, however.

The permanent kidneys develop from two different sources: (1) the metanephric diverticulum or ureteric bud and (2) the metanephric mesoderm (Figure 63-3). The ureteric bud gives rise to the ureter, renal pelvis, calyces, and collecting tubules. The collecting tubule is also derived from the ureteric bud. The major and minor calyces are developed from these collecting tubules.

The ends of the tubules form metanephric vesicles. The ends of these tubules are invaginated by an ingrowth of the fine blood vessels, the glomerulus, to form a double-layered cup called the glomerular capsule, or Bowman's capsule. The renal corpuscle (glomerulus and capsule) and its associated tubules form a nephron. Each distal convoluted tubule contacts an arched collecting tubule, and then the tubules become confluent, forming a uriniferous tubule. Each uriniferous tubule consists of two parts: a nephron and a collecting tubule.

The arterial vascular supply to the kidneys comes from the arteries that arise from the aorta. Usually these vessels disappear when the kidneys ascend, but some of them may persist, which accounts for the variations that can be found in the renal arteries. At least 25% of adult kidneys have two to four renal arteries.

The kidneys initially lie very close together in the pelvis. Gradually they migrate into the abdomen and become separated from one another (Figure 63-4). They normally complete this migration by the 9th week of gestation. In some cases, one of the kidneys may remain in the pelvic cavity while the other migrates into the posterior flank of the abdomen. With sonography, the identification of a **pelvic kidney** may be seen with adequate bladder dilation and may appear in females as a pelvic mass.

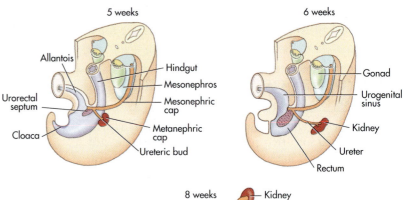

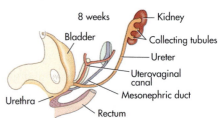

FIGURE 63-2 Early embryologic development of the urinary system.

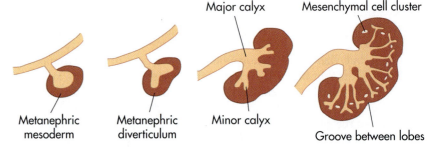

FIGURE 63-3 Developing kidney in weeks 5 through 8.

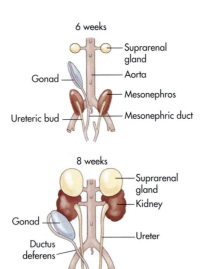

FIGURE 63-4 The kidneys begin in the pelvis with gradual migration into the abdomen.

Development of the Urinary Bladder

The fetal urinary bladder is derived from the hindgut derivative known as the urogenital sinus (see Figure 63-2). The caudal ends of the mesonephric ducts open into the cloaca, and parts of them are gradually absorbed into the wall of the urinary bladder. This development causes the ureters (derived from the ureteric buds) and the mesonephric ducts to enter the bladder separately.

Although the kidneys migrate upward, the orifices of the ureters move cranially, and the primordia of the ejaculatory ducts (derived from the mesonephric ducts) move toward one another and enter the prostatic part of the urethra. The epithelium of the female urethra and most of the epithelium of the male urethra are derived from the endoderm of the urogenital sinus.

Development of the External Genitalia

Although the early development of the external genitalia is similar for both sexes, distinguishing sexual characteristics begin during the 9th week and external genital organs are fully differentiated by the 12th week of gestation (Figure 63-5). In the 4th week, a genital tubercle develops at the cranial end of the cloacal membrane. Labioscrotal swellings and urogenital folds develop on either side of this membrane. The genital tubercle elongates to form a phallus, which is similar in both sexes. The hormonal changes cause further development of the male and female reproductive system (Figure 63-6).

Development of the Male External Genitalia. The fetal testes produce androgens that cause the masculinization of the external genitalia. The phallus elongates

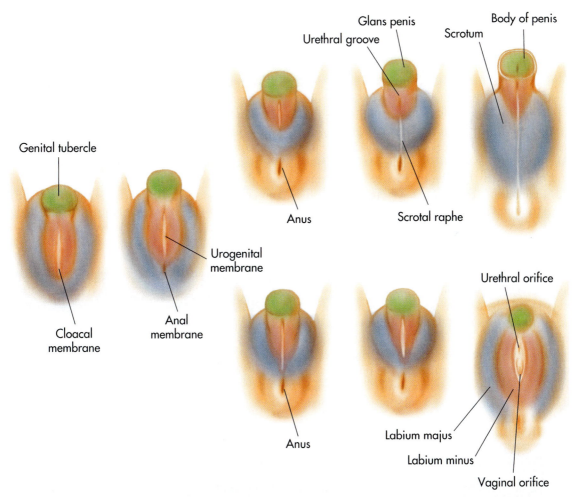

FIGURE 63-5 Sexual characteristics begin to develop during the 9th week and are fully differentiated by the 12th week.

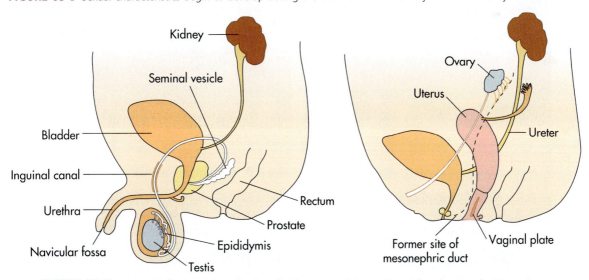

FIGURE 63-6 Hormonal changes cause further development of the male and female reproductive systems.

to form the penis. This sonographic finding is known as the "turtle sign." The urogenital folds fuse on the ventral surface of the penis to form the spongy urethra. The labioscrotal swellings grow toward the median plane and fuse to form the scrotum. The line of fusion of the labioscrotal folds is called the scrotal raphe.

Development of the Female External Genitalia. Both the urethra and vagina open into the urogenital sinus, the vestibule of the vagina. The urogenital folds become the labia minora, the labioscrotal swellings become the labia majora, and the phallus becomes the clitoris.

SONOGRAPHIC EVALUATION OF THE UROGENITAL SYSTEM

The Kidneys

The kidneys should be evaluated by assessing their anatomy, texture, and size. With transvaginal sonography, the fetal kidneys have been documented as early as 9 weeks of gestation. By 12 weeks of gestation, at least 86% of the fetal kidneys may be imaged. The fetal kidneys and bladder may be seen by 13 weeks of gestation. At this time period, the kidneys appear as bilateral hyperechoic structures in the paravertebral regions. At approximately 15 weeks of gestation, the overall echogenicity will decrease and the renal pelvis may be seen as sonolucent areas within the central kidney. As the fetal age advances, fat deposits in the perinephric and sinus regions become visible. Beginning at 18 weeks of gestation, kidneys should be documented in all fetuses sonographically. Between 18 and 20 weeks of gestation, the kidneys are slightly hyperechoic with regard to surrounding tissues (i.e., bowel and paravertebral tissues). By 25 weeks it is possible to distinguish the renal cortex from the medulla, outline the renal capsule clearly, and see a central echogenic area in the renal sinus region (Box

63-1). Sonographically this would appear as a relatively homogeneous renal cortex and parenchyma, hypoechoic pyramids and calyces, and anechoic renal pelvis (Figure 63-7).

The kidneys can be imaged in the sagittal, transverse, or coronal planes. The size of the fetal kidneys may be assessed by measuring the length, width, and height (anterior/posterior diameter) of the kidney (Table 63-1). In both the sagittal and transverse view, the kidneys can be best visualized with the fetal spine situated anteriorly on the screen. In the sagittal plane, kidney length and anterior/posterior (AP) measurements can be obtained (Figure 63-8). This involves measuring the length of the kidney from the upper to lower pole. Careful attention

---

BOX 63-1 Sonographic Evaluation of the Urogenital System

- Bladder: assess presence and size
- Kidneys: assess presence, number, position, appearance (texture)
- Collecting system: assess if normal or dilated; if dilated, look for level and cause of obstruction, whether it is unilateral or bilateral
- Fetal gender

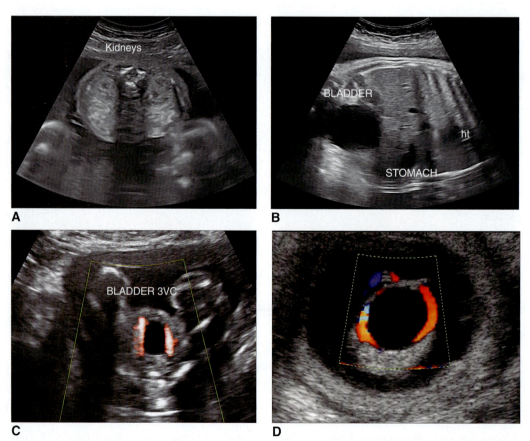

FIGURE 63-7 A, Normal kidneys in the transverse view located on either side of the fetal spine. The anterior position of the spine provides optimal resolution for evaluating the kidneys. **B,** The anechoic bladder is noted caudal in the fetal body as it relates to the anechoic fetal stomach. *ht,* heart. **C,** The bladder is noted lying low within the pelvis. Color Doppler reveals arterial blood flow on each side of the bladder supporting the findings of a three-vessel cord. **D,** An obstructed fetal bladder is noted in an early second-trimester fetus. Color Doppler reveals the presence of a three-vessel cord.

Age (weeks)	Kidney Thickness (mm)			Kidney Width (mm)			Kidney Length (mm)			Kidney Volume (cm³)		
	5th	50th	95th	5th	50th	95th	5th	50th	95th	5th	50th	95th
16	2	6	10	6	10	13	7	13	18	—	0.4	2.6
17	3	7	11	6	10	14	10	15	20	—	0.6	2.8
18	4	8	12	6	10	14	12	17	22	—	0.7	2.9
19	5	9	13	7	10	14	14	19	24	—	0.9	3.1
20	6	10	13	7	11	15	15	21	26	—	1.1	3.3
21	6	10	14	8	12	15	17	22	28	—	1.4	3.6
22	7	11	15	8	12	16	19	24	29	—	1.7	3.9
23	8	12	16	9	13	17	21	26	31	—	2.1	4.3
24	9	13	17	10	14	18	22	28	33	0.3	2.5	4.7
25	10	14	18	11	15	19	24	29	34	0.8	3.0	5.2
26	11	15	19	12	16	19	25	31	36	1.3	3.5	5.7
27	11	15	19	12	16	20	27	32	37	1.9	4.1	6.3
28	12	16	20	13	17	21	28	33	38	2.5	4.7	6.9
29	13	17	21	14	18	22	29	35	40	3.2	5.4	7.6
30	14	18	22	15	19	23	31	36	41	3.9	6.1	8.3
31	14	18	22	16	20	24	32	37	42	4.6	6.8	9.0
32	15	19	23	17	20	24	33	38	43	5.4	7.5	9.7
33	16	20	23	17	21	25	34	39	44	6.1	8.3	10.5
34	16	20	24	18	22	26	35	40	45	6.8	9.0	11.2
35	17	21	25	18	22	26	35	41	46	7.4	9.6	11.8
36	17	21	25	19	23	27	36	41	47	8.1	10.2	12.4
37	18	22	26	19	23	27	37	42	47	8.6	10.8	13.0
38	18	22	26	19	23	27	37	43	48	9.0	11.2	13.4
39	19	23	27	19	23	27	38	43	48	9.4	11.6	13.8
40	19	23	27	19	23	27	38	44	49	9.6	11.8	14.0

TABLE 63-1 Kidney Dimensions: Normal Values

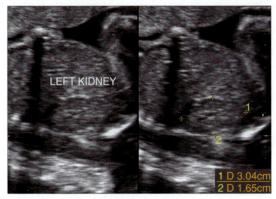

FIGURE 63-8 A length measurement of the left kidney is 3.04 cm. This is in normal range for the 30-week fetus. The length of a normal kidney reflects the approximate gestational age for the fetus.

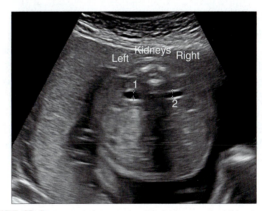

FIGURE 63-9 A normal amount of fluid is noted within the renal pelvis. Anterior posterior diameters reflect the amount of pyelectasis.

should be made not to include the adrenal gland. The length of the kidney closely correlates with the gestational age of the fetus. The transverse view allows the sonographer to view both kidneys simultaneously. The kidneys are circular structures lying on each side of the spine. In this view, both kidneys can be evaluated and compared for echogenicity, width size, and renal pelvis size. The renal pelvis, if visible, may be measured in their anterior-posterior diameter when the fetal spine is toward the maternal anterior wall (Figure 63-9). The upper limit of normal is 4 mm up to the third trimester and 7 mm

from the third trimester until term. It is important to remember that a small amount of urine may be seen in the renal pelvis in the normal fetus. On coronal images, the kidneys are bordered medially by the psoas muscles and superiorly by the hypoechoic adrenal glands.

Ureters, Bladder, and Urethra

The normal fetal ureters are usually not seen, but a normal bladder should always be seen in fetuses. The ureters typically measure less than 1 to 2 mm in diameter and should not be filled with anechoic fluid. These characteristics make them difficult to visualize under normal conditions. However, slight dilatation of the ureter may be visible at the renal pelvis and urine jets may be seen in the bladder where the ureters enter. The urethra, like the ureters, is usually unidentifiable in the normal fetus.

The bladder is imaged as a rounded echo-free area located centrally in the pelvis. There is no specific bladder measurement usually applied; however, documentation of the bladder filling and emptying is important. Sonographers should identify the fetal bladder early in the ultrasound examination to make sure adequate fluid is present. If no bladder is seen or the bladder appears too large, the sonographer should reevaluate the bladder at the end of the examination. This is done in part because the fetal bladder usually takes at least 30 minutes to fill and empty. The normal bladder wall can be measured and should be thin in a normal fetus. The wall is normally 2 mm or less and is best measured at the level of the umbilical artery.

External Genitalia

Determination of the fetal gender should be documented with the presence of other abnormalities or in cases in which the external organ does not meet the sonographic criteria for a male or female. It is extremely important that the sonographer utilize specific sonographic criteria to determine gender. The inability to visualize the penis and scrotum should not be used as the deciding factor for identifying a female fetus.

In the majority of fetuses, the external genitalia can be differentiated in the second trimester. In the first trimester, differentiation is hard to determine because of the protrusion of the external genital tubercle. The genital tubercle will appear the same in the male and female fetus. In the second trimester, identification of the female fetus should only be determined when the major and minor labia are seen. Visualization of the labia is often called the "hamburger" sign (Figure 63-10, A). The use of 3D/4D image has proved helpful as well (Figure 63-10, B). The male fetus in the second trimester is determined by the visualization of the penis and scrotal sac, also known as the "turtle sign" (Figure 63-10, C). The testes are not visible within the scrotal sac until approximately 28 weeks of gestation.

Amniotic Fluid

Amniotic fluid is a critical marker in the assessment of renal function. The fetal kidneys begin to excrete urine after the 11th week but do not become the major contributor of fetal urine (and hence of amniotic fluid volume) until 14 to 16 weeks of pregnancy. Therefore, the observation of normal amniotic fluid volume before this time will not exclude the possibility of renal agenesis (absent kidneys).

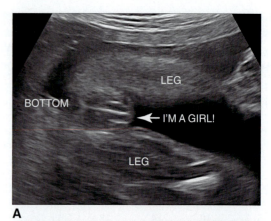

A

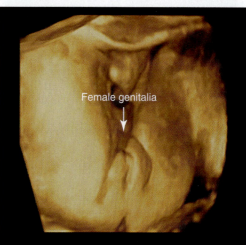

B

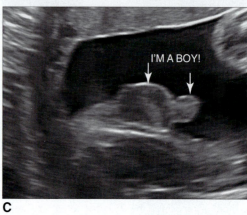

C

FIGURE 63-10 A, Echogenic lines of the major labia and minor labia reflect the "hamburger sign" in this female fetus. **B,** Utilization of 3D/4D technology aids in the visualization of the female genitalia. **C,** The scrotum and penis of this male fetus is clearly appreciated.

SONOGRAPHIC FINDINGS SUGGESTING ABNORMALITIES OF THE UROGENITAL SYSTEM

This section is intended to stimulate the sonographer's mind in how to think through any abnormality that may be seen. Sonographers should be encouraged to critically think through their images and document supporting evidence that would aid in diagnosis. This section outlines sonographic findings that suggest abnormalities of the urogenital system. Detailed descriptions of each of the pathologic conditions mentioned here may be found in separate sections that follow.

Dilation of Any Part of the Urinary Tract

Obstructions of the urinary system may originate anywhere along the urinary tract. One sonographic feature of the dilatation is anechoic enlargement of the affected area (Figure 63-11, *A*). The consequences and

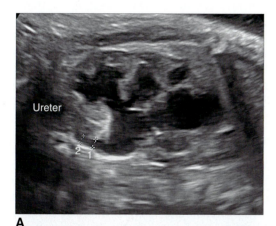

A

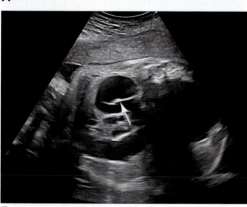

B

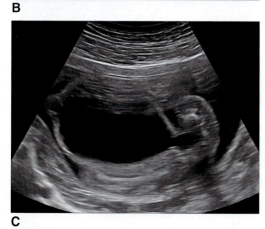

C

FIGURE 63-11 A, The kidney in this fetus reflects dilatation of the ureter, renal pelvis, and calyces. **B,** This image reveals a dilated tortuous ureter. **C,** The signature "keyhole" sign is noted in this enlarged bladder and urethra.

sonographic findings of an obstruction depend on the origin of the blockage. For example, in fetuses with a urethral obstruction, such as complete posterior urethral valve obstruction, urine is unable to pass through the urethra and into the amniotic fluid. Consequently, urine backs up in the posterior urethra, bladder, and ureters and often extends to the kidneys (hydronephrosis).

If dilatation of the renal collecting system is present, either hydronephrosis or reflux should be considered. Complete sonographic evaluation of the kidney, ureter, and bladder should be made to help determine the level of the obstruction causing the dilatation. The level of obstruction is determined by the degree of dilatation of the renal pelvis and ureter. When the entire renal collecting system is involved, a simple hydronephrosis is usually the cause. Obstruction of the ureteropelvic junction shows dilation of the renal pelvis, whereas ureteric dilation suggests either a ureterovesical junction obstruction or reflux (Figure 63-11, *B*). Ureterovesical reflux may also cause bilateral hydronephrosis. When the hydronephrosis is bilateral, the possibility of bladder outlet obstruction should be considered. The sonographer should look for dilated ureters, thickened (hypertrophied) bladder wall, and dilation of the posterior urethra (Figure 63-11, *C*). Lastly, analysis of the renal parenchyma should be made in the presence of hydronephrosis. If an echogenic cortex is present with subcapsular cysts, secondary renal dysplasia and poor function of the affected kidney may be present. In cases of urethral obstruction and bilateral renal dysplasia, oligohydramnios is typically noted after 16 weeks of gestation.

Dilation of the posterior urethra is highly suspicious for an obstructive process, such as posterior urethral valve syndrome, known as the "keyhole sign" of the urinary bladder on sonography, as the dilated bladder has the shape of a keyhole superior to the obstructed urethra (see Figure 63-11, *C*). Both kidneys will appear with severe hydronephrosis (late stages may appear with dysplastic changes), oligohydramnios will be present, the stomach will not be seen, and both ureters will be dilated. The **posterior urethral valve** occurs only in male fetuses and is manifested by the presence of a valve in the posterior urethra.

Hydronephrosis in Only One Pole of the Kidney

Duplication of the renal collecting system is common. It usually occurs in females and is not typically diagnosed in utero. The duplication occurs during embryology in which two ureteral buds are formed. The term *moiety* is often used to describe the two parts of the kidney. The degree of duplication will vary: two renal pelves are noted with two ureters each entering the bladder; two renal pelves join together high to form one ureter; or two renal pelves with two ureters join in the abdominopelvic cavity before bladder insertion.

In most cases the upper pole is susceptible to obstruction whereas the lower pole is susceptible to reflux. In utero the sonogram may reveal an enlarged kidney, but the presence of hydronephrosis located high in the kidney rather than midway is an indication of possible obstruction related to duplication. The bladder should be carefully examined for the presence of a **ureterocele**. Ureteroceles are commonly associated with duplicated collecting systems and appear as an anechoic cystic structure within the bladder.

Renal Cyst

If macroscopic cysts are present in one kidney, careful assessment of the adjacent kidney should be made. Do not confuse multicystic renal disease with hydronephrosis. The multicystic kidney shows a large central cyst with multiple small noncommunicating peripheral cysts. In hydronephrosis involving the calyces, the appearance is similar, but these cysts communicate with one another. If a single large cyst is found, it most likely represents a simple renal cyst.

Enlarged Echogenic Kidneys

When the kidneys appear enlarged and echogenic, the sonographer should consider a form of polycystic disease, trisomy 13, or Meckel-Gruber syndrome. In cases of congenital polycystic diseases, a thorough review of family history should be completed. In infantile polycystic renal disease, oligohydramnios may be present, whereas normal amniotic fluid volumes are seen with adult polycystic disease. In cases of syndrome association, a complete obstetrical sonogram will most likely reveal other findings related to the syndrome.

Kidney Not Seen

Both kidneys should be visualized adjacent to the spine. The sonographer should look for a pelvic kidney and the absence of one or both kidneys. The evaluation of the fetal pelvis should be made to aid in determination of the presence of an ectopic pelvic kidney. It is possible to have unilateral renal agenesis or bilateral renal agenesis. In unilateral agenesis, the contralateral kidney is usually quite large as a result of compensating for the absent kidney. If both kidneys are absent, the bladder will not be seen, the stomach will not be seen and severe oligohydramnios is evident. However, early in the first trimester the oligohydramnios may not be apparent and the stomach may be visible. The use of color Doppler is sometimes helpful to determine the location of the renal vessels leading into the kidney or lack of kidney.

Bladder Not Seen

Failure to observe the bladder may indicate a severe renal abnormality when accompanied by oligohydramnios.

BOX 63-2	Renal Abnormalities

- Renal agenesis
- Multicystic renal dysplasia
- Congenital hydronephrosis
- Renal duplication
- Pelvic kidney
- Horseshoe kidney
- Infantile polycystic kidney disease
- Adult polycystic kidney disease
- Meckel-Gruber syndrome

When obstruction occurs at the level of the urethra, the bladder wall becomes hypertrophied. The presence of ureteral jets may be assessed in the fetus to rule out obstruction. Utilizing color Doppler over the area of the bladder, near the base, will aid in the visualization of ureteral jets. The presence of ureteral jets streaming into the bladder indicates that the ureter is not obstructed.

Anechoic, Tortuous Pelvic Mass

When the ureters are pathologically dilated, they become visible as tortuous cystic masses in the midportion of the lower fetal pelvis. Abnormally dilated ureters are referred to as **hydroureters** and may be traced into the kidney and bladder (see Figure 63-11, *B*). Careful attention should be made not to mistake the dilated ureter for bowel. In cases of unilateral ureter obstruction, the amniotic fluid will most likely be low to normal, but if both ureters are obstructed, oligohydramnios will be present.

Abnormal Amniotic Fluid Volume

Amniotic fluid volume is a significant factor in predicting outcome. Box 63-2 lists common renal abnormalities. In fetuses with severe renal disease, amniotic fluid is reduced, and in the most severe malformations, it is virtually absent. When severe oligohydramnios is found, usually both kidneys or ureters and the urethra are malformed. Unilateral obstructions may yield a normal amount of amniotic fluid because the contralateral kidney produces urine. Conversely, hydramnios may be present with some renal disorders, such as mesoblastic nephroma and unilateral renal obstruction.

ABNORMALITIES OF THE URINARY TRACT

Renal malformations may be divided into two categories: (1) those involving congenital malformation and (2) those resulting from an obstructive process. The consequences of renal malformations vary depending on the type of lesion and extent of obstruction (Figure 63-12). The recognition of urinary tract anomalies is of significant clinical concern because several fetal conditions are

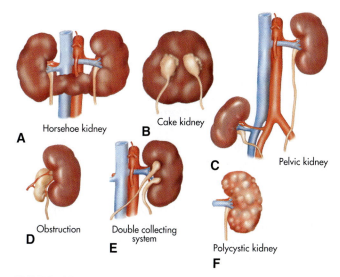

FIGURE 63-12 Variations of the kidney. **A,** Horseshoe kidney shown as two kidneys connected by an isthmus anterior to the aorta and inferior vena cava. **B,** "Cake" kidney that has failed to divide with a double collecting system. **C,** Pelvic kidney with one kidney in the normal retroperitoneal position. **D,** Extrarenal pelvis. **E,** Double collecting system. **F,** Polycystic kidney.

incompatible with life. Recognition of lethal or treatable renal anomalies is necessary to ensure appropriate clinical and therapeutic management.

CONGENITAL MALFORMATIONS OF THE KIDNEYS

Renal Agenesis

Etiology. Complete absence of the kidney(s) is known as **renal agenesis.** This condition occurs when the ureteric buds fail to develop or when they degenerate before they can induce the metanephric mesoderm to form nephrons.

Clinical Findings and Prognosis. Prognosis is dependent on unilateral or bilateral involvement of the kidneys as well as associated abnormalities. In the diagnosis of renal agenesis, acquiring a complete clinical history and a thorough examination of all fetal structures is critical. Family members should be screened for renal abnormalities to rule out the possibility of autosomal dominant inheritance. Clinical history should include documentation of possible cocaine usage and maternal diabetes. Both have been linked to renal agenesis.

Bilateral renal agenesis is a lethal disorder because of renal insufficiency and hypoplasia of the lungs. The absence of amniotic fluid plays a role in the underdevelopment of the fetal lungs. In cases of unilateral agenesis, the presence of at least one functioning kidney contributes to excellent survival rates. Therefore, unilateral agenesis carries a good prognosis, especially with appropriate urologic follow-up. Bilateral agenesis occurs in 1 in 3000 to 1 in 10,000 births and the male-to-female ratio is 2.5:1. Unilateral agenesis is more common and

has been estimated to occur in 1 in 600 to 1000 births with a male-to-female ratio of 1:1.

Bilateral renal agenesis is often referred to as **Potter's syndrome.** Infants born with bilateral renal agenesis exhibit Potter's facies (flat nose, recessed chin, abnormal ears, and wide-set eyes) and abnormal or malpositioned limbs. These deformities are caused by the lack of amniotic fluid. Under normal conditions, amniotic fluid protects the fetus from the walls of the uterus allowing fetal structures such as the extremities to open and close. In cases of oligohydramnios, the uterine walls place pressure on the fetus and the fetal extremities are typically held in limited positions leading to abnormal development.

Other fetal anomalies found in association with bilateral renal agenesis include cardiac defects and musculoskeletal disorders (sirenomelia, absent radius and fibula, anomalies of the digits, sacral agenesis, diaphragmatic hernia, and cleft palate). Central nervous system anomalies include hydrocephalus, meningocele, cephalocele, holoprosencephaly, anencephaly, and microcephaly. Gastrointestinal anomalies include duodenal atresia, imperforate anus, tracheoesophageal fistula, malrotation, and omphalocele. The sonographer should understand that most of these malformations are not detected prenatally because of poor visualization resulting from anhydramnios (complete lack of amniotic fluid). Unilateral agenesis may be associated with uterine anomalies in females and testicular hypoplasia, agenesis, or **hypospadias** in males. It should also be noted that there is a high incidence of abnormalities in the functioning kidney, specifically vesicoureteral reflux.

Sonographic Findings. Sonographic findings are dependent on unilateral or bilateral renal agenesis. In both cases the kidney or kidneys are not visualized (Figure 63-13). Careful examination of the abdominopelvic region must be completed to rule out a possible ectopic or pelvic kidney. Color Doppler can be used to delineate the renal vessels and the attachment to the aorta in the area of the kidneys. In the renal fossa of the absent kidney(s), the adrenal gland may mimic the kidney. The adrenal gland will appear hypoechoic with an echogenic center and in a flattened or lying-down position.

In bilateral renal agenesis, the kidney(s) and bladder are not visualized sonographically (Figure 63-14 and Box 63-3). The presence or absence of the urinary bladder will determine if the kidneys are present or not. It has been noted that nonvisualization of the urinary bladder during 1 hour of consistent scanning is considered a sonographic sign of renal agenesis. One of the major signs is the absence of or severely decreased (oligohydramnios) levels of urine. This is a direct result of urine not being produced. It is important to remember that in the early stages of renal agenesis (before 15 to 18 weeks), amniotic fluid may be visible because it is produced from other fetal sources. Also verify that the patient has not experienced rupture of the membranes.

In unilateral renal agenesis, the contralateral kidney may be hypertrophied to compensate for the absent kidney (see Figure 63-13, *B*). Therefore, the length of the kidney present will be greater than the gestational age. The bladder will be visualized and adequate amounts of amniotic fluid are produced.

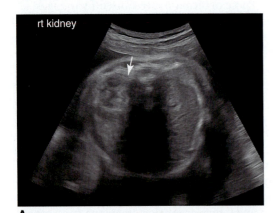

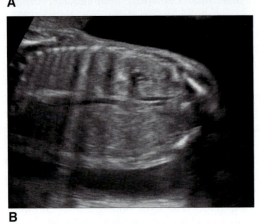

FIGURE 63-13 **A,** Transverse view of the fetal kidneys in this 31-week fetus reveals visualization of the right kidney without visualization of the left kidney at the same level. **B,** This sagittal view of the same fetus supports the empty renal fossa on the left.

Horseshoe Kidneys

Etiology. A **horseshoe kidney** forms when the inferior poles of the kidney fuse while they are in the pelvis. This fusion may occur in 1 to 4 of 1000 births and is two to three times more common in males (see Figure 63-12).

Clinical Findings and Prognosis. Horseshoe kidneys may be found as an isolated anomaly or in association with other anomalies or syndromes. They have a frequency of approximately 1 in 450 births. Isolated horseshoe kidneys carry good prognosis but are often associated with other renal conditions. The prevalence of kidney stones, urinary tract infections, and hydronephrosis as well as reflux is common in cases of horseshoe kidneys. The presence of other abnormalities directly affects the outcome of the fetus. Anomalies occurring with horseshoe kidneys include central nervous system disorders, cardiac abnormalities, or urogenital abnormalities. The incidence of trisomy 18 and 45X is also increased.

Sonographic Findings. The horseshoe kidney is the fusion of the lower poles of both kidneys. In general, horseshoe kidneys are difficult to diagnosis in utero. The

BOX 63-3	Sonographic Findings in Renal Agenesis

- Severe oligohydramnios after 13 to 15 weeks' menstrual age
- Persistent absence of urine in fetal bladder (observe for period of 1 hour)
- Failure to visualize kidneys or renal arteries (use color flow to outline renal arteries)
- Abnormally small thorax
  Note: Difficulties arise when oligohydramnios is present or when fetus is in breech presentation. Be careful not to mistake bowel or adrenal gland for kidneys. An empty bladder may be due to other impaired renal function problems.

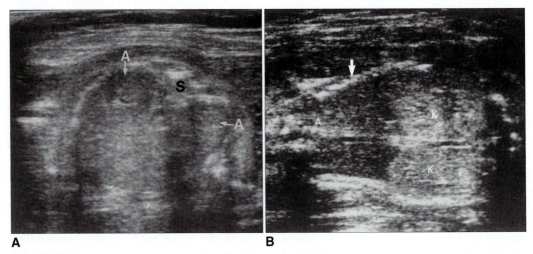

FIGURE 63-14 **A,** Renal agenesis in a 29-week fetus showing enlarged adrenal glands *(A)* occupying the renal spaces. Oligohydramnios and an absent bladder confirmed the diagnosis. **B,** Infantile polycystic kidney disease shown with enlarged and dense kidneys *(K)*. Note the enhanced transmission of sound through the kidneys because of the dilated cystic tubules. Oligohydramnios and absent bladder were coexisting findings.

bridge of tissue connecting the lower poles must be demonstrated for accurate diagnosis. There are several sonographic clues that may indicate a horseshoe kidney. The transverse images of the fetal abdomen demonstrate an abnormal lie of the kidney. If the spine is down, the connecting isthmus may be seen anterior to the aorta. In the sagittal and coronal views, clear delineation of the inferior pole of the kidney is not well seen and the kidneys may appear oblique.

Renal Ectopia

Etiology. As discussed before, the kidneys initially lie close together in the pelvis. Gradually they migrate into the abdomen and become separated from one another. They normally complete this migration by the 9th week of gestation. In some cases, one of the kidneys may remain in the pelvic cavity while the other migrates into the posterior flank of the abdomen.

Clinical Findings and Prognosis. Ectopic kidney(s) occurs when the kidney lies outside of its normal position in the renal fossa, usually in the area of the pelvis (see Figure 63-12). Occasional crossed ectopia will occur. In crossed ectopia both kidneys may be fused or appear to be fused because they are located on the same side of the body (considered a form of horseshoe kidney). The cross-fused ectopic kidney lies on the opposite side of the abdomen relative to its ureteral insertion into the bladder. The kidneys are usually fused together and are found usually on the right side of the abdomen. In rare incidences the kidney may be located in the thoracic cavity, more commonly on the left side.

Prognosis for ectopic kidneys is based on acquired complications or in association with other anomalies. Ectopic kidneys can have complications of dilatation or dysplasia. Associated anomalies include skeletal, cardiovascular, gynecologic, and gastrointestinal abnormalities.

Sonographic Findings. Sonography will demonstrate absence of the kidney in its normal position, with the adrenal gland filling the space of the renal fossa. The abnormally located kidney will typically be smaller and rotated obliquely or horizontal. If the kidney is located in the pelvis, it is typically found lying superior to the bladder or adjacent to the iliac wing (Figure 63-15). In cases of crossed-fused ectopic kidneys, both kidneys will appear on the same side; therefore, kidney measurements will demonstrate an enlarged bilobed kidney.

Exstrophy of the Bladder

Etiology. Exstrophy of the bladder is characterized by the protrusion of the posterior wall of the urinary bladder, which contains the trigone of the bladder and the ureteric orifices. Exstrophy of the bladder is caused by the defective closure of the inferior part of the anterior abdominal wall during the 4th week of gestation.

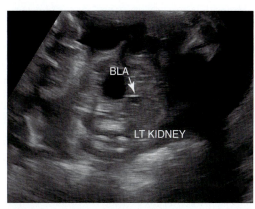

FIGURE 63-15 The left kidney was not seen in its normal location in this 23-week fetus. Further evaluation of the fetus identified the left kidney adjacent to the bladder in the lower pelvis. *BLA,* Bladder.

As a result of this defect, no muscle or connective tissue forms in the anterior abdominal wall to cover the urinary bladder, and therefore the bladder is formed external to the abdominal wall.

Clinical Findings and Prognosis. Exstrophy of the bladder occurs primarily in males and the incidence is 1 in 30,000 births. It is most likely of sporadic occurrence and isolated. Laboratory markers will reveal an elevated maternal serum alpha-fetoprotein (MSAFP). Genitalia malformations are commonly seen, such as undescended testes or anterior displaced scrotum and a small penis with **epispadias** in males or a cleft clitoris in the female. Multiple surgical procedures are required to correct the bladder abnormality as well as other associated genital anomalies. Urinary continence is restored in the majority of cases.

Sonographic Findings. A fluid-filled bladder is not visualized, but normal kidneys and amniotic fluid are evident. A small irregular mass representing the everted atrophied bladder is identified in the lower abdomen below the umbilical cord insertion (Figure 63-16). The sonographer should note the cord insertion is abnormally low when this anomaly is present. A sagittal view of the abdominal pelvic region of the fetus will reveal an anterior mass that appears as a mound of soft tissue. A transverse view of the pelvic bones will demonstrate widening of the iliac crest. It is important to differentiate this from **cloacal exstrophy.** In this condition the bladder findings are the same. However, large and small intestine are included in the anterior wall mass as well as multiple other anomalies.

Urachal Abnormalities

Etiology. Early in development, the urinary bladder is continuous with the allantois. The allantois regresses to become a fibrous cord known as the urachus. This cord, or ligament, extends from the apex of the bladder to the umbilicus. If the lumen of the allantois persists while the urachus forms, a urachal fistula develops, which causes

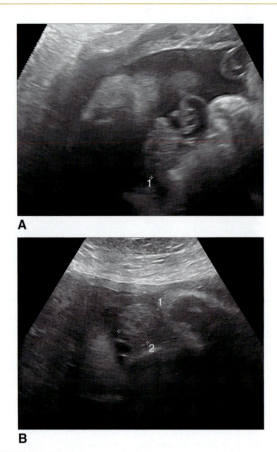

FIGURE 63-16 **A,** A 33-week female fetus presents with a soft tissue mass anterior to the area of the bladder. **B,** The mass was seen in both sagittal and transverse views. No bladder was documented sonographically. The patient presented with bladder exstrophy at birth.

urine to drain from the bladder to the umbilicus. If only a small part of the lumen of the allantois persists, it is called an **urachal cyst,** or a vesicoallantoic cyst. If a larger portion of the lumen persists, it may cause a urachal sinus to develop that may open at the umbilicus or into the urinary bladder. In this case, the term *patent urachus* is often used.

Clinical Findings and Prognosis. Urachal abnormalities are sporadic in occurrence and uncommon but, when seen, are more common in males. Association with posterior urethral valves and prune-belly syndrome has been documented, but structural anomalies are uncommon. After the fetus is born, urine discharge or drainage from the umbilicus is frequently noted. However, it is possible for the urachal cyst to rupture in utero into the cord or amniotic fluid. In either case the urachal remnant is surgically removed.

Sonographic Findings. Sonographically an anechoic cyst is usually seen within the base of the umbilical cord. The cyst can be visualized communicating with the bladder. The amniotic fluid level and kidneys typically appear normal. However, hydronephrosis has been noted as the result of reflux in patients with urachal abnormalities (Figure 63-17). It has also been identified that the cystic mass will change size along with emptying of the bladder (see Figure 63-17, C). For instance, the cystic mass may become larger as the fetus urinates from the bladder as a result of reflux into the allantoic canal.

RENAL CYSTIC DISEASE

Renal cystic disease is a heterogeneous group of heritable, developmental, and acquired disorders. The diseases

FIGURE 63-17 **A,** In this transverse image, bilateral pyelectasis is noted as well as an enlarged bladder at the level of the kidneys. **B,** Upon sagittal view, the bladder appeared abnormal in shape with the cranial end becoming narrow. **C,** Continuous scanning of the bladder indicated a change in shape and size of the abnormal bladder with fetal urination. **D,** With the aid of 3D/4D technology, the diagnosis of a urachal abnormality was clearly seen.

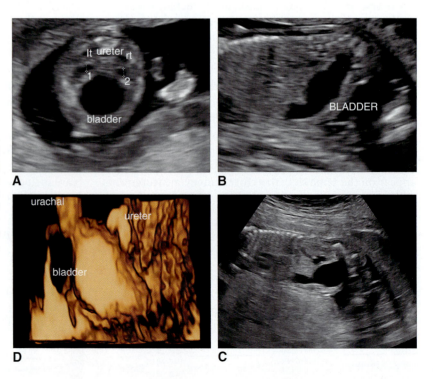

have been categorized in many ways, for instance, the Potter's classification or **Potter's sequence** is used to describe diseases that are associated with renal failure, oligohydramnios, and Potter's facies (Box 63-4); dividing the diseases into groups of hereditary versus nonhereditary; and dividing the diseases by dysplastic kidney, hereditary cyst, and nondysplastic nonhereditary cyst. There are also a number of very rare syndromes associated with renal cystic disease as outlined in Table 63-2 that are included in some classifications but not in others. This section will identify numerous types of renal cystic disease without using a classification system.

Infantile Polycystic Kidney Disease

Etiology. Infantile polycystic kidney disease (IPKD), or autosomal recessive polycystic kidney disease (ARPKD), is an autosomal-recessive congenital disorder that affects both fetal kidneys and liver. The disorder is characterized by the development of small cysts in both kidneys and

---

BOX 63-4	**Renal Cystic Disease**

Potter's Type I: Sonographic Findings in Infantile Polycystic Kidney Disease
- Progressive renal enlargement
- Echogenic renal parenchyma
- Empty bladder and oligohydramnios

Potter's Type II: Sonographic Findings in Adult Multicystic Dysplastic Kidney
- Multiple noncommunicating cysts of variable size
- No distinct renal pelvis
- No distinct renal parenchyma
- Renal size may be normal, hypoplastic, or enlarged
- Severe oligohydramnios if bilateral

Potter's Type III: Sonographic Findings in Adult Polycystic Kidney Disease
- Large kidneys with hyperechoic parenchyma
- Size may be asymmetric
- Genetic link

Potter's Type IV: Sonographic Findings in Obstructive Cystic Disease
- Small, echogenic kidneys
- Cortical peripheral cysts
- Bilateral disease: "keyhole bladder," bilateral hydronephrosis, thick-walled bladder, severe oligohydramnios

---

liver cysts. The cysts in the kidney are thought to be caused by tubular malformation and ectasia of the collecting ducts. The distal collecting ducts are typically affected more than the proximal ducts because of their earlier development. The malformation results in cystic dilatation of the renal tubules measuring 1 to 2 mm, usually arranged in a symmetrical pattern leading to overall enlargement of the kidneys. The formation of the cysts results in tubulointerstitial damage resulting in tubular dysfunction and fibrosis. Eventually renal failure will occur because of the replacement of normal tissue by enlarged nonfunctioning collecting tubules.

Clinical Findings and Prognosis. This disease has varying presentations, affects 1 in 40,000 to 50,000 births, and is associated with a 25% recurrence rate. Varying presentations include different types such as the perinatal form and the juvenile form. In view of the high recurrence rate and dismal prognosis in severe IPKD, recognition of this defect is important. IPKD may occur as part of a genetic syndrome, such as Meckel-Gruber syndrome or trisomy 13. The most severe forms of IPKD are found prenatally and are associated with renal failure, oligohydramnios, and an absent urinary bladder. In some cases the kidneys are so massive that they fill the entire abdomen. Prognosis depends on the severity of the renal disease. Most fetuses diagnosed in utero will be stillborn or die early in the neonatal period because of renal failure and lung hypoplasia. It is rare for a fetus to survive the first year of life.

Sonographic Findings. In this disease, the collecting tubules of the kidney are microscopically dilated. Sonographically, individual cysts are not identified; instead the kidneys are massively enlarged because of hundreds of dilated tubules (Figure 63-18). Enlargement of the kidneys may not occur until the 24th week of gestation; therefore, serial studies of at-risk fetuses are recommended. It is not uncommon for the kidneys to measure above the 90% percentile in length and width. This enlargement will lead to an abdominal circumference that is large for the gestational age.

Enhanced renal tissue echogenicity is characteristic because of the multiple interfaces created by the dilated cystic tubules. Oligohydramnios and a small or absent bladder are present. The oligohydramnios may not be evident until after 15 to 18 weeks of gestation. Liver cysts and fibrosis may or may not be visualized.

TABLE 63-2	**Syndromes Associated with Cystic Renal Disease**

Syndrome	Clinical Findings
Meckel-Gruber syndrome	Large echogenic kidneys, polydactyly, encephalocele
Patau's syndrome (trisomy 13)	Large echogenic kidneys, polydactyly, holoprosencephaly, facial clefting
Beckwith-Wiedemann syndrome	Large echogenic kidneys, macrosomia, hepatosplenomegaly, macroglossia, omphalocele
Jeune syndrome	Echogenic kidneys, dwarfism, small thorax
Short rib polydactyly syndrome	Large echogenic kidneys, dwarfism, polydactyly, small thorax
Laurence-Moon syndrome (Bardet-Biedl syndrome)	Cystic kidneys, hypotonicity, limb contractures, congenital cataracts, hypoplastic corpus callosum, heterotopias

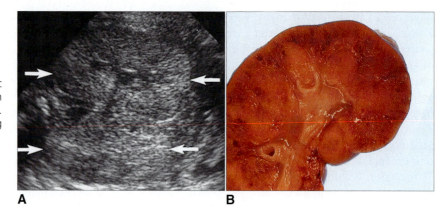

FIGURE 63-18 Autosomal recessive polycystic kidney disease. **A,** Kidneys are enlarged with increased echogenicity at 27 weeks of gestation. **B,** Gross pathology of the disease showing diffuse microscopic cysts.

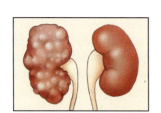

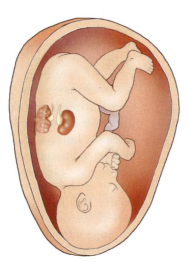

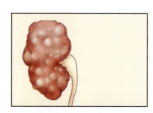

Contralateral mild to moderate pelvocaliectasis

Contralateral renal agenesis
Severe hypoplasia
Severe oligohydramnios
Lethal

Bilateral multicystic dysplastic kidneys
Severe oligohydramnios
Lethal

FIGURE 63-19 Multicystic dysplastic kidney disease may be unilateral, bilateral, or associated with contralateral renal agenesis. Although the affected kidney typically produces very little urine, it may change in size throughout gestation. Because the contralateral kidney is the only potentially functional kidney, it must be examined carefully.

Multicystic Dysplastic Kidney Disease

Etiology. Congenital **multicystic dysplastic kidney disease (MCDK)** is characterized by multiple, smooth-walled, nonfunctioning, noncommunicating cysts of variable size and number. In this condition, renal tissue is replaced by cysts of varying sizes that are found throughout the kidney. The entire kidney or only a portion of the kidney may be affected. Between the cysts, renal stroma may be present; normal renal tissue is absent. The ureter and renal pelvis may be atretic, and the renal artery is hypoplastic or absent. The condition is thought to result from early obstruction uropathy or abnormal development of the metanephric mesoderm and the ureteric bud. The affected kidney is nonfunctional.

Clinical Findings and Prognosis. Multicystic dysplastic kidney disease is the most common form of renal cystic disease in childhood and represents one of the most common abdominal masses in the neonate. The incidence is 1 of 3000 births, and the disease is found more often in males than in females. Research has also concluded a link with maternal diabetes.

Although most cases are unilateral, nearly one quarter of the cases are bilateral. Associated abnormalities may involve the contralateral kidney, heart, central nervous system, extremities, and gastrointestinal syndromes. Many syndromes also been identified in associations with MCDK; Meckel Gruber, Apert, Zellweger, and short rib polydactyly represent only a few.

The prognosis for infants with multicystic kidney disease varies based on the prenatal findings (Figure 63-19). In isolated cases of unilateral involvement, the disease will regress with time and disappear, or a small collection of cysts with a calcified border will be present in the renal fossa (Figure 63-20). If the kidney appears to be interfering with other organs, such as bowel, it can be surgically removed. If only a segment of the kidney is involved, renal insufficiency may result. When both kidneys are found to be multicystic, oligohydramnios and an absent bladder are expected, a lethal condition

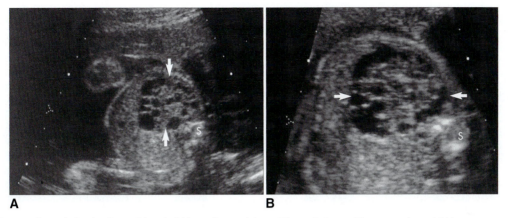

FIGURE 63-20 **A,** Unilateral dysplastic multicystic kidney *(arrows)* in a 25-week fetus. The contralateral kidney appeared normal with adequate amniotic fluid volume. A single umbilical artery was identified. *S,* Spine. **B,** In the same fetus, a magnified view of the dysplastic kidney *(arrows)*.

exists for the neonate. This is also true when one kidney is multicystic and the other absent.

▨ **Sonographic Findings.** In the midtrimester ultrasound scan, the fetus with multicystic renal dysplasia will present with at least one kidney, demonstrating multiple cysts of varying size that may affect a part of or the entire kidney (Figure 63-21). The cysts typically start at the periphery and appear small. Over time the cyst will enlarge and more cysts will develop in the hilum. Echogenic stroma may be visible between the cysts. The overall size of the kidney may be enlarged, resulting in possible enlargement of the abdominal circumference. Kidney borders are difficult to define because of the distorted renal outline and absence of significant renal parenchyma (Figure 63-22, *A*). If only one kidney is affected, the contralateral kidney may be enlarged as a result of compensatory hypertrophy. The contralateral kidney should be carefully evaluated for renal anomalies. The bladder and amniotic fluid volume are usually within normal limits (Figure 63-22, *B*). When the condition is bilateral, there is oligohydramnios and absence of the bladder. Because of the progression of this disease, over time the nonfunctioning kidney will decrease in size. However, this process may not be evident until after birth.

Adult Dominant Polycystic Kidney Disease

Etiology. Congenital adult (autosomal) dominant polycystic kidney disease (ADPKD) is associated with cystic dilation of the nephrons and of the collecting tubule walls in both kidneys. It is thought to be caused by a defective gene that does not allow for normal epithelial cell development. The result is cystic development of the cortex and medulla. The cysts typically do not enlarge or impair renal function until adulthood.

Clinical Findings and Prognosis. APKD has an incidence of 1 in 1000 births and is the most common of the hereditary renal cystic diseases with a recurrence risk of 50%. The manifestations of the disease typically

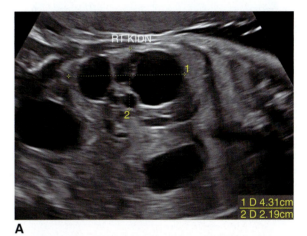

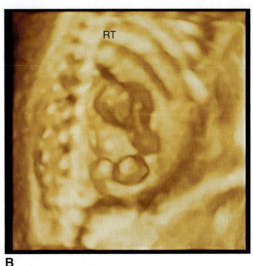

FIGURE 63-21 **A,** A unilateral multicystc dysplastic kidney is identified with multiple cysts of varying sizes throughout the kidney. The kidneys are enlarged, measuring 4.31 cm for this 28-week fetus. **B,** The cysts of the kidney are clearly seen utilizing 3D technology. The lack of the cysts communicating with each other helps to differentiate it for hydronephrosis.

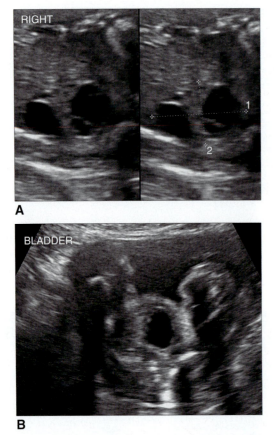

A

B

FIGURE 63-22 **A,** In this case of multicystic dysplastic kidney, the cysts are enlarged, creating the inability to clearly delineate the borders of the kidney. **B,** Only one kidney in this fetus is affected, so visualization of a normal bladder is clearly seen.

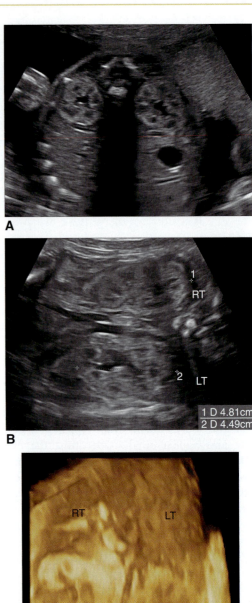

A

B

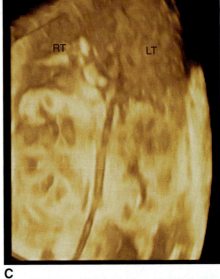

C

FIGURE 63-23 **A,** This 25 week female fetus presented with a known family history of adult polycystic kidney disease including the mother. The transverse view of the kidneys demonstrates symmetrical enlarged echogenic kidneys. **B,** In a follow-up sonogram at 35 weeks of gestation, the enlargement is clearly seen in the longitudinal images of the kidneys. The kidneys measure 4.81 cm and 4.49 cm. **C,** The use of advanced technology aids in visualizing the kidneys.

develop in adulthood, but the disease may be diagnosed in a fetus when there is a family history of polycystic kidneys, liver, or both. Conversely, visualization of bilateral enlargement of the kidneys may prompt a renal and liver workup in the parents to exclude this disorder. Associated anomalies include cysts (liver, spleen, and pancreas), cardiac malformations, pyloric stenosis, and skeletal anomalies. It should be noted that extrarenal cysts are typically only identified in the adult.

Prognosis for prenatal diagnosis of APKD is dependent on the progression of cyst development leading to renal failure. In some cases the cyst development is rapid with renal failure apparent at birth, and in other cases the cyst development is slow with progression to hypertension and ultimately end-stage renal failure. If a sibling has been affected, the outcome may be easier to predict. Renal dialysis with eventual renal transplant is required in cases of bilateral renal failure.

Sonographic Findings. The sonographic appearance is similar to autosomal recessive polycystic renal disease in that the kidneys are symmetrically enlarged and echogenic. The bladder is usually present and amniotic fluid volume is normal. The corticomedullary junction may appear accentuated or indistinct (Figure 63-23).

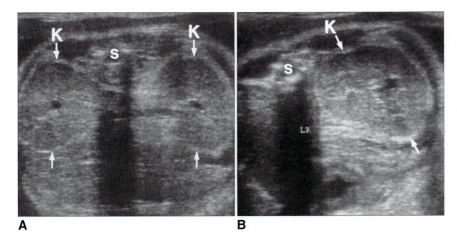

FIGURE 63-24 **A,** Bilateral renal enlargement of the kidneys *(K, arrows)* in a 32-week fetus with Beckwith-Wiedemann syndrome (congenital visceromegaly of organs, which may present with or without an omphalocele). Both kidneys occupy more than half of the abdomen. *s,* Spine. **B,** In the same fetus, a sagittal view shows an enlarged left kidney *(K, arrow)*.

Occasionally, macroscopic cysts within the echogenic kidneys are seen. This condition is nearly always bilateral.

Because of the rarity of diagnosing this disease in utero, it is often confused with other diseases that present with similar sonographic appearance. The appearance of bilateral echogenic kidney enlargement may be found in association with a syndrome, such as Beckwith-Wiedemann syndrome. This syndrome presents with visceromegaly of many organs (Figure 63-24). The urinary bladder is usually present. The corticomedullary junction may appear accentuated or be indistinct. Meckel-Gruber syndrome is associated with the presence of bilateral renal cystic disease, but with Meckel-Gruber syndrome, additional anomalies such as encephalocele, polydactyly, and severe oligohydramnios are present.

Obstructive Cystic Dysplasia

Etiology. In obstructive cystic dysplasia, renal dysplasia occurs secondary to kidney obstruction in the first or early second trimester of pregnancy. The long-standing obstruction leads to the development of fibrosis and cystic replacement of the renal tissue (Figure 63-25). Unilateral disease can be caused by a ureteropelvic or ureterovesical junction obstruction. Severe obstruction from an ureterocele can cause dysplasia in an upper pole of a duplex kidney. Bilateral obstructive dysplasia is caused by severe bladder outlet obstruction, usually **urethral atresia** or posterior urethral valves.

Clinical Findings and Prognosis. The incidence is 1 in 8000 births, although this is difficult to determine because only a small number of obstructive kidneys progress to renal dysplasia. Because of the variety of causes of this disease, anomaly associations are variable. The prognosis depends on unilateral or bilateral involvement. Bilateral involvement would indicate a poor outcome as a result of renal failure and lung hypoplasia. Unilateral involvement may vary from normal outcome to dependence on associated anomalies or the presence of anomalies affecting the functioning kidney.

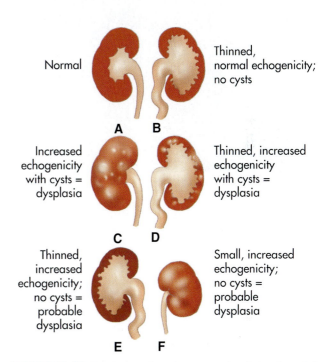

FIGURE 63-25 Renal parenchymal responses to obstruction. **A,** In distal urinary tract obstruction without reflux, the kidneys may remain normal. **B,** Pyelocaliectasis may thin the renal parenchyma. **C,** Cystic dysplasia may occur with renal cysts and fibrosis (increased echogenicity) and cease to function (lack of pyelocaliectasis). **D,** Cystic dysplasia may occur with persistent pyelocaliectasis. **E,** Increased renal echogenicity with visible cysts suggests, but is not diagnostic of, dysplasia. **F,** A small, echogenic kidney without pyelocaliectasis is also suggestive, but not diagnostic, of dysplasia.

▶ **Sonographic Findings.** Early sonographic findings may only be hydronephrosis or hydroureter, depending on the level of obstruction. The kidney will most likely appear enlarged during this time. Early signs of dysplasia include the presence of hydronephrosis with cortical cysts. The cortical cyst will not communicate with the anechoic cystic-like appearance of the hydronephrosis. As the kidney slowly stops functioning, the renal cortex becomes completely dysplastic and replaced with the

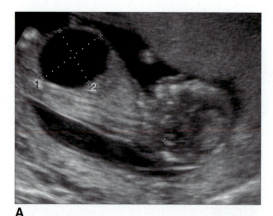

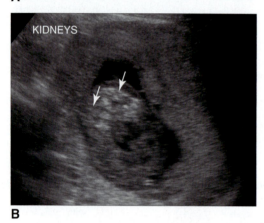

FIGURE 63-26 **A,** A bladder outlet obstruction was suspected in this 14-week fetus. **B,** The kidneys were later seen as very small and echogenic (*arrows*). The renal dysplasia was a result of the early onset of obstruction that led to renal compromise.

OBSTRUCTIVE URINARY TRACT ABNORMALITIES

The urinary tract may be obstructed either at the junction of the ureter entering the renal pelvis (ureteropelvic junction [UPJ]), at the junction of the ureter where it enters the bladder (ureterovesical junction [UVJ]), or at the level of the urethra (**megacystis**). The degree of obstruction will depend on the gestational age at which the obstruction began (see Figure 63-25). If the obstruction is early, a multicystic kidney may develop. If the obstruction occurs in the first or second trimester, cystic dysplasia may result. Late obstruction produces hydronephrosis. The term *pelviectasis* is commonly used in conjunction with hydronephrosis. However, *pyelectasis* refers to dilatation of the renal pelvis without dilatation

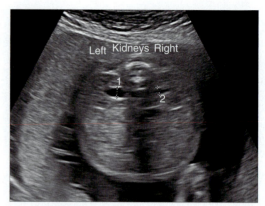

FIGURE 63-27 Mild pyelectasis is noted in both kidneys of this fetus diagnosed with Down syndrome.

BOX 63-5	Anterior Posterior Diameter Measurement of the Renal Pelvis

- Intrapelvic diameter greater than 7 mm is consider mild hydronephrosis.
- Intrapelvic diameter measuring 7 to 15 mm is consider moderate hydronephrosis.
- Intrapelvic diameter measuring greater than 15 mm is considered marked dilatation or severe hydronephrosis.

of the calyces, and *hydronephrosis* refers to dilatation of the renal pelvis and calyces.

Hydronephrosis

Etiology. Dilation of the renal pelvis occurs in response to a blockage of urine at some junction in the urinary system. Hydronephrosis commonly occurs when there is an obstruction in the ureter, bladder, or urethra. Hydronephrosis is generally the end result of an obstruction at a lower level in the urinary tract. Fetal hydronephrosis may occur as a unilateral or bilateral process. Unilateral renal hydronephrosis commonly results from an obstruction at the junction of the renal pelvis and the ureter.
Clinical Findings and Prognosis. Fetal hydronephrosis is the most common fetal anomaly. Findings suggesting hydronephrosis include an abnormal intrapelvic anterior posterior (AP) diameter measurement. Although this measurement will fluctuate with gestational age, if a measurement is greater than 4 to 4.5 mm before the third trimester or greater than 7 mm after the third trimester is found, the kidney should be followed with serial examinations (Box 63-5). Another useful guide is that if the measurement exceeds one third of the renal diameter, follow-up should be considered. In cases in which **pyelectasis** is diagnosed, the fetus should be carefully examined for anomalies associated with aneuploidy. Mild pyelectasis is a common feature associated with Down syndrome (Figure 63-27).

The prognosis of a fetus with hydronephrosis depends on the severity and cause. When considering severity

multiple cortical cysts. The dysplastic kidney will appear small and echogenic with cortical peripheral cysts (Figure 63-26). If only one kidney is affected, the bladder and amniotic fluid level will be within normal limits. If the disease is bilateral, a bladder outlet obstruction ("keyhole sign of urinary bladder") may be apparent as well as severe oligohydramnios.

without relating to cause or dysplasia, mild hydronephrosis has been found to resolve antenatally or postnatally without surgical intervention. Cases of moderate to severe hydronephrosis have resolved antenatally and postnatally, although surgical correction is common. In cases in which the hydronephrosis is related to a specific cause and no dysplasia is evident, surgical correction is required. In some cases when a fetus has unilateral obstruction of the urinary tract, early delivery of the fetus is often warranted to salvage the normal kidney. The common finding of renal dysplasia following obstruction is represented by cystic changes within the renal tissue. Renal dysplasia often leads to renal failure of all or part of the kidney.

Sonographic Findings. The sonographic appearance of urinary tract obstruction varies depending on the site and extent of blockage (Figure 63-28). It is extremely important that a true cross section plane through the mid renal pelvis be obtained for measuring the AP diameter of the anechoic pelvis. A transverse view of the abdomen with the spine located anteriorly is optimal. Oblique or off-axis images lead to erroneous measurements.

The dilated anechoic renal pelvis is centrally located and distended with urine. If only the pelvis is seen, the term *pyelectasis* is used. Hydronephrosis will be identified with a dilatation of the renal pelvis and calyces. The sonographic appearance of the surrounding parenchymal tissue will appear within normal limits. However, depending on the degree of dilatation, the parenchyma may appear thin. If dysplasia is evident, cystic replacement of the renal tissue will be evident.

Based on the severity and cause of the hydronephrosis, the bladder and amniotic fluid level will vary. Further investigation into the sonographic findings associated with these causes will follow in the next section.

Ureteropelvic Junction Obstruction

Etiology. Ureteropelvic junction (UPJ) obstruction occurs at the junction between the renal pelvis and ureter.

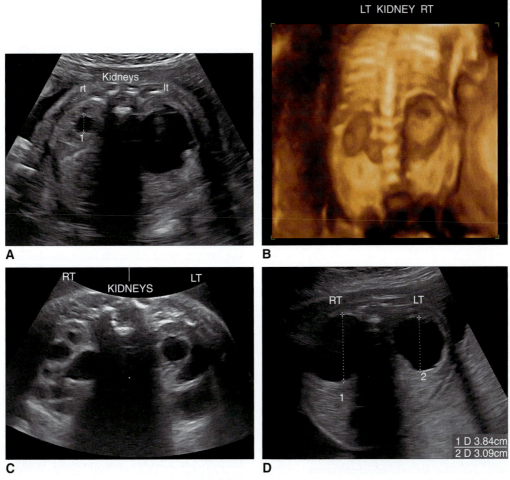

FIGURE 63-28 A, In this image, mild hydronephrosis is noted in the right kidney and severe hydronephrosis is seen in the left kidney. **B,** 3D technology clearly identifies the round cystic structure in the renal pelvis connecting to ureters. **C,** In this case of hydronephrosis, both the renal pelvis and the connecting calyces are seen. **D,** This fetus presents with bilateral severe hydronephrosis. Notice the thinning of the renal tissue.

The obstruction results in a backup of urine into the renal pelvis and calyces. The causes of UPJ obstructions include abnormal bends or kinks in the ureter, adhesions, abnormal valves in the ureter, abnormal outlet shape at the ureteropelvic junction, or absence of the longitudinal muscle that is imperative for the normal excretion of urine from the kidney.

Clinical Findings and Prognosis. Ureteropelvic junction obstruction is the most common reason for hydronephrosis in the neonate. It is more common in males and is usually unilateral. Only half of these disorders are found during early childhood; therefore, early prenatal detection may improve long-term renal function. Uteropelvic junction obstruction is usually a unilateral defect, and amniotic fluid remains normal because of the normal contralateral kidney. Bilateral ureteropelvic junction obstruction is uncommon. Anomalies associated with this disorder may involve the presence of a urinoma. Prognosis for UPJ obstruction is determined by the degree of renal impairment caused by the obstruction. Serial sonograms are performed to document progression of obstruction as well as amniotic fluid levels. Most cases do not require early delivery unless there is evidence of severe bilateral obstruction with oligohydramnios. Neonates will typically receive antibiotics and a complete urologic examination.

Sonographic Findings. Sonographically, there is a collection of anechoic urine located medially within the renal pelvis that communicates with the calyces (caliectasis) (Figure 63-29). The renal pelvis may take on a bullet shape that is surrounded by dilated or normal calyces. The renal cortex, ureter, bladder, and amniotic fluid are usually normal in cases of unilateral involvement. Ureteropelvic junction obstruction may be severe, leading to distended calyces and renal cortex reduction. In cases of severe obstruction, the affected kidney should be evaluated for sonographic features associated with dysplasia.

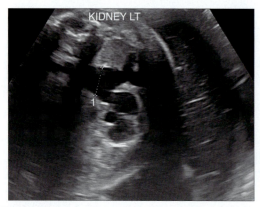

FIGURE 63-29 In this image, the renal pelvis and calyces are clearly seen connecting. Identifying the connection between the pelvis and calyces should be used to differentiate the anechoic areas from renal cysts.

Ureterovesical Junction Obstruction

Etiology. Ureterovesical junction (UVJ) obstruction commonly presents with dilation of the lower end of the ureter. The obstruction leads to the back up of urine in the kidney (hydronephrosis) and an enlarged, urine-filled ureter (**megaureter**). Megaureter may result from a primary ureteral defect (stenotic ureteral valves or fibrosis) or may arise secondary to obstruction at another level, causing reflux or backward flow of urine. In the majority of cases, the cause is the distal portion of the ureter being aperistaltic (primary megaureter). Under normal conditions, constant muscular contractions of the ureter are responsible for moving the urine from the kidney to the bladder. Therefore, if a segment of the ureter is aperistaltic, it lacks the ability to compress those muscles. The constant contractions are disrupted, which leads to the inability of urine to be moved into the bladder at a constant normal rate. UVJ obstruction has also been found to result from an ectopic ureterocele within the bladder, causing obstruction of the upper pole of the kidney. (This condition is discussed in the next section.)

Clinical Findings and Prognosis. UVJ obstruction is more common in males, is unilateral, and is of sporadic incidence. Bilateral involvement has been reported. It is not uncommon for other abnormalities to be found in the affected kidney. Duplication of the renal collecting system is common and may be diagnosed prenatally. In approximately 25% of cases, the contralateral kidney will present with anomalies. One of the most important components in the diagnosis of UVJ obstruction is to determine whether the obstruction is associated with retrograde flow of urine from the bladder back to the ureter (reflux). Definitive diagnosis is made only after delivery with the aid of a voiding cystourethrogram (VCU) examination.

The prognosis for infants with UVJ obstruction is good regardless of whether it is associated with a refluxing ureter or a nonrefluxing ureter. Like other renal obstructions, the prognosis depends on the degree of renal impairment caused by the obstruction. Surgical correction may be required in some cases to help prevent further renal damage.

Sonographic Findings. The affected kidney is visualized with anechoic dilation of the renal pelvis and tortuous fluid filled dilated ureter (Figure 63-30). Careful attention should be paid to differentiate dilated bowel from the dilated ureter. If the ureter is dilated, it should appear anechoic, whereas the bowel will appear with low-level echoes. The bladder and amniotic fluid volume are normal in cases involving only one kidney. If both kidneys are affected, the amniotic fluid volume may be reduced.

If renal duplication is identified, a dilated upper renal pole is observed with a normal lower pole. In cases of reflux, sonography may reveal changes in the AP

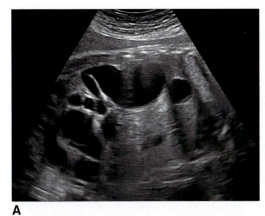

A

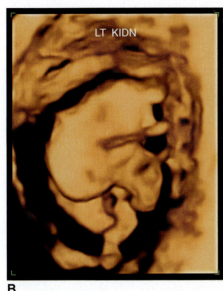

LT KIDN

B

FIGURE 63-30 A, In this image of a UVJ obstruction, the dilated renal pelvis is seen communicating with a dilated tortuous renal ureter. **B,** A rendered 3D image further supports the degree of dilatation of the renal pelvis and ureter.

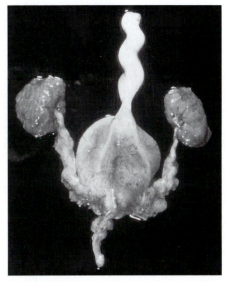

FIGURE 63-31 Pathologic specimen of obstructed urinary tract showing bladder enlargement, hydroureters, and bilateral hydronephrosis in posterior urethral valve syndrome.

diameter measurements of the renal pelvis. These changes may represent the presence of reflux.

Posterior Urethral Valve Obstruction

Etiology. Posterior urethral valve (PUV) obstruction results in hydronephrosis, hydroureters, or dilation of the bladder and posterior urethra (Figures 63-31). The obstruction is produced by an abnormal congenital membrane within the posterior urethra. The membrane is thought to be valvelike and derived from Wolffian duct tissue. The congenital malformation results in the inability of urine to pass through the urethra and into the amniotic fluid. The degree of obstruction can be complete, partial, or intermittent.

Clinical Findings and Prognosis. PUV obstruction is considered the most common urethral anomaly and in males is the most common cause of infravesical

obstruction. The obstruction causes a backup of urine in the bladder, ureter, and, in the most severe cases, the kidneys. Because this anomaly is developed during embryologic stages, obstruction is apparent throughout the pregnancy and leads to impaired renal function and dysplasia. Fetal renal function may be assessed by aspirating urine from an obstructed bladder (Figure 63-32). Cystic dysplasia and poor renal function are suggested when sodium, chloride, and osmolality are unusually elevated. The prognosis is typically poor in cases of complete obstruction because of the high association of renal failure and pulmonary hypoplasia when oligohydramnios is present. When the urinary tract is completely blocked, severe oligohydramnios and the Potter sequence occur. If the fetus survives birth, it is common for it to develop chronic renal failure. Intrauterine therapeutic procedures have been utilized. Intrauterine decompression of an obstructed urinary tract (posterior urethral valve syndrome), which includes draining of the bladder and adding fluid to the amniotic sac, has been performed to relieve the obstruction and allow expansion of the lungs to prevent pulmonary hypoplasia. In some cases, an indwelling bladder shunt is inserted to relieve the obstruction, which sometimes improves chances for survival (Figure 63-33). The shunt drains the blocked urine into the amniotic fluid, allowing the fetal lungs to develop.

Bladder rupture and kidney rupture have occurred in cases where the pressure from the obstruction was too high. In those cases, fetal ascites or perirenal urinomas may develop. The prognosis for patients with partial and intermittent obstruction depends on the severity of renal function and associated oligohydramnios.

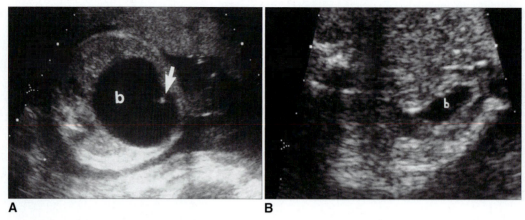

A   B

FIGURE 63-32 A, In this fetus, bladder aspiration was performed to assess kidney function. Note the needle *(arrow)* within the bladder *(b)*. **B,** After urine aspiration, decompression of the bladder *(b)* occurred. Note the thickened bladder wall. Laboratory analysis of osmolality, sodium, potassium, and chloride levels indicates favorable renal function. Bilateral reflux was diagnosed after birth.

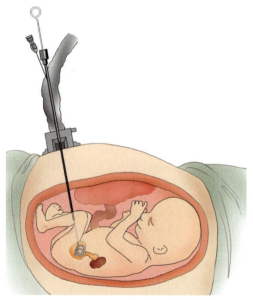

FIGURE 63-33 Schematic showing initial steps in a bladder shunt procedure.

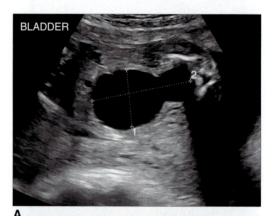

A

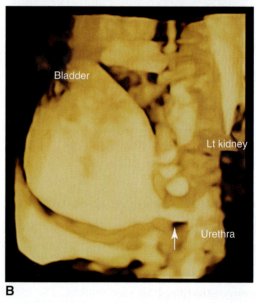

B

FIGURE 63-34 A, The keyhole sign is clearly depicted in this fetus with posterior urethral valve obstruction. **B,** The additional imaging of the bladder with advanced technology enables the sonographer to view the enlarged bladder in relation to the kidney and urethra.

Sonographic Findings. Sonographic features most commonly seen with PUV include severe bladder dilatation, massive hydronephrosis with dysplastic changes seen in the renal tissue, dilated tortuous ureters, and oligohydramnios. The bladder wall is severely thickened with a dilated posterior urethra—the "keyhole sign" (Figure 63-34). If the kidneys have become dysplastic, the sonographic features include an anechoic dilated bladder that occupies the abdomen, mild hydronephrosis, and small echogenic kidneys (Figure 63-35). It is possible for the bladder to rupture in utero because of the pressure of the fluid. In these cases, ascites or hydrops is present; the bladder appears to be of normal size; there is moderate hydronephrosis and little to no amniotic fluid. Intermittent posterior urethral valve obstruction may occur with a normal amount of amniotic fluid. Diminishing fluid volume and increased hydronephrosis may prompt early delivery.

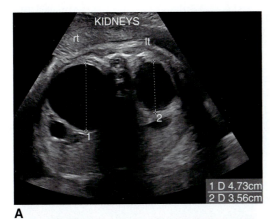

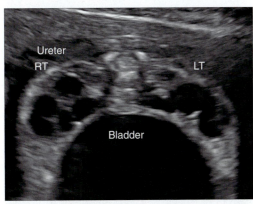

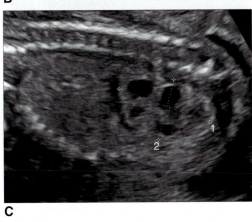

FIGURE 63-35 **A,** The kidneys will both appear with severe hydronephrosis in the early stages of posterior valve obstruction. **B,** The severe hydronephrosis will eventually lead to cystic replacement of renal tissue. **C,** Once dysplasia occurs, the renal function is impaired, resulting in small echogenic kidneys.

Anterior Urethral Valves

Etiology. This congenital defect results in obstruction of the anterior urethral valve in males. Valves are located in multiple locations in the anterior urethra. An exact cause of obstruction is unclear. In some cases, however, it is thought to be caused by abnormal tissue growth, dilated periurethral glands, and proximal and distal urethra formation failure.

Clinical Findings and Prognosis. Anterior urethral valves are rare and either are an isolated finding or are found in conjunction with a diverticulum. The degree of obstruction varies owing to a range of clinical findings such as bilateral hydronephrosis with dilated ureters, end stage renal disease, and bladder rupture. Most cases present after birth with clinical symptoms of a weak urinary stream. VCU examinations are used to make the definitive diagnosis. Prognosis is good with endoscopic resection of the abnormal valve. Other surgeries may be required if other abnormalities are identified. However, like other obstructed lesions, the prognosis will vary depending on the degree of renal impairment.

Sonographic Findings. Dilated anechoic urethra is seen proximal to the valve. The valve is usually not appreciated in obstetric examinations. Utilization of 3D technology can be helpful in determining the extent of the obstruction within the urethra. The obstruction may be complete, partial, or intermittent (Figure 63-36). The amount of amniotic fluid present and the degree of dilatation of the collecting system and ureter will vary from normal to severe. It should be noted that the obstruction may not be apparent until late in gestation.

Prune-Belly Syndrome

Etiology. Prune-belly syndrome is recognized by three features: cryptorchidism, agenesis, or hypoplasia of abdominal wall muscle and dilatation of the collecting system. It is thought to result from an embryologic defect of the mesoderm or as a urethral obstruction malformation complex. In the latter case, the muscle defects are thought to be caused by the dilatation of the collecting system.

Clinical Findings and Prognosis. This syndrome is often referred to as Eagle-Barrett syndrome. It is a rare condition seen mostly in males. The association with males is thought to be due to the complex development of the male urethra. The prognosis depends on renal function. In cases where normal amniotic fluid levels are apparent, the prognosis is typically good. However, most cases are associated with early obstruction, which leads to renal dysplasia and hypoplasia of the lungs. Other anomalies that may also be present and adversely affect the prognosis are microcolon, intestinal malrotation, and cardiac anomalies.

Sonographic Findings. The bladder appears anechoic, large and thin walled. The prostatic urethra in males may be enlarged, mimicking the features of PUV obstruction, but the "keyhole" sign will not be seen. Both kidneys appear with hydronephrosis with possible dysplasia. The ureters are dilated and tortuous. The ureters may appear as numerous cystic lesions within the distended abdominal cavity. Oligohydramnios is usually apparent. The abdomen is extremely distended compared with the small thoracic cavity. The sonographic documentation of

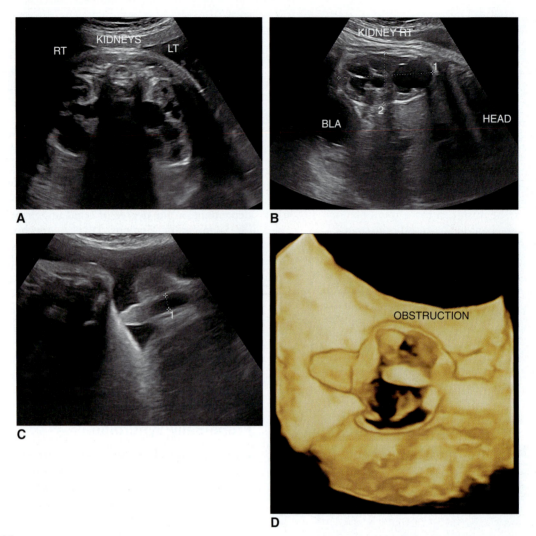

FIGURE 63-36 A male fetus presented with a rare case of obstructed anterior urethral valves. Previous sonograms did not indicate hydronephrosis, an abnormal bladder, or polyhydramnios. All fetal structure appeared normal up to 36 weeks of gestation. **A,** At 38 weeks of gestation the fetus presented with bilateral hydronephrosis. **B,** The renal parenchyma appeared normal surrounding the dilated pelvis and calyces. **C,** Close examination of the male penis revealed an anechoic area within the penis, suggesting obstruction of urine flow at the distal end of the urethra. **D,** With the aid of 3D technology, the obstruction was clearly identified. Findings of anterior urethral valve obstruction were made upon delivery.

absent or hypoplastic abdominal muscles and undescended testicles is often difficult (Box 63-6).

OTHER URINARY ANOMALIES

Ureterocele

Etiology. A ureterocele is a cystic dilation of the intravesical (bladder) segment of the distal ureter. It is commonly found in cases of duplex collecting systems and is associated with upper pole moiety. The ureter attached to the ureterocele in a duplex collecting system drains the upper pole of the kidney as it enters the bladder in a more medial and caudal position (ectopic ureter). The ureter typically inserts into an ectopic location on the bladder and can easily become obstructed. The lower pole of the duplicated kidneys is more prone to reflux and the upper pole more prone to obstruction. The

BOX 63-6	Sonographic Findings in Prune-Belly Syndrome

- Absent abdominal musculature
- Undescended testes
- Large urinary bladder
- Dilated prostatic urethra
- Dilated and tortuous ureters
- Kidneys can be normal, hydronephrotic, or dysplastic

hydronephrotic, nonfunctioning upper pole may cause downward displacement of the lower pole calyces.
Clinical Findings and Prognosis. Females are more likely to present with ureteroceles in the presence of renal duplication. Ureteroceles can occur with normal renal collecting system development, and in these cases males are more likely to be affected. Ureteroceles may also

appear bilaterally. The prognosis for an infant diagnosed with an isolated ureterocele and good renal function is excellent with surgical correction. In cases of duplication where the upper pole has become impaired, surgical removal of the upper pole (partial nephrectomy) and the attached accessory ureter is required. Resection or drainage of the ureterocele is also required.

Sonographic Findings. The sonographic appearance of a ureterocele is that of an anechoic cystic mass surrounded by a thin echogenic membrane within the bladder (Figure 63-37). It is best visualized when the bladder is somewhat full. If the bladder is empty, the ureterocele may be mistaken for a small bladder, and in cases in which the bladder is too full, the ureterocele may be compressed. Therefore, the bladder should be evaluated multiple times through the examination.

If a duplex kidney is associated, the kidney will typically appear with hydronephrosis of the upper pole. However, it is not uncommon to see urine collection in the lower pole as a result of reflux (Figure 63-38, *A* and *B*). The ureter associated with the ureterocele is commonly dilated, tortuous, and connects to the bladder in an abnormal location. Because this abnormality is associated with

the splitting of the embryologic buds, a duplication of the vessels may be apparent. The use of color Doppler can aid in this finding (Figure 63-38, *C* and *D*). The amniotic fluid level is typically normal. However, ureterocele may obstruct the bladder or be associated with renal impairment leading to oligohydramnios.

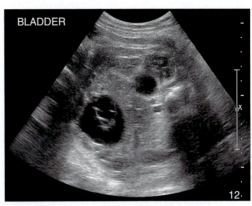

FIGURE 63-37 An anechoic mass surrounded by an echogenic rim is identified as a ureterocele in this patient with an obstructed upper pole of the right kidney.

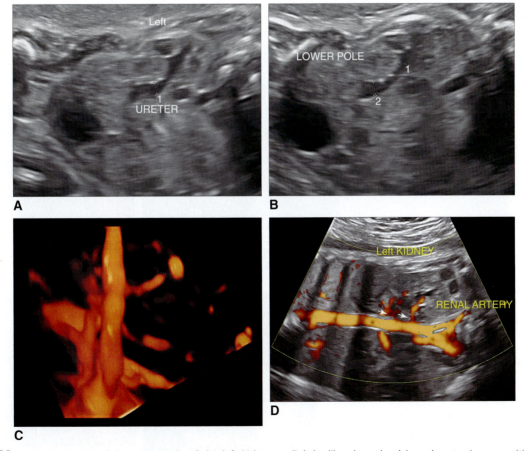

FIGURE 63-38 A, In this image of the upper pole of the left kidney, a slightly dilated renal pelvis and ureter is seen exiting the kidney. **B,** In the same kidney, a slightly dilated renal pelvis and ureter is seen exiting the lower pole of the left kidney. **C,** Power Doppler along with 3D technology was utilized to aid in the visualization of the renal arteries. The image reveals two left renal arteries. The arteries were each traced to the left kidney, one entered at the upper pole and the other at the lower pole. **D,** A coronal view with power Doppler easily identified the duplicated renal arteries.

Renal Tumors

Tumors of the fetal kidney are rare. It is often difficult to differentiate lung, liver, renal, and adrenal tumors in utero. For the purpose of this section, some of the renal and adrenal tumors documented in utero will be discussed.

Etiology. The most common renal tumor is a mesoblastic nephroma. Also known as a hamartoma, it is a benign tumor composed of a collection of oddly arranged tissue indigenous to the area (Figure 63-39). Wilms' tumor is a malignant tumor thought to be derived from abnormal renal cells; it is more commonly seen in females (Figure 63-40). The neuroblastoma of the adrenal gland is a malignant tumor that develops from nerve tissue in the adrenal gland.

Clinical Findings and Prognosis. Although renal tumors are rare, there is an associated risk of tumor

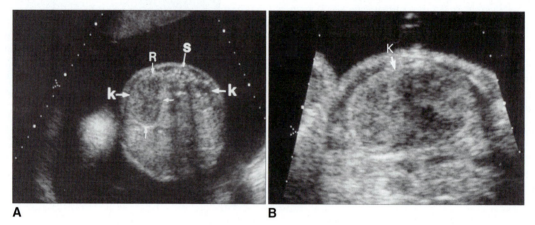

FIGURE 63-39 A, Mesoblastic nephroma in a 32-week fetus showing obvious enlargement of the right kidney *(k, arrows) (R)* compared with the left kidney *(k)*. Hydramnios was observed. *S,* Spine. **B,** In the same fetus the encapsulated and solid appearance of the nephroma *(K)* was observed. The nephroma was removed within a few days of birth.

FIGURE 63-40 A, This fetus presents with a solid abdominal mass in the area of the left kidney. The right kidney appears within normal limits. **B,** The left kidney could not be clearly seen. The solid mass was large and extended from the stomach to the fetal bladder. **C,** Rendering of the mass determined the mass was inferior to the diaphragm. **D,** Color Doppler revealed internal vascularity within the mass. Upon delivery, a biopsy of the mass revealed Wilms' tumor.

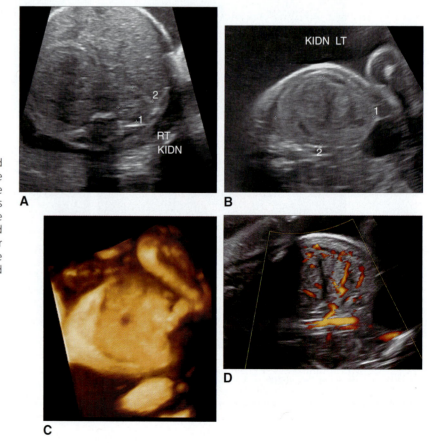

BOX 63-7 | Sonographic Findings of Renal Tumors

Mesoblastic nephroma. Large, single, solid mass originating from the kidney; appears isoechoic or hyperechoic to kidney parenchyma.
Wilms' tumor. Solid or partially cystic.
Neuroblastoma. Varying echo patterns (usually echogenic) with diffuse vascularity and possibly liver metastasis.

development in certain syndromes. These syndromes include Beckwith-Wiedemann, Perlman, and Drash. In cases of mesoblastic nephroma, the opposite kidney is usually normal; therefore, with surgical removal of the affected kidney, prognosis is excellent. Renal tumors typically appear more commonly in males and are benign. The prognosis for Wilms' tumor is good with early resection. Neuroblastomas usually present in the third trimester and occur more often on the right side. If the mass is solid, it will likely metastasize to the liver in utero. If the mass is large or metastasis is evident, fetal hydrops is likely to develop. Polyhydramnios is a typical finding with these tumors. The patient may undergo therapeutic amnioreductions to prevent preterm labor or as a result of maternal clinical symptoms.

Sonographic Findings. Masses in the kidney should be suspected when the contour of the kidney is distorted or replaced by a mass and the pelvicaliceal echoes are absent (Box 63-7). Polyhydramnios is a typical manifestation, as are enlarged abdominal circumference measurements.

CONGENITAL MALFORMATIONS OF THE GENITAL SYSTEM

Although congenital malformations of the genital system are rare, the sonographic team may be requested to determine the gender of the fetus when a gender-linked disorder is considered (i.e., hemophilia or aqueductal stenosis). Because these conditions usually occur in male fetuses, identification of male genitalia aids in counseling and diagnostic testing. Likewise, the demonstration of abnormal fetal genitalia may indicate syndromes of the endocrine and genital systems. In the female, positive identification of the labia is as essential to the diagnosis as demonstration of the penis and scrotum is in the male.

Hydrocele

Etiology. Hydroceles occur in the male fetus and are seen as an accumulation of serous fluid surrounding the testicle, resulting from a communication with the peritoneal cavity.
Clinical Findings and Prognosis. Hydroceles may occur unilaterally or bilaterally and are generally benign.

They can be identified as simple or complex. Complex hydroceles have been identified secondary to hemorrhage, infarction, or torsion of the testes. In the majority of cases of simple hydroceles, the testes are normal and the hydrocele will resolve after birth. Hydroceles have been reported in cases of hydrops.

Sonographic Findings. With a scrotal scan, simple hydroceles appear as anechoic fluid surrounding or partially surrounding the testes. Echogenicities present within the fluid indicate a complex hydrocele.

Undescended Testicles

Etiology. The gonads eventually descend from the abdomen to the pelvis. As this occurs, a diverticulum of the peritoneum, the processus vaginalis, protrudes through the anterior abdominal wall to form the primordium of the inguinal canal. The processus vaginalis is attached to a ligament that extends from the caudal pole of the gonad to the labioscrotal swelling.

In the male, the testes remain near the deep inguinal rings until the 28th week. They descend through the inguinal canals and enter the scrotum before birth. If the descent is interrupted or stopped, the testes will remain located within the inguinal canal. This condition is called undescended testes, or **cryptorchidism.** The distal part of the processus vaginalis persists as the tunica vaginalis of the testis. In the female, the ligament attaches to the uterus to form the ovarium ligament and the round ligament.
Clinical Findings and Prognosis. Undescended testicles are associated with risk of torsion and development of cancer. However, the risks are significantly lowered if the testes are surgically placed within the scrotum sac early in childhood.

Sonographic Findings. The scrotal sac will appear void of testicular tissue. Small amounts of anechoic fluid will likely be evident in the scrotum. In utero diagnosis of the testes within the inguinal canal is difficult.

Ambiguous Genitalia

Etiology. *Ambiguous genitalia* is the sonographic finding that describes the inability to delineate fetal gender. Several congenital malformations contribute to this finding. The malformations typically result from chromosomal defects or abnormal hormone levels:

- *True hermaphroditism.* This is a rare condition in which both ovarian and testicular tissues are present. The internal and external genitalia are variable. Most fetuses will have a normal karyotype, but some are mosaics (46,XX/46,XY). Determination of fetal gender may be critical in establishing a correct diagnosis (see Figure 59-40).
- *Female pseudohermaphrodism.* The female fetus with pseudohermaphrodism has a 46,XX karyotype. The most common cause is congenital virilizing adrenal

hyperplasia that causes masculinization of the external genitalia (enlarged clitoris, abnormalities of the urogenital sinus, and partial fusion of the labia majora).

- *Male pseudohermaphrodism.* The male fetus with pseudohermaphroditism has testes and a 46,XY karyotype. There can be variable external and internal genitalia depending on the development of the penis and genital ducts.

Clinical Findings and Prognosis. The sonographer must be careful diagnosing ambiguous genitalia because penile and clitoral size may vary in the normal fetus. Genetic amniocentesis is needed for karyotyping to determine the genetic makeup. Chromosomal abnormalities associated with ambiguous genitalia include trisomy 13, triploidy, and certain deletions and translocation. Other associations include cloacal malformation and adrenogenital syndrome. Surgery may be required to repair associated abnormalities or for cosmetic concerns.

Sonographic Findings. Sonographically the key signs to investigate for gender are absent. In many cases an abnormally small penis is hard to differentiate from the enlarged clitoris, or a bifid scrotum may appear as enlarged labia (Figure 63-41).

OTHER PELVIC MASSES

Hydrometrocolpos

Etiology. Obstruction of the uterus and vagina that results in collections of fluid is referred to **hydrometro-colpos**. The obstruction has numerous causes, such as atresia of the vagina or cervix, imperforate hymen or abnormal membranes within the vaginal lumen.

Clinical Findings and Prognosis. Hydrometrocolpos has been noted in conjunction with a double uterus and septated vagina (vagina divided by a septum into two components), cloacal malformations, renal agenesis, and as part of a syndrome. The fluid collection may be so large that it extends into the abdominal cavity or may cause compression of the ureters and hydronephrosis of the kidneys. The prognosis depends on other abnormalities present; the malformation itself can be surgically corrected.

Sonographic Findings. Hydrometrocolpos appears as a hypoechoic "cystlike" ovoid mass posterior to the bladder in the area of the uterus. These masses may be predominantly cystic, may contain midlevel echoes, or may have fluid-debris levels. Echoes within these masses may result from mucous secretions.

Fetal Ovarian Cyst

Etiology. The ovarian mass results from maternal hormonal stimulation and is usually benign. The cysts typically represent normal functional ovarian cysts.

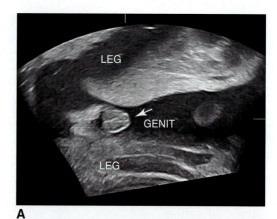
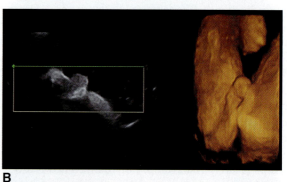
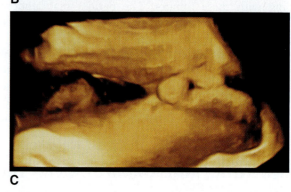

FIGURE 63-41 **A,** A clear delineation of external genitalia could not be made in this third-trimester fetus. **B** and **C,** Further evaluation with 3D and 4D technology did not provide additional information regarding clear support of male or female external genitalia.

Clinical Findings and Prognosis. Ovarian cysts represent the most common cystic mass in female fetuses. They range in size from small to large and are usually located on one side of the abdomen or lower pelvis. They can be unilateral or bilateral and are often confused with other masses. Differential considerations include a mesenteric cyst, a urachal cyst, or an enteric duplication. Most cysts will regress either in utero or during the postnatal period. However, complications have been documented. The mass may twist on itself, which may lead to torsion, rupture, or intestinal obstruction. Treatment is dependent on associated complications.

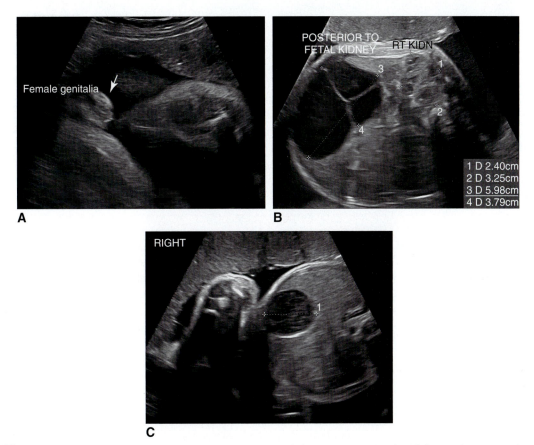

FIGURE 63-42 A-C, Ovarian cyst may appear anechoic or hypoechoic. If the cyst is associated with hemorrhage or torsion, sonographic features may include a complex or solid appearance.

◢ **Sonographic Findings.** A **fetal ovarian cyst** may appear anechoic or hypoechoic. If the cyst is associated with hemorrhage or torsion, sonographic features may include a complex or solid appearance (Figure 63-42).

ACKNOWLEDGEMENTS

Thanks to Roy Bors-Koefoed, MD; Janet Thweatt, BHS, RT(R), RDMS; Patricia Williams, RDMS; Christina Taff, BHS, RDMS; and Terri Vest RN, RDMS, for their contribution of sonographic images for this chapter.

The Fetal Skeleton

Charlotte G. Henningsen

OBJECTIVES

On completion of this chapter, you should be able to:
- Describe in detail the embryology of the fetal skeleton
- Describe the variety of musculoskeletal anomalies that can occur in the fetus
- Differentiate sonographically among the most common skeletal dysplasias
- List limb abnormalities and the anomalies that are associated with specific defects

OUTLINE

EMBRYOLOGY OF THE FETAL SKELETON

The majority of the musculoskeletal system forms from the primitive mesoderm arising from mesenchymal cells that are the embryonic connective tissue. These cells arise from different regions of the body. The vertebral column and ribs arise from the somites, and the limbs arise from the lateral plate mesoderm. The formation of the head is more complex in that the cranial bones that form the roof and base of the skull arise from mesenchymal cells of the primitive mesoderm, but the facial bones actually arise from mesenchymal cells arising from the neural crest, which is ectodermal in origin. The skeleton initially appears as cartilaginous structures that later undergo ossification.

Limb development begins the 26th or 27th day after conception with the appearance of upper limb buds. Lower extremity development begins 2 days later. Although the stages of development for the upper and lower extremities are the same, lower extremity development continues to lag behind that of the upper extremities. Initially the limbs have a paddle shape with a ridge of thickened ectoderm, known as the apical ectodermal ridge, at the apex of each bud. Digital rays begin to differentiate from the apical ectodermal ridge around day 41 through a process of cell death of the ridge between the digits. The fingers are distinctly evident by day 49, although they are still webbed, and by the eighth week of development the fingers are longer. The development of the feet and toes is essentially complete by the ninth week, although the soles of the feet are still turned inward at this time.

Anomalies of the skeletal system often result from genetic factors, though the cause may be unknown or be the result of environmental factors, including drug or mechanical effects.

ABNORMALITIES OF THE SKELETON

Skeletal dysplasia is the term used to describe abnormal growth and density of cartilage and bone, and the incidence is 1 in 4000 to 5000 births in the United States. Dwarfism is the condition of a disproportionately short stature; it occurs secondary to a skeletal dysplasia. There are more than 100 types of skeletal dysplasias, and not all of them are amenable to sonographic detection. The perinatal team may be able to isolate a skeletal dysplasia when abnormal skeletal structures are observed, such as bone shortening or hypomineralization.

Some skeletal dysplasias are incompatible with life. The lethal forms characteristically are extremely severe in their prenatal appearance, as with severe micromelia.

Nonlethal skeletal dysplasias tend to manifest in a milder form. The sonographer should become familiar with the sonographic characteristics of the more common skeletal dysplasias that can be diagnosed in utero.

There are multiple anomalies of the musculoskeletal system that may be identified with ultrasound. Many of these osteochondrodysplasias have similar features, although often there are distinguishing features that can lead to a diagnosis. A list of short-limb skeletal dysplasias, ultrasound characteristics, and their distinguishing features are listed in Table 64-1.

Sonographic Evaluation of Skeletal Dysplasias

The patient whose fetus is at risk for a skeletal dysplasia is commonly referred to a maternal-fetal center for genetic counseling and a targeted ultrasound. Although many skeletal dysplasias are inherited, sporadic occurrences and new mutations do occur, so it is important to screen for skeletal dysplasias as part of every obstetric ultrasound examination. Most prenatally diagnosed skeletal dysplasias occur in association with polyhydramnios or other fetal anomalies or when there is a risk for recurrence.

When a skeletal dysplasia is suspected, the protocol of the obstetric ultrasound examination should be adjusted to include the following criteria:

1. Assess limb shortening. All long bones should be measured. A skeletal dysplasia is suspected when limb lengths fall more than two standard deviations below the mean (Tables 64-2 and 64-3).
2. Assess bone contour. Thickness, abnormal bowing or curvature, fractures, and a ribbon-like appearance should be noted.
3. Estimate degree of ossification. Decreased attenuation of the bones with decreased shadowing suggests hypomineralization. Special attention should be focused toward this assessment of the cranium, spine, ribs, and long bones.
4. Evaluate the thoracic circumference and shape. A long, narrow chest or a bell-shaped chest may be indicative of specific dysplasias.
5. Survey for coexistent hand and foot anomalies, such as talipes and polydactyly.
6. Evaluate the face and profile for facial clefts, frontal bossing, micrognathia, hypertelorism, and other facial anomalies that may be associated with skeletal dysplasias.

TABLE 64-1	Osteochondrodysplasia Findings	
Anomaly	**Sonographic Findings**	**Distinguishing Characteristics**
Thanatophoric dysplasia	Severe micromelia Macrocephaly Cloverleaf skull Narrow thorax	Cloverleaf skull
Achondrogenesis	Severe micromelia Macrocephaly Poor ossification of spine, skull Short thorax	Decreased ossification Severity of limb shortening
Achondroplasia	Rhizomelia Macrocephaly Trident hands	Rhizomelic shortening Trident hands
Camptomelic dysplasia	Hypoplastic fibulas Long bone bowing Micrognathia Small thorax Talipes	Fibular hypoplasia Bowing affects lower extremities
Osteogenesis imperfecta (type II)	Severe micromelia Generalized hypomineralization Narrow thorax Multiple fractures	Normal head size Hypomineralization of skull Multiple fractures
Short-rib polydactyly syndrome	Micromelia Narrow thorax Facial cleft Polydactyly	Facial anomalies Polydactyly
Hypophosphatasia	Mild limb shortening Narrow thorax Limb fractures and bowing	Hypomineralization of skull Fractures

TABLE 64-2	Length of the Bones of the Leg: Normal Values						

Week No.	Tibia Percentile				Fibula Percentile		
	5th	50th	95th		5th	50th	95th
12	—	7	—	:	—	6	—
13	—	10	—	:	—	9	—
14	7	12	17	:	6	12	19
15	9	15	20	—:—	9	15	21
16	12	17	22	:	13	18	23
17	15	20	25	:	13	21	28
18	17	22	27	:	15	23	31
19	20	25	30	:	19	26	33
20	22	27	33	:	21	28	36
21	25	30	35	:	24	31	37
22	27	32	38	:	27	33	39
23	30	35	40	:	28	35	42
24	32	37	42	:	29	37	45
25	34	40	45	—:—	34	40	45
26	37	42	47	:	36	42	47
27	39	44	49	:	37	44	50
28	41	46	51	:	38	45	53
29	43	48	53	:	41	47	54
30	45	50	55	:	43	49	56
31	47	52	57	:	42	51	59
32	48	54	59	:	42	52	63
33	50	55	60	:	46	54	62
34	52	57	62	:	46	55	65
35	53	58	64	—:—	51	57	62
36	55	60	65	:	54	58	63
37	56	61	67	:	54	59	65
38	58	63	68	:	56	61	65
39	59	64	69	:	56	62	67
40	61	66	71	:	59	63	67
	mm	mm	mm		mm	mm	mm

From Jeanty P, Romero R, editors: *Obstetrical ultrasound,* New York, 1984, McGraw-Hill.

7. Survey for other associated anomalies, such as hydrocephaly, heart defects, and nonimmune hydrops.

The manifestation of skeletal dysplasias varies based on the specific dysplasia, and three-dimensional ultrasound may aid in the diagnosis. First-trimester assessment may present with an increased nuchal translucency, and chorionic villus sampling may provide important diagnostic information regarding the type of skeletal dysplasia. Additionally, long bones are affected in different patterns (Figure 64-1) according to the dysplasia. Rhizomelia is shortening of the proximal bone segment (humerus and femur). Mesomelia refers to shortening of the middle segments (radius/ulna and tibia/fibula). Micromelia describes the shortening of the entire extremity. Sonographic examination of the long bones should include an assessment to define whether there is segmental shortening or micromelia, because this will aid in the diagnosis. Three-dimensional evaluation may provide further definition of the abnormality.

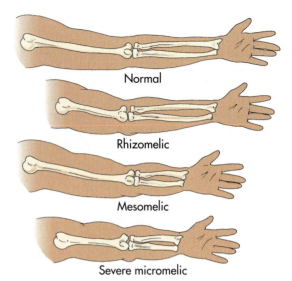

FIGURE 64-1 Varieties of short-limb dysplasia according to the affected bones. Rhizomelic dysplasia is characterized by shortening of the proximal long bones (humerus and femur). Mesomelic dysplasia is described as shortening of the distal extremities (radius/ulna and tibia/fibula). Severe micromelia produces shortening of both proximal and distal extremities.

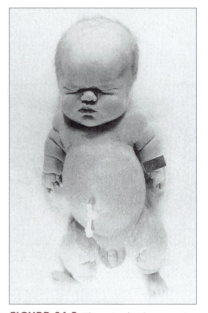

FIGURE 64-2 Thanatophoric neonate.

Thanatophoric Dysplasia

Thanatophoric dysplasia is the most common lethal skeletal dysplasia and occurs in 1 in 4000 to 10,000 births (Figure 64-2). The term *thanatophoric* comes from the Greek word *thanatos,* which means *death personified.* The two main subdivisions of thanatophoric dysplasia are types I and II. Type I is characterized by short, curved femurs and flat vertebral bodies. Type II is characterized by straight, short femurs, flat vertebral bodies, and a cloverleaf skull. Most cases of thanatophoric dysplasia are sporadic occurrences and the result of mutations in

TABLE 64-3	Length of the Bones of the Arm: Normal Values						
		Ulna Percentile				Radius Percentile		
Week No.		5th	50th	95th		5th	50th	95th
12	:	—	7	—	:	—	7	—
13	:	5	10	15	:	6	10	14
14	:	8	13	18	:	8	13	17
15	—:—	11	16	21	—:—	11	15	20
16	:	13	18	23	:	13	18	22
17	:	16	21	26	:	14	20	26
18	:	19	24	29	:	15	22	29
19	:	21	26	31	:	20	24	29
20	:	24	29	34	:	22	27	32
21	:	26	31	36	:	24	29	33
22	:	28	33	38	:	27	31	34
23	:	31	36	41	:	26	32	39
24	:	33	38	43	:	26	34	42
25	—:—	35	40	45	—:—	31	36	41
26	:	37	42	47	:	32	37	43
27	:	39	44	49	:	33	39	45
28	:	41	46	51	:	33	40	48
29	:	43	48	53	:	36	42	47
30	:	44	49	54	:	36	43	49
31	:	46	51	56	:	38	44	50
32	:	48	53	58	:	37	45	53
33	:	49	54	59	:	41	46	51
34	:	51	56	61	:	40	47	53
35	—:—	52	57	62	—:—	41	48	54
36	:	53	58	63	:	39	48	57
37	:	55	60	65	:	45	49	53
38	:	56	61	66	:	45	49	54
39	:	57	62	67	:	45	50	54
40	:	58	63	68	:	46	50	55
	mm	mm	mm	mm	mm			

From Jeanty P, Romero R, editors: *Obstetrical ultrasound,* New York, 1984, McGraw-Hill.

the fibroblast growth factor receptor 3 (FGFR3) gene. Prenatal molecular analysis can aid in making the definitive diagnosis.

The prognosis for thanatophoric dysplasia is extremely grim. It is considered a lethal anomaly, with most infants dying shortly after birth as a result of pulmonary hypoplasia, which results from the narrow thorax.

Sonographic Findings. The sonographic features of thanatophoric dysplasia include the following:

- Severe micromelia (Figure 64-3, *A* and *B*), especially of the proximal bones (rhizomelia)
- Cloverleaf deformity (Kleeblattschädel skull), which occurs as a result of premature **craniosynostosis** and may be associated with agenesis of the corpus callosum
- Narrow thorax with shortened ribs (Figure 64-3, *C* and *D*)
- Protuberant abdomen
- Frontal bossing (bulging forehead)
- Hypertelorism (widely spaced eyes)
- Flat vertebral bodies (platyspondyly)

Other sonographic findings that may be associated with thanatophoric dysplasia include severe polyhydramnios, hydrocephalus, and nonimmune hydrops.

Achondroplasia

Achondroplasia is the most common nonlethal skeletal dysplasia and occurs in 2.53 of every 100,000 births. It results from decreased endochondral bone formation, which produces short, squat bones. It is most commonly the result of a spontaneous mutation but can also be transmitted in an autosomal fashion. Advanced paternal age increases the risk for this dysplasia.

The prognosis for achondroplasia depends on the form. **Heterozygous achondroplasia,** inherited from one parent, has a good survival rate with normal intelligence and a normal life span. Health problems may include neurologic complications that may require orthopedic or neurologic surgical intervention. **Homozygous achondroplasia,** inherited from two parents, is considered lethal, with most infants dying shortly after birth from

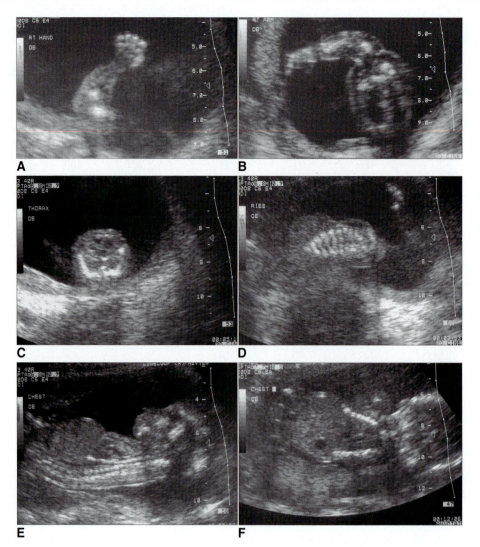

FIGURE 64-3 Lethal skeletal dysplasia consistent with thanatophoric dysplasia at a gestational age of 18 weeks, 1 day. **A** and **B,** The right arm demonstrates micromelia. The lower extremities were also short, with the femurs measuring a gestational age of 14 weeks. **C,** The thorax was very narrow. **D,** The ribs were short. The abdomen was protuberant **(E)** and compared with the narrow thorax **(F)** gives the appearance of a champagne cork.

respiratory complications. With this form, sonographic findings are more severe and include a narrow thorax.

🔖 **Sonographic Findings.** The sonographic features of achondroplasia may not be evident until after 22 weeks of gestation, when biometry becomes abnormal. Ultrasound-guided chorionic villus sampling may aid in the diagnosis in the first trimester for parents with this genetic disorder, and amniocentesis may also be utilized. Sonographic findings include the following:

- Rhizomelia
- Macrocephaly
- Trident hands (short proximal and middle phalanges)
- A depressed nasal bridge
- Frontal bossing
- Mild ventriculomegaly may be identified

Achondrogenesis

Achondrogenesis is a rare, lethal skeletal dysplasia occurring in 1 of 40,000 fetuses. It is caused by cartilage abnormalities that result in abnormal bone formation and hypomineralization. The two types of achondrogenesis are types I (Parenti-Fraccaro) and II (Langer-Saldino). Type I is considered more severe and is transmitted in an autosomal recessive mode, whereas type II is less severe, more common, and is the result of a spontaneous mutation.

The prognosis for achondrogenesis is grim. It is a lethal abnormality with infants either being stillborn or dying shortly after birth from pulmonary hypoplasia.

🔖 **Sonographic Findings.** The sonographic features (Figure 64-4) of achondrogenesis include the following:

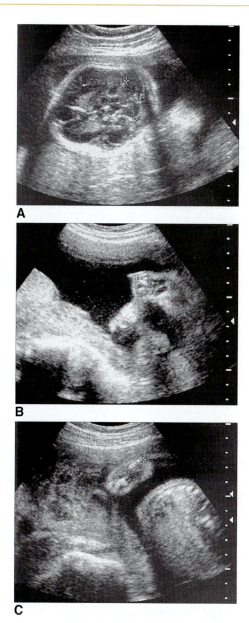

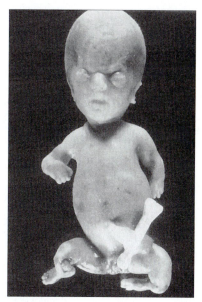

FIGURE 64-5 Postmortem photograph of neonate with osteogenesis imperfecta (type II).

FIGURE 64-4 This fetus at 24 weeks' gestation presented with decreased ossification that was noted in the spine and (A) calvarium, which was compressible. Severe micromelia is evidenced in the (B) femur and (C) humerus, where the measurement was consistent with 13 weeks' gestation. Achondrogenesis was diagnosed following delivery, and the baby died shortly thereafter.

- Severe micromelia
- Decreased or absent ossification of the spine
- Macrocephaly
- Short trunk
- Short thorax and short ribs
- Micrognathia
- Polyhydramnios
- Hydrops possibly identified

Osteogenesis Imperfecta

Osteogenesis imperfecta is a rare disorder of collagen production leading to brittle bones; manifestations in the teeth, skin, and ligaments; and blue sclera. There are four classifications, types I to IV. Types I and IV are the mildest forms, and it would be unlikely that a diagnosis would be made in utero. Types I and IV are transmitted in an autosomal-dominant fashion. Type III is a severe form that may be transmitted in an autosomal-dominant or autosomal-recessive manner. Type II (Figure 64-5) is considered the most severe form of osteogenesis imperfecta, having a lethal outcome. It has a prevalence of 1 to 2 per 100,000 births and is inherited in autosomal-dominant or autosomal recessive fashion or may result from a spontaneous mutation.

The prognosis for osteogenesis imperfecta depends on the type. Children with types I and IV may have multiple fractures during childhood and may be short. Type I children may also suffer with kyphoscoliosis and deafness. Because of the severity of the brittle bones and multiple fractures, osteogenesis imperfecta type III may produce significant handicaps with progressive deformities of the long bones and spine. Infants with type II usually die shortly after birth because of respiratory complications.

Sonographic Findings. Osteogenesis imperfecta has presented with an increased nuchal translucency in the first trimester of pregnancy. Other more specific sonographic features of osteogenesis imperfecta type II include the following:

- Generalized hypomineralization of the bones, especially the calvarium (Figure 64-6)
- Multiple fractures of the long bones, ribs, and spine (Figures 64-7 and 64-8)
- Narrow thorax (see Figure 64-6, A)
- Micromelia

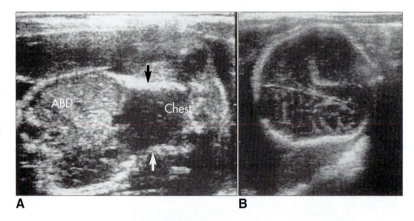

FIGURE 64-6 A, In this fetus with osteogenesis imperfecta (type II), a small thoracic cavity *(arrows)* is shown. *ABD,* Abdomen. **B,** In the same fetus, hypomineralization of the skull is evident. Note the improved resolution of brain anatomy because of the lack of calvarial calcification.

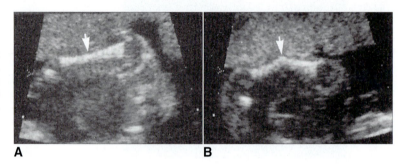

FIGURE 64-7 Images of both femurs in a 22-week fetus. **A,** The femur *(arrow)* is normal compared with **B,** in which a femoral fracture *(arrow)* is shown. Other long bones appeared normal in length and contour. There was hypomineralization of the spine. Osteogenesis imperfecta type I or IV is considered.

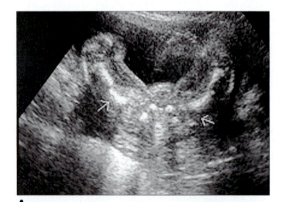

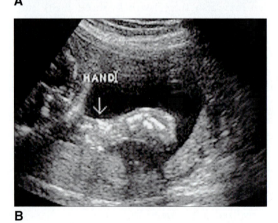

FIGURE 64-8 A, Bilateral fractured femora in a fetus with osteogenesis imperfecta (type II). **B,** In the same fetus, fractures of the ulna and radius are demonstrated.

In addition to these findings, brain structures are clearly visualized because of the hypomineralization of the calvarium. The calvarium will also be compressible. The multiple fractures that have occurred during the course of pregnancy may leave the bones bowed, thickened, and sharply angulated. Polyhydramnios may also be evident.

The sonographic features of osteogenesis imperfecta type III are similar to those of type II, though it is less severe.

Congenital Hypophosphatasia

Congenital **hypophosphatasia** is a condition that presents with diffuse hypomineralization of the bone caused by an alkaline phosphatase deficiency. The occurrence rate is 1 per 100,000 births. It is an inherited condition transmitted in an autosomal-recessive manner. Congenital hypophosphatasia may have features similar to osteogenesis imperfecta and achondrogenesis. Diagnosis can be confirmed with alkaline phosphatase assay, which can be achieved through fetal blood sampling or chorionic villus sampling, or through DNA analysis.

Congenital hypophosphatasia is a lethal disorder, with death usually occurring shortly after birth as a result of respiratory complications.

Sonographic Findings. The sonographic features of congenital hypophosphatasia include the following:

- Diffuse hypomineralization of the bones
- Moderate to severe micromelia
- Extremities that may be bowed, fractured, or absent

- Poorly ossified cranium with well-visualized brain structures
- Small thoracic cavity

Diastrophic Dysplasia

Diastrophic dysplasia is a rare disorder characterized by micromelia, talipes, cleft palate, micrognathia, scoliosis, short stature, earlobe deformities, and hand abnormalities (Figure 64-9). It is inherited in an autosomal-recessive pattern, and the mutation has been mapped to the long arm of chromosome 5. It has been reported with a significant increased frequency in the Finnish population.

The prognosis for diastrophic dysplasia is variable. There is an increase in infant mortality because of respiratory complications related to the micrognathia and kyphoscoliosis. This is not a lethal disorder, with most patients having a normal life span and normal intelligence. Adult height is usually less than 4 feet, and orthopedic abnormalities can cause significant handicaps.

▌ **Sonographic Findings.** The sonographic features of diastrophic dysplasia include the following:

- Micromelia (Figure 64-10)
- Talipes
- Fixed abducted thumb (hitchhiker thumb; see Figure 64-10, *B*)
- Scoliosis
- Talipes (clubfoot)
- Micrognathia (small chin)
- Cleft palate

Camptomelic Dysplasia

Camptomelic (bent bone) dysplasia is a group of lethal skeletal dysplasias that are characterized by bowing of the long bones. This rare, short-limbed dysplasia occurs in 1 per 150,000 births. Most cases occur as a spontaneous mutation, but camptomelic dysplasia is also inherited in an autosomal-recessive pattern.

Camptomelic dysplasia is considered a lethal anomaly, with most infants dying in the neonatal period because of pulmonary hypoplasia. Infants surviving the neonatal period usually die within the first year of life and suffer

with respiratory and feeding problems, are developmentally delayed, and are mentally retarded.

▌ **Sonographic Findings.** The sonographic features of camptomelic dysplasia include the following:

- Bowing of the long bones with the lower extremities affected most severely (Figures 64-11 and 64-12)
- Small thorax
- Hypoplastic fibulas
- Hypoplastic scapulae
- Hypertelorism
- Cleft palate
- Micrognathia
- Talipes (Figures 64-13 and 64-14)
- Hydrocephalus
- Polyhydramnios
- Hydronephrosis

Roberts' Syndrome

Roberts' syndrome is a rare autosomal-recessive disorder characterized by phocomelia and facial anomalies. It is

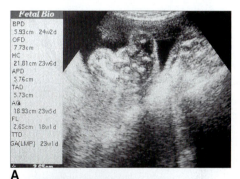

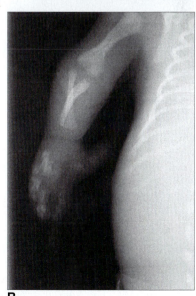

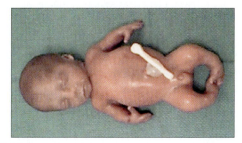

FIGURE 64-9 Postmortem photograph of a fetus with diastrophic dysplasia.

FIGURE 64-10 Diastrophic dysplasia imaged at 23 weeks and 1 day. **A,** Micromelia is demonstrated in this femur measuring 18 weeks, 1 day. The thoracic circumference was also small. **B,** Postmortem radiograph demonstrates the "hitchhiker thumb."

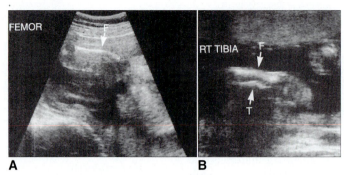

FIGURE 64-11 A, Camptomelic dysplasia and Swyer syndrome in a 20-week fetus with femoral bowing *(F)* found bilaterally. The femoral lengths were normal. **B,** In the same fetus, the tibias *(T)* were short and hypoplastic with sharp anterior bowing of the midshaft of the bone. Distal bowing was also observed. The fibulas *(F)* were hypoplastic and bowed. The upper extremities were normal in length without bowing or angulation. Bilateral hydronephrosis was observed. Examination of the neonate and radiologic findings (see Figure 64-12) confirmed the diagnosis of camptomelic dysplasia. Gonadal dysgenesis (female internal and external genitalia with a male karyotype) was consistent with Swyer syndrome. The neonate had other characteristic signs of the disorder, including tall and narrow hypomineralized ischial bones, absent pubic bone ossification, receding chin, hypoplastic cervical vertebrae, elongated clavicles, hypoplastic scapulae, and flexion abnormalities of the feet.

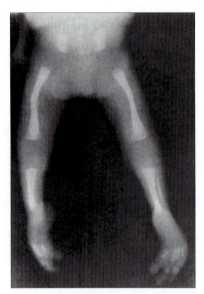

FIGURE 64-12 Radiograph of neonate shown in Figures 64-11, 64-13, and 64-14 with camptomelic dysplasia and Swyer syndrome. The radiograph demonstrates the lower extremity deformities, including anterior lateral bowing of the femurs at the midshaft. Both tibias are short, with sharp anterior bowing at midshaft and mild bowing at the distal ends. The fibulas are hypoplastic and bowed. Minimal ischial ossification and absent mineralization of the pubic bone are shown.

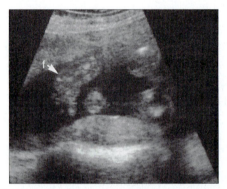

FIGURE 64-13 In the fetus with camptomelic dysplasia and Swyer syndrome, as shown in Figures 64-11, 64-12, and 64-14, abnormal plantar flexion of the feet is shown. The feet *(f)* are notably supinated, with curvature to the soles of the feet. The toes are plantar flexed, with the great toes separated by flexion.

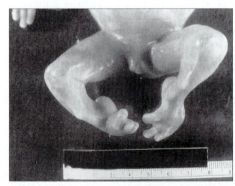

FIGURE 64-14 Postmortem photograph of the neonate shown in Figures 64-11, 64-12, and 64-13, with camptomelic dysplasia and Swyer syndrome. Note the markedly angulated lower legs with protrusion of the tibia anteriorly at the midshaft. The fibulas were hypoplastic and bowed. The feet, as shown in Figure 64-13, are abnormally rotated with prominent heels (rocker-bottom feet).

also known as a pseudothalidomide syndrome. Roberts' syndrome may present with associated chromosomal abnormalities.

The prognosis for Roberts' syndrome is poor. Stillbirth and infant mortality are common. Survivors are growth-restricted and have severe mental retardation.

Sonographic Findings. The sonographic features of Roberts' syndrome include the following:

- Phocomelia with the upper extremities more severely affected

- Bilateral cleft lip and palate
- Hypertelorism
- Microcephaly
- Cardiovascular, renal, and gastrointestinal anomalies may be identified

Short-Rib Polydactyly Syndrome

Short-rib polydactyly syndrome is a lethal skeletal dysplasia characterized by short ribs, short limbs, and **polydactyly**, with a prevalence of 1 in 200,000 births. There have been four primary types of this dysplasia defined, which are inherited in an autosomal-recessive manner. Type I is also known as Saldino-Noonan syndrome; type II is also known as Majewski syndrome; and type III is known as Naumoff syndrome. Type IV, Beemer-Langer dysplasia, was included in this group of short-rib dysplasias in the 1992 International Classification of Osteochondrodysplasias, and there have been a total of seven types of short-rib polydactyly syndrome classified in the literature.

Short-rib polydactyly syndrome is considered a lethal anomaly. Most infants die shortly after birth as a result of pulmonary hypoplasia.

Sonographic Findings. Common sonographic features of short-rib polydactyly syndrome include the following:

- Narrow thorax with short ribs
- Polydactyly (Figure 64-15)
- Micromelia
- Midline facial cleft

Other sonographic findings associated with short-rib dysplasias include anomalies of the central nervous system, cardiovascular system, and genitourinary tract. Polyhydramnios may also be identified. Saldino-Noonan and Naumoff syndromes are usually not associated with cleft lip and palate, and polydactyly may not always be present in Beemer-Langer dysplasia.

Jeune's Syndrome

Jeune's syndrome, also known as asphyxiating thoracic dysplasia, is a skeletal dysplasia characterized by a very narrow thorax. The prevalence of Jeune's syndrome is 1 in 100,000 to 130,000 births, and it is inherited in an autosomal-recessive manner. Two types of Jeune's syndrome have been described, and there is a range of

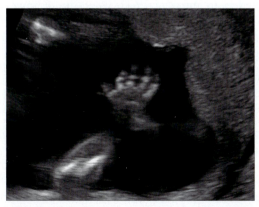

FIGURE 64-15 Polydactyly of the fetal hands is identified.

severity with the most severe form resulting in death because of pulmonary hypoplasia, which results from the narrow thorax.

Sonographic Findings. The sonographic features of Jeune's syndrome include the following:

- Small thorax
- Rhizomelia
- Renal dysplasia
- Polydactyly (less common)

Ellis-van Creveld Syndrome

Ellis-van Creveld syndrome is also known as chondroectodermal dysplasia. The prevalence is 1 in 60,000 births, with an increased frequency in the Amish community estimated to be up to 1 in 5000 births. It is inherited in an autosomal-recessive pattern.

Ellis-van Creveld syndrome may present with a narrow thorax, causing pulmonary hypoplasia, and heart defects, the most common of which is the atrial septal defect (ASD). Approximately one half of these patients will die during infancy from cardiorespiratory complications. Other features identified with this syndrome include abnormal teeth, hypoplastic nails, and thin hair. Survivors have normal intellect and are short in stature.

Sonographic Findings. The sonographic features of Ellis-van Creveld include the following:

- Limb shortening
- Narrow thorax
- Polydactyly (see Figure 64-15)
- Heart defects (50%)

Caudal Regression Syndrome/Sirenomelia

Caudal regression syndrome (CRS) includes a range of malformations of the caudal end of the neural tube. Sirenomelia is an anomaly in which there is fusion of the lower extremities. Sirenomelia had been traditionally considered an extreme form of CRS but it is currently thought to be a separate disorder. The overall incidence of CRS is unknown; the incidence of sirenomelia is reported to be 1 in 60,000 births, with a male prevalence of 2.7 to 1.

The cause of CRS is not completely understood, although it has been associated with diabetes. Genetic factors have also been linked with this disorder. Vascular hypoperfusion is thought to be a causative factor in sirenomelia, with a single umbilical artery commonly associated that may divert blood flow to the caudal end. Sirenomelia is also associated with monozygotic twinning and with cocaine use.

The prognosis for caudal regression syndrome depends on the severity and the associated anomalies. Neurologic and orthopedic evaluations with their interventional techniques can help to reduce and correct deformities and minimize handicaps. Sirenomelia is considered a lethal anomaly because of the severe renal anomalies that result in oligohydramnios and pulmonary hypoplasia.

▸ **Sonographic Findings.** Sonographic features of caudal regression syndrome include the following:

- Sacral agenesis (Figure 64-16)
- Talipes
- Abnormal lumbar vertebrae, pelvic abnormalities, and contractures or decreased movement of the lower extremities may also be seen

Sonographic features of sirenomelia include the following:

- Variable fusion of the lower extremities (Figure 64-17)
- Bilateral renal agenesis
- Oligohydramnios
- Single umbilical artery

When severe oligohydramnios is present, a confident diagnosis with ultrasound may be difficult. Amnioinfusion, three-dimensional sonography, and magnetic resonance imaging may be used to evaluate the severity of anomalies.

VACTERL Association

The VACTERL association is a group of anomalies that may occur together. In this sporadic group of anomalies,

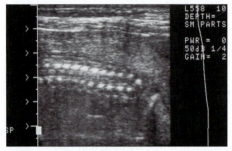

FIGURE 64-16 Sacral agenesis noted at 21 weeks of gestation. Note the lack of tapering usually seen in the lumbosacral area.

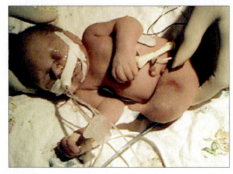

FIGURE 64-17 A neonate with sirenomelia. Note the fusion of the lower extremities. There was also bilateral renal agenesis, and the infant died shortly after birth. This was a twin pregnancy, and the other infant was normal.

*v*ertebral defects, *a*nal atresia, *c*ardiac anomalies, *t*racheo*e*sophageal fistula, *r*enal anomalies, and *l*imb dysplasia may occur in combination. For the VACTERL association to be considered, three of these features must be identified. A single umbilical artery may also be identified. When the VACTERL association is seen with accompanying hydrocephalus, it has been termed VACTERL-H syndrome. The VACTERL association with concurrent sirenomelia has also been reported.

Postural Anomalies

The normal development of the fetus requires movement. There are multiple events that can cause a decrease in fetal movement, including oligohydramnios, multiple gestations, and congenital uterine anomalies. Decreased movement may also be due to an abnormality of the fetal nerves, connective tissue, or musculature. These fetal conditions may not only cause a decrease or absence of fetal movement, but they may also result in abnormal contractures and postural deformities.

Arthrogryposis Multiplex Congenita. Arthrogryposis multiplex congenita is a condition marked by severe contractures of the extremities because of abnormal innervation and disorders of the muscles and connective tissue. It represents a group of disorders that may be inherited or sporadic.

▸ **Sonographic Findings.** The sonographic findings for arthrogryposis include the following:

- Rigid extremities
- Flexed arms
- Hyperextension of the knees
- Clenched hands
- Talipes

Polyhydramnios or oligohydramnios may accompany this anomaly, as can anomalies of the central nervous system. Other defects that may be associated include facial and renal anomalies. Additionally, fetal seizures have been identified in fetuses with arthrogryposis.

Lethal Multiple Pterygium Syndrome. Lethal multiple pterygium syndrome is characterized by webbing across the joints and multiple contractures. It is usually inherited in an autosomal-recessive fashion; however, an X-linked mode of inheritance has also been reported.

▸ **Sonographic Findings.** The sonographic findings for pterygium syndrome include the following:

- Limb contractures
- Webbing across joints
- Cystic hygroma

Micrognathia, renal anomalies, hydrops, and polyhydramnios are also associated with this syndrome.

Pena-Shokeir Syndrome. Pena-Shokeir syndrome is characterized by abnormal joint contractures, facial abnormalities, polyhydramnios, intrauterine growth restriction, and pulmonary hypoplasia. This syndrome may be inherited in an autosomal-recessive manner or as a sporadic occurrence. Pena-Shokeir syndrome and trisomy 18 have similar features, so karyotyping should be offered.

Sonographic Findings. The sonographic findings of Pena-Shokeir (Figure 64-18) include the following:

- Limb abnormalities such as contractures, clenched hands, talipes, and rocker-bottom feet
- Facial abnormalities, including micrognathia and cleft palate

Polyhydramnios and hydrops may also be identified.

OTHER LIMB ABNORMALITIES

Hand and foot abnormalities may occur with skeletal dysplasias, as part of a chromosomal syndrome, or as an isolated event. Amputation defects may be identified as total or partial absence and may be associated with amniotic band syndrome. Congenital absence of one or more extremities (amelia) may be observed prenatally (Figure 64-19).

Hand anomalies may include missing digits, fused digits (syndactyly) (Figure 64-20), or a split hand (lobster-claw deformity) (Figure 64-21). Extra digits

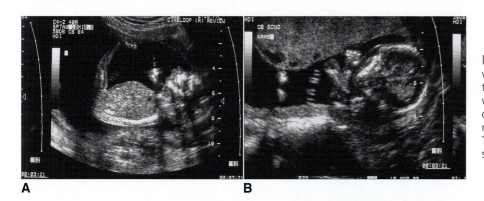

A   **B**

FIGURE 64-18 A, An ultrasound at 19 weeks of gestation revealed rigid legs with the knees hyperextended. **B,** The arms were contracted and crossed over the chest with hands clenched. Polyhydramnios and micrognathia were also noted. The primary diagnosis was Pena-Shokeir syndrome.

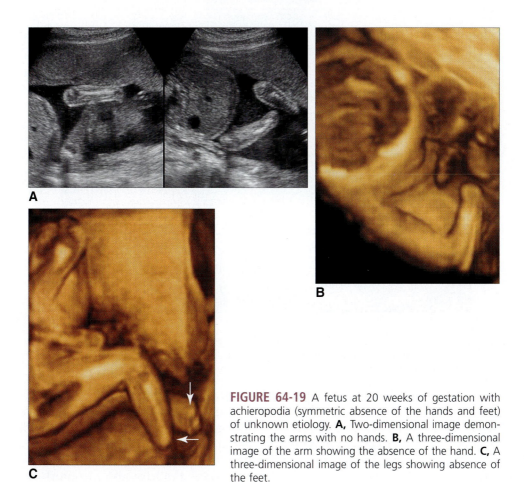

A   **B**   **C**

FIGURE 64-19 A fetus at 20 weeks of gestation with achieropodia (symmetric absence of the hands and feet) of unknown etiology. **A,** Two-dimensional image demonstrating the arms with no hands. **B,** A three-dimensional image of the arm showing the absence of the hand. **C,** A three-dimensional image of the legs showing absence of the feet.

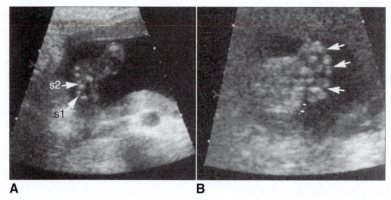

FIGURE 64-20 **A,** Polysyndactyly in a fetus with Carpenter's syndrome. There was webbing (syndactyly) of the first and second toes *(s1)* and of the third and fourth toes *(s2)*. Six toes were present (polydactyly). **B,** In the same fetus, scans of the toes *(arrows)* show malalignment of the phalanges. Other sonographic findings included craniosynostosis, ventriculomegaly, and umbilical hernia.

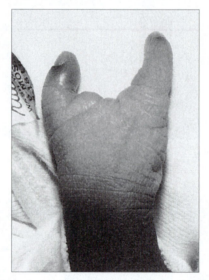

FIGURE 64-21 Pathologic specimen showing a split-hand deformity (ectrodactyly).

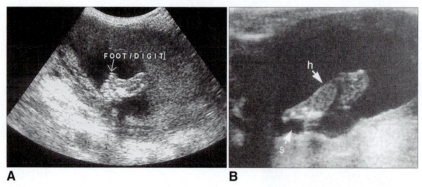

FIGURE 64-22 **A,** Polydactyly is identified in the foot of a fetus. **B,** The foot of a fetus with trisomy 18 was split (ectrodactyly). Note the splaying of the toes *(s)* and malalignment of the metatarsals. Coexisting anomalies included a septal cardiac defect, bilateral choroid plexus cysts, polydactyly, hydramnios, and growth restriction. Autopsy was declined. *h*, Heel.

(polydactyly) may be isolated or part of a syndrome or chromosomal anomaly (Figures 64-22 to 64-24). Overlapping digits (clinodactyly) and clenched hands (see Figure 64-23B) may also be a feature of a syndrome or chromosomal anomaly.

Radial ray defects include hypoplasia or aplasia of the radius and thumb. Radial ray defects (Figure 64-25) are associated with chromosomal anomalies, such as trisomies 13 and 18 and the VACTERL association. Numerous syndromes have also presented with an absent or

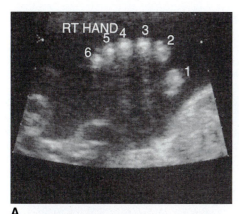

A

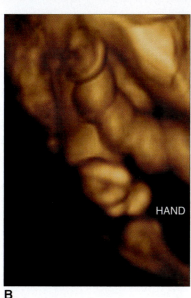

B

FIGURE 64-23 **A,** Polydactyly (six fingers) in a 26-week fetus with multiple congenital anomalies, including micromelic dwarfism and semilobar holoprosencephaly. A normal karyotype was found by amniocentesis, but genetic evaluation after birth suggested pseudotrisomy 13 (an autosomal-recessive condition). **B,** A different fetus with clenched hands and overlapping digits in which chromosomal analysis revealed trisomy 18.

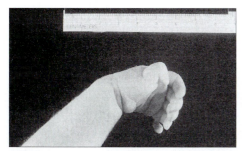

FIGURE 64-24 Polydactyly of a hand shown in a neonate.

hypoplastic radius and thumb, including Holt-Oram syndrome and thrombocytopenia with absent radii (TAR) syndrome (Figure 64-26). Ulnar ray anomalies can also occur.

Clubfoot, also known as talipes, describes deformities of the foot and ankle. It occurs in approximately 1 to 3

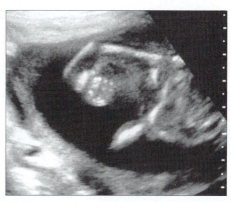

FIGURE 64-25 A radial ray defect in a fetus that also presented with anencephaly and tetralogy of Fallot. A chromosomal anomaly was suspected.

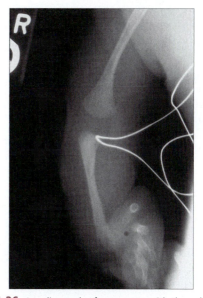

FIGURE 64-26 A radiograph of a neonate with thrombocytopenia with absent radii (TAR) syndrome. Note the absence of the radius in the arm and the turned-back hand.

in 1000 live births. There is a male predominance, and half of the cases of clubfoot are unilateral.

The majority of cases of talipes are idiopathic and isolated findings. Talipes may be associated with chromosomal anomalies, syndromes, musculoskeletal disorders, and spina bifida. It has also been associated with exposure to tubocurarine, sodium aminopterin, and lead poisoning. Clubfoot has also been identified with oligohydramnios and in multiple gestations. Because of the numerous anomalies that may be identified, karyotyping should be offered.

Clubfoot may be identified sonographically when there is persistent abnormal inversion of the foot perpendicular to the lower leg (Figure 64-27).

Rocker-bottom foot is characterized by a prominent heel and a convex sole. It has been associated with

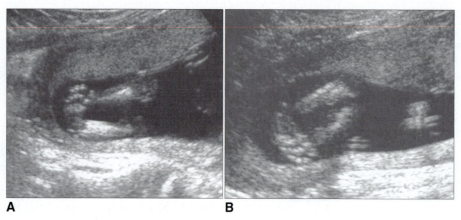

FIGURE 64-27 Bilateral talipes is identified in this fetus. The right **(A)** and left **(B)** feet are both noted to be medially inverted. The patient and her grandmother also had histories of talipes.

multiple syndromes and chromosomal anomalies, especially trisomy 18.

ACKNOWLEDGMENTS

I would like to acknowledge the sonographers Maria Roman, Lucy Burgos, Jamie Prieto, and Lori Sisk at the Maternal Fetal Center, Orlando, Florida, for continually sharing their interesting cases with me so that I am able to share a piece of their knowledge. I would also like to thank the perinatologist Dr. Fuentes for allowing me to continue to expand my skills and knowledge under his mentoring.

abdominal circumference (AC) measurement at the level of the stomach, left portal vein, and left umbilical vein

abruptio placentae bleeding from a normally situated placenta as a result of its complete or partial detachment from the maternal wall after the 20th week of gestation

achondrogenesis lethal autosomal-recessive short-limb dwarfism marked by long bone and trunk shortening, decreased echogenicity of the bones and spine, and flipper-like appendages

achondroplasia a defect in the development of cartilage at the epiphyseal centers of the long bones producing short, square bones

acquisition method of collecting patient anatomy as a series of slices which are then processed and stored for display as 3D volume data

acrania condition associated with anencephaly in which there is complete or partial absence of the cranial bones

adenomyosis benign invasive growth of the endometrium that may cause heavy, painful menstrual bleeding

adnexa structure or tissue next to or near another related structure; the ovaries and the fallopian tubes are adnexa of the uterus

age range analysis (ARA) fetal parameter's size and proportionality expressed as age

allantoic duct elongated duct that contributes to the development of the umbilical cord and placenta during the first trimester

alobar holoprosencephaly most severe form of holoprosencephaly, characterized by a single common ventricle and malformed brain; orbital anomalies range from fused orbits to hypotelorism, with frequent nasal anomalies and clefting of the lip and palate

alpha-fetoprotein (AFP) protein manufactured by the fetus, which can be studied in amniotic fluid and maternal serum; elevations of alpha-fetoprotein may indicate fetal anomalies (neural tube, abdominal wall, gastrointestinal), multiple gestations, or incorrect patient dates; decreased levels may be associated with chromosomal abnormalities

amaurosis fugax transient partial or complete loss of vision in one eye

amenorrhea the absence of menstruation

amniocentesis transabdominal removal of amniotic fluid from the amniotic cavity using ultrasound; amniotic fluid studies are performed to determine fetal karyotype, lung maturity, and Rh condition

amnion smooth membrane enclosing the fetus and amniotic fluid; it is loosely fused with the outer chorionic membrane except at the placental insertion of the umbilical cord, where the amnion is contiguous with the membranes surrounding the umbilical cord

amniotic band syndrome multiple fibrous strands of amnion that develop in utero that may entangle fetal parts to cause amputations or malformations of the fetus

amniotic cavity cavity in which the fetus exists that forms early in gestation and surrounds the embryo; amniotic fluid fills the cavity to protect the embryo and fetus

amniotic fluid produced by the umbilical cord and membranes, the fetal lung, skin, and kidneys

amniotic fluid index (AFI) sum of the four quadrants of amniotic fluid; the uterus is divided into four quadrants; each "quadrant" is evaluated with the transducer perpendicular to the table in the deepest vertical pocket without fetal parts; the four quadrants are added together to determine the amniotic fluid index

anasarca severe generalized massive edema often seen with fetal hydrops

androgen substance that stimulates the development of male characteristics, such as the hormones testosterone and androsterone

anembryonic pregnancy (blighted ovum) gestational sac without an embryo

anencephaly neural tube defect where absence of the brain, including the cerebrum, the cerebellum and basal ganglia, may be present; this abnormality is incompatible with life

aneuploidy fetal syndromes associated with an abnormal number of chromosomes

anophthalmia absent eyes

anophthalmos absence of one (cyclops) or both eyes

anteflexed position of the uterus when the uterine fundus bends forward toward the cervix

anterior cerebral artery (ACA) smaller of the two terminal branches of the internal carotid artery

anterior communicating artery (ACoA) a short vessel that connects the anterior cerebral arteries at the interhemispheric fissure

anterior tibial artery artery that begins at the popliteal artery and travels down the lateral calf in the anterior compartment to the level of the ankle

anterior tibial veins veins that drain blood from the dorsum of the foot and anterior compartment of the calf

anteverted position of the uterus when the fundus is tipped slightly forward

aortic stenosis abnormal development of the cusps of the aortic valve that results in thickened and domed leaflets

apex of ventricle the ventricles of the heart come to a point called the *apex*; normally the apex is directed toward the left hip

aphasia inability to communicate by speech or writing

arcuate vessels small vessels found along the periphery of the uterus

arhinia absence of the nose

ascites abnormal serous fluid collection found in the abdomen or pelvis

Asherman's syndrome acquired uterine condition characterized by the presence of intrauterine scars or synechiae

asphyxiating thoracic dystrophy significantly narrow diameter of the chest in a fetus

asplenia no development of splenic tissue

assisted reproductive technology (ART) technologies employed using male and female gametes to assist the infertility patient to become pregnant; these methods include in vitro fertilization, gamete intrafallopian transfer, zygote intrafallopian transfer, and artificial insemination

ataxia   impaired ability to coordinate movement, especially disturbances in gait

atrial septal defect   communication between the right and left atrium that persists after birth

atrioventricular block   block of transmission of the electrical impulse from the atria to the ventricles (may be 2:1 or 3:1 block)

atrioventricular node   area of specialized cardiac muscle that receives the cardiac impulse from the sinoatrial node and conducts it to the atrioventricular bundles

atrioventricular septal defect (AVSD)   defect that occurs when the endocardial cushion fails to fuse in the center of the heart

atrioventricular valve   valve located between the atria and ventricle

atrium of the lateral ventricles   the portion of the cerebral ventricular system where the lateral lobes, temporal lobes, and occipital lobes connect; located posterior and lateral to the thalami

augmentation   increase in blood flow velocity with distal limb compression or with the release of proximal limb compression

automatic acquisition   collection of patient anatomy as a series of slices without having to manually move the probe during the acquisition process

autonomy   self-governing or self-directing freedom and especially moral independence; the right of persons to choose and to have their choices respected

average age (AA)   average of multiple fetal parameters' age

axillary artery   continuation of the subclavian artery

axillary vein   vein that begins where the basilic vein joins the brachial vein in the upper arm and terminates beneath the clavicle at the outer border of the first rib

Baker's cyst   synovial fluid collection that can be found in the popliteal fossa or upper posterior calf, associated with synovial fluid drainage

banana sign   the shape of the cerebellum when a spinal defect is present (cerebellum is pulled downward into the foramen magnum)

basal plate   the maternal surface of the placenta that lies contiguous with the decidua basalis

basilar artery (BA)   artery formed by the union of the two vertebral arteries

basilic vein   vein that originates on the small finger side of the dorsum of the hand

battledore placenta   marginal or eccentric insertion of the umbilical cord into the placenta

Beckwith-Wiedemann syndrome   hereditary disorder transmitted as an autosomal recessive trait; clinical manifestations include umbilical hernia (exomphalos), macroglossia, and gigantism, often accompanied by visceromegaly and dysplasia of the renal medulla; also called exophthalmos-macroglossia-gigantism (EMG) syndrome

beneficence   bringing about good by maximizing benefits and minimizing possible harm

bicuspid aortic valve   congenital abnormality characterized by two leaflets instead of the normal three leaflets, with asymmetric cusps

binocular distance (BD)   measurement that includes both fetal orbits at the same time to predict gestational age

biophysical profile (BPP)   assessment of fetus to determine fetal well-being; includes evaluation of cardiac non-stress test, fetal breathing movement, gross fetal body movements, fetal tone, and amniotic fluid volume

biparietal diameter (BPD)   fetal transverse cranial diameter at the level of the thalamus and cavum septum pellucidum

blighted ovum   see **anembryonic pregnancy**

bowel herniation   during the first trimester, the bowel normally herniates outside the abdominal cavity between 8 and 12 weeks

brachial artery   continuation of the axillary artery

brachycephaly   fetal head is elongated in the transverse diameter and shortened in the anteroposterior diameter

branchial cleft cyst   a cystic defect that arises from the primitive branchial apparatus

Braxton-Hicks contractions   spontaneous painless uterine contractions described originally as a sign of pregnancy; they occur from the first trimester to the end of pregnancy

breech   indicates the fetal head is toward the fundus of the uterus

broad ligament   broad fold of peritoneum draped over the fallopian tubes, uterus, and ovaries

bronchogenic cyst   most common lung cyst detected prenatally

bronchopulmonary sequestration   extrapulmonary tissue is present within the pleural lung sac (intralobar) or connected to the inferior border of the lung within its own pleural sac (extralobar)

bruit   noise caused by tissue vibration produced by turbulence

bulbus cordis   primitive chamber that forms the right ventricle

cardinal ligament   wide bands of fibromuscular tissue arising from the lateral aspects of the cervix and inserting along the lateral pelvic floor

cardiomyopathy   disease of the myocardial muscle layer of the heart that causes the heart to dilate secondary to regurgitation and also affects cardiac function

caudal regression syndrome   lack of development of the lower limbs (may occur in the fetus of a diabetic mother)

cavernosal artery   supplies the corpus cavernosum with blood in the penis

cavum septum pellucidum   a cavity within the septum pellucidum in the anterior midportion of the fetal brain

cebocephaly   form of holoprosencephaly characterized by a common ventricle, hypotelorism, and a nose with a single nostril

cephalic vein   vein that begins on the thumb side of the dorsum of the hand

cephalocele   protrusion of the brain from the cranial cavity

cerclage   suturing of the ligatures around the cervix uteri to treat cervical incompetence during pregnancy

cerebral vasospasm   vasoconstriction of the arteries

cerebrovascular accident (CVA)   abnormal condition of the brain characterized by occlusion by an embolus, thrombus, or cerebrovascular hemorrhage or vasospasm, resulting in ischemia of brain tissues normally perfused by the damaged vessels

cervical polyp hyperplastic protrusion of the epithelium of the cervix; may be broad based or pedunculated

cervical stenosis acquired condition with obstruction of the cervical canal

cervix inferior segment of the uterus; more than 3.5 cm long during normal pregnancy, decreases in length during labor

Chlamydia trachomatis organism that causes a great variety of diseases, including genital infections in men and women

choledochal cyst cystic growth on the common bile duct

cholelithiasis gallstones

chorioamnionitis bacterial infection of the fetal membranes usually the result of an ascent of the infection from the vagina

chorion cellular, outermost extraembryonic membrane composed of trophoblast lined with mesoderm; it develops villi about 2 weeks after fertilization, is vascularized by allantoic vessels a week later, gives rise to the placenta, and persists until birth

chorion frondosum the portion of the chorion that develops into the fetal portion of the placenta

chorionic cavity surrounds the amniotic cavity; the yolk sac is between the chorion and amnion

chorionic plate that part of the chorionic membrane that covers the placenta

chorionic sac see gestational sac

chorionic villi microscopic vascular projections from the chorion that combine with the maternal uterine tissue to form the placenta

chorionic villus sampling (CVS) invasive diagnostic genetic testing that involves sampling zygotic cells from developing placental tissue

choroid plexus echogenic tissue within the lateral ventricles that produces CNS fluid and that is seen prominently during second trimester fetal sonography

circle of Willis vascular network at the base of the brain

circummarginate placenta condition in which the chorionic plate of the placenta is smaller than the basal plate, with a flat interface between the fetal membranes and the placenta

circumvallate placenta condition in which the chorionic plate of the placenta is smaller than the basal plate; the margin is raised with a rolled edge

cisterna magna a posterior fossa cistern that contains CSF

claudication walking-induced muscular discomfort of the calf, thigh, hip, or buttock caused by ischemia

cloacal exstrophy complex malformation involving lower limb anomalies, spinal defect, anal atresia, and lower abdominal wall defect below the cord insertion that involves exstrophy of the bladder and protrusion of the intestines

coarctation of the aorta narrowing in the aortic arch (discrete, long segment, or tubular), usually at the level of the left subclavian artery near the insertion of the ductus arteriosus or as a shelflike protrusion in the isthmus of the arch

coccygeus muscles muscles that form the floor of the pelvis

collateral pathway pathway that develops because of vessel obstruction; smaller side branches of the vessel provide alternative flow pathways

color flow mapping (CFM) ability to display blood flow in multiple colors depending on the velocity, direction of flow, and extent of turbulence

common carotid artery (CCA) artery that rises from the aortic arch to supply blood to the head and neck

common femoral vein (CFV) vein formed by the confluence of the profunda femoris and the superficial femoral veins; also receives the greater saphenous vein

common iliac vein vein formed by the confluence of the internal and external iliac veins

complete abortion complete removal of all products of conception, including the placenta

confidentiality the nondisclosure of certain information except to another authorized person

congenital bronchial atresia pulmonary anomaly that results from the focal obliteration of a segment of the bronchial lumen

congenital cystic adenomatoid malformation (CCAM) abnormality in the formation of the bronchial tree with secondary overgrowth of mesenchymal tissue from arrested bronchial development

congenital diaphragmatic hernia (CDH) opening in the pleuroperitoneal membrane that develops in the first trimester

conjoined twins monozygotic twins physically joined by varying degrees; condition that occurs when the division of the egg occurs after 13 days

continuous murmur heart murmur that begins in systole and continues without interruption through the time of the second heart sound into all or part of diastole

continuous wave probe probe with which sound is continuously emitted from one transducer and continuously received by a second transducer

cornu, cornua any projection like a horn; refers to the fundus of the uterus where the fallopian tube arises

coronal plane refers to horizontal plane through the longitudinal axis of the body to image structures from anterior to posterior

corpus callosum a narrow band of compact tissue forming a solid covering over the roof of the third ventricle and connecting the hemispheres of the brain

corpus cavernosum the two columns of tissue in the penis that fill with blood to create an erection

corpus luteum yellow body formed from the Graafian follicle after ovulation that produces estrogen and progesterone

corpus luteum cyst small endocrine structure that develops within a ruptured ovarian follicle and secretes progesterone and estrogen to prevent menses should fertilization occur

corrected transposition of the great arteries congenital heart defect; right and left atrium are connected to the morphologic left and right ventricle, respectively, and the great arteries are transposed

corticosteroids drugs administered to pregnant women to help accelerate fetal lung maturity

cor triatriatum heart defect that occurs when the left atrial cavity is partitioned into two parts; pulmonary veins drain into an accessory left atrial chamber proximal to the right of the thorax

craniosynostosis early ossification of the calvarium with destruction of the sutures; hypertelorism frequently found in association; sonographically, the fetal cranium may appear brachycephalic

crown-rump length (CRL) most accurate measurement for determining gestational age in the first trimester

cryptorchidism failure of the testes to descend into the scrotum

curettage scraping with a curet to remove the contents of the uterus

cyclopia severe form of holoprosencephaly characterized by a common ventricle, fusion of the orbits with one or two eyes present, and a proboscis (maldeveloped cylindrical nose)

cystadenocarcinoma a malignant tumor that forms cysts

cystadenoma benign adenoma containing cysts

cystic fibrosis congenital condition marked by mucous buildup within the lungs and other areas of the body

cystic hygroma dilation of jugular lymph sacs (axillary or inguinal) because of improper drainage of the lymphatic system into the venous system; large, septated hygromas are frequently associated with Turner's and Down syndromes, congestive heart failure, and fetal demise in utero; isolated hygromas may occur as solitary lesions at birth; they may be part of a general condition, lymphangiectasis, or a benign focal process

dacryocystocele cystic dilation of the lacrimal sac at the nasocanthal angle

decidua basalis the part of the decidua that unites with the chorion to form the placenta

decidua capsularis the part of the decidua that surrounds the chorionic sac

deep femoral vein vein that travels with the profunda femoris artery to unite with the superficial femoral vein to form the common femoral vein

depolarization describes the electrical activity that triggers contraction of the heart muscle

dermoid benign tumor composed of hair, muscle, teeth, and fat

dextrocardia heart defect in which the heart is in the right chest with the apex pointed to the right of the thorax

dextroposition condition in which the heart is located in the right side of the chest and the cardiac apex points medially or to the left

diamniotic multiple pregnancy with two amniotic sacs

diastole part of the cardiac cycle in which the ventricles are filling with blood; the tricuspid and mitral valves are open during this time

diastolic murmur heart murmur that begins with or after the time of the second heart sound and ends at or before the time of the first heart sound

dichorionic multiple pregnancy with two chorionic sacs

diplopia double vision

dizygotic twins that arise from two separately fertilized ova

dolichocephaly fetal head is shortened in the transverse plane and elongated in the anteroposterior plane

Doppler frequency red blood cells move from a lower-frequency sound source at rest toward a higher-frequency

sound source; change in frequency is called the Doppler shift in frequency

dorsalis pedis artery continuation of the anterior tibial artery on the top of the foot

double decidual sac sign interface between the decidua capsularis and the echogenic, highly vascular surface on the opposite side of the endometrial cavity

ductal constriction heart defect that occurs when flow is diverted from the ductus secondary to tricuspid or pulmonary atresia or secondary to maternal medications given to stop early contractions

ductus arteriosus communicating structure that carries oxygenated blood from the pulmonary artery to the descending aorta; closes after birth

ductus venosus vascular structure within the fetal liver that connects the umbilical vein to the inferior vena cava and allows oxygenated blood to bypass the liver and return directly to the heart

duodenal atresia complete blockage at the pyloric sphincter

duodenal stenosis narrowing of the pyloric sphincter

dysarthria difficulty with speech because of impairment of the tongue or muscles essential to speech

dysmenorrhea pain associated with menstruation

dysphagia inability or difficulty in swallowing

Ebstein's anomaly abnormal apical displacement of the septal leaflet of the tricuspid valve toward the apex of the right ventricle; the right ventricle above this leaflet becomes the "atrialized" chamber

echogenic intracardiac focus (EIF) an echo within a fetal heart chamber that is as bright (echogenic) as bone and persists despite changes in the sonographic plane

eclampsia coma and seizures in the second- and third-trimester patient secondary to pregnancy-induced hypertension

ectocervix a portion of the canal of the uterine cervix that is lined with squamous epithelium

ectopic pregnancy pregnancy occurring outside the uterine cavity

electrocardiography method of recording the electrical activity generated by the heart muscle

embryo conceptus to the end of the 9th week of gestation

embryo transfer a technique that follows IVF in which the fertilized ova are injected into the uterus through the cervix

embryonic age (conception age) age of embryo stated as time from date of conception

embryonic heart rate (EHR) the heart rate before the early 9th week of gestation

embryonic period time between 4 and 10 weeks of gestation

encephalocele protrusion of the brain through a cranial fissure

endocardium inner layer of the heart wall

endometrial carcinoma malignancy characterized by abnormal thickening of the endometrial cavity; usually presents with irregular bleeding in perimenopausal and postmenopausal women

endometrial hyperplasia benign condition that results from estrogen stimulation to the endometrium without the influence of progestin; frequent cause of bleeding (especially in postmenopausal women)

endometrial polyp pedunculated or sessile well-defined mass attached to the endometrial cavity

endometrioma localized tumor of endometriosis most frequently found in the ovary, cul-de-sac, rectovaginal septum, and peritoneal surface of the posterior wall of the uterus

endometriosis condition that occurs when functioning endometrial tissue invades sites outside the uterus

endometritis infection within the endometrium of the uterus

endometrium inner lining of the uterine cavity that appears echogenic to hypoechoic on ultrasound, depending on the menstrual cycle

epicardium outer layer of the heart wall

epignathus teratoma located in the oropharynx

epispadias abnormal congenital opening of the male urethra on the top side of the penis

esophageal atresia congenital hypoplasia of the esophagus; usually associated with a tracheoesophageal fistula

esophageal stenosis narrowing of the esophagus, usually in the distal third segment

estimated fetal weight (EFW) incorporation of all fetal growth parameters (biparietal diameter, head circumference, abdominal circumference, femur, and humeral length)

estrogen steroidal hormone secreted by the theca interna and granulose cells of the ovarian follicle that stimulates the development of the female reproductive structures and secondary sexual characteristics; promotes the growth of the endometrial tissue during the proliferative phase of the menstrual cycle

ethics the study of what is good and bad and of moral duty and obligation; systematic reflection on an analysis of morality

exencephaly abnormal condition in which the brain is located outside the cranium

exophthalmia abnormal protrusion of the eyeball

exstrophy of the bladder protrusion of the posterior wall of the urinary bladder, which contains the trigone of the bladder and the ureteric orifices

external carotid artery (ECA) smaller of the two terminal branches of the common carotid artery

external iliac vein single vein that travels with the artery beginning at the level of the inguinal ligament; it is joined with the internal iliac vein to become the common iliac vein

false knots of the umbilical cord occurs when blood vessels are longer than the cord; they fold on themselves and produce nodulations on the surface of the cord

false pelvis portion of the pelvic cavity that is above the pelvic brim, bounded posteriorly by the lumbar vertebrae, laterally by the iliac fossae and iliacus muscles, and anteriorly by the lower anterior abdominal wall

femoral artery artery that courses the length of the thigh through Hunter's canal and terminates at the opening of the adductor magnus muscle

femoral veins upper part of the venous drainage system of the lower extremity found in the upper thigh and groin that empties into the inferior vena cava at the level of the diaphragm

femur length (FL) measurement from the femoral head to the distal end of the femur

fetal cystic hygroma malformation of the lymphatic system that leads to single or multiloculated lymph-filled cavities around the neck

fetal goiter (thyromegaly) enlargement of the thyroid gland

fetal hydronephrosis dilated renal pelvis in the fetus; most common fetal anomaly

fetal ovarian cyst ovarian mass that results from maternal hormone stimulation and is usually benign

fetus papyraceus fetal death that occurs after the fetus has reached a certain growth that is too large to resorb into the uterus

follicle-stimulating hormone (FSH) hormone secreted by the anterior pituitary gland that stimulates the growth and maturation of graafian follicles in the ovary

follicular cyst benign cyst within the ovary that may occur and disappear on a cyclic basis

foramen of Bochdalek type of diaphragmatic defect that occurs posterior and lateral in the diaphragm; usually found in the left side

foramen of Morgagni diaphragmatic hernia that occurs anterior and medial in the diaphragm and may communicate with the pericardial sac

foramen ovale opening between the free edge of the septum secundum and the dorsal wall of the atrium; also termed *fossae ovale*

frontal bossing protrusion or bulging of the forehead

functional cyst cyst resulting from the normal function of the ovary

Gartner's duct cyst small cyst within the vagina

gastrocnemius veins paired veins that lie in the medial and lateral gastrocnemius muscles and terminate into the popliteal vein

gastroschisis congenital defective opening in the wall of the abdomen just to the right of the umbilical cord; bowel and other organs may protrude outside the abdomen from this opening

genetic sonogram adjusting an individual patient's risk assessment for aneuploidy based on the presence or absence of sonographic markers

gestational (menstrual) age length of pregnancy defined in the United States as the number of weeks from first day of last normal menstrual period (LNMP)

gestational sac structure lined by the chorion that normally implants within the uterine decidua and contains the developing embryo

gestational sac diameter measurement used in the first trimester to estimate appropriate gestational age with menstrual dates

gestational trophoblastic disease condition in which trophoblastic tissue overtakes the pregnancy and propagates throughout the uterine cavity; may be partial or complete

gonadotropin a hormonal substance that stimulates the function of the testes and ovaries

gonadotropin-releasing hormone (GnRH) hormone secreted by the hypothalamus that stimulates the release of the follicle-stimulating hormone and luteinizing hormone by the anterior pituitary gland

gravidity (G) total number of pregnancies

greater saphenous vein   originates on the dorsum of the foot and ascends anterior to the medial malleolus and along the anteromedial side of the calf and thigh; joins the common femoral vein in the proximal thigh

growth-adjusted sonar age (GASA)   method whereby the fetus is categorized into small, average, or large growth percentile

haustral folds   one of the sacculations of the colon caused by longitudinal bands that are shorter than the gut

hemangioma of the cord   vascular tumor within the umbilical cord

hematometra   obstruction of the uterus or vagina characterized by an accumulation of blood

hemianopsia   partial loss of the visual field

hemifacial microsomia   abnormal smallness of one side of the face

hemiparesis   unilateral partial or complete paralysis

hemopoiesis   production and development of blood cells

hermaphroditism   condition in which both ovarian and testicular tissues are present

heterotopic pregnancy   simultaneous intrauterine and extrauterine pregnancy

heterozygous achondroplasia   short-limb dysplasia that manifests in the second trimester of pregnancy; conversion abnormality of cartilage to bone affecting the epiphyseal growth centers; extremities are markedly shortened at birth with a normal trunk and frequent enlargement of the head

Hirschsprung's disease (congenital megacolon)   congenital disorder in which there is abnormal innervations of the large intestine

holoprosencephaly   failure of forebrain to divide into two cerebral hemispheres, resulting in a single large ventricle with varying amounts of cerebral cortex; has been known to occur with trisomies 13, 15, and 18

homozygous achondroplasia   short-limb dwarfism affecting fetuses of achondroplastic parents

horseshoe kidney   forms when the inferior poles of the kidney fuse while they are in the pelvis

human chorionic gonadotropin (hCG)   a glycoprotein secreted from placental trophoblastic cells; this chemical component is found in maternal serum and urine when pregnant

humeral length   measurement from the humeral head to the distal end of the humerus

hydatidiform mole   benign form of gestational trophoblastic disease in which there is partial or complete conversion of the chorionic villi into grapelike vesicles; villi are avascular and there is trophoblastic proliferation; condition may result in malignant trophoblastic disease

hydramnios   increased amount of amniotic fluid

hydranencephaly   congenital absence of the cerebral hemispheres because of an occlusion of the carotid arteries; midbrain structures are present, and fluid replaces cerebral tissue

hydrocephalus   ventriculomegaly in the neonate; abnormal accumulation of cerebrospinal fluid within the cerebral ventricles, resulting in compression and, frequently, destruction of the brain

hydrometra   obstruction of the uterus or vagina characterized by an accumulation of fluid

hydrometrocolpos   collection of fluid in the vagina and uterus

hydrops fetalis   fluid occurring in at least two areas in the fetus: pleural effusion, pericardial effusion, ascites, or skin edema

hydrosalpinx   fluid within the fallopian tube

hydroureters   dilated ureters

hyperechoic bowel   increased echogenicity of the bowel associated with aneuploidy risk and fetal pathology

hyperemesis gravidarum   excessive vomiting that leads to dehydration and electrolyte imbalance

hypertelorism   abnormally wide-spaced orbits usually found in conjunction with congenital anomalies and mental retardation

hypophosphatasia   congenital condition characterized by decreased mineralization of the bones resulting in "ribbonlike" and bowed limbs, underossified cranium, and compression of the chest; early death often occurs

hypoplasia   underdevelopment of a tissue, organ, or body

hypoplastic left heart syndrome   underdevelopment of the left ventricle with aortic or mitral atresia; left ventricle very thickened compared with right ventricle

hypoplastic right heart syndrome   underdevelopment of the right ventricular outflow tract secondary to pulmonary stenosis

hypospadias   abnormal congenital opening of the male urethra on the undersurface of the penis

hypotelorism   abnormally closely spaced orbits; association with holoprosencephaly, chromosomal and central nervous system disorders, and cleft palate

iliacus muscles   paired muscles that form the lateral wall of the pelvis

iliopectineal line   bony ridge of the inner surface of the ilium and pubic bones that divides the true and false pelves

immune hydrops   accumulation of abnormal fluid collections caused by rhesus incompatibility

incompetent cervix   condition in which the cervix dilates silently during the second trimester; without intervention, the membranes bulge through the cervix, rupture, and the fetus drops out, resulting in a premature delivery

incomplete spontaneous abortion   loss of pregnancy with products of conception remaining in the uterus

infantile polycystic kidney disease (IPKD)   autosomal recessive disease that affects the fetal kidneys and liver; the kidneys are enlarged and echogenic on ultrasound

inferior vena cava   largest abdominal vessel formed by the union of the common iliac veins; flows posterior to the liver to enter the right atrium of the heart; supplies the right atrium of the heart along the posterior lateral wall

informed consent   providing complete information and ensuring comprehension and voluntary consent by patient or subject to a required or experimental medical procedure

iniencephaly   rare neural tube defect in which the brain tissue protrudes through a fissure in the occiput, so that the brain and spinal cord occupy a single cavity

innominate artery   first branch artery from the aortic arch

innominate veins   veins that follow these courses: on the right, courses vertically downward to join the left innominate vein below the first rib to form the superior vena cava; on the left, courses from left chest beneath the sternum to join the right innominate vein; the left innominate vein is longer than the right

integrity   adherence to moral and ethical principles

internal carotid artery (ICA)   larger of the two terminal branches of the common carotid artery that arises from the common carotid artery to supply the anterior brain and meninges

internal iliac vein   single vein that travels with the internal iliac artery; drains the pelvis

internal os   inner surface of the cervical os

interstitial pregnancy   pregnancy occurring in the fallopian tube near the cornu of the uterus; also known as *cornual pregnancy*

intramural leiomyoma   most common type of leiomyoma; deforms the myometrium

intrauterine contraceptive device (IUCD)   device inserted into the endometrial cavity to prevent pregnancy

intrauterine growth restriction (IUGR)   reduce growth rate (symmetrical IUGR) or abnormal growth pattern (asymmetrical IUGR) of the fetus; results in a small for gestational age (SGA) infant

intrauterine insemination   the introduction of semen into the vagina or uterus by mechanical or instrumental means rather than by sexual intercourse

introitus   an opening or entrance into a canal or cavity, as the vagina

in vitro fertilization (IVF)   a method of fertilizing the human ova outside the body by collecting the mature ova and placing them in a dish with a sample of spermatozoa

ischemic rest pain   symptom of critical ischemia of the distal limb when the patient is at rest

jejunoileal atresia   blockage of the jejunum and ileal bowel segments that appears as multiple cystic structures within the fetal abdomen

justice   the ethical principle that requires fair distribution of benefits and burdens; an injustice occurs when a benefit to which a person is entitled is withheld or when a burden is unfairly imposed

large for gestational age (LGA)   fetus measures larger than would be expected for dates (diabetic fetus)

last menstrual period (LMP)   the first day of the LMP is used as a start date for human pregnancies

lateral ventricles   the largest portion of the ventricular system in the fetal cranium

left atrium   filling chamber of the heart

left ventricle   pumping chamber of the heart

leiomyoma   most common benign gynecologic tumor in women during their reproductive years

lemon sign   sonographic sign of frontal bones collapsing inward; occurs with spina bifida

lesser saphenous vein   vein that originates on the dorsum of the foot and ascends posterior to the lateral malleolus and runs along the midline of the posterior calf; vein terminates as it joins the popliteal vein

levator ani muscles   a pair of muscles that form the floor of the pelvis

levocardia   normal position of the heart in the left chest with the cardiac apex pointed to the left

levoposition   condition in which the heart is displaced further toward the left chest

ligamentum venosum   fibrous remains of the ductus venosus from fetal circulation

likelihood ratio   the probability that a fetus exhibiting a specific finding will be affected by a specific condition; likelihood ratios in pregnancy are typically used to predict risk for aneuploidy

limb–body wall complex   anomaly with large cranial defects, facial cleft, large body wall defects, and limb abnormalities

lower uterine segment   thin expanded lower portion of the uterus at the junction of the internal os and sacrum that forms in the last trimester of pregnancy

luteinizing hormone (LH)   secreted by the anterior pituitary gland to stimulate ovulation and induce luteinization of the ruptured follicle to form the corpus luteum

lymphangiectasia   dilation of a lymph node

macrocephaly   enlargement of the fetal cranium as a result of ventriculomegaly

macroglossia   hypertrophied tongue seen persistently protruding outside the fetal mouth

macrosomia   birth weight greater than 4000 g or above the 90th percentile for the estimated gestational age; these infants have fat deposition in the subcutaneous tissues

main pulmonary artery   main artery that carries blood from the right ventricle to the lungs

manual acquisition   original 3D method of collecting anatomy requiring the sonographer to manually slide the probe along the patient's skin to collect anatomy as a series of slices

maternal serum alpha-fetoprotein (MSAFP)   one of several biochemical tests used to assess fetal risk for aneuploidy or fetal defect; a component of the "quad screen," the normal value of MSAFP varies with gestational age, so assessment of gestational age is essential to the accurate interpretation of results

maternal serum quad screen   test of maternal serum biochemical levels in the second trimester: human chorionic gonadotropin (hCG), alpha-fetoprotein (AFP), estriol, and inhibin A

maximum vertical pocket   method to determine the amount of amniotic fluid; pocket less than 2 cm may indicate oligohydramnios; greater than 8 cm indicates polyhydramnios; this method is used more often in multiple gestation pregnancy

mean velocity   velocity based on the time average of the outline velocity (maximum velocity envelope)

Meckel's diverticulum   congenital sac or blind pouch found in the lower portion of the ileum; a remnant of the proximal part of the yolk stalk

meconium ileus   small-bowel disorder marked by the presence of thick echogenic meconium in the distal ileum

megacystitis   the level of the urethra where the urinary tract may become obstructed

megaureter   dilation of the lower end of the ureter; the common presentation of ureterovesical junction obstruction

Meigs' syndrome   benign tumor of the ovary associated with ascites and pleural effusion

membranous or velamentous insertion of the cord   insertion of the cord into the membranes before it enters the placenta

menarche   onset of menstruation; state after reaching puberty in which menses occur normally every 27 to 28 days

meningocele   open spinal defect characterized by protrusion of the spinal meninges

meningomyelocele   open spinal defect characterized by protrusion of meninges and spinal cord through the defect, usually within a meningeal sac

menopause   cessation of menstruation

menorrhagia   abnormally heavy or long periods

menses   periodic flow of blood and cellular debris that occurs during menstruation

menstrual age   gestational age of the fetus determined from the first day of the last normal menstrual period (LMP) to the point at which the pregnancy is being assessed

menstruation   days 1 to 4 of the menstrual cycle; endometrial canal appears as hypoechoic central line representing blood and tissue

mesocardia   atypical location of the heart in the middle of the chest with the cardiac apex pointing toward the midline

mesosalpinx   upper portion of the broad ligament that encloses the fallopian tubes

mesovarium   posterior portion of the broad ligament that is drawn out to enclose and hold the ovary in place

metrorrhea   irregular, acyclic bleeding

microcephaly   head smaller than the body

micrognathia   abnormally small chin; commonly associated with other fetal anomalies

microphthalmos   small eyes

middle cerebral artery (MCA)   large terminal branch of the internal carotid artery

midline echo complex (the falx)   widest transverse diameter of the skull; proper level to measure the biparietal diameter

mirror view   displays simultaneous rendered volume images from four different perspectives in real time

mitral atresia   (congenital mitral stenosis) abnormal development of the mitral leaflet that may lead to the development of a hypoplastic left ventricle

mitral regurgitation   failure of the leaflets to close completely, allowing blood to leak backward into the left atrium during systole

mitral valve   atrioventricular valve between the left atrium and left ventricle

molar pregnancy   also known as gestational trophoblastic disease; abnormal proliferation of trophoblastic cells in the first trimester

monoamniotic   multiple pregnancy with one amniotic sac

monochorionic   multiple pregnancy with one chorionic sac

monozygotic   twins that arise from a single fertilized egg that divides to produce two identical fetuses

morality   the protection of cherished values that relate to how persons interact and live in peace

mucinous cystadenocarcinoma   malignant tumor of the ovary with multilocular cysts

mucinous cystadenoma   benign tumor of the ovary that contains thin-walled, multilocular cysts

multiplanar display   demonstrates anatomy as three simultaneous orthogonal scan planes (longitudinal, transverse, and coronal)

multiple dysplastic kidney disease (MCDK)   multiple cysts replace normal renal tissue throughout the kidney, usually causing renal obstruction

multislice view   displays 3D anatomy as a series of sequential parallel images similar in display format to that of CT and MRI

murmur   (of the heart) relatively prolonged series of auditory vibrations of varying intensity (loudness), frequency (pitch), quality, configuration, and duration; the murmur is produced by structural changes or hemodynamic events in the heart or blood vessels

myocarditis   cardiac disease process of necrosis and destruction of myocardial cells as well as inflammatory infiltrate

myocardium   thick contractile middle layer of the heart

myometritis   infection within the myometrium of the uterus

myometrium   middle layer of the uterine cavity that appears very homogeneous with sonography

nabothian cyst   benign tiny cyst within the cervix

nomogram   written representation by graphs, diagrams or charts of the relationship between numerical variables

nonimmune hydrops (NIH)   group of conditions in which hydrops is present in the fetus but not a result of fetomaternal blood group incompatibility

nonmaleficence   refrain from harming oneself or others

Non-stress test (NST)   test that utilizes Doptone (a brand of Doppler instrumentation used in obstetric examinations) to record the fetal heart rate and its reactivity to the stress of uterine contraction

normal situs   typical position of the abdominal organs with the liver and IVC on the right, stomach on left, and the heart apex directed toward the left

nuchal cord   condition that occurs when the cord is wrapped around the fetal neck

nuchal lucency   increased thickness in the nuchal fold area in the back of the neck associated with trisomy 21

nuchal skin fold   the thickness of the fetal skin at the back of the fetal neck that may be visualized and measured between 16 and 20 weeks' gestational age to assess aneuploidy risk

nuchal translucency   a collection of fluid that extends behind the fetal neck and along the spine in the first trimester

oblique view   two-dimensional drawing of an object with "forced" depth to represent a third dimension; from its inception, 2D ultrasound has dictated documentation of anatomy and pathology in two orthogonal planes, usually longitudinal and transverse

oblique view extended (OVIX)   similar to oblique view but displays the corresponding volume slice instead of the corresponding planar image

obturator internus muscle   arises from the anterolateral pelvic wall surrounding the obturator foramen to insert on the greater trochanter of the femur

oculodentodigital dysplasia   underdevelopment of the eyes, fingers, and mouth

oligohydramnios   insufficient amount of amniotic fluid

oligomenorrhea   abnormally light menstrual periods

omphalocele   congenital anterior abdominal wall defect in which abdominal organs (liver, bowel, stomach) are atypically located within the umbilical cord and protrude outside the wall; highly associated with cardiac, central nervous system, renal, and chromosomal anomalies; it develops when there is a midline defect of the abdominal muscles, fascia, and skin

omphalomesenteric cyst   cystic lesion of the umbilical cord

oocyte   primordial or incompletely developed ovum

oophoritis   infection within the ovary

ophthalmic artery   first branch of the internal carotid artery

osteogenesis imperfecta   metabolic disorder affecting the fetal collagen system that leads to varying forms of bone disease; intrauterine bone fractures, shortened long bones, poorly mineralized calvaria, and compression of the chest found in type II forms

otocephaly   underdevelopment of the jaw that causes the ears to be located close together toward the front of the neck

ovarian carcinoma   malignant tumor of the ovary that may spread beyond the ovary and metastasize to other organs via the peritoneal channels

ovarian cyst   cyst of the ovary that may be found in the fetus; results from maternal hormone stimulation and is usually benign

ovarian hyperstimulation syndrome (OHS)   a syndrome that presents sonographically as enlarged ovaries with multiple cysts, abdominal ascites, and pleural effusions; often seen in patients who have undergone ovulation induction following the administration of follicle-stimulating hormone or a GnRH analogue followed by hCG

ovarian ligament   paired ligament that extends from the inferior/medial pole of the ovary to the uterine cornua

ovarian torsion   partial or complete rotation of the ovarian pedicle on its axis

ovulation induction therapy   controlled ovarian stimulation with clomiphene citrate or parenterally administered gonadotropins

ovum   the female egg

oxycephaly   the condition of having a relatively high cranial vault with a peaked appearance; it is caused by molding of the cranium, which exaggerates the vertical axis, or in more severe cases by premature closure of the coronal, sagittal, and lambdoidal sutures

parametritis   infection within the uterine serosa and broad ligaments

paraovarian cyst   cystic structure that lies adjacent to the ovary

parity   number of live births

partial anomalous pulmonary venous return   condition in which the pulmonary veins do not all enter into the left atrial cavity

partial situs inversus   reversal of the heart or the abdominal organs (dextrocardia or liver on the left, stomach on the right)

patent ductus arteriosus   open communication between the pulmonary artery and descending aorta that does not constrict after birth

pelvic inflammatory disease (PID)   all-inclusive term for all pelvic infections (endometritis, salpingitis, hydrosalpinx, pyosalpinx, and tuboovarian abscess)

pelvic kidney   location of the kidney when the kidney does not migrate upward into the retroperitoneal space

pentalogy of Cantrell   rare anomaly with five defects: omphalocele, ectopic heart, lower sternum, anterior diaphragm, and diaphragmatic pericardium

perforating veins   veins that connect the superficial and deep venous systems

pericardial effusion   abnormal collection of fluid surrounding the epicardial layer of the heart

pericardium   sac surrounding the heart, reflecting off the great arteries

perimetrium   serous membrane enveloping the uterus; also called the *serosa*

periovarian inflammation   enlarged ovaries with multiple cysts and indistinct margins

peristalsis   movement of the bowel

peroneal veins   veins that drain blood from the lateral lower leg

phenylketonuria (PKU)   hereditary disease caused by failure to oxidize an amino acid (phenylalanine) to tyrosine, because of a defective enzyme; if PKU is not treated early, mental retardation can develop

Pierre Robin syndrome   micrognathia and abnormal smallness of the tongue usually with a cleft palate

piriformis muscle   muscle that arises from the sacrum between the pelvic sacral foramina and the gluteal surface of the ilium

placenta   organ of communication where nutrition and products of metabolism are interchanged between the fetal and maternal blood systems; forms from the chorion frondosum with a maternal decidual contribution

placenta accreta   growth of the chorionic villi to the myometrium; it does not penetrate through the myometrium

placenta increta   growth of the chorionic villi deep into the myometrium

placenta percreta   growth of the chorionic villi through the myometrium to the uterine serosa

placenta previa   placental implantation that encroaches upon the lower uterine segment; the placenta presents first in late pregnancy and bleeding is inevitable

placental grade   technique of grading the placenta for maturity

placental insufficiency   abnormal condition of pregnancy manifested by a restricted rate of fetal and uterine growth; one or more placental abnormalities cause dysfunction of maternal-placental or fetal-placental circulation

placental migration   movement of the placenta as the uterus enlarges the placenta; a low-lying placenta may move out of the lower uterine segment in the second trimester

platycephaly   flattening of the vertex of the skull; it is often associated with cranial molding and compensatory exaggeration of the biparietal diameter

pleural effusion (hydrothorax) accumulation of fluid within the thoracic cavity

polycystic ovarian syndrome (PCOS) endocrine disorder associated with chronic anovulation

polydactyly anomalies of the hands or feet in which there is an addition of a digit; may be found in association with certain skeletal dysplasias

polyhydramnios excessive amount of amniotic fluid

polymenorrhea an abnormally frequent recurrence of the menstrual cycle; a menstrual cycle of less than 21 days

polysplenia more than one spleen; associated with cardiac malformations

popliteal artery artery that begins at the opening of the adductor magnus muscle and travels behind the knee in the popliteal fossa

popliteal vein vein that originates from the confluence of the anterior tibial veins and posterior and peroneal veins

posterior arch vein main tributary of the greater saphenous vein

posterior cerebral artery (PCA) artery that originates from the terminal basilar artery and courses anteriorly and laterally

posterior communicating artery (PCoA) courses posteriorly and medially from the internal carotid artery to join the posterior cerebral artery

posterior tibial veins veins that originate from the plantar veins of the foot and drain blood from the posterior lower leg

posterior urethral valve occurs only in male fetuses; manifested by the presence of a valve in the posterior urethra

postterm fetus born later than the 42-week gestational period

Potter's sequence term used to describe renal diseases other than renal agenesis that result in renal failure and facial or structural abnormalities caused by oligohydramnios

Potter's syndrome characterized by a group of findings associated with oligohydramnios and renal failure or bilateral renal agenesis; findings include abnormally positioned extremities, wide-set eyes, and broad nasal bridge

Pourcelot resistive index Doppler measurement that takes the highest systolic peak minus the highest diastolic peak divided by the highest systolic peak

preeclampsia complication of pregnancy characterized by increasing hypertension, proteinuria, and edema

pregnancy-induced hypertension (PIH) elevation of maternal blood pressure that may put the fetus at risk

premature atrial and ventricular contractions fetal cardiac arrhythmia resulting from extrasystoles and ectopic beats

premature rupture of the membranes (PROM) leaking or breaking of the amniotic membranes causing the loss of amniotic fluid, which may lead to premature delivery or infection

premenarche time period in young girls before the onset of menstruation

preterm fetus born earlier than the normal 38- to 42-week gestational period

primary yolk sac first site of formation of red blood cells that will nourish the embryo

proboscis a cylindrical protuberance of the face that in cyclopia or ethmocephaly represents the nose

profunda femoris artery artery posterior and lateral to the superficial femoral artery

progesterone steroidal hormone produced by the corpus luteum that helps prepare and maintain the endometrium for the arrival and implantation of an embryo

proliferative phase (early) days 5 to 9 of the menstrual cycle; endometrium appears as a single thin stripe with a hypoechoic halo encompassing it; creates the "three-line sign"

proliferative phase (late) days 10 to 14 of the menstrual cycle; ovulation occurs. The endometrium increases in thickness and echogenicity

prune belly syndrome dilation of the fetal abdomen secondary to severe bilateral hydronephrosis and fetal ascites; fetus also has oligohydramnios and pulmonary hypoplasia

pseudoaneurysm perivascular collection (hematoma) that communicates with an artery or a graft and has pulsating blood entering the collection

pseudoascites sonolucent band near the fetal anterior abdominal wall seen in the fetus over 18 weeks (does not outline the falciform ligament or bowel as ascites will)

pseudogestational sac decidual reaction with fluid occurring within the uterus in a patient with an ectopic pregnancy

psoas major muscle begins at the level of the hilum of the kidneys and extends inferiorly along both sides of the spine into the pelvis

pulmonary embolism (PE) blockage of the pulmonary circulation by a thrombus or other matter; may lead to death if blockage of pulmonary blood flow is significant

pulmonary hypoplasia underdeveloped lungs with resultant reduction in lung volume; secondary to prolonged oligohydramnios or as a consequence of a small thoracic cavity

pulmonary sequestration extra pulmonary tissue is present within the pleural lung sac (intralobar) or connected to the inferior border of the lung within its own pleural sac (extralobar)

pulmonary stenosis Abnormal pulmonary valve characterized by thickened, domed leaflets that restrict the amount of blood flowing from the right ventricle to the pulmonary artery to the lungs

pulmonary veins four pulmonary veins bring blood from the lungs back into the posterior wall of the left atrium; there are two upper (right and left) and two lower (right and left) pulmonary veins

pulsatility index (PI) Doppler measurement that uses peak systole minus peak diastole divided by the mean

pulsed wave Doppler type of Doppler used in most fetal examinations; the transducer has the ability to both send and receive Doppler signals

pulsed wave transducer single crystal that sends and receives sound intermittently; a pulse of sound is emitted from the transducer, which also receives the returning signal

pyelectasis mild dilation of the renal pelvis

pyometra obstruction of the uterus or vagina characterized by an accumulation of pus

pyosalpinx retained pus within the inflamed fallopian tube

radial artery branch of the brachial artery that runs parallel to the ulnar artery in the forearm

Raynaud's phenomenon intermittent digital ischemia in response to cold or emotional stress (primary) or caused by vascular occlusion or stenosis to the digits (secondary)

reactive hyperemia alternative method to stress the peripheral arterial circulation

rectouterine pouch (pouch of Douglas) area in the pelvic cavity between the rectum and the uterus where free fluid can accumulate; also known as the *posterior cul-de-sac*

renal agenesis renal system fails to develop

repolarization describes electrical activity just before the relaxation phase of cardiac muscle activity

resistive index peak systole minus peak diastole divided by peak systole (S-D/S = 5 RI); an RI of 0.7 or less indicates good perfusion; an RI of 0.7 or higher indicates decreased perfusion

respect for persons incorporates both respect for the autonomy of individuals and the requirement to protect those with diminished autonomy

respiratory phasicity change in blood flow velocity with respiration

retroflexed position of the uterus when the uterine fundus bends posteriorly upon the cervix

retroverted position of the uterus when the fundus is tipped posteriorly

reversible ischemic neurologic deficit (RIND) cerebral infarct that lasts longer than 24 hours but less than 72 hours

Rh blood group system of antigens that may be found on the surface of red blood cells; when the Rh factor is present, the blood type is Rh positive; when the Rh antigen is absent, the blood type is Rh negative; a pregnant woman who is Rh negative may become sensitized by the blood of an Rh positive fetus; in subsequent pregnancies, if the fetus is Rh positive, the Rh antibodies produced in maternal blood may cross over the placenta and destroy fetal cells, causing erythroblastosis fetalis

right atrium filling chamber of the heart

right ventricle pumping chamber of the heart that sends blood into the pulmonary artery

round ligaments paired ligaments that originate at the uterine cornua, anterior to the fallopian tubes, and course anterolaterally within the broad ligament to insert into the fascia of the labia majora

sagittal plane refers to a vertical plane through the longitudinal axis of the body that divides it into two portions

salpingitis infection within the fallopian tubes

scoliosis abnormal lateral curvature of the spine

secondary yolk sac sac formed at 23 days when the primary yolk sac is pinched off by the extra embryonic coelom

secretory (luteal) phase days 15 to 28 of the menstrual cycle; the endometrium is at its greatest thickness and echogenicity, with posterior enhancement

semilunar valve valve located in the aortic or pulmonic artery

septum primum first part of the atrial septum to grow from the dorsal wall of the primitive atrium; fuses with the endocardial cushions

septum secundum part of the atrial septum that grows into the atrium to the right of the septum primum

serous cystadenocarcinoma most common type of ovarian carcinoma; may be bilateral with multilocular cysts

serous cystadenoma second most common benign tumor of the ovary; unilocular or multilocular

simple ovarian cyst smooth, well-defined cystic structure that is filled completely with fluid

single umbilical artery condition of one umbilical cord instead of two; it has a high association with congenital anomalies

single ventricle congenital anomaly in which there are two atria but only one ventricular chamber, which receives both the mitral and tricuspid valves

sinoatrial node forms in the wall of the sinus venosus near its opening into the right atrium

situs inversus heart and abdominal organs are completely reversed

small for gestational age (SGA) a normal fetus that measures smaller than would be expected for dates

soleal sinuses large venous reservoirs that lie in the soleus muscle and empty into the posterior tibial or peroneal veins

sonohysterography technique that uses a catheter inserted into the endometrial cavity with the instillation of saline solution or contrast medium to fill the endometrial cavity for the purpose of demonstrating abnormalities within the cavity or uterine tubes; also called *saline-infused sonography (SIS)*

space of Retzius located between the anterior bladder wall and the pubic symphysis; contains extraperitoneal fat

spatial temporal imaging correlation (STIC) used to collect a greater amount of cardiac anatomic data using a longer acquisition time (12 to 15 seconds)

Spaulding's sign overlapping of the skull bones; results in fetal death

spectral analysis waveform graphic display of the flow velocity over time

spina bifida neural tube defect of the spine in which the dorsal vertebrae (vertebral arches) fail to fuse together, allowing the protrusion of meninges or spinal cord through the defect; two types exist: spina bifida occulta (skin-covered defect of the spine without protrusion of meninges or cord) and spina bifida cystica (open spinal defect marked by sac containing protruding meninges or cord)

spina bifida occulta closed defect of the spine without protrusion of meninges or spinal cord; alpha-fetoprotein analysis will not detect these lesions

spontaneous flow is present without augmentation

spontaneous pregnancy loss (SPL) another term for a missed abortion or miscarriage

squamous cell carcinoma most common type of cervical cancer

strabismus eye disorder in which optic axes cannot be directed to the same object

striations parallel longitudinal lines commonly seen in muscle tissue when imaged sonographically; appear as hyperechoic parallel lines running in the long axis of the hypoechoic muscle tissue

subclavian artery artery that originates at the inner border of the scalenus anterior and travels beneath the clavicle to the outer border of the first rib to become the axillary artery

subclavian steal syndrome characterized by symptoms of brain stem ischemia associated with a stenosis or occlusion of the left subclavian, innominate, or right subclavian artery proximal to the origin of the vertebral artery

subclavian vein continuation of the axillary vein; joins the internal jugular vein to form the innominate vein

submandibular window window formed when the transducer is placed at the angle of the mandible and angled slightly medially and cephalad toward the carotid canal

submucosal leiomyoma type of leiomyoma found to deform the endometrial cavity and cause heavy or irregular menses

suboccipital window window formed when the transducer is placed on the posterior aspect of the neck inferior to the nuchal crest

subpulmonic stenosis occurs when a membrane or muscle bundle obstructs the outflow tract into the pulmonary artery

subserosal leiomyoma type of leiomyoma that may become pedunculated and appear as an extrauterine mass

succenturiate placenta one or more accessory lobes connected to the body of the placenta by blood vessels

superior vena cava vessel receiving venous return from the head and upper extremities into the upper posterior medial wall of the right atrium

superior vesical arteries after birth the umbilical arteries become the superior vesical arteries

supravalvular pulmonic stenosis abnormal narrowing in the main pulmonary artery superior to the valve opening

supraventricular tachyarrhythmias abnormal rhythms above 200 beats per minute with a normal sinus conduction rate of 1:1

surface epithelial-stromal tumors gynecologic tumors that arise from the surface epithelium and cover the ovary and the underlying stroma

suspensory (infundibulopelvic) ligament paired ligaments that extend from the infundibulum of the fallopian tube and the lateral aspect of the ovary to the lateral pelvic wall

syncope loss of consciousness and postural tone; fainting

systemic lupus erythematosus (SLE) inflammatory disease involving multiple organ systems; fetus of a mother with SLE may develop heart block and pericardial effusion

systole part of the cardiac cycle in which the ventricles are pumping blood through the outflow tract into the pulmonary artery or the aorta

systolic murmur heart murmur that begins with or after the time of the first heart sound and ends at or before the time of the second heart sound

systolic to diastolic (S/D) ratio Doppler determination of the peak systolic velocity divided by the peak diastolic velocity

tamoxifen antiestrogen drug used in treating some carcinomas of the breast

teratoma solid tumor

tetralogy of Fallot a congenital anomaly consisting of four defects: membranous ventricular septal defect, overriding of the aorta, right ventricular hypertrophy, and pulmonary stenosis

thanatophoric dysplasia lethal short-limb dwarfism characterized by a marked reduction in the length of the long bones, pear-shaped chest, soft-tissue redundancy, and frequently clover-leaf skull deformity and ventriculomegaly

theca-lutein cysts multilocular cysts that occur in patients with hyperstimulation (hydatidiform mole and infertility patients)

thoracic outlet syndrome (TOS) changes in arterial blood flow to the arms related to intermittent compression of the proximal arteries

tibial-peroneal trunk arterial branch that exits after the anterior tibial artery and bifurcates into the posterior tibial artery and the peroneal artery

TORCH acronym originally coined from the first letters of Toxoplasmosis, Rubella, Cytomegalovirus, and Herpesvirus type 2; the *O* stands for other transplacental infections

total anomalous pulmonary venous return (TAPVR) condition in which the pulmonary veins do not return at all into the left atrial cavity; the veins may return into the right atrial cavity or into a chamber posterior to the left atrial cavity

transient ischemic attack (TIA) episode of cerebrovascular insufficiency, usually associated with partial occlusion of a cerebral artery by an atherosclerotic plaque or an embolus

translabial across, or through, the labia

transorbital window transducer is placed on the closed eyelid

transperineal across, or through, the perineum

transposition of the great arteries failure of the truncus arteriosus to complete its rotation during the first trimester; causes the pulmonary artery to arise from the left ventricle and the aorta to arise from the pulmonary artery (blue baby at birth)

transtemporal window transducer is placed on the temporal bone cephalad to the zygomatic arch anterior to the ear

transvaginal (TV) transducer high-frequency transducer that is inserted into the vaginal canal to obtain better definition of first-trimester pregnancy

transverse lie description of the fetus lying transversely (horizontally) across the abdomen

Treacher Collins syndrome underdevelopment of the jaw and cheek bone and abnormal ears

tricuspid atresia underdevelopment of the tricuspid valve (usually associated with hypoplasia of the right ventricle and pulmonary stenosis)

tricuspid valve atrioventricular valve found between the right atrium and right ventricle

trigonocephaly premature closure of the metopic suture

trimester a 40-week pregnancy is divided into three 13-week periods from the first day of the last normal menstrual period; first trimester: weeks 1 through 13; second trimester: weeks 14 through 27; third trimester: week 28 to term

true knots of the umbilical cord arise from fetal movements and are more likely to develop during early pregnancy when relatively more amniotic fluid is present and greater fetal movement occurs; true knots are associated with advanced maternal age, multiparity, and long umbilical cords

true (minor) pelvis found below the brim of the pelvis; the cavity of the minor pelvis is continuous at the pelvic brim with the cavity of the major pelvis

truncus arteriosus common arterial trunk that divides into the aorta and pulmonary artery; congenital heart lesion in which only one great artery arises from the base of the heart

tuboovarian abscess (TOA) infection that involves the fallopian tube and the ovary

tuboovarian complex fusion of the inflamed dilated fallopian tube and ovary

Turner's syndrome nonlethal congenital endocrine disorder caused by failure of the ovaries to respond to pituitary hormone; chromosomal makeup is 45 XO instead of the normal 46 XX or XY; cystic hygroma is often seen in affected fetuses in the first trimester; survivors tend to be short in stature with low-set ears, webbing of the neck, shield-shaped chest, and infertility

twin-to-twin transfusion syndrome (TTS) monozygotic twin pregnancy with single placenta and arteriovenous shunt within the placenta; the donor twin becomes anemic and growth restricted with oligohydramnios; the recipient twin may develop hydrops and polyhydramnios

ulnar artery branch of the brachial artery that runs parallel to the radial artery in the forearm

umbilical cord connecting lifeline between the fetus and placenta; it contains two umbilical arteries and one umbilical vein encased in Wharton's jelly

umbilical herniation failure of the anterior abdominal wall to close completely at the level of the umbilicus

urachal cyst small part of the lumen of the allantois that persists while the urachus forms

ureterocele congenital outpouching of the distal ureter into the bladder

ureteropelvic junction (UPJ) junction of the ureter entering the renal pelvis; most common site of obstruction

ureterovesical junction (UVJ) junction where the ureter enters the bladder

urethral atresia lack of development of the urethra; condition that causes a massively distended bladder (prune belly)

uterosacral ligaments posterior portion of the cardinal ligament that extends from the cervix to the sacrum

VACTERL *v*ertebral abnormalities, *a*nal atresia, *c*ardiac abnormalities, *t*racheoesophageal fistula, and *r*enal and *l*imb abnormalities; VATER excludes cardiac and limb anomalies

valve fold of intima that temporarily closes to permit blood flow in one direction only

varicose veins dilated, elongated, tortuous superficial veins

vasa previa occurs when the intramembranous vessels course across the internal cervical os

velamentous placenta cord insertion on the membranes

ventricular septal defect defect in the ventricular septum that provides communication between the right and left chambers of the heart; most common congenital lesion in the heart

ventriculomegaly abnormal accumulation of cerebrospinal fluid within the cerebral ventricles resulting in dilation of the ventricles without enlargement of the cranium; compression of developing brain tissue and brain damage may result; commonly associated with additional fetal anomalies

veracity truthfulness, honesty

vertebral artery branches of the subclavian artery that merge to form the basilar artery

vertex position of fetus with head down in the uterus

vertigo sensation of having objects move about the person or sensation of moving around in space

vesicouterine pouch pouch formed by the deflection of the peritoneum from the bladder to the uterus

volume slice displays seven sequential 3D rendered volume images simultaneously

voxels three-dimensional pixels that have assigned grayscale values depending upon the strength (amplitude) of the returning 2D echoes

Wharton's jelly mucoid connective tissue that surrounds the umbilical vessels

yolk sac circular structure within the gestational sac seen on ultrasound between 4 and 10 weeks of gestational age; supplies nutrition, facilitates waste removal, and is the origin of early hematopoietic stem cells in the embryo; it lies between the chorion and the amnion

yolk stalk the umbilical duct connecting the yolk sac with the embryo

zygote products of conception from fertilization through implantation; the zygotic stage of pregnancy lasts for approximately 12 days after conception

Aehlert B: *Mosby's comprehensive pediatric emergency care*, St. Louis, 2007, Mosby
Figure 3-25, *A*

Chapleau W, Pons PT: *Emergency medical technician: making the difference*, St. Louis, 2007, Mosby/JEMS
Figure 3-25, *B*

Chervenak FA and others: Fetal cystic hygroma: cause and natural history, *N Eng J Med* 309:822, 1985
Figure 58-39, *A*

Damjanov I, Linder J: *Pathology: a color atlas*, St. Louis, 2000, Mosby
Figures 9-6; 9-13; 10-29; 10-33; 10-35; 10-46; 10-53; 10-56; 10-61; 10-64; 10-66; 11-18; 11-22; 11-33; 11-40; 11-48; 12-7; 12-23; 12-24; 12-29; 12-32; 12-33; 12-36; 12-37; 12-39; 12-40; 12-44; 15-14; 15-16; 20-18; 22-7; 22-13; 22-15; 22-17; 22-18; 22-20; 22-22; 22-24; 22-25; 25-26; 25-31; 25-34; 25-40; 25-46; 26-12; 26-22, *C*; 26-25, *C*; 27-11; 27-15, 42-21, *A*; 42-24; 42-29, *A*; 42-30; 42-31; 42-34

England MA: *Color atlas of life before birth*, St Louis, 1983, Mosby
Figure 47-14, *A*

Hadlock FP, Shah YP, Kanon DJ, Lindsey JV: Fetal crown-rump length: reevaluation of relation to menstrual age (5–18 weeks) with high resolution real time US, *Radiology* 182:501, 1992
Figures 47-26, 47-28

Henningsen C: *Clinical guide to ultrasonography*, St. Louis, 2004, Mosby
Figures 14-52, *A*, *B*; 14-53, *A*, *B*; 21-29, *A-F* (modified); 25-27; 25-29, *A-C*; 25-32, *A-D*; 25-35, *A*, *B*; 26-13; 29-12, *A*, *B*; 29-16, *A*, *B*; 29-23, *A-C*; 53-13; 53-20; 53-25, *A*, *B*; 53-28; 59-13; 59-32, *A*, *B*; 59-38, *A*, *B*; 59-45, *A*, *B*; 64-4, *A-C*; 64-8, *A*, *B*; 64-22, *A*

Kremkau FW: Principles and instrumentation. In Merritt CRB, editor: Doppler color imaging, New York, 1992, Churchill Livingstone
Figure 6-31

Kremkau FW: *Principles and pitfalls of real-time color-flow imaging*. In Bernstein EF, editor: *Vascular diagnosis*, ed 4, St Louis, 1993, Mosby
Figures 6-28, *A-C*; 6-29, *A-E*; 6-33

Kremkau FW: *Semin Roentgenol* 27:6–16, 1992
Figures 6-25, 6-27, *B*

Kremkau FW, Taylor KJW: *J Ultrasound Med* 5:227, 1986
Figure 6-6

Kremkau FW: J *Vasc Technol* 15:265–266, 1991. Reprinted with permission by the Society for Vascular Ultrasound (SVU).
Figure 6-27, *C*

Maternal Fetal Medicine Foundation, Washington, D. C.
Figure 47-30 (redrawn)

Mayden KL and others: Cystic adenomatoid malformation in the fetus: Ultrasound evaluation, *Am J Obstet Gynecol* 148:349, 1984.
Figure 60-8, *A*, *B*

McMinn RMH: *Functional and clinical anatomy*, St. Louis, 1999, Mosby
Figures 13-1, *A-D*; 13-24; 16-17; 17-1, *A-D*; 17-24; 20-25, *A*; 25-1; 25-2; 25-4; 25-5; 29-1; 29-2; 29-4; 29-5

Nyberg DA et al, editors: *Transvaginal ultrasound*, Mosby, 1992, St. Louis
Figure 41-33

Nyberg DA, Mahony BS, Pretorius DH, editors: *Diagnostic ultrasound of fetal anomalies: text and atlas*, St Louis, 1990, Mosby
Figure 53-23

Potter PA, Perry AG, *Fundamentals of nursing*, ed 7, St. Louis, 2009, Mosby
Figures 3-3, *A*; 3-6, *A*, *B*; 3-9, *B*; 3-12, *A-C*; 3-13; 3-14; 3-18, *B*; 3-20, *A-E*

Queenan JT: *Modern management of the Rh problem*, ed 2, Hagerstown, PA, 1977, Harper & Row Medical. http://lwww.com
Figure 52-8

Rumack C, Wilson S, Charboneau W: *Diagnostic ultrasound*, ed 4, St Louis, 2011, Mosby
Figures 21-30; 21-41, *A*, *B*; 21-43, *A*, *B*; 21-44, *A*, *B*; 25-36, *A*, *B*; 25-38, *A*, *B*; 25-39, *A-C*; 27-3; 29-8; 29-9, *A*, *B*; 29-10, *A*, *B*; 29-11; 29-13, *A*, *B*; 29-15; 29-18, *A-C*; 30-6, *A*; 30-7, *A-F*; 30-8, *A*, *B*; 30-12, *A-C*; 30-13, *A-G*; 30-16, *A-C*; 41-20; 41-25; 42-9; 42-13; 42-15; 42-20; 48-14; 59-22; 63-18

Taylor KJW, Holland S: *Radiology* 174:297–307, 1990.
Figure 6-23, *A-E*

Thibodeau GA, Patton KT: *The human body in health and disease*, ed 5, St Louis, 2010, Mosby
Figure 7-4

Young AP: *Kinn's the administrative medical assistant: an applied learning approach*, ed 7, Philadelphia, 2011, Saunders
Figures 3-1; 3-2; 3-3, *B*; 3-5, *A*; 3-21; 3-22; 3-24

AAA	abdominal aortic aneurysm	
AB	abortion	
ABI	ankle-brachial index	
AC	abdominal circumference; acromioclavicular (joint)	
ACA	anterior cerebral artery	
AcoA	anterior communicating artery	
ACOG	American College of Obstetrics and Gynecology	
ACR	American College of Radiology	
ACTH	andrenocorticotropic hormone	
AD	autosomal dominant	
ADPKD	autosomal-dominant polycystic kidney disease	
AE	acoustic emission	
AFAFP	amniotic fluid alpha-fetoprotein	
AFI	amniotic fluid index	
AFP	alpha-fetoprotein	
AFV	amniotic fluid volume	
AI	aortic insufficiency	
AIDS	acquired immunodeficiency syndrome	
AIUM	American Institute of Ultrasound in Medicine	
ALH	atypical lobular hyperplasia	
ALK PHOS	alkaline phosphatase	
ALT	alanine aminotransferase	
AMA	American Medical Association; against medical advice	
Amb	ambulatory	
AP	anteroposterior	
Appy	appendectomy	
AR	autosomal recessive	
ARDS	adult respiratory distress syndrome; acute respiratory distress syndrome	
ARPKD	autosomal-recessive polycystic kidney disease	
ART	assisted reproductive technology	
AS	aortic stenosis	
ASAP	as soon as possible	
ASD	atrial septal defect	
AST	aspartate aminotransferase	
AT	acceleration time	
ATN	acute tubular necrosis	
AV	atrioventricular	
AVF	arterio-venous fistula	
AVM	arteriovenous malformation	
AVSD	artrioventricular septal defect	
BA	basilar artery	
BD	biocular distance	

Bi-RADS	Breast Imaging and Reporting Data Systems
BPD	biparietal diameter
BPP	biophysical profile
BSE	breast self-examination
BUN	blood urea nitrogen
bx	biopsy
CA	calcium; cancer; celiac axis
CABG	coronary artery bypass graft
CAD	coronary artery disease
CBD	common bile duct
CBE	clinical breast examination
CBF	cerebral blood flow
CCA	common carotid artery
CD	common duct
CES	contrast-enhanced sonography
CFA	common femoral artery
CFI	color flow imaging
CFM	color flow mapping
CHD	congestive heart disease; congenital heart disease
CHF	congestive heart failure
CI	cardiac index; cephalic index
CK	creatine kinase
CL	caudate lobe
CNS	central nervous system
CO_2	carbon dioxide
COPD	chronic obstructive pulmonary disease
Cr	creatinine
CRL	crown-rump length
CSF	cerebrospinal fluid
CSP	cavum septum pellucidum
CT	computed tomography
CVA	cerebrovascular accident
CVS	chorionic villus sampling
CW	continuous wave
Cx	cervix
D&C	dilation and curettage
dB	decibel
DCIS	ductal carcinoma in situ
DDH	developmental displacement of hip
DFE	distal femoral epiphyseal (ossification)
DFV	deep femoral vein
DM	diabetes mellitus
DOB	date of birth
DVT	deep vein thrombosis
DWM	Dandy-Walker malformation
dx	diagnosis
ECA	external carotid artery
ECG	electrocardiogram

EDC	expected date of confinement
EDD	expected date of delivery
EFW	estimated fetal weight
ERCP	endoscopic retrograde cholangiopancreatography
ESP	early systolic peak
ETOH	alcohol
FAST	focused assessment with sonography for trauma
FBM	fetal breathing movements
FCC	fibrocystic condition
FL	fetal length; falciform ligament
FM	fetal movement
FMD	fibromuscular dysplasia
FNA	fine needle aspiration
FNH	focal nodular hyperplasia
FSH	follicle-stimulating hormone
FT	fetal tone
FUO	fever of unknown origin
GASA	growth-adjusted sonar age
GB	gallbladder
GDA	gastroduodenal artery
GI	gastrointestinal
GIFT	gamete intrafallopian transfer
GSHI	gray scale harmonic imaging
GSV	greater saphenous vein
GSW	gunshot wound
GU	genitourinary
GYN	gynecology
HC	head circumference
HCC	hepatocellular carcinoma
hCG	human chorionic gonadotropin
Hgb	hemoglobin
HI	harmonic imaging
HIV	human immunodeficiency virus
HLHS	hypoplastic left heart syndrome
hPL	human placental lactogen
HPS	hypertrophic pyloric stenosis
HV	hepatic veins
Hx	history
Hz	Hertz
IA	iliac arteries
IAE	induced acoustic emission
ICA	internal carotid artery
IDC	invasive ductal carcinoma
IDC-NOS	infiltrating ductal carcinomanot otherwise specified
IDDM	insulin-dependent diabetes mellitus
IHF	interhemispheric fissure
IJV	internal jugular vein
IMA	inferior mesenteric artery
INR	international normalized ratio